For Deneige (at 30) and Andrew
and Jeremy (at 28) and Alison.

May you continue to retain your illusion of control.

ANXIETY AND ITS DISORDERS

Anxiety and Its Disorders

The Nature and Treatment of Anxiety and Panic

Second Edition

David H. Barlow

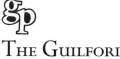

THE GUILFORD PRESS

New York   London

© 2002 The Guilford Press
A Division of Guilford Publications, Inc.
72 Spring Street, New York, NY 10012
www.guilford.com

Printed in the United States of America

This book is printed on acid-free paper.

Last digit is print number: 9 8 7 6 5 4 3 2 1

Library of Congress Cataloging-in-Publication Data

Barlow, David H.
    Anxiety and its disorders : the nature and treatment of anxiety and panic / David H. Barlow.—2nd ed.
      p. ; cm.
    Includes bibliographical references and index.
    ISBN 1-57230-430-8
    1. Anxiety. I. Title.
    [DNLM: 1. Anxiety Disorders. WM 172 B258a 2002]
RC531 .B28 2002
616.82'223—dc21   2001040754

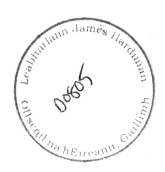

About the Author

David H. Barlow received his PhD from the University of Vermont in 1969 and has published over 400 articles and chapters and over 20 books, mostly in the area of anxiety disorders, sexual problems, and clinical research methodology.

Dr. Barlow was formerly Professor of Psychiatry at the University of Mississippi Medical Center and Professor of Psychiatry and Psychology at Brown University, and founded clinical psychology internships in both settings. He was also Distinguished Professor in the Department of Psychology at the University at Albany, State University of New York at Albany. Currently, he is Professor of Psychology, Research Professor of Psychiatry, Director of Clinical Training Programs, and Director of the Center for Anxiety and Related Disorders at Boston University.

Dr. Barlow is the recipient of the 2000 American Psychological Association (APA) Distinguished Scientific Award for the Applications of Psychology. He is also the recipient of the First Annual Science Dissemination Award from the Society for a Science of Clinical Psychology of the APA, and recipient of the 2000 Distinguished Scientific Contribution Award from the Society of Clinical Psychology of the APA. He received an award in appreciation of outstanding achievements from the General Hospital of the Chinese People's Liberation Army, Beijing, China, with an appointment as Honorary Visiting Professor of Clinical Psychology. Other awards include Career Contribution Awards from the Massachusetts and California Psychological Associations and a MERIT award from the National Institute of Mental Health for long-term contributions to the clinical research effort. He is Past-President of the Society for Clinical Psychology and the Association for Advancement of Behavior Therapy, and is currently Editor of the Journal *Clinical Psychology: Science and Practice*. He was also a member of the DSM-IV Task Force of the American Psychiatric Association and was Co-Chair of the Work Group for revising the anxiety disorder categories. He is also a Diplomate in Clinical Psychology of the American Board of Professional Psychology and maintains a private practice.

Contributing Authors

Martin M. Antony, PhD, Anxiety Treatment and Research Centre, St. Joseph's Hospital, Hamilton, Ontario, Canada; Department of Psychiatry and Behavioural Neurosciences, McMaster University, Hamilton, Ontario, Canada

Timothy A. Brown, PsyD, Center for Anxiety and Related Disorders, Department of Psychology, Boston University, Boston, MA

Terence M. Keane, PhD, National Center for PTSD in Boston; Boston Veterans Administration Healthcare System; Departments of Psychiatry and Psychology, Boston University, Boston, MA

Stefan G. Hofmann, PhD, Assistant Professor of Psychology, Center for Anxiety and Related Disorders, Department of Psychology, Boston University, Boston, MA

Susan M. Orsillo, PhD, Boston Veterans Administration Healthcare System; Center for Anxiety and Related Disorders, Department of Psychology, Boston University, Boston, MA

Lizabeth Roemer, PhD, University of Massachusetts at Boston; Center for Anxiety and Related Disorders, Department of Psychology, Boston University, Boston, MA

Gail Steketee, PhD, School of Social Work, Boston University, Boston, MA

Kamila S. White, PhD, Center for Anxiety and Related Disorders, Department of Psychology, Boston University, Boston, MA

Preface

To provide some background on the genesis of this book, first published in 1988, it seems worthwhile to revisit a few paragraphs from the preface to the first edition. At that time I observed:

> "This tale grew in the telling," as J.R.R. Tolkein put it. After years of research and practice, it seemed a straightforward enough task to write a book on the nature and treatment of anxiety disorders. The surge of interest in these disorders during the past 5 years sparked rapid-fire advances in both psychological and pharmacological treatments, and I felt that such a book would be timely. After reviewing these advances, I planned to describe newly developed treatments for the anxiety disorders at our Center for Stress and Anxiety Disorders in Albany that take into account innovations from around the world. These treatments would be described in the framework of anxiety disorders as defined and described in the revisions to DSM-III. I told my publisher that I would have it for him in 12 to 18 months.
>
> During this time, our own treatments changed dramatically as exciting new discoveries emerged from our research center and elsewhere on the nature and treatment of panic. These developments seemed to require, at the very least, a full explication of the nature of anxiety and panic based on these new developments. But these developments could not be described adequately without putting them in the framework of current theoretical conceptions of anxiety in general. I found that repeating tried and true theories of anxiety proved totally inadequate, since new conceptual approaches, ranging from neurobiological to social-constructivist, have appeared only in the past 2 years. These models are beginning to affect our view of anxiety. And then there is the mystery of panic!
>
> This confusing combination of new and old perspectives on anxiety and panic led inexorably to a consideration of the nature of emotion. The book stood still for a half a year while I absorbed once again the views of emotion theorists and attempted to integrate our rapidly emerging clinical knowledge of anxiety and panic with the old and distinguished tradition of emotion theory dating back to Darwin over 100 years ago. For anxiety disorders, in the last analysis, are emotional disorders. It became increasingly clear that it was impossible to say something fresh about emotional disorders without considering the traditions of emotion theory.
>
> At this point, I started working backward, rewriting the book from the point of view of the accumulated wisdom of emotion theory. After the integration of relevant recent developments in cognitive science and neuroscience, what emerged was a new model of panic and anxiety with implications for treatment. These theories and concepts were then integrated with newly developed treatment protocols for the various anxiety disorders. Only then was I able to write the book I intended.

In writing this second edition I had the good fortune to be subjected to some of my own illusions of control. First, with the prospect of revising the book rather than writing it anew, and with the privilege of spending the 1997–1998 year at the Center for Advanced Studies in Behavioral Sciences in Palo Alto, California, I thought I could finish the book in a year and a half and have it to my publisher in the late fall of 1998. As with the first edition, I was off by 2 years! The explosion of knowledge in epidemiology and phenomenology, as well as in cognitive, behavioral, and neurological science, made it clear that I would be lucky to finish even the first half of the book in 3 years' time.

With my closest colleagues at Boston University and the Center for Anxiety and Related Disorders (CARD), where I relocated in the fall of 1996, we devised a plan that in the second edition we would collaborate on the chapter on classification of anxiety disorders, as well as the last six chapters devoted to the nature, assessment, and treatment of each individual anxiety disorder. Those chapters apply the theory explicated in the first part of the book. Since all of the collaborating individuals are either current colleagues at Boston University and CARD, or in the case of Martin M. Antony, a former (stellar) student who is now an international authority in his own right, a full integration and continuity of the ideas throughout the book was ensured. As I sit here putting the finishing touches on this massive effort, it seems very possible to me that I may owe my own sanity to my good friends and close collaborators, each of whom has achieved a more important mastery of his or her individual topic than I would have ever hoped to do alone. To Timothy A. Brown, Kamila S. White, Martin M. Antony, Terence M. Keane, Stefan G. Hofmann, Lizabeth Roemer, Susan M. Orsillo, and Gail Steketee, my deepest and most sincere gratitude. The book is better for their efforts.

There is one less chapter in this edition (15) than in the first edition, but there have been conceptual and structural changes in three chapters. Given enormous advances in our knowledge of the process and nature of anxiety, this topic is now accorded its own chapter (Chapter 3). This chapter follows Chapter 1, on the experience of anxiety, which is considerably rewritten and updated, and Chapter 2, on fear, anxiety, and theories of emotion, which summarizes the burgeoning literature on emotion theory as it may apply to emotional disorders. Chapters 4, 5, and 6, on the phenomenon of panic, provoking panic in the laboratory, and neurobiological aspects of anxiety and panic, respectively, remain unchanged in title but enormously changed in content. Chapters 7 and 8 integrate the preceding information and update my theoretical approaches to the origins of fear and panic and the origins of anxiety, respectively.

To accommodate all of this additional information, the first edition's Chapter 8, on the process of fear and anxiety reduction, had to be dropped, although many of its ideas on applying the principles of emotion theory to our new psychological and pharmacological interventions can be found in the later clinical chapters of this new edition. After Chapter 9, which covers classification, the last six chapters are devoted to the individual clinical anxiety disorders, including and combining two chapters from the first edition, on panic disorder, into one.

Much of what was hypothesized in the first edition concerning the nature and treatment of anxiety has been borne out in the ensuing 14 years, while other suggestions have proven considerably off-base. During the 1990s, the centrality of emotion theory as a legitimate basis for the investigation of emotional disorders was recognized, and the study of emotion from a variety of perspectives has been reinvigorated. The uniqueness of the phenomenon of panic, first recognized by Donald Klein, has been reaffirmed vis-à-vis the related but distinct emotion of anxiety, and the functional relationship of these two emotions, first suggested in the first edition of this book, have become the basis for some of the criteria for anxiety disorders in DSM-IV. The provocation of panic in the laboratory, a subject of considerable controversy at the end of the 1980s, has been confirmed by leading neurobiological investigators to be mediated largely by psychological factors in some recent seminal studies; this also confirms a suggestion made in the first edition. And the sense of a lack of control, rooted deep in early experience, as the core of anxiety has received increasing support in both animal and human models.

On the other hand, conceptions of the process of worry postulated in the first edition have changed considerably, based on the pioneering work of Thomas Borkovec, Rudolph Hoehn-Saric, and their colleagues as detailed in Chapter 3. Advances in the last decade have also altered my opinions on the classifications of anxiety and related disorders, as I have recognized the overarching importance of broad dimensions of negative affect and neuroticism. From the point of view of treatment, the role of interoceptive exposure, initially described in the first edition of this book, has broadened and deepened considerably. We also approach situational exposure in some important new ways.

Many readers were intrigued with my dedication in the first edition to my children, then teenagers, a dedication I have altered only slightly in this edition to happily accommodate our son-in-law and daughter-in-law. The "illusion of control" mentioned there refers, of course, to a fundamental psychological characteristic that contributes substantially to physical and mental health, an idea that has received increasing support and is described in some detail in Chapter 8. I am deeply appreciative of comments I have received from readers, not only on the dedication but all aspects of the book. Many of these concepts have assisted me greatly in advancing my own thinking.

Since my own style of research has always been collaborative, this book owes much to all of my colleagues and students over the years who have worked with me to develop these ideas. I take full responsibility for the fact that the ideas and thoughts of those individuals may not have been represented exactly as they intended. Nevertheless, in most cases their contributions will be recognizable.

A special thanks to Michelle Craske, my colleague for over 15 years, who continues to amaze me with her capacity for work and creativity. Thanks also to Sue Mineka and Mark Bouton, with whom I spent a very enjoyable year at the Center for Advanced Studies. I can only say that the Center was as heavenly as we all thought it would be. My thanks again to Janet Klosko and Patty Coakley, who made important contributions to the more literary initiatives attempted in Chapter 1. Beyond these individuals, other colleagues on the faculty here at Boston University have provided me with the benefit of their thinking, including David Spiegel, Henry Marcucella, Fabio Idrobo, and Kim Saudino. To my administrative assistants Bette Selwyn, who began the book, and Rebekah Morris, who demonstrated her uncanny ability to find missing references while finishing the book, I express my admiration and deepest appreciation. To my wife, Beverly, enduring the nights, weekends, and "vacations" I spent working on the book, my gratitude and love for her patience. And to my copyeditor, Marie Sprayberry, who saw and considered carefully every word of the first edition, and now has accomplished the same task with the second edition, my appreciation for her remarkable talent and attention to detail.

And finally, as I bring this edition to a close with no expectations whatsoever of attempting this Herculean task again, I look with enthusiasm to the next generation of investigators who will share my excitement in continuing to unravel the mysteries of anxiety.

DAVID H. BARLOW

Contents

CHAPTER 1

The Experience of Anxiety

Shadow of Intelligence or Specter of Death?

In our society, individuals spend billions of dollars yearly to rid themselves of anxiety. The costs of visits to primary care physicians, and the utilization of health care services in general by individuals with anxiety disorders, are double what they are for those without anxiety disorders, even if the latter are physically ill (Simon, Ormel, Von Korff, & Barlow, 1995). Many take away prescriptions from their physicians for various drugs to treat anxiety, making these drugs among the most widely used in the world. For these individuals, anxiety is a curse—something they could live without. But could we all live without anxiety? Many of our most prominent philosophers, psychologists, and psychiatrists think not. Some think that it serves a protective function. For others, it is at the very root of what it means to be human. Still others believe that our very ability to adapt and plan for the future depends on anxiety. Consider the thoughts of the well-known early psychologist Howard Liddell:

> The planning function of the nervous system, in the course of evolution, has culminated in the appearance of ideas, values, and pleasures—the unique manifestations of man's social living. Man, alone, can plan for the distant future and can experience the retrospective pleasures of achievement. Man, alone, can be happy. But man, alone, can be worried and anxious. Sherrington once said that posture accompanies movement as a shadow. I have come to believe that anxiety accompanies intellectual activity as its shadow and that the more we know of the nature of anxiety, the more we will know of intellect. (Liddell, 1949, p. 185)

Is anxiety the shadow of intelligence? Or is anxiety the overwhelming specter of death and nothingness? The hypothetical advantages of being anxious are considered first.

THE SHADOW OF INTELLIGENCE

Survival

Since women reportedly suffer disproportionately from the pathological effects of anxiety, it is fitting that one of the most eloquent and lucid portrayals of the experience of anxiety comes from a woman. In a short story by M. F. K. Fisher entitled "The Wind Chill

1

Factor,"[1] the character Mrs. Thayer is staying alone in a friend's cottage on the ocean during a brutal winter blizzard. The blizzard has been raging for days; nevertheless, Mrs. Thayer is warm, comfortable, and unconcerned with possible consequences of the storm as she drifts off to sleep.

> A little after four, an extraordinary thing happened to her. From deep and comfortable dreamings she was wrenched into the conscious world, as cruelly as if she had been grabbed by the long hairs of her head. Her heart had changed its slow, quiet beat and bumped in her rib cage like a rabbit's. Her breath was caught in a kind of net in her throat, not going in and down fast enough. She touched her body and it was hot, but her palms felt clammy and stuck to her.
>
> Within a few seconds she knew that she was in a state—perhaps dangerous—of pure panic. It had nothing to do with physical fear, as far as she could tell. She was not afraid of being alone, or of being on the dunes in a storm. She was not afraid of bodily attack, rape, all that. She was simply in panic, or what Frenchmen home from the Sahara used to call *le cafard affolé*. (p. 162)

At this point, Mrs. Thayer experiences an urge to flee that is among the most fundamental and ancient in the behavioral repertoire of living organisms.

> This is amazing, she said. This is indescribable. It is here. I shall survive it or else run out howling across the dunes and die soon in the waves and the wind. Such a choice seemed very close and sweet, for her feeling was almost intolerably wishful of escape from the noise. It was above and against and around her, and she felt that it was invading her spirit. This is dangerous indeed, she said, and I must try not to run outside. That is a suicide wish, and weak. I must try to breathe more slowly, and perhaps swallow something to get back my more familiar rhythms. She was speaking slowly to her whole self, with silent but precise enunciation. (p. 162)

Is this experience Liddell's shadow of intelligence? Is there anything intelligent or even useful in an unbearably strong urge to flee the warmth and security of a safe shelter to run headlong into a raging sea? Paradoxically, there probably is, and this tendency may well have been responsible for the survival of the species. But is it only humans who can experience "anxiety" in this way? According to the naturalist Charles Darwin, certainly not.

> With all or almost all animals, even with birds, Terror causes the body to tremble. The skin becomes pale, sweat breaks out, and hair bristles. The secretions of the alimentary canal and of the kidneys are increased, and they are involuntarily voided, owing to the relaxation of the sphincter muscles, as is known to be the case with man, and as I have seen with cattle, dogs, cats, and monkeys. The breathing is hurried. The heart beats quickly, wildly, and violently; but whether it pumps the blood more efficiently through the body may be doubted, for the surface seems bloodless and the strength of the muscles soon fails. . . . The mental faculties are much disturbed. Utter prostration soon follows, and even fainting. A terrified canary-bird has been seen not only to tremble and to turn white about the base of the bill, but to faint; and I once caught a robin in a room, which fainted so completely, that for a time I thought it was dead. (Darwin, 1872, p. 77)

---

[1]Fisher, M. F. K. The wind chill factor or, a problem of mind and matter. In *As They Were* by M. F. K. Fisher. Copyright 1982 by M. F. K. Fisher. Reprinted by permission of Alfred A. Knopf, Inc. Originally appeared in *The New Yorker*. Page numbers of excerpted passages refer to those in S. Cahill (Ed.), *Women and Fiction 2: Short Stories by and about Women* (pp. 160–166). New York: New American Library, 1978.

Darwin may have developed a keen interest in these responses for a very good reason. It now seems clear that Darwin himself suffered the ravages of terror in the form of panic attacks, and that these attacks and the resulting agoraphobia kept him close to home, working with an all-consuming passion on his most famous works *On the Origin of Species by Means of Natural Selection* and *The Expression of the Emotions in Man and Animals* (Barloon & Noyes, 1997).

How can this elemental response be useful? As every student in introductory psychology knows, this behavior and the overwhelming emotion associated with it represent the organism's alarm reaction to potentially life-threatening emergencies. The almost reflexive urge to escape or, alternatively, to stand and engage the threat ("fight or flight") seems clearly a behavioral tendency that has been selectively favored in an evolutionary sense. Organisms without this capacity undoubtedly were overwhelmed by the welter of emergencies when the species was young. Organisms able to respond quickly and efficiently to life-threatening situations survived and won the day.

On close inspection, the specific functional contributions of various components of this biological survival mechanism seem clear (Cannon, 1927). Activation of the cardiovascular system is one of the major components. Typically, peripheral blood vessels constrict, thereby raising arterial pressure and decreasing blood flow to the extremities. Excess blood is redirected to the skeletal muscles that can be used to defend oneself in a struggle. Blood pooled in the torso is more available to vital organs that may be needed in an emergency. Often people seem "white with fear"; that is, they blanch with fear as a result of decreased blood flow to the skin. Trembling with fear may be the result of shivering and perhaps piloerection, in which body hairs stand erect to conserve heat during periods of vasoconstriction. These defensive adjustments can also produce the commonly observed "hot" and "cold" spells. Breathing becomes more rapid and usually deeper to provide necessary oxygen to rapidly circulating blood. This increased blood circulation carries oxygen to the brain, where cognitive processes and sensory functions are stimulated. An increased amount of glucose (sugar) is also released from the liver into the bloodstream to further energize various crucial muscles and organs, including the brain. Pupils dilate, presumably to allow a better view of the situation. Hearing becomes more acute, and digestive activity is suspended, resulting in a reduced flow of saliva (the "dry mouth" of fear). There is often pressure to urinate, to defecate, and occasionally to vomit. In the short term, voiding will further prepare the organism for concentrated action and activity; in the longer term, vomiting and diarrhea may be reflexive reactions protecting against the danger of absorption of noxious substances (Beck & Emery with Greenberg, 1985; Nesse, 1987; Stein & Bouwer, 1997).

Is this mobilization of the organism for fighting or escaping the only behavior associated with our ancient alarm system? It seems not. Consider the following case from our files: A young physician in radiology was attending an Ingemar Bergman movie one evening. The camera focused suddenly on massive bleeding from one character in an unexpected context. The physician slumped over. His companion thought he might be napping, although he had seemed quite interested in the movie to that point. When the physician came to, he was very shaken, realizing that he had fainted unexpectedly. Even more disconcerting was the fact that his faint was due to the sight of blood. In fact, throughout medical school, he had often noticed feeling uneasy in the presence of blood, but had "steeled" himself to the occasion. In all likelihood, he had employed various muscle-tensing strategies that maintain or increase blood pressure (Öst & Sterner, 1987; Antony, Craske, & Barlow, 1995b; Craske, Antony, & Barlow, 1997) (see Chapter 11). In any case, he remained sufficiently uncomfortable to choose a specialty where contact with blood was minimized. After the Bergman film, his discomfort escalated to a full phobic reaction, causing the avoidance of any situation where he might encounter blood.

Fainting, of course, requires a very different physiological response from that required by fighting or fleeing. Instead of the sustained sympathetically innervated surges in cardiovascular function that are associated with the usual alarm reaction, marked decreases in heart rate and blood pressure precede fainting (Page, 1994). Could this also be an adaptive response? Very clearly it could, and it probably was such a response under conditions that existed in millenia past. When under attack, those who responded to injury and bleeding with a dramatic drop in blood pressure—thereby minimizing blood loss and the danger of shock—were far more likely to survive the attack than those who did not. Today this behavioral action tendency is maladaptively present in the large numbers of individuals with extreme fears of blood, injury, and injection (see Chapter 11).

But what of Darwin's robin, which presumably did not see blood, but nevertheless fainted so completely when caught that Darwin thought it was dead? Is this the same reaction as that described above? Probably not. In recent years, investigators have rediscovered an archaic response that seems to be yet another action tendency associated with alarm reactions in specific situations. When in the presence of an approaching predator, and particularly when in direct contact with a predator, most species will initially evidence the agitation associated with fight or flight. This reaction may be followed immediately by a very different response similar to paralysis, but characterized by waxy flexibility. These animals look as if they were dead, as did Darwin's robin. In fact, this is the "playing dead" or "freezing" response so often seen in animals in the wild under attack. Investigators in this area refer to the response as "tonic immobility" (Gallup, 1974) and differentiate it from the temporary motionless response exhibited by many animals preceding their attempts to flee from a predator seen at a distance (Woodruff & Lippincott, 1976). But investigators have determined that tonic immobility is not a volitional or strategic strategy on the part of the animal. Rather, this response represents another ancient behavioral reaction with obvious survival value. For the large number of predators for which attack is triggered and maintained by movement, freezing is an effective antidote that prevents further attack and increases the victim's chances of survival.

This response may have important biological implications for human anxiety, as outlined in Chapter 6. But investigators concerned with human anxiety have showed little interest in tonic immobility, since it has not been thought to occur in humans. Now it seems we may have overlooked a tragic but obvious example of this reaction in humans. During brutal rapes, many women report feeling paralyzed. Comments such as "I felt trembling and cold—I went limp," or "My body felt paralyzed," or "My body went absolutely stiff," reflect this paralytic state. This may be analogous to the muscular rigidity and motor inhibition evidenced by animals during tonic immobility following manual restraint. Loss of consciousness does not occur, since the victim can later relate events that occurred during the attack. Some victims have reported feeling "freezing cold," which may reflect the characteristic decrease in body temperature of immobile animals. Many survivors of rape also report feeling completely numb or insensitive to pain during the ordeal; this may be similar to the analgesic effects of immobility observed in animals. Burgess and Holmstrom (1976) reported that 22 out of 34 rape survivors demonstrated physical paralysis at some point during the encounter. The similarities between tonic immobility and rape-induced paralysis have been outlined by Suarez and Gallup (1979) and are found in Table 1.1.

It is not clear that the survival response of freezing obviates some of the dangers of rape. One could speculate that freezing decreases the risk of injury from physical aggres-

TABLE 1.1. Similarities between Tonic Immobility and Rape-Induced Paralysis

Tonic immobility	Rape-induced paralysis
Profound motor inhibition	Inability to move
Parkinsonian-like tremors	Body shaking
Suppressed vocal behavior	Inability to call out or scream
No loss of consciousness	Recall for details of the attack
Apparent analgesia	Numbness and insensitivity to pain
Reduced core temperature	Sensation of feeling cold
Abrupt onset and termination	Sudden onset and remission of paralysis
Aggressive reactions at termination	Attempts to attack the rapist following recovery

Note. From Suarez and Gallup (1979). Copyright 1979 by *The Psychological Record*. Reprinted by permission.

sion. Furthermore, restricted movement cues may reduce sexual arousal in the rapist (Suarez & Gallup, 1979). But recognizing that rape survivors are paralyzed or tonically immobile could prevent a tragic interpretation by many authorities, who have assumed in the past that a survivor is somehow acquiescing to the rape.

The Sound of the Wind

If these responses are termed "anxiety," and one considers it "intelligent" to avoid threats successfully, then anxiety may be the shadow of intelligence. But most would not consider this behavior to be "intelligent" in the sense of a complex rational response. Nevertheless, it shares something of Howard Liddell's conception, in that it is adaptive, useful, and indispensable.

But there is something very mysterious about the fictional Mrs. Thayer's experience that does not fit the Darwinian scenario. "It had nothing to do with physical fear, as far as she could tell. She was not afraid of being alone, or of being on the dunes in a storm. She was not afraid of bodily attack, rape, all that" (Fisher, 1978, p. 162). The threat in her own mind is not the storm or being alone, but the urge to flee itself: "This is dangerous indeed, she said, and I must try not to run outside. That is a suicide wish, and weak" (p. 162). But the "suicide wish" is more than a flirtation with death running through her head in the form of frightening thoughts. There are other components to this threat emanating from within her own body:

> The sound of the wind, for her, had been going sideways exactly on a line with the far horizon of the Atlantic for days, nights—too long. It was in her bowels and suddenly they were loosened, and later, again to her surprise, she threw up. She told herself dizzily that the rhythm of the wind had bound her around, and that now she was defying it, but it kept on howling. (p. 165)

How does one cope with this human experience where the threat is internal and the consequence is death? With great difficulty, Mrs. Thayer struggles to walk to the kitchen, where she takes two aspirins and a mug of warm milk. Ritualistically, she remembers advice that during periods of deep stress one should drink the liquid in three slow sips, wait 5 minutes before taking three more sips, and so on. After the medicine and the rituals, she turns to other, more psychological methods of coping:

She pulled every trick out of the bagful she had collected during her long life with neurotics. She brushed her hair firmly, and all the while her heart kept ticking against her ribs and she felt so sick that she could scarcely lift her arm. She tried to say some nursery rhymes and the Twenty-third Psalm, but with no other result than an impatient titter. She sipped the dreadful sweet milk. She prayed to those two pills she had swallowed. (p. 163)

But at the last she turns to the great arbiter of all human difficulties, one's own reason.

For a time, as the aspirin and the warm milk seemed to slow down her limitless dread (Dread of what? Not that the roof would fly off, that she was alone, that she might die . . .), she made herself talk reasonably to what was pulling and trembling and flickering in her spirit. She was a doctor—or, rather, an unwitting bystander caught in some kind of disaster, forced to be cool and wise with one of the victims, perhaps a child bleeding toward death or an old man pinned under a truck wheel. She talked quietly to this helpless, shocked soul fluttering in its poor body. She was strong and calm. All the while, she knew cynically that she was nonexistent except in the need thrust upon her, and that the victim would either die or recover and forget her dramatic saintliness before the ambulance had come.

"Listen to your breathing," she said coolly. "You are not badly hurt. Soon you will feel all right. Sip this. It will make the pain go away. Lift your head now, and breathe slowly. You are not really in trouble." And so on. Whenever the other part of Mrs. Thayer, the threatened part, let her mind slip back to the horror of an imminent breaking with all reason—and then, so then, out the door it would be final—the kindly stranger seemed to sense it in the eyeballs and the pulse as she bent over the body and spoke more firmly: "Now hold the cup. You can. I know you can. You will be all right." (p. 164)

Mrs. Thayer perseveres and later decides that the pills, helped by the warm drink, have worked. She concludes that her mind has not failed her as she attempts to distract herself with the Twenty-third Psalm and convince herself that "she would never have run out like a beast, to die quickly on the dunes" (p. 165). Later she reflects on her experience.

In another two hours everything was all right inwardly in her, except that she was languid, as if she had lain two weeks in a fever. The panic that had seized her bones and spirit faded fast, once routed. She was left wan and bemused. Never had she been afraid—that is, of tangibles like cold and sand and wind. She was not afraid, as far as she knew, of dying either fast or slowly. It was, she decided precisely, a question of sound. If the storm had not lasted so long, with its noise so much into her, into her brain and muscles . . . If this had been a kind of mating, it was without joy.

. . . And during the late afternoon while she dozed with a deep, soft detachment, the sound abated and then died, and she was lost in the sweet dream life of a delivered woman. (p. 166)

Terms and Meanings

Mrs. Thayer's experience, and her methods of coping both during and after the experience, illustrate what is essential and mysterious about the human emotion we call anxiety. Is it really the wind that causes Mrs. Thayer's panic? Or is the search for causes necessitated by some fundamental human quality that cannot let events such as this go unexplained? Is it better that she find a cause, even if incorrect, than that she not search at all?

In fact, speculation concerning cues has played a pivotal role in theorizing about anxiety over the years. Many early theorists, among them Kierkegaard and Freud, based definitions and distinctions of "fear" and "anxiety" on the presence or absence of cues. For most, one important distinction became prominent: "Fear" was seen as a reaction to a specific, observable danger, while "anxiety" was seen as a diffuse, objectless apprehension. Theorizing about anxiety, then, involved a search for "hidden" cues that was not unlike Mrs. Thayer's speculations on the sound of the wind. This distinction between fear and anxiety produced the rich theoretical framework that still underlies much of our thinking on the development of psychopathology. Standard definitions of "fear" and "anxiety" in dictionaries and introductory psychology textbooks continue to refer to the presence or absence of identifiable cues as the essential distinction. The ascendance of direct behavioral approaches to treating fears and phobias began to change that, however (Wolpe, 1958). Behavior therapy assumed that all anxiety has clear identifiable cues, although some cues are more diffuse than others (e.g., patterns of light and dark). The distinction between "fear" and "anxiety" became blurred for many, and these terms have until recently been equated in psychology and psychiatry.

But terminology describing experiences such as Mrs. Thayer's is more varied and confusing than the hypothetical distinction between fear and anxiety. Among many terms in common use in the English language today are "anxiety, fear," "dread," "phobia," "fright," "panic," and "apprehensiveness." Each of these terms is often qualified with such words as "acute," "morbid," "generalized," "diffuse," and so forth to provide different shades of meaning. In addition, no student of anxiety reflecting on terminology can omit the German word *angst*. Although difficult to translate, this word forms the basis for much of our thinking about the role of anxiety in psychopathology, since it was the word used by both Kierkegaard and Freud. For Kierkegaard, *angst* would be both "dread" and "anxiety"; however, sometimes one is used in English translations of Kierkegaard and sometimes the other. For Freud, *angst* came to reflect the notion of anxiety without an identifiable object. Rather, *angst* was a vague apprehension about the future (although the theoretical significance focused on the present and the past). When anxiety had an object, Freud also preferred the word *furcht* (fear). Although "anxiety" is the word with which we are now familiar, Sir Aubrey Lewis (1980) suggests that a more precise translation of *angst* would be "agony," "dread," "fright," "terror," "consternation," "alarm," or "apprehension." Essentially, the word *angst* signifies a far more shattering emotion than the English word "anxiety," which is often used as synonymous with "concern." As Lewis (1980) points out, the relevant root word passed down from Greek and Latin is *angh*, which refers literally in Latin to the concept of narrowness or constriction. Various derivatives of this root have evolved differently in different Western languages, as one can see by examining the number of words in English with the *angh* root. Among these are "anxiety," "anguish," and "anger."

The profusion of meanings and flavors surrounding the key words *angst*, "anxiety," and "dread"; the somewhat different usages in different languages; and the imprecision resulting from translations of seminal works have all resulted in an understandable vagueness surrounding the term "anxiety" in English. The short history of the usage of the term in psychopathology has produced even less precision. In recent years, "anxiety" has been used to refer to emotional states such as doubt, boredom, mental conflict, disappointment, bashfulness, and feelings of unreality. Various cognitive deficits, such as lack of concentration, are also labeled "anxiety." In addition, the term has been inextricably bound up with the variety of terms describing depressive emotional states. The emergence of theoretical and descriptive qualifiers (e.g., "unconscious," "conscious," "cognitive," "somatic," "free-floating," "bound," "signal") produces further confusion. For this reason, the difficulty in settling on precise distinctions among the anxiety-related terms in English is not surprising.

This state of confusion has caused some to propose that we drop the word altogether, since it is so imprecise as to be unscientific (Sarbin, 1964). In fact, Sarbin and other social constructivists such as Hallam (1985) have proposed new ways of thinking about the concept. For example, Hallam has suggested that anxiety is essentially a lay construct that can refer to vastly different cognitive and somatic points of reference from person to person. For social constructivists, anxiety is best considered a metaphor. For the moment, I forgo my own definitions of the crucial terms "anxiety," "fear," "panic," "apprehension," and so on; I elaborate on these terms at appropriate points in later chapters.

Being and Preparing

Mrs. Thayer can find no reason for her panic until deciding, upon reflection, that the cause is the incessant sound of the storm. For this reason, many would say that her experience is one of anxiety rather than fear, although since the 1980s many would employ the term "panic" as she herself does. But what could be the purpose of this experience? If Darwinian fear and panic facilitate survival, what is the purpose of "anxiety" in the traditional usage of the term, where there is nothing to fear? Philosophers preoccupied with a search for cues have often decided that there is something very valuable indeed in this experience, which may lead one, in an ironic way, to a greater sense of fulfillment and actualization.

Kierkegaard (1844/1944) was one of the first to make this suggestion when he decided that the source of anxiety is deep within the individual. Anxiety, thought Kierkegaard, is rooted not just in a fear of death, but in a fear of nonexistence, nonbeing, or nothingness. Only through recognizing and confronting this fear of becoming nothing—only through the threat of dissolution of the self—can one truly discover the essence of being. Only through this experience can one achieve a clear distinction of the self from other objects or from nonbeing.

Other well-known theorists and clinicians have settled on a similar cause for diffuse and objectless anxiety. For example, Rollo May (1979) has proposed:

> [Anxiety is] the apprehension cued off by a threat to some value that the individual holds essential to his existence as a personality. The threat may be to physical life (a threat of death), or to psychological existence (the loss of freedom, meaninglessness). Or the threat may be to some other value which one identifies with one's existence (patriotism, the love of another person, "success," etc.). (p. 180)

In the sense that this confrontation results in a higher level of existence and a greater appreciation of what it is to be alive, this may represent the shadow of intelligence, and the purpose and meaning of anxiety.

As Freud saw it, *angst* can be cued by activation of elemental threats to the child, which are stored deep in memory and elicited in the adult by a variety of learned associations (Freud, 1926/1959; Michels, Frances, & Shear, 1985; Shear, Cooper, Klerman, & Busch, 1993). In this sense, anxiety is related to the persistence of remembered danger situations that seemed real at an earlier stage of development. For example, the developmentally immature fears of castration or separation may be activated by the emergence of an associated wish or by the occurrence of a symbolically linked situation currently present in one's environment. Anxiety functions to warn of a potential danger situation and triggers the recruitment of internal psychological and/or external protective mechanisms. The institution of effective psychological defense mechanisms serves the adaptive purposes of protecting the integrity of the individual and allowing a higher and more mature level of functioning. Anxiety may also be adaptive in recruiting help from others when there is real danger. Sometimes defensive reactions are inadequate and lead to symptom formation. These may include phobic or compulsive symptoms that are symbolically related to the unconscious wishes or fears that have generated the anxiety. Self-defeating aspects of anxiety are further elaborated below.

Freud would view the raging storm and incessant noise of Mrs. Thayer's blizzard as providing sensory stimuli indicative of a real threat. Anxiety occurs in reaction to the possibility of being overwhelmed by this threat and rendered helpless. The sense of ultimate separation and isolation one can only experience alone in a blizzard may also elicit memories of childhood fears of separation. For Mrs. Thayer, this dual challenge leads to the emergence of unmanageable levels of anxiety and a strong primitive urge to find some human contact.

But even these popular and still current ideas probably do not capture Liddell's (1949) meaning when he talked of anxiety as the shadow of intelligence. Although Liddell was talking of human experience, his scientific explorations concerned the development of pathological anxiety in animals. In his most famous experiments, he produced what came to be called "experimental neurosis" (see Chapter 8). One consequence of experimental neurosis is that animals become more vigilant concerning future threats. Liddell theorized that vigilance has positive consequences in addition to simply helping the animal to notice more quickly the next threat to its well-being. He observed that vigilant animals seem to be conditioned or to learn more easily. Vigilance, therefore, which Liddell supposed to be the animal counterpart of anxiety, may produce more learning and therefore more intelligent animals. But it is the type of learning that is particularly important. The vigilant animal, occupied as it is with future threat, is concerned with what is going to happen in the immediate future. In a very elementary sense, the animal is planning for that future by taking an orientation to the future best characterized by the question "What happens next?". The planning function is apparent. In humans, this is extremely adaptive. Liddell suggested that effective planning for the future and the retrospective enjoyment of past achievements are the means by which human beings construct culture. The capacity to experience anxiety and the capacity to plan are therefore two sides of the same coin. It is in this sense that anxiety accompanies intellectual activity as its shadow.

Anyone who has succeeded at any task, however small, has probably experienced some aspect of this fascinating and mysterious quality of anxiety. For we have known for almost 100 years that our physical and intellectual performance is driven and enhanced by the experience of anxiety, at least up to a point. In 1908, Yerkes and Dodson demonstrated this in the laboratory by showing that the performance of animals on a simple task was better if they were made "moderately anxious" than if they were experiencing no anxiety at all. Since that time, similar observations have been made concerning human performance in a wide variety of situations and contexts. Without anxiety, little would be accomplished. The performance of athletes, entertainers, executives, artisans, and students would suffer; creativity would diminish; crops might not be planted. And we would all achieve that idyllic state long sought after in our fast-paced society of whiling away our lives under a shade tree. This would be as deadly for the species as nuclear war.

In summary, several centuries of thought from very diverse sources have emphasized the importance of anxiety to creativity, intelligence, and survival itself. But it is unlikely that Mrs. Thayer, trapped in her cottage on the ocean at the height of a storm, comes to consider it a growth experience. For her in her fictional setting, as well as for countless millions of individuals in the course of their everyday existence, it is a dramatic life-and-death struggle with the ever-present possibility that death may win out. And there is evidence that death does win out on occasion, as a result of the cumulative consequences of anxiety.

THE SPECTER OF DEATH

The Neurotic Paradox

In 1950, O. Hobart Mowrer described a mystery:

> [It is] the absolutely central problem in neurosis and therapy. Most simply formulated, it is a paradox—the paradox of behavior which is at one and the same time self-perpetuating and self-defeating! . . . Common sense holds that a normal, sensible man, or even a beast to the limits of his intelligence, will weigh and balance the consequences of his acts: if the net effect is favorable, the action producing it will be perpetuated; and if the net effect is unfavorable, the action producing it will be inhibited, abandoned. In neurosis, however, one sees actions which have predominently unfavorable consequences; yet they persist over a period of months, years, or a lifetime. (p. 486)

This paradox is seen daily in clinics all over the world. Consider the case of John Madden, the well-known American sports announcer and former professional football coach, who has written widely about his anxiety and uses it in a humorous manner in several television commercials. Although Madden has overcome the stigma and embarrassment that would be keenly felt by any 6'4", 260-pound former football player whose business is to be tough and courageous, he has not overcome the anxiety itself. Rather than taking a few hours to fly from New York to San Francisco to announce the next football game, he must spend the better part of his week on a train going across the country. In fact, his fears are not limited to planes, but extend to all claustrophobic situations.

Although Madden was always tense in planes, he originally thought of his tension as a reaction to altitude, probably the symptoms of an inner ear infection. When he realized that his anxiety began before the plane took off, but after the stewardess closed the door, he questioned his previous diagnosis. One day while flying across the country, he experienced a particularly severe panic attack, left the plane at a stop halfway across the United States, and never flew again.

John Madden and countless millions of other individuals suffering from anxiety-based disorders are well aware that there is little or nothing to fear in the situations they find so difficult. Therefore, in Mowrer's terms, Madden should have long since weighed the consequences of his acts and decided that, since flying is the safest way to travel, it would be in his best interest to fly in order to save himself time and help maintain his lucrative career. And yet he does not and cannot abandon his self-defeating behavior. One might say that if Madden at least attempted to fly, he would learn something that does not seem amenable to the rational force of persuasion by either himself or others—namely, that flying is safe. But we know from years of clinical and scientific experience that even forced exposure to difficult situations does not always resolve the paradox.

The self-defeating nature of anxiety and its consequences is dramatically elaborated in psychoanalytic theory. Freud saw anxiety as the psychic reaction to danger. A situation can be defined as dangerous if it threatens a person with helplessness in the face of threat. Dangers regarding the external world lead to realistic anxiety, and dangers to conscience result in moral anxiety; however, dangers surrounding the strength of the passions lead to neurotic anxiety. Neurotic anxiety originates from an inner instinctual wish that is associated with a reactivation of an infantile fear situation. The generation of anxiety in any of these spheres leads to the institution of a defense mechanism. All forms of anxiety occur in normal individuals. In the process of development, individuals learn to modify and modulate the expression of anxiety from its most disruptive intense form to an unnoticeable form called "signal anxiety." Signal anxiety is imperceptible to the person experiencing it, and serves the sole purpose of rapidly and efficiently triggering a defensive reaction. Thus normal anxiety is limited in intensity and duration, and is associated with adaptive defenses. Anxiety is self-defeating or pathological when it is noticeable, intense, disruptive, and paralyzing, or when it triggers self-defeating defensive processes, also called "symptoms." Phobic and obsessive symptoms are especially common in reaction to anxiety. These symptoms represent an insufficient attempt at warding off a danger situation, and typically incorporate elements of the danger. For example, a dog phobia may develop in connection with the activation of an infantile fear of castration. The fear is displaced, but the aggressive component is retained.

In the world of Freud, we confront our infantile modes of psychological functioning. Pathological anxiety emerges in connection with some of our deepest and darkest instincts. Before Freud, the embodiment of good and evil and of urges and prohibitions was conceived of as external and spiritual, usually in the guise of demons confronting the forces of good. Since Freud, we ourselves have become the battleground of these forces, and we are inexorably caught up in the battle, sometimes for better and sometimes for worse.

Mortality

If anxiety, in the minds of some, is apprehension over confronting nothingness, consider the consequences of severe anxiety, which result occasionally in physical destruction or death. Consider the man with fears of choking so severe that he consumes only strained and blended food; the results may be malnourishment, loss of teeth, and eventually death. Or consider the woman with obsessive–compulsive disorder (OCD) who ritualistically washes and disinfects her arms and legs for the better part of her waking day; the results may be massive abrasions, bleeding, and scabbing.

Cardiovascular Disease

Whereas self-defeating behavior associated with anxiety may occasionally produce death, the long-term consequences of anxiety itself may hasten the dreaded confrontation with nothingness. Long-term follow-up studies of both inpatients (Coryell, Noyes, & Clancy, 1982) and outpatients (Coryell, Noyes, & House, 1986) found a greater-than-expected mortality rate in patients with original diagnoses of anxiety disorders, particularly panic disorder. This excess mortality rate was attributed primarily to cardiovascular disease and suicide. Interestingly, excess mortality due to cardiovascular disease in these studies was limited to males with panic disorder. Expected death rates for females with panic disorder from cardiovascular disease were within normal range.

More recent prospective studies, with larger groups of males, confirm this frightening finding. In the first of these studies, Kawachi, Colditz, et al. (1994) examined over time a large group of over 33,000 male health professionals between the ages of 42 and 77, to assess the relationship between anxiety and the risk of coronary heart disease. Data were obtained from a large-scale study of normative aging. Men with the highest levels of phobic anxiety had a level of risk for fatal coronary heart disease three times higher than that of men with lower levels of anxiety. More importantly, the relative risk was limited to men experiencing sudden cardiac death as opposed to nonsudden coronary death. In fact, men with the highest levels of phobic anxiety had a relative risk of sudden death six times that of men with the lowest anxiety levels. In a second study, the relationship between symptoms of anxiety and coronary heart disease in over 2,200 male community residents aged 21 through 80 revealed an increased risk of fatal coronary heart disease that was almost five times that of males with few or no anxiety symptoms. It is significant that this elevated risk ratio was present even after confounding variables (family history of heart disease, smoking, blood pressure, etc.) were controlled for. One possible mechanism by which anxiety might influence cardiac function is decreased heart rate variability in anxious individuals, which can result in ventricular arrhythmias (Kawachi, Sparrow, Vokonas, & Weiss, 1995; Zaubler & Katon, 1996). Findings suggesting the relationship between decreased heart rate variability and anxiety are becoming more robust (Yeragani et al., 1995) and are discussed in more detail in Chapter 6.

Suicide

Death by suicide is an event most often associated with depression. But Coryell et al. (1986) found that the frequency of suicide in patients with anxiety disorders was equal to the frequency in matched groups suffering from depression. Why would people who are anxious kill themselves? Coryell et al. (1986) speculated that patients diagnosed with anxiety disorders may subsequently develop major depression or alcoholism as a complication. They thought it possible that earlier studies had overlooked the occurrence of suicide in anxious patients because they noticed only the subsequent complication of alcoholism or depression. But if alcoholism or depression is a consequence of anxiety, than the long road to suicide may begin with anxiety. This intriguing early study was not widely noted.

But a subsequent study, published by Myrna Weissman and her colleagues in the *New England Journal of Medicine*, attracted international attention from public health communities, this study noted that, based on data from a community survey—the Epidemiologic Catchment Area (ECA), study described in more detail below—some 20% of patients with panic disorder had made a suicide attempt at some point during their lives (Weissman, Klerman, Markowitz, & Ouellette, 1989). This finding was alarming to clinicians who treated panic disorder. Weissman et al. (1989) also agreed with Coryell et al. (1986) that the risks of suicide in patients with panic disorder were comparable to those associated with major depression. In a subsequent report (Johnson, Weissman, & Klerman, 1990), the investigators were very careful to analyze panic disorder either with or without comorbid diagnoses such as depression or substance abuse, and found that the risks of suicide were substantially elevated even in patients *without* these cormorbid disorders.

This finding then became very controversial, since clinicians had difficulty confirming the presence of suicidal risk in patients with panic disorder under their care. For example, my colleagues and I (Friedman, Jones, Chernen, & Barlow, 1992) and Beck, Steer, Sanderson, and Skeie (1991) examined hundreds of patients with panic disorder in outpatient clinics, and did not find a suicidal risk that seemed to be associated exclusively with panic disorder. That is, any suicidal risks (e.g., suicidal attempts or ideation) seemed to be present only in those patients with additional disorders (such as comorbid borderline personality disorder, in which suicidal attempts are a prominent characteristic). For example, Beck et al. (1991) reported that in their last 900 outpatients with panic disorder, all suicide attempts were attributed to a comorbid depressive disorder. This was in direct contradiction to the large community study reported by Weissman et al. (1989).

What accounts for these marked discrepancies? Of course, the method of assessment and type of interview used in the studies differed considerably, as did the populations studied. Individuals in the ECA study came from a random sample of the community. The clinical samples consisted of patients seeking treatment. Thus it is possible that the ECA study may have included individuals who not only were untreated for panic disorder, but also were unaware of the possibility of treatment for this disorder. As a result, they might have become hopeless and begun to think about suicide. All patients at the clinics, on the other hand, were properly diagnosed and about to receive treatment. On the other hand, Beck et al. (1991) and our group (Friedman et al., 1992) also checked for lifetime suicide attempts in the clinical samples and did not find elevated risk at any time, which would include periods prior to seeking treatment. Also, Hornig and McNally (1995) looked more closely at the original ECA data from Weissman and colleagues' studies, and suggested after additional analyses that elevated risk of suicide was associated with comorbid diagnoses, if the data on comorbidity were analyzed in the aggregate rather than by individual comorbid disorder.

The discrepancy remains something of a mystery, but other studies have now appeared that continue to alarm clinicians. For example, Noyes (1991) reviewed a number of early studies, many examining the relationships of suicide attempts to anxiety disorders in general, and concluded there was an elevated risk. In a large and important study, Allgulander and Lavori (1991) examined over 3,000 inpatients in Sweden with "pure" anxiety neurosis (i.e., without comorbid depressive or other diagnoses). They concluded that the risk of completed suicide in these patients was as high as that in persons with depression. In a follow-up study, Allgulander (1994) expanded his inquiry to almost 10,000 patients with anxiety disorders and concluded that the risk for completing suicide before the age of 45 years among men and women with anxiety disorders without any other psychiatric diagnoses was between 4.9 and 6.7 times that of the risk in the general population. Examining the issue from another perspective, Norton, Rockman, Luy, and Marion (1993) noted that patients with substance use disorders and accompanying panic disorder were at substantially more risk for attempting suicide than those individuals with substance use disorders without panic disorder—a finding also reported by Hornig and McNally (1995). Although many questions remain, and further analyses are required, evidence is converging that the experience of anxiety and panic may increase the probability of ending one's life.

Anxiety and Substance Abuse/Dependence

Suicide may be an extreme consequence of the experience of anxiety, but evidence indicates that another type of self-destructive behavior is not. A series of investigations suggests that the relationship of substance use disorders, particularly alcohol abuse and dependence, to anxiety disorders is startlingly high. In an early study, Quitkin, Rifkin, Kaplan, and Klein (1972) reported in some detail on 10 patients with anxiety disorders who also suffered severe complications from drug and alcohol dependence. The important suggestion by Quitkin et al. (1972) was that patients presenting with substance dependence may well be self-medicating an anxiety disorder. Thus any treatment program for individuals with alcohol or other substance use disorders must target this anxiety if the program is to be successful, as well as if it is to prevent relapse.

Although this has always been a common clinical observation, a study by Mullaney and Trippett (1979) attracted new attention to this potentially severe complication of anxiety. They discovered that 33% of 102 individuals with alcohol dependence also had severe, disabling agoraphobia and/or social phobia. In addition, another 35% had mild versions of the same phobias. Thus over 60% of a large group of patients admitted to an alcoholism treatment unit presented with identifiable anxiety disorders of varying severity (in this case, phobias). Smail, Stockwell, Canter, and Hodgson (1984) explored this same question in a particularly systematic and skillful way. They found similar although somewhat less dramatic results. Specifically, 18% of a group of 60 patients presenting with alcohol dependence also presented with severe agoraphobia and/or social phobia, with another 35% evidencing mild versions of the same phobias. Once again, over half (53%) of a group of individuals dependent on alcohol had identifiable phobic disorders.

Since that time, studies using even more conservative criteria have also reported a rather high range from 25% to 45% of patients with severe alcohol use problems presenting with one or more anxiety disorders (e.g., Chambless, Cherney, Caputo, & Rheinstein, 1987; Kushner, Sher, & Beitman, 1990; Mullan, Gurling, Oppenheim, & Murray, 1986; Bowen, Cipywnyk, D'Arcy, & Keegan, 1984; Powell, Penick, Othmer, Bingham, & Rice, 1982; Weiss & Rosenberg, 1985). In addition, Cox, Norton, Dorward, and Fergusson (1989) found that over 50% of a group of inpatients with alcohol-related diagnoses reported at least one panic attack in the prior 3 weeks. Over 80% of these patients reported using alcohol to self-medicate their panic attacks.

The above-mentioned studies looked at the incidence of anxiety disorders in individuals diagnosed with alcohol-related disorders. Another approach involves examining the incidence of alcoholism in patients diagnosed as having an anxiety disorder. Otto, Pollack, Sachs, O'Neil, and Rosenbaum (1992) found that 24% of 100 patients with panic disorder presented with a history of alcohol dependence. Thyer, Parrish, et al. (1986) found that 27 out of 156 patients with anxiety disorders, or 17.3%, scored in the "alcoholic" range on the Michigan Alcoholism Screening Test. Bibb and Chambless (1986) also found that from 10% to 20% of individuals with agoraphobia were misusing alcohol.

The obvious question is this: Which comes first, the anxiety or the substance use problem? Several investigators have looked at this issue, and the evidence emerging suggests that a complex relationship exists (Kushner, Sher, & Beitman, 1990; Kushner, Abrams, & Borchardt, 2000). Some retrospective studies indicate that severe anxiety precedes the onset of drinking or substance misuse in most cases (Chambless et al., 1987; Mullaney & Trippett, 1979; Smail et al., 1984). Other studies suggests that alcoholism consistently predates the development of anxiety (Mullan et al., 1986; Kushner, Sher, & Beitman, 1990).

The thoughtful review by Kushner, Sher, and Beitman (1990) of studies done prior to that time suggests that part of the answer for these discrepant results may be due to different patterns of alcohol use problems associated with specific anxiety disorders. In the phobic disorders (particularly agoraphobia and social phobia), alcohol use problems appear more likely to follow the development of the disorders and to begin, perhaps, with attempts to self-medicate the phobic and anxiety symptoms. Disorders without substantial phobic components (such as panic disorder and generalized anxiety disorder [GAD]), on the other hand, may be more likely to be a consequence of excessive consumption of alcohol. Kushner, Sher, and Beitman (1990) also reported that the incidence of alcohol use problems was higher in patients with phobic disorders than in patients with anxiety disorders without substantial phobic components. In a later review, Kushner et al. (2000) confirmed that anxiety disorders and alcohol use disorders can each serve to initiate the other, and that anxiety contributes to maintenance and relapse of alcohol use disorders.

Thus a number of studies have demonstrated elevated incidence of alcohol use problems in patients with anxiety disorders, particularly phobic disorders; and studies have also suggested a higher incidence of anxiety and panic in populations suffering from substance use problems. But the figures differ substantially from study to study, as well as between community samples assessed though proper epidemiological methods and clinical samples. Some investigators reviewing the literature even found little evidence of an increased risk of true anxiety disorders among individuals with alcohol dependence, concluding that most prior studies suffered from faulty methodology (Schuckit & Hesselbrock, 1994). More recently, however, a major study reported by leading epidemiologists from around the world has shed some light on the complexities and contradictions reported above.

Swendsen et al. (1998) examined the comorbidity of alcoholism with anxiety and depressive disorders in four different epidemiological investigations conducted in diverse geographic sites. This study is noteworthy because the four epidemiological investigations are well known for having used "state-of-the-art" methodology, and because the results were relatively consistent in different parts of the world. This consistency affords the first definitive answers to questions on the relationship of substance abuse and dependence to anxiety and depressive disorders noted above.

The four epidemiological studies utilized were the ECA study mentioned above, which sampled over 12,000 community residents in five different geographical areas in the United States (excluding institutionalized individuals); the National Comorbidity Survey (NCS), a sophisticated probability sample of over 8,000 noninstitutionalized community residents; an epidemiological study of Puerto Rico, which consisted of a stratified sample of the entire island, yielding over 1,500 eligible residents; and a cohort study of young adults in Zurich, Switzerland, where almost 600 residents of the canton of Zurich were interviewed. Data for the comorbidity of alcoholism with specific anxiety or depressive disorders are presented in Table 1.2. These data clearly indicate that the probability (the odds ratio) of presenting with alcohol abuse or dependence within the past 12 months is two to three times greater if individuals have also had a depressive or anxiety disorder at some point in their lives than if they haven't. These odds ratios represent statistically significant elevations of risk. Furthermore, these ratios are probably underestimates, since GAD, OCD, and posttraumatic stress disorder (PTSD) were not included in these analyses.

Swendsen et al. (1998) also attempted to ascertain the order of onset of alcoholism in relation to anxiety or depressive disorders. This analysis confirmed the findings of Kushner, Sher, and Beitman (1990), in that no consistent or distinctive pattern was observed concerning the onset of alcoholism relative to the nonphobic disorders of major depression, dysthymia, or panic disorder; that is, sometimes alcoholism came first, and at other times the anxiety or depressive disorder came first. In contrast, there was strong evidence that phobias preceded the development of alcohol abuse or dependence. These data are clearly presented in Table 1.3. Values are provided for the proportion of subjects with the onset of alcoholism either preceding, concomitant to, or postdating the onset of anxiety or depressive disorders. For example, for comorbid depressive disorders and alcoholism in the ECA study, 45% of the comorbid sample developed alcoholism first, 10% developed the disorders at the same time, and 45% developed the depressive disorders first. For phobias and alcoholism in the ECA study, on the other hand, 13.1% developed the alcoholism first, and 83% developed the phobic disorders first.

The investigators conclude that since alcoholism, anxiety disorders, and depressive disorders are the most frequent psychological disorders in community samples, the fact that they frequently co-occur is of considerable concern to clinicians and public health officials. Furthermore, whereas the order of onset of alcoholism and nonphobic anxiety or depressive disorders is inconsistent, a strong relationship emerges for alcoholism following the onset of phobic disorders. Thus panic disorder or GAD could occur either as a consequence of alcoholism, or subsequent to attempts to self-medicate panic and anxiety. For phobic disorders,

TABLE 1.2. Odds Ratios of Previous 12–Month Alcohol Abuse/Dependence Comorbidity with Lifetime Depressive and Anxiety Disorders, Accounting for Age, Gender, and Education (Weighted Data)

	ECA		NCS		Puerto Rico		Zurich	
	OR	95% CI	OR	95% CI	OR	95% CI	OR	95% CI
Comorbidity of alcohol abuse and/or dependence with . . .								
Major depression	3.01*	2.89–3.12	2.27*	1.73–2.99	1.25	0.46–3.41	4.77*	1.72–13.22
Dysthymia	1.67*	1.58–1.71	2.45*	1.19–5.06	1.36	0.42–4.40	4.53	0.86–23.95
Any depressive disorder[a]	2.68*	2.63–2.90	2.28*	1.70–3.06	2.88	0.82–10.09	4.48*	1.38–14.53
Agoraphobia	2.67*	2.57–2.78	2.57*	1.55–4.28	2.91*	1.23–6.90	7.84*	2.07–29.73
Simple phobia	1.95*	1.91–1.99	2.91*	2.08–4.06	1.79	0.84–3.86	3.27	0.99–10.82
Social phobia	1.81*	1.01–3.26	2.20*	1.49–3.25	0.87	0.12–10.98	2.96	0.32–27.09
Any phobia[b]	1.95*	1.92–1.99	2.40*	1.79–3.22	3.46*	1.85–6.48	4.23*	1.05–17.01
Panic disorder	4.06*	3.90–4.22	1.21	0.77–1.90	0.40	0.49–12.68	4.08	0.79–21.18
Any anxiety disorder[c]	2.10*	2.06–2.14	2.38*	1.77–3.19	3.26*	1.78–5.99	2.32*	1.02–5.29

Note. OR, odds ratio; CI, confidence interval. Swendsen et al. (1998). Copyright 1998 by W. B. Saunders Company. Reprinted by permission.
[a]Any major depression or dysthymia.
[b]Any agoraphobia, simple phobia, or social phobia.
[c]Any agoraphobia, simple phobia, social phobia, or panic disorder.
*$p < .05$(two-tailed).

on the other hand, the self-medication hypothesis receives strong support and underscores the risk in phobic disorders of developing substance abuse or dependence.

Patients with anxiety disorders who also suffer from alcohol abuse or dependence generally present with more severe anxiety (Chambless et al., 1987; Woodruff, Guze, & Clayton, 1972). Periods of abstinence seem to result in a general improvement in fear and anxiety in many patients (e.g., Stockwell, Smail, Hodgson, & Canter, 1984). Thus, contrary to myth, alcohol does not necessarily reduce anxiety and fear in the long term, and may in fact worsen it (Thyer & Curtis, 1984). Whether anxiety disorders precede substance use disorders or follow them, the alcohol (or drug) use seems to have a deleterious effect on mood, creating a vicious cycle. (Kushner et al., 2000; Kushner, Sher, & Erickson, 1999). This finding is very clearly underscored in the epidemiological data from Swendsen et al. (1998). Table 1.4 presents increases in symptoms of anxiety and depression associated with comorbid alcohol abuse or dependence. Although there was little or no impact of alcoholism on the symptoms of phobic disorders, comorbid alcoholism increased other depressive and anxiety symptoms substantially in some cases. Conversely, the presence of any anxiety or depressive disorder was significantly associated with moderate increases in the number of symptoms of alcohol abuse or dependence. Among the anxiety disorders, this effect was most notable for panic disorder, with an increase of 0.48 (ECA) or 0.60 (NCS) in the number of alcohol symptoms over what would be expected from alcohol abuse or dependence alone.

A recent prospective study, the first of its kind, has confirmed that the odds of developing a comorbid anxiety disorder in the context of an existing alcohol use disorder (alcohol use disorder leading to anxiety disorder) or vice versa (anxiety disorder leading to alcohol use disorder) are 3.5 to 5 times what they would be in the absence of a preexisting disorder (Kushner, Sher, & Erickson, 1999).

TABLE 1.3. Retrospective Estimates for Order of Onset of Alcohol Abuse/Dependence with Anxiety and Depressive Disorders

Age of onset	Depressive disorders[a]			Phobias[b]			Panic		
	ECA	NCS	Puerto Rico	ECA	NCS	Puerto Rico	ECA	NCS	Puerto Rico
A < B	45.0%	54.9%	40.0%	13.1%	19.0%	27.3%	45.2%	62.3%	33.3%
A = B	10.0%	10.7%	20.0%	3.2%	4.2%	9.1%	10.2%	5.1%	16.7%
A > B	45.0%	34.4%	40.0%	83.0%	76.7%	63.6%	44.5%	32.7%	50.0%
Total no.	174	441	15	315	585	33	23	96	6

Note. A, alcoholism; B, index disorder. From Swendsen et al. (1998). Copyright 1998 by W. B. Saunders Company. Reprinted by permission.
[a]Any major depression or dysthymia.
[b]Any agoraphobia, simple phobia, or social phobia.

Thus anxiety and panic, when self-medicated with alcohol, result in an ever-increasing downward self-destructive spiral—not only from the effects of alcohol (or drug) addiction, but also from the exacerbating effects of the drugs on the anxiety and panic. (Kushner et al., 2000). It may be this complication, along with the development of helplessness and depression, that leads to the increased risk of suicide in patients with anxiety (Coryell et al., 1986; Norton et al., 1993).

Furthermore, alcohol is not the only substance that has a notable association with anxiety. There is a growing literature on the strong association between the use of cocaine and at least one anxiety disorder: panic disorder (Louie et al., 1996; Bystritsky, Ackerman, & Pasnau, 1991). In one report (Louie et al., 1996), 86 patients reported developing panic attacks after significant usage of cocaine. But the more frightening finding was that full-blown panic disorder continued long after cessation of cocaine use and misuse. Thus panic attacks seem related to both the use of cocaine and the abrupt cessation of its use (almost 20% of patients reported that they were worse immediately after stopping the cocaine), and panic disorder and associated anxiety may linger after cessation of use. The experience of these individuals shows that anxiety and panic are a very heavy price indeed to pay for the momentary pleasure associated with cocaine.

Surgery

Substance abuse or dependence is often a self-initiated attempt to cope with the unbearable experience of anxiety. In its most severe form, the paralysis and self-destruction associated with anxiety have led to equally dramatic attempts on the part of concerned health care practitioners to alleviate this suffering. Among the more desperate efforts is neurosurgery (sometimes called "psychosurgery," since the goal is to treat psychological disorders) (Jenike et al., 1991; Marks, Birley, & Gelder, 1966; Sachdev, Hay, & Cumming, 1992; Smith & Kiloh, 1980). As with any major surgical procedure, death can be a complication. Causes of death are most often cerebral hemorrhage or edema, although the trend toward more precise and limited lesions has greatly decreased the risk of serious side effects. Neurosurgical procedures as treatments for anxiety disorders, mostly severe OCD, have been reported in the literature on thousands of patients (e.g., Smith & Kiloh, 1980).

TABLE 1.4. Increase in Disorder Symptoms Associated with Comorbid Alcohol Abuse/Dependence

Study site	Class of symptoms	Metric regression coefficient	95% CI
ECA	Major depression	.96*	0.87–1.05
	Dysthymia	1.00*	0.91–1.09
	Panic	.35*	0.29–0.42
	Agoraphobia	.01	0.00–0.02
	Simple phobia	.01	-01–0.03
	Social phobia	.00	0.00–0.01
	Any phobia[a]	.04*	0.01–0.07
	Any anxiety[b]	.59*	0.49–0.69
NCS	Major depression	.81*	0.71–0.91
	Dysthymia	1.00*	0.90–1.10
	Panic	.48*	0.36–0.60
	Agoraphobia	.07*	0.03–0.11
	Simple phobia	.07*	0.03–0.11
	Social phobia	.15*	0.09–0.21
	Any phobia[a]	.25*	0.15–0.35
	Any anxiety[b]	.58*	0.40–0.76

Note. Global model df (ECA) = 5, 12,708; global model df (NCS) = 6, 8,091. From Swendsen et al. (1998). Copyright 1998 by W. B. Saunders Company. Reprinted by permission.
[a]Any agoraphobia, simple phobia, or social phobia.
[b]Any agoraphobia, simple phobia, social phobia, or panic disorder.
*$p < .05$(two-tailed).

Although rare in the United States and the United Kingdom, these therapeutic procedures are fairly standard in some countries. It is probably safe to conclude that hundreds of thousands of patients have consented to this type of surgical treatment, most often after all other treatments have failed.

Surgical procedures have become very sophisticated in recent years. For OCD, cingulotomy and orbito-medial lesions are now the most common procedures. Jenike et al. (1991) and Sachdev et al. (1992) found that between 25% and 40% of patients with very severe and intractable OCD evidenced some clinically useful improvement (see Chapter 15).

PREVALENCE AND COURSE

Anxiety kills relatively few people, but many more would welcome death as an alternative to the paralysis and suffering resulting from anxiety in its severe forms. For decades, studies have shown that millions of individuals each year seek help for what is broadly construed as "anxiety" or "nervousness." Statistics compiled from the offices of front-line primary care practitioners startle even the most jaded experts in the area. In an early study from the state of Virginia, investigators surveying the reasons why patients sought out their local physicians found that hypertension, cuts and bruises, and sore throats ranked right behind a general medical checkup as the most common reasons motivating a visit. Close behind these common maladies was "anxiety," ranking well ahead of even bad colds or bronchitis (Marsland, Wood, & Mayo, 1976). Another early survey documented that one of every five primary care patients was taking benzodiazepines (Wells, Goldberg, Brook, & Leake, 1986). This kind of information explains the high utilization of health care and high costs of anxiety in primary care settings (e.g., Greenberg et al., 1999; Simon et al., 1995). In fact, one recent study documented that over 50% of the estimated $1,500+ cost per individual suffering from anxiety in the United States was attributed to utilization of primary care services (Greenberg et al., 1999).

Is everyone with a complaint of "anxiety" or "nerves" who seeks out a local physician or health care practitioner really suffering from anxiety? Does everyone who takes minor tranquilizers have a clearly defined anxiety disorder? Most clinicians and investigators would guess that these millions of individuals do not present with clearly identifiable anxiety disorders, but rather with some vague combination of stress, adjustment to difficult family or work situations, or other temporary problems (e.g., difficulty sleeping). For years it was impossible actually to ascertain the number of these individuals presenting with anxiety disorders. Recently, however, epidemiologists have begun to undertake this arduous task, culminating in two of the most ambitious studies of the prevalence of mental disorders ever undertaken.

Before these studies are described, it is interesting to put the numbers in context. One of the first studies using sophisticated, up-to-date sampling techniques to estimate the distribution of fears and phobias in the general population was undertaken by Agras, Sylvester, and Oliveau (1969). They conducted a probability sample of the household population of a small city in the United States (Burlington, Vermont), and they interviewed the 325 individuals who made up the sample. From this study, the estimated total prevalence of phobias was 7.7%, but only 0.02% presented with phobias severe enough to result in an absence from work or the inability to manage common household tasks. The investigators diagnosed 0.06% of the sample, or 6 out of 1,000, as having agoraphobia. Many more individuals, approaching 50% of the population, presented with mild fears of objects or situations (snakes, heights, storms, etc.).

Another important finding from this study was that phobias ran a prolonged course: Most often an individual, once he or she developed a phobia, had that phobia in at least a mild form for a lifetime. Figure 1.1 shows the rates of incidence (the beginning of the phobia) and prevalence (the presence of the phobia) at various ages within the population. The findings on the prolonged course of phobias were confirmed in a later follow-up study: Agras, Chapin, and Oliveau (1972) found very little improvement in individuals with untreated phobias followed 5 years after the original study, particularly if they were 20 years old or older and if their phobias were more generalized. More recent data supporting this finding are presented below (Goisman et al., 1998). In fact, a distinguishing feature of anxiety disorders and major depressive episodes is that depression tends to remit temporarily whether treated or not—usually in a matter of months, with 9 months the average duration (Barlow & Durand, 1999). Anxiety disorders, on the other hand, tend to be chronic and to remain present in somewhat less severe form even if successfully treated (Noyes & Clancy, 1976; Noyes, Clancy, Hoenk, & Slymen, 1980; Yonkers, Warshaw, Massion, & Keller, 1996; Roy-Byrne & Cowley, 1995).

Two very important developments made more sophisticated and wide-ranging epidemiological efforts possible. First, diagnostic criteria for anxiety disorders were specified in much more detail, allowing more certain identification of the various anxiety

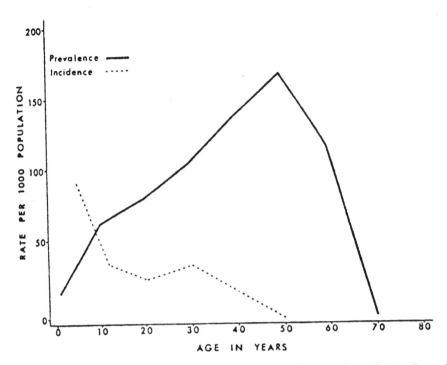

FIGURE 1.1. Incidence and prevalence rates for phobias within the general population. From Agras, Sylvester, and Oliveau (1969). Copyright 1969 by Grune & Stratton. Reprinted by permission.

disorders. Second, semistructured interviews were devised to insure that all investigators would cover the same essential points when interviewing for the presence of anxiety (or other) disorders (see Chapter 9). These developments permitted a more standardized and objective approach to the question of the frequency of specific clinical anxiety disorders in the population.

Data from the ECA study, sponsored by the National Institute of Mental Health and described above, were collected in five different sites around the United States beginning in 1980. The sample population size in each site was approximately 300,000. Approximately 12,000 individuals across sites were interviewed. A semistructured interview that yielded *Diagnostic and Statistical Manual of Mental Disorders*, third edition (DSM-III) anxiety disorder diagnoses was employed by lay individuals trained to administer this interview. Some of the results for panic and phobic disorders from the first wave of interviews are presented in Tables 1.5 and 1.6. These tables present results for panic disorder and the three phobic disorders broken down by sex and ethnicity. Agoraphobia, in Table 1.5, refers to agoraphobia with and without panic attacks according to the older DSM-III criteria. Table 1.5 provides data for lifetime prevalence only for the phobic disorders. As one can see from both tables, females in this study evidenced panic and phobic disorders at about twice the rate of males. From the second wave of the ECA study, we also have an estimate of the lifetime prevalence of DSM-III GAD of 4.0% (Blazer, Hughes, George, Schwartz, & Boyer, 1991).

The second major epidemiological study, the NCS, referred to above, interviewed a random sample of over 8,000 noninstitutionalized individuals in the United States. Since this was a later study, DSM-III-R diagnoses were utilized. Data indicating the prevalence

TABLE 1.5. Lifetime Prevalence[a] of Phobia Subtypes by Sex and Ethnicity, in Percentages (Standard Errors in Parentheses)

	Sample Size[b]	Lifetime Prevalence of . . .		
		Agoraphobia	Simple phobia	Social phobia
Total	14,436	5.63 (0.29)	11.25 (0.40)	2.73 (0.20)
Both sexes				
White	8,501	5.21 (0.31)	10.35 (0.42)	2.68 (0.22)
Black	4,185	9.19 (1.13)	19.70 (1.55)	3.39 (0.71)
Hispanic	1,526	5.37 (1.22)	9.63 (1.59)	2.46 (0.84)
Men				
All groups	6,212	3.18 (0.32)	7.75 (0.49)	2.53 (0.29)
White	3,694	2.85 (0.33)	7.12 (0.51)	2.71 (0.32)
Black	1,630	5.81 (1.35)	14.06 (2.01)	1.87 (0.78)
Hispanic	733	2.90 (1.29)	6.33 (1.88)	1.66 (0.99)
Women				
All groups	8,224	7.86 (0.47)	14.45 (0.61)	2.91 (0.29)
White	4,807	7.38 (0.50)	13.30 (0.65)	2.65 (0.31)
Black	2,555	12.00 (1.71)	24.38 (2.27)	4.66 (1.11)
Hispanic	753	7.74 (2.02)	12.79 (2.52)	3.21 (1.33)

Note. From Eaton, Dryman, and Weissman (1991). Copyright 1991 by The Free Press. Reprinted by permission.
[a]Four sites' combined respondents (Baltimore, St. Louis, Durham, Los Angeles) weighted to the U.S. general population by age, sex, and ethnicity.
[b]Sample sizes given are for agoraphobia. For simple phobia, the total sample was 14,429, and for social phobia, the total was 14,400.

of anxiety disorders in this study, for both the last 12 months and over the course of a lifetime broken down by gender, are presented in Table 1.7. Notice that the total for anxiety disorders over the past 12 months was 17.2% with 24.9% reporting a lifetime occurrence of one of the anxiety disorders included in this report. And this total does not include data for PTSD or OCD.

Despite these exclusions, anxiety disorders were more prevalent than any other class of disorders in the NCS. For example, the 12-month prevalence for mood disorders was 11.3%. For substance use disorders, the prevalence was also 11.3%. The investigators point out that the higher ratio of 12-month to lifetime anxiety disorder prevalence indirectly suggests that these disorders are more chronic than either mood disorders or substance use disorders. In a later report, Kessler, Sonnega, Bromet, Hughes, and Nelson (1995) estimated the lifetime prevalence of PTSD in the NCS at 7.8%.

Direct comparisons of the ECA and NCS results are interesting but somewhat imprecise, given the different diagnostic criteria and somewhat different methodology. Lifetime prevalence for the phobic disorders provides an interesting example. For agoraphobia with and without panic attacks, the prevalence was 5.63% in the ECA study and 6.7% in the NCS. For social phobia, the very discrepant results were 2.73% in the ECA study and 13.3% in the NCS. For simple phobia (now known as specific phobia), the almost identical results were 11.25% in the ECA study and 11.3% in the NCS (Eaton, Dryman, & Weissman, 1991; Magee, Eaton, Wittchen, McGonagle, & Kessler, 1996). Recently, D. Regier,

TABLE 1.6. Prevalence of Panic Disorder by Sex and Ethnicity

| | Sample size | Prevalence in percentages (SE) | | |
		One-month	One-year	Lifetime
Total	19,498[a]	0.53 (.07)	0.91 (.10)	1.57 (.13)
Both sexes				
White	12,968	0.50 (.08)	0.90 (.11)	1.62 (.14)
Black	4,668	0.64 (.26)	1.00 (.32)	1.31 (.37)
Hispanic	1,604	0.51 (.32)	0.66 (.36)	0.87 (.41)
Men				
All groups	8,375	0.35 (.09)	0.58 (.11)	0.99 (.15)
White	5,573	0.33 (.09)	0.58 (.12)	1.02 (.16)
Black	1,855	0.27 (.25)	0.57 (.36)	0.57 (.36)
Hispanic	818	0.31 (.36)	0.32 (.36)	0.41 (.41)
Women				
All groups	11,123	0.69 (.12)	1.22 (.16)	2.10 (.21)
White	7,395	0.65 (.13)	1.20 (.17)	2.17 (.23)
Black	2,813	0.94 (.42)	1.37 (.51)	1.93 (.60)
Hispanic	786	0.69 (.52)	1.00 (.62)	1.31 (.71)

Note. From Eaton, Dryman, and Weissman Edited (1991). Copyright 1991 by The Free Press. Reprinted by permission.
[a]For lifetime prevalence, the total sample size was 19,501. These three additional cases were also included in the calculation of lifetime prevalence for the subgroups.

W. Narrow, and D. Rae (personal communication, 2000) have prepared a best estimate of the prevalence of anxiety (and mood) disorders from these two major surveys (see Table 1.8). These data represent the most accurate estimates to date of the prevalence of anxiety disorders.

These are startling figures. Among many mysteries and paradoxes present in these data, one will notice first that estimates of the prevalence of anxiety disorders in the population have risen from the Agras et al. (1969) study to the ECA study to the NCS. What could account for these differences in estimates of prevalence? Possibly it was the way the questions were asked. For example, in the Agras et al. (1969) study, very conservative criteria were used. But it seems unlikely that this could account for all of the difference. In both the ECA study and the NCS, as noted above, lengthy semistructured interviews and specific, reliable, diagnostic definitions were employed. These factors, when combined with the enormous numbers of people involved, tend to make one more confident in these data. Over time, there has also been an enormous increase in awareness of the problem of anxiety disorders, although once again it is hard to see how this could account for absolute increases in the prevalence of the problem. Are anxiety disorders increasing? For the time being, we do not know.

In any case, these startling statistics have established one overriding fact: Anxiety disorders represent the single largest mental health problem in the country. The prevalence of anxiety disorders in the ECA study surpassed that of any other mental health disorder (including substance use disorders)—even before one considers data for GAD or PTSD, which were not included in the first wave of ECA interviews, or PTSD and OCD, which were not

TABLE 1.7. Lifetime and 12-Month Prevalence of DSM-III-R Anxiety Disorders

	Male				Female				Total			
	Lifetime		12-month		Lifetime		12-month		Lifetime		12-month	
Disorders	%	SE	%	SE	%	SE	%	SE	%	SE	%	SE
Panic disorder	2.0	0.3	1.3	0.3	5.0	1.4	3.2	0.4	3.5	0.3	2.3	0.3
Agoraphobia w/o panic disorder	3.5	0.4	1.7	0.3	7.0	0.6	3.8	0.4	5.3	0.4	2.8	0.3
Social phobia	11.1	0.8	6.6	0.4	15.5	1.0	9.1	0.7	13.3	0.7	7.9	0.4
Simple phobia	6.7	0.5	4.4	0.5	15.7	1.1	13.2	0.9	11.3	0.6	8.8	0.5
Generalized anxiety disorder	3.6	0.5	2.0	0.3	6.6	0.5	4.3	0.4	5.1	0.3	3.1	0.3
Any anxiety disorder	19.2	0.9	11.8	0.6	30.5	1.2	22.6	0.1	24.9	0.8	17.2	0.7

Note. Adapted from Kessler et al. (1994). Copyright 1994 by the American Medicial Association. Adapted by permission.

included in the first report on the NCS. Even the more limited category of phobic disorders alone is the most frequent mental health disorder category in women and the second most frequent in men, following only substance use disorders in the ECA study. Similar results are evident in the NCS. In view of the information reviewed above on the relationship of alcohol abuse or dependence and anxiety disorders, it is also very possible that a large proportion of individuals suffering from substance abuse or dependence are continuing to medicate an underlying phobic disorder, thus further inflating prevalence figures.

Anxiety disorders are particularly prevalent in primary care settings. Spitzer et al. (1995) surveyed primary care settings and reported that fully 18% of patients in these settings reported either panic disorder, GAD, or anxiety symptoms that approximated these disorders. These figures specifically excluded the much larger phobia category. A large World Health Organization (WHO) study of mental disorders in primary care settings also found rates of approximately 10% for panic disorder with and without agoraphobia and GAD in primary care settings around the world (Sartorius, Ustun, Lecrubier, & Wittchen, 1996). Furthermore, it is important to note that certain patterns of physical symptoms presenting in primary care medical settings are highly associated with a subsequent diagnosis of panic disorder. For example, as reviewed in detail in Chapter 4, patients with chest pain and normal coronary arteries (noncardiac chest pain) meet criteria for panic disorder approximately 40% of the time (Katon et al., 1988). Other unexplained physical symptoms that often meet criteria for panic disorder upon further examination include palpitations (45% of the time), unexplained faintness (20%), irritable bowel syndrome (40%), and unexplained vertigo and dizziness (20%) (Roy-Byrne & Katon, 2000). As noted above, patients with anxiety disorders also seek out medical specialists in disproportionate numbers. It is interesting to note that patients with GAD most often end up seeing gastroenterologists, whereas patients with panic disorder tend to see neurologists and otolaryngologists (Kennedy & Schwab, 1997). Anxiety disorders are also strongly associated with chronic respiratory illness (Perna, Bertani, Polito, Columbo, & Bellodi, 1997; Pollack, Kradin, et al., 1996), gastrointestinal symptoms, and vestibular abnormalities (Roy-Byrne & Katon, 2000) (see Chapter 4).

TABLE 1.8. Best-Estimate 1-Year Prevalence based on ECA and NCS Data (Ages 18–54)

	ECA prevalence (%)	NCS prevalence (%)	Best estimate[a](%)
Any anxiety disorder	13.1	18.7	16.4
Simple phobia	8.3	8.6	8.3
Social phobia	2.0	7.4	2.0
Agoraphobia	4.9	3.7	4.9
GAD	(1.5)[b]	3.4	3.4
Panic disorder	1.6	2.2	1.6
OCD	2.4	(0.9)[b]	2.4
PTSD	(1.9)[b]	3.6	3.6
Any Mood disorder	7.1	11.1	7.1
MD episode	6.5	10.1	6.5
MD disorder	5.3	8.9	5.3
Dysthymia	1.6	2.5	1.6
Bipolar I	1.1	1.3	1.1
Bipolar II	0.6	0.2	0.6

Note. MD, major depression. From D. Regier, W. Narrow, and D. Rae (personal communication, 2000). Used by permission of the authors.

[a]In developing best-estimate 1-year prevalence rates from the two studies, a conservative procedure was followed that had previously been used in an independent scientific analysis comparing these two data sets (Andrews, 1995). For any mood disorder and any anxiety disorder, the lower estimate of the two surveys was selected, which for these data was the ECA. The best-estimate rates for the individual mood and anxiety disorders were then chosen from the ECA only, in order to maintain the relationships between the individual disorders. For other disorders that were not covered in both surveys, the available estimate was used.

[b]Number in parentheses indicates the prevalence of the disorder without any comorbidity. These rates were calculated using the NCS data for GAD and PTSD, and the ECA data for OCD. The rates were not used in calculating the "any anxiety disorder" totals for the ECA and NCS columns. The unduplicated GAD and PTSD rates were added to the best-estimate total for any anxiety disorder (3.3%).

As noted above, it has also become very clear in the past several years that anxiety disorders are chronic, and may last for decades or even a lifetime in the absence of effective treatment. Indirect estimates on chronicity from the NCS have been presented above. Marks and Lader (1973) reviewed a series of early studies conducted in the 1950s and 1960s surveying the long-term course of "anxiety neuroses," and found that although some subjects showed some improvement over the course of time, the majority continued to be symptomatic following a chronic and recurrent course over many years. Keller and Baker (1992) reviewed a number of studies completed since the 1970s suggesting similar findings in follow-up periods ranging from 3 to 8 years. In one of the best known of these studies, Noyes et al. (1980) followed 112 patients with anxiety disorders for 4 to 9 years. Eighty-eight percent of this group continued to experience mild to moderate symptoms during this time period. In the Agras et al. (1972) study described above, 43% of subjects with phobia showed some improvement or recovered, but 53% were either unchanged or worse over a 5-year period. Pollack et al. (1990) followed 100 patients with panic disorder prospectively and observed high rates of chronicity; specifically, only 19% of those with extensive phobic avoidance had had at least a 2-month period of remission since the onset of their disorder. Katschnig and Amering (1994) followed a sample of 220 patients with panic disorder naturalistically for 2–6 years after completion of a course of pharmacological treatment. Although 31% recovered and retained their gains during the follow-up period, the remaining 69% demonstrated continued symptomatology over this period of time, with fully 19% of the sample evidencing a severe and chronic course.

In the most ambitious study of its type to date, Martin Keller and colleagues are continuing to conduct a prospective naturalistic and longitudinal study charting the course and outcome of selected anxiety disorders. This study, known as the Harvard–Brown Anxiety Disorder Research Program (Keller, 1994), has already yielded important data. For example, Hirschfeld (1996), analyzing data from this study, observed that during the first 22 months following the onset of an episode, only 18% of patients with panic disorder and agoraphobia, and about 43% of those with panic disorder without agoraphobia, had recovered; by contrast, approximately 80% of those with major depressive disorder had recovered (see Figure 1.2). As of 1997, over 700 initial interviews had been completed, and data on chronicity and relapse are quickly accumulating (M. B. Keller, personal communication July 27, 2000). Some of these data are presented in Table 1.9, which shows that the remission rates for the index anxiety disorders (i.e., panic disorder with and without agoraphobia, agoraphobia without panic disorder, social phobia, and GAD) were uniformly low after 5 years, with the possible exception of uncomplicated panic disorder. But even with panic disorder, there was a 37% probability of remaining in the intake episode after 5 years of prospective follow-up. Relapse rates following a complete recovery were more variable, with relapse rates for panic disorder both with and without agoraphobia very high, and relapse rates for social phobia and GAD somewhat lower, although the numbers were relatively small in these categories. Particularly interesting was a cumulative probability of remission after 2 years of 25% for GAD and 18% for social phobia (and only 28% after 5 years for social phobia). Goisman et al. (1998), analyzing data from this same study, found that the mean length of an episode of specific phobia reported at time of intake was over 22 years! These findings make it very clear that, in addition to being the most prevalent class of mental disorders in the population at large, anxiety disorders are also among the most chronic. This fact has important public health implica-

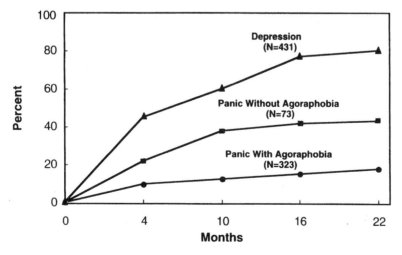

FIGURE 1.2. Recovery from episodes of panic disorder or depression. Data sources: Keller and Baker (1992), Keller et al. (1992). From Hirschfeld (1996). Copyright 1996 by the Guilford Press. Reprinted by permission.

TABLE 1.9. Cumulative Probabilities of Remission and Relapse from the Intake Episode for the Index Disorders

Time	Panic disorder		Panic disorder w/agoraphobia		Agoraphobia only		Social phobia		Generalized anxiety disorder	
	Prob. remission ($n = 77$)	Prob. relapse ($n = 44$)	Prob. remission ($n = 338$)	Prob. relapse ($n = 110$)	Prob. remission ($n = 26$)	Prob. relapse ($n = 7$)	Prob. remission ($n = 160$)	Prob. relapse ($n = 42$)	Prob. remission ($n = 167$)	Prob. relapse ($n = 61$)
1 year	.40	.39	.10	.41	.12	N/A[a]	.12	.08	.16	.12
2 years	.57	.55	.23	.55	.17	.18	.16	.25	.21	
3 years	.58	.58	.29	.64	.17	.26	.16	.28	.27	
4 years	.63	.33	.31	.27	.37					
5 years	.63	.35	.31	.28	.47					

Note. From Keller (2000). Reprinted by permission of the author.
[a]There were too few subjects to estimate relapse rates.

tions pertaining to the costs, both financial and human, of anxiety disorders in our society (see below).

Anxiety disorders do, however, tend to diminish somewhat with increasing age (Flint, 1994). The prevalence of anxiety disorders expressed as a percentage in elderly subjects, as contrasted to subjects of all ages (based on a reanalysis of the ECA data), is presented in Table 1.10. Notice that the prevalence of phobic disorders, panic disorder, and OCD shows a consistent drop across each disorder, as do all anxiety disorders in the aggregate. Notice also that the decline is proportionally similar.

THE HUMAN COSTS OF ANXIETY DISORDERS

With high prevalence and chronicity, one would expect that anxiety disorders would be associated with substantial costs to individuals and to our health care system, not only in terms of money but in lost productivity and reductions in quality of living. The actual expenses, however, dwarf even the most pessimistic estimates (Greenberg et al., 1999; Hofmann & Barlow, 1999). For example, in recent years anxiety disorders accounted for approximately 31% of total costs of mental health care, compared to 22% for mood disorders and 20% for schizophrenia (Rice & Miller, 1993). DuPont et al. (1996) estimated these costs in 1990 at $46.6 billion out of a total expenditure on mental illness of $147.8 billion that year, or 31.5% of the total. These costs included not only the direct cost of services, but also indirect costs of lost productivity.

In the most comprehensive study to date, Greenberg et al. (1999) calculated the annual economic burden of anxiety disorders in the United States in a particularly detailed manner. They estimated the annual cost of anxiety disorders to be approximately $42.3 billion in the United States in 1990, or $1,542 per sufferer. Notice that their estimate is slightly lower than the estimate by DuPont et al. (1996), due to improved methodology. A breakdown of these costs is presented in Figure 1.3. Notice that the costs are largely attributable to direct treatment by a mental health professional, whereas 10% of the costs are due to indirect workplace costs, most of it attributable to lost productivity as opposed to absenteeism. Fully 54% of the costs are associated with excess utilization of primary health care services.

TABLE 1.10 Prevalence of Anxiety Disorders in Elderly Subjects and Combined Age Groups, and Peak Prevalence in the ECA Study

	All anxiety disorders			Phobic disorder			Panic disorder			Obsessive–compulsive disorder		
	M	F	Total	M	F	Total	M	F	Total	M	F	Total
Subjects aged ≥65	3.6	6.8	5.5	2.9	6.1	4.8	0.0	0.2	0.1	0.7	0.9	0.8
Subjects of all ages	4.7	9.7	7.3	3.8	8.4	6.2	0.3	0.7	0.5	1.1	1.5	1.3
Peak	4.7	11.7	8.3	3.5	10.2	6.9	0.3	1.1	0.7	1.2	1.9	1.8

Note. M, males; F, females. From Flint (1994). Copyright 1994 by the American Psychiatric Association. Reprinted by permission.

The relative costs of individual anxiety disorders, in terms of the utilization of services and workplace costs, are shown in Table 1.11. As is evident in this table, the greatest costs were associated with panic disorder and PTSD, but all anxiety disorders except specific phobia were associated with substantial impairment in the workplace.

Markowitz, Weissman, Ouellette, Lish, and Klerman (1989) and Leon, Portera, and Weissman (1995) evaluated the quality of life among individuals with anxiety disorders in the ECA study. Leon et al. (1995) found that individuals with anxiety disorders (panic disorder, OCD, phobias) had elevated rates of financial dependence and unemployment (as reflected in disability payments, welfare, and unemployment compensation), compared to patients without anxiety disorders. Among patients with panic disorder alone, 68% of females and 60% of males with panic disorder were unemployed at the time of the evaluation. Twenty-nine percent of female patients and 25% of male patients were chronically unemployed for 5 years or more. Studying patients with panic disorder, Markowitz et al. (1989) found that both their physical and emotional health were poorer than those of controls without panic disorder or depression; the patients' rates of alcohol and drug misuse were high as well. Rates of health care utilization were likewise significantly higher, as

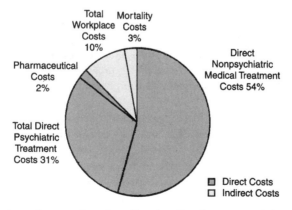

FIGURE 1.3. Distribution of costs of anxiety disorder. Total costs equal $42.3 billion per year in 1990 U.S. dollars. From Greenberg et al. (1999). Copyright 1999 by Physicians Postgraduate Press. Reprinted by permission.

TABLE 1.11. Risk Factors for Service Usage and Adverse Workplace Outcomes

Variable	PTSD	Panic disorder	Agoraphobia	GAD	Social phobia	Specific phobia
Direct psychiatric medical service utilization						
Hospitalization	▲		▲		●	
Physicians						
Family doctors	▲	▲	●	▲		
Psychiatrists	▲	▲	▲		●	
Psychologists	▲	●		●		●
Other specialists (e.g., gynecologists, cardiologists)	▲		▲	▲		
Other						
Social workers	▲	▲	●			
Counselors	▲	▲				
Nurses/therapists	●	▲	▲	●	●	
Other professionals	●	●			●	
Indirect workplace outcomes						
Work loss (absenteeism)		●	●	●	●	
Work cutback days	▲	▲		▲	▲	
Number of categories with significant or large impact	10	9	7	6	6	1
Number of categories with significant impact	8	6	4	3	1	0

Note. Triangles indicate statistically significant impact at the 5% level; circles indicate large odds ratio was obtained, but above the 5% level of significance. From Greenberg et al. (1999). Copyright 1999 by Physicians Postgraduate Press. Reprinted by permission.

reflected in patterns of medical care alone and psychiatric care alone, as well as in visits to the emergency room. For example, 28% of individuals with panic disorder had visited the emergency room during the previous 12 months, compared to 2% of the controls without panic disorder or depression. Forty-three percent of the patients with panic disorder had utilized both psychiatric and medical care in the previous 12 months, compared to only 4% of the controls.

Using ECA data, Boyd (1986) has discovered that an individual with panic disorder is more likely to seek professional help than an individual with schizophrenia or any other mental disorder. Furthermore, the high prevalence of panic attacks associated with other mental disorders may be one of the primary reasons why many patients with other disorders seek treatment. Boyd speculates that the overwhelming sensations of panic and the associated thoughts of death and dying may be the motivating factors in this enormous utilization of health care resources. In addition, we now know with some certainty that many of these patients end up in the offices of cardiologists (Roy-Byrne & Katon, 2000). For example, Beitman, Lamberti, et al. (1987) found that a high proportion of cardiac patients who complained of chest pain, but who had angiographically normal coronary arteries, met criteria for panic disorder. Patients with panic disorder have a long history of seeking out cardiologists (see Chapter 4).

As noted at the beginning of the chapter, the overall health care costs for individuals with anxiety disorders utilizing health care services are double what they are for those without anxiety disorders, regardless of the latter's physical illness. (Simon et al., 1995). In an important study, Sherbourne, Wells, Meredith, Jackson, and Camp (1996) studied the health-related quality of life in patients with chronic medical diseases such as diabetes, heart disease, and hypertension as a function of whether such patients presented with comorbid anxiety disorders or not. Patients receiving general medical care with comorbid anxiety were functioning at lower levels of well-being than those without comorbid anxiety disorders. In particular, patients with hypertension and diabetes who had comorbid anxiety were as debilitated as patients with heart disease, and this diminished quality of life persisted over the 2-year course of the study.

A recent study of patients presenting in general medical settings with well-defined anxious symptoms that did not meet criteria for disorders demonstrated a fourfold increase in disability when compared to patients not reporting anxious symptoms (18 vs. 4.8 bed days) (Marcus, Olfson, Pincus, Shear, & Zarin, 1997). Roy-Byrne et al. (1999) showed that patients in primary care settings diagnosed with panic disorder had higher rates of visits to the physician and visits to the emergency room, compared to similar primary care patients without a psychiatric diagnosis.

Studies are now beginning to appear on the cost savings of effectively treating anxiety disorders. For example, a study from Spain suggests a cost offset effect of 94% following 12 months of drug treatment for panic disorder (Salvador-Carulla, Segui, Fernandez-Cano, & Canet, 1995). Specifically, the total direct costs of health care use during the year prior compared to the year after the diagnosis was made (and treatment begun) were $29,158 and $46,256, respectively (since the cost of treatment itself was factored in), whereas the indirect costs of lost productivity were $65,643 and $13,883, respectively. Thus not treating a disorder is substantially more expensive than providing appropriate treatment. This is particularly true if indirect costs are high, and if treatments are efficacious and cost-effective.

IS ANXIETY A FEMALE DISORDER?

Everyone experiences anxiety and fear, and phobias are found all over the world. But phobias in particular, and other anxiety disorders to a lesser extent, have one very peculiar characteristic: a selective association with being female, as is evident in the epidemiological data presented earlier in this chapter. For example, individuals who suffer from a phobia of insects or small animals severe enough to keep them from moving to rural areas, or even visiting friends in areas where small animals or insects might be present, are almost certain to be female—as are 90% of the people with this particular phobia (Craske et al., 1996). Data from a large survey conducted by the WHO in primary care settings revealed a consistently high proportion of women with panic disorder with or without agoraphobia (odds ratio, 1.63; 95% confidence intervals, 1.18–2.20). And this was consistent around the world (Gater et al., 1998). Odds ratios for GAD were also high, although the variation was greater in centers around the world, suggesting a stronger influence of local cultural factors on the gender imbalance in GAD. Similarly, a large sample of over 1,000 adolescents who had either experienced an anxiety disorder at some time in their lives, or not, revealed a strong preponderance of females among those experiencing an anxiety disorder. Furthermore, this preponderance emerged early in life: Retrospective data indicated that by the age of 6, females were already twice as likely to have experienced an anxiety disorder than males (Lewinsohn, Gotlib, Lewinsohn, Seeley, & Allen, 1998). It is also notable that depression is largely a female disorder, and fascinating explanations for the overwhelming preponderance of anxiety and depression among females are explored in Chapter 8. Gender ratios for individual anxiety disorders, and possible reasons for gender imbalances where they exist, are taken up in the chapters devoted to specific disorders.

ANXIETY ACROSS CULTURES

By all accounts, the shadow of intelligence or the specter of death that is the experience of anxiety should be universally present across cultures and species. For purposes of both survival in the Darwinian sense, and effective planning for the future as posited by Liddell, evolution should favor members of a species who are anxious. But excesses of any valuable trait exist in certain individuals. Is anxiety in its pathological expression present in other cultures? If so, are the forms of the disorder the same as those found in Western culture? Consider the following case.

Several years ago, a 31-year-old married Inuit male presented at the Alaska native health service complaining that he was "very nervous." Although Inuit was his native language, he spoke English well enough to communicate about his problem in that language. He reported that he had begun to feel nervous over 3 years earlier. Now he stayed at home most of the time, particularly in winter, when he felt worse. Since the men of his village were responsible for hunting, fishing, and carrying water or ice to the house with dog teams or snowmobiles, he was relying increasingly on other villagers, relatives, and public assistance for his contribution to these activities. Going out alone made him feel worse unless he went with his wife. Since she herself had a chronic physical illness, she was seldom able to venture away from home. However, since his condition had deteriorated substantially, both had decided that it was necessary to undertake the 50-mile journey to the hospital by snowmobile! He had no idea what caused his problem, but speculated that it might be connected with an episode of flu several years previously (Hudson, 1981). At the beginning of the 20th century, Danish travelers to Greenland reported observing a condition in which Inuit hunters, alone in kayaks on a perfectly still sea for hours on end waiting for seals to emerge, would experience sudden breathing difficulties and racing heartrate. Subsequently, these hunters would be unable to venture far from their villages. This condition was referred to as "kayak angst" (Katschnig, 1999).

It would seem that both the Inuit man in Alaska and the Inuit hunters in Greenland suffered from the same disorder so frequently encountered in cities and suburbs of the Western world—namely, panic attacks with agoraphobia. That this occurs despite overwhelming differences between cultures is noteworthy. Nevertheless, preliminary conclusions from cross-cultural investigations suggest that what seems to be anxiety in one culture may take many different forms in other cultures. The expression of emotion in general is well known to be culturally determined. The intensity of emotion expressed by southern European and Mediterranean cultures compared to northern European cultures is legendary. Thus it is not surprising that emotional disorders are expressed differently, even if some common biological or etiological roots exist. What is surprising is how very differently anxiety presents in other cultures.

Koro

In 1967, a wave of severe anxiety swept Singapore. Numerous males, particularly among the large ethnic Chinese population, presented with anxiety so acute that they could be said to be in a state of panic (Ngui, 1969; Tan, 1969, 1980). Each expressed an overwhelming fear that his sexual organs were retracting into his abdomen. These individuals believed that when the organ totally retracted, death would result. Screams for help usually resulted in assistance from the family and the community. This assistance might take the form of the construction of various contraptions to prevent the genitals from retracting. Usually the anxiety subsided in a few hours (Tan, 1980). Recurrences also passed quickly, particularly if support was available in the community. These individuals were suffering from *koro*, a syndrome often encountered in that culture. This syndrome is less frequent in women, where it takes the form of fear of retraction of the nipples, the breasts, or occasionally the labia. Patients presenting with *koro* usually relate the onset of their condition to some sexual misdemeanor occurring in their past (Tan, 1980).

Pa-Leng

Pa-leng, also found in Chinese cultures, is sometimes labeled "frigophobia" or "fear of the cold." Individuals with this problem present with cold, clammy hands; tachycardia; dry mouth; and other related somatic symptoms. Like *koro*, *pa-leng* can only be understood in the context of traditional ideas—in this case, the traditional Chinese notions of *yin* and *yang* (Tan, 1980). Chinese medicine holds that there must be a balance of the *yin* and *yang* forces within the human body for health to be maintained. *Yin* represents the cold, dark, windy, energy-sapping aspects of life; *yang* refers to the bright, warm, energy-producing aspect of life. In both *koro* and *pa-leng*, the presenting symptoms are associated with an excess of *yin*. In *pa-leng*, individuals present with a morbid fear of the cold. They ruminate over further loss of body heat, which may be a threat to life. Closely associated with this fear of the cold is a fear of wind. Sufferers from *pa-leng* wear several layers of clothing even on a hot day to keep out wind and cold. Complaints of belching and flatulence may reflect the presence of too much wind, and therefore too much *yin* in the body.

Kyol Goeu, Orthostatic Panic, and "Sore Neck" among the Khmer

Devon Hinton, a psychiatrist/anthropologist, and his colleagues have recently described a fascinating manifestation of panic disorder among Khmer refugees in the United States. This inquiry began with the observation of a very high rate of panic disorder, as diagnosed using a valid adaptation of the Structured Clinical Interview for DSM-IV panic model, for Cambodian refugees. Specifically, 60% of 89 patients surveyed at two psychiatric clinics presented with current panic disorder. A substantial percentage of these panic attacks were associated with orthostatic dizziness and "sore neck" (Hinton, Ba, Peou, & Um, 2000). What Hinton's group discovered (Hinton, Um, & Ba, in press-a, in press-b) is that the Khmer concept of *kyol goeu*, or "wind overload," mediates the focus of catastrophic cognitions on certain bodily sensations. Specifically, the Khmer conceptualize their bodies as containing vessels that carry blood and wind (this is somewhat similar to the Chinese conception of *yin* and *yang*). The most important of these vessels are located in the limbs and neck. When a person is healthy, blood and wind are able to flow without interruption; stress or disease on the other hand, blocks these vessels. These blockages result in increased bodily wind, which in turn gives rise to a variety of bodily symptoms. For example, somatic symptoms of anxiety such as trembling, weakness, or fatigue are often described as *jok*, which means literally to "plug up, as with a cork."

These blockages have dire consequences, according to cultural idioms. Among the most severe include the possibility of the bursting of vessels in the neck, as wind attempts to move upward toward the head, which may result in death. If wind arrives at the head, it may swirl in the cranium, causing dizziness and feelings of fainting. Thus the attention of the Khmer seems selectively focused on symptoms of dizziness and slight perturbations of circulation in the area of the neck. Panic attacks are triggered by these specific interoceptive symptoms. The Khmer have devised a "test" of their physical (mental) health: The degree of dizziness registered upon quickly standing up reveals the strength or weakness of the body. That is, excessive orthostatic hypotension (or the exacerbation of these sensations by self-focused attention) is a sign of disorder that may signify imminent death. Thus, these symptoms frequently trigger panic attacks and, ultimately, panic disorder.

In summary, what Hinton et al. (in press-a, in press-b) seem to have demonstrated is a classic example of panic disorder—with the sudden rush of associated sympathetic symptoms, feelings of impending doom, and so forth, as well as anxiety focused on these sensations. These symptoms are experienced and described in a culturally distinct manner. Failure to understand this cultural idiom would quickly lead to a misdiagnosis and inappropriate treatment.

Heart Distress

In Iran, a frequently encountered disorder is referred to as "heart distress" (Good & Kleinman, 1985). Individuals experiencing palpitations or other sensations in their hearts interpret them within the framework of symbolic meanings peculiar to the culture of Iran. But the focus is almost always on somatic symptoms associated with the heart around which a disorder is constructed. Western observers studying this phenomenon find that in some instances patients with heart distress would fit into the Western category of depression, while other cases would more clearly be cases of anxiety, particularly panic disorder.

Fright Disorders and Voodoo Death

Heart distress contrasts with "fright disorders," which have their origins in observable fear reactions or exaggerated startle responses. Subsequent emotional disorders are ascribed to experiences of extreme fright. In fact, a wide variety of behavioral and emotional problems can be attributed to fright in various cultures, including hysterical conversion symptoms and temporary psychotic episodes. Nevertheless, the predominant expression seems to be similar to Western anxiety disorders. Many examples of fright disorders exist in different cultures. For example, *susto* in Latin American cultures is characterized by various anxiety-based symptoms (irritability, insomnia, phobias, the somatic symptoms of sweating and tachycardia, etc.). The causes of *susto* also lie in sudden fright, black magic, or witchcraft—in particular, the "evil eye," prominently mentioned in fright disorders around the world (Good & Kleinman, 1985; Tan, 1980). In Iranian culture, both "fright disorders" and "heart distress" are terms used to refer, for the most part, to symptoms of emotional disorders. But in fright disorders the cause is attributed to an event in the social environment. In heart distress, the particular symptom itself becomes the focus and cause of the disorder.

In what may be the ultimate specter of death, it seems that some individuals in certain cultures are scared to death. Black magic or the "evil eye" is associated with this event; this suggests that death may be an occasional complication of certain fright disorders in some cultures. Cannon (1942), examining the phenomenon of voodoo death, suggested that the sentence of death by a medicine man may create intolerable autonomic arousal with little opportunity for effective action. Ultimately, this results in damage to internal organs and death.

Shinkeishitsu

The clinical presentation of what seem to be anxiety disorders in Japan is best subsumed under the clinical label of *shinkeishitsu*. In general, the word *shinkeishitsu* refers to a broad category of people who might be referred to as "neurotic" in the West. For example, these individuals are perfectionistic, are extremely self-conscious, and become concerned quickly and easily over particular somatic or social issues. *Shinkeishitsu* was elaborated in some detail by the famous Japanese psychiatrist Shoma Morita, who subsequently formed his own school of psychotherapy. A good summary of the clinical presentation of *shinkeishitsu* is presented by Reynolds (1976):

> Morita therapists view the neurotic as a person with a particularly strong need to live a full life, perfectionistic tendencies, and extreme self-consciousness. . . . This person encounters some unpleasant event that focuses his attention on a particular problem; blushing, headaches, and constipation are typical examples. He becomes quite concerned about the problem and he becomes increasingly conscious of its effect on his life. He becomes caught in a spiral of attention and sensitivity which produces a sort of obsessive self consciousness. His efforts to overcome the problem directly by his will serve only to exacerbate his fixation. By the time he arrives at a Morita therapy clinic, such a person is generally very shy and sensitive; he is unable to function socially, preferring to spend his life in his room withdrawn from the world outside. He is immobilized by the storm of counterconflicts and pressures raging within his psyche. (pp. 9–10)

The crucial issue of self-focused attention or self-preoccupation, seemingly so much a part of *shinkeishitsu*, is taken up in some detail in Chapter 3.

There are three subcategories of *shinkeishitsu*. The first is described as the obsessive phobic form, which seems to account for about 50% of individuals with this disorder in Japan. This form would seem closely related to social phobia in Western culture. These people have a strong fear of looking people in the eye and are afraid that some aspect of their personal presentation (e.g., blushing, stuttering, body odor, etc.) will appear reprehensible. This condition is more usually known as *taijin kyofusho* and is distinct in one very fundamental way from social phobia as it exists in Western countries. That is, the individual with *taijin kyofusho* in Japan and other East Asian cultures is afraid of offending others, whereas the person with social phobia in Western cultures becomes anxious at the possibility of being scrutinized by others and embarrassed (Chang, 1997; Kleinknecht, Dinnel, Kleinknecht, Hiruma, & Harada, 1997).

Individuals with the neurasthenic form display strong hypochondriacal symptoms, poor concentration, and feelings of shyness. This category accounts for approximately 25% of individuals with shinkeishitsu. Finally, anxiety states, which seem descriptively very close to panic attacks, account for approximately 10% of these patients. This problem usually begins with some sort of heart palpitation or other somatic symptom. The remaining 15% do not fall neatly into one of these three categories.

Panic Disorder in African Americans and Hispanic Americans

As in other countries, prevalence rates of anxiety disorders, such as panic disorder, are similar among different ethnic groups in the United States, including African Americans and Hispanic Americans. Furthermore, black and white patients with panic disorder show no significant differences in symptoms (Friedman, Paradis, & Hatch, 1994). It is important to note, however, that hypertension is a frequent concomitant of anxiety disorders such as panic disorder in African American patients (Neal-Barnett & Smith, 1997; Neal, Nagle-Rich, & Smucker, 1994; Neal & Turner, 1991).

A phenomenon similar to panic in Hispanic Americans, particularly those from the Caribbean, is called *ataque de nervios* (Liebowitz et al., 1994). The symptoms of an *ataque* comprise most of the symptoms of a classical panic attack, but may also include such manifestations as shouting uncontrollably or bursting into tears. Finally, there is a fascinating condition referred to as "isolated sleep paralysis" that seems to have a strong cultural contribution and is described in more detail in Chapter 4. Isolated sleep paralysis, which occurs during the transitional state between sleep and waking, is experienced as a surge of terror accompanied by an inability to move, and occasionally by vivid hallucinations. The incidence of isolated sleep paralysis is significantly higher in African Americans with panic disorder (59.6%) than in other groups such as European Americans with panic disorder (7.5%) (Paradis, Friedman, & Hatch, 1997), for reasons that are not entirely clear.

Anxiety across Cultures: Conclusions

It is certainly not easy to map the symptoms and features of anxiety as we know them in the West onto other cultures. It seems clear that the experience of anxiety exists in nearly all cultures and subcultures, but that this experience is articulated in culture-specific idioms. Various interpretations of the experience of anxiety from culture to culture affect its course, the specific aspects of its presentation (i.e., which symptoms are focused on), and various methods for resolving it. For example, attempts to treat various emotional disorders in China by Western pharmacological techniques have been relatively unsuccessful, since patients believe that the causes of their emotional disorders are fully attributable to stresses at work, separation from their families or homes, or other environmental stressors. Thus treatment with Western medicines does not produce a resolution of the experience of illness for many of these patients (Good & Kleinman, 1985).

The overwhelming finding from cross-cultural studies is that the somatic manifestation of emotional disorders is the prominent expression of anxiety in countries and cultures other than those of the European-influenced West. Furthermore, this chronic somatization as a function of stress or other causes may take quite different forms from culture to culture. The preoccupation with sexual symptoms in Chinese cultures has been mentioned in the context of *koro*. Administering standardized checklists of anxiety symptoms to different cultures produces similar overall levels of "anxiety" from culture to culture, but the emphasis is on very different symptoms. Responses to a symptom checklist in a cross-national study were collected by Inkeles (1983) and are presented in Table 1.12. To take one example from this table, the overall percentage of symptoms endorsed is relatively similar in Israel and Nigeria, but awareness of rapid heart rate, shortness of breath, or complaints of "nervousness" are represented very differently in those two cultures.

In Saudi Arabia, OCD is approximately as prevalent as in other countries, but the content of the obsessions and the nature of the compulsions differ somewhat. The themes of obsessions are predominantly related to religious practices, specifically prayers and/or

TABLE 1.12. **Responses to Symptom Checklist in a Cross-National Study**

	India	Chile	Israel	Nigeria
Average percentage of symptoms per country	24	29	22	28
Individual symptoms (%)				
Trouble sleeping	54	23	37	21
Nervousness	48	36	27	9
Heart beating	13	24	13	45
Shortness of breath	8	15	6	32
Disturbing dreams	21	22	35	48

Note. From Inkeles (1983). Copyright 1983 by Columbia University Press. Reprinted by permission.

the associated washings that accompany the prayers (Mahgoub & Abdel-Hafeiz, 1991). In other cultures, including Western cultures, religion is a less common obsessional theme. The Saudi culture also seems to influence the nature of compulsions, since cleaning compulsions are more common than in the West. These cultural differences seem closely related to strong Muslim beliefs and religious practices.

In summary, some individuals in all cultures seem apprehensive, worried, fearful, and aroused, and make attributions concerning their worries and arousal. Furthermore, the prevalence of many anxiety disorders seems relatively consistent around the world. For example, in Lesotho (an African nation), the prevalences of both panic disorder and GAD are equal to or greater than their prevalences in North America (Hollifield, Katon, Spain, & Pule, 1990). In one of the more comprehensive studies to date, prevalence rates for panic disorder were remarkably similar in the mainland United States, Canada, Puerto Rico, New Zealand, and Korea, with only Taiwan showing somewhat lower rates (Horwath & Weissman, 1997). But the object of worry or apprehension, the source of fear, and the specific attributions these individuals make are culture-specific and have marked implications for classification, course, and treatment. One should not expect an anxious Chinese individual in Malaysia to be concerned over confronting nothingness, or to be amenable to attributing anxiety either to unconscious instinctual wishes or to alterations in sensitivity of serotonergic receptors. The experience of anxiety seems to be culturally determined, even if the occurrence of basic negative affect and most anxiety disorders is universal (see Chapter 2). With the enormous difficulties in defining "anxiety" even in Western cultures, it is not surprising that problems increase across cultures. This makes an investigation into the basic nature of anxiety all the more compelling.

THE MYSTERIES OF ANXIETY

The mysteries of anxiety are legion. How can an emotion with which most of us are intimately familiar be at once so common and yet so diffuse and vague? Does the experience of fainting at the sight of blood or entering a seemingly involuntary state of paralysis when under attack really have anything in common with the forebodings concerning the welfare of our family, our occupation, or our finances, with which we are often preoccupied? Why are women strikingly more afflicted with anxiety in Western cultures, while males seek out treatment in equally remarkable numbers in Eastern cultures? Why do individuals around the world continue to engage in self-defeating, self-destructive behavior when they are perfectly able to verbalize a rational course of action and behavior that would be life-enhancing and rewarding? Finally, what is it in us that seems to necessitate an obsessive search for causes of our unpleasant and occasionally unbearable negative emotional experiences? Could this be the source of major cross-cultural differences? Does the sound of the wind in a cabin on the ocean or the terror of imagining one's genitals retracting result in the same experience, or is the experience itself somehow very different? Is anxiety really just a metaphor for such a heterogeneous human experience that the term no longer deserves to exist, as suggested by the social constructivists (e.g., Hallam, 1985)? Or is there really a universal experience that deserves a common name? Is it the specter of death that is universal about the experience of anxiety, whether it be separation from a loved one, confrontation with nothingness, voodoo death, or overwhelming *yin*? Or is it the shadow of intelligence, which drives individuals and cultures to higher levels of achievement? To answer these and all of the mysteries of anxiety, we must first explore what is basic about the nature of anxiety itself.

CHAPTER 2

Fear, Anxiety, and Theories of Emotion

If the scientific study of human behavior has been characterized by mind–body dualism, the study of emotion has been the primary battlefield. In this way, studying emotion is much like experiencing emotion. One is continually buffeted by the variety of creative but conflicting ideas concerning this elusive phenomenon. For over 100 years, the development of biological and psychological views of emotion have progressed—sometimes in tandem, but more often independently. Even in this age of astounding progress in the understanding of human behavior, entire books continue to appear concentrating on either the psychological or the biological view of emotion, without any reference whatsoever to the alternative intellectual tradition.

If the experience of emotion is Lewis Carroll's Wonderland, anxiety is the Red Queen. Always a future threat, often an unbearably overwhelming present danger, the Red Queen dominates Wonderland in the same way the study of anxiety has dominated emotions. For this reason, it is difficult to consider the nature of anxiety without placing anxiety firmly in the context of what we know about emotion in general.

The tradition surrounding the study of emotion continues to be influenced by such intellectual giants as Darwin, James, and Cannon. Most theorists now agree that emotion consists of several components. Only one of these components is the actual subjective experience of affect, although the experience of affect defines emotion for most of us. Affect is reported as a variety of rich and diverse feeling states ("happiness," "sadness," "anger," "surprise," "joy," "melancholy," etc.). Terms such as these are strongly represented in our common expressive and literary heritage. In our own experience, these terms have been elaborated into subtle variations that greatly enrich our appreciation of what it is to be human. But knowledge of affect relies on introspection, and an uncertain, qualitative type of introspection at that. As such, it is a slippery subject for science. Other components of the emotional system are more suitable for scientific inquiry, and therefore have been emphasized.

In addition to the subjective experience of affect, emotion is also considered to be fundamentally a set of expressive behaviors, an integrated neurobiological response, and a cognitive perception or appraisal. For most of the last 100 years, investigators steeped in a particular tradition concentrated on one component or another, such as the behavioral, neurobiological, or cognitive aspects of emotion. Since these traditions in the study of emotion undergird approaches to the study of anxiety, they were reviewed in some detail in the first edition of this book.

Over the last decade, the study of emotion has become more integrative (e.g., Ekman & Davidson, 1994; Lang, 1994a). Thus only summaries of past traditions in the study of emotion begin this chapter, followed by brief descriptions of prominent models of anxiety that map closely onto these specific traditions in emotion theory. Theories of anxiety are also elaborated in theories of personality, where anxiety is conceptualized as a personality trait. "Trait," in this context, refers to a disposition to behave anxiously with some consistency over time or across situations. For example, the most popular measure of trait anxiety, the State–Trait Anxiety Inventory (Spielberger, Gorsuch, & Lushene, 1970), simply asks subjects whether they feel anxious much of the time ("trait") as opposed to at that moment ("state"). Therefore, the present review of models of anxiety integrates state and trait approaches.

The chapter ends with a description of yet another approach to studying emotion—an approach relying on a dimensional analysis—after considering more recent integrative theories of emotion. Knowledge of the great traditions in the study of emotion, and their derivative models of anxiety, continues to have a direct bearing on the study of anxiety and fear; such knowledge provides an important foundation for the theoretical and clinical expositions in this book.

EMOTION AS BEHAVIOR

The first great tradition in studying emotional behavior was initiated by Charles Darwin, in a book entitled *The Expression of the Emotions in Man and Animals* (1872). Building on a tradition dating back to Aristotle, Darwin emphasized behavioral expression, including facial expression, as the fundamental aspect of emotion. Darwin's legacy is alive and well today, and continues to have a strong influence on the field, due to the breadth and depth of supporting experimental evidence (e.g., Ekman & Davidson, 1994). Despite this long tradition, the implications of evidence from this area of study have been ignored for the most part by psychopathologists and clinicians investigating emotional disorders.

The underlying premise of the study of expressive behavior and its function is that emotions are innate patterns of reaction and responding that have evolved in many life forms because of their functional significance. Although clearly modifiable by learning and maturation, these basic patterns of emotion are present in humans and animals at birth, and show a remarkable consistency both within and across species (Izard, 1977). Since the primary means of expressing oneself in both animals and humans are nonverbal postures and facial expressions, these objective behaviors have become one focus of study. Several different lines of evidence have been used to support the centrality of expressive behavior (Izard, 1977; Izard & Blumberg, 1985; Plutchik, 1980). Among these are the abovementioned consistencies in emotional expressions across many species of animals. In addition, Darwin pointed out that in humans, emotional expressions are similar at different ages. Infants express emotions in much the same way as adults, before the necessary learning required for this expression can possibly have taken place. Darwin also made the intriguing observation that subtle, emotional expressions as represented in facial expressions are the same in those born blind as in those who are normally sighted, and that many emotional expressions are present in a similar fashion across different cultures and races. These statements continue to receive strong support (Ekman, 1994; Izard, 1994).

The primary function or adaptive value of emotional behavior includes not only preparation for action, but also communication from one member of the species to another. For example, the function of the emotion of fear seems clearly to prepare the animal for immediate and decisive action—usually running away or fighting. But the expression of fear also communicates danger to other animals and therefore affects their chance for survival, enabling observers to respond more quickly to a threat they might not have anticipated. The expression of many emotions has the same communicative or signal value. The underlying assumption of this expressive-behavioral approach is that basic patterns of emotion differ from one another in fundamental ways, and various behavioral and psychopathological data support this proposition (Izard, 1994; Schwartz, Weinburger, & Singer, 1981; Izard & Youngstrom, 1996; Ekman, Levenson, & Friesen, 1983; Rusalova, Izard, & Simonov, 1975; Schwartz, Fair, Salt, Mandel, & Klerman, 1976).

The Development of Emotions in Young Children

Another important line of evidence supporting the "innateness" of emotion comes from the study of the development of emotions in young children (Lewis, 1993). Emotion theorists studying developmental processes have noted the emergence of seemingly innate emotional responses at very specific points in development. At 3 months, the facial expression of infants during certain emotional states begins to show a remarkable consistency with adult facial expressions reflecting the same emotion (Emde, 1980; Emde, Kligman, Reich, & Wade, 1978; Lewis, 1993). These emotions and facial expressions in infants also seem to be consistent across cultures (Bowlby, 1973; Izard, 1971, 1991). The functional value of the expression of emotion in infants is particularly evident, in that parents rely on these emotional expressions to guide their interaction with an infant and gauge the needs of the child. Since language is not available at this time, an understanding of nonverbal expressive behavior is really the sole means of communication, and its adaptive value is readily apparent.

The emergence of emotional expressions such as the smile and cry has been a focus of investigation by developmentalists (e.g., Emde, Gaensbauer, & Harmon, 1976). Particularly interesting for those concerned with adult anxiety is the emergence of what have been termed "stranger distress" and "separation distress" (Bowlby, 1973; Campbell, 1986). Emde et al. (1976) suggest that these two forms of distress are separate phenomena. Specifically, stranger distress appears in some infants between 7 and 9 months of age, with a mean age of onset at approximately 8 months and a peak at about 9 months of age. As suggested by the means, the onset is rapid (often within 1 month), decreasing rather rapidly after that. Stranger distress is characterized by fearful expressions, crying, and attempts to escape in the presence of a "stranger," who may in fact be a grandmother or other relative the infant has not seen for some time.

On the other hand, separation distress (specifically, distress at separation from the mother) seems to begin somewhat earlier in some infants, at approximately 4 months, and increases gradually and sporadically; it reaches a peak at about 13–18 months and declines thereafter. Early theorists thought that stranger distress might reflect a fear of losing the mother, but careful observational studies suggest that this is not the case. To take just one example, many infants show stranger distress, although they have not yet developed separation distress and show no reaction to the mother's leaving. Because of these very different patterns of development and a variety of other evidence, separation distress and stranger distress seem very different phenomena. Birds and mammals also seem to show stranger distress. Specifically, these species will begin to flee from strange species or certain visual configurations at very specific points in their development. It is likely that stranger distress occurs across species, although the development of this response occurs somewhat later as one moves up the phylogenetic scale (or, more accurately, as neuronal organization becomes more complex). The approximate times of appearance of this flight reaction in different species have been organized by Emde et al. (1976) and are presented in Table 2.1 as adapted by Plutchik (1980).

In any case, Emde et al. (1976) suggest that the development of stranger distress indicates the emergence of a coherent fear system in humans between 7 and 9 months of age, and later observations confirm this time frame (Lewis, 1993). Based on their observations of emotional development in infants, they conclude that this response has an innate basis; that it appears universally across cultures; that it has the same course in congenitally blind infants; and that it occurs in greater synchrony in monozygotic twins than in dizygotic twins. Furthermore, there is no evidence that learning has an effect on the emergence of this response. On the other hand, contextual factors, such as presence or absence of the mother, do seem to affect the expression of the response.

In addition, it seems that fear of strangers is but one example of specific fear that occurs to many stimuli at this point in time. If this is so, then stranger distress is the first and primary expression of pure fear, and it should be recognized as such by psychopathologists looking for developmental precursors to adult anxiety disorders. This observation becomes important in the discussion of the origins of fear and panic in Chapter 7.

The Primacy of Affect

The reemergence of the expressive-behavioral tradition in basic psychology, if not psychopathology, has been represented by Zajonc's reiteration of the primacy of affect (Zajonc, 1980, 1984). Noting that affect is usually considered postcognitive by most contemporary theorists, he suggests the opposite. Specifically, he speculates that affect and cognition are under the control of separate and partially independent systems—a premise that is receiving increasing experimental support (Barnard & Teasdale, 1991; LeDoux, 1996; Lang, Davis, & Öhman, 2000; Öhman, 1999). This information in turn influences ongoing perceptual and evaluative processes. Zajonc also suggests that affective responses are "effortless, inescapable, irrevocable, holistic, more difficult to verbalize yet easy to communicate and to understand" (1980, p. 169). Although this article sparked healthy controversy in the literature over the primacy of affect versus the primacy of cognition when it was published (Lazarus, 1984; Zajonc, 1984), more importantly, it served to reawaken the sleeping giant of innate emotions.

TABLE 2.1. Approximate Time of Appearance of Flight Reactions in Different Species

Species	Time of appearance
Birds	24 hours
Cats	5 weeks
Dogs	5–7 weeks
Monkeys	2–3 months
Chimpanzees	4–6 months
Humans	7–9 months

Note. Adapted by Plutchik (1980) from Emde, Gaensbauer, and Harmon (1976). Copyright 1976 by International Universities Press, Inc. Adapted by permission.

Emotion as the Sensation of Bodily Changes: The James–Lange Theory

A related approach to emotions—one familiar to everyone who has read an introductory psychology textbook—was first proposed by William James (1890). Subsequent work by a Danish physiologist named C. Carl Lange suggesting a similar (but not identical) idea resulted in the conceptualization known as the "James–Lange theory." The basic premise of their ideas was that behavioral and bodily changes, which differ from emotion to emotion, occur as a response to some antecedent event, and that the sensation or "feeling" of these bodily changes is elicited by the behavioral and bodily changes. James pointed out that this sequence is contrary to the more common-sense view, in which an emotion occurs because the perception of a situation gives rise to a conscious "feeling" of emotion, which is then followed by various bodily changes or behaviors. "Bodily changes," for the most part, refer to visceral or psychophysiological changes (heart rate increases, temperature changes, etc.) of which the person can be aware.

In fact, this approach is similar to and compatible with evolutionary behavioral conceptions of emotions, although a slightly different emphasis appears (see below). Within the James–Lange conception, the idea that basic emotions exist that differ from each other and have functional adaptive value is consistent with behavioral theories. What James did was to emphasize visceral reactions as one of the primary components of emotion, while at the same time noting the importance of the subjective experience of affect—a combination largely ignored by early evolutionary theorists.

Unfortunately, evidence quickly accumulated that emotions can be experienced, expressed, and felt, without the types of visceral physiological changes thought so important by James. Most of the evidence for this observation revolved around examples where autonomic reactivity was disconnected, sometimes surgically, from the remainder of the nervous system; nevertheless, emotional experience and behavior were not diminished. For example, in 1929 Walter Cannon reported that when no visceral sensory impulses whatsoever were available to animals after surgical disconnection, they were still able to show typical emotion-related behavior. Various additional arguments have been mustered against this conception of emotion (Lang, 1994a; Plutchik, 1980). Neoevolutionary theorists have attempted to answer this objection by noting that the whole variety of sensory experience, including feedback from the motor components of expressive behavior in addition to any visceral changes, contributes to the affective component of emotion—a position James himself would take (Lang, 1994a).

FEAR AND ANXIETY AS EXPRESSED BEHAVIOR

In the neoevolutionary approach, fear is considered a basic, fundamental, discrete emotion that is universally present across ages, cultures, races, and species. Few would disagree that this emotion, whether innate or not, is universal and has a clear functional value in the evolutionary sense. But for all the clarity with which discrete-emotion theorists conceptualize fear as a basic, individual emotion, "anxiety" has been considered both different from discrete emotions and at the same time something very vague, imprecise, and muddled.

For example, Izard (1977) has viewed anxiety as a hybrid or blend of a number of emotions, although fear is admittedly dominant in the blend. The basic emotions most commonly considered to combine with fear to make up anxiety include distress/sadness, anger, shame, guilt, and interest/excitement. Furthermore, anxiety, according to Izard's view, may assume a different blend across time and situations. For example, in one instance, fear, distress, and anger may be the blend referred to as "anxiety" by the individual; in another instance, shame and guilt may be combined with fear. Naturally, such combinations make it difficult indeed to talk of anxiety in a precise way. Nevertheless, anxiety is considered to be a blend of fundamental, innate emotions, each of which is modified by learning and experience. Individuals may learn to associate discrete emotions such as fear with a large number of cognitive and situational factors, including the evocation of other, related emotions.

According to Izard (1977; Izard & Blumberg, 1985), the development of an anxious personality results from the interaction of learning with basic emotions, resulting in stable affective–cognitive structures that are trait-like. These "traits" result from the repeated occurrence of particular patterns of affective–cognitive interactions. Izard and other neo-evolutionary theorists allow for biologically determined "emotion thresholds," which contribute to the frequency or intensity of an emotion or a blend of emotions, and to its perception as a personality trait. In keeping with Izard's differential-emotion theory, however, biological emotion thresholds are specific to one emotion or another, rather than contributing to a general trait of emotionality. This combination of factors, then, is thought to account for the development of an "anxious" personality. Although fear is a basic innate emotion, an anxious personality for the most part is learned. But Izard (1977) concludes that anxiety, because of this vagueness, "can never obtain the requisite precision to guide definitive scientific investigation" (p. 378). As noted in Chapter 1, many clinicians have been unaccustomed to making distinctions between fear and anxiety, and generally have paid little attention to fear and anxiety as conceptualized by the emotion theorists.

EMOTION AS BIOLOGY

A truly different tradition in the study of emotion was initiated by Walter Cannon (1929), who viewed emotion as primarily a brain function. After dismissing the James–Lange theory, Cannon's creative and influential research centered on the process of "extirpation of parts," or surgical removal of various areas of the brain in animals. Cannon found, among other things, that removal of part or all of the cerebral cortex seemed to release emotions. Therefore, the cortex, by and large, was not thought to be directly involved in emotion except to serve a controlling function. Rather, the site of emotion was thought to be the hypothalamus, which, when destroyed, resulted in a dramatic elimination of most of the components of emotion. Essentially, Cannon reasoned that the subjective experience of affect, as well as expressive behavior and any associated bodily changes, is a function of activity in the hypothalamus.

A long and distinguished series of investigators have attempted to understand emotion in terms of brain processes that are active during emotional states. Much of the early activity centered on the limbic system (e.g., MacLean, 1963), although other areas of the brain have also been involved. For years, the primary research methodology continued to be extirpation of various sections of the brain, with changes in emotional responses subsequently observed. In later years, more precise electrical stimulation of various areas of the brain was correlated with emotional behavior. The goal of brain ablation and stimulation studies was to locate specific neuroanatomical areas associated with each emotion. This was a fruitful and useful line of research in previous decades, although current research focuses as much on brain function as brain structure (e.g., Lang et al., 2000). In any case, even this early research suggested that areas of the brain associated with emotional expression are generally more phylogenetically ancient and primitive, and that there may be direct neurobiological connections between these ancient areas and the retina, which allow emotional activation without intermediation of the higher cognitive processes (Moore, 1973; Zajonc, 1984; LeDoux, 1987; Izard, 1992). This finding, in particular, has received empirical support, as scientists have discovered multiple cortical and subcortical pathways to emotional activation (LeDoux, 1996; Lang et al., 2000). These brain areas are also shared to a great extent with other, more primitive species. Many of these species do not possess cortical areas associated with higher cognitive processes. This fact seems to account for observations from the behavioral evolutionary tradition of the universality of emotions across species.

Subsequent research revealed that no easy answers were forthcoming on the precise site of various emotions, since stimulation of the same area under somewhat different conditions may produce different emotional (and nonemotional) responses. Conversely, stimulating somewhat different areas may produce similar emotional responses at different points of time (Izard, 1977; Panksepp, 1982; Plutchik, 1980). As noted above, more recent advances in neuroscience have focused attention on specific neurotransmitter and neuromodulator systems and their relationship to emotions. With this new emphasis has come the realization that fine-grained neuroanatomical exploration will never offer a full explanation, even at a basic neurobiological level, of the workings of emotions (Lang, 1994b; Gray & McNaughton, 1996; LeDoux, 1995, 1996).

Within the biological tradition of study, the notion that emotional responses are distinct and separate remains largely intact. Although Cannon (1929) assumed that emotional "arousal" is a unitary phenomenon, with different levels of arousal accounting for the different emotions, most modern neurobiologists seek different neurotransmitter systems involving multiple areas of the brain as possibly underlying the variety of emotions or dimensions of positive and negative affect. Although no firm evidence is yet available, there are some promising leads. (A review of research relevant to anxiety within this context is presented in Chapter 6.)

Of course, some neurobiological theorists concentrate on biological processes and tend to ignore issues involving the antecedents to emotions and the perception that begins the emotional process. This tendency, along with the ever-present danger of reducing a complex human response such as emotion to its chemical and cellular components, has kept many biological theorists less than fully aware of advances in alternative approaches to emotions—a state of affairs that, unfortunately, characterizes the study of emotion in general. As Lazarus (1984) pointed out almost 20 years ago, no less an authority on the neurobiology of emotion and behavior than Sperry (1982) despaired of finding specific anatomical sites or neurobiological systems exclusively associated with one or another emotion.

ANXIETY AS BIOLOGY

Over the years, a number of theorists have concentrated on the neurobiological basis of anxiety in formulating theoretical models of anxiety and inhibition. Although the focus on research has shifted from a solely neuroanatomical perspective to one combining neuroanatomy with receptor physiology, biochemistry, and brain function, the emphasis, dating back to Cannon, on emotion (and therefore anxiety) as a neurobiological event remains. New developments, and data on genetic, psychophysiological, and neurobiological views of anxiety, are presented in some detail in Chapter 6. However, at this point it is useful to consider briefly several trait models of anxiety that are based on biological theorizing, since these theories on personality or temperament have played a significant role in our thinking about anxiety.

Eysenck's Introverted Neuroticism

What is undoubtedly the most widely known biological theory of personality was originated and elaborated by Hans Eysenck (1967, 1981). Eysenck based his theory on different levels or intensities of cortical arousal. He suggested that positive or pleasant emotions are associated with moderate levels of arousal; negative or unpleasant emotions are associated with arousal that is either too high or too low. This state of affairs motivates individuals to seek moderate levels of arousal and avoid the extremes. However, since individuals differ markedly in their resting level of arousal, which is biologically determined, consistent and lasting differences in behavior appear as a direct result of levels of arousability. Specifically, individuals with relatively low levels of cortical arousal (due to a chronic low level of reactivity of the ascending reticular activating system) tend to seek out higher optimal levels of cortical arousal and greater amounts of stimulation. People in this group are "extraverted." "Introverted" persons, on the other hand, find their optimal levels of arousal at much lower levels of stimulation.

The other well-known axis in Eysenck's theory, which is of more interest to us here, has a construct called "neuroticism" at one end and one termed "stability" at the other end. The underlying biological factor associated with this dimension of personality is thought to be autonomic nervous system reactivity, which feeds back to influence limbic system activity. Neurotic individuals possess the characteristic of intense autonomic nervous system activity and very slow rates of habituation. These axes, presented in Figure 2.1,

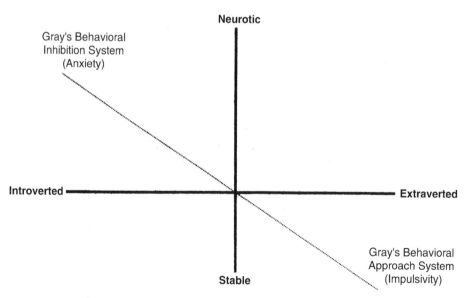

FIGURE 2.1. Eysenck's introversion–extraversion and neuroticism–stability axes, with Gray's anxiety–impulsivity axis superimposed. Adapted from Eysenck (1967). Copyright 1967 by Charles C Thomas. Adapted by permission.

have appeared for decades in textbooks on psychopathology. Eysenck's theory has had a profound influence, and some newer theories reviewed below are based on Eysenck's work.

Although Eysenck's theory is a modern personality theory that attempts to encompass the full range of behavior, the close relationship of this approach to biological theorizing on emotion, and its direct relationship to Cannon's (1929) views on emotion, are apparent. Thus emotion in general, and anxiety in particular, are seen as resulting largely from the interaction of individual traits of cortical arousal and autonomic nervous system reactivity with influence from the limbic system. Anxious individuals tend to have both high resting levels of cortical arousal and high autonomic nervous system reactivity. Unlike Cannon, of course, Eysenck was a pioneer in advocating the interacting role of learning and conditioning in the formation and expression of these personality traits, as well as in the alleviation of psychopathology arising from extremes of these biological traits. In propagating these notions, Eysenck (1960) became one of the founders of behavior therapy.

Gray's Behavioral Inhibition System

One of the foremost theorists of the neurobiological basis of anxiety is Jeffrey Gray, whose careful experimentation in his animal laboratories and subsequent creative theorizing are mentioned frequently in this book. Rather than relying on the increasingly untenable concept of differential intensity of arousal (see Chapter 6), Gray (1982; Gray & McNaughton, 1996) has proposed that personality and emotions are determined by three different affective–motivational systems. The primary system in his model is the behavioral inhibition system (BIS), which consists of the septal area, the hippocampus, and the Papez circuit. This system includes neocortical inputs to the septo-hippocampal system, dopaminergic ascending input to the prefrontal cortex, cholinergic ascending input to the septo-hippocampal system, noradrenergic input to the hypothalamus, and the descending noradrenergic fibers of the locus ceruleus. After specific stimulus input (particularly signals of punishment, nonreward, and novelty), the BIS suppresses ongoing behavior and redirects attention toward the relevant stimuli. In Gray's view, an active and sensitive BIS that reacts to signals of novelty or punishment with exaggerated inhibition is the biological basis of anxiety. A complementary system involving the medial forebrain bundle responds to signals of rewards and nonpunishment (safety signals) by facilitating approach (the behavioral approach system). These two systems, then, regulate much of the organism's behavior. As Gray (1982, 1985) points out, what he has done is to emphasize a new dimension or axis, one end of which falls between Eysenck's introversion and neuroticism (see Figure 2.1). Thus the trait of "anxiety" falls 45 degrees from either introversion or neuroticism. Individuals with an active BIS (i.e., anxious individuals) reflect a combination of Eysenck's introversion and neuroticism. On the other hand, people with an active behavioral approach system, which is sometimes referred to as "impulsivity," reflect a combination of extraversion and stability. Gray's new axis is superimposed on Eysenck's axes in Figure 2.1.

A third system, the fight–flight system (FFS), responds to unconditioned punishment (especially pain) and unconditioned frustrative nonreward by defensive aggression and/or unconditioned escape behavior (Gray, 1991; Gray & McNaughton, 1996). In contrast to the BIS, the FFS is characterized by surges of autonomic arousal and the associated action tendencies of escape, active avoidance, or defensive aggression. This system is organized in the central periaqueductal gray and the medial hypothalamus, with descending control by the amygdala. Inputs and outputs for the BIS and the FFS are shown in Figure 2.2. That there seem to be two fundamentally distinct, albeit related, systems underlying anxiety on the one hand (BIS) and fear or panic on the other (FFS) is taken up below.

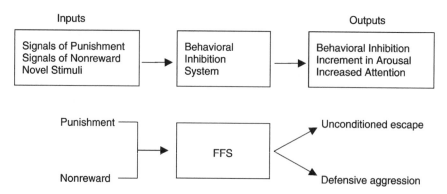

FIGURE 2.2. Inputs and outputs for the BIS and FFS. From Gray and McNaughton (1996). Copyright 1996 by University of Nebraska Press. Reprinted by permission.

Kagan's Behavioral Inhibition

In the 1980s, Jerome Kagan and his colleagues (Kagan, 1989, 1994; Kagan & Snidman, 1991, 1999; Kagan, Snidman, & Arcus, 1992; Kagan, Reznick, & Snidman, 1988) reported that approximately 15–20% of 2-year-old European American children reacted to novelty or strangers in a characteristic manner. Most typically, the children would tend to withdraw from the unfamiliar person or setting and seek comfort from somebody well known to them, such as a parent. In addition, they would look fearful and distressed, suppress any ongoing play or social behavior, and refrain from interacting at all with the unfamiliar object or setting or from vocalizing or smiling. Kagan's group also noticed that a greater percentage of children (approximately 30–35%) tended to display a behavioral profile on the other extreme of the continuum—characterized by relatively rapid approach to unfamiliar people or objects, accompanied by spontaneous vocalization and smiling. Interestingly, about 75% of children characterized as possessing one of these two behavioral profiles retained some aspects of that identifiable profile into their eighth year (Kagan et al., 1988) indicating remarkable stability. Kagan (1989) termed these profiles "temperaments," to reflect his conclusion that the behavioral clusters have a relatively stable biological base in the organism's genotype. On the other hand, he has also observed that the environment is clearly capable of modifying these biologically based tendencies. Table 2.2 presents a summary of observed differences between infants judged to be "high-reactive" (inhibited) at 4 months and infants who were "low-reactive," followed into their eighth year (Kagan & Snidman, 1999).

Kagan has noted a variety of physiological correlates of behavioral inhibition, including increased salivary cortisol levels and muscle tension, high and stable heart rates, greater dilation of the pupils, and elevated urinary catecholamine levels. He attributes these temperamental variations to biological predispositions—specifically, reactivity of several brain circuits originating in the amygdala. He presupposes that because these brain circuits are associated with motor activity and distress calls in animals, variation in the same behavior in young infants might also reflect variability in thresholds in these brain circuits (Kagan et al., 1992). Kagan also cites work by Davidson (1992) and Fox (1991) showing that inhibited children evidence greater activation of alpha activity in the right frontal area of the brain as measured by electroencephalographic methods, in contrast to uninhibited children, who show greater activity in the left frontal area. Kagan et al. (1992) note that these results are consistent with emerging evidence that the right hemisphere is more strongly associated with negative affect than the left. Interestingly, as mentioned in Chapter 6, right-

TABLE 2.2. Differences between High-Reactive and Low-Reactive Infants from 14 Months to 7.5 Years

Variable	High-reactive[a]	Low-reactive[a]	
Mean fear at 14 months	4.2	2.5	$t(286) = 11.1, p < .001$
	(2.4)	(1.6)	
Mean fear at 21 months	3.4	2.0	$t(243) = 4.67, p < .001$
	(2.5)	(1.9)	
Mean spontaneous comments at 4.5 years	40.7	53.7	$t(191) = 1.96, p < .05$
	(39.3)	(47.5)	
Mean smiles at 4.5 years	17.8	27.7	$t(191) = 3.69, p < .01$
	(15.3)	(19.3)	
Percent inhibited with peers at 4.5 years	46%	10%	$\left.\right\}\chi^2(1) = 35.5, p < .001$
Percent uninhibited with peers at 4.5 years	27%	67%	
Mean spontaneous comments at 7.5 years	19.6	32.8	$t(109) = 2.37, p < .01$
	(27.9)	(30.3)	
Mean smiles at 7.5 years	14.4	22.0	$t(109) = 1.97, p < .05$
	(18.2)	(21.5)	
Percent with anxious symptoms at 7.5 years	45%	15%	$\chi^2(2) = 12.8, p < .01$

Note. From Kagan and Snidman (1999). Copyright 1999 by The Society of Biological Psychiatry. Reprinted by permission.
[a]Numbers in parentheses are standard deviations.

side anterior cerebral hemispheric activation in adults may indicate a chronic vulnerability to adult anxiety and depression (Davidson, 1993b).

Kagan believes that this temperament has a strong heritable component, which he estimates at approximately .50 (Robinson, Kagan, Reznick, & Corley, 1992). Others who have carefully calculated the heritability of various temperaments in children make somewhat lower estimates in the range of .30 to .50 (e.g., Saudino & Cherny, 2001). Once again, Kagan readily acknowledges the importance of environment in activating and modulating this temperament (Kagan, 1997; Kagan, Snidman, & Arcus, 1998). In fact, he prefers to conceptualize this temperamental bias as "constraining" the probability of developing a consistently fearless and spontaneous profile, rather than as determining an anxious or introverted phenotype (Kagan & Snidman, 1999). Nevertheless, he believes that its biological basis (which is most likely to be lower thresholds of reactivity in brain circuits originating in the amygdala) should be considered a qualitatively different disposition, rather than one on a dimension from inhibited to uninhibited (Kagan & Snidman, 1991). He cites a variety of evidence supporting this view, including different profiles of physical features such as eye color and width of face, in addition to different physiologies. Specifically, Kagan finds a greater proportion of inhibited children among those with the more Nordic characteristics of blue eyes and blond hair—a finding he attributes to fundamental evolutionarily influenced neurobiological development in the brain (e.g., Rosenberg, & Kagan, 1987; Kagan, 1994).

Work on this temperament is increasingly influential among those studying the nature and development of anxiety. Several studies now show a connection between this temperament and the development of anxiety disorders. For example, children possessing this temperament are at increased risk for developing multiple anxiety disorders themselves later in childhood (Biederman et al., 1993; Hirshfeld et al., 1992). In addition, Rosenbaum, Biederman, Hirshfeld, Bolduc, and Chaloff (1991) have found that first-degree relatives of behaviorally inhibited children present with a significantly elevated pattern of anxiety disorders themselves, compared to the relatives of uninhibited children. Reviewing the evidence in the literature, Turner, Beidel, and Wolff (1996) concur that behavioral inhibition can now be construed as a risk factor for the development of later anxiety disorders in children.

This interesting theory is stimulating considerable research on the biological origins of anxiety at this time. However, the relationships of behavioral inhibition to other similar temperaments, traits, or anxiety-related phenomena have yet to be clearly articulated. Kagan himself notes that behavioral inhibition overlaps considerably with Eysenck's trait of introversion, although behavioral inhibition is defined more precisely and probably describes only a subset of those who would meet criteria for introversion. Similarly, behavioral inhibition has much in common with the concepts of separation anxiety and stranger distress (described earlier in this chapter as more specific emotional responses), both of which seem to have a strong biological and neoevolutionary basis. Others (e.g., Plomin & Stocker, 1989) have commented that the term "behavioral inhibition" may not be an accurate descriptor of this trait. They point out that infants (in contrast to 2-year-olds) are not "inhibiting" behavior in the usual sense. Rather, they are specifically inhibiting their play behavior because they are fearful or distressed in novel situations. For example, among the behaviors coded in rating behavioral inhibition are sobbing, vocalizing distress, and clinging to the mother. These authors suggest that "emotionality" forms a substantial component of this temperament, which might bring it closer to Eysenck's neuroticism (Plomin & Stocker, 1989).

It is also important to note that in a study by Biederman et al. (1990), only 30% of children who clearly met criteria for behavioral inhibition early in life went on to develop an anxiety disorder. This fact, along with the malleability of this temperament as clearly outlined by Kagan (e.g., Kagan & Snidman, 1991), lends perspective to the contribution of this seemingly biological vulnerability to the development of anxiety in adult life, and supports Kagan's notion of the "constraining" rather than "determining" role of this temperament.

EMOTION AS COGNITION

The most recent and, in a way, the most radical approach to emotion can be characterized as cognitive. Although many investigators and theorists have proposed explanations of emotions emphasizing cognitive factors, two approaches continue to stand out.

Appraisal Theory

The first approach, which came to be known as "appraisal theory," can be said to have originated in 1962 with publication of the well-known experiment by Schachter and Singer. Concluding that there is little evidence that emotions are associated with differential patterns of arousal as suggested by Cannon, Schachter and Singer asserted that generalized arousal may be reported differently, depending on the context. That is, noticing arousal, individuals may appraise the context to determine an appropriate label for the arousal. If one were aroused while jumping out of a plane without a parachute, the arousal would be described as fear, while the same level of arousal during sexual relations would be described as love. The essential step in understanding emotion is, then, the process of appraising the context and attributing a causal relationship following the perception of a generalized, undifferentiated arousal state.

This hypothesized sequence of events proved to be an exciting and thought-provoking theory that generated considerable discussion and experimentation over the decades. Nevertheless, it became apparent early that there was little evidence to support this theory in its entirety (e.g., Reisenzein, 1983), and contradictory evidence soon became available. One of the most cogent criticisms was provided by Maslach (1979a, 1979b), who concluded that any differences found in the original Schachter and Singer (1962) experiment were very weak, and that even those differences were experimentally confounded. In addition, several attempts were made to replicate the original experiment, without success (Marshall, 1976; Marshall & Zimbardo, 1979). These replication attempts found that unexplained arousal is perceived negatively, regardless of the environmental cues. For example, arousal will not be attributed to happiness or love simply because that is the context. Although the tendency to perceive unexplained arousal negatively does not support an attribution theory of emotion in general, it is a finding that becomes important when models of psychopathological anxiety are considered later in this chapter and in Chapter 8. Other objections focused on the asynchrony of arousal from other aspects of emotion. Ever since the early experiments by Walter Cannon, investigators have demonstrated time and again that emotional behavior and reports of emotion can occur in the absence of arousal. What is probably the best-known restatement of this old fact was made by Peter Lang (1968), who observed that the three response systems involved in anxiety—behavior, verbal report, and physiological arousal—are only loosely correlated. The implication of this restatement, confirmed early and often, was that reports and behavior associated with anxiety can occur in the absence of arousal (e.g., Barlow & Mavissakalian, 1981).

Richard S. Lazarus (Lazarus, 1968, 1991; Lazarus, Averill, & Opton, 1970) also developed an early theory of emotions involving cognitive appraisal. Specifically, changes in the environment are appraised in terms of their potential impact on the individual. For example, one may appraise a gun as dangerous and thus experience fear. Although this approach is rich and complex, and considers emotion as an adaptive behavior, the emphasis is clearly on cognitive appraisal of events as the primary determinant of the type and quality of an emotional response. This work put a necessary emphasis on an aspect of emotion often ignored by other theories—the initial perception, as well as cognitive elaborations of that perception.

Nevertheless, several problems arose with Lazarus's early formulations. For example, one difficulty encountered by appraisal models is the phenomenon of irrational emotions. It is common for an individual either to report an emotional experience that is recognized as irrational ("There was no reason for me to feel that way"), or at least to be unable to verbalize any rational appraisal preceding the emotional response, despite careful inquiry. Appraisal theorists have some difficulty handling this event, usually resorting to an "out-of-awareness" or unconscious process, which is difficult to test.

Of course, depending on how broadly "appraisal" is defined, it is possible that a very basic type of appraisal, closely connected with an initial perception, does precede emotion. For example, as reviewed below (e.g., Derryberry & Rothbart, 1984; MacLeod, Mathews, & Tata, 1986; McNally, 1996; Mathews, 1997; Lang et al., 2000), it appears that information is perceived and processed out of awareness. Furthermore, cognitive sets or expectancies can markedly alter the expression of even the most intense of emotions (see Chapter 5). Therefore, cognitive-appraisal theories may be much closer to biobehavioral theories citing the primacy of affect (e.g., Zajonc, 1984) than one might think. Differences may simply revolve around definitional elaborations of "appraisal." For example, does any perception of a stimulus qualify as a basic form of appraisal, (including the processing of information in DNA molecules), or do appraisals have to involve conscious, rational elaboration of settings and consequences? In any case, cognitive-appraisal approaches generated a proportionately large amount of interest among clinical investigators and clinicians working with emotional disorders in the 1970s and 1980s, particularly those interested in cognitive therapy for emotional disorders.

ANXIETY AS COGNITION

Clinicians working with anxiety disorders have been particularly interested in attribution and appraisal theories, with their intuitively appealing description of the relationship of cognitive processing to emotion. Therapy, in this context, becomes a process of directly attacking maladaptive appraisals and attributions centering on danger or threat. A number of individuals have considered creatively the role of cognition in anxiety, but the primary theorists in this area over the years have been George Mandler (e.g., 1984); Charles D. Spielberger (1985); Irwin G. Sarason (1985); Aaron T. Beck (e.g., Beck, 1993; Beck & Emery with Greenberg, 1985; Beck & Clark, 1997); and, representing a constructionist viewpoint, Richard Hallam (1985).

Mandler's Interruption Theory

Mandler (1975, 1984) highlights a process whereby ongoing cognitive activity is interrupted. This interruption produces a diffuse autonomic discharge. The autonomic discharge results in detailed appraisal of the source of the interruption, which is then evaluated either positively or negatively, depending on the results of the appraisal and the relationship of this appraisal to the intensity of the autonomic arousal. Naturally, if the arousal is very high, and the deduction as a result of the appraisal is that some sort of a threat to the individual is involved, then the resulting emotions will be fear and anxiety. The assumptions of this approach are that arousal is relatively undifferentiated, and that the burden of emotional formation is on the cognitive process of appraisal following the interruption. Thus Mandler adopts the basic premises of appraisal, but emphasizes in a more focused way the initial stimulus event.

Spielberger's State–Trait Model

A different model has been proposed and elaborated by Spielberger (1966, 1972, 1979, 1985). This model, presented in Figure 2.3, has contributed a number of terms and concepts to our current vocabulary. Spielberger is one of the few cognitive theorists who, as evidenced in his state–trait conceptualization, considers anxiety as a personality trait. State anxiety is considered to be a transitory emotional state, whereas the disposition to experience state anxiety frequently or to be "anxiety-prone" is considered a personality trait (trait anxiety). In the model (see Figure 2.3), external stressors as well as internal stimuli will be appraised in such a way as either to produce anxiety or not. In part, this appraisal will be a function of one's level of trait anxiety. As one can see, the most critical point of this process is, once again, the act of appraisal. State–trait notions have proved useful in distinguishing common anxiety reactions from more frequent, intense, and consistent anxiety, although the causes of these individual differences in trait anxiety are unknown. As with all appraisal theories, there is some difficulty in handling irrational anxiety.

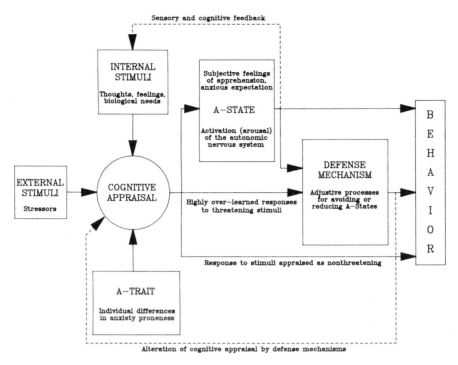

FIGURE 2.3. A state–trait–process model of anxiety. The model posits two anxiety constructs, state anxiety (A-State) and trait anxiety (A-Trait), and specifies the relationships between these constructs, external and internal stressors, cognitive appraisal of threat, and psychological defense mechanisms. From Spielberger (1972). Copyright 1972 by Academic Press. Reprinted by permission.

Beck's Cognitive Schemata

A cognitive approach with a different emphasis from that of appraisal theory is advocated in the pioneering work of Beck (e.g., Beck et al., 1985; Beck, 1993; Beck & Clark, 1997). Beck recognizes emotions in general and anxiety in particular as complex biopsychosocial responses with important evolutionary, biological, affective, and cognitive components. Beck fully appreciates the fact that most basic emotions are innate, survival-oriented responses to an environment that has changed greatly over the course of evolution. For example, he suggests that the behavioral expression and action set associated with fear, which was adaptive during the millenia when human beings were hunter–gatherers, may no longer be appropriate when threats and danger are primarily psychological rather than physical. It is under conditions where emotions are inappropriate, exaggerated, or disordered that Beck begins to emphasize the importance of cognitive factors. Thus Beck's theorizing is confined largely to instances where danger is misperceived or exaggerated.

More specifically, the locus of the problem in the anxiety disorders is not in the affective system, but in hypervalent cognitive "schemata" where reality is continually interpreted as dangerous. Information about one's self, the world, and the future (the "cognitive triad") is continually processed in a distorted way as dangerous. Consequently, states of anxiety are associated with (automatic) thoughts and images relevant to danger. For Beck, these automatic thoughts and images, resulting from distorted information processing, trigger inappropriate motor, physiological, and affective components of the anxiety response.

Therapy is directed at altering these automatic thoughts and the underlying schemata responsible for distorted processing of information. This approach is not really a theory of anxiety, but rather a theory of anxiety disorders, since Beck would agree that anxiety and fear continue to be adaptive under some circumstances.

Unlike previous models, this approach does not depend on conscious rational appraisal, but is closer to a "verbal-mediational" model of learning. The cause of anxiety lies in faulty processing of information, rather than a clear, on-the-spot, rational perception of threat. This twist begins to circumvent the difficulties that other cognitive approaches have with irrational anxiety, since the automatic thoughts present within the irrational hypervalent schemata are not always obvious to the individual. It is not at all unusual for anxious patients to report that their fears are irrational, but this knowledge does not stop continuous thoughts of threat and impending doom. Of course, if "not obvious" comes to mean "not open to scientific scrutiny of any kind," then the theory will be incapable of disconfirmation and will die the slow death of other theories with this fault. Fortunately for the theory, this does not seem to be the case.

There is evidence (reviewed below) that anxious patients do selectively perceive threat more often than nonanxious patients, and that automatic thoughts of threat are present if the antecedents of anxiety are systematically monitored (McNally, 1996; Mathews, 1997). There is also the beginnings of some evidence that inappropriate habitual cognitive schemata do precede emotional disorders—an issue that is important to the integrity of this model (Chorpita & Barlow, 1998; see Chapter 8). Of course, it is possible that automatic thoughts and anxious cognitions are simply by-products of the disordered emotional response, with the cause of both phenomena lying elsewhere (Bouton, Mineka, & Barlow, 2001). Nevertheless, Beck's thinking and his early attempts at integrating the vast diversity of information concerning anxiety from different points of view are extremely valuable. These efforts have already guided a new generation of research and clinical practice, and it seems certain that this influence will continue to grow.

Hallam's Theory of Anxiety as a Personal Construct

Hallam's (1985) approach emanates from a somewhat different tradition than do other theories of anxiety, but remains cognitive in its epistemological underpinnings. This model is also relevant to the context of the definitional problems with anxiety discussed in Chapter 1. Basing his thinking on the work of the social constructivists, Hallam concludes that anxiety can never have scientific status, since it is essentially a multireferential lay construct. Hallam's conclusion about the nature of anxiety comes surprisingly close to Izard's neoevolutionary view.

In the great tradition of constructivist thinking, Hallam suggests that anxiety (and panic) is basically a metaphor based on a construing of certain combinations of events by an individual. These events may include, but may not be limited to, a client's beliefs, linguistic skills, purposes, and concurrent identity problems. The important question for constructivists is what causes the individual to report anxiety. As Hallam (1985) points out, "the most positive contribution a social constructivist position has to offer is to dissuade researchers from regarding these real life problems as reflecting an underlying emotion of anxiety or, even less helpful, an anxiety disorder" (p. xiv).

Constructivist positions have always seemed very extreme to clinicians and clinical researchers accustomed to dealing daily with people suffering from anxiety. However, by emphasizing how the individual construes his or her world in the context of situations where anxiety is often reported, Hallam has introduced an additional theoretical issue that may prove to be important in elucidating the basis of anxiety complaints. To paraphrase Hallam, one of the most important errors preventing us from advancing our knowledge about anxiety and panic (or any emotion, for that matter) is our inability to consider it as a multireferential lay construct. Based on the evolution of convenient but vague terms from everyday conversation, our conception of anxiety has changed from anxiety as a metaphor to anxiety as an actual entity encapsulated within the organism. For accurate reports on its nature, this entity needs only to be carefully observed and reported by the individual (since it is not observable by others). These reports of anxiety are treated as if they are (imperfect) observations of this entity. In fact, according to Hallam (1985), various antecedents and internal (e.g., somatic) and external consequences are functionally related to reports of anxiety, but always in a complex way. Among these referents are specific and contextual environmental events, sensory feedback from autonomic and other somatic processes, overt and covert behavior (e.g., escape, facial expressions), and combinations of these classes of referents, as well as cognitive schemata representing beliefs and attributions of causality. The undeniable point that Hallam hammers home is that any or all of these referents may be present without an individual's reporting panic (or anxiety), and certainly without an individual's requesting treatment for the same. Rather, the individual, as an agent, construes these referents in such a way that anxiety is reported. Only by untangling the functional relationship of these many referents in a given individual, in the context of how he or she construes them, can we say anything about the nature of anxiety.

Hallam's ideas are not nearly as radical as they might seem; furthermore, as noted above, they have an intriguing similarity to Izard's (1977; Izard & Blumberg, 1985) conception of anxiety. Any approach based on cognitive appraisal is in some sense constructivist, but Hallam elegantly takes it to a logical extreme. Hallam is certainly not saying that anxiety and anxiety disorders do not exist, but rather that a variety of biological and cognitive factors may be functionally related to reports of anxiety in a given individual, and that these factors differ across individuals and within individuals over time. Once again, the important questions for Hallam are the following: What factors are functionally related to reports of anxiety in an individual? What would be the critical processes involved in changing the individual's construction of those events that are associated with considerable suffering and are reported as anxiety?

Although constructivist positions have not been influential, these points of view deserve consideration. For example, as discussed in Chapter 8, a number of individuals experience marked psychophysiological events (with accompanying behavioral events) that meet criteria for anxiety or panic, but do not *report* the experience of anything even remotely resembling these emotions. Others may report being "anxious" when careful inquiry reveals a state closer to fatigue or exhaustion, according to the definitions and conceptions of most people.

MODERN EMOTION SCIENCE: INTEGRATION

Recent Work by Izard and Others

In the 1990s, the study of emotion once again caught fire after a period of relative dormancy in the last half of the 20th century. Common to these new approaches is a general recognition of what is distinct about emotions and their function (Gross, 1999). As Öhman (1996, 1999; Lang et al., 2000) points out, the function of emotions, in this sense, can be understood as a clever means, guided by evolution, to insure that we do what we have to do to pass on our genes successfully to coming generations. In other words, emotions are now conceptualized by most theorists as fundamental action tendencies whose purpose is to motivate behavior related to survival of the species. Some of these behaviors or action tendencies include preparing for, avoiding, and escaping potentially dangerous life-threatening events, which are at the heart of the emotions of fear and anxiety, and constitute the focus of the major part of this book. Other "emotional" behaviors include seeking protection and support from fellow members of the species, gaining access to sexual partners and subsequently engaging in sexual relations, and caring for offspring.

It now seems self-evident that the burden of this very important aspect of human functioning cannot be relegated to neurobiological, behavioral, or cognitive systems in isolation. Of necessity, emotions must involve an important integration of these response systems while retaining their qualitatively distinct nature. Most theorists now see the necessity for an integrationist perspective on emotions encompassing neurobiological, behavioral, and cognitive subsystems. For example, Carroll Izard in his more recent work outlines a multisystem model of emotion activation (Izard, 1993, 1994; Izard & Youngstrom, 1996), in which he proposes that humans generate emotions in a number of different ways. In addition to neural processes and cognitive systems underlying emotional expression, he also specifies the salience of sensory–motor and motivational systems in activating emotions. In this conceptualization, neural processes involve specific neurotransmitter activity along various brain circuits. Emotional activation due to efferent motor messages that occur during various facial expressions, postures, and behavioral action tendencies comprises the sensory–motor system. Typical physiological drives such as hunger, thirst, and sex contribute to emotional expression through the motivational system; various appraisals, evaluations, and attributions stimulate emotions through the cognitive system. Most importantly, Izard now conceptualizes these four subsystems as interacting in a loose hierarchical system, and he hypothesizes that a variety of environmental contingencies and trait-like individual differences combine to produce the richness of emotional experience. Other important emotion theorists such as Lazarus (1995), best known for articulating cognitive processes in emotion as noted above, now endorse a biological universality of emotional processing, while allowing that this phenomenon is of course subject to cultural variations.

Integrative emotion theorists such as John Teasdale (e.g., Barnard & Teasdale, 1991; Teasdale, 1993) and Howard Leventhal (Leventhal, 1991) have also proposed hierarchical integrative models that make important contributions. For example, Barnard and Teasdale (1991) formulated their own conceptualization of emotional processing, which they refer to as "interacting cognitive subsystems," emphasizing the information-processing aspects of emotional responding. Like most modern theorists of emotion, Barnard and Teasdale note that emotions can be elicited and processed out of awareness, and they distinguish the processing of information that produces "emotional or intuitive belief" or "knowing with the heart" from more intellectual beliefs or rational knowing. Teasdale (1993) also proposes that some of the most effective ways of changing maladaptive emotions may include the direct alteration of emotional behavior, such as changing avoidant responses or facial expressions.

Lang's Bioinformational Theory of Emotion

Peter Lang's bioinformational theory of emotion is perhaps the most prominent integrative theory of emotion and anxiety (e.g., Lang, 1978, 1979, 1984, 1985, 1994b, 1995; Lang, Bradley, & Cuthbert, 1998). This theory conceptualizes emotion as action tendencies stored in memory and accessed in a variety of ways, all of which involve the processing of information. Despite the importance of considering the dimensional aspects of emotion, Lang considers the essential core of emotion to be behavioral acts or broad response dispositions that occur in specific stimulus contexts. These stimulus contexts define the function and direction of the act (e.g., fight–escape, etc.). These emotional dispositions or acts are likened to software in a computer. The "data file" of these acts includes not only stimulus information (which prompts action), but also response propositions that are appropriate, such as avoidance and underlying physiological reactivity. "Response propositions" are data in the form of statements relevant to response components of the emotion stored in long-term memory. "Meaning propositions," wherein the stimulus information and response propositions are interpreted, are also part of the data file and essentially define an event's significance. For example, in a phobic situation, stimulus information is recognition of the frightening object. Response propositions are relevant responses, such as avoidance and elevated physiological responding to prepare for the emergency. But meaning propositions tie these two together. For example, meaning propositions may include the following statement: "In this situation, that thing is unpredictable and dangerous, and my responding indicates that I'm afraid." Lang rejects the long-held view that images are basically "pictures in the mind" or iconic representations in storage, and that imagining involves the inward perceiving of these images. Lang cites Pylyshyn (1973), who suggested that images in the brain are more like elaborated descriptions. In short, the image is a functionally organized, finite set of propositions.

Since data structures are stored in memory as propositions more or less strongly associated, the entire network is conceptual and accessed by information-processing mechanisms. The likelihood of accessing an emotion is increased by presenting information that maximizes the number of propositions matched. For example, if one hears mention of a fearful object (or sexual object or anger-producing object), this may or may not be sufficient to activate the entire emotional prototype. But if one is face to face with the object and the context is correct, *and* one is already physically aroused from exercise, *and* the appropriate emotional (fear, anger, or sex) meaning propositions have been primed (perhaps through unrelated conversation), then the chance of accessing the full emotional response is maximal.

Lang recognizes that all emotional expression exists along several dimensions. One dimension is arousal, from low to high; a second involves valence, from pleasant to unpleasant. A third possible dimension is control (or lack of it). (A dimensional approach to emotion and anxiety is considered in more detail below.) Consideration of the dimensions of emotion has much to do with differentiating emotional networks from other knowledge structures in the brain. Emotion networks are directly connected to the brain's primary motivational systems. These are systems with marked evolutionary significance whose function is to activate behaviors that are basic to survival. In addition, these motivational systems are associated with predominant brain circuits that are, in an important sense, "hard-wired." Based on a variety of prior work, Lang supposes that the motivational structure of emotion can be divided into an appetitive system (associated with pleasant emotions) and a defensive system (associated with unpleasant emotions). Pleasant emotions are an integral component of important appetitive behaviors, such as eating, drinking, sexual activity, and other nurturant behaviors. The significance of this motivational system is apparent. Unpleasant emotions are associated with a strong defensive system motivating protection from threat or danger. Emotion networks, then, have important connections to this primitive motivational circuitry, which once again distinguishes these emotion networks from other knowledge networks reflecting nonemotional associations.

For our purposes, emotion networks representing fear- and anxiety-related behavior incorporate a defensive motivational circuit. The behavioral output from these emotional networks may vary depending on the environmental context, but it includes (1) defensive immobility, reflected in the commonly observed freezing and hypervigiliance responses; and (2) defensive action as reflected in the flight-or-fight response (depending on context) in the presence of imminent attack. These two broad action tendencies mirror Gray's BIS and FFS, although Lang assumes somewhat different neural circuitry associated with these action tendencies. Other outputs from the defensive motivational system include the startle response, and automatic responding such as increase in blood pressure and heart rate (Lang, Bradley, & Cuthbert, 1998).

From the dimensional point of view, then, this defensive emotion network reflects a high level of intensity on the arousal dimension and a high level of unpleasantness on the valence dimension. Following the work of Davis (1997), Lang has focused much of his recent research on the phenomenon of startle potentiation, which seems to be one common output of the defensive motivational system. Activation of this defensive system is associated with an incrementally stronger startle response, making the startle response a convenient objective marker of this system. Thus much of Lang's attention in recent years has been devoted to exploring the parameters of this startle response (e.g., Bradley, Cuthbert, & Lang, 1996; Lang, Bradley, & Cuthbert, 1990).

In any case, fear and anxiety are behavior programs existing in memory (much like computer programs), comprising stimulus, response, and meaning structures. These emotions are integral parts of the defensive motivational system. In addition, these emotional programs must be fully accessed if any important therapeutic change is to occur. In other words, to modify fear or anxiety, the individual must first become fearful or anxious. The fundamental strategy of treatment is to "process" information comprising the emotional image, and the emotional image is, for Lang, the prototype fear image stored in long-term memory. This "template" can be elicited for emotional processing in a variety of ways, either imaginal or in vivo, but all aspects of it should be processed for successful therapy. This processing may make possible the formation of a new response prototype preliminary to overt behavior change. This new prototype would contain a less anxious or nonanxious response to the stimulus propositions (Rachman, 1980; Foa & Kozak, 1986).

This creative and carefully thought-out theory avoids the difficulty of discordance that confronts the theory of discrete emotions, since weak or incomplete matching of propositions may only access part of the response. The evolutionary behavioral theorists, on the other hand, would suggest that a fundamental, innate discrete emotion is always present in its entirety, albeit at varying levels of intensity.

Lang does not elaborate on the origin of emotions, but presumably emotional prototypes are, by and large, learned and reflect the variety of emotional responding that may emerge from interaction of the defensive motivational system with environmental context and other individual differences. He does admit to the possibility that some stimulus propositions are innate, and therefore more likely to evoke a strong emotional response. Examples may include "prepared" fear stimuli such as snakes and spiders, or perhaps various sexual postures. But most emotional networks and specific emotional responses are thought to be the products of experience and conditioning rather than of innate neurocircuitry, which is more characteristic of basic motivational systems. This approach also bypasses the requirement of an intervening cognitive appraisal, which produces difficulty for appraisal theorists. That is, emotional responses are directly accessed without intervening appraisal if enough propositions are matched. Of course, meaning propositions, which are basically interpretations, come very close to the concept of attribution as elaborated by Schachter (1964); however, attributions are seen as simply one type of propositions among many, not as necessary antecedents.

Perhaps most significant from the point of view of cognitive science, the scientific exploration of this process does not depend on self-report of experiential thought or feeling. Self-reports can be influenced by conditions that distort the underlying information-processing sequence. Bioelectric recording is seen as a more direct, contemporaneous method of examining bioinformational processing without the distortions of self-report. It is direct because emotion is considered an action set that generates efferent output, whether the behavior is actually expressed or not. That is, experiencing fear will produce physiology associated with avoidance responding, whether one actually avoids the feared object or not.

Interestingly, this theory requires an ultimate concordance of the various response systems constituting an emotion (at least a strongly coherent emotion) somewhere deep in memory structure, even if this concordance is not always apparent upon expression—or, more accurately, even if all components of the emotion are not accessed, or the context does not allow the occurrence of a particular component (e.g., aggressive attack during a business meeting). In view of the existing data on discordance and Lang's own pioneering conceptualization of these data, this requirement still demands a leap of faith for the time being. On the other hand, as Lang (1985, 1994a) argues, some emotions may be more coherent and "tighter" in their structures; once such emotions are accessed, an "all-or-none" type of response occurs, including all response components. Other emotions may be much more diffuse, with a great deal of fluidity among affective response structures. Thus many stimuli may partially access these more fluid structures, although not as intensely and with greater discordance. Lang considers "generalized" anxiety as one possible example of this more fluid, diffuse affective state.

Summary of Integrative Models

In summary, based on modern integrative models of emotion such as Lang's, emotions are a unique aspect of our experience associated with fundamentally important activities for us as individual members of a species. In addition to the experiential "feel" of emotional experience, which seems to be associated with their motivational function, emotions also reflect more primitive and at times "irrational" patterns of behavior strongly associated with subcortical brain functioning. These behavior patterns often occur out of awareness. Recent brain imaging studies confirm the existence of subcortical emotional circuits and their distinction from more cortical inputs associated with awareness and rational appraisals. These more cortically based circuits, in turn, seem to represent knowledge networks (in Lang's model) that are not necessarily tied to fundamental motivational systems (Öhman, Flykt, & Lundqvist, 2000; Öhman & Soares, 1994, 1998). Nevertheless, emotional expression must be studied in the context of a comprehensive interaction of neurobiological, behavioral, and cognitive response systems—a position now espoused by almost all modern emotion theorists. This viewpoint is increasingly evident among the newest breed of emotion theorists, who are beginning to apply emerging principles from an integrative study of emotion to emotional disorders (e.g., Gross, 1999; Gross & Munoz, 1995; Kring & Bachorowski, 1999).

THE DIMENSIONS OF EMOTION

A survey of different theoretical traditions illuminates the variety of approaches one can take in attempting to understand emotion in general, or specific emotions such as fear in particular. The development of a consensus on the basic components of emotion permits the coordinated study and measurement of emotion. But only a thorough analysis of the basic dimensions shared by all emotions allows a complete theoretical elaboration of the nature of emotion. For that reason, careful consideration of the dimensions of emotion finds its way into leading theoretical analyses from several different traditions (e.g., Izard, 1977; Lang, 1984; Lang, Cuthbert, & Bradley, 1998).

An important consequence of a dimensional analysis is a greater specification of the nature of individual emotions, such as fear, anger, or love. By contrasting these emotions or mood states with affective states that are often closely related, such as depression, one can begin to see what is essential about fear and anxiety. Finally, specifying the critical dimensions of anxiety has important implications for the etiology and treatment of anxiety disorders.

Much of the serious inquiry into dimensions of emotion thus far has focused on subjective experience. The primary method of studying the subjective experience of emotion relies on self-report, using the variety of affect-laden adjectives available from the richness of language. As noted above, self-report, particularly retrospective report, is subject to a variety of distortions resulting from inadequacies of memory, contrast effects, and repression. Nevertheless, in everyday life, one of the most common personal interactions is to ask someone "How are you?" or "How are you feeling?" and to receive a similar question in return. This common question has become an important part of the self-monitoring of disordered emotional states. Patients with emotional disorders are asked while in specific situations or at specific times to rate a particular affect, such as depression, anxiety, or anger, along levels of intensity (Barlow, 2001). Using this approach, some investigators have attempted a semantic mapping of the world of emotions. The purpose of this semantic mapping is to ascertain basic emotional expressions based on self-report, and to examine the dimensions of affect shared by all emotions. Similarities or differences in discretely described emotions can then be determined by their relationship to one another in the context of the major dimensions of emotion.

The primary measurement tools in this type of research are adjective checklists. Subjects check adjectives that are judged to describe their current emotional state or their long-term emotional dispositions. Major instruments include the Multiple Affect Adjective Checklist (Zuckerman & Lubin, 1965), the Profile of Mood States (McNair, Lorr, & Droppleman, 1971), the Mood Adjective Checklist (Nowlis & Nowlis, 1956), and the Positive and Negative Affect Scale (Watson, Clark, & Tellegen, 1988). The primary analytic tools for determining relevant discrete emotions as well as overall dimensions of affect have been sophisticated correlational procedures, such as factor analysis and related cluster-analytic techniques. When stable emotional dispositions are the subject of inquiry or measurement, rather than moment-to-moment emotional states, the study of mood becomes the study of personality (e.g., Watson & Clark, 1984; Watson, Clark, & Harkness, 1994).

Despite the identification of discrete emotions through factor-analytic work, over the years researchers investigating dimensions of personality and emotion have consistently narrowed down the possibilities to two or three major bipolar dimensions (e.g., Eysenck, 1961; Russell, 1980; Russell & Carroll, 1999; Wundt, 1896). Eysenck has put most of the emphasis on two discrete, orthogonal axes, as noted earlier. Most investigators have concluded that this arrangement puts an undue burden on the specification of one axis that comprises emotion or personality. For that reason, a consensus has developed that the best way to represent the factors emerging from these factor-analytic studies is a circumplex model (Plutchik, 1980; Plutchik & Conte, 1997).

In a circumplex model, various emotions are placed circularly in order to reflect their relationship to other dimensions of affect, as well as their opposites to be found on the other side of the circle. Emotions that are highly positively correlated will be found close to each other, while negatively correlated emotions will be found on opposite sides of the circle (e.g., see Figure 2.4, below). One of the best-known early examples of a circumplex model was proposed by Freedman, Leary, Ossorio, and Coffey (1951) and later elaborated for its clinical relevance by Timothy Leary (1957). For example, distributed along one side of the circle are "critical," "punitive," and "rejecting," while on the opposite side are "loving," "cooperative," and "trustful," and so on around the circumplex. Circumplex models are perfectly amenable to identification, description, and "plotting" of discrete emotions through factor-analytic techniques. Indeed, Izard and his colleagues, using adjective checklists, identified (and therefore validated, in Izard's view) the 10 fundamental discrete emotions emerging from expressive-behavioral studies (Izard, Kagan, & Zajonc, 1984). Furthermore, facial expressions can be arranged in a circumplex model corresponding to descriptive adjectives.

Russell's Circumplex

Nevertheless, analyses of the dimensions of affect such as Russell's (1980; Russell & Carroll, 1999) have identified two axes within the circumplex that account for the major proportion of the variance in attempts to ascertain dimensions of emotion. The first of these axes can be termed "activation," with high activity or arousal at one end and low activity or calmness at the other. Russell also includes "valence," which refers to a bipolar dimension of pleasure–displeasure. Russell and Mehrabian (1977) identified a third dimension that accounts for somewhat less of the variance, but would seem to be important in making certain discriminations among emotions. This dimension is termed "dominance–submission." But they put it more descriptively as feelings of lack of control versus feelings of influence or being in control. After studying this dimension further, Russell (1980) concluded that dominance–submission is not really an affect, but a strong cognitive correlate of emotion. That is, control is a perceived consequence of an emotion, rather than an emotion per se. Nevertheless, the perception of control may be particularly important within the emotion of anxiety, since perceptions of control under high arousal and negative valence (unpleasurably high arousal) may discriminate, for example, between anger and anxiety. People who are angry may feel unpleasantly aroused but in control of the situation or dominant, whereas anxious people may feel not in control and submissive, helpless, or vulnerable.

Tellegen's Circumplex

One of the most creative and sophisticated researchers in the area of personality has proposed a variation on this circumplex of emotion, which organizes the data somewhat differently from previous models but seems to fit the (self-report) data quite well. Starting with a long representative list of adjectives from current self-rating inventories for mood, Auke Tellegen (1985) replicated the primary discrete-emotion factors found by Izard and others; however, he also demonstrated, as did Russell (1980) before him, that the item intercorrelations were dominated by two large dimensions. These dimensions repeatedly emerged from studies of different groups of subjects tested on the same occasion, or of the same group of subjects tested periodically over periods of time ranging up to 3 months (e.g., Zevon & Tellegen, 1982). This latter method is particularly convincing, since it avoids the problem of retrospective distortion.

Tellegen (1985) has also found that arranging the emotional descriptors emerging from these two major factors in a circumplex proves most satisfactory in terms of describing their relationship. Thus the circle is divided into eight sections, since correlations have yielded consistent descriptors that fit into these eight sections. The two major factors are labeled in a straightforward manner: "positive affect" and "negative affect." The full circumplex model is presented in Figure 2.4. This emphasis differs a bit from earlier descriptions, where "arousal" and "valence" axes have been highlighted (e.g., Russell, 1980). But the term "engagement," appearing in the upper right quadrant, is preferred by Tellegen over the term "arousal," resulting in an engagement–disengagement axis. "Engagement" refers to the same clustering of adjectives previously called "arousal." The "valence" dimension, also identified by others, is termed "pleasantness–unpleasantness" in this circumplex. Arousal (or engagement) and valence (or pleasantness–unpleasantness) are therefore found as diagonal axes in this circumplex. However, Tellegen notes that he prefers emphasizing the axes of positive and negative affect, for several reasons. He suggests that they conform more closely to the factor-analytic data, as well as to major personality factors discussed below. In addition—and more importantly, from our point of view—this configuration has had substantial impact on the study of emotion (e.g., Lang, Cuthbert, & Bradley, 1998) and has proven useful in studying emotional disorders (e.g., Brown, Chorpita, & Barlow, 1998; see Chapter 8). Some controversy does continue, however, regarding whether positive and negative affect are orthogonal or independent, or represent different positions on the same dimension, as thought by Russell and Carroll (1999). In fact, Peter Salovey and colleagues argue quite persuasively that positive and negative affect are not orthogonal,

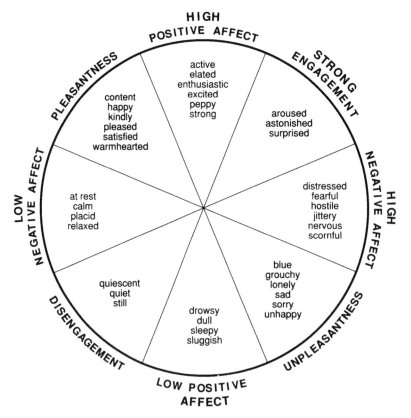

FIGURE 2.4. The two-factor structure of self-rated mood. From Tellegen (1985). Copyright 1985 by Lawrence Erlbaum Associates. Reprinted by permission.

and thus that the data of Tellegen and colleagues do not really support independence of these affective states. In addition, they believe with Russell and Carroll (1999) that emphasizing the axes of "pleasantness–unpleasantness" (valence) and "arousal–calm" provides a better fit for the data (Green, Goldman, & Salovey, 1993; Green & Salovey, 1999; Green, Salovey, & Truax, 1999).

THE DIMENSIONS OF ANXIETY AND DEPRESSION

With the foregoing overview of the dimensions of emotion, it is now possible to consider anxiety from a dimensional point of view. More specifically, how does anxiety relate to discrete emotions, as well as to more general dimensions of affect? Since all theorists (and therapists) agree that anxiety and depression are closely related, a more specific version of this question is as follows: What are the dimensions of anxiety and depression, and how do they differ?

This is a particularly good way to begin an examination of the nature of anxiety, since this question has been extremely troublesome to basic-emotion theorists and clinical practitioners, who have found distinctions difficult to identify (Clark & Watson, 1991; Kendall & Watson, 1989). Many clinicians over the years defaulted to a clinical syndrome that came to be known as "mixed anxiety–depression," in an attempt to better characterize this state of affairs (Zinbarg & Barlow, 1991; Zinbarg et al., 1994, 1998).

Early evidence reflecting this overlap was presented by Dobson (1985), who calculated correlations between a number of anxiety and depression self-rating scales, such as the State–Trait Anxiety Inventory (Spielberger et al., 1970) and the Zung Self-Rating Depression Scale (Zung, 1965). The correlation among anxiety scales was .66; among depression scales, it was .69; and between anxiety and depression scales, it was .61. The amount of shared variance for each correlation was very high, ranging from .37 to .47. This degree of shared variance suggested that these questionnaires were not useful in measuring the intensity of two different affective states, anxiety and depression; rather, they were measuring the same or very similar affective states. Breslau (1985) found a similar lack of discriminability in the Center for Epidemiologic Studies Depression Scale, a widely used depression rating scale.

Lee Anna Clark and David Watson (two students of Auke Tellegen) have developed what they term a "tripartite" model, and research generated from this heuristic has shed considerable light on the nature of anxiety and closely related affective states, such as depression. Basically, Clark and Watson (e.g., Clark & Watson, 1991; L. A. Clark, Watson, & Mineka, 1994; Watson, Clark, et al., 1995; Watson, Weber, et al., 1995; Mineka, Watson, & Clark, 1998) have concluded that anxiety and depression share a significant but nonspecific component of generalized distress termed "negative affect." Symptoms of anxious or depressed mood, poor concentration, sleep disturbances, or irritability are examples of negative affective symptoms shared by anxiety and depression. However, a related concept, "positive affect," must also be considered for a full understanding of anxiety and depression. Specifically, in addition to high negative affect, depression is characterized by low positive affect (e.g., inability to experience any pleasure [anhedonia], combined with cognitive and motor slowing). This component contributes an identifiable proportion of variance to depression but not to anxiety. The third corner of the triangle of the tripartite model is physiological hyperarousal, which until recently was thought to be more strongly associated with anxiety than with depression. More recent research, in fact, has suggested that this construct plays a more complex and specific role in anxious and depressive phenomena than do the more fundamental concepts of positive and negative affect. These developments are discussed in more detail in Chapter 3.

Over the last decade, sophisticated studies have emerged supporting the general structure of the tripartite model (e.g., Joiner, 1996; Joiner, Catanzaro, & Laurent, 1996; Joiner et al., 1999; Watson, Clark, et al., 1995). In fact, the dimension of negative affect, representing as it does nonspecific distress or unpleasant emotionality, is key to an understanding of the nature of anxiety and depression, and plays an important role in theories of emotion reviewed above. For example, negative affect is considered a basic dimension in Lang's defensive motivational system or Gray's BIS. Thus negative affect may represent a crucial vulnerability factor for the development of the somewhat more elaborated affective states of anxiety and depression.

To return to dimensional analyses of emotion, Russell's (1980) early findings and conclusions regarding control become important. Control, or lack of control, assumes a position of sufficient strength to appear in factor analyses of self-report ratings of affect adjectives. Since the various negative emotional states that share high engagement or activation are close together in any circumplex, it is possible that what distinguishes a report of anxiety from a report of anger or even interest is a sense of lack of control. In this sense anger and hostility are closer to fear and anxiety than to depression, since in any dimensional scheme of emotion states, both are negative affective states that share action tendencies of engagement with supporting physiology. This fact may have important implications for differentiating anxiety and stress disorders, as outlined in Chapter 8.

In any case, this sense of uncontrollability is associated with a number of important phenomena. Among these is a decrease in valence or pleasure associated with the affective state. Another effect is a marked shift in attention from the object of interest to salient material or events congruent with apprehensiveness and anxiety, as well as to one's own affective response to these events (see Chapter 3). For a sense of control (or lack of it) is a construct with primarily internal referents. As noted above, this interruption/shift in attention constitutes an integral part of many theories of anxiety, including biological and cognitive theories (Gray & McNaughton, 1996; Mandler, 1984). The anticipated uncontrollability is future-oriented rather than something that actually happens. In other words, it is not present danger, but a vague sense of future danger, which is due to a sense of impending uncontrollability combined with distorted and unadaptive shifts in allocation of attention.

SUMMARY AND CONCLUSIONS

At the beginning of the 21st century, emotion has assumed its rightful position alongside cognition and behavior as proper subject matter for psychological science. Among the reasons for this new emphasis on the study of the structure and function of emotion is a coming together and integration of the three grand traditions in the study of emotion that have dominated the field for over a century. Detailed inquiry into the distinct components of emotion—expressive-behavioral, neurobiological, and cognitive—has resulted in a deeper understanding of these fundamental components, as well as a more integrative view of the nature of emotion, which rejects the idea that these components can somehow exist in splendid isolation. Dimensional study of the experience of emotion has complemented this inquiry by highlighting both what is common and what is unique among the varieties of emotional experience. This inquiry, in turn, paves the way for more detailed analyses of the varieties of emotional experience.

With these developments, the mysteries of anxiety are gradually giving way to a new appreciation of the varieties of behavioral patterns associated with our defensive motivational system. Perhaps most important is a recognition of substantial and fundamental differences in the behavioral expression of anxiety on the one hand and fear on the other, which has only recently come to light as alluded to above. The intimate dance of these two action tendencies within the defensive motivational system can be observed not only at the level of behavior and cognition, but also in closely related but unique brain circuits underlying these action tendencies (see Chapter 6).

It also seems clear that a fuller understanding of the components of emotion contributes to an appreciation of the origins of specific emotions such as anxiety and fear. Strong biological contributions conveyed to us as part of our genetic endowment seem to create at least one set of vulnerabilities that set the stage for the subsequent appearance of anxiety. Crucial work identifying fundamental temperaments such as Kagan's behavioral inhibition, and the moderation of these temperaments by experience, will ultimately lead us to a fuller understanding of gene–environment interactional models of the development of anxiety and fear. Basic cognitive structures seem to represent a second, more psychological vulnerability to experience anxiety and fear, emanating, perhaps, from early experience. These cognitive filters process day-to-day events through the dark glass of danger and threat, and manifest themselves in commonly observed cognitive distortions. A full discussion of vulnerabilities contributing to the development of anxiety and its disorders appears in Chapter 8.

Dimensional analyses of the specific experience of anxiety have revealed much about the structure of this emotion and its relation to closely related emotions, such as depression, fear, and excitement. The mix of affective and cognitive dimensions, with emphasis on affective valence, arousal, and a relative sense of controllability, has done much to identify what is unique about anxiety. With this foundation of current perspectives on emotion, it is now possible to delve deeper into the mysteries of anxiety by examining the structure and process of this enigmatic emotional state.

CHAPTER 3

The Nature
of Anxious Apprehension

In Chapter 2, I have concluded that anxiety can best be characterized as a unique, coherent cognitive–affective structure within the defensive motivational system. In the first edition of this book (Barlow, 1988), I developed a model of the structure of various components of anxiety and their interaction. At the heart of this structure is a sense of uncontrollability focused largely on possible future threat, danger, or other potentially negative events. Thus this state can be roughly characterized as a state of helplessness, because of a perceived inability to predict, control, or obtain desired results or outcomes in certain upcoming personally salient situations or contexts. This negative affective state is accompanied by a shift in attention to what would be primarily a self-focus or a state of self-preoccupation in which evaluation of one's (inadequate) capabilities to deal with the threat is prominent. Accompanying this negative affective state is a strong physiological or somatic component that may reflect activation of distinct brain circuits associated with engagement of the corticotropin-releasing factor (CRF) system and Gray's behavioral inhibition system (BIS) (Sullivan, Kent, & Coplan, 2000; Gray & McNaughton, 1996: Chorpita & Barlow, 1998) (see Chapter 6). This somatic state may be the physiological substrate of "readiness," which may underlie a state of preparation to counteract helplessness. Vigilance (hypervigilance) is another characteristic of anxiety that suggests readiness and preparation to deal with potentially negative events. If one were to put anxiety into words, one might say, "That terrible event could happen again, and I might not be able to deal with it, but I've got to be ready to try." For these reasons, I have suggested that a better and more precise term for anxiety might be "anxious apprehension." This conveys the notion that anxiety is a *future-oriented* mood state in which one is ready or prepared to attempt to cope with upcoming negative events. Another term often paired with "anxiety" is "anticipatory." But in the present definition, all anxiety is anticipatory, so this qualifying adjective does not appear again. "Anxiety" or "anxious apprehension" also allows a clear discrimination from "panic" or "fear"—terms that have often been categorized under the general rubric of "anxiety" in the past. The process of anxiety as described above is presented in Figure 3.1.

It is important to remember that I consider the construct shown in Figure 3.1 to be composed of a number of coherent, closely related affective and cognitive components. In this model, a variety of "cues" or "propositions," to use the terms of Lang (1985, 1994a, 1994b), would be sufficient to evoke anxious apprehension. Importantly, this process could occur without the necessity of a conscious, rational appraisal. For example, one might expe-

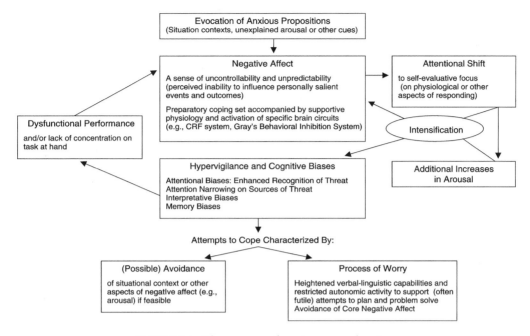

FIGURE 3.1. The process of anxious apprehension.

rience anxiety without realizing the specific trigger or cue, such as an object or situation that "represents" an earlier trauma, or an internal somatic sensation. These cues may be broad-based or very narrow. An example of a narrow set of cues is the case of test anxiety or sexual dysfunction, in which cues signaling the necessity of imminent performance evoke a state of anxious apprehension, with its associated heightened tension, elevated arousal, and negative valence. This state in turn is associated with a shift in attention to a self-evaluative focus (or a rapidly shifting focus of attention from an external, potentially threatening context to internal self-evaluative content). Evidence suggests that this shift to a self-focused attentional state further increases arousal and negative affect, thus forming its own small positive feedback loop. This subsystem is also represented in Figure 3.1.

Continuing on in the larger system or feedback loop, attention narrows to sources of threat or danger, setting the stage for additional distortions in the processing of information through either attentional or interpretive biases, reflecting preexisting hypervalent cognitive schemata. In any case, one becomes hypervigilant for cues or stimuli associated with sources of anxious apprehension. This process in humans is analogous to, and may represent, Gray's (1987; Gray & McNaughton, 1996) "stop, look, and listen" state of behavioral inhibition, although the actual state of inhibition is not so readily apparent in clinical examples of human anxiety as it is in animals. At sufficient intensity, this process results in disruption of concentration and performance. The process of anxiety is seldom pathological, even when intense, until it becomes chronic.

When anxiety becomes chronic, one or both of two prominent consequences of the process of anxiety develop in an attempt to cope with negative affect and its triggers. First, a tendency to avoid entering a state of anxious apprehension is always present. This tendency becomes more pronounced and observable, depending on the severity or intensity of the state, and on the specificity of the contextual cues that set the occasion for anxious apprehension. Thus test-anxious individuals will avoid tests to the extent that this is possible, and sexually dysfunctional individuals will eventually avoid sex. But this rather maladaptive coping skill may not be available to individuals whose anxious apprehension has diffused to many different situational contexts (or, more accurately in Langian terms, across many different "networks in memory"). In these individuals, subtle avoidance behaviors, rituals, or "superstitious" behaviors may become established (see Chapter 14). Second, worry that is driven by the process of anxiety and that (at intense levels) is very difficult to control (Brown, Dowdall, Côté, & Barlow, 1994) seems best construed as an additional (and most often futile) attempt to cope with chronic anxiety. In the fourth edition of the *Diagnostic and Statistical Manual of Mental Disorders* (DSM-IV), lack of control over the worry process is a defining feature of generalized anxiety disorder (GAD) (Brown, Barlow, & Liebowitz, 1994). Worry, or concern over future events, is of course not problematic and may even be adaptive under some circumstances, unless it is so driven by anxiety that it becomes intense and uncontrollable. It is in this sense that worry can become chronic and maladaptive. Chronic anxiety is also characterized by persistent central nervous system tension and arousal (Sullivan et al., 2000; Gray & McNaughton, 1996; Chorpita & Barlow, 1998), which seem to reflect the consequences of a state of perpetual readiness to confront danger. The characterization of avoidance and worry as closely related and maladaptive attempts to cope with the process of chronic anxious apprehension is a clarification and elaboration to my working model of anxious apprehension that is new to this edition, but is supported by research described below.

It is important to understand that this is an illustration of the process of chronic anxious apprehension, not a description of the etiology of anxiety. Much of the empirical data underlying the development of our conceptions of anxiety or anxious apprehension come from research on sexuality and sexual dysfunction conducted over the years in our Sexuality Research Program. Several years of programmatic research into the factors that maintain sexual dysfunction have helped to illustrate the roles of affect, cognition, and their interaction, with implications for the way anxiety works (e.g., Barlow, 1986; Cranston-Cuebas & Barlow, 1990; Barlow, Chorpita, & Turovsky, 1996). Before these new developments are discussed, it may be helpful to describe the context of sexuality research from which these data emerged.

ANXIOUS APPREHENSION IN SEXUAL DYSFUNCTION

Anxiety and Sexual Arousal

For years, writers of virtually every theoretical persuasion believed that "anxiety" plays a substantial role in the development and maintenance of sexual dysfunction for both men and women. For example, Fenichel (1945) considered anxiety to be a contributing factor to the development of the various types of sexual dysfunctions in both men and women. Masters and Johnson (1970) underlined the importance of performance fears and fears of inadequacy as major factors in individuals and couples experiencing sexual dysfunctions. Kaplan (1974) also gave fear of failure to perform adequately a primary role in the development of sexual anxieties, and added other fears (e.g., demands for performance on the part of the partner and excessive need to please partners) to the list of sexual anxieties. Sexual anxieties are seen as preventing an individual from experiencing sexual arousal, and, in fact, as inhibiting autonomic nervous system functioning to such an extent that physiological arousal is inhibited (Kaplan, 1974). In both Masters and Johnson's and Kaplan's conceptualizations, a major task of therapy is overcoming performance fears and feelings of sexual inadequacy, as well as treating other sources of sexual anxiety.

In a similar vein, as early as 1958 Wolpe suggested the use of systematic desensitization in the treatment of sexual dysfunctions, with the elimination of anxiety as the goal of treatment. This is familiar ground for most clinicians, particularly those who have ever dealt with sexual dysfunctions. People with these problems report the signs and symptoms of anxiety, and most treatments are aimed at reducing this anxiety (or determining the cause of it).

In fact, this state of affairs is an example of a situation common to our clinical science, in which facts that have been available for years simply do not support these assumptions. As early as 1943 Ramsey surveyed adolescent boys and reported that approximately 50% of the boys noted erections from some type of nonerotic stimulus or context. These nonerotic responses usually involved elements of fear, excitement, or other nonsexual emotional situations. They included events such as accidents, near-accidents, being chased by the police, fear of being punished, and so forth.

Sarrel and Masters (1982) reported a series of startling and gruesome events that are difficult to believe if one assumes that anxiety inhibits sexual arousal. These gruesome events involved rape, but not the unfortunately familiar scenario of men raping women. Rather, gangs of women accosted a number of men and demanded that they have sexual relations, threatening them at knifepoint or with other weapons if they failed. Under these circumstances the men reported not only achieving erection, but the ability to perform repeatedly (although they did suffer severe emotional consequences, forcing them to seek clinical assistance).

For anyone who has worked with patients suffering from paraphilias or sexual deviations, particularly exhibitionism or voyeurism, the association between fear and sexual arousal is evident. Many of these individuals are unable to become sexually aroused without first experiencing fear or anxiety over the possibility of being apprehended or otherwise threatened in some way (Beck & Barlow, 1984). Nor is the relationship of fear and sexual arousal limited to humans. Barfield and Sachs (1968) observed similar phenomena in rats.

Some of the more interesting experiments on the relationship between anxiety and sexual arousal (or attraction) have come from social psychologists. In one of the best examples, Dutton and Aron (1974) arranged to interview male students who had just crossed a rickety suspension bridge, thereby evoking some mild fear or anxiety, and compared them to students who had not crossed the bridge. Both groups of male students were then interviewed by an attractive female student. Students who had crossed the bridge, and therefore had become mildly "anxious," reported more sexual material in a projective test designed to assess this issue without the subjects' being aware of it than students who had not crossed the bridge. In addition, they called the female student (who had provided them with her telephone number on a pretext) and asked for a date significantly more times than subjects in the comparison group did! The conclusion of Dutton and Aron (1974), and other social psychologists approaching the issue from a somewhat different perspective (e.g., Berscheid & Walster, 1974; Brehm, Gatz, Goethals, McCrimmon, & Ward, 1978; Riordan, 1979), was that experimentally induced anxiety can increase interpersonal or sexual attraction.

At this point investigators began to examine the relationship of anxiety and sexual arousal directly in the laboratory. Hoon, Wincze, and Hoon (1977), as part of a larger study, conducted an empirical investigation of Wolpe's (1958) concept of reciprocal inhibition. Sexually functional women were shown a 2-minute film sequence that consisted of either "neutral" (travelogue scenes) or "noxious" (scenes of automobile accidents) content. Immediately following the film clip, subjects in each group were exposed to a sexually explicit film segment. This design allowed a test of Wolpe's (1958) contention that anxiety and sexual arousal are mutually inhibitory responses. It was hypothesized that sexual arousal following preexposure to a noxious stimulus (evoking sympathetic arousal such as increased heart rate) would be lower than that following preexposure to a neutral stimulus (which would evoke parasympathetic arousal, or relaxation), due to sympathetic inhibition of sexual arousal in the former condition. Surprisingly, results indicated the converse. Sexual arousal (operationalized as vaginal blood volume increases) was significantly greater in those women who had been preexposed to the anxiety-producing as opposed to the neutral film. Interestingly, when the order of film presentation was reversed (erotic preexposure to either a neutral or noxious stimulus film), sexual arousal was lower during the anxiety-producing segment. My colleagues and I (Wolchik et al., 1980) obtained similar results with a sample of sexually functional men.

In response to these findings, Wolpe (1978) suggested that the anxiety preexposure paradigm did not provide an adequate test of the reciprocal inhibition theory. He stated that one could not assume the "perseverative effects" (p. 453) of noxious preexposure, and therefore that increases in sexual arousal subsequent to an anxiety-producing event such as a film (as in the Hoon et al. [1977] investigation) might be due to an "emotional state of relief" (p. 453) rather than a facilitatory effect of anxiety.

To address the possibility that "anxiety relief" might have been playing a role in the Hoon et al. (1977) study, we evaluated these ideas more rigorously with sexual arousal in normal male volunteers (Barlow, Sakheim, & Beck, 1983). The purpose of this experiment was to find out, under controlled laboratory conditions, the effects of inducing "anxiety" simultaneous with sexual arousal. Anxiety was manipulated by shock threat during an explicit erotic film. Before the actual experiment was begun, the tolerance level of all subjects to a painful but harmless electric shock to the forearm was determined, and the subjects were told that this would be used in the experiment. Each subject experienced three different experimental conditions administered in a counterbalanced fashion. Each condition was signaled by a different light above the video screen the subject was watching. In the first condition, a light signaled that no shock would occur. This was the control condition. In the second condition, subjects were told that there was a 60% chance that they would receive a shock while they watched the erotic film. This condition was termed "noncontingent shock threat," since there was no indication that the shock threat would have anything to do whatsoever with the subjects' behavior. In the third condition, however, subjects were told that there was a 60% chance they would receive a shock if they did not achieve at least as large an erection as the average male in our laboratory. This condition was termed, quite appropriately, "contingent shock threat." In fact, subjects were never actually shocked during the experiment, but postexperimental assessment indicated that they thought they would be and were appropriately "anxious." Rather than decreasing sexual arousal, the results indicated that the noncontingent shock threat increased sexual arousal when compared to no shock threat. But, in an unexpected development, the contingent shock threat also increased sexual arousal when compared to no shock threat. In fact, this condition produced the highest overall sexual arousal! The data are presented in Figure 3.2. Thus performance demand not only did not interfere with sexual arousal, but actually increased it! This revelation made an investigation of the reaction of sexually dysfunctional men to this same paradigm all the more important. Indeed, results from other early reports suggested that such males did more poorly under shock threat (e.g., Beck, Barlow, Sakheim, & Abrahamson, 1984, 1987; Bruce & Barlow, 1990)—a topic to which I return below.

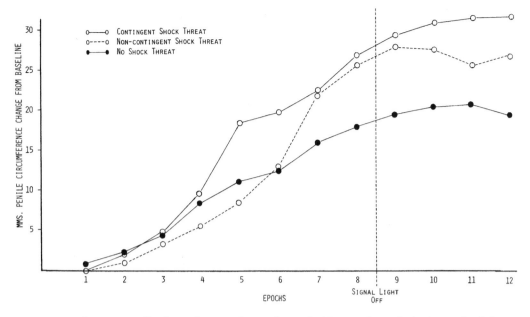

FIGURE 3.2. Average penile circumference change for each 15-second epoch during each of three conditions: no shock threat, noncontingent shock threat, and contingent shock threat. From "Anxiety Increases Sexual Arousal" by D. H. Barlow, D. K., Sakheim, and J. G. Beck, 1983, *Journal of Abnormal Psychology, 92*, 49–54. Copyright 1983 by the American Psychological Association. Reprinted with permission.

More recently, several investigators have extended the analysis of this phenomenon in women. For example, Meston and Gorzalka (1996) attempted to isolate the effects of sympathetic nervous system (SNS) activation by using exercise films as their manipulation. Thus sexually functional women and women with different types of sexual dysfunctions exercised vigorously to a standardized criterion prior to watching an erotic film. Exercise significantly increased both vaginal pulse amplitude and vaginal blood volume responses, but *not* subjective reports of sexual arousal to erotic stimuli, in sexually functional women and women with low sexual desire (but not inorgasmic women) compared to a no-exercise control condition. These authors noted that the exercise condition would not be equivalent to the shock threat performance demand condition in the studies mentioned above (i.e., Bruce & Barlow, 1990), since cognitive components of anxiety focused on voluntary threat or performance inadequacy were not present.

In addition, in another important series of replications, Palace (Palace & Gorzalka, 1990; Palace, 1995) demonstrated increased arousal in both sexually functional women and a group of women with mixed sexual dysfunctions. Palace used a paradigm similar to the Hoon et al. (1977) procedure, where viewing either a neutral film or an "impending danger" film preceded the erotic stimulus. Only the "impending danger" film produced increased arousal, and this response was also restricted to physiological measures compared to subjective reports. Thus the paradigm was not directly comparable to the results we obtained with males who had sexual dysfunction (Barlow, Sakheim, & Beck, 1983). Once again no simultaneous "performance demand" was present, and arousal increased in all groups.

Together with the information reviewed above from the social-psychological and developmental literature, it seems that emotions can "transfer," such that eliciting one emotion simultaneously with a second makes the second more "intense" (Zillmann, 1983b). Meston and Gorzalka's (1996) findings suggest that SNS activation is this component of emotion that transfers. Another possibility in our studies is that shock threat "motivated" our sexually functional subjects to higher levels of performance. Postexperimental inquiry seemed to support this interpretation, since several subjects made comments such as "I didn't want any part of that shock, so I really concentrated on the film." Nevertheless, sexual arousal increased almost as much in the noncontingent condition, where presumably no motivational factors were present. Thus it would seem that emotion transfer (or the SNS activation within emotion) accounts for the majority of the effect.

Emotion transfer is a relatively common theme in theories of emotion—particularly in more cognitive theories (see Chapter 2), where appraisal of physiological arousal and the context in which this arousal occurs plays an important role in emotional expression. One can also rely on a Langian analysis, also supported by Zillmann (1983b), by suggesting that the experimental conditions gave a "boost" to the response propositions involved in sexual arousal, thereby producing more successful accessing of sexual arousal. For present purposes, though, it is probably not necessary to consider whether an elementary type of appraisal occurred. It is enough to note that arousal transferred and increased in an additive way, but only for functional subjects in our studies evaluating "performance demand," not for those who were already sexually dysfunctional. What could have caused such marked differences in the way the males in our studies responded to the same experimental conditions?

Cognitive Interference

Since emotion seems to have transferred between anxiety and sexual arousal very nicely in our sexually functional subjects, what was happening to our sexually dysfunctional patients? It would seem that something was interfering with the transfer of emotion, but it was difficult to conceive of the nature of this interference. A close examination of ongoing cognitive processes, particularly in the manner in which they might interfere with sexual activity, seemed an obvious place to start.

In fact, we had known for some time that cognitive factors can interfere with sexual arousal, and some of these cognitive factors had been isolated. For example, Briddell et al. (1978) and Lansky and Wilson (1981) reported that inducing various expectancy sets in a systematic way seems to influence arousal. Another body of research indicated that males are capable of suppressing their arousal during erotic stimulation if asked to do so (e.g., Abel, Blanchard, & Barlow, 1981). When suppression occurs, presumably the mechanism by which subjects suppress erections is self-distraction or a shift in attention. Geer and Fuhr (1976) tested this idea directly in normal volunteers, using a "dichotic listening" device: while listening to erotic audiotapes in one ear, subjects were required to listen to increasingly distracting cognitive tasks in the other ear. Sexual arousal decreased as the complexity of the distracting task increased.

To examine the effects of distraction more closely, we tested the effects of neutral distraction (listening to audiotapes portraying a nonsexual passage from a popular novel) on both sexually dysfunctional patients and age-matched sexually functional volunteers (Abrahamson, Barlow, Sakheim, Beck, & Athanasiou, 1985). Subjects viewed an erotic film while listening to the distracting audiotapes and were told they would be questioned on material from the audiotapes after the experiment. This was contrasted to a condition where distraction was not present. Both groups achieved adequate and equivalent levels of penile responding under the no-distraction condition. The normal volunteers evidenced significant detumescence during distraction. But, in a surprising development, our sexually dysfunctional patients were not affected by distraction and maintained tumescence; if anything, their arousal increased a bit during the distracting condition. The data are presented in Figure 3.3. Although dysfunctional patients usually showed slightly less sexual arousal than functional subjects did in our laboratory, it was not unusual for subjects with psychogenic erectile dysfunction (who had been carefully screened to exclude any cases of sexual dysfunction with organic components, such as vascular problems) to demonstrate substantial arousal under these benign laboratory conditions. What was surprising was the marked difference in the response of these two groups to distraction; it was particularly puzzling, because clinicians working with these patients have long observed that distraction while trying to perform sexually seems to be a major difficulty that individuals with a dysfunction encounter. This paradox is discussed further below.

There is also evidence that a variety of alternative performance demand conditions are capable of decreasing arousal. For example, when sexually dysfunctional patients and sexual functional volunteers both watched an erotic film of a woman who was obviously highly aroused, compared to an erotic film where the woman did not appear sexually aroused, interesting differences emerged. The sexually functional volunteers showed substantial arousal to the erotic film where the woman was not aroused, but this arousal increased significantly when they perceived the woman as aroused. On the other hand, the

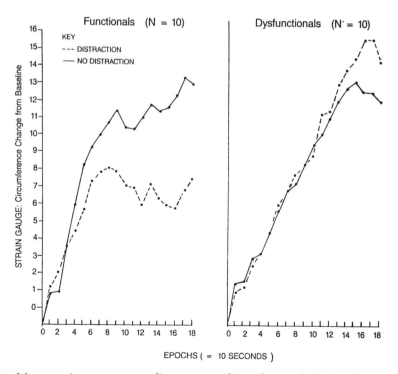

FIGURE 3.3. Mean strain gauge responding across subjects by epoch during distraction and no distraction: Sexually functional (left) versus sexually dysfunctional (right) subjects. From Abrahamson, Barlow, Sakheim, Beck, and Athanasiou (1985). Copyright 1985 by the Association for Advancement of Behavior Therapy. Reprinted by permission.

sexually dysfunctional patients showed less arousal if they perceived that the woman was highly aroused, compared to a film where she was not aroused (Abrahamson, Barlow, Beck, Sakheim, & Kelly, 1985; Beck, Barlow, & Sakheim, 1983). What seemed to be happening was that the highly responsive woman elicited performance-related concerns, which were "distracting" to our patients. The volunteers, on the other hand, attended to and concentrated on the erotic cues under either condition.

Our preliminary conclusions from these and related experiments (cf. Barlow, 1986) suggested that our sexually dysfunctional patients were also subject to the strong influence of distraction, but that the distracting influences differed in terms of their effects on patients and sexually functional volunteers. The volunteers showed marked decrements in their arousal under the influence of neutral off-task types of distracting influences, but demonstrated marked increases in arousal under conditions of performance demand. Our patients, on the other hand, could accommodate the neutral distraction quite easily, even showing some disinhibition, but were markedly affected by the influence of performance demand. This performance demand condition seemed to cue a variety of self-evaluative thoughts concerning internal physiology, as well as the strong possibility of failure to perform and subsequent humiliation. Such thoughts were strong, salient, or "hot" cognitions with an intense negative affective tone, and they seemed impervious to rational intervention or the simple effects of persuasion. In other words, they seemed to be an integral part of a basic, automatic, instantaneous, cognitive–affective response.

One reason for the strength of this cognitive–affective process may have emerged, at least partially, from the next series of experiments, which targeted the relationship of cognition and affect in this group of patients. In one experiment, sexually functional volunteers were presented with erotic audiotapes simultaneous with four levels of shock threat: no shock, half tolerance, tolerance, and twice tolerance (Beck et al., 1987). As a further check on their level of attention to the audiotapes, a sentence recognition task administered with signal detection methodology was carried out immediately following presentation of the stimuli. Essentially, the results indicated that shock threat lowered sexual responding, particularly during half tolerance and tolerance shock; however, during the twice-tolerance condition, sexual responding returned somewhat and approached responding under the no-shock condition. Performance on the sentence recognition task improved during half tolerance and tolerance shock, and then deteriorated somewhat during the twice-tolerance condition. Thus performance on the sentence recognition task formed an inverted U-shaped function under increasing intensities of shock threat, as one can see in Figure 3.4.

This finding, of course, is as old as the Yerkes–Dodson law (Anderson, 1990; Yerkes & Dodson, 1908) referred to in Chapter 1; that is, efficiency of performance (in this case, on the sentence recognition task) will increase, up to a point, under conditions of arousal (in this case, shock threat). Particularly interesting, however, was the effect of our experimental condition on the process of sexual arousal. As one can see in Figure 3.4, sexual arousal essentially mirrored this inverted U. The better subjects did on the sentence recognition task (presumably as a function of greater attention to the sentences), the less sexual arousal they demonstrated. In our previous shock threat experiments we did not have this type of task, and therefore these effects were not observed. Our initial conclusion was that "anxiety" induced by shock threat will improve performance or concentration in an inverted U-shaped function; however, if the focus of attention is nonsexual, sexual arousal will suffer proportionally. What would the implication of this finding be for our dysfunctional patients? In these patients, as the reader will remember, anxiety or shock threat seemed to interfere with sexual arousal, even when no overt alternative focus of attention was available. Therefore, it was possible that the dysfunctional patients were already focusing on

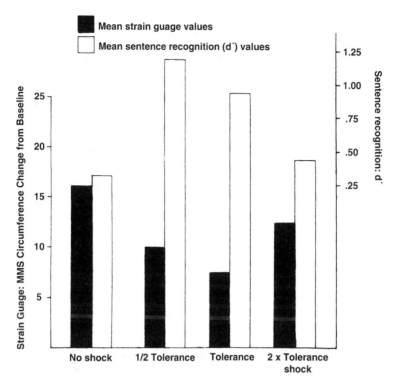

FIGURE 3.4. Mean strain gauge responding averaged across stimulus duration, and mean sentence recognition values, during four shock threat conditions. From Beck, Barlow, Sakheim, and Abrahamson (1987). Copyright 1987 by the Society for Psychophysiological Research, Inc. Reprinted by permission.

or attending to something other than erotic cues. Increasing levels of "anxiety," then, evidently sharpened and increased the efficiency of their focus of attention. Unfortunately, this other-directed focus occurred at the expense of sexual arousal. Evidence that this was happening was present in the distraction studies described above and in some subsequent, rather complex experiments (Beck & Barlow, 1986a, 1986b).

Another experiment from our laboratory seemed to confirm this differential focus of attention between groups (J. C. Jones, Bruce, & Barlow, 1986). Sexually dysfunctional and age-matched sexually functional volunteers both viewed erotic films under the four levels of shock threat described above. The primary finding to emerge was that the volunteers showed increased sexual arousal in an inverted U-shaped function as intensity of shock threat increased (up to full tolerance level), but the patients showed decreased arousal in a normal U-shaped function. In other words, the sexual arousal pattern of these two groups under these experimental conditions mirrored each other. This outcome seemed to confirm that the volunteers and the patients were attending to different cues: For our dysfunctional patients, the cues were nonsexual.

Therefore, the preliminary evidence suggested that our sexually functional volunteers did worse (i.e., evidence lower sexual arousal) when given a task that removed their focus somewhat from the direct processing of erotic cues. But, to return to the paradox mentioned above, the intriguing finding not yet discussed fully here is that our sexually dysfunctional patients either showed no effect or did slightly better when distracted from processing erotic cues by a neutral, off-task distraction, such as readings from popular novels. On the other hand, performance-related sexual demands seemed to "distract" our patients, and the presence of increasing levels of anxiety during performance demand further decreased sexual arousal, probably by enhancing concentration on the nonerotic content of their attentional focus. Presumably, as suggested above, this focus centered on internal physiology (including erectile response); on performance-related concerns; and on apprehension of scrutiny, failure, and ridicule.

But introducing a competing nonerotic task for our dysfunctional subjects, such as counting numbers or listening to neutral stories, did not reduce sexual arousal and in some cases disinhibited it slightly. It was possible that the shift in allocation of attention produced by counting numbers or listening to stories while watching an erotic film had the effect of taking the patients' minds off the performance-related concerns ("hot cognitions") that so occupied their attention. Of course, it was unclear that this reallocation of attention would ever lead to functional levels of performance, since the allocation of attention still remained relatively split, but it was an interesting possibility.

Cognitive and Affective Differences

Several other differences between our sexually dysfunctional patients and age-matched sexually functional volunteers emerged in these early experiments that contributed to our conception of the specifics of the coherent cognitive–affective structure now referred to as "anxious apprehension." First, these two groups had different affective responses in a sexual context. As might be expected, patients evidenced substantial negative affect in a sexual context, whereas the volunteers reported generally positive affective responses (according to affect adjective checklist items). For these patients, negative affect was situationally specific to the sexual context, and may well have been a result of expectancies of inadequate responding or inability to control responding. An intriguing possibility is that negative affective responses predate sexual dysfunction and contribute to its etiology. For example, Donn Byrne (1977, 1983a, 1983b) investigated personality variables that were dispositional in terms of adequate responding to erotic cues. The trait that emerged fell along the dimension he termed "erotophilia–erotophobia." The negative affective responses of sexually dysfunctional men placed them within the erotophobic end of the dimension, and it is interesting that Byrne chose the term "-phobic." These men may have been psychologically vulnerable to sexual dysfunction in some ways outlined below. For example, the effects of successful manipulation of negative affect (Mitchell, DiBartolo, Brown, & Barlow, 1998) described below, as well as instigation of internal attribution for erectile failure in otherwise normal subjects (Weisberg, Brown, Wincze, & Barlow, 2001) would seem to support this assertion. In any case, negative affective responses may contribute to an avoidance of erotic cues, and thereby may facilitate the cognitive interference produced by focusing on nonerotic cues.

In a more recent study testing the effects of positive and negative mood on sexual arousal, we (Mitchell et al., 1998) induced both positive and negative mood through well-established musical mood induction procedures in a group of 24 sexually functional males. Compared to both baseline and a neutral control condition, positive mood resulted in increased objective arousal, as measured by penile strain gauge measures as well as increased reports of subjective arousal. In contrast, negative mood significantly lowered objective sexual arousal, with a trend toward lowered subjective arousal. These results suggest that affect alone, independently of other contextual factors, affects sexual arousal in both negative and positive directions. Meisler and Carey (1991) found similar significant decreases in objective sexual arousal in sexually functional men following another mood induction technique.

It is not clear what mediates this response, but one possibility is that overall arousal is lower in the context of negative affect or depression, and thus that less is available for transfer to sexual arousal than in positive affective states. In fact, Rowland, Cooper, and Heiman (1995) indicated that positive affect was significantly greater for sexually functional than for dysfunctional males during periods of erotic stimulation, but not during the baseline period.

Also, our male patients with psychogenic sexual dysfunctions have consistently underreported their actual levels of sexual arousal. That is, at the same level of erectile response, these patients have reported far less sexual arousal than either sexually functional men or patients with organogenic sexual dysfunctions (Sakheim, Barlow, Abrahamson, & Beck, 1987). This has also been true for dysfunctional women (Morokoff & Heiman, 1980).

In an interesting preliminary report, this inaccurate perception of arousal seemed to extend to estimates of personal control over arousal. That is, when patients and sexually functional volunteers were asked to suppress their arousal, both groups did so, but the volunteers reported success, whereas the patients seemed unaware that they were successfully suppressing arousal and were unable to report any means by which they were, or might be able to, control their sexual arousal. In the minds of these patients, then, a sexual context, particularly one in which performance might be required, brought forth strong negative affective responding and perceptions of lack of control over their sexual responding (Barlow, 1986; Mitchell, Marten, Williams, & Barlow, 1990).

A MODEL OF ANXIOUS APPREHENSION IN SEXUAL DYSFUNCTION

Although experiments dealing with sexual dysfunction may seem far afield from anxiety, they are in fact extremely relevant. All evidence suggests that sexual dysfunction falls quite neatly into the category of social phobia, as implied by Byrne's "erotophobic" trait. Sarason and colleagues, in a rigorous and systematic series of early studies on test anxiety later extended to other areas of performance, have isolated what seems to be a similar process (Sarason, 1982, 1984, 1985; Sarason, Pierce, & Sarason, 1996). Specifically, level of autonomic arousal seems unrelated to eventual performance on tests; rather, the amount of distracting cognitive activity regarding the possibility and the consequences of failure seems directly related to poor test performance. Furthermore, highly test-anxious students do worse under conditions that increase distracting cognitive activity, such as shifts in focus of attention to self-evaluative concerns (Carver, Peterson, Follansbee, & Scheier, 1983; see below), whereas students low in anxiety do better under these conditions. Other parallels are outlined elsewhere (Beck & Barlow, 1986b).

Of course, test anxiety and sexual dysfunction are only two small examples of contexts where the process of anxiety is operative. But they are particularly suitable for experimental analysis, because the responses or behavioral outputs directly affected by anxiety are quantifiable (test scores and sexual arousal). Therefore, one can "input" any one of the hypothetical elements of the cognitive–affective structure of anxiety, either singly or in combination, and examine carefully the effects on subsequent behavior.

Based on our group's early studies in the 1980s, I constructed a "minimodel" of the processes operating in sexual dysfunction (Barlow, 1986, 1988). This model is presented in Figure 3.5. Basically, in this model the perception of a sexual context—particularly the possibility of having to perform—elicits negative affective responding, including perceptions of lack of control or inability to obtain desired results. At this point a critical shift of

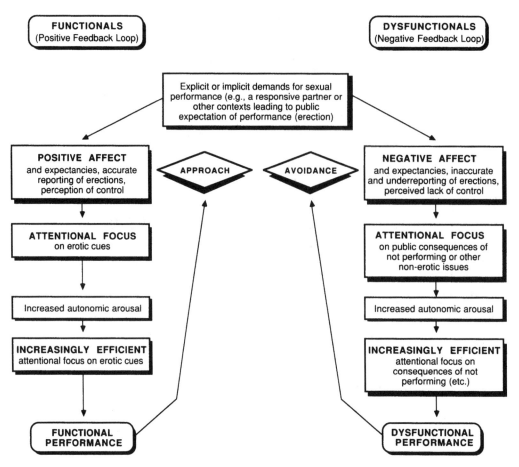

FIGURE 3.5. Model of inhibited sexual excitement. From "Causes of Sexual Dysfunction: The Role of Anxiety and Cognitive Interference" by D. H. Barlow, 1986, *Journal of Consulting and Clinical Psychology*, *54*, 140–148. Copyright 1986 by the American Psychological Association. Reprinted with permission.

attention occurs from an external focus (on erotic material, in this instance) to a more internal self-evaluative focus; at least, a negative self-evaluative focus becomes more salient. The increasing arousal associated with this affective structure narrows attention in the manner described by basic research on attention narrowing. But the focus of attention is on negatively affective self-evaluative statements and/or the autonomic signs and symptoms of arousal itself. Since increasing arousal insures an increasingly efficient focus or "narrowing of attention," the negative affective content (in this case, aspects of the sexual response and the consequences of failure during sexual performance) becomes even more salient or "hot." At this point, these patients may actually become distracted from what they are doing, which in the worst instances interferes with performance (as is the case with sexual dysfunction and test anxiety). It was this model that led to the theoretical construction encompassing the process of anxious apprehension generally, presented in Figure 3.1. What follows is a more detailed exploration of research supporting the process of anxious apprehension, as well as some updating of the model based on more recent research.

THE PROCESS OF ANXIOUS APPREHENSION

Self-Focused Attention

An important component of this model relies on concepts of attentional capacity (Baddeley, 1986). Specifically, as just noted, I theorized that increasing threat serves to narrow attention and increase concentration on a particular focus. I hypothesized that in the sexual context the focus for individuals with dysfunction is on performance concerns, such as "I'm not getting aroused." This internal focus of attention and the resulting increases in anxiety-related arousal lead to decreased tumescence (because erotic material is not processed). For sexually functional individuals, by contrast, attention is more efficiently focused externally on the erotic material. Although this hypothesis regarding differential attentional allocation was originally only inferential (i.e., no measures of attention were taken), post hoc examination of thought content in a replication of the Abrahamson, Barlow, Sakheim, et al. (1985) research suggested that distraction *did* increase off-task thinking for functional subjects, but *not* for dysfunctional subjects (Bruce & Barlow, 1990).

Thus, by inference, dysfunctional subjects maintain a pathological attentional process that is focused internally on concern about performance-related failure. Neutral distraction somehow redirects attention *away* from this self-focus, and thereby allows a somewhat greater processing of on-task stimuli (in this case, erotic material). On the other hand, negative affect in this model, as induced by the shock threat or mood induction experiments, serves to increase arousal and to narrow the focus of attention either internally or externally, ultimately interfering with information-processing resources.

This tendency toward self-focus seems to be an important, although largely overlooked, component of the cognitive–affective structure of anxious apprehension. Fortunately, basic social-psychological research with sexually functional volunteers has elucidated some of the issues involved in this process.

Since the advent of biofeedback, we have been aware that it is possible for individuals to discriminate changes in autonomic activity with an unexpected degree of accuracy (Blanchard & Epstein, 1977; Schwartz, 1976). Why, then, are people usually so poor at ascertaining their internal state? Zillmann (1983a, 1983b) has suggested, on the basis of the biofeedback literature, that it has nothing to do with abilities to perceive internal changes, which obviously are highly developed. Rather, people do not use these capacities at anywhere near their full potential. As Shapiro (1974) pointed out, there may well be a very good reason for this. Specifically, the relative lack of attention to (or limitations in awareness of) internal events may have been functionally adaptive in an evolutionary sense. Placing a limit on awareness of internal events may have reduced an important source of distraction to ongoing external activity. In other words, humans functioning in past millennia as hunter–gatherers, or today in the home or the office, would be far less efficient if people were distracted continually by a welter of internal stimuli to which they fully attended. Consider how quickly external efficiency breaks down when various types of internal events force themselves into awareness: (1) angina and other pain; (2) the sensations arising from the urge to eliminate waste products; (3) hunger; (4) triggering of the cough or sneeze reflex; (5) fever. Nevertheless, people's abilities to monitor their own functioning closely at all times remain, and the way in which this capacity is exercised may play a role in the development and maintenance of emotional disorders.

Basic research (e.g., Kahneman, 1973; Baddeley, 1986) has demonstrated that attention has several properties. It can be concentrated or diffused over a number of contexts. It can also be characterized by more or less vigilance, alertness, or effort (Scheier, Carver, & Matthews, 1983). Some of these qualities undoubtedly are related to the amount of arousal associated with attention. For example, arousal seems to result in attention narrowing, as described in Chapter 2. Social psychologists (e.g., Duval & Wicklund, 1972; Scheier et al., 1983; Carver & Scheier, 1991; Schwarzer & Wicklund, 1991) have determined that human beings have a limited amount of attention to allocate, and that although attentional capacity may vary somewhat over time, a mutual antagonism exists between a focus on the self and a focus on the environment. In other words, the amount of attention directed to external events or tasks limits proportionately the amount of attention directed to internal events. Furthermore, shifts of attention from external focus to self-focus can be reliably manipulated or cued. In the laboratories of social psychologists, mirrors have been used to turn attention inward, but any environmental cue may prompt a shift to self-focused attention through learning. Duval and Wicklund (1972) first systematized these observations into a theory of objective self-awareness.

One of the major cues resulting in a shift to self-focused attention is the perception, or increased awareness of, physiological sensations. For example, in an interesting basic experiment, Wegner and Giuliano (1980) manipulated general arousal in their subjects by having them either lie down and relax, sit in a chair, or run in place; they then presented the subjects with a form containing a series of sentences with words missing. The results indicated that subjects who had experienced and noted marked arousal (after running in place) chose more self-relevant words to complete the sentences, whereas those who relaxed chose fewer self-relevant words. Fenigstein and Carver (1978) came to a similar conclusion in an experiment on false heart rate feedback. It seems that making physiological sensations salient causes individuals to reflect more intensely about themselves in general, drawing their attention to affective qualities, values, standards of behavior, and self-critical judgments (Duval & Wicklund, 1972). In view of these results with rather weak manipulations, one can only wonder about the effect of attention of the dramatic, intense physiological sensations associated with false alarms (see Chapter 7).

Several results of this important work on self-focused attention are relevant to present purposes. First, as with any human trait, individuals seem to vary in their disposition to be self-attentive, as measured by psychometically sound questionnaires (e.g., Carver & Scheier, 1981, 1991; Scheier & Carver, 1983). Examining the effects of self-attention (either measured as a disposition at any one time or experimentally manipulated in the laboratory through mirrors or other devices), investigators have demonstrated that self-focused attention greatly increases sensitivity to bodily sensations and other aspects of internal experience. Furthermore, this sensitivity to bodily sensations quickly spreads to other aspects of the self, such as self-evaluative concerns. In basic research, "self-focused attention" refers to matching one's behavior to preordained standards and often coming up short. In normal subjects, attention to the self can have some potentially positive consequences. For example, subjects high in a disposition to be self-attentive or subjects experimentally manipulated to be high in self-attentiveness will be much less susceptible to the suggestibility inherent in placebo manipulations. If given a placebo and told that it will make them aroused, alert, and excitable, self-attentive subjects will be less susceptible to the suggestion than will more externally directed subjects. Data directly bearing on this proposition are presented below.

But the most important consequences of direction of attention in the context of emotional disorders concern its effect on emotion. Experimental provocation of various emotions in the laboratory is experienced as more intense by individuals with a greater disposition to self-focus than by those with a greater disposition to external focus. This does not, of course, imply support for the James–Lange notion that perception of physiological or other internal sensations is the trigger for emotional experience. Rather, this notion is consistent with most emotion theories, including expressive-behavioral formulations. That is, a self-directed focus and the resulting increased sensitivity to physiological or proprioceptive sensations are likely to result in greater subjective intensity of emotional experience after the emotion has been elicited. Evidence that the attentional shift to a self-focus follows initial arousal or affect comes from several early experiments (e.g., Carver, Blaney, & Scheier, 1979; Wegner & Guiliano, 1980). Of course, a small negative feedback loop within the larger loop is created by the intensifying of arousal and negative affect that follows the shift in attention to self-focus. This small feedback loop is also represented in Figure 3.1. One additional important consequence of self-focused attention is a failure to habituate to external stimuli while in this attentional mode (Scheier et al., 1983). This aspect of self-focused attention has substantial implications for anxiety reduction strategies.

Focusing on Sensations versus Affect

A final step in the process of self-focused attention relevant to emotional disorders concerns different aspects of internal experience to which attention can be allocated in concentrated, selective ways. Two important aspects attracting attention are the stimulus sensations associated with the experience and the emotional or affective components of the experience. In a classic experiment, Leventhal, Brown, Shachan, and Engquist (1979) instructed normal volunteers to immerse their hands in cold water (the "cold pressor test") while periodically assessing their emotional distress. Subjects also reported on strength of physical sensations during the test. Among the number of instructional sets administered to these subjects before they immersed their hands were two that emphasized either the precise stimulus qualities to expect (e.g., cold, tingling, numbness) or the emotional distress they would experience (e.g., apprehension, "butterflies," tension, weakness). Subjects concentrating on the rather mechanical aspects of physical stimulus and response sensation reported less distress and less intense emotional aspects of the experience. As Scheier et al. (1983) pointed out, it is likely that concentration on the emotional aspect of an experience also leads to further sympathetic discharge. This finding is consistent with earlier work on intensification of the emotional state through self-focused attention.

To return to my colleagues' and my work on sexual dysfunction, there are some additional interesting parallels (Beck & Barlow, 1986a, 1986b). In one experiment, sexually dysfunctional patients and age-matched sexually functional controls were instructed either to focus on their sensations or feelings of arousal while watching an erotic film, or to focus more objectively on how much genital response they were achieving "as if from an outsider's perspective." The latter instructional set was meant to reproduce as closely as possible the concept of "spectatoring," mentioned so often in the literature on sexual dysfunction as a possible maintaining factor. These instructional sets were delivered under either the threat of contingent shock described above ("There is a 60% chance you'll be shocked if you are not as aroused as the average subject") or no threat. Sexually functional subjects were distracted by these "spectatoring" instructions, and shock threat seemed to intensify the effects of the distracting instructions for these subjects by reducing arousal. Once again, this was not the case for sexually dysfunctional patients, who surprised us by showing their highest levels of arousal when the "spectatoring" instructions were accompanied by shock threat. Thus, whether functional subjects were told to focus on the content of a neutral story while watching an erotic film (see Figure 3.3) or some other nonaffective stimuli, attention to erotic cues and resulting sexual arousal suffered. But for dysfunctional subjects, attending to a neutral story did not reduce arousal and may actually have disinhibited it slightly (see Figure 3.3), as did attending to other nonaffective stimuli in another study (Cranston-Cuebas & Barlow, 1990). Here is the paradox once again. But when subjects in the experiment just described were asked to attend to affect and feelings, different results were observed. Dysfunctional subjects evidenced some negative affect and generally seemed to distance themselves slightly from the situation. Functional subjects, on the other hand, were subjectively involved and interested (Beck & Barlow, 1986b).

In view of these findings, it is possible once again that the mechanical spectator focus for the dysfunctional subjects in this experiment took their minds off the negative, self-evaluative aspects of their affect or distress associated with sexual functioning, and thus facilitated sexual responding! In fact, careful examination of their focus of attention suggested that the dysfunctional subjects tended to drift back to the erotic film significantly more than the functional subjects did during the "spectatoring" condition. It was almost as if having something else to focus on during the film allowed them somehow to bypass their negative affect regarding this situation. Thus a shift to self-focused attention seems critical; however, after this shift occurs, focusing on negative affect or distress rather than mechanical stimulus contexts seems implicated in emotional disorders.

In summary, self-focused attention seems to increase perception of internal states. If one experiences an affective state, this state can be intensified by subsequent self-focused attention. However, in a more ambiguous situation, the direction of self-attention can be allocated either to the stimulus configurations (as well as other operational aspects of the context) or to the affective qualities of the experience. This latter focus seems particularly salient if the affective, self-evaluative qualities involve distress of some sort (Scheier et al., 1983). Parallels in clinical research exist, which are discussed at greater length below. For example, Rapee (1986), in an experiment described in Chapter 5, found that panic was all but eliminated during a laboratory provocation experiment if the panic patients were told in great detail about the specific sensory experiences associated with CO_2 inhalation. During the trial, presumably, the patients focused attention on these sensations at the expense of the affective or distress components of the experience.

Implications for Clinical Disorders

The implications of self-focused attention for anxiety and related disorders are suggested in several analogue studies. In one experiment, subjects with snake phobia approached a snake either in the presence of a mirror or with no mirror. In a second experiment, subjects high and low in self-consciousness were threatened with electric shock on a pretext. In both experiments (Scheier, Carver, & Gibbons, 1981), self-directed attention intensified fear and resulted in stronger and more rapid avoidance behavior. Similar findings are apparent in other analogue studies. For example, individuals who are high in self-consciousness react more negatively in terms of affect to negative events such as failure (e.g., Hull & Young, 1983).

Evidence also now exists on the deleterious effects of self-focused attention from studies of individuals with a focus of anxiety other than sexual difficulties. For example, Hope, Heimberg, and Klein (1990) studied undergraduates with social and evaluative anxiety, who did not meet criteria for social phobia, in a series of interactions with peers. These individuals were then required to recall various details of social interactions, such as the content of the conversation or what the other person was wearing. Socially anxious individuals recalled less information from the encounters and made more errors than less anxious subjects, presumably because they were focusing internally and were less able to process details of the external task.

Sheila Woody (1996), in a well-designed experiment, studied patients with social phobia who were instructed to present speeches before a small audience. She describes it as follows:

> Two participants with social phobia, Client A and Client B, stood together in front of an audience of 4 staff members from the hospital in which the clinic was based. The staff members were men and women of varying ages. The entire procedure was videotaped for subsequent rating by observers. An experimenter randomly assigned speech roles to each of the participants: In this example, Client A performed the speaker role, and Client B took the passive role. For the experimental task, Client A made two consecutive speeches. The content of the speeches was anxious bodily sensations, cognitions, and emotions, but the person who was the focus of the speech varied for each trial. In the first trial, the content of A's speech focused on her own current experience: her bodily sensations, cognitions, emotions. For the second trial, A's speech was about Client B: his apparent bodily sensations, cognitions, and emotions.
>
> Because this was an unusual social task, every speaker received a list of a series of prompts to use as a guide for both speeches. These prompts included positive and negative emotions, thoughts, and bodily sensations or outward signs of anxiety. Speakers typically used their partners' outward physical cues to help them make the speech about the passive client. (Woody, 1996, p. 63)

Ratings of anxiety were taken either as each individual delivered his or her speech (active condition) or while each patient observed the other individual delivering the speech (passive condition). Of course, speaking about one's own reactions, or hearing someone else speak about one's own reactions, is a manipulation that increases self-focused attention. The results are presented in Figure 3.6. Self-focused attention increased both self-ratings and observer ratings of anxiety during the speech, as predicted.

Borden, Lowenbraun, Wolff, and Jones (1993) evaluated 19 patients with panic disorder and 20 normal controls for the presence of self-focused attention under a variety of conditions. These conditions included baseline recording, followed by a 15-minute period of relaxation, and finally 4 minutes of a mild mental stressor consisting of the "serial 7's" task (subtracting 7's sequentially from a large number). Results suggested significantly higher self-focus for the patients than for the controls. During the relatively unstructured baseline and relaxation periods, the patients with panic disorder experienced heightened focus upon internal physical sensations. During the serial 7's task, the patients remained self-focused, but shifted this self-focus somewhat to a greater awareness of their behavior.

Finally, Panayiotou and Vrana (1998) evaluated 25 males with high social anxiety and 30 males with low social anxiety on a digit recall task where subjects either were told or were not told that they would be evaluated on the task. Half of the trials were performed under self-focused conditions. In the remaining trials, subjects were instructed to focus on the task. Self-focus led to a larger startle response among the socially anxious individuals (reflecting heightened anxiety; see Chapter 2) and, when combined with evaluation, led to poorer results in recall among all subjects.

These findings have parallels in the literature on depression (Ingram, 1990; Schwarzer & Wicklund, 1991). Musson and Alloy (1988) suggested, after reviewing a large body of literature, that there is a strong relationship between self-directed attention and the affective, behavioral, and cognitive characteristics of depression, and that distraction *reduces the negative consequences of both depression and self-focus*. For example, Miller (1975) reviewed a variety of evidence demonstrating that external distraction leads to improve-

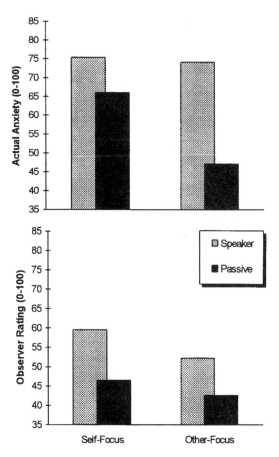

FIGURE 3.6. Self-focused attention and speaking. From "Effects of Focus of Attention on Anxiety Levels and Social Performance of Individuals with Social Phobia" by S. R. Woody, 1996, *Journal of Abnormal Psychology, 105,* 61–69. Copyright 1996 by the American Psychological Association. Reprinted by permission.

ment in the performance of depressed individuals on motor and speed tests. This finding seemed to parallel the effects of distraction on arousal in our sexually dysfunctional patients. Ingram (1990), after reviewing the literature on self-focused attention, extended the conceptualization of self-focused attention as a vulnerability to increased anxiety and depression.

Is an Exaggerated External Focus of Attention Pathological?

The findings reviewed above also suggest a crucial distinction between "normal" and "pathological" anxiety. Before any type of performance, including most of the challenges we confront daily, an adaptive human response includes physical and mental preparation. The essence of this response consists of arousal and preparation to cope, which, as shown in Chapter 1 and above, improve performance.

Sometimes this response is termed a "stress response" (see Chapter 6). This is also Liddell's (1949) "shadow of intelligence," described in Chapter 1. According to our data, as well as this experimental tradition, preparatory increases in arousal are not in themselves pathological. What is pathological is the associated shift in attention to a negatively valenced, self-evaluative, off-task focus that seems to be an integral part of the cognitive–affective structure of anxiety. This negative self-evaluative focus and disruption of attention is in large part responsible for decreases in performance. This attentional shift in turn contributes to a vicious cycle of anxious apprehension, in which increasing anxiety leads to further attentional shifts, increased performance deficits, and subsequent spiraling of arousal.

But how do nonanxious individuals experience arousal—particularly the arousal that accompanies important challenges, such as major speeches or other critical events? Athletes and professional performers often discuss preperformance "jitters" and debate whether it's "excitement" or "nerves." Arousal-related concepts such as "butterflies in the stomach" are sometimes construed positively as signifying a state of preparedness, but are often experienced as unpleasant. But when the performance or game begins, this preparatory arousal (however it is construed) is often translated into effective action, as is the case with almost all professional athletes and performers. For this to happen, attention has to be focused fully and completely on the task at hand. Without this attentional shift to external events, professional performers would be like our sexually dysfunctional patients, unable to concentrate and ultimately unable to perform. Other factors contributing to the process of anxious apprehension are discussed further below.

The importance of self-focused attention is also highlighted by considering the possible consequences of an exaggerated, exclusively external focus of attention. Scheier et al. (1983) have made some particularly interesting observations in this regard on the association between focus of attention and stress, using the Type A personality construct as an example. They have speculated, with some supporting evidence, that an important component of the Type A personality construct is a very strong external focus of attention. These individuals exert control over their world and the stressors in it by concentrating fully on the task at hand. This results in a marked decrease in the amount of attention available for internal focus and a subsequent lack of sensitivity to internal bodily events (low anxiety sensitivity).

One consequence of attentional focus is that driven, externally focused personalities seek out medical assistance less often for real physical problems, including pain associated with myocardial infarction or other stress-related physical conditions. These conditions would be noticed and attended to by individuals with a greater facility for shifting to an internal focus. Suls and Fletcher (1985b) confirmed that individuals lower in self-consciousness become ill more often, probably as a result of internal insensitivity. This suggests that either an exaggerated internal or an exaggerated external focus of attention may be pathological under certain circumstances. Suls and Fletcher (1985a) have characterized these operations as "avoidant" and "nonavoidant" strategies for coping with stress.

In any case, a very interesting and perhaps essential difference between stress and anxiety disorders is suggested—a difference that has perplexed clinical investigators for years. It is possible that individuals with some specific stress disorders are characterized by an external focus of attention and a perception of control over events in the environment. Therefore, they experience few if any of the affective qualities that accompany anxious self-preoccupation in connection with stressful experiences. On the other hand, stress-prone individuals evidence physical breakdowns based on organ or system vulnerability because of their relative insensitivity to the beginnings of symptoms associated with these physical conditions. Patients with chronic anxious apprehension have learned to attend very early to internal sensations in general, and have become preoccupied with the affective qualities of these sensations. Thus, for them, otherwise normal life events evoke self-focused attention and a cycle of anxious apprehension.

This self-evaluative focus most likely becomes integrated with the response propositions of anxiety as time goes on. It may not be conceptually correct to separate evaluative self-focus from the cognitive representations of anxious apprehension, as implied in Figure 3.1, despite the evidence that a shift to self-focus initially follows arousal or affect. But I continue to consider it separately here, since this particular feature of anxious apprehension has implications for therapy.

Conclusions about Self-Focused Attention

To refer once again to Figure 3.1, the results summarized above on self-focused attention suggest that situational cues associated with negative affect result in a shift from an external to an internal focus of attention directed to somatic sensations, as well as the affective and self-evaluative components of the context, which results in further increases in arousal, and so on. The affective and self-evaluative focus seems most heavily implicated in deteriorating performance and further increases in arousal and anxiety. As with most advances in science, however, the findings have proven to be less clear-cut than seemed apparent, in light of additional data collected in the context of studying interoceptive awareness.

Interoceptive Awareness

A subsequent study from our work on sexual dysfunction seemed to contradict attentional allocation hypotheses concerning the deleterious effects of self-focused attention. We (Abrahamson, Barlow, & Abrahamson, 1989) used a genital feedback paradigm developed in our laboratory to attempt to examine self-focused attention. Sexually dysfunctional and sexually functional male subjects each viewed erotic film segments during three conditions. These conditions differed in that an adjacent video monitor showed either live genital feedback (obtained from a video camera focused on the subjects' genitals), a variable-length straight line, or no stimulus. The feedback condition required each subject to give a rating of the percentage of full erection he had at the moment based on the feedback, and to indicate whether the erection was sufficient for sexual intercourse. This was, in a sense, the ultimate extension of the prototypical "mirror" manipulation used in self-focused attention paradigms, in which viewing oneself increases self-focus (e.g., Ingram, 1990; Scheier et al., 1983). During the neutral distracting condition, the subject was instructed to give a rating of the length of the line as a percentage of a standard line, and to judge whether the presented line was the same width or narrower than a standard line shown previously. This task was intended to control for the amount of "cognitive work" performed in the feedback condition.

The data, which are shown in Figure 3.7, demonstrated that the distracting condition involving self-focused attention (focusing on one's genitals) had a markedly different effect on the two groups, in contrast to a neutral distracting condition requiring about the same amount of cognitive effort. That is, self-focused attention produced the highest overall penile circumference levels for sexually functional subjects. Sexually dysfunctional subjects, on the other hand, demonstrated their lowest level of arousal during the self-focused attention condition. Neutral distraction had very little effect in either group, unlike the results from the distraction paradigm discussed above (see Figure 3.3), probably because the distraction stimulus was insufficiently demanding. Thus the inference from these re-

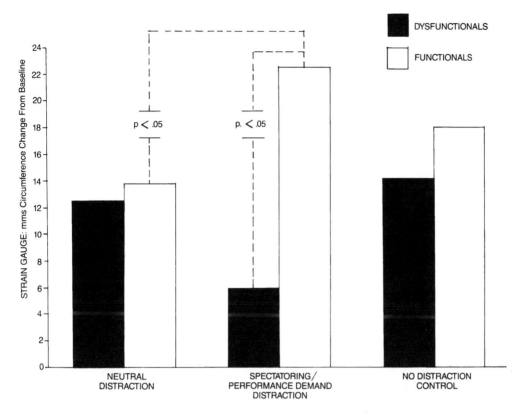

FIGURE 3.7. Average maximum penile circumference change from baseline: Group × condition. From "Differential Effects of Performance Demand and Distraction on Sexually Functional and Dysfunctional Males" by D. J. Abrahamson, D. H. Barlow, and L. S. Abrahamson, 1989, *Journal of Abnormal Psychology*, *98*, 241–247. Copyright 1989 by the American Psychological Association. Reprinted with permission.

sults is that the process of self-focused attention seems specifically associated with erectile dysfunction, but the effects *may not* be due to a fully occupied attentional capacity associated with self-focused attention. I suggest some other possibilities below.

These results on self-focused attention also contradict another set of data suggesting that sexually dysfunctional individuals are *not* focusing attention inward or internally. For example, in one paradigm utilized in years past in our laboratory, male subjects were required to monitor their erectile response continuously with a "cognitive lever" (e.g., Wincze, Venditti, Barlow, & Mavissakalian, 1980). Subjects were trained to move this cognitive lever at points between 0 and 100, based on their own estimates of their percentage of full erection. Rather than focus closely on their genital (non)response at the expense of attending to external erotic cues, a consistent and strong set of results from our laboratory (e.g., Sakheim, Barlow, Abrahamson, & Beck, 1987) demonstrated that at the same levels of erectile responding, sexually dysfunctional subjects *underestimated* their erections, whereas functional subjects were more accurate. Other studies also evidenced this effect very clearly (Abrahamson, Barlow, Sakheim, et al., 1985; Abrahamson et al., 1989). Interestingly, in the latter study, dysfunctional subjects characteristically reported lower arousal when their erection levels were more substantial; when erection levels were near 0, functional subjects reported accurately, but dysfunctional subjects inaccurately reported the presence of some erectile response. In fact, the correlation between our continuous subjective measure and genital responding for functional subjects was .61, compared with only .32 for dysfunctional subjects (Abrahamson et al., 1989). The fact that our dysfunctional subjects were inaccurate in judging their erectile response *suggested* that, although preoccupied with their performance, these subjects were either *not* allocating attention to their genital functioning, or possibly somehow distorting information from an attentional focus on genital functioning. Thus we were faced with seemingly conflicting data sets suggesting, on the one hand, that self-focused attention on erectile performance is associated specifically with dysfunctional sexuality, but that sexually dysfunctional individuals are monitoring their performance less accurately. This quandary suggested that self-focused attention and interoceptive awareness, though frequently conflated, may actually represent rather different constructs. We addressed this notion in subsequent research.

Misattribution

Several years ago, we produced and replicated one of the more remarkable findings in the history of our Sexuality Research Program (Cranston-Cuebas & Barlow, 1995; Cranston-Cuebas, Barlow, Mitchell, & Athanasiou, 1993). To provide some background, in a classic experiment, Storms and Nisbett (1970) produced a reverse placebo effect in subjects with insomnia by providing them with placebo pills at bedtime, describing the pills as either increasing or decreasing arousal. Surprisingly, subjects fell asleep faster after receiving the placebo pill with instructions that it would *increase* arousal. Conversely, subjects fell asleep more slowly after receiving a pill they thought would *decrease* their arousal. Brockner and Swap (1983) suggested that this reverse placebo effect was most likely to occur in those subjects who were more interoceptively aware, through their comparison of sensations with the externally provided information about the pill's effects as noted earlier. That is, subjects who found themselves less aroused than they expected fell asleep more quickly, and vice versa. In a replication of Storms and Nisbett's (1970) original investigation, using additional measures of private body consciousness (Miller, Murphy, & Buss, 1981) and private self-consciousness (Fenigstein, Scheier, & Buss, 1975), this relationship between high private body consciousness and a reverse placebo was confirmed (Brockner & Swap, 1983).

We adapted this paradigm to research with sexually functional and dysfunctional subjects (Cranston-Cuebas et al., 1993). In this paradigm, functional and dysfunctional males viewed sexually explicit films following ingestion of three placebo pills in a repeated measures design. The pills were described to subjects as an erection "enhancement" pill, an erection "detraction" pill, and a "placebo" pill. Consistent with predictions derived from a misattribution hypothesis, the sexually functional subjects' erectile responding evidenced a clear reverse placebo effect. That is, erectile responding in the "detraction" condition was significantly *greater* than responding in either the enhancement or placebo conditions. The latter conditions did not differ significantly from one another. Interestingly, analysis of subjective ratings of arousal indicated *no significant differences* among conditions. Therefore, these data do not represent the classic misattribution effect for functional subjects, since previous reports in the social-psychological literature illustrated changes in *reports* of emotional state through provision of alternative labels for physiological arousal. In our experiment, changes were effected in *actual physiological responding* through a similar manipulation. On the other hand, the sexually dysfunctional subjects, rather than demonstrating a reverse placebo effect, evidenced a clear direct placebo effect. That is, dysfunctional subjects evidenced significantly lower erectile responding under the detraction condition, although there were no significant differences under enhancement and placebo conditions. Once again, the dysfunctional subjects evidenced *no effects* on self-reports of arousal as a result of pill manipulation.

Thus, according to Brockner and Swap's (1983) interpretation, our dysfunctional subjects may have evidenced a direct placebo effect as a result of their being relatively *unaware* of their internal bodily sensations. This lack of internal awareness would have precluded a discovery of the discrepancy between internally and externally provided information (upon which the reverse placebo effect is presumably predicated). This, of course, is in agreement with our data indicating that dysfunctional males are relatively *unaware* of their erectile response and provide low or inaccurate estimates of their erectile response on the cognitive lever. But it seems, on the face of it, contradictory to the literature on self-focused attention mentioned above.

We completed a replication of these findings with functional males (Cranston-Cuebas & Barlow, 1995) in which, specifically, 50 sexually functional men viewed three sexually explicit films following ingestion of a placebo pill described as either an erection "enhancement" pill or an erection "detraction" pill. The first condition was a control condition that replicated the Cranston-Cuebas et al. (1993) investigation, but used a between-subjects design. The second and third conditions (presented in counterbalanced order) were attentional focus task conditions: "Erotic focus" required that subjects tally (by pushing a button) specified erotic elements appearing in the film; "nonerotic focus" required that subjects tally specified nonerotic elements. Results from the first (control) condition replicated the reverse placebo effect observed in the Cranston-Cuebas et al. (1993) study, with significantly greater erectile responding for subjects in the detraction pill group than in the enhancement pill group. More importantly, the Cranston-Cuebas and Barlow (1995) study added prestimulus reports concerning subjects' expectations for how they would be affected by the pills, thus allowing the beginnings of a causal relationship to be drawn between subjects' misattribution to the pills and their patterns of erectile response. Subjects' expectations were in line with the experimental manipulation and could not account for the results. These manipulations were aided by elaborate pretrial procedures, including "instant" urinalysis. As in the previous investigation, there were no effects of groups or conditions on either subjects' feelings of sexual arousal (as measured by the cognitive lever) or their reported levels of erection. Thus our manipulation directly affected erectile response while bypassing "perception" of arousal.

Contrary to expectation, the attentional focus tasks employed did not redirect subjects' attentional focus sufficiently to reverse patterns of erectile response. Questionnaire analyses revealed that while subjects scoring high on the Private Body Consciousness Scale and those having high strain correlations between strain gauge and cognitive lever results (reflecting accurate estimates of erectile response) followed the group pattern (i.e., the reverse placebo effect), those subjects scoring higher on a small group of items reflecting a more general state of negative affect regarding bodily concerns (which we labeled "hypochondriasis") evidenced a direct placebo effect. These subjects' erectile response patterns were more similar to those of dysfunctional men than to those of functional men. This finding, although preliminary at this time, may shed some light on the discrepancy between the seeming *lack* of self-focused attention in our dysfunctional groups (as reflected in the lack of a reverse placebo effect and inaccurate estimates of erectile response) and the hypothesized increase in self-focused attention among other groups with high negative affect (Ingram, 1990).

To summarize, it may be that a negatively affective attentional process focusing on somatic functioning and other self-evaluative concerns, combined with a tendency to avoid direct observation of one's functioning (lack of accurate interoceptive awareness or interoceptive focus), may characterize psychopathology associated with anxiety and other related disorders. In other words, self-focused attention as reflected in a pathological and affectively laden worry process may be fundamentally an avoidant technique (Borkovec, 1994a; Brown, Barlow, & Liebowitz, 1994; Roemer & Borkovec, 1993) that is orthogonal to accurate interoceptive awareness or focus. In any case, these results are consistent with more recent data indicating that our sexually dysfunctional patients score significantly lower in private body self-consciousness than do our functional patients.

Interoceptive Awareness in Anxious Patients

We have begun to examine these constructs more directly in anxious patients. Clinical observations over the years have indicated that patients with anxiety disorders, particularly panic disorder, seem to evidence great awareness of internal bodily states and are constantly vigilant for any somatic changes that might signal the beginning of the next panic attack. Thus it has been assumed that patients with anxiety can perceive their bodily state more accurately than other subjects can (e.g., Tyrer, 1973, 1976). Several studies have confirmed that patients do report higher awareness of bodily sensations than controls do (e.g., King, Margraf, Ehlers, & Maddock, 1986; Ehlers & Breuer, 1992). More recently, Schmidt, Lerew, and Trakowski (1997) constructed a brief scale, the Body Vigilance Scale, to measure the tendency to attend differentially to somatic sensations, and reported that this tendency is distributed normally in a nonclinical sample. In addition, this scale discriminates patients with panic disorder from patients with social phobia when attention to panic symptoms are specifically assessed. Schmidt, Lerew, and Trakowski (1997) are careful to distinguish this "increased attention" hypothesis from an enhanced ability to perceive somatic sensation accurately (interoceptive accuracy).

Ehlers and Breuer (1992, Study 2) specifically evaluated "interoceptive accuracy" by having a number of patients with anxiety disorders, as well as normal control subjects, estimate their heart rate. Specifically, Ehlers and Breuer (1992) compared 65 patients with panic disorder, 50 patients with infrequent panic who did not meet criteria for panic disorder, and 27 patients with specific phobias to 46 normal control subjects. Generally, the results indicated that patients with panic disorder were more accurate in perceiving their heartbeats than were patients with specific phobias, patients with infrequent panic, or control subjects. In a related replication in the same report (Ehlers & Breuer, 1992, Study 3), in which groups of patients with GAD and depression were included, patients with panic disorder were once again better at perceiving their heartbeats than were patients with depression. But patients with GAD were also more accurate and did not differ from patients with panic disorder. These results have been replicated in normal subjects with high anxiety sensitivity scores compared to subjects with low scores (Sturges & Goelsch, 1996), and in subjects with infrequent panic compared to subjects with no panic (Zoellner & Craske, 1999).

These results have been difficult to replicate in other clinical settings, however. We (Antony, Brown, et al., 1995) tested patients with panic disorder, patients with social phobia, and normal controls, utilizing the same paradigm in which subjects were asked to count heartbeats. In this experiment, the perceptual accuracy of the groups was tested not only at rest, but also following a period of strenuous exercise consisting of repeated step-ups. The results are presented in Figure 3.8. Contrary to the results in Ehlers and Breuer (1992), the data from this experiment suggested that the patients with panic disorder were no more accurate in counting their heartbeats than the patients with social phobia or

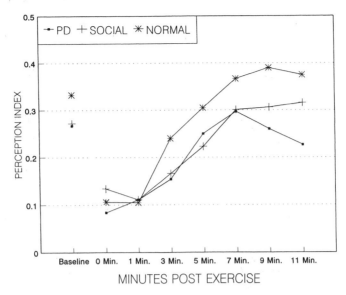

FIGURE 3.8. Accuracy of heartbeat estimations by subjects with panic disorder (PD), subjects with social phobia (Social), and nonanxious controls (Normal): Baseline (average across trials) and postexercise phase 2 (lower values indicate greater accuracy). Reprinted from Anthony, Brown, Craske, Barlow, Mitchell, and Meadows (1995), copyright 1995, with permission from Excerpta Medica Inc.

nonanxious subjects, although the means were in the expected direction. Nevertheless, subsequent analyses suggested that even these mean effects were illusory, since differences accounted for only 3% of the variance. Some subjects, however, became more accurate as heart rate increased due to exercise. Furthermore, we examined possible changes in cardiac awareness in patients with panic disorder following successful cognitive-behavioral treatment (Antony, Meadows, Brown, & Barlow, 1994). Despite significant reductions in panic attacks and related symptomatology, cardiac awareness did not change on average, although some individual subjects showed dramatic changes in both directions, reflecting either greatly increased awareness or greatly decreased awareness. Ehlers and Breuer (1996) report a similar finding, which they attributed at the time to the fact that good interoception is a stable interindividual difference.

Ehlers and Breuer (1996) provide a thoughtful summary of the studies mentioned above, as well as related studies on ambulatory monitoring of heart rate in patients with anxiety disorders. Two conclusions seem possible. It is very clear that patients with anxiety disorders (and perhaps other related disorders, such as depression and somatoform disorders) evidence increased self-focused attention to bodily sensations and other aspects of their behavior, and that this is accompanied by affectively laden self-evaluative concerns. However, the evidence on whether these individuals accurately perceive somatic responding such as heart rate as measured objectively—that is, whether they display interoceptive accuracy—is relatively weak. As Ehlers and Breuer (1996) point out, patients with infrequent panic do not seem to differ from controls in either ambulatory or laboratory assessment of heartbeat perception, and the results from patients with panic disorder depend on the paradigms used. For example, during 24-hour ambulatory monitoring, reports of heart rate elevations relate only weakly to objectively measured elevations in heart rate, as reviewed in Chapter 5. In the laboratory, positive results are available only from one paradigm (a mental tracking paradigm in which subjects are asked to count their heartbeats silently without taking their pulses), and even then the results are heavily dependent on instructions given to the subjects (Ehlers & Breuer, 1996). Furthermore, the effect size in these studies is quite small.

Using alternative procedures such as ambulatory monitoring, Barsky, Cleary, Sarnie, and Ruskin (1994) actually found that patients with panic disorder who reported palpitations were less accurate in reporting arrhythmias (as detected by Holter monitor recordings) than a group of patients who also reported palpitations but without a lifetime history of panic disorder. Pauli et al. (1991) also compared patients with panic disorder and control subjects during 24-hour ambulatory monitoring of heart rate. Interestingly, they found that the groups did not differ in their ability to detect significant cardiac events as measured objectively by ambulatory monitoring, but that the patients with panic disorder became more anxious than the control subjects when they did (rightly or wrongly) detect these events. In an additional report examining the ability of patients with panic disorder and healthy control subjects to detect increasing concentrations of CO_2, Rapee (1994b) examined the possibility that patients would detect increases more accurately because of the increased somatic sensations associated with this task. Once again, patients with panic disorder were no better than controls at detecting increased levels of CO_2 during the task, which does not support the notion of greater objective interoceptive accuracy.

In any case, based on the well-done and well-reasoned reports from Ehlers and her colleagues, it is not yet clear that the objective assessment of interoceptive accuracy for brief periods in the laboratory is related in any meaningful way to the state of anxiety. As Ehlers and Breuer (1996) point out, the ability to perceive heart rate accurately is distributed normally in the population, and it does not seem to change after successful treatment (as one would expect if this skill were inherently related to anxious apprehension). Contrast this to self-focused attentional processes, which do seem responsive to treatment (e.g., Hofmann, 2000a; Schmidt, Lerew, & Trakowski, 1997). Following up these conclusions, van der Does, Antony, Ehlers, and Barsky (2000) pooled 709 participants from seven studies and confirmed that accurate interoception is uncommon even in patients with anxiety disorders, although it is somewhat more prevalent in such patients than in nonanxious controls.

In conclusion, it does seem clear—both from studies of patients with sexual dysfunctions and from research on patients with anxiety and related disorders—that these individuals are hypervigilant for and differentially attend to *perceptions* of the occurrence of somatic sensations and other self-evaluative concerns, which result in a spiral of arousal and increasing anxiety. It is also clear that these reports are often inaccurate perceptions or misperceptions of objective reality. The fact that some patients with anxiety disorders may be somewhat more accurate in reporting heart rate as measured objectively in the laboratory for brief periods of time under certain conditions seems a contradictory finding, but it may be an unimportant and unrelated phenomenon that is also unreliable, pending further study. Nevertheless, studies of interoceptive accuracy—not only accuracy about heart rate in patients with panic disorder and other anxiety disorders, but accuracy about a the variety of somatic symptoms (including sexual arousal) in sexually dysfunctional patients—should continue to prove a very interesting and important area of inquiry.

Illusions of Control and Psychological Vulnerabilities

The "minimodel" of sexual functioning (Barlow, 1986) proposes that sexually functional and dysfunctional men enter a sexual situation with differential expectancies for their performance: Dysfunctional individuals expect to perform poorly, and functional individuals expect to perform well. Results from the misattribution experiments discussed above (Cranston-Cuebas et al., 1993; Cranston-Cuebas & Barlow, 1995) and other studies from our laboratory, may indicate that sexually functional subjects have a resistance to the formation of these negative expectancies. Specifically, the detraction manipulation ("This pill will interfere with erectile response") may be viewed as creating a context in which one might predict that subjects would form negative expectancies regarding their sexual performance. Under this condition, however, sexually functional subjects experienced their greatest arousal. In contrast, sexually dysfunctional subjects were most aroused under the enhancement condition. Thus providing them with positive expectancies from an external source seemed to aid in their arousal.

One of our initial studies found that sexually functional subjects overlooked small decrements in their performance and failed to report decreases in their physiological arousal (Abrahamson, Barlow, Sakheim, et al., 1985; Mitchell et al., 1990). This finding has also been interpreted to suggest that sexually functional men may demonstrate an "illusion of control" (Abrahamson, Barlow, Sakheim, et al., 1985) by ignoring evidence that might support negative expectancies of performance. In contrast, since sexually dysfunctional men tend to underreport their physiological arousal (Sakheim et al., 1987), we might conclude that such men maintain negative expectancies of performance.

Findings from another pilot study (Weisberg, Sbrocco, & Barlow, 1994) also support the possibility that functional individuals retain an illusion of control regarding sexual performance. Fantasy use, or the ability to form vivid mental representations, has repeatedly been found to be important for the voluntary control of sexual arousal (e.g., Stock & Geer, 1982). Because sexually dysfunctional subjects have reported feeling they have less control over their arousal (Mitchell et al., 1990) and also report less use of fantasy in sexual situations (Marten & Barlow, 1991; Weisberg et al., 1994), the relationship among imagery ability, fantasy content, and voluntary arousal was explored (Weisberg et al., 1994). Sexually functional male subjects were asked to engage in either a fantasy in which they would not be able to attain and maintain an erection, or a fantasy in which their performance was satisfactory. Surprisingly, there were no differences in arousal between fantasy groups. Sexually functional subjects who were asked to create a fantasy in which they experienced sexual difficulties evidenced as much penile tumescence and subjective arousal as subjects asked to engage in a fantasy in which no problems occurred. Examination of the written fantasies of subjects in the "negative" fantasy condition revealed that their fantasies included accounts of sexual problems, according to the instructions, but that these problems were not the focus of the fantasies. In other words, these subjects created arousing fantasies in which problems occurred (such as detumescence), but these were not dwelled upon or were fantasized as being only temporary.

In a related experiment (Bach, Brown, & Barlow, 1999), we examined the effects of low efficacy expectancies for obtaining adequate erectile responses on subsequent sexual arousal in sexually functional men. Twenty-six males were randomly assigned to either a false-negative-feedback group or a no-feedback group. After viewing several erotic films, the participants in the false-feedback group were told that their responses were less than those of the average participant in our laboratory. The control group received no such feedback. The instructions were credible to the subjects, since efficacy expectations were considerably lower when the feedback group viewed a third erotic film, as was physiological response measured by the penile strain gauge. Despite these effects on physiological arousal, and counter to predictions, the false feedback *did not* lead to a decline in either subjective arousal or an increase in negative affect. Thus a self-focus on potential inadequate responding *did* lower physiological sexual arousal, consistent with the model in Figure 3.2. But the fact that this false-feedback condition was *not* associated with changes in subjective arousal, self-estimates of arousal, or negative affect once again suggests that sexually functional males may have an illusion-of-control mentality. That is, by ignoring or discounting occasional decrements in erectile response, functional males may retain an illusion of control over their responding, and thus protect themselves from subsequent difficulties.

Overall, it appears that sexually functional men maintain positive expectancies for their performance, despite experimental attempts to manipulate this (Cranston-Cuebas et al., 1993; Cranston-Cuebas & Barlow, 1995; Weisberg et al., 1994) and despite physiological evidence that their performance has decreased (Abrahamson, Barlow, Sakheim, et al., 1985; Mitchell et al., 1990). In contrast, sexually dysfunctional men underreport their erections (Sakheim et al., 1987), maintaining negative expectancies of their performance except when provided with external sources of confidence (Cranston-Cuebas et al., 1993).

These findings have parallels in social-psychological research, where findings from a variety of studies suggest that individuals often avoid accurate knowledge about themselves, and will often sustain inaccurate knowledge if the truth is threatening in some way (Gibbons, 1991; Thompson, Armstrong, & Thomas, 1998; Thompson, 1999). In an early study, Sackheim and Gur (1979) reported that answering "no" to questions that should be universally true, such as "Have you ever doubted your sexual adequacy?" or "Have you ever thought your parents hated you?", was negatively correlated with depression and neuroticism. In other words, this "self-deception" may be a characteristic of mental health. In a classic experiment, Alloy and Abramson (1979) found that individuals with depressed mood, even if this mood was induced experimentally in the laboratory, demonstrated a more realistic assessment of their ability to control an outcome than did individuals with normal mood who evidenced an unrealistic assessment, or, illusion of control. In a study with results resembling the Weisberg et al. (1994) and Bach et al. (1999) studies described above, Alloy and Clements (1992) found that subjects who displayed greater illusion of control in a laboratory task experience less negative mood after a failure on the task, but also were less likely to get depressed months later after experiencing negative life events than subjects with less illusion of control. Taylor and Brown (1988, 1994) and Taylor, Kemeny, Reed, Bower, and Grunewald (2000) have documented the large number of findings from social-psychological experimentation supporting the adaptive effects of retaining an illusion of control on both mental and physical health.

Since it seems clear that sexually functional individuals without problems maintain an illusion of control when confronted with occasional difficulties and failures, which serves a protective function, it is tempting to conclude that clinical patients are somehow lacking this illusion of control, and that this deficit predates the onset of any difficulties. This formulation would, of course, be consistent with a diathesis–stress model of etiology, and is supported by other evidence to be reviewed in Chapters 7 and 8. Nevertheless, one that conclusion cannot be drawn at this point, since none of the studies reported above assessed sexually dysfunctional patients *prior* to the onset of their difficulties. Thus it could be that the robust set of findings in our clinically anxious patients—including negative expectancies for performance, a self-focus on negative evaluative components of their response, and inaccurate observations of their responding—all may have been consequences of the development of a clinically significant disorder. But the weight of the evidence reviewed later suggests otherwise. That is, the developing web of evidence points to the existence of psychological vulnerability that predates the beginnings of a specific clinically significant problem. Some tantalizing evidence in support of this suggestion has now emerged from our research.

In a follow-up study to the Bach et al. (1999) research that employed a similar paradigm, attributions for perceived erectile failure were manipulated following a similar bogus feedback condition (Weisberg et al., 2001). Specifically, 52 young men with normal sexual functioning viewed similar sexually explicit films while wearing a penile strain gauge. Once again, all men were told that they did not become as aroused as the typical study participant, but they were then given either an external, fluctuating attribution (i.e., "The films must have been very poor quality") or an internal, constant attribution (i.e., "It seems from questionnaires you filled out that maybe you have a type of belief about sex that sometimes makes it difficult to get aroused here in our lab") as the cause of their poor erectile performance. All participants then viewed a third film to examine responsivity under the differing attributions.

The results indicated that subjects given the external, fluctuating attribution showed greater physiological and subjective sexual arousal during a third film than did participants given the internal, constant attribution. In addition, negative affect and perceptions of erectile control negatively influenced sexual arousal during the third film. These results suggest that after an occasion of erectile difficulty, the cause to which the difficulty is attributed, the degree of negative affect experienced, and the degree of perceived erectile control all seem to influence future sexual functioning. Thus the results suggest that in the context of negative affect and somewhat lower perceived control, direct manipulation of attributions may diminish to a certain degree the illusion of control that exists in otherwise functional individuals, since both objective and subjective sexual arousal were somewhat lower in our subjects under these conditions.

These findings from the Sexuality Research Program have altered and extended some of my thinking contributing to the model of anxious apprehension presented in Figure 3.1. My focus is now less on attentional allocation within an overall model of attentional capacity, and more on the antecedents, components, and consequences of a sense of uncontrollability with which one anticipates future events. That is, one could easily interpret the negative expectancies seemingly present in our patient populations as reflecting this profound sense of a lack of control over upcoming situations and responses. In the case of our sexually dysfunctional patients, this sense of uncontrollability and unpredictability is focused on erectile responding; in the case of patients with panic disorder, it is focused on the next unpredictable panic attack (see Chapter 10); and so on. An in-depth discussion of programmatic research on the nature and development of a sense of controllability, and the relationship of these findings to the development of anxiety, constitutes the better part of Chapter 8.

In addition, as noted in the first edition of this book (Barlow, 1988) and above, it may not be conceptually correct to separate evaluative self-focus or self-preoccupation from the cognitive and emotional representations of anxiety (as depicted in Figure 3.1). It does seem clear, however, that affectively laden self-preoccupation serves to increase further the intensity of anxious apprehension and the arousal associated with it. Of course, this self-focused attention is likely to become very much integrated with anxiety over time as anxiety becomes chronic. That is, unexplained arousal and anxiety may initially trigger a shift to self-focused attention in vulnerable individuals, but eventually self-focused attention becomes an integral part of the core of anxiety. Thus individuals caught up with the uncontrollability of upcoming negative events are trapped in a never-ending cycle of self-evaluative focus or "neurotic self-preoccupation." Despite the seeming interrelatedness of the cognitive and emotional representations of anxious apprehension, as represented by a sense of uncontrollability and a negative self-evaluative focus, it is still useful to highlight and articulate self-focused attention in any model of anxiety, since this particular component of anxious apprehension has implications for therapy (Barlow, 1991a).

Hypervigilance and Cognitive Bias

When the first edition of this book (Barlow, 1988) was published, the paradigms of cognitive science had just begun to be applied to the processing of information in anxiety and its disorders (e.g., MacLeod, Mathews, & Tata, 1986). Traditionally, the attributes of cognitive processing associated with anxiety have been subsumed under the umbrella of a generalized hypervigilance for threat-related stimuli, where attention is narrowed and tightly focused on possible sources of threat. A phenomenon observed in numerous experiments with different purposes and methodologies over the past 40 years involves what has been called "narrowing of attention" during emotional arousal. Easterbrook (1959) was one of the first to describe this process. He suggested that narrowing of attention is a preoccupation with mood-congruent material during emotional reactivity that varies as a function of the intensity of the emotion: The more intense the emotion, the narrower the attention. Specifically, the number of cues utilized decreases as emotional intensity increases. One becomes preoccupied with the central mood-congruent cues as intensity of mood increases, at the expense of concurrent attention to external stimuli. Stimuli relevant to the emotion become more salient, whereas mood-incongruent or irrelevant stimuli are allocated less and less attention.

This phenomenon was verified in a number of early experiments (e.g., Callaway & Stone, 1960; McNamara & Fisch, 1964). Some investigators suggested that extreme cue restriction results in decreased processing efficacy and impaired performance. For example, Korchin (1964) suggested that at the most intense levels of arousal, attention is characterized by distractibility and disarray. That is, since the individual loses the broader perspective, he or she is unable to respond adaptively. This seems similar to, and may account for, the Yerkes–Dodson law (Yerkes & Dodson, 1908), where performance relates to arousal in an inverted U-shaped function. According to this law, performance initially increases and then decreases as arousal reaches maximal levels. Thus narrowing of attention and its consequence may explain the Yerkes–Dodson law.

Investigation in the 1980s began to elucidate a bias in individuals with anxiety to differentially detect, perceive, and process anxiety-related cues (Burgess et al, 1981; Parkinson & Rachman, 1981c; MacLeod et al., 1986). This line of research received a substantial impetus from the influential work of Aaron T. Beck (e.g., Beck & Emery with Greenberg, 1985). Beck theorized the existence of a hypervalent cognitive schema in which reality is often interpreted or processed as threatening or dangerous; this schema acts as a trait-like source of vulnerability for the development of anxiety and its disorders. Beck noted early that these appraisals need not be "conscious" or "rational." Thus much research over the past several years has been focused on (1) characterizing the cognitive manifestations of hypervigilance, and (2) ascertaining whether this biased processing of information predates the development of clinical disorders.

In the past decade, cognitive scientists have explored these processes in more detail, utilizing a variety of clever experimental paradigms. Data from these paradigms have begun to suggest that biases reflecting anxious apprehension occur both explicitly and implicitly (out of awareness) in individuals experiencing anxiety (Eysenck, 1992; Mathews, 1997; Mathews & MacLeod, 1994). McNally (1996, 1999) subdivides cognitive bias relevant to the experience of anxiety into four distinctive categories: interoceptive acuity bias, attentional bias, memory bias, and interpretative bias. Having considered interoceptive acuity phenomena above, I now focus on the latter categories.

Attentional Bias

Data from our own experiments on attentional direction and capacity in the context of sexually functional and dysfunctional individuals have been described above. To summarize briefly, it seems that sexually dysfunctional individuals are hypervigilant for, and differentially attend to, perceptions of the occurrence of bodily sensations and other self-evaluative concerns. Experiments more directly testing the notion that individuals with anxiety selectively attend to potentially threatening information have come from several ingenious paradigms, all of which extend the early work on attention narrowing.

In the dichotic listening paradigm described earlier (e.g., Abrahamson, Barlow, Sakheim, et al., 1985), words that represent areas of threat, danger, or concern are presented in one ear (perhaps imbedded in music or other messages), while distracting information that the individual is asked to recall is presented in the other ear. A series of experiments have demonstrated that patients with anxiety are better able to detect idiosyncratic anxiety-relevant words than are nonanxious controls (e.g., Foa & McNally, 1986; Mathews & MacLeod, 1986). MacLeod (1991), however, has criticized dichotic listening methods as perhaps a nonspecific test of attentional bias that does rule out other competing hypotheses. These would include the tendency to respond more often with anxiety-related answers when presented with an ambiguous task.

In perhaps the most popular cognitive paradigm, the "Stroop test" (Williams, Mathews, & MacLeod, 1996), participants are requested to name the color of the ink in which a word is printed while attempting to ignore the word itself. In studies of individuals with anxiety, both anxiety-provoking and neutral words are typically presented sequentially for a brief time in different colors. If the individuals take longer to name the color of an anxiety relevant word, the notion is that they are selectively attending to the content of the word, which delays their ability to describe its color accurately. For example, Chen, Lewin, and Craske (1996) examined Stroop interference for individuals with fears of spiders, both while the individuals were at rest and while they were in a stressful situation where they were anticipating approaching a spider. In both conditions, these individuals showed more interference for spider-related words than did control subjects who were not fearful of spiders.

In general, this paradigm has successfully measured differential allocation of attention to threat-specific words in a variety of anxiety disorders, such as rape-related words in rape-induced posttraumatic stress disorder (Foa, Feske, Murdock, Kozak, & McCarthy, 1991). Similarly, socially anxious individuals respond differentially to words reflecting evaluation and other aspects of social anxiety, compared to control subjects (Mattia, Heimberg, & Hope, 1993; McNeil, Ries, Taylor, et al., 1995). With a few exceptions, patients with panic disorder seem to respond differentially to words depicting potentially dangerous bodily sensations or the possibility of having a heart attack, collapsing, or the like, compared to individuals without panic disorder (e.g., Hope, Rapee, Heimberg, & Dombeck, 1990; Ehlers, Margraf, Davies, & Roth, 1988). Other studies have shown this specificity for GAD (Mogg, Bradley, Williams, & Mathews, 1993). In a particularly interesting variation, some investigators have "masked" words in the Stroop task (i.e., the words are presented for too short a time to be consciously perceived), but they continue to find the same type of response reflecting a cognitive bias for threat-related words (e.g., Bradley, Mogg,

Millar, & White, 1995; van den Hout, Tenney, Huygens, & de Jong, 1997). Nevertheless, some have criticized the Stroop test as reflecting emotionality in general rather than threat-specific attentional bias. For example, positive words can sometimes elicit the same type of interference as negative words (McNally, 1996), although not all studies have reported this finding (Maidenberg, Chen, Craske, Bohn, & Bystritsky, 1996). Other studies have reported the occasional nonspecificity of the Stroop task with anxious patients, who tend to respond with interference to a variety of emotionally threatening stimuli (Craske, 1999).

The final paradigm utilized with some frequency is the "dot probe detection task." In this paradigm individuals are presented with pairs of words, usually on a computer screen, and are instructed to read out loud the top word in each pair. Occasionally, one of the words will be threatening. Subjects are (usually) instructed to press a button whenever they see a dot replacing one of the words on the screen. The notion here is that anxious subjects will display selective attention by pressing the button more quickly when the dot replaces a threat word as compared to a neutral word.

This paradigm has been used successfully by Asmundson, Sandler, Wilson, and Walker (1992) and McNally, Hornig, Otto, and Pollack (1997) with patients who have panic disorder. Dot probe detection procedures has also produced relevant findings in patients with obsessive–compulsive disorder (Tata, Leibowitz, Prunty, Cameron, & Pickering, 1996). This paradigm has produced similar results with threat words, presented just at or below the level of awareness, suggesting that these attentional biases are preconscious (Mogg et al., 1993). However, as with all cognitive paradigms, these results are sometimes difficult to replicate (Asmundson & Stein, 1994–1995; McNally, 1999).

Generally, the accumulated evidence of the last two decades supports the existence of attentional bias and hypervigilance toward threatening cues in anxious individuals using a variety of paradigms. But the parameters of this attentional bias have not yet been fully worked out, and alternative explanations that could account for some of these feelings have not been ruled out.

Memory Bias

In the first edition of this book, I described the beginnings of an important line of research suggesting that subjects' abilities to retrieve important information from memory are often facilitated if their current mood is congruent with their mood at the time the information was originally encoded (Bower, 1981; Gilligan & Bower, 1984; Teasdale, 1983). Although subsequent research has not supported this particular model (Mathews & MacLeod, 1994), Bower's work with depression in this area did much to spark more cognitive scientific approaches to the interaction of cognition and emotion. However, at the time of the first edition, studies in this area had not been able to demonstrate memory bias in clinically anxious patients (e.g., Mogg, Mathews, & Weinman, 1987).

Since that time, a number of studies have attempted to elucidate the nature of memory biases in individuals with demonstrable anxiety. Generally, studies in this area examine either "explicit memory" biases or "implicit memory" biases. Explicit memory, of course, concerns the retrieval of information of which the subject is fully aware. The notion here is that patients with anxiety disorders report continual preoccupation with anxiety- and danger-related themes, even in the absence of objective "triggers" of some type. This implies that memory for threatening cognitions is highly accessible in these patients and is easily prompted or "primed" by any number of internal or external cues. Tests of explicit memory involve an active attempt to retrieve this information, usually by recall or recognition, but the results have been decidedly mixed. Cloitre, Shear, Cancienne, and Zeitlein

(1994), presented word pairs to patients with panic disorder and several control groups. The word pairs were such that either one or both words in each pair were threatening, positive, or neutral. Subjects were asked to read the word pairs aloud and attend to the degree to which they were related. Later, when they were asked to recall these words, patients with panic disorder remembered more threat-related words compared to the control groups. Nevertheless, the majority of studies have been unable to find improved memory for anxiety-related information, despite elegant experimental manipulations (Cloitre, Cancienne, Heimberg, Holt, & Liebowitz, 1995; Rapee, 1994a; MacLeod & McLaughlin, 1995; Mogg, Gardner, Stavrou, & Golombok, 1992).

In fact, more favorable evidence supporting the existence of memory bias is found in tests of implicit memory. Implicit memory is generally measured by changes in performance as a result of prior exposure to information, regardless of the individual's awareness of this information. Thus Pauli et al. (1997) examined the ability of 15 patients with panic disorder to identify at a later time words depicting threatening bodily sensations or conditions (compared to nonthreatening nonsomatic words) presented very quickly on a tachistoscope. These results were compared to those of 15 healthy control subjects. The speed of presentation was set at the threshold with which each subject could correctly identify 50% of the neutral words. The results indicated that patients with panic disorder identified more threatening somatic words than neutral words. Furthermore, these words evoked significantly more event-related brain potential cortical responses, suggesting that these words not only were selectively processed, but carried greater affective valence than neutral words. Nevertheless, a number of studies have not been able to produce differential implicit memory in either patients with anxiety disorders (e.g., Rapee, McCallum, Melville, Ravenscroft, & Rodney, 1994) or nonclinically anxious subjects (Nugent & Mineka, 1994). Thus the evidence suggests that memory biases may be present, particularly implicit biases; however, the results are elusive, and relatively weak when present.

Interpretative Bias

Perhaps the most interesting paradigm for examining cognitive bias examines the tendency for patients with anxiety disorders to differentially interpret ambiguous material as threatening. Here the evidence supporting the existence of cognitive bias is somewhat stronger than it is for memory distortions. Clark et al. (1997) utilized a well-investigated method described by Butler and Mathews (1983) for assessing interpretative bias, in which subjects are presented with written ambiguous scenarios that could be interpreted as either threatening or nonthreatening. For example, patients with panic disorder may read a scenario in which they have carried out a number of routine activities, some of them involving mild exertion, and notice their hearts beating faster. After reading the scenario, subjects are asked to quickly judge the possible reasons for increased heart rate. Although most subjects may think that the effects would be the results of physical exertion, patients with panic disorder may think of having a heart attack or the like. In social anxiety, the scenario may be that someone delivering a speech notices four people dozing off to sleep in the audience. Most individuals may assume that these individuals are tired and probably should not have come to the talk. A socially anxious individual will interpret the same situation as reflecting negative evaluation of his or her speech.

Utilizing this paradigm, Clark et al. (1997) found that patients with panic disorder were particularly prone to interpreting ambiguous situations in which they noticed a sudden increase in some aspect of their physical functioning (breathing rate or heart rate) as threatening, compared to patients with other anxiety disorders. Other studies using similar procedures have found the same general pattern of results (McNally & Foa, 1987; Kamieniecki, Wade, & Tsourtos, 1997). Furthermore, this interpretive bias seems specific to the focus of anxiety in patients presenting with anxiety disorders, at least in some studies. For example, in the Clark et al. (1997) study, patients with panic disorder interpreted only ambiguously occurring physical sensations as threatening, and not other more general ambiguous threat scenarios. Other studies have found similar biases in patients with GAD compared to normal control subjects (Eysenck, Mogg, May, Richards, & Mathews, 1991; Butler & Mathews, 1983), and for individuals with social phobia (Wells & Clark, 1997).

Finally, Chan and Lovibond (1996) utilized a somewhat different paradigm to assess a similar interpretive cognitive bias. They assessed college students with differing levels of trait anxiety during an experiment in which subjects were presented with two types of stimuli: a noise, and the same noise combined with pictures of flowers. The noise alone was always followed by a shock, whereas the noise-and-flower stimulus was never followed by a shock. Nevertheless, individuals with high trait anxiety expected shock a significantly greater proportion of the time when presented with the noise-and-flower combination, compared to individuals with less anxiety; they thereby showed a tendency to "interpret" this ambiguous stimulus as more threatening.

Conclusions about Cognitive Bias

The sum of the evidence suggests that cognitive bias reflecting hypervigilance clearly exists in patients with anxiety disorders and in other individuals scoring high on various measures of anxiety. The data suggest that attentional and interpretative biases reflecting the immediate detection of potential danger and threat are stronger than memory biases, particularly explicit memory bias, which involves actively retrieving threatening material from memory. In fact, Williams, Watts, MacLeod, and Mathews (1988) have suggested in an influential book that explicit memory of threatening cues may actually be avoided in individuals with high anxiety, suggesting a process that has come to be known as "seek to avoid." In other words, individuals with anxiety are far better than nonanxious individuals at detecting threatening stimuli, but then mobilize their resources to avoid the stimuli insofar as possible. This includes avoiding representations of the threatening stimuli stored in memory, or other cognitive strategies in which these stimuli are processed more elaborately.

Reflecting back on the seeming paradox of high self-focused attention and negative evaluation in anxious individuals, but only weak evidence for their perceiving internal functioning accurately (interoceptive accuracy), it is possible to interpret this seeming paradox with the "seek to avoid" heuristic. That is, patients with panic disorder, for example, are quick to detect threatening bodily sensations, particularly in a context where this is likely to occur; however, they then divert their attention away from these sensations, making them somewhat less accurate (or no more accurate than normal) in judging the rate or extent of the response. Similarly, in our sexually dysfunctional patients, attention is quickly focused inward in a negative-affect-laden self-evaluative mode, but further attentional resources are diverted away from actually monitoring sexual responsivity, such as erectile response.

In any case, these cognitive biases share another interesting feature: Almost without exception, they seem to reflect the presence of anxiety (and its disorders), forming a psychological "marker" of anxiety. Furthermore, these biases successfully resolve with treatment. However, there is little evidence to date that these cognitive biases are enduring traits that may reflect preexisting psychological vulnerabilities to develop severe anxiety or anxiety disorders; at least, there is little evidence from studies utilizing the paradigms described above. Evidence from other sources, however, may be more relevant to detecting preexisting psychological vulnerabilities manifesting as cognitive biases. This evidence is reviewed in Chapter 8.

Worry

While investigating the nature and treatment of insomnia in the 1970s, Thomas Borkovec observed that psychologically based insomnia was associated with uncontrollable cognitive intrusions. In severe cases, these intrusions would interfere with the ability to go to sleep or remain sleeping. Although the content might be logical and related to ongoing activities of the day, such as problems at home or at the office, the setting for considering these issues was entirely inappropriate. To Borkovec and his colleagues (e.g., Borkovec, 1979), these cognitions seemed to have the quality of being "driven" by some process totally out of the control of the individuals suffering from insomnia. On the basis of these important observations, Borkovec began studying such individuals, whom he called "chronic worriers" (Borkovec, 1985a; Borkovec, Robinson, Pruzinsky, & DePree, 1983).

In so doing, Borkovec and his colleagues observed a driven, unending process in which their subjects with chronic worry entertained a stream of thoughts regarding possible negative or traumatic events in their future and ways in which they might deal with them. They also noted that these subjects never reached solutions in terms of possible methods of dealing with the future "what-if" possibilities, but that the process continued in any case.

The beginnings of more structured empirical studies comparing worriers and nonworriers in the 1980s revealed that distraction and difficulty in "shutting off" worry activity were among the most noticeable discriminators of severe worry associated with anxiety. Pruzinsky and Borkovec (1983) also found that subjects with chronic worry were significantly more depressed and anxious than subjects without such worry on general affect questionnaires. This finding is interesting, since the former subjects were chosen strictly on the basis of frequent worrying, rather than on criteria reflecting severity of depression or anxiety. They also had more difficulty with attention control on the Imaginal Process Inventory (Singer & Antrobus, 1972), and evidenced more interference with performance (Borkovec, Shadick, & Hopkins, 1991).

At this point in the hypothetical process of anxious apprehension, then, worry is the point at which "hot" cognitions, driven by spiraling arousal, attain a life of their own—traveling beyond the volitional control of individuals as anxiety becomes chronic. Worry may seem, on the face of it, a perfectly reasonable activity in view of one or another ongoing situations that may need attention. Worry may even provide the illusion of taking some action in regard to a foreboding future. This would be consistent with the strong preparatory set and supportive physiology that seem to be essential components of anxiety. For this reason, there seems to be a reinforcing and therefore self-perpetuating quality to worry (Borkovec et al., 1991), which relates to attempts to cope and regain control. More recent conceptualizations, reviewed below, argue convincingly that worry is best considered an attempted coping mechanism that actually serves to avoid the threatening emotional core of anxiety (Craske, 1999), thereby functioning as a negative reinforcer. Thus worry seems to be reinforcing on both a conscious level, with the illusion that one is planning effectively for the future (Freeston, Rhéaume, Letarte, Dugas, & Ladouceur, 1994), and on an unconscious level, in that one is avoiding the processing of core affective themes. But in fact worry as a coping mechanism, conscious or unconscious, is nonfunctional: Eventually, concentration and ongoing activities are disrupted. The logical antidote, the refocusing of attention of external tasks, is usually out of the individual's reach.

During the past decade, the study of the process of worry has burgeoned (e.g., Davey & Tallis, 1994). In Chapter 1, I have referred to the classic comments of Howard Liddell (1949) describing anxiety as the "shadow of intelligence." By this he was referring to the human proclivity to look to the future in an attempt to plan for potentially difficult or threatening events. The process most closely associated with this planning function is worry. In the first edition of this book (and as noted above), I suggested that the principal function of worry is to prepare to attempt to cope with future threat, and most theorists over the years have more or less agreed with this position (Gray, 1982; Mathews, 1990; Eysenck, 1992). As such, worry can be a normal and adaptive process that can become unadaptive or pathological if carried to extremes. Thus, like many other psychopathological features, the process of worry seems to move along a dimension or continuum from normal to pathological, and it is sometimes difficult to draw the boundary. Various features have been assessed with the potential to assist in differentiating normal and pathological worry. These include content of worry, pervasiveness of worry, interference with functioning as a result of worry, and the degree of perceived control over the worry process.

Since pathological worry has become the nosological cardinal feature of one of the anxiety disorders, GAD (see Chapters 9 and 14), many studies examining the process of worry and the attributes of pathological versus nonpathological worry have included patients with GAD.

Regarding themes of worry, one of our studies examined the most commonly reported spheres of worry among 22 patients with GAD (Sanderson & Barlow, 1990). The areas that served as the principal foci of worry were family, finances, work, and illness. More importantly, patients with GAD reported more worry about minor matters than other clinically anxious groups. In a follow-up study (Craske, Rapee, Jackel, & Barlow, 1989), patients with GAD again reported worrying more about miscellaneous minor matters than nonanxious individuals did. They also worried most about illness and least about finances, compared to normal participants, who reported worrying most about work and least about illness. Roemer, Molina, and Borkovec (1997) also noted that patients with GAD reported worrying about a greater number of topics than a control group without significant clinical anxiety; consistent with previous studies, their worry often centered on what were considered to be minor matters. Thus pathological worry is more pervasive and more often focused on what are consensually agreed to be minor matters that simply don't deserve the degree of intellectual and emotional effort put forth. Pathological worry also occupies a greater amount of one's day than more normal worry does. We (Sanderson & Barlow, 1990) reported that 19 out of 22 patients with GAD reported feeling tense, anxious, and worried for 50% or more of a typical day. In the follow-up study (Craske, Rapee, et al., 1989), we reported that the percentage of the day spent worrying was significantly higher for patients with GAD than for nonanxious controls.

Perhaps most importantly, individuals suffering the effects of pathological worry consistently report this process as being "out of control," meaning that it is difficult if not impossible to stop this runaway, intense cognitive process in these individuals. Contrast this to nonpathological worry, where individuals seem able to allocate certain amounts of time to the process before going on to other things (Brown, 1997; Brown, Barlow, & Liebowitz, 1994). This aspect of the worry process has been evaluated as a crucial distinguishing feature in assigning the diagnosis of GAD in DSM-IV (Brown, Barlow, & Liebowitz, 1994). In addition, pathological worry seems to interfere more substantially with daily functioning than more "normal" worry does (Borkovec et al., 1991).

It also seems clear that the normal worry process can be a successful problem-solving activity (Davey, 1994a), but only if not accompanied by significant anxiety. Specifically,

Davey (1993a, 1993b) found that worry was associated with a range of problem-focused coping abilities only after levels of trait anxiety were parceled out. In other words, worry and trait anxiety contributed unique sources of variance, in that worry was positively correlated, and trait anxiety negatively correlated, with cognitive coping and problem solving. Ladouceur, Blais, Freeston, and Dugas (1998) and Davey (1994d) have both noted that one of the problems with pathological worry does not seem to be that problem-solving abilities are absent; rather, the presence of anxiety reduces perceived control over problem-solving abilities, resulting in less confidence that the process will be fruitful. Anxiety also results in decreased ability to focus specifically on the problem at hand. These studies suggest a theme to which I return below: the partial independence of the process of worry from anxiety (Davey, Hampton, Farrell, & Davidson, 1992).

Tom Borkovec and his colleagues (e.g., Borkovec, 1994a) have integrated research findings from around the world and proposed a creative and useful theory that suggests a somewhat different role for the process and function of worry than I suggested in the first edition of this book. Specifically, Borkovec has conceptualized worry as principally verbal or semantic activity that actually serves to prevent the full experience of anxiety- or fear-provoking stimuli when anxiety becomes chronic, as alluded to above. That is, the arousal driven, attention occupying the verbal/linguistic process of worry effectively suppresses the full experience of the negative emotional state of anxiety. As such, it prevents the processing of these emotions, and all of their stimulus, response, and meaning propositions, to use the terminology of Peter Lang (see Chapter 2). In addition, the process of worry is associated with a distinctive psychophysiological process in which autonomic arousal, particularly sympathetic arousal, is substantially restricted; this probably reflects, once again, the inability of the individual to experience the SNS component of fear and anxiety in its fullest sense. Rather, individuals engaged in pathological worry can best be characterized from a psychophysiological point of view as evidencing heightened parasympathetic activity or low vagal tone (see Chapter 6).

A variety of evidence has accumulated over the years to support these propositions. For example, individuals engaging in the process of worry report having more thoughts than images (Borkovec & Inz, 1990; Borkovec, 1994a). This phenomenon seems to be true of nonpathological worry as well as more clinical worry (Borkovec, 1994a; Freeston, Dugas, & Ladouceur, 1996; Tallis, Davey, & Capuzzo, 1994). In one interesting experiment demonstrating this phenomenon, Rapee (1993) instructed his subjects to engage in the worry process while also continuously engaging in tasks that used either primarily verbal components of working memory or primarily visual and spatial components. Only the activity tapping verbal components of working memory seemed to interfere with the worry process, highlighting once again the verbal/linguistic nature of worry. Bergman and Craske (1994) also reported that individuals worrying about an upcoming public speaking task shifted from primarily visualizing a neutral scene to engaging in more verbal/linguistic activity as they began worrying about their upcoming speech.

The functional relationship first suggested by Borkovec (e.g., Borkovec & Inz, 1990) is that the worry process, by preventing full access to the structure of anxiety, suppresses negative affect. This may account for the (negatively) reinforcing qualities that I noted in the first edition of this book. Restricted SNS responding supports this analysis. Freeston, Dugas, and Ladouceur (1996) have noted that stronger endorsement of thoughts during the worry process correlates positively with reduced autonomic hyperactivity. In individuals evidencing more pathological worry, such as those with GAD, the principal finding is one of decreased autonomic flexibility and reduced heart rate variability. This pychophysiological process is described in some detail in Chapter 6. But the notion, once again, is that this autonomic inflexibility reflects a successful avoidance of the experience of anxiety.

By anticipating and planning for future negative events, the process of worry may also reduce the seeming unpredictability and uncontrollability of these events—a process that is known to heighten the aversiveness of these events (Mathews, 1990; Eysenck, 1992). In this way, too, the process of worry can be negatively reinforcing (Roemer & Borkovec, 1993). In addition, as suggested by Craske (1999), the suppression of strong autonomic arousal may well allow for more productive cognitive planning and problem solving. In support of this notion, several studies have found increased left-hemisphere activation (as measured by electroencephalographic recordings) compared to right-hemisphere activation during the worry process. Of course, left-hemisphere activity is associated with verbal/linguistic activity, while right-hemisphere activation is associated with more visual/experiential processing of information associated with higher autonomic activity. Findings of differential hemispheric activity favoring the left hemisphere in anxious subjects have also been reported by Heller, Nitschke, Etienne, and Miller (1997).

In view of these findings, Craske (1999) has argued persuasively that worry is not synonymous with anxious apprehension; rather, it is a closely associated consequence of anxious apprehension that may be an attempt at coping with this process for many individuals. Her reasoning is based on findings that, despite high correlations between trait anxiety and worry (e.g., Tallis, Eysenck, & Mathews, 1992b), further analysis indicates that worry and anxiety account for unique sources of variance (Davey et al., 1992). There is also much evidence that anxious apprehension, at least as experienced acutely, is associated with autonomic arousal relative to baseline conditions, whereas the process of worry as an integral component of more chronic anxiety, as just reviewed, is associated with autonomic suppression. Our work, reviewed in Chapter 6 (e.g., Holden & Barlow, 1986; see Figure 6.2), shows elevated sympathetic responding when individuals are anticipating confrontation with feared situations compared to baseline levels of responding, particularly if these baseline measures are taken after confrontation such that further anticipatory anxiety is not present. Various studies of individuals with nonclinical anxiety demonstrate elevated autonomic responding in anticipation of a challenging or threatening event. Once again, this is in contrast to the worry process associated with chronic anxiety, which is characterized by a high but stable and inflexible autonomic response.

In addition to these seeming psychophysiological differences, Craske (1999) also supposes that cognitive processing may become less elaborate as one moves from a state of worry over possible upcoming negative events, to a state of anticipatory anxiety when these events are more imminent, and finally to a state of fear or panic when danger or threat is actually present and cognitive activity is at a minimum (Fredrikson et al., 1993). This arrangement is diagrammed in Figure 3.9.

In summary, the evidence at this point supports the notion that the process of worry is perhaps best considered an independent process that may be either an adaptive, or failed, attempt to cope with intending threat or danger and associated with chronic anxious apprehension, depending on the intensity of the worry process. As anxiety increases and becomes chronic, so does the process of worry (at least in some individuals), until pathological levels of each process are attained. At this point, the process of worry is an out-of-control, unadaptive process that interferes with performance and becomes the principal feature of at least one anxiety disorder, GAD. At the same time, worry itself can become the focus of anxious apprehension, as reflected in the DSM-IV criteria for GAD, and in Adrian Wells's concept of "meta-worry" (Wells, 1994a; Wells & Papageorgiou, 1998a). We return to this issue in Chapter 14.

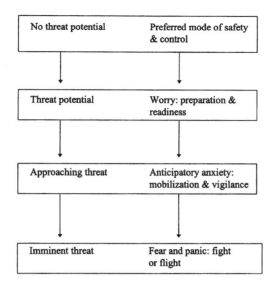

FIGURE 3.9. Relationship of worry, anxious apprehension, and fear (panic). From Craske (1999). Copyright 1999 by Westview Press. Reprinted by permission.

Evidence supporting the partial independence of the process of worry, in turn, requires alterations to the model of the process of anxious apprehension presented in the first edition of this book as described above. These alterations are presented in Figure 3.1. In this new depiction, worry precedes entry into the anxious apprehension cycle, consistent with Craske's conceptualizations. At the same time, it must be remembered that these two processes are highly related and often intricately bound up in a spiraling pathological process that makes them phenomenologically inseparable in their most severe presentation. Nevertheless, the worry process seems to best represent Liddell's (1949) planning function, as he envisioned, over 50 years ago. When it works as seemingly intended, this strategy can assist the individual in warding off future threat by actively planning for future threat or danger, thereby preventing entry into the anxious apprehension cycle.

ANXIETY VERSUS FEAR

The process of anxiety, then, is that of a coherent cognitive–affective structure consisting of a negative feedback cycle characterized to varying degrees by a sense of both internal and external events proceeding in an unpredictable, uncontrollable fashion, accompanied by a supportive physiology and increasingly well-established patterns of brain activation (brain circuits; see Chapter 6). This process is also characterized by maladaptive shifts in attention to an internal, negative self-evaluative focus; a number of cognitive biases reflecting hypervigilance for threat and danger; and, at intense levels, dysfunctional performance. Avoidance and worry are intricately bound up in this cycle, but when anxiety becomes chronic, they are fundamentally failed coping mechanisms.

It does not make sense to say that anxiety as a coherent system "begins" with activation of specific brain circuits, or perceptions of threat or uncontrollability, or attentional shifts. Each facet of anxiety is part of a whole and is difficult to study out of context. The origins of anxiety and anxiety disorders are more fully explicated in Chapter 8.

Now that research and theory on the nature of anxiety have been reviewed, it is important to consider potentially important differences between the emotions of anxiety and fear, alluded to throughout the chapter. Neoevolutionary emotion theorists inform us that fear is a distinct and basic emotion, and human experience in general would seem to validate this. Fear is a primitive alarm in response to present danger, characterized by strong arousal and action tendencies. By contrast, anxiety seems best characterized as a future-orientated emotion, characterized by perceptions of uncontrollability and unpredictability over potentially aversive events and a rapid shift in attention to the focus of potentially dangerous events or one's own affective response to these events. Gray and McNaughton (1996) have theorized on two partially independent brain systems undergirding these two emotions, the BIS and the fight–flight system (FFS; see Chapter 2). Lang talks of discriminatively different outputs from his defensive motivational system: active defense (fight or flight) on the one hand, and behavioral "freezing" on the other. Other theorists make similar discriminations.

If the clinical manifestation of anxiety is a behavioral interruption and a refocusing of attention on possible sources of future threat or danger ("It could happen again, and I might not be able to deal with it, but I've got to be ready to try"), then what is the clinical manifestation of fear? In my view this clinical manifestation is panic, and panic is the unadulterated, ancient, possibly innate alarm system human beings call "fear." Before the etiology of anxiety and its disorders can be discussed, therefore, it is necessary to consider the phenomenon of panic.

CHAPTER 4

The Phenomenon of Panic

I was 25 when I had my first attack. It was a few weeks after I'd come home from the hospital. I had had my appendix out. The surgery had gone well, and I wasn't in any danger, which is why I don't understand what happened. But one night I went to sleep and I woke up a few hours later—I'm not sure how long—but I woke up with this vague feeling of apprehension. Mostly I remember how my heart started pounding. And my chest hurt; it felt like someone was standing on my chest. I was so scared. I was sure that I was dying—that I was having a heart attack. And I felt kind of queer, as if I were detached from the experience. It seemed like my bedroom was covered with a haze. I ran to my sister's room, but I felt like I was a puppet or a robot who was under the control of somebody else while I was running. I think I scared her almost as much as I was frightened myself. She called an ambulance.

This description was offered by a patient of ours. Compare this to an earlier account of an anxiety attack that "erupts into consciousness without being called forth by any train of thought":

An anxiety attack may consist of a feeling of anxiety alone, without any associated ideas, or accompanied by the interpretation that is nearest to hand such as ideas of the extinction of life, or a stroke, or the threat of madness . . . or the feeling of anxiety may have linked to it a disturbance of one or more of the bodily functions—such as respiration, heart action, vaso-motor innervation or glandular activity. From this combination the patient picks out in par-ticular now one, now another, factor. He complains of "spasms of the heart," "difficulty in breathing," "outbreaks of sweating" . . . and such like; and in his description, the feeling of anxiety often recedes into the background. (Freud, 1895/1940, p. 86)

The roots of the experience of panic are deeply embedded in our cultural myths. The Greek god Pan, the god of nature, resided in the countryside, presiding over rivers, woods, streams, and the various grazing animals. But Pan did not fit the popular image of a god: He was very short, with legs resembling those of a goat, and he was very ugly. Unfortu-nately for ancient Greeks traveling through the countryside, Pan had a habit of napping in a small cave or thicket near the road. When disturbed from his nap by a passer-by, he would let out a blood-curdling scream that was said to make one's hair stand on end. Pan's scream was so intense that many a terrified traveler died. This sudden, overwhelming terror or fright came to be known as "panic," and on occasion Pan would use his unique talent to vanquish his foes. Even the other gods were subject to his terror and at his mercy.

Although Pan has faded deep into myth, his power is experienced daily by millions. In fact, panic is so common, so widespread, and so much a part of our experience that we have managed to overlook its importance. In lay terms, "panicking" is a part of our lives, usually occurring before some deadline that seems impossible to make, or at points when one is suddenly faced with danger. But the importance of the phenomenon of panic is such that increasing our understanding is essential if we are to solve the many puzzles surrounding anxiety disorders. In addition, we now know that a full understanding of other major psychological disorders, such as depression, somatoform disorders (e.g., hypochondriasis), and stress disorders, may be difficult without first understanding panic. While we have learned much in the last decade, we still have much to learn about the phenomenon of panic.

WHAT IS PANIC?

Fear and Panic

As reviewed in Chapter 2, many emotion theorists, such as Carroll Izard (e.g., Izard, 1992; Izard & Blumberg, 1985; see also Ekman, 1992), suggest that fear is a distinct, primitive basic emotion. Or, according to Peter Lang's conceptualization (e.g., Lang, 1994a, 1994b, 1995), it is a tightly organized component of our defensive motivational system that is fundamentally a behavioral act. Fear is associated with intense neurobiological and cognitive features. Fear occurs when we are directly and imminently threatened—whether by marauding tribes or wild animals, which was so often the case for our distant ancestors living in caves, or more modern-day dangers, such as an out-of-control vehicle bearing down on us. The action tendency at the heart of this emotion is the well-known "fight-or-flight" response. It is of course essential that this response be instantaneous, because the survival of the organism may depend on it. This is Cannon's (1929) "emergency response" or "alarm reaction." Most theorists would agree that this response is evolutionarily favored, ancient, and found far down the phylogenetic scale. Subjectively, the response is characterized by an overwhelming urge to escape, often expressed as "I've got to get out of here." This subjective urge seems to reflect the basic action tendency of fear, which is escape.

In a dangerous context, the emotion of fear mobilizes us physically and cognitively for quick action and sometimes "superhuman" efforts. Although running away or escaping is the most common behavioral manifestation of fear, occasionally directed action to counter the threat is apparent, such as attacking a predator, or single-handedly lifting an automobile so that a child trapped underneath can escape. As I suggested in the first edition of this book (Barlow, 1988), sometimes these actions are counterproductive, as in the case of a drowning victim's vainly struggling when a rational response would be to lie still and attempt to float.

What is the clinical manifestation of fear? In my view, the summation of developmental and phenomenological evidence to date suggests that the clinical manifestation of the basic emotion of fear is most evident in panic attacks. In addition to a strong autonomic surge, patients experiencing a panic attack report extreme fear and terror, thoughts of dying, and an overwhelming behavioral urge to escape or "get out of here." For patients with panic disorder, these urges may be irrational and counterproductive, as in an urge to escape an important business meeting or family gathering. These urges have important consequences. For instance, many avoid, if at all possible, situations where this strong emotional urge to act might be blocked (e.g., dentists' or beauty salon chairs, or formal social gatherings such as churches or movie theaters, where sudden escape would attract attention and be embarrassing). An often-replicated finding from research on basic emotions is that the intensity of the emotion increases if the action tendency is blocked (e.g., Izard, 1977). The further intensification of the panic attack may contribute to phobic avoidance in patients with anxiety disorders.

Additional data also support the equivalence of fear and panic. Most investigators would suppose that the reaction of individuals with specific phobia when confronting their phobic object represents the prototype for a strong fear reaction. But data collected in our clinic and elsewhere show no important differences between the reaction experienced by individuals with specific phobia upon confronting their feared object or situation, and the panic attacks experienced by patients with panic disorder who did not report a "cue" for their attack (Barlow, 1988; Barlow et al., 1985; Craske, 1991; Margraf, Taylor, Ehlers, Roth, & Agras, 1987; Street, Craske, & Barlow, 1989). These findings and others are responsible for the essential definitional equivalence of these concepts in the *Diagnostic and Statistical Manual of Mental Disorders*, fourth edition (DSM-IV; American Psychiatric Association, 1994), in which an unexpected (uncued) panic attack occurring in the context of panic disorder differs from a "situationally based" panic attack occurring in the context of specific phobia only in the presence of a cue.

One noted theorist, Donald Klein, presumes that at least some panic attacks differ from fear in that they represent a "suffocation alarm" associated with a centrally based CO_2 sensitivity (Klein, 1993; see Chapters 5 and 6). But neither symptom profiles nor neurobiological functioning (e.g., CO_2 sensitivity, hypothalamic–pituitary–adrenocortical axis responding) suggests that these differences between panic and fear exist.

In summary, people experiencing a specific fear response on the one hand, or a panic attack on the other, report very similar subjective experiences, including symptomatology; experience similar behavioral tendencies to escape; and seem to experience similar underlying neurobiological processes. Thus a growing web of evidence supports the equivalence of fear and panic. But at this time the evidence is still largely phenomenological, and much more work is needed on a more precise analysis of fear and panic, particularly at a neurobiological level.

The Presentation of Panic

Much of our increased attention to the concept of panic resulted from the description of panic first appearing in DSM-III (American Psychiatric Association, 1980), where it was defined as "the sudden onset of intense apprehension, fear, or terror, often associated with feelings of impending doom" (p. 230). "Sudden onset" has come to mean 10 minutes during which panic will reach a peak, and this temporal criterion has been included in subsequent revisions of DSM (e.g., DSM-IV; American Psychiatric Association, 1994).

A second important part of the definition is the list of symptoms constituting a panic attack. Most of these symptoms are physical or somatic expressions of panic, such as palpitations or dizziness. DSM-III listed 12 symptoms and specified that at least 4 must be present to label the event a true or "full-blown" panic attack. In DSM-III-R, 14 symptoms were listed. This was accomplished by adding 1 (nausea or abdominal distress) and by breaking down the 12th symptom listed in DSM-III (fear of dying, going crazy, or doing something uncontrolled during an attack) into two symptoms: fear of dying, and fear of losing control or going crazy. This allowed a bit more precision in identifying the characteristic physical symptoms as well as the cognitive expression of dread (going crazy or dying) with which an individual may present during a panic attack. DSM-IV retained this list, but combined the somatic symptoms of faintness with dizziness, lightheadedness, or unsteady feelings to arrive at a list of 13 symptoms. The 13 symptoms from DSM-IV are listed in Table 4.1. Once again, the individual must report having a panic characterized by "the sudden onset of intense apprehension" and so on, and must report at least 4 of these symptoms.

These symptoms were originally developed largely through the clinical experience of investigators working with the anxiety disorders. Clinical experience (as well as more systematic collections of reports of symptoms) also tells us that different individuals may experience different combinations of the symptoms, and that the same person may report a slightly different mix of symptoms from one panic attack to another (Rapee, Craske, & Barlow, 1990). Typically, patients who are experiencing panic attacks report far more than the minimum number of four symptoms specified in DSM-IV (Fyer & Rassnick, 1990). Several years ago my colleagues and I asked a large group of patients to indicate symptoms each of them experienced during their typical or most recent panic. Table 4.2 illustrates the number and percentage of a group of 41 patients with DSM-III agoraphobia with panic attacks who endorsed each of the 12 DSM-III symptoms. For purposes of comparison, corresponding data from a group of 55 patients with DSM-III-R panic disorder with agoraphobia are also presented.

As one can see from the table, most of these patients reported the physical symptoms of palpitations, dizziness, and trembling. Shortness of breath (dyspnea), sweating, faintness, and hot and cold flashes were also common. Choking, paresthesias, feelings of unreality, and chest pain were somewhat less common, although the percentage endorsing the last symptom was quite different between groups. No fewer than 90% of the first group reported a fear of dying, going crazy, or losing control. When these cognitive symptoms were broken down according to DSM-III-R, more patients endorsed the fear of losing control, although the percentage endorsing one or the other was close to 100%. It should be noted that since these descriptions were taken mostly from the patients' "typical" panics, the specific number of symptoms associated with any one discrete panic attack may have been somewhat less.

Another approach to this issue is to examine relative intensity of symptoms. Ley (1985) also interviewed a group of patients with DSM-III agoraphobia with panic attacks, and chronicled their symptom reports by ranking the symptoms on the basis of intensity. He

---

TABLE 4.1. DSM-IV Panic Attack Criteria

[A panic attack is a] discrete period of intense fear or discomfort, in which at least four (or more) of the following symptoms developed abruptly and reached a peak within 10 minutes:

(1) palpitations, pounding heart, or accelerated heart rate
(2) sweating
(3) trembling or shaking
(4) sensations of shortness of breath or smothering
(5) feeling of choking
(6) chest pain or discomfort
(7) nausea or abdominal distress
(8) feeling dizzy, unsteady, lightheaded, or faint
(9) derealization (feelings of unreality) or depersonalization (being detached from oneself)
(10) fear of losing control or going crazy
(11) fear of dying
(12) paresthesias (numbness or tingling sensations)
(13) chills or hot flushes

Note. Reprinted with permission from the *Diagnostic and Statistical Manual of Mental Disorders*, Fourth Edition. Copyright 1994 American Psychiatric Association.

TABLE 4.2. Number and Percentage of 41 Patients with DSM-III Agoraphobia with Panic Attacks, and 55 Patients with DSM-III-R Panic Disorder with Agoraphobia, Reporting Each of the Panic Symptoms

Symptom	DSM-III agoraphobia with panic attacks (n = 41)		DSM-III-R panic disorder with agoraphobia (n = 55)	
	Number	%	Number	%
Dyspnea	37	90	41	75
Palpitations	40	98	48	87
Chest pain	31	76	21	38
Choking	30	73	28	50
Dizziness	39	95	48	87
Unreality	28	68	31	57
Paresthesias	26	63	32	58
Hot or cold flashes	35	85	40	74
Sweating	35	93	38	70
Faintness	31	76	37	68
Trembling	36	88	47	86
Fear of dying, going crazy, losing control	37	90		
(DSM-III-R:)				
Abdominal distress			30	56
Fear of dying			29	52
Fear of going crazy, losing control			42	76

then compared his group's rankings with those for the 41 patients with DSM-III agoraphobia described above. This list, appearing in Table 4.3, demonstrates a strikingly similar patterning of the intensity with which these symptoms were reported.

The prominence of the cognitive symptoms (fear of dying; fear of losing control or going crazy), in terms of both relative frequency and relative intensity, caused investigators to carefully consider the role of these symptoms in the definition of panic attacks and panic disorder for DSM-IV. In DSM-III and DSM-III-R, these symptoms were either one or two items in a much longer list, and patients needed only to meet a minimum of four symptoms to meet criteria for a panic attack. Thus DSM-III or DSM-III-R did not require the presence of a cognitive symptom as part of the four-symptom criterion for panic. Additional research (Agras, 1990) suggested that these symptoms might be made more central to the definition of a panic attack. This suggestion was reinforced by subsequent research, which continued to show that the vast majority of patients with panic disorder reported catastrophic cognitions associated with panic (e.g., 95% in Brown, Marten, & Barlow, 1996). Other research suggested that the presence of these thoughts often differentiates individuals with panic disorder from patients with other anxiety disorders and individuals with nonclinical panic (e.g., Rapee, Sanderson, McCauley, & Di Nardo, 1992). Finally, these symptoms have some utility in predicting agoraphobic avoidance (Agras, 1990; Clark, 1990; Craske & Barlow, 1988). Thus the stipulation was added to the DSM-IV criteria for panic disorder that "at least one of the attacks has been followed by one month (or more) of . . . (b) worry about the implications of the attack or its consequences (e.g., losing control, having a heart attack, "going crazy")" (American Psychiatric Association, 1994, p. 402). Although other criteria can be substituted for this stipulation, such as a signifi-

TABLE 4.3. Rank Orders of the Intensity of Symptoms Experienced by Patients with Agoraphobia during Panic Attacks

Symptoms	Ley's rank	Barlow's rank	Composite rank
Fear of dying, etc.	1	2	1
Palpitations	3	1	2
Trembling	2	4	3
Dyspnea	4	5.5	4
Dizziness	7	3	5
Hot or cold flashes	6	5.5	6
Faintness	8.5	7	7
Unreality	5	11	8
Sweating	8.5	8	9
Chest pain	10	10	10.5
Choking	11	9	10.5
Paresthesias	12	12	12

Note. From Ley (1985). Copyright 1985 by Pergamon Journals, Ltd. Reprinted by permission.

cant change in behavior related to the attacks, it is clear that the overwhelming majority of patients report these cognitive symptoms.

Nevertheless, my colleagues and I have suggested elsewhere that although the presence of cognitive symptoms is very useful in a definition of panic disorder, it need not be essential to the definition of a panic attack. For example, these cognitive symptoms are not particularly evident in the panic attacks experienced by individuals with other anxiety disorders, such as specific phobia (Craske, Zarate, Burton, & Barlow, 1993). Thus it is possible that these cognitive symptoms, which are really personal attributions concerning the cause or consequence of the attack, may be viewed as epiphenomenal to the experience of panic. This conclusion is also supported by data from prospective studies of panic attacks in patients with panic disorder, in which the attribution concerning dying seemed to be a product of the intensity of the attack rather than an associated symptom of the attack (Basoglu, Marks, & Sengun, 1992) or in which these cognitions were not identified at all (Kenardy, Fried, Kraemer, & Taylor, 1992). At the present time, these cognitive symptoms seem very useful in defining panic disorder, but do not seem inherently necessary as a definition of panic attack (Barlow, Brown, & Craske, 1994).

The DSM-IV Task Force also examined the utility of requiring a minimum number of somatic symptoms in the definition of panic attacks. This examination was stimulated by the finding noted above that specific symptoms are inconsistently reported across attacks. For example, we (Rapee, Craske, & Barlow, 1990) observed that less than one symptom was experienced consistently across panic attacks by the average subject in our study of 62 patients with panic disorder. Also, symptom report does not appear to correlate well with physiological measures. For example, some studies show that subjects with panic disorder report more hyperventilatory symptomatology than do patients with other anxiety disorders, despite equivalence in objective measures of overbreathing, such as arterial CO_2 pressure (pCO_2) (e.g., Holt & Andrews, 1989b; Rapee, Brown, Antony, & Barlow, 1992). Nevertheless, very few patients report fewer than four symptoms associated with their attacks (Fyer & Rassnick, 1990), and there seemed no reason to change this criterion.

Another important issue is to determine whether the somatic panic symptoms are unique among a larger set of somatic symptoms in defining panic attacks, or simply a subset of reportable somatic symptoms for a group of somatically hypersensitive patients. For example, King, Margraf, Ehlers, and Maddock (1986) reported that patients with panic disorder indiscriminately endorsed a large number of somatic symptoms, many of which were seemingly unrelated to the experience of panic. On the other hand, Goetz et al. (1989) added a number of irrelevant somatic symptoms to a clinical rating inventory used to rate panic attacks provoked by lactate infusions in the laboratory, and found that these additional items did not differentiate patients with lactate-induced panic attacks from patients without such attacks (whereas the core panic symptoms did, at least in ratings of intensity). The majority of phenomenological studies of panic suggest that the characteristic sympathetic surge as reflected in the somatic symptom set defining panic attacks accurately reflects the nature of this reaction, although there is wide variability from individual to individual (Barlow et al., 1994).

Limited-Symptom Attacks

Clinicians have identified what seems to be another variety of panic attack, which meets all the criteria for panic mentioned above with one exception: Fewer than four symptoms are reported. In DSM-IV, these experiences are called "limited-symptom attacks." There is now evidence that these attacks are aptly named, since on the whole they are rated by patients as less intense than major attacks (Taylor et al., 1986). For example, while monitoring panics for 6 days in a group of 12 patients with panic disorder, Taylor et al. (1986) noted that 8 out of 33 panic attacks would be classified as minor or limited-symptom attacks. Nevertheless, these limited-symptom attacks were rated by patients at an average intensity of 2.5 (compared to 3.9 for major attacks) on a scale of 0–10, and they were associated with an average heart rate increase of 17.3 beats per minute (BPM), as compared to an increase of 49.2 BPM for major attacks. On the other hand, certain types of limited-symptom attacks can be very intense. For example, my colleagues and I interviewed a woman who reported that her initial panic episode consisted of two specific symptoms: diarrhea and excessive perspiration. Following that first episode, a typical agoraphobic pattern emerged in which she would avoid going out as much as possible. Her greatest fear was that the diarrhea and sweating would suddenly recur (which would occasionally happen). Thus, when she did go out, she would always check for the availability of bathrooms, and would only begin to feel more comfortable when she had easy access to a bathroom. She was also particularly conscientious about applying antiperspirants and so forth. This woman soon learned the location of every bathroom along her frequented routes in the small city in which she lived.

Functionally, this type of limited-symptom attack seems to serve the same purpose as a full panic attack. That is, it has the same consequences (see Chapter 2). However, in our clinical experience, this type of attack is relatively rare in the absence of major panic attacks. For example, in a series of 1,455 individuals with agoraphobia we have seen, only 9 reported having had these limited attacks without ever having experienced a major attack.

On the basis of these findings, we have delineated two types of limited-symptom attacks. The first type represents experiences of individuals who have had severe attacks and have subsequently developed panic disorder. Consistent with research evidence (e.g., Rapee, Craske, & Barlow, 1990), these patients present with full panic attacks (i.e., four or more symptoms) interspersed with a series of minor "attacks" involving reports of fewer than four symptoms. These limited-symptom attacks may be subjective anxiety (conditioned by prior panics) without an actual physiological surge. The second type of limited-symptom attack is an isolated but severe somatic symptom, which leads to agoraphobic avoidance, as described above.

In summary, panic attacks are described by individuals as sudden bursts of emotion consisting of a large number of somatic symptoms, accompanied often by feelings of dying and/or losing control. The symptoms are relatively consistent, on the average, across people experiencing panic; however, individual panic attacks may present with a different "mix" or number of symptoms and may vary in intensity. The reports clearly resemble the primitive alarm of fear described in Chapter 1 (Cannon, 1927; Darwin, 1872). Although these reports seem to describe a unique event, do more objective measurement procedures support these reports?

The Psychophysiology of Panic

Panic during Psychophysiological Monitoring in a Clinic

Several years ago, my colleagues and I recorded detailed physiological changes preceding and accompanying "spontaneous" panic attacks in two patients who happened to be undergoing psychophysiological monitoring at the time (Cohen, Barlow, & Blanchard, 1985). These panic attacks were unexpected by the patients and certainly unexpected by us. Interestingly, both attacks occurred while the patients were engaging in relaxation—one during a psychophysiological assessment, and the other during a biofeedback-assisted relaxation training session. Why relaxation might provoke a panic is a fascinating issue taken up later in this volume (see Chapters 5 and 14). Because these serendipitous data provide part of the answer to the question "What is panic?", the two patients and their data are presented in some detail here.

The first patient was a 33-year-old female who, interestingly, was diagnosed as having generalized anxiety disorder (GAD; see Chapter 14). She is referred to here as "Mary." She presented to our Anxiety Disorders Clinic at the State University of New York at Albany with primary complaints of chronic tension, irritability, palpitations, faintness, and an inability to relax. Prior to her seeking treatment at our clinic, she had been treated by her family physician for irritable bowel syndrome. She reported experiencing occasional panic attacks, but not of sufficient frequency to meet the criteria for panic disorder.

The panic attack described here occurred while Mary was undergoing a pretreatment psychophysiological assessment. After a 10-minute period of adaptation to the laboratory, a 4-minute baseline was recorded. Next, Mary was instructed to relax first her whole body, and then her face and forehead. The panic attack occurred during this relaxation period. Following the attack, after a few minutes of reassurance by the experimenter, she was able to resume the assessment. In later phases of the assessment she was required to perform a series of stressor tasks, including mental arithmetic, stressful imagery, and the cold pressor test, which involved submerging her hand in a bucket of ice-cold water for as long as she could; she completed these tasks with little difficulty. At the end of the session, when asked to rate her anxiety levels during each phase of the assessment, she reported having felt the most relaxed during the relaxation phase, just prior to her panic attack. She also reported slight nausea associated with the relaxation, however.

The second subject was a 34-year-old female, "Jill," who was being treated for panic disorder. She reported experiencing many of her panic attacks in stressful situations. On occasion, however, they would occur at times when she felt carefree and relaxed, although usually shortly following a period of increased stress. For example, she recalled a recent panic attack that had occurred in a restaurant. She had been very tense and pressured, attempting to dress her children and see to it that her family arrived at the restaurant in time for their reservation. She was fearful that her increased tension would precipitate an attack in the restaurant, but after finally settling down and ordering her meal, she remembered thinking, "Everything is all right now; I made it." As she began to relax and enjoy her meal, she experienced an intense panic attack.

The panic described here occurred during Jill's third biofeedback treatment session, in which she was being taught to relax her muscles. Prior to beginning biofeedback training, she had practiced progressive relaxation for several weeks. She had made good progress, although on several occasions she had experienced slight dizziness during her practice. In this particular session, a 4-minute baseline was recorded, after which she was instructed to begin relaxation.

Physiological changes for both subjects from the start of the recording session through the onset and peak of the panic attacks are presented in Figure 4.1 for Mary and in Figure 4.2 for Jill. In each case, physiological recording ceased at the time the therapist entered the room to comfort and reassure the patient. Since the panics occurred during relaxation, and thus did not represent a separate phase of the procedure, their onset is indicated by the broken line on the figures.

The figures show remarkably similar changes for Mary and Jill. During the relaxation phase, up to the onset of the panic attacks, both Mary and Jill were relaxing nicely as indicated by decreases in heart rate and frontalis electromyography (EMG). Mary showed a mean heart rate decrease of 4 BPM and a mean EMG decrease of 2.4 μV. Jill's heart rate dropped 2 BPM, while her EMG level declined 5.5 μV. These heart rate decreases were followed by abrupt increases during the panic attack, reaching a level of tachycardia within 1 minute for Mary and 2 minutes for Jill. EMG measures during the panics also showed increases for both patients. Hand surface temperature showed minimal changes, but the pattern was consistent for both Mary and Jill (i.e., decreases during relaxation were followed by increases during panics). Particularly striking are the magnitude of the increases and the abruptness with which they occurred. Mary's heart rate increased about 40 BPM within 1 minute and Jill's increased over 50 BPM within 2 minutes, while both of them were relaxing!

Lader and Mathews (1970) observed a similar pattern of physiological responses from three patients who were also undergoing physiological assessment but panicked part way through. In each case these panics were unexpected, although patients were experiencing various levels of anxiety during the assessment. In at least one case, however, the patient reported that she was "coming to" from a state of mild drowsiness when the panic occurred. This may have been similar to Jill's and Mary's situation. The attacks were also over in several minutes for Lader and Mathews's patients, prompting them to speculate on innate inhibitory physiological mechanisms that must have been present to cause such a rapid decrease in the panic.

Panic during Ambulatory Psychophysiological Monitoring

Subsequently, clinicians and clinical investigators began to monitor patients who were vulnerable to panic attacks as they went about their day-to-day affairs. This was made possible by advances in technology allowing relatively unobtrusive physiological monitoring on a 24-hour basis. Furthermore, this allowed the investigators to see whether naturally occurring panic attacks would look the same as those captured in the laboratories. For example, Robert Freedman and his colleagues in Detroit (Freedman, Ianni, Ettedgui,

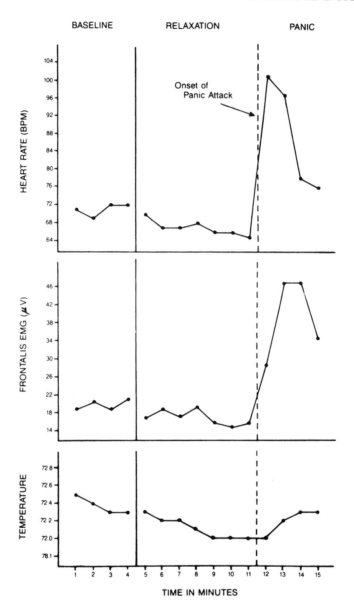

FIGURE 4.1. Physiological changes for Subject 1 ("Mary") from the start of the recording session through the onset and peak of the panic attack. From "The Psychophysiology of Relaxation-Associated Panic Attacks" by A. S. Cohen, D. H. Barlow, and E. B. Blanchard, 1985, *Journal of Abnormal Psychology, 94,* 96–101. Copyright 1985 by the American Psychological Association. Reprinted with permission.

& Puthezhath, 1985) monitored patients with panic disorder over a period of 2 days, and "caught" five patients having one or more panic attacks. Increases in heart rate and changes in other physiological indicators were substantial, but the attacks were essentially over in 5 minutes, as were the laboratory attacks described above.

   One of the difficulties in identifying naturally occurring panic attacks is that people wearing ambulatory physiological monitors are engaging in their usual and customary

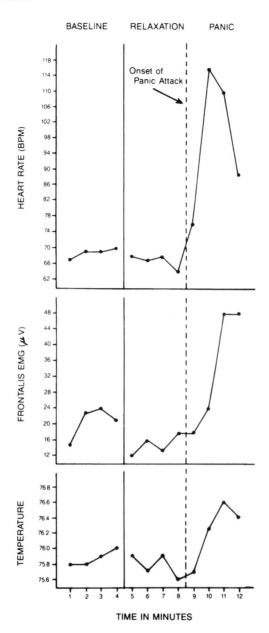

FIGURE 4.2. Physiological changes for Subject 2 ("Jill") from the start of the recording session through the onset and peak of the panic attack. From "The Psychophysiology of Relaxation-Associated Panic Attacks" by A. S. Cohen, D. H. Barlow, and E. B. Blanchard, 1985, *Journal of Abnormal Psychology, 94,* 96–101. Copyright 1985 by the American Psychological Association. Reprinted with permission.

routines, most of which involve some sort of physical activity. Distinguishing the proportion of a sudden physiological change that is due to a sudden increase in physical activity or exercise from the proportion that may be due to panic is a sophisticated task—one that C. Barr Taylor and his associates at Stanford began to undertake in the 1980s (Taylor et al., 1986; Taylor, Telch, & Haavek, 1983). In an early study (Taylor et al., 1983), they observed that the high heart rate noted from several patients during self-reported panic attacks was confounded by the fact that the patients were physically very active at the time. They devised a statistical program to separate out heart rate increases due to panic attacks from those due to physical activity. Essentially, this procedure specifies heart rate increases over and above what may be expected from the physical activity ongoing at the time.

In an important study, Taylor et al. (1986) then monitored 12 patients with panic disorder and 12 matched subjects without panic disorder for 6 days, 24 hours a day. They proved that naturally occurring panic attacks could be identified on the basis of abrupt elevations in heart rate that could not be attributed to physical activity. Data from one of their patients, for whom heart rate and activity levels were monitored concurrently, are presented in Figure 4.3. The physiological signature was very similar to that observed previously in the laboratories. Average heart rate increase from the start of the panic to the peak was 38.6 BPM. Heart rate reached its peak in an average of 4 minutes. Patients reported that the entire episode lasted an average of 15.8 minutes. But according to the criteria developed by Taylor et al., the panic, as measured by heart rate, lasted a mean of 20.2 minutes from beginning to end. Although these values were slightly longer than durations reported in the laboratory, the reassurance of an experienced therapist was not present during these naturally occurring panics. Finally, the time of day associated with the greatest

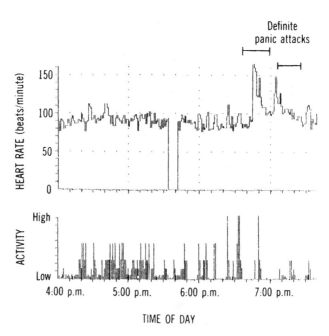

FIGURE 4.3. Heart rate and activity level during two definite panic attacks. From Taylor et al. (1986). Copyright 1986 by the American Psychiatric Association. Reprinted by permission.

frequency of "spontaneous" panic attack was 1:30 to 3:30 A.M., while the patients were in bed and presumably relaxed! The fascinating phenomenon of nocturnal panic is examined below.

At least two features of this important study raise perplexing questions. First, approximately 40% of the major panic attacks reported by these patients were not accompanied by heart rate changes that were different from what would be expected during normal activity. Nevertheless, patients reported an adequate number of panic symptoms to meet criteria. Since heart rate elevations during "typical" panic are very marked (see Figures 4.1 and 4.2), and since these patients were not necessarily exercising vigorously, there appeared to be a phenomenon that was identified by these patients as "panic" but that was not accompanied by characteristic physiological responding. On the other hand, panic attacks that were accompanied by heart rate increases were rated as more intense (a mean of 4.7 on a scale of 0–7) than those not accompanied by heart rate increases (a mean of 3.3 on the same scale).

Second, when Taylor et al. (1986) examined the 24-hour physiological records, they found a large number of otherwise unexplainable heart rate elevations (not due to activity) that would have met the criteria for the most severe panic attack, but were not in any way labeled "panic" by the patients. What this indicates is that marked heart rate elevations alone are not a good indicator of panic in the absence of the subjective experience of the symptoms.

Since that study, a number of additional investigations have confirmed the occurrence of reports of panic attacks in the absence of heart rate elevations or other signs of autonomic activation (Hofmann & Barlow, 1996; Lint, Taylor, Fried-Behar, & Kenardy, 1995; Shear et al., 1992). For example, in the Lint et al. (1995) study, ambulatory monitoring data were collected from 10 women with panic disorder over a period of 5 days. The authors recorded a total of 96 instances of elevated heart rate (tachycardia), but only 12 of these events were clearly associated with panic attacks, and 84 occurred in the absence of reports of panic. In addition, 11 panic attacks were reported that were not associated with elevated heart rate. In addition, Gorman et al. (1983) blocked absolute increases in heart rate with beta-blockers, but noted the report of panic attacks (although relative increases from a dampened baseline of heart rate were observed). This finding would seem to be evidence against designating an absolute indication of peripheral physiological surge as necessary in any definition of panic. Indeed, if the biological base of emotion is in the limbic system, and if panic is an emotion, perhaps fear (Barlow, 1988), then one might not expect a one-to-one correspondence between central and peripheral responding. This lack of correspondence was demonstrated years ago by Cannon (1929) in his refutation of the specifics of the James–Lange theory of emotion.

The Taylor et al. (1986) data and subsequent replications resulted in an increased awareness of the importance of determining how patients construe somatic symptoms. For example, panic may be a unique event. But once panic disorder develops, patients may become extremely sensitive to all somatic sensations originally associated with panic. They may then overreport these symptoms and exaggerate their significance. These issues become very important as the nature of panic is elaborated on below.

Finally, the Taylor et al. (1986) study provides a fascinating look at what happens to normal people who find themselves in situations that are very stressful—situations that many of us have experienced. In one case, one of Taylor et al.'s subjects without panic disorder had been working on a suicide prevention line for the first time and received her first call. On examination, her heart rate pattern met the criteria for a severe panic, but she reported only one symptom (feeling anxious and tense), rather than the three required in this study to meet the criteria for panic attack. Another woman reported two situations in which she reported that she "panicked." In the first, her young child suddenly ran out into the middle of the street. In the second situation, she was driving to the shopping mall when another car came speeding along and appeared to be about to crash into her. There were no heart rate changes during either of these episodes that could be attributed to anxiety, and she reported only one instead of three or more symptoms in each instance. Not one of Taylor's 12 subjects without panic disorder ever met the criteria for a panic attack combining both required heart rate elevations and reports of three or more symptoms. What happened to the alarm reaction described in Chapter 1? Is this reaction representative of individuals suddenly experiencing the emotion of fear? A variety of evidence suggests that it is not (see Chapter 2). But this limited sampling of three events in two individuals clearly underlines the need for larger-scale investigations into this issue utilizing new technological advances. In fact, an expanded analysis with 19 control subjects (Margraf et al., 1987) suggested that panic and anxiety episodes do appear very similar in presenting symptoms to those of patients. Differences occurred only in frequency and intensity of the events.

Nocturnal Panic

As noted above, Taylor et al. (1986) found that the greatest frequency of panic attacks occurred between 1:30 and 3:30 A.M. Perhaps no experience is more terrifying than panicking while sleeping, as illustrated by the report of the patient at the beginning of the chapter. Approximately 25% of all individuals with panic disorder presenting at the Anxiety Disorders Clinic at Albany reported the experience of at least one nocturnal panic attack. In an early study, we assessed a group of 41 individuals who had experienced nocturnal panic (Barlow & Craske, 1988b). These people gave affirmative answers to the question "Are there times when you awake from sleep in a panic?" They were then questioned specifically about the duration of such panics, amount of sleep before onset of panics, symptom intensity, and differences between nocturnal and daytime panics. The majority of nocturnal panics occurred within 1–4 hours of sleep onset (especially between the second and third hours), the time during which slow-wave sleep is most prevalent. This is the same time frame reported by Taylor et al. (1986).

Of the 41 patients with nocturnal panic we assessed (Barlow & Craske, 1988b), 43% reported that the first symptom they noticed upon awakening was cognitive (e.g., fear of losing control, dying, or going crazy), whereas 57% reported that their first symptom upon awakening was somatic (e.g., a racing heart). In regard to symptom severity, 54% reported that their nocturnal panics were more severe than their daytime panics, 25% said that they were less severe, and 21% said that they were of equal severity. In regard to symptom frequency, 46% reported that they experienced more symptoms during nocturnal panic than during the day, 21% reported fewer symptoms at night, and 33% said that there were an equal number of symptoms. Nocturnal panic lasted an average of 24.6 minutes, with a range of 1–180 minutes.

Since this early study, additional data have been collected on the nature of nocturnal panic attacks, primarily by Michelle Craske and her colleagues (Craske & Rowe, 1997b; Craske, 1999). We now know from sleep laboratory studies that nocturnal panics tend to occur in non-rapid-eye-movement (non-REM) sleep. Specifically, nocturnal panics occur most often during the transition into slow-wave sleep (between late Stage 2 and early Stage 3 sleep) (Hauri, Friedman, & Ravaris, 1989; Craske & Rowe, 1997b). Consistent with our early study (Craske & Barlow, 1989), approximately 50% (44–71%) of patients with panic disorder report having experienced nocturnal panic attacks at least once (e.g., Uhde, 1994; Craske, 1999), and 18–45% of individuals with panic disorder experience nocturnal panics on a regular basis (Craske & Rowe, 1997b). There is also some evidence that patients with panic disorder who experience nocturnal panic have more severe attacks than their counterparts who do not experience nocturnal panic. For example, individuals experiencing nocturnal panic report more severe and more frequent daytime panic attacks (Craske & Barlow, 1989) and evidence substantially more comorbidity, particularly with GAD, social phobia, and major depression (Labbate, Pollack, Otto, Langenauer, & Rosenbaum, 1994). Individuals with nocturnal panics in the Labbate et al. study were also more likely to have experienced anxiety during childhood and had an earlier onset of their panic disorder than their counterparts without nocturnal panic attacks. Even college students without a clinical anxiety disorder are more likely to report nocturnal panics as a function of being more physiologically reactive and evidencing a greater wariness of unexplained bodily sensations (Craske & Kreuger, 1990). Perhaps because of this, some individuals with nocturnal panic attacks are afraid to go to sleep at night!

What causes nocturnal panic? Before possible answers to this question are examined, it is important to distinguish nocturnal panic from other disruptions of sleep. As noted above, nocturnal panics do not occur during REM sleep, which rules out nightmares or other dreamlike activity as a cause of nocturnal panic. REM sleep also typically occurs much later in the sleep cycle than nocturnal panic attacks do. This is consistent with reports of patients who note that they do not remember dreaming anything after waking from a nocturnal panic.

On occasion, nocturnal panics are mistaken for a breathing disorder called "sleep apnea," which is an interruption of breathing during sleep that resembles the sensation of suffocation. The causes of sleep apnea may be central or peripheral. If peripheral, the causes are most often found in morbid obesity or other physical characteristics that interfere with respiration while sleeping. Sleep apnea must be ruled out in individuals suspected of experiencing nocturnal panic attacks, but several factors suggest that sleep apnea is rarely a contributing factor. First, the concentration of nocturnal panic in the early part of the sleep cycle is inconsistent with the repeating cycle of sleep apnea throughout the night, which is characterized by apnea, arousal, resumption of breathing, and sleep once again. Also, obesity is frequently associated with apnea, but not selectively with nocturnal panic.

"Sleep terrors" or "night terrors" are other disruptions of sleep that resemble panic attacks. Such an event, occurring most often in children, is typically manifested by a child's awakening with the fear that something or someone is chasing him or her around the room. It is very common for children experiencing night terrors to scream and actually get out of bed as if something were after them. However, they very seldom wake up and typically do not remember the event. Sleep terrors also tend to occur during a later stage of sleep (Stage 4 sleep), a stage that is associated with sleepwalking.

Finally, there is the fascinating condition called "isolated sleep paralysis," described in Chapter 1, that seems culturally determined. As noted in Chapter 1, isolated sleep paralysis occurs during the transitional state between sleep and waking. It is during this period that the individual reports being unable to move and experiencing a surge of terror that resembles a panic attack, occasionally accompanied by vivid hallucinations. The interesting differential association with ethnic groups has been described in Chapter 1. The "paralysis" seems to be due to the fact that those individuals are still in REM sleep as they begin to awake, and therefore continue to experience the motor constriction associated with REM sleep. As an aside, it seems that this phenomenon is also responsible for the experience of many individuals who report memories of having been abducted by aliens. The paralysis and images of bright lights reported by these individuals almost always occur during this stage of sleep (R. J. McNally, personal communication, April 2000).

In the context of this information, scientists have examined both biological and psychological contributions to nocturnal panic attacks. For example, some investigators have proposed that nocturnal panics may result from hypersensitive centrally based CO_2 receptors. This biological abnormality may in turn cause hyperventilation, extreme hypercapnia, and chronic hyperventilation (e.g., Ley, 1988). Preliminary studies testing this hypothesis, however, have found no evidence of CO_2 hypersensitivity or chronic hyperventilation in either laboratory settings (Craske & Barlow, 1990) or during the course of sleep (Hauri et al., 1989). Hauri et al. (1989) and Hauri, Friedman, Ravares, and Fisher (1985) both noted increased large movements during the sleep of individuals experiencing nocturnal panic, compared to the sleep of both normal controls and a group of individuals with "psychophysiological" insomnia. Uhde (1994) has suggested that increased movement during sleep may actually be a defensive reaction against falling into a state of deep relaxation that seems to trigger nocturnal panics. This is perfectly consistent with our own interpretation of causes of nocturnal panics as depending on increased vigilance for potentially dangerous bodily sensations.

In an important study examining potential psychological triggers for nocturnal panic, Craske and Freed (1995) assured a group of 18 individuals with panic disorder and nocturnal panic attacks that any experience of physiological arousal during sleep was perfectly normal, and that they should expect such experiences from time to time. A control group of 18 patients with nocturnal panic received no such assurances. Both groups were then subjected to a series of audio signals during sleep that ostensibly indicated increased autonomic arousal. The subjects who were not reassured of the harmlessness and safety of increased autonomic arousal awoke with more self-reported distress and panic, and reported a variety of anxious symptoms, compared to their reassured counterparts (see Table 4.4). This finding is consistent with the notion that we are all perfectly capable of processing information during sleep, even the depth of slow-wave or delta-wave sleep, particularly information that may signal something dangerous or salient in our environment. If unexpected bodily sensations associated with prior panic attacks become signals for danger and the objects of vigilance, one would expect to find an increased frequency of various somatic sensations prior to the occurrence of nocturnal panic attacks. This is just what has been found in sleep laboratories, where respiratory changes, increased body movements, heart rate accelerations, and increased sweat gland activity have all been observed just prior to nocturnal attacks and subsequent awakening (Craske, 1993; Hauri et al., 1989; Craske & Rowe, 1997b). Craske and Rowe have constructed a model of factors contributing to the maintenance of nocturnal panic attacks, which is presented in Figure 4.4.

It is also interesting that slow-wave sleep tends to be associated with reduced eye movements, lowered blood pressure, and reduced heart rate and respiration. These are also the common characteristics of wakeful relaxation. It is therefore tempting to make a connection between nocturnal panic and relaxation-associated panic as described above (Cohen et al., 1985). Relaxation is known to be associated with cognitive, physiological, or sensory side effects that may be perceived as unpleasant (Heide & Borkovec, 1984). For example, a patient may become alarmed by a decreasing heart rate that occurs during relaxation—a cue to which the panic-prone patient is very sensitive, and which may therefore trigger a panic attack (see Chapter 5). Similarly, as noted above, a sleeping individual may be oblivious to his or her environment, but may remain attuned to personally significant stimuli. For example, a mother may be undisturbed by the noise of a loud truck driving past her house, but may awaken to the sound of her baby crying. Thus relaxation-associated panics and nocturnal panics may be closely related.

TABLE 4.4. Reactions of Patients with Panic Disorder Who Had Nocturnal Panic Attacks, and of Matched Healthy Controls, to Audio Signals That Ostensibly Measured Autonomic Arousal during Sleep

	Group			
	Nocturnal panic (n = 18)		Control (n = 18)	
Measure	M	SD	M	SD
Anxiety rating (0–8)				
ER	1.1	1.4	1.3	1.2
UN	4.5	1.8	2.7	1.6
Sum of symptom ratings (0–52)				
ER	2.1	2.0	4.0	4.9
UN	11.7	7.7	4.3	4.7
Latency to press event button (min)				
ER	28.1	16.6	37.3	9.1
UN	27.3	17.1	34.3	11.6
	%		%	
Abrupt awakening				
ER	22		11	
UN	44		11	
Abrupt symptoms				
ER	22		0	
UN	67		11	
Abrupt fear				
ER	11		0	
UN	44		0	
Panic				
ER	11		0	
UN	44		0	

Note. Panic disorder patients who were led to believe that the signals were unexpected and who were not given reassuring information about arousal during sleep (UN) were more anxious and symptomatic and were more likely to waken with abrupt fear and panic than patients who were led to believe that the signals were to be expected and who were given reassuring information about arousal during sleep (ER). Fewer differences existed between control participants. From "Expectations about Arousal and Nocturnal Panic" by M. G. Craske and S. Freed, 1995, *Journal of Abnormal Psychology, 104,* 567–575. Copyright 1995 by the American Psychological Association. Reprinted with permission.

A Definition of Panic

In the process of constructing the anxiety disorders section of DSM-IV, we struggled with appropriate definitions of panic attacks that would incorporate not only the cognitive and somatic symptoms reviewed above, but also other features of this alarm response that make it unique (Barlow et al., 1994). Prospective studies have determined that subjective "intensity" is a dimension that successfully discriminates panic from other, more tonic emotional states such as anxiety (e.g., Başoğlu et al., 1992), although intensity alone would not be a marker for panic (Freedman et al., 1985). Furthermore, a few individuals do not report fear or terror, although all panics are associated with reports of intense discomfort. I discuss "nonfearful" panic attacks below.

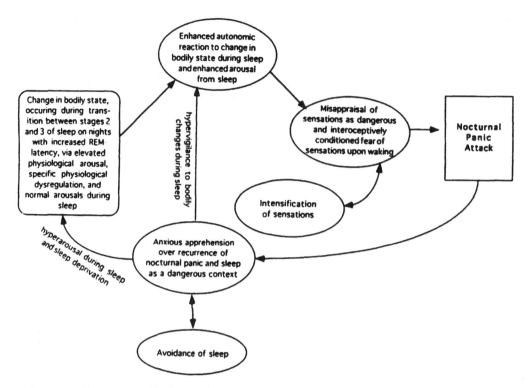

FIGURE 4.4. Factors contributing to the persistence of nocturnal panic attacks in panic disorder. From Craske and Rowe (1997b). Copyright 1997 by Oxford University Press. Reprinted by permission.

Abruptness, among other characteristics, seems to distinguish panic from anxiety and thus may be a crucial element to any definition of panic. The addition of abruptness as an essential criterion of panic would be consistent with the conception of panic as an emotional "alarm" prompting immediate action (fight or flight). Accordingly, it would be inappropriate to plot average values of anxiety across participants over a relatively long period of time, because this would confound panic and anticipatory anxiety. It may be that only subjects showing an instantaneous alarm reaction, both subjectively and physiologically peaking within 3–5 minutes, can be said to be experiencing panic (as in Figure 4.1). Indeed, most naturally occurring attacks, serendipitously recorded, look much like those in Figure 4.1 in terms of rapid and abrupt surges peaking in 1–4 minutes (e.g., Freedman et al., 1985; Lader & Mathews, 1970; Taylor et al., 1986). Difficulties arise when we consider including more objective physiological indices, such as heart rate increases or hyperventilation, as an essential component in any definition of panic. Numerous studies have clearly indicated that panic is often accompanied by sudden heart rate increases (e.g., Cohen et al., 1985; Kenardy, Evans, & Oei, 1988; Lader & Mathews, 1970; Taylor et al., 1983). These increases are not only reported subjectively, but are also measured objectively in ambulatory monitoring studies (Kenardy et al., 1988; Lint et al., 1995; Taylor et al., 1986). Nevertheless, it is also very clear that abrupt physiological surges in isolation are quite common and have no implications for a definition of panic. More problematic are patients' clear reports of a sudden surge of fear or terror in the absence of physiological indices of this event, as reviewed above (Kenardy et al., 1988; Lint et al., 1995). Among physiological indices, heart rate alone may not prove to be the best marker of panic in all cases. Perhaps a combination of measures, including heart rate and pCO_2, and possibly other physiological indicators of an alarm response, might prove to be useful. For example, objective assessment of panic attacks using respiratory or transcutaneous CO_2 level may prove helpful in this regard (Hibbert, 1986; Pilsbury & Hibbert, 1987). Of course, these physiological indicators may be impractical to measure in most clinical settings. We should recognize that the peripheral manifestation of what is almost certainly a central process may be inhibited or otherwise discordant with a strong subjective experience of panic. Nevertheless, the data from Figures 4.1 and 4.2 and the other data reviewed above indicate that the prototypical panic is accompanied by these surges, and therefore that these surges should form part of a specific and conservative, although perhaps less sensitive, research definition of panic. Ley (1992), in an interesting comment, also concluded that a much narrower definition of "classic" panic attacks should be based in part on objectively measured increases in physiological indices, although he emphasized respiratory measures, consistent with his view of the importance of hyperventilation in panic.

The study of emotion has produced wide agreement that emotions are expressed in three response systems: subjective, physiological, and behavioral (Lang, 1968). This principle must be considered when defining panic, and therefore the behavioral component must also be an important part of any precise definition of panic. A clear behavioral expression of panic would be an overwhelming urge to escape a situation, usually followed by the escape behavior itself. This would be consistent with models viewing panic as activation of the fight-or-flight emotional system (Barlow, 1991a; Gray & McNaughton, 1996). Moreover, this behavior differs from the common anticipatory phobic avoidance that develops secondary to panic. Ley (1992) comes to a similar conclusion from a different perspective. Clinically, most patients with panic disorder report overwhelming, if irrational, urges to escape during their panic attacks. These urges become a salient part of their experience. For instance, many avoid situations where this strong emotional urge to act might be blocked (e.g., in formal social gatherings or in dentists' or beauty salon chairs). Although known only through clinical observations at present (and self-reports of these urges and resulting escape behavior), the behavioral component of panic attacks may well be the experience of this overwhelming urge to escape. Future research may demonstrate that the behavioral component contributes more to the definition of panic than does the component involving objectively measured, peripheral physiological surges.

In summary, the typical panic attack seems to be a unique psychological event characterized by feelings of apprehension, terror, or impending doom; a report of four (or more) somatic symptoms or fears of losing control or dying; and a clear and pressing urge to escape or flee. Often these attacks are also accompanied by heart rate elevations of approximately 40 BPM that cannot be accounted for by physical exercise. In these cases, panic seems a clear example of the ancient alarm reaction of fear (Darwin, 1872). Occasionally, these attacks may be "limited," in that fewer than four symptoms are reported and/or they are not accompanied by marked elevation in physiological measures. These "limited" attacks are often, but not always, rated as less intense. Finally, some patients report panic in the absence of any clear biological markers, such as rapid elevation in physiological responding. It is possible that these patients have become sensitized to any number of somatic and cognitive events formerly associated with panic, and that these events are now "construed" as panic by the patients. In any case, with the dramatic presentation of this terrifying event, it is surprising that we have recognized its significance only recently.

CONCEPTIONS OF PANIC IN TIMES PAST

In view of the nature and significance of panic, why was it not recognized earlier? The answer is that it *was* recognized and given a variety of names, many of which depicted hypothetical causes of this sudden burst of emotion. In fact, attacks have been observed and reported for hundreds of years, but the significance of panic was overlooked. Instead, the phenomenon was integrated into various theories of pathology, both psychological and physical.

As indicated at the beginning of this chapter, one does not have to look beyond Freud for a cogent description of panic. Freud accomplished the unique and singular task of integrating almost every facet of human behavior and emotion into an all-encompassing theory. Whatever one thinks of his theoretical constructs, his extraordinary intellectual achievement rests in his ability to integrate, on a conceptual level, so much of our experience. The experience of anxiety is no exception, and because of their prominence within psychoanalytic theory, Freud's views on anxiety and panic are particularly interesting from a historical perspective.

Freud actually distinguished three types of anxiety. In 1917 he noted differences among free-floating or generalized anxiety, which he referred to as "expectant anxiety"; "phobic anxiety," or anxiety that only occurs in specific situations; and "anxiety attacks." On the basis of his descriptions, these "anxiety attacks" would be called "panic" today (Freud, 1917/1963). In fact, even earlier in 1895, he seemed to describe very clearly the process of the development of agoraphobia when he stated, "In the case of agoraphobia, etc., we often find *the recollection of an anxiety attack*; and what the patient actually fears is the occurrence of such an attack under the special conditions in which he believes he cannot escape it" (1895/1962, p. 81; Freud's italics). Unfortunately, as Klein (1983) points out, Freud's clear observations eventually became blurred by the heavy theoretical baggage that his constructs of anxiety carried, and by 1932 these distinctions had been largely lost.

A more interesting but completely different view of the phenomenon arose over the years within the field of medicine and the subspecialty of cardiology in particular. For example, in 1871, DaCosta described a syndrome he encountered in a series of 300 patients he saw during the Civil War in the United States. This syndrome was characterized by palpitations, dizziness, and so on, and originated without any clear cause. DaCosta called it "irritable heart." In England during World War I, Lewis (1917) described a condition he referred to as "effort syndrome," which in fact seemed to be a collection of the same symptoms observed by DaCosta during the American Civil War. Lewis called it "effort syndrome" because he observed this problem in a large series of soldiers who developed the syndrome during physical exertion associated with their combat activities. He noted that this problem seemed to occur in those soldiers with "constitutional weaknesses," either nervous or physical, or in those "played out" by exposure and strain. His early reference to stress as a precipitant is still interesting (see Chapter 6). It is also interesting, in light of recent theories, that he suspected blood acidosis produced by changes in CO_2 or lactate acid levels as playing a role in the genesis of these attacks (see Chapter 5).

From somewhat different points of view, Oppenheim (1918) and Cohen and White, conducting epidemiological work in the 1940s and 1950s (Cohen, Badal, Kilpatrick, Reid, & White, 1951; Cohen & White, 1950), referred to seemingly the same syndrome as "neurocirculatory asthenia." This was the old term for anxiety states with marked cardiovascular features.

In the meantime, Roth (1959, 1960) identified a separate syndrome, which he and his colleagues termed the "phobic anxiety–depersonalization syndrome." In a particularly perceptive analysis of 135 patients with this syndrome, Roth (1959) suggested that the phenomenon of depersonalization, and the underlying psychophysiology of the regulation of awareness associated with depersonalization, might be important keys to the disorder. But his major contribution was to set off this group of patients, who presented very clearly with panic attacks, in a nosological way from "those with anxiety neurosis," who were not fully described in his papers but most probably presented with generalized anxiety. The distinction between panic and generalized anxiety has since become a subject of intense study.

Various other labels have been used over the decades to refer to what seems to be the same disorder. These include "vasoregulatory asthenia," "nervous tachycardia," "vasomotor neurosis," and "nervous exhaustion" (Cohen & White, 1950).

THE "UNIQUENESS" OF PANIC

Is the psychological experience of panic a truly unique event? To be unique, it should be qualitatively different from the more usual generalized anxiety with which we are all so familiar. As we observed above, panic has always attracted attention in the clinical literature, but usually these experiences were described as "anxiety attacks"; the implication was that these experiences were simply manifestations of intense anxiety.

Donald Klein and Pharmacological Dissection

As is so often the case in science, the initial suggestion that panic might be qualitatively different was based on an insightful clinical hunch. This clinical hunch was then bolstered by a line of research that came to be called "pharmacological dissection." In fact, this approach provided only weak evidence supporting panic as a qualitatively different experience. Nevertheless, this clinical hunch and the subsequent research it generated opened up other more direct and powerful lines of investigation, from which we have learned much about the nature of panic.

In 1959, when individuals with agoraphobias were still called "schizophrenics" by most clinicians because of their severe symptoms and marked social impairment, Donald Klein began studying the then new and unmarketed drug imipramine. Although expecting a stimulant effect, he found, much to his surprise, that imipramine first caused sedation in depressed patients, followed after several weeks by marked improvement in mood. At this time, Klein had a number of patients on his unit who, in retrospect, were experiencing panic attacks. Since these patients were not responding to other forms of psychotherapy or drug therapy, Klein decided to try imipramine—not because of any prior scientific findings indicating that it would be effective, but rather, "it was more a case of our not knowing what else to do for them, and thinking that perhaps this strange new safe agent with peculiar tranquilizing powers might work" (Klein, 1981, p. 237). Initially, patients, ward staff, nurses, and therapists noted no improvement whatsoever from these drugs. But after several weeks the nurses observed that the patients had stopped running to the nurses' station with protests of dying or losing control. When asked, the patients said that they'd stopped running to the nurses' station because they had learned that the nurses couldn't do anything for them!

Klein published these clinical results in 1962 (Klein & Fink, 1962), and reported on a small double-blind study in 1964 (Klein, 1964). In this double-blind study, which was part of a larger study, 14 patients who had been described as having "affective disorders" were reclassified as having "phobic anxiety reactions," based on a retrospective diagnostic review. Of these, 6 received placebo, 7 received imipramine, and 1 received chlorpromazine. The patient on chlorpromazine had the poorest response of any of the 14 and actually deteriorated somewhat. However, based on global clinical ratings by two psychiatrists, the 7 on imipramine improved more than the 6 receiving placebo.

Although panic was not specifically measured in this very early study, Klein's clinical observations were that the drug reduced or eliminated panic attacks, but did nothing for the chronic anticipatory anxiety continuously present, which seemed to keep the patients from leaving a safe place or a safe person. As Klein concluded,

> [T]he panic attack was much more severe than the chronic anxiety, but one could hardly believe that the panic attack was simply the quantitative extreme of chronic anxiety since imipramine could dispel the apparently worse anxiety, but had little effect on the chronic minor form. Again, this implied a qualitative discontinuity between these two distressing affects that had initially seemed so similar. (1981, p. 239)

Thus Klein noted that imipramine had a very specific effect on panic attacks, and therefore panic attacks were "dissected" from generalized chronic or anticipatory anxiety as a qualitatively different state.

Unfortunately, inferring something about the nature of a psychopathological state by observing treatment effects is a very weak experimental approach, subject to a logical fallacy (*post hoc ergo propter hoc*, or "the result implies the cause"). The weakness of this experimental approach becomes an issue again when the nature of panic is explored further below. But, nevertheless, this type of evidence was suggestive and was found again in the following experiment, conducted from a somewhat different vantage point.

Psychological Dissection

The purpose of one preliminary experiment in our clinic at Albany was to evaluate the effects of psychosocial treatments on intense anxiety that included but was not limited to panic episodes (Waddell, Barlow, & O'Brien, 1984). Three patients with panic disorder were treated with a combination treatment, consisting of a cognitive therapy phase followed by a phase combining cognitive therapy and relaxation training. The phases were introduced in a staggered fashion, so that each therapeutic phase was started for different patients at different times in a multiple-baseline-across-subjects experimental design format (Barlow & Hersen, 1984). This allowed us to observe specific effects of therapeutic procedures as they were introduced to each patient. The patients recorded both number and duration of episodes of "heightened or intense" anxiety and panic, using detailed self-monitoring forms devised for this purpose. In addition, they recorded ratings of chronic background anxiety (not necessarily associated with periods of intense anxiety and panic) four times a day. All patients demonstrated a marked decrease in the number and duration of episodes of intense anxiety and panic—an improvement that was maintained at a 3-month follow-up. However, two patients showed a clear increase in background anxiety at the same time that episodes of intense anxiety were lessening during the combined treatment phase. For the third patient, chronic background anxiety decreased in synchrony with episodes of panic.

This experiment suffered from the same logical flaws as the early work in pharmacological dissection, since it would be tempting to conclude from these results that there are two different types of anxiety. In addition, results from only three subjects were reported, and only two of them showed the "split" in their recordings of panic versus chronic background anxiety. In fact, most treatment outcome data for patients with panic disorder show clear reductions in both panic attacks and anxiety. It is possible that certain treatments (both psychological and pharmacological) are effective for anxiety in some patients only when anxiety is "intense," but that this intense anxiety or panic does not differ in any real qualitative way from less intense anxiety. Despite their weaknesses, these results were also suggestive, and paved the way for more direct comparisons of panic and anxiety.

Direct Phenomenological Comparisons of Panic and Anxiety

Further supporting evidence for differences between anxiety and panic came from some of the early studies described previously in this chapter, where both anxiety and panic were monitored during day-to-day activities. For example, Taylor et al. (1986) had patients wear ambulatory devices to record both anticipatory anxiety and panic in the manner described earlier over a period of 6 days. In each of eight periods of intense anticipatory anxiety, heart rate remained relatively stable, and was significantly lower than heart rate recorded during panic attacks. Heart rate averaged 89.2 BPM during anticipatory anxiety, as compared to 108.2 BPM during spontaneous panic attacks. These differences in heart rate occurred in spite of the fact that subjective ratings of intensity during the two types of anxiety were virtually identical.

In a similar vein, Freedman et al. (1985) measured heart rate during self-reported panic attacks and also observed heart rate during "control periods," in which anxiety was reported as equally intense, but was not labeled as panic. For example, if a panic attack was rated at an intensity of 80 on a scale of 0–100, the investigators examined heart rate at another time when the patient also reported anxiety to be at an intensity of 80 but did not report a panic attack. Presumably, these control periods represented anticipatory or generalized anxiety. Abrupt heart rate elevations did not occur during these control periods. This is illustrated for several patients in Figure 4.5.

These studies were useful, since they showed that a direct comparison of panic and anxiety in the same patients is possible. Another line of evidence comes from studies comparing groups of patients with diagnoses of GAD or panic disorder, most usually on various questionnaire measures. This is a weaker approach, since patients with panic disorder also experience marked anticipatory or generalized anxiety. Nevertheless, some interesting information is available from these sources.

In our clinic, an early series of patients with panic disorder evidenced a stronger somatic component to their anxiety than did patients with GAD on questionnaire measures of anxiety (Barlow, Cohen, et al., 1984). Subjects with panic disorder scored significantly higher on the Somatic scale of the Cognitive and Somatic Anxiety Questionnaire (panic disorder mean = 23.9; GAD mean = 15.50; $t = 2.91$, $p < .02$). Scores on the Cognitive scale, on the other hand, did not differ, although the mean score was slightly higher for subjects with GAD (panic disorder mean = 17.55; GAD mean = 18.38). Hoehn-Saric (1981) compared 15 patients with GAD to 36 patients with mixed anxiety disorders who were suffering from panic attacks. Scores on a variety of questionnaires, including the Somatic Symptom Scale, the Eysenck Personality Inventory, and the State–Trait Anxiety Inventory, were compared. Essentially no differences emerged between the groups, with the exception of scores on the Somatic Symptom Scale. Patients with panic attacks scored significantly higher on this scale, indicating more intense and more severe somatic signs of anxiety (e.g., muscle tension, respiratory symptoms, palpitations, etc.).

Other studies have replicated this finding by demonstrating a stronger somatic presentation in patients with panic disorder than in patients with GAD (Anderson, Noyes,

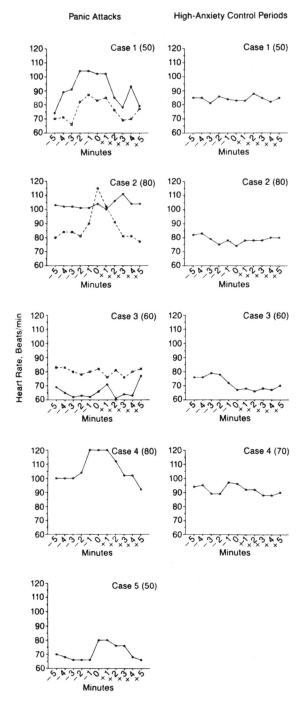

FIGURE 4.5. Heart rates during panic attacks and high-anxiety control periods. Anxiety ratings are shown in parentheses after case numbers. Solid lines represent first attack; dotted lines, second attack. From Freedman, Ianni, Ettedgui, and Puthezhath (1985). Copyright 1985 by the American Medical Association. Reprinted by permission.

& Crowe, 1984; Rapee, 1985). The lack of differences observed on measures of "general" anxiety such as the State–Trait Anxiety Inventory in these studies is interesting, since patients suffering primarily from panic do not score higher on these scales, as might be the case if panic disorder were simply a more intense version of GAD. In fact, Rapee (1985) reported in an early study that patients with panic disorder in Australia scored lower than patients with GAD on the Taylor Manifest Anxiety Scale.

More recently, Peter Lang and his associates found a different pattern of psychophysiological responses in a group of individuals with specific phobias, such as animal phobias, compared to individuals with more diffuse anxiety disorders (McNeil, Vrana, Melamed, Cuthbert, & Lang, 1993). That is, patients with specific phobias showed a marked visceral response to phobic stimuli, which the authors associated with a fearful and escape-oriented action tendency. More generally anxious patients, on the other hand, seemed oriented toward passive avoidance, restlessness, negative self-talk, and worry. Patients with panic also present with a different pattern of cognitions and cognitive activity than do patients with anxiety but without panic (Hibbert, 1984; Rapee, 1985). This pattern of catastrophic thoughts concerning present danger (dying, losing control, etc.) certainly fits with the notion of panic as the ancient emotion of fear. Of course, these differences may be epiphenomenal, reflecting defining characteristics of patients falling into this category rather than something fundamental about panic. For example, the tendency for patients with panic disorder to overreport and exaggerate somatic symptoms has been mentioned above.

On the other hand, Craske (1999) reviews evidence highlighting a potential distinction between anxiety and panic (fear) in information processing. Several reports have noted that processing of information may actually decrease substantially at the height of intense fear, perhaps because the cognitions associated with this fundamental and ancient emotion are elementary and automatic, in contrast to the more complex information processing associated with anxiety (Watts, Trezise, & Sharrock, 1986; Goldsmith, 1994). In fact, S. L. Williams, Kinney, Harap, and Liebmann (1997) noted that few, if any, cognitions reflecting danger or extreme threat are present during actual periods of exposure to highly fearful situations.

Clear phenomenological distinctions between fear and anxiety are also present in the emotional expressions of individuals without psychological disorders. For example, we (Craske, Brown, Meadows, & Barlow, 1995) monitored commonly reported emotional episodes of sadness, panic, anger, and excitement that occurred for no apparent reason (uncued) in a large group of college students. From 10% to 34% of the sample reported instances of these well-defined acute emotional experiences, but a much smaller percentage reported a more pervasive anxiety or distress associated with these emotions. Similar findings have been obtained in factor-analytic work on emotional expression in normal populations. For example, as mentioned in Chapter 2, Tellegen (1982, 1985) in constructing his circumplex of emotion found that factors associated with fear on the one hand or anxiety on the other loaded on orthogonal higher order factors. Ollendick, Yule, and Ollier (1991) studying children found that items on a fear scale are relatively homogeneous and load on factors that are clearly distinct from items shared by anxiety and depression scales. It is also clear that these two factors are not only seemingly independent but also relate in very different ways to other anxiety disorders and depression. For example, recent structural equation modeling and factor analyses of symptomatology in clinically anxious patients in the context of work exploring the dimensions of anxiety and depression, as reviewed in Chapter 3, has uncovered, among other things, two separable factors. One is characterized by strong autonomic arousal, which seems best described as panic; the other is characterized by apprehension and worry accompanied by tension, which are best described as anxiety (Brown, Chorpita, & Barlow, 1998; Mineka, Watson, & Clark, 1998; Zinbarg & Barlow, 1996). Anxiety, a principal component of GAD, is very closely related to depression. The strong autonomic arousal characteristic of panic, on the other hand, is substantially restricted in patients with GAD (Borkovec, 1994a; Hoehn-Saric, McLeod, & Zimmerli, 1989; Brown et al., 1998).

Perhaps the strongest supporting data on the uniqueness of panic comes from an increasingly strong web of neurobiological evidence supporting the existence of at least two negative emotional states occupying different brain circuits, reviewed in some detail in Chapter 6. This includes the observation of different patterns of regional brain activity associated with anxious apprehension on the one hand, and panic on the other (Heller, Nitschke, Etienne, & Miller, 1997).

In summary, there is strong but not yet definitive evidence that panic is a unique event distinguishable from anxiety on the basis of presenting characteristics, neurobiology, and functional analyses.

THE UBIQUITY OF PANIC

Panic across Different Diagnostic Categories

In view of the distinctive presentation of panic, it is important to determine the prevalence of panic across different diagnostic categories. Panic attacks were first observed, of course, in the context of panic disorder where attacks occurred in an unexpected fashion without identifiable cues (thus the term "spontaneous"). To determine the prevalence of panic across various diagnostic categories, we examined for panic attacks in 108 consecutive patients meeting DSM-III anxiety or affective disorder diagnoses in an early study (Barlow et al., 1985), using a semistructured interview, the Anxiety Disorders Interview Schedule (ADIS; Di Nardo, O'Brien, Barlow, Waddell, & Blanchard, 1983) (see Chapter 9).

During each interview, patients were asked about the occurrence of any panic attacks and about their onset and frequency. Specifically, each patient was asked, "Have you had times when you felt a sudden rush of intense fear or anxiety or feelings of impending doom?" If the patient admitted to having had a panic attack, he or she was then asked about each of the 12 symptoms of panic attacks listed in DSM-III. Questions centered on presence or absence and degree of intensity of each symptom, using a typical or the most recent attack as a point of reference. Each symptom was rated by the interviewer on a 5-point scale of severity (0 = "absent," 4 = "very severe"). "Spontaneity" of the panic attack was ascertained by careful questioning regarding the circumstances surrounding the panic, as well as whether the panic was expected or not.

Table 4.5 lists the frequencies of primary diagnoses represented by the sample, along with the mean age and sex distribution for each diagnostic category. Also included in this table are the percentages of each subgroup who reported having had a panic attack and the percentage who met the DSM-III criteria for panic disorder. A "report of panic" meant that the patients answered "yes" to the question "Have you ever had times when you felt a sudden rush of intense fear or anxiety or feelings of impending doom?" "Diagnosis met except for panic frequency" meant that the patients reported panic and also reported at least 4 of the 12 symptoms listed as associated with panic in DSM-III. "Diagnosis on

TABLE 4.5. Sample Descriptors and Incidence of Panic across Diagnostic Categories

Variable	Agoraphobia with panic	Social phobia	Simple phobia	Panic disorder	GAD	Obsessive–compulsive	Major depressive episode	Statistical comparison
Men (n)	2	10	2	6	8	2	1	
Women (n)	39	9	5	11	4	4	5	
Mean age (in years)	36.2_{ab}	28.8_a	44.6_{bc}	34.8_a	36.1_{ab}	28.5_a	46.3_c	$F(6, 101) = 4.64**$
Reports of panic (%)	98	89	100	100	83	83	83	$\chi^2 (6, n = 108) = 7.27$
Diagnosis met except for panic frequency (%)	98	84	85	100	75	83	83	$\chi^2 (6, n = 108) = 9.50$
Diagnosis on DSM-III panic criteria (%)	74	50	33	82	29	t	t	$\chi^2 (6, n = 108) = 14.67*$

Note. Categories sharing subscripts are not significantly different by Duncan's multiple-range test. t, n's were too low to analyze because of missing data on panic frequency. However, for the 3 obsessive–compulsives and 3 depressed patients for whom we had complete data, 100% met the criteria. GAD, generalized anxiety disorder. From Barlow, D. H., Vermilyea, J. A., Blanchard, E. B., Vermilyea, B. B., Di Nardo, P. A., & Cerny, J. A. (1985). The phenomenon of panic. *Journal of Abnormal Psychology, 94,* 320–328. Copyright 1985 by the American Psychological Association. Reprinted by permission.

*p < .03.

**p < .001.

DSM-III panic criteria" meant that the patients reported panic, met the 4 symptom criteria, and reported at least three panics in a 3-week period.

Six patients eventually received a consensus diagnosis of major depressive disorder. Of course, these patients did not represent a random sample of major depression, since they were referred to our clinic for problems with anxiety. Nevertheless, their data are included for comparison purposes.

From Table 4.5, it is clear that panic was a ubiquitous problem among these patients with anxiety disorders: At least 83% of patients in each diagnostic category reported at least one panic attack. Furthermore, almost all patients reporting a panic attack (a sudden rush of intense fear) also endorsed at least 4 of the 12 symptoms necessary to meet the DSM-III definition of panic. Only in regard to the frequency criteria did differences among diagnostic groups emerge: The percentages of patients with social phobia, simple phobia, and GAD who met the frequency criteria were markedly lower than the percentage with panic disorder. The apparent anomaly in Table 4.5, whereby only 82% of patients with a diagnosis of panic disorder met the full DSM-III criteria, was an artifact of the methods used (see Barlow et al., 1985). Further analyses in this study of number of symptoms or symptom severity of panic attacks among diagnostic groups revealed no important differences. Thus this early report suggested that some attacks are unique psychopathological events that are common occurrences in any number of disorders. Since that time, numerous studies have confirmed the ubiquity of panic and its essential nature across different diagnostic groups, with important differences occurring only in triggers or cues for the attacks (e.g., Craske, 1991, 1999).

Other early studies observed a high prevalence of panic attacks in mood disorders. For example, Leckman, Weissman, Merikangas, Pauls, and Prusoff (1983), using DSM-III criteria, reanalyzed data from a large group of 133 patients with major depressive disorder and found that nearly 25% met the criteria for panic disorder or agoraphobia with panic attacks. Since the criterion for panic disorder was a very strict one of six panics in a 6-week period, this was a very high percentage. Breier, Charney, and Heninger (1984) noted that over 80% of their depressed patients reported panic attacks. In a study from our clinic at Albany that was designed to answer this question, the percentage of patients with DSM-III affective disorders who presented with panic was approximately 50% (Benshoof, 1987). Subsequent studies have repeatedly confirmed these findings (Brown & Barlow, 1992; Brown, Antony, & Barlow, 1995). Whether patients with mood disorders experience panic attacks or not may have important implications for classification (see Chapter 9).

Evidence on the ubiquity of panic also exists in psychiatric disorders other than anxiety and mood disorders. Boyd (1986) extracted information from the large Epidemiologic Catchment Area study (reviewed in Chapter 1) on the percentage of patients with different diagnoses who reported at least one panic attack in the last 6 months. The results are presented in Table 4.6. The results varied widely across sites, but the rates were very high for a number of disorders. In our own center at Boston University, efforts are underway to treat panic attacks in individuals with schizophrenia, where panic greatly complicates the clinical picture (Hofmann, Bufka, Brady, DuRand, & Goff, 2000).

DSM-IV has implicitly recognized the ubiquity of panic by noting that panic attacks may accompany withdrawal from substances such as barbiturates, intoxication due to caffeine or amphetamines, and so on. More importantly, DSM-IV has pointed out the now well-known fact that panic attacks occur in the context of specific or social phobias, although only in the phobic situation. That is, there are clear "cues" for the panic attacks. For this reason, descriptions and definitions of panic attacks are separated from defini-

TABLE 4.6. Prevalence of Panic Attacks among Subjects with Other Diagnoses in Five Sites: Weighted Data (in Percents)

Diagnostic Interview Schedule	New Haven 1980–1981 ($n = 5,034$)	Baltimore 1981–1982 ($n = 3,481$)	St. Louis 1981–1982 ($n = 3,004$)	Durham, NC 1982–1983 ($n = 3,921$)	Los Angeles 1983–1984 ($n = 3,132$)
Somatization	44	—[a]	34	49	—[a]
Schizophrenia	28	35	62	33	63
Major depressive episode	39	25	42	24	25
Mania	41	18	53	31	19
Dysthymia	21	19	8	8	15
Obsessive–compulsive	35	25	32	24	23
Antisocial personality	30	27	13	6	9
Phobia	26	13	28	12	23
Alcohol abuse or dependence	6	12	10	6	7
Drug abuse or dependence	17	12	9	6	6
Cognitive impairment (severe)	2	6	5	1	2

Note. From Boyd (1986).
[a]There were too few cases to make a stable estimate.

tions of any one disorder, and placed in the anxiety disorder section prior to descriptions of criteria for specific anxiety disorders.

Nonfearful Panic

Panic is also astonishingly prevalent in the offices of nonpsychiatric medical specialists, as indicated in several early reports. Beitman, DeRosear, Basha, Flaker, and Corcoran (1987) discovered that 40% of a group of cardiology patients with nonanginal chest pain evidenced clear panic attacks. Katon, Vitaliano, Russo, Jones, and Anderson (1987) reported that 36% of 195 primary care patients were diagnosed with panic disorder. Klonoff, Polefrone, Dambrocia, and Nochomovitz (1986) reported that the problem was sufficiently pervasive among patients with chronic obstructive pulmonary disease that the American Lung Association had published a self-help book for these patients on managing panic.

More recent reports confirm these early findings. For example, a number of reports have focused attention on a group of subjects defined in the literature as having "nonfearful panic disorder" (NFPD). Many patients with NFPD present to cardiologists with chest pain without cardiac pathology, and report what seem to be physiological attacks without subjective fear or without cognitive symptoms or attributions such as dying, going crazy, or losing control (Beitman, DeRosear, et al., 1987; Kushner & Beitman, 1990; Kushner, Beitman, & Bartels, 1990). These patients seem to experience distress or anxiety over these out-of-the-blue events, because they subsequently seek help. However, this anxiety or distress is focused very narrowly on chest pain (or related symptoms) and does not generalize to other somatic sensations (Beck, Berisford, Taegtmeyer, & Bennett, 1990; Beck, Taegtmeyer, Berisford, & Bennett, 1989).

One must be cautious in considering nonfearful panics, because the features of these phenomena that overlap with panic attacks (i.e., marked autonomic surge and brief rise time) are shared by other emotional states as well (e.g., anger, excitement; cf. Fava, Anderson, & Rosenbaum, 1990). An interesting direction for future study would be to examine whether subjects with NFPD experience surges that are at least partially connected with other emotions (e.g., anger), and that subsequently produce distress and result in consultation with a cardiologist. For example, whereas other similarities have been noted between NFPD and panic disorder (e.g., associated symptomatology and familial aggregation; see Kushner & Beitman, 1990, for a review), these similarities may well be a function of emotionality in general rather than of panic attacks per se (cf. Barlow, 1988; Eysenck, 1970).

However, a more trivial explanation seems likely. These individuals, who do not report panic or associated negative attributions (e.g., fear of dying or going crazy), nevertheless report behavioral changes consistent with fear and anxiety. For example, the DSM-IV field trial on panic disorder identified a group of patients who otherwise met criteria for panic disorder, but who reported no anxiety over future panics or negative attributions concerning panics. All of these patients were found in primary care settings. Despite not reporting anxiety over future panic, each patient had changed his or her behavior immediately after experiencing panic. Many developed mild escape or avoidance behavior; some became preoccupied and somewhat withdrawn from their families; and so on. For this reason, Criterion A in DSM-IV was altered to cover these individuals by noting that panic was followed by "a significant change in behavior related to the attacks" (p. 402). Thus, whereas the overwhelming majority of patients meeting criteria for panic disorder report anxiety over a subsequent attack or negative attributions concerning the "implications of the attack or its consequences" (p. 402), a small minority, particularly among patients in primary care settings, would meet DSM-IV criteria by virtue of the behavior change criterion. Therefore, NFPD may represent another example of asynchrony among response systems where self-report of fear and anxiety is disconnected from behavior and physiology (although discomfort is reported).

Nonclinical Panic

Studies from around the world are converging to suggest that occasional panic attacks are also relatively frequent in the general population. The first study to suggest this was reported by Norton, Harrison, Hauch, and Rhodes (1985), who administered questionnaires to 186 presumably normal young adults. Fully 34.4% of these subjects reported having had one or more panic attacks in the past year. The percentage reporting more frequent attacks during the past year decreased markedly. For example, of this 34.4%, 17.2% reported two or more attacks in the past year; 11.3% reported three to four panic attacks; and 6% reported five or more attacks in the past year. In the past 3 weeks, 17.2% reported experiencing one panic attack, while 4.8% (nine subjects) reported two panic attacks in the past week—a frequency that met DSM-III criteria for panic disorder. In addition, 2.1% (four subjects) reported avoiding some activities or situations because of panic attacks.

One interesting facet of these data is that the number reporting panic attacks that would meet clinical criteria was very close to (and even a little bit less than) what we might expect, given the epidemiological investigations reviewed in Chapter 1 (e.g., Myers et al., 1984; Kessler et al, 1994). This fact, as well as subsequent replication, lends credence to these data. These individuals with nonclinical panic also reported significantly more depression, anxiety, and phobic anxiety on the well-known and often used Hopkins Symptom Checklist 90 (Derogatis, Lipman, & Covi, 1973) than those who had never panicked.

It is also interesting to observe that these individuals with nonclinical panic seemed to experience fewer symptoms and less severe symptoms during their panics than patients. For example, two-thirds of those with infrequent panic experienced 6 symptoms or fewer, whereas two-thirds of the patients in clinical samples described earlier reported 10 or more symptoms. In addition, patients reported average symptom severity ratings of 5.5 on a scale of 0–8, while the average symptom severity score of those with nonclinical panic was 3.0. Of course, as Norton, Harrison, et al. (1985) suggest, some of these people might progress later into full-blown panic disorder and increase the number of symptoms they would report, as well as their ratings of symptom severity.

Although the assessment of the presence or absence of panic attacks by questionnaire can be justifiably criticized, more careful assessment of 24 of these nonclinical subjects who reported panic by structured interview revealed that 22 met DSM-III criteria for panic attacks (but not necessarily panic disorder). The remaining two subjects actually reported experiencing intense nonpanic anxiety (Harrison, 1985). This finding also supports the validity of these data.

In a cross-validation study reported by Norton, Dorward, and Cox (1986), 256 subjects completed a variety of questionnaires, including a more sophisticated questionnaire than was utilized in the first study. This questionnaire assessed not only the presence or absence of panic attacks, but severity, temporal factors associated with the attacks, whether the attacks were predictable or unpredictable, and so on. Once again, individuals with nonclinical panic scored significantly higher than those without panic on general anxiety and depression as measured by a number of scales, such as the State–Trait Anxiety Inventory, the Beck Depression Inventory, and the Anxiety and Depression subscales of the Profile of Mood States. Closely replicating the first study, 35.9% (or 92 subjects) reported experiencing one or more panic attacks in the past year, with 22.6% experiencing one or more panic attacks within the past 3 weeks. Other data were also comparable to those of the first report, and both sets of data are presented in Table 4.7.

This replication provided new information regarding the situations in which individuals with nonclinical panic reported experiencing panic attacks. Situations most frequently associated with panic attacks were as follows: public speaking, mentioned by 55.2% of all those with panic; interpersonal conflict, mentioned by 46.6%; periods of high stress, mentioned by 54.5%; and tests and exams, mentioned by 77.3%. In addition, 27.6% of the subjects reported experiencing panic attacks totally out of the blue, or, in other words, without any identifiable precipitant whatsoever. Smaller percentages reported panics during sleep (13.8%) and during relaxation (8.6%). Number and severity of symptoms were similar to those found in the earlier study.

TABLE 4.7. Panic in the Normal Population

	Norton, Harrison, Hauch, & Rhodes (1985)(n = 186)	Norton, Dorward, & Cox (1986)(n = 256)
One or more panics in last year	34.4%	35.9%
Panic frequency last year		
1–2	17.2%	
3–4	11.3%	
5+	6.0%	
Panic frequency last 3 weeks		
1	17.2%	12.5%
2	4.8%	7.0%
3+	2.1%	3.1%

Similar data on the prevalence of panic in the general population have been reported by Salge, Beck, and Logan (1988) and by Norton, Cox, and Malan (1992), who reviewed over 20 studies. Survey data from our clinic at Albany (Rapee, Ancis, & Barlow, 1988) suggest that approximately 14% of the population has experienced uncued, unexpected, "spontaneous" panic. This figure is in close agreement with data collected by Wittchen and Essau (1991) in Germany for this type of panic. Somewhat lower figures for uncued, unexpected panic have more recently been reported for young adolescent girls by Hayward et al. (1997).

Another factor that builds confidence in the validity of these findings concerning the high rates of panic in the general population is evidence on the aggregation of panic and other psychopathology in the families of individuals with nonclinical, infrequent panic. For example, Norton et al. (1986) found that a significantly greater proportion of those with such panic than of those without panic reported fathers, mothers, brothers, and sisters who had had panic attacks. These findings are particularly strong, since the results were statistically significant for each class of relatives, rather than just in the aggregate. These data resemble results demonstrating a high familial aggregation of panic in the families of patients with panic disorder (see Chapter 5). For example, Crowe, Noyes, Pauls, and Slymen (1983) found that 25% of first-order relatives of patients with panic disorder also met DSM-III criteria for panic disorder. An additional 30% experienced infrequent panic attacks. In Norton et al. (1986), approximately 30% of first-order relatives were reported to experience panic. The data from Crowe et al. (1983) also attest to the seemingly high prevalence of panic in the population at large.

In summary, individuals with nonclinical panic tend to report fewer or less intense attacks, and, more importantly, little or no worry or anxiety over having another attack (Telch, Brouillard, Telch, Agras, & Taylor, 1989). However, the validity of these observations is mitigated by the fact that very few studies have examined (or have adequately assessed) the phenomenon of panic in nonclinical samples.

Although many studies have noted that the panics reported by nonclinical subjects share marked phenomenological similarities to the panics of clinical patients (e.g., Brown & Cash, 1989, 1990; Norton et al., 1986), consideration of the literature on nonclinical panic is limited by several facts. First, the procedures used to classify subjects as having or not having such panic have frequently failed to distinguish adequately the various types of panic (e.g., situationally bound [cued] or unexpected [uncued]). Second, nonclinical studies have failed to separate adequately subjects experiencing panic from those experiencing forms of anxiety that could be misclassified as panic (cf. Brown & Cash, 1989). This latter difficulty has stemmed largely from the absence of strict criteria defining panic (e.g., lack of a rise time criterion, the use of yes–no classifications without assessing the presence of a marked autonomic surge accompanied by a report of fear, etc.) and retrospective reporting. Moreover, variations in the method of assessment have significantly affected the observed prevalence rates of nonclinical panic. For example, whereas questionnaire studies have found the past-year prevalence of unexpected (uncued) panic to be in the 10–15% range (e.g., Donnell & McNally, 1990; Rapee, Ancis, & Barlow, 1988; Telch, Brouillard, et al, 1989), studies using structured interviews have observed much lower prevalence rates (e.g., Brown & Deagle, 1992). Of 171 subjects who were administered a validated structured interview to assess panic, Brown and Deagle (1992) found that only 4 (2.3%) had experienced an unexpected (uncued) panic in the prior year, although measurement procedures in this study differed from other studies in ways that may have influenced the results.

DESCRIPTORS OF PANIC: CUED VERSUS UNCUED
AND EXPECTED VERSUS UNEXPECTED

The DSM-IV defines three types of panic attacks: "unexpected (uncued)," "situationally predisposed," and "situationally bound (cued)." This represents the first formal typology of panic in the DSM system, and is meant to be a user-friendly amalgamation of prior suggestions for panic typologies (Klein & Klein, 1989; Barlow, 1988).

Differences between unexpected (uncued) panics and situationally bound (cued) panics have been examined. Following up on earlier reports (e.g., Barlow et al., 1985; Thyer & Himle, 1987), we (Craske et al., 1993) compared symptom endorsement rates for unexpected (uncued) panics and situationally bound (cued) panics in a sample of patients with panic disorder. Some differences were noted in the two types of panic, with unexpected panics associated with significantly higher symptom endorsement ratios.

Rapee, Sanderson, et al. (1992) examined the symptoms of the typical unexpected (uncued) panic attacks reported by 55 patients DSM-III-R panic disorder, and compared these with the symptoms reported by a group of 65 patients with other DSM-III-R anxiety disorders (i.e, patients with either simple phobia, social phobia, or obsessive–compulsive disorder) as accompanying panic upon exposure to their feared cue. Relative to the latter group, patients with panic disorder were more likely to report the following symptoms: fear of dying, fear of going crazy or losing control, paresthesias, dizziness, faintness, unreality, and shortness of breath. Symptom intensity ratings did not differ between groups. In a second study in this report, Rapee, Sanderson, et al. (1992) examined 90 patients with DSM-III-R panic disorder who had a coexisting DSM-III-R diagnosis of social phobia, simple phobia, or obsessive–compulsive disorder, to evaluate symptom profile differences of the panic attacks of patients who experienced both unexpected (uncued) and situationally bound panic. Within this group of patients, differences in the frequency of report occurred for only three symptoms (i.e., fear of dying, fear of going crazy or losing control, and paresthesias), which were reported more frequently as associated with unexpected (uncued) panic attacks. However, unexpected (uncued) panics were also associated with higher symptom intensity ratings for the symptoms of dizziness and trembling. The authors concluded that an attentional bias for interceptive cues, or possibly certain physiological differences (i.e., the tendency to hyperventilate), may have accounted for differences in symptom report between patients with panic disorder and patients with anxiety disorders who did not report unexpected (uncued) panic attacks.

Unfortunately, these data are based on retrospective report. In addition, Rapee, Sanderson, et al. (1992) noted, for example, that the groups without panic disorder were not asked to distinguish their symptoms when fearful in the presence of the phobic cue from those experienced in anticipation of confronting the feared object or situation. Thus it is uncertain whether the symptoms reported by this group were those accompanying panic as opposed to those associated with anticipatory anxiety. Moreover, in data from concurrent self-monitoring (Street et al., 1989), no significant differences have emerged within groups of patients with panic disorder, in either cognitive or somatic symptoms among different categories of panic associated with panic disorder itself. In other words, the types of panic occurring within panic disorder were phenomenologically identical. However, situationally bound (cued) panics tended to be rated as somewhat more severe. In the Margraf et al. (1987) study, and also most recently in a study by Garssen, de Beurs, et al. (1996), situationally bound (cued) or situationally predisposed attacks were also rated as somewhat more severe, but otherwise phenomenologically similar. In this report, severely disturbing cognitions (but not somatic symptoms) tended to be reported more frequently during situational attacks than during unexpected panics.

One study compared panic attacks occurring within panic disorder with panic attacks occurring within DSM-III simple phobias during behavioral approach tests. Rachman, Levitt, and Lopatka (1987) administered 69 exposure trials to 20 patients with panic disorder. Thirty (43.5%) of the trials resulted in a panic attack. In corresponding trials with patients who had claustrophobia, situationally bound (cued) or predisposed panic attacks occurred during 50 (36%) of 140 trials. Interestingly, subjects with claustrophobia tended to report dyspnea, choking, dizziness, and fears of dying and gong crazy more frequently than did patients with panic disorder. Subjects with panic disorder, on the other hand, tended to report palpitations, hot flashes, and trembling more frequently than did subjects with claustrophobia. Nevertheless, the overall patterns of panic frequency and symptom report were relatively similar, with few systematic differences. However, no temporal criterion for panic, or specification of response systems, was incorporated into Rachman and colleagues' study. In an extensive review, Craske (1991) suggested that situationally bound (cued) panic attacks occurring in the context of a specific phobia do not differ from unexpected (uncued) attacks except for the presence or absence of a cue, as reported by the patient. There have been no developments in the last several years to change that conclusion.

Thus it is safe to say that if any differences exist among types of panic attacks, they are very small in terms of the presenting characteristics of the panic attacks themselves. All attacks seem to represent the basic emotion of fear firing at an inappropriate time. Nevertheless, whether a cue is perceived or not by the patient may have important functional implications. But the causes or maintaining factors of panic attacks, whether cued or uncued, are only speculations based on the descriptive data provided in this chapter. All we can say for certain at this point is that panic itself seems a distinctive event based on presenting characteristics, with clear topographical differences from anxiety. One important way to learn more about the nature and cause of panic is to produce it experimentally in the laboratory. It is to this rich area of clinical investigation that I now turn.

CHAPTER 5

Provoking Panic in the Laboratory

If one can produce a psychological or biological phenomenon in the laboratory, one can begin to talk about the cause of that phenomenon. On the other hand, what appears at first blush to be the immediate cause may be misleading. From all available evidence, it seems that we can produce panic in the laboratory. Furthermore, investigators have been provoking panic in the laboratory for over 80 years. A report of a patient's reactions during an early well-done study (Lindemann & Finesinger, 1938) illustrates a typical panic provocation session. In fact, this patient was administered two antagonistic substances approximately 1 month apart: adrenaline, with marked sympathetic effects, and mecholyl (i.e., acetylcholine), with primarily parasympathetic effects. An account of both sessions provides an interesting contrast that has renewed importance for current theorizing on the nature of panic.[1]

[The subject was a] 42-year-old white, American, college graduate who was treated in the [outpatient department] because of attacks of anxiety which [have] troubled him frequently during the last ten years. The attacks occurred whenever he tried to walk long distances alone, when he attempted to use a bus or train alone, [and] when he attempted to drive the car alone. He then was seized by a sensation of panic, intense fear that his heart might stop, that he might drop dead the next moment, or that he might disintegrate in some way. He felt weak in his knees, dizzy, and had a feeling of fullness and oppression in his upper abdomen. He was keenly aware of his heart, which seemed to pound but not to race. Occasionally he broke out in perspiration. The first of these attacks occurred suddenly when he was sitting in a movie, watching a vaudeville act in which a box containing a living woman was supposedly sawed into pieces, the woman appearing without injury afterwards. At that time the patient, for a moment, thought he was going to become blind, left the theatre in a panic and for the next few weeks was in a state of almost continuous fear which gradually changed into a state of greater calm except for the situations described above. He had to give up his job, as a successful business man, and is now working on a [Works Progress Administration] project.

The physical examination showed no abnormal findings. The neurological examination was negative. The pulse rate was at about 70, blood pressure 140/80. The vasomotor reactions were not abnormal. The hands were usually warm and slightly moist. On March 7, 1936, this patient was observed under the influence of adrenaline. At 11:33 he received a preliminary injection of

[1]From Lindemann, F., & Finesinger, J. E. (1938). The effect of adrenaline and mecholyl in states of anxiety in psychoneurotic patients. *American Journal of Psychiatry. 95*, 353–370. Copyright 1938 by the American Psychiatric Association. Reprinted by permission.

1 cc. of saline before the injection of adrenaline at 11:40. Two minutes later he asked what made the heart beat differently, "If I put the diaphragm out it seems to stop the palpitation." After 4 minutes he noticed that his hands were sweaty. "I suppose that is nervousness but there is no real difference." After 6 minutes he still insisted there was no difference in his feelings but reported that he was quivery all over as though he were shivering when cold, "Shivering as if I were waiting for a street car on a cold night." After 7 minutes one noticed a gross tremor of his hands. After 9 minutes the patient stated that his heart was pounding and he still felt a quivering in his thighs. He had a slight feeling of insecurity in his legs. The patient did not seem anxious at all. He reminisced about former attacks of anxiety. After 17 minutes he seemed thirsty and asked for a glass of milk. Standing up he still had the sensation of shivering in the knees. From then on one noticed that the patient was rather self-absorbed and did not talk much. After 37 minutes he became impatient, "How much longer is it going to last, Doctor? I am getting hungry. The shivering is wearing off. The pounding is still there but not so bad." From then on he became more talkative again.

It must be noted that under the influence of adrenaline the patient reported about the typical sensations of shivering and about heart pounding, but that he had no attack of anxiety.

On April 11 he received mecholyl. During the preliminary period he stated that he felt good, noticed no difference in his feelings. At 11:32 the injection was started. 15 mgs. were injected in the course of 5 minutes. After 2 minutes the patient appeared alarmed, frightened, was restless and wanted to get up. He rose from the bed, held on to the examiner as if in a state of panic, "I feel terrible. Don't you see that I have cold perspiration all over? Must you go on?" Then he continued, "Am I going to die? I feel very uncomfortable, really very weak. Sweat is pouring all over me." The patient had a flushed face and was perspiring. Patient laughed in a curious manner several times. After 5 minutes he began to feel chilly, "I'm awfully afraid," and began to cry, "I'm soaking wet all over. My nose is running. I feel as if I had gotten a cold in a couple of minutes." After 9 minutes he continued, "This is the most powerful stuff you ever gave me. I don't want to have anything like that ever again." Turning directly toward the experimenter, he addressed him, "Why should you have inflicted this upon me? I have manifested kindness and for all the kindness I seem to get an illness and have to suffer. Look at the water coming off my body. I have a headache too." After 12 minutes the patient's panic reaction seemed to abate and he became very talkative. He kept in close contact with the examiner and continued, "Let me explain to you. When you put that needle in I don't know what happened. I worked myself up to a pitch of fear. That is the way the fear comes on me. I start thinking about it and it manifests itself. It works itself to a panicky feeling. Suddenly the fear came. All that fear came to my mind, as if something was working itself to a climax. You don't know when it is going to stop. Just panicky." The patient appeared like a person who was greatly perturbed and eagerly trying to figure out something that puzzled him. He continued, "My heart did not pound at all, yet I had that panic. Standing up I was not dizzy but weak. It was working up somehow to a peak. I wasn't going to faint. It was just a cross between panic and calm, as if you were gradually going to rise right up. This seems to be leading . . . losing my integrity." During these words the patient seemed somewhat hostile, "I thought you were cruel and punishing me. You are cruel. You just kept on." After 25 minutes he appeared more relieved. He began to joke, remained very talkative, reported the story of how he came to see a doctor. After 33 minutes he was somewhat more silent, complained about a chill going up and down his legs. He continued, "I think I have had all the sensations that I have had in my condition in that one medicine. There was a fear of fainting, a feeling that the heart was going to stop, a terrible panic, the feeling of alarm, the sensation of losing my equilibrium. I lost the sense of control, of contact with the world, as if something was radically wrong and it came so naturally, it came so suddenly." "I'm laboring under the idea that there wasn't any medicine in there at all. You were waiting so long. You said, 'This won't hurt.' Perhaps the response came entirely through my concentration on the needle. I was more alarmed than anything else, just like a man being blindfolded and being told he is going to be branded. Then he is touched with a piece of ice and he thinks he is branded. I think it is just because it took so long. If there was really . . . it washes out of my argument, and then the medicine did what you expected anyway." After 60 minutes the patient was more quiet. He said, "It's all over now, I guess." (pp. 357–362)

Since this experiment, thousands of patients have experienced the terror of panic in the laboratory. (The fact that this patient reacted unexpectedly to mecholyl rather than adrenaline is just one of many puzzles taken up in this chapter.) But determination of the cause of panic remains elusive. Various procedures have been used to produce panic or panic-like symptoms. The panicogenic qualities of many of these operations were discovered quite by accident, opening up new avenues of investigation into the nature of panic.

The experimental provocation of panic by whatever means deepens our understanding of the nature of panic. At the same time, these procedures undermine many current assumptions and raise important new questions. In this chapter, the major procedures for provoking panic are described. Some of these techniques involve biochemical infusions; others involve stimulating respiratory systems in a direct way. Panic can also be elicited by a number of other procedures. I review each in turn. From the 1960s through the 1980s, the major focus was on the consequences of sodium lactate infusions. In the 1990s, biological investigators largely shifted their attention to respiratory system abnormalities. Putative mechanisms of action associated with each procedure, according to current thinking, are reviewed and integrated. Commonalities among seemingly diverse provocation procedures suggest factors that might maintain panic attacks in susceptible individuals. These in turn contribute to a comprehensive theory of the origins of panic and anxiety disorders, which is outlined in Chapters 7 and 8.

Of course, methodological issues confound this field of study. Early studies had not yet recognized, or defined, the phenomenon of panic. Later studies utilized widely differing definitions of panic, some of which would not cross current thresholds of severity. Issues in defining panic have been reviewed in detail in Chapter 4, and early definitional problems with laboratory provocation procedures were reviewed in detail in the first edition of this book (Barlow, 1988). More recently, investigators have utilized more up-to-date measures that assess reports of both cognitive and somatic symptoms, similarity to naturally occurring panic, and the presence of an abrupt surge, all at sufficient levels of severity. With this sophisticated assessment battery, laboratory provocation procedures such as lactate and CO_2 challenges would seem to produce "panic attacks" that are sufficiently realistic to prove valuable sources of information on the nature of panic (Goetz, Klein, & Gorman, 1994; Sanderson & Wetzler, 1990). Of course, physiological and neurobiological correlates of panic are distorted somewhat by the particular substances utilized in the challenge, making these indices less useful.

BIOCHEMICAL PROVOCATION

Substances Used in Biochemical Provocation Studies

The laboratory provocation of panic by biochemical or pharmacological agents has aroused considerable interest, particularly during the last two decades. But these procedures for provoking panic and anxiety have a lengthy and extensive history (Shear, 1986; Wamboldt & Insel, 1988). Among the various substances utilized over the years are epinephrine (or adrenaline), isoproterenol, and yohimbine, all of which are directly implicated in noradrenergic functioning. Other substances include agonists for the neuropeptide cholecystokinin (CCK), such as CCK in its tetrapeptide form (CCK-4) or pentagastrin; flumazenil, a benzodiazepine antagonist; metachlorophenylpiperazine (mCCP), a serotonin agonist; caffeine; and sodium lactate.

Adrenaline or Epinephrine

One of the earliest studies in which an attempt was made to provoke panic in the laboratory is noteworthy, since the methods employed are nearly identical to those employed
today in studies of this type. In 1919, Wearn and Sturgis injected 5 mg of adrenaline into
army recruits suffering from the "irritable heart syndrome." As noted in Chapter 4, this
seems to have been one of the terms used to describe panic attacks and panic disorder during
World War I. What makes this study important is that Wearn and Sturgis injected control
subjects in a similar fashion, making this one of the few early studies to use a control group.
In the patients with "irritable heart," symptoms characteristic of their acute anxiety reactions occurred and were reported. These included the typical panic symptoms of palpitations, dizziness, and tachycardia. Control subjects also manifested some physiological
symptoms, although less pronounced, but reported little or no "anxiety."

In fact, Breggin in 1964 reviewed what was by then a very extensive literature on
adrenaline infusions, consisting of at least 24 separate studies over the intervening 45 years.
Naturally, not all were controlled studies, and most suffered from a lack of clear definitions of patients and reactions. Furthermore, the "adrenaline" used in the early studies
was a poorly defined mixture of epinephrine and norepinephrine (Wamboldt & Insel, 1988).
But Breggin (1964) reported consistent support for the early Wearn and Sturgis (1919)
results. In study after study, subjects who developed acute anxiety during the infusions
had a past history of recurrent anxiety reactions characterized by sudden high levels of
arousal and anxiety. On the other hand, subjects without this history did not experience
intense anxiety during infusions, according to their own reports as well as observations by
the experimenters. These subjects would report on occasion that they were feeling "as if"
they might be anxious, in that they would experience physiological reactions without subjective feelings of fear or dread. In his lengthy and perceptive review, Breggin (1964) noted
another factor that seemed to influence the extent of the anxiety (panic) reaction during
the infusions. He referred to this variable as "environmental cues." By this, he meant cues
in the situation that made it possible or likely for subjects to attribute their strong emotional reaction to one emotion or another, such as fear, anger, or elation. For example if a
situation was made to seem more "dangerous" through the use of "awe inspiring monitoring apparatus and a large number of observers including psychiatrists" (p. 560), then
more marked fear or anxiety responses could be expected. This observation, of course, was
suggested by the then relatively new findings on the possible importance of attributing an
emotional state to the context of the situation one happens to be in (Schachter & Singer,
1962). As noted in Chapter 2, this particular theory has not survived intact, but Breggin's
general impressions have received substantial experimental support, as described in some
detail below.

The biological effects of epinephrine are relatively well mapped out. Epinephrine
is, of course, an endogenous catecholamine secreted through the adrenal medulla that
produces wide-ranging peripheral arousal. It stimulates both alpha- and beta-adrenergic
receptors.

Naturally, there is some question whether these early studies with adrenaline or epinephrine were actually provoking panic. Since current diagnostic conventions were not
available, it is not possible to know for certain; however, from descriptions provided in
many of these early studies (including the Lindemann & Finesinger [1938] study, quoted
above), it would seem that major panic attacks were occurring. For example, in the first
study (Wearn & Sturgis, 1919), the soliders with "irritable heart" suffered the "acute anxiety
reaction" that brought them to the clinic in the first place. These attacks were character-

ized by cardiovascular instability, dizziness, and fatigue, as well as by the subjective psychological symptoms of anxiety and dread. This pattern of symptoms, along with the observation of the similarity of these laboratory "panics" to naturally occurring anxiety attacks, largely fulfills even the more stringent current definitions of laboratory panic. In view of the possible relevance of this work, it is surprising that few studies on adrenaline or epinephrine have been reported since 1965. Among these few, van Zijderveld and colleagues (van Zijderveld, van Doornen, Orlebeke, & Snieder, 1992; van Zijderveld et al., 1993) replicated the production of somatic symptoms without arousal in normal subjects, and produced "full-blown" panic attacks in 8 out of 12 patients with panic disorder (van Zijderveld et al., 1997).

Isoproterenol

Frohlich, Tarazi, and Duston (1969) infused isoproterenol into 15 patients who were complaining of panic-like symptoms. Reactions in this group were compared to those patients with hypertension and of normotensive controls who were also infused. In 9 out of the 14 patients with panic-like symptoms, "isoproterenol evoked an hysterical outburst, almost uncontrollable" (p. 4). Once again, subjects in the control groups experienced some increases in physiological measures, but no subjective feelings of anxiety. Consistent with previous patients, they reported feeling "as if" they were anxious. Easton and Sherman (1976) also produced what seemed to be clear panic attacks with isoproterenol infusions in five patients suffering from panic-like symptoms.

Rainey et al. (1984) compared the effects of isoproterenol with those of sodium lactate in patients with established diagnoses of panic disorder. This early study was one of the few that has directly compared two panicogenic substances. Eleven patients with panic disorder and 10 control subjects received lactate and isoproterenol, as well as a placebo consisting of a 5% glucose solution. The authors reported that 10 of the 11 patients with panic disorder and 3 of the 10 control subjects experienced a panic attack during lactate. During isoproterenol infusion, 8 of the 11 patients and 2 of the 10 control subjects experienced panic. Four of the patients and none of the control subjects panicked during the glucose placebo infusion. The patients rated their panic attacks during both lactate and isoproterenol as very much like their naturally occurring panic attacks. Overall, lactate panics were rated as somewhat more intense than isoproterenol panics. In a later report from this group, 66% of 86 patients with panic disorder met criteria for panic attacks during isoproterenol infusion, compared to 9% of 95 control subjects. Only 16% (14 of 86) of the same patients panicked during a placebo infusion (Pohl, Yeragani, Balon, Ortiz, & Aleem, 1990).

There is some question about the overall "severity" of these attacks. The Research Diagnostic Criteria definition of panic was used rather than the *Diagnostic and Statistical Manual of Mental Disorders* (DSM) definition; the former allows for a less severe burst of emotion. In contrast to the studies described above, Nesse, Cameron, Curtis, McCann, and Huber-Smith (1984) did not observe any panic attacks in a group of eight patients and six controls infused with isoproterenol. However, the isoproterenol infusions were part of a long 4-hour protocol that also included a variety of exercise and rest conditions. Few, if any, systematic controlled studies on isoproterenol have appeared since these early reports.

Isoproterenol is particularly interesting, since it selectively stimulates only beta-adrenergic receptor sites. As such, it acts more specifically than epinephrine, although still at a peripheral level. This becomes important when the effects of drugs that block beta-adrenergic receptor sites (beta-blockers) on panic are reviewed.

Yohimbine

Yohimbine, an alpha-adrenergic antagonist, has also been used to provoke panic. Yohimbine is one of the few biochemical agents of its type capable of crossing the blood–brain barrier and acting centrally, probably in an area of the midbrain called the locus ceruleus. The locus ceruleus has been implicated in studies of anxiety and panic for over 25 years. This makes investigation of yohimbine important from the perspective of mechanisms of action of panic provocation (see below).

In 1961, Holmberg and Gershon injected patients carrying a variety of diagnoses with yohimbine and compared their reactions to those of control subjects similarly injected. The reactions they noted in this early study included perspiration, pupillary dilation, flushing, a rise in heart rate and blood pressure, trembling, and "irritableness." In a later study, Garfield, Gershon, Sletten, Sundland, and Ballows (1967) injected yohimbine as well as epinephrine into "schizophrenic" and "nonschizophrenic" patients. They concluded that the presentation of symptoms, particularly in terms of the combination of physiological and psychological aspects of anxiety, indicated that yohimbine produced more intense and realistic clinical anxiety than did epinephrine.

Although these early studies suffered from a rather global definition of "anxiety" and marked heterogeneity in the patient populations, later studies were more sophisticated. Charney, Heninger, and Breier (1984) compared the reactions of 39 patients with clear DSM-III diagnoses of either agoraphobia with panic attacks or panic disorder to those of 20 healthy subjects. All subjects were injected not only with yohimbine, but also with placebo. Both physiological and psychological reactions were examined. During yohimbine injections, patients rated themselves as significantly more anxious and nervous, and reported that their reaction was similar in quality to that experienced during naturally occurring panic attacks. Patients also experienced marked increases in somatic symptoms, such as palpitations, hot and cold flashes, tremors, blood pressure, and pulse rate. Consistent with the results of other infusion studies, control subjects reported mild increases in somatic symptoms that were not accompanied by psychological symptoms such as subjective reports of nervousness or anxiety. Despite these interesting results, yohimbine has received little experimental attention in recent years.

Caffeine

It is no secret to millions of people throughout the world who drink coffee that caffeine results in increased alertness and attention. In general, caffeine seems to act as an antagonist of adenosine, a neuromodulator that influences the noradrenergic system. Specifically, caffeine antagonizes the action of adenosine by blocking adenosine receptors and preventing adenosine from inhibiting release of norepinephrine. Thus caffeine indirectly increases norepinephrine and arousal. Nevertheless, surveys of caffeine consumption and the effects of caffeine suggest marked individual differences in response to this drug. For example, early studies suggested that the personality characteristics of neuroticism or introversion (see Chapter 2) seem to relate to caffeine consumption. In one study, individuals with both neuroticism and introversion drank less coffee than comparison groups, particularly under stressful conditions (Bartol, 1975). These findings with nonpatients have raised questions about the effects of caffeine in patients with anxiety disorders.

Boulenger, Uhde, Wolff, and Post (1984) surveyed caffeine consumption as well as self-rated anxiety and depression in a series of patients with clear diagnoses of panic disorder or major depressive disorder. These patients were compared to well-matched control groups. They found that patients with panic disorder (but not depressed patients or normal controls) reported levels of self-rated anxiety and depression that correlated with their degree of caffeine consumption: The more caffeine, the more anxiety. In fact, patients with panic disorder had a marked sensitivity to the effects of even one cup of coffee. The experience of drinking coffee was judged to be aversive by these patients. Of the 30 patients with panic disorder, 20 had stopped drinking coffee, compared to only 5 of the 23 depressed patients. Of the 20 patients with panic who had given up coffee, 11 mentioned central nervous system stimulation as the reason for stopping, and 2 more mentioned gastrointestinal symptoms. Similar results were reported by Lee, Cameron, and Greden (1985).

Of course, survey research differs markedly from the infusion studies discussed above. Thus investigators began to observe directly the ingestion of caffeine in patients with panic disorder versus controls. After some preliminary studies (e.g., Uhde, Boulenger, Vittone, Siever, & Post, 1985), Charney, Heninger, and Jatlow (1985) administered 10 mg/kg of caffeine orally to 21 patients meeting DSM-III criteria for agoraphobia with panic attacks or panic disorder, as well as 17 healthy subjects. Of the patients, 71% "panicked" in that they reported marked increases in subjective anxiety, as well as somatic signs of anxiety. They also judged that these attacks were similar to panic experienced naturally. Smaller numbers of control subjects reported increases in subjective anxiety (approximately 25%), and none "panicked." Similarly, control subjects evidenced smaller increases in somatic symptoms when compared to patients. Higher baseline ratings were also evident on somatic symptoms for patients before ingestion of caffeine. Beck and Berisford (1992) compared responses among 21 patients with panic disorder and 18 matched normal controls to a somewhat smaller dosage of caffeine (250 mg) or placebo. Although the dosage was not designed to produce panic, 4 patients panicked, compared to none in the control group. The patients also reported a significant increase in subjective anxiety (but not physiological indices of anxiety) during caffeine induction but not during placebo conditions. Interestingly, these results did not covary with the report of physical symptoms. That is, subjective reports of anxiety (culminating in panic in some individuals) did not seem to be a function of increased production of somatic symptoms.

In one additional study (Bruce, Scott, Shine, & Lader, 1992), the authors reported that the panicogenic or anxiogenic effects of caffeine were not specifically related to panic disorder, since patients with generalized anxiety disorder (GAD) reacted with at least as much anxiety, if not more anxiety, than patients with panic disorder. Patterns of comorbidity were not reported, so the possibility exists that patients with GAD had panic attacks somewhere in the picture. Extending this investigatory line to nonclinical subjects, Telch, Silverman, and Schmidt (1996) reported that subjects with high scores on the Anxiety Sensitivity Index (Reiss, Peterson, Gursky, & McNally, 1986; Taylor, 1999) responded with more anxiety to caffeine ingestion than subjects with low scores on this index. This suggests that responses to provocation procedures, like those to other challenge procedures, may lie on a continuum as a function of underlying traits or temperaments.

Cholecystokinin

CCK is a neuropeptide that acts as a neurotransmitter in brain regions that are important in the production of panic symptoms, such as the limbic area and the brain stem (Bradwejn et al., 1994). Infusions of forms of CCK, such as CCK in its tetrapeptide form (CCK-4) or pentapeptide form (pentagastrin), have been shown to provoke panic in a number of studies (Abelson, Nesse, & Vinik, 1994). For example, Abelson and Nesse (1994) noted the occurrence of panic attacks in 7 out of 10 patients infused with pentagastrin, compared to 0 out of 10 control subjects with no disorder. Bradwejn, Koszycki, and Shriqui (1991) reported that 25 µg of CCK-4 produced panic attacks in 17% (2 out of 12) control subjects, compared to 91% (10 out of 11) patients with panic disorder. A slightly higher dose of 50 µg produced panic in 100% of the same group of patients infused, compared to 47% in the control group. More recently, a number of investigators have shown that CCK-induced panic attacks are blocked or attenuated by antipanic medications—including imipramine (Bradwejn & Koszycki, 1994) and several selective serotonin reuptake inhibitors (SSRIs), such as fluvoxamine (van Megan, Westenberg, & den Boer, 1997) and citalopram (Shilik, Aluoja, Vasar, & Bradwejn, 1997). These medications have similar effects to other CCK receptor antagonists (Bradwejn et al., 1994).

Interestingly, a more recent report (Flint et al., 1998) suggests that reactions to CCK-4 are attenuated in older subjects, which parallels the observed attenuation of anxiety and panic in general in elderly populations (as described in Chapter 1). Recent studies have also characterized responses to CCK-4 in healthy volunteers (Koszycki, Zacharko, LeMelledo, & Bradwejn, 1998; Bradwejn, LeGrand, Koszycki, Bates, & Bourin, 1998). Generally, among normal subjects, those who panic in response to CCK-4 evidence a more robust neurobiological response than those who do not panic, particularly in terms of cardiovascular and hormonal (hypothalamic–pituitary–adrenocortical [HPA] axis) function. CCK-4 also produces marked changes in respiration in healthy volunteers (Bradwejn et al., 1998). This response profile is more similar to naturally occurring panic than that produced by some other substances. For all of these reasons, research on CCK-4 as a provocateur of panic has been more active during the 1990s than research on other pharmacological agents has been.

Flumazenil and mCCP

To give some indication of the variety of agents utilized in panic provocation studies, I now review two additional diverse substances utilized to successfully provoke panic. Nutt, Glue, Lawson, and Wilson (1990) administered flumazenil, a benzodiazepine antagonist, to 10 patients with panic disorder and 10 healthy control subjects. Eight of 10 patients experienced a sudden panic attack, compared to none in the control group. Although the patients reported these experiences to be very much like their naturally occurring panics, they did note one exception: a lack of marked respiratory distress and dyspnea. Woods, Charney, Silver, Krystal, and Heninger (1991) reported similar results and interpret these findings as consistent with altered benzodiazepine receptor function in patients with panic disorder. In view of the substantial role that has been suggested for the benzodiazepine system in the production of anxiety and panic over the past several decades, it is somewhat surprising that there has not been more research on substances interacting with this system to provoke anxiety and panic.

Other studies have examined the possible panicogenic effects of mCCP, a serotonin agonist that selectively affects HPA axis functioning. Several studies have observed some tendency of mCCP to selectively provoke panic in patients with panic disorder (Charney, Woods, Goodman, & Heninger, 1987; Kahn, Wetzler, van Praag, Asnis, & Strauman, 1988; Klein, Zohar, Geraci, Murphy, & Uhde, 1991). Once again, in view of the proven efficacy of SSRIs in the treatment of panic disorder, it is somewhat surprising that research involving the serotonergic system has not been pursued more vigorously in the provocation literature. However, Coplan, Gorman, and Klein (1992) suggest that panic attacks provoked in this way differ in many ways from lactate- and CO_2-induced panic (as well as naturally occurring panics), due to differential action on the HPA axis and the lack of a sudden "crescendo" of symptoms, which seems to make serotonergically based responding from provocation to be more like generalized anxiety than panic.

Lactate

In the context of a long history of research on infusions of various types with anxious patients, one of the more important studies in terms of its impact was not reported until 1967. At that time, Pitts and McClure (1967) observed that standard exercise had produced characteristic anxiety symptoms in several previous studies (Cohen & White, 1950; Holmgren & Strom, 1959; Jones & Mellersh, 1946; Linko, 1950). They hypothesized, as had other investigators, that the anxiety symptoms found in these studies might have been due to an extremely rapid rise of blood lactate acid occurring as a consequence of the exercise. Pitts and McClure concluded that the lactate ion itself may produce anxiety attacks in susceptible persons. Pilot work revealed that all nine patients with "anxiety neurosis" who were tested developed typical anxiety attacks during lactate infusion. In a subsequent double-blind study, 14 patients and 10 normal controls were infused with lactate, as well as with a modified lactate infusion containing a calcium ion, and a third infusion consisting of only glucose. Of the 14 patients, 13 reported an anxiety attack similar to their naturally occurring attacks during the lactate infusion; 2 of the 10 control subjects also reported panic attacks. Less intense anxiety was experienced during the modified lactate infusion. Neither patients nor controls reported any particular response to the glucose. The investigators hypothesized that the lactate ion may cause panic attacks through alkalinization of the blood. They also noted that the effects observed could have been due to "nonspecific stress" (Pitts & McClure, 1967).

This study, more than any other, generated interest in the possibility of uncovering the nature of panic attacks through this methodology. Since that time, over 20 studies describing lactate infusion with anxious patients have been reported. For example, similar results were reported in early studies by Fink, Taylor, and Volavka (1970), Bonn, Harrison, and Rees (1971), and Kelly, Mitchel-Heggs, and Sherman (1971). In the 1980s, more studies of lactate infusion began to appear (Liebowitz et al., 1984; Ehlers et al., 1986).

Even monkeys have not escaped the effects of lactate. Friedman, Sunderland, and Rosenblum (1988) administered lactate to primates. According to behavioral ratings made by evaluators who were unaware of the experimental conditions, lactate, compared to a placebo, produced intense circumscribed emotions in monkeys that differed from a generalized arousal response. The emotional response most closely resembled fear!

Cowley and Arana (1990) carefully reviewed all studies of sodium lactate infusion prior to 1990 in the context of diagnostic sensitivity and specificity when patients with panic disorder were compared to nonpsychiatric control subjects, and to patients with psychiatric disorders other than panic disorder. Rates of successful panic provocation across different groups are presented in Table 5.1. For purposes of comparison, Cowley and Arana summarized panic provocation rates from four different groups: (1) patients with panic disorder; (2) nonpsychiatric controls; and patients with psychiatric disorders other than panic disorder who (3) either reported panic attacks somewhere in the diagnostic picture, or (4) did not. The principal diagnoses of patients *with* panic attacks who did not meet criteria for panic disorder, among the four studies reporting such results, included patients with depression, posttraumatic stress disorder, or infrequent panic attacks not sufficient to meet DSM criteria. The principal diagnoses of patients without panic attacks in the picture included various forms of depression, bulimia nervosa, GAD, obsessive–compulsive dis-

TABLE 5.1. Lactate Provocation across Diagnostic Groups

	n	Response Rate: No. (%) of subjects
Panic disorder	338	227 (67%)
Other psychiatric disorders with coexisting panic attacks	61	34 (56%)
Other psychiatric disorders without panic attacks	92	9 (10%)
Nonpsychiatric controls	140	17 (13%)

Note. From Cowley and Arana (1990). Copyright 1990 by American Medical Association. Reprinted by permission.

order, and social phobia. As one can see, across all studies, 67% of patients with panic disorder experienced a panic attack during lactate infusion. This compared to 56% of patients without panic disorder who reported occasional panic attacks; 10% of patients with other disorders with no reports of panic attacks; and 13% of nonpsychiatric controls.

Cowley and Arana (1990) reported that lactate-induced panic had a sensitivity of 67% and a specificity of 89% in differentiating patients with panic disorder from nonpsychiatric control groups in these studies. However, the authors noted that lactate-induced panic was not specific for panic disorder, but rather for the phenomenon of panic attacks regardless of coexisting diagnosis. Patients with other principal diagnoses with panic attacks somewhere in the picture, or even with panic attacks as infrequent as once a year, responded to lactate at a rate similar to those with panic disorder. Similarly, in summarizing several decades of work from the active group at the New York State Psychiatric Institute, Coplan, Goetz, et al. (1998) noted that of 170 patients receiving lactate infusion, 101 (51%) met conservative criteria for experiencing a panic attack during infusion. This compared to only 1 out of 44 normal healthy volunteer controls who panicked.

Mechanisms of Biochemically Provoked Panic

As noted above, one of the major difficulties precluding clear interpretations in early studies involves the definition of panic. At first blush this would not seem to be a problem, in view of the distinctive appearance of a panic attack, but the difficulties presented in defining a panic attack have been fully described in Chapter 4. Thus, early studies, in particular, suffered from variable and inconsistent definitions of panic.

Nevertheless, in view of the relative consistency with which lactate, caffeine, isoproterenol, yohimbine, CCK, epinephrine, and other substances provoke panic, speculation has focused over the last several decades on the underlying neurobiological mechanisms associated with panic attacks. As Coplan and Klein (1996) point out, the diversity of agents capable of provoking panic would seem to imply that panic attacks can be triggered through a variety of fundamentally different mechanisms. Nevertheless, the search has centered on finding a common biological denominator. But this finding has proven elusive. The very different pathways to panic have never been better illustrated than in the early and largely overlooked study by Lindemann and Finesinger (1938) comparing the effects of adrenaline with one of its antagonists, mecholyl (i.e., acetylcholine). Lindemann and Finesinger's report was one of the long series of studies investigating the effects of adrenaline on individuals with "anxiety attacks." Consistent with most of these reports, adrenaline provoked "anxiety attacks" in 11 of 20 patients. That these patients clearly seemed to be suffering from what we would now call "panic disorder" is also evidenced in the case report from this study presented at the beginning of this chapter. However, in a very elegant methodological twist, the investigators also administered acetylcholine in a counterbalanced fashion to these patients. Acetylcholine is antagonistic to adrenaline, with primary parasympathetic rather than sympathetic activation. The investigators were very careful to record not only physiological responses such as heart rate, but also detailed cognitive and somatic reactions to the injection. In addition, they encouraged simultaneous verbalization about the experience, as is evident in the case report. Despite the limited apparatus available at the time, this methodology still ranks among the most sophisticated laboratory provocation studies.

Adrenaline, of course, produced the usual sympathetic constellation of physiological responses. Acetylcholine, on the other hand, produced quite a different effect, including vasodilation of the face and excessive perspiration. The results indicated that out of 20 patients, 6 panicked with adrenaline but not with acetylcholine; 5 patients panicked with acetylcholine but not adrenaline; both drugs activated a panic attack in 5 patients; and neither of the drugs activated panic in 4 patients.

The following select examples represent some of the major efforts to identify common biological denominators over the past several decades. Although some theories are no longer tenable, a brief review of these ideas provides perspective on current thinking, and illustrates very nicely the slow but inexorable progress of science.

Hypocalcemia

In 1967, Pitts and McClure put forth a new conception of the "cause" of panic, as noted above. They suggested that anxiety symptoms may be related to hypocalcemia produced by excess lactate. They suggested that one may find in these patients "a defect in aerobic or anerobic metabolism resulting in excess lactate production, a defect in calcium metabolism or some combination of these" (p. 1335). Grosz and Farmer (1969) criticized these notions on several grounds. First, they pointed out that anxiety can occur without high blood lactate concentrations, and conversely that high blood lactate levels may be present without accompanying anxiety. In addition, lactate infusions produce metabolic alkalosis, but lactate produced by exercise shifts the acid-based balance of the body to metabolic acidosis. Finally, they noted that the rise in lactate produced by infusions should cause only a very small change in ionized calcium. In fact, Pitts and Alan (1979) themselves confirmed this notion in a later experiment when they demonstrated that infusions of a powerful calcium chelator, strong enough to produce symptoms of tetany in patients with panic, did not induce panic attacks.

As an alternative hypothesis, Grosz and Farmer (1969) suggested that sodium bicarbonate levels rise with lactate infusions and that the accompanying state of hyperventilation may cause feelings of discomfort. In a subsequent study, Grosz and Farmer (1972) repeated the Pitts and McClure (1967) experiment with the addition of an infusion of sodium bicarbonate. Both infusions produced marked anxiety, but neither was associated with a rise in blood lactate. Unfortunately, Grosz and Farmer (1972) infused only nonpatients, not patients suffering from anxiety disorders. But Gorman et al. (1989) infused patients with panic disorder with either sodium lactate or sodium bicarbonate and found that 13 of 22 subjects panicked in response to lactate, compared to 9 of 20 subjects in response to bicarbonate. The authors concluded that hyperventilation and subsequent hypocapnia appeared to be the common denominator in lactate- and bicarbonate-induced panic. With these experiments, the hypocalcemia hypothesis suffered an early demise, although the role of breathing irregularities is continuing to receive increased attention as a panicogenic mechanism.

With the fate of the hypocalcemia hypothesis sealed, a number of other specific biological mechanisms proposed as underlying laboratory-provoked panic were suggested and ruled out, such as metabolic alkalosis, or abnormalities in pyruvate and phosphate (Nutt & Lawson, 1992). Several additional hypotheses were formulated in the context of lactate-provoked panic that seemingly were applicable to other substances capable of provoking panic. Two of the most intriguing possibilities centered on beta-adrenergic hypersensitivity and central CO_2 chemoreceptor hypersensitivity.

Beta-Adrenergic Hypersensitivity

Beta-adrenergic hypersensitivity and other related theories focusing on peripheral arousal mechanisms as biological mediators of panic attracted considerable attention in the 1980s. For example, epinephrine is an endogenous catecholamine that stimulates both alpha- and beta-adrenergic receptors. Isoproterenol infusions, on the other hand, are thought to selectively stimulate beta-adrenergic receptors. Both of these infusions seemingly produced panic in some subjects but not in others. One obvious experiment was to block beta-adrenergic receptors during infusion with panicogenic substances and ascertain whether patients panicked or not. In an early study, Gorman et al. (1983) administered propranolol, which lowers beta-adrenergic sensitivity (i.e., it is a beta-blocker), to six patients who previously had panicked when infused with sodium lactate. In all six cases, panic attacks occurred during lactate infusion, despite pretreatment infusion with propranolol. Examination of the data in Figure 5.1 shows that heart rate was in fact reduced by preinfusion with propranolol in the group receiving it, as one would expect from this beta-blocker, although heart rate did increase during the lactate infusion. But because heart rate had dropped initially, there was little or no heart rate increase over baseline values in the group receiving propranolol. And yet all patients reported panic. The fact that reports of panic can occur without absolute increases in heart rate has been described in Chapter 4 (e.g.. Taylor et al., 1986).

On the basis of these data, both Rainey, Ettedgui, Pohl, and Bridges (1985) and Gorman and Klein (1985) initially suggested that lactate and isoproterenol infusions must produce panic by different biological mechanisms. That is, in view of the ineffectiveness of propranolol in blocking lactate-induced panic, lactate must not operate by the mechanism of beta-adrenergic hypersensitivity. Studies that directly tested the effects of beta-blockers in samples of patients with panic disorder also produced mixed and weak (clinical) results in reducing panic attacks or other symptoms of panic disorder (Pohl et al., 1990). In fact, subsequent research has strongly suggested that no peripheral biochemical or physiological change serves as a special trigger in panic provocation experiments. Rather, biochemically-induced panic attacks appear to be primarily a central nervous system phenomenon with inconsistent peripheral sequelae. This leaves unanswered questions on the panicogenic neurobiological mechanism of isoproterenol, or other peripherally acting agents, unless indirect effects of these substances on respiration are contributory.

Central CO_2 Chemoreceptor Sensitivity

In their early review of the biochemical and physiological correlates of lactate provocation, Liebowitz, Gorman, Fyer, Levitt, et al. (1985) pointed out that lactate metabolism produces CO_2, which freely crosses the blood–brain barrier. Thus, lactate infusion may produce transient cerebral CO_2 elevation, even though peripheral partial pressure of CO_2 (pCO_2) falls because of the hyperventilation that occurs during lactate infusions. Thus CO_2 increases centrally (hypercapnia) but decreases peripherally (hypocapnia).

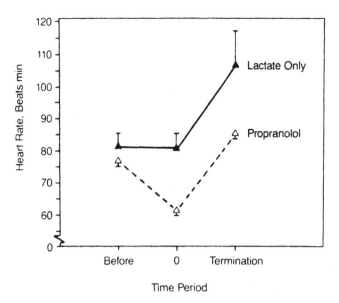

FIGURE 5.1. Comparison of effect on mean heart rate of 5% dextrose–sodium lactate and propranolol hydrochloride–sodium lactate in six subjects. Vertical lines indicate plus or minus the *SEM*. From Gorman et al. (1983). Copyright 1983 by the American Medical Association. Reprinted by permission.

Since CO_2 is a locus ceruleus stimulant (Elam, Yoa, Thorén, & Svensson, 1981; Wamboldt & Insel, 1988; Gorman & Papp, 1990), it was thought that increases in central CO_2 produced by lactate infusion might also stimulate locus ceruleus activity in the same manner as yohimbine. Thus it was hypothesized that lactate and yohimbine may be provoking panic in fundamentally the same manner, both acting centrally rather than peripherally. In addition, there is evidence that the central CO_2 hypersensitivity hypothesis may accommodate other panicogenic agents, such as caffeine (e.g., Papp, Klein, & Gorman, 1993).

Also, as Liebowitz, Gorman, Fyer, Levitt, et al. (1985) pointed out in a particularly cogent observation, increased central nervous system CO_2 drives respiration, which may give patients with panic the feeling of being "out of control." Thus it is this feeling of being "out of control" that may be the common denominator in the provocation of panic (for more on this, see below).

Despite the seeming parsimony of this mechanism of action, subsequent research points to the fact that elevated central CO_2 *cannot* account for the effects of lactate. For example, Gorman et al. (1990) compared sodium L-lactate (which, as noted above, is metabolized to CO_2 and crosses the blood–brain barrier) to sodium D-lactate (which is not metabolized to CO_2). Nevertheless, both substances triggered panic attacks in approximately equal proportions of patients. In a subsequent experiment, Coplan, Sharman, et al. (1992) administered sodium lactate to nonhuman primates and examined the effects on lactate and CO_2 levels. Despite the usual and the characteristic peripheral biochemical effects of infused sodium lactate, no increases in central lactate or CO_2 levels were observed. The authors conclude that the panicogenic effects of lactate must be due to other factors such as cognitive misevaluation of peripheral somatic sensations. In fact, and as reviewed below, it now seems that the phenomena occurring just *before* the lactate infusion—particularly elevations of anticipatory anxiety, HPA axis activity, and hyperventilation—are more robust predictors of subsequent panic attacks during lactate infusion (Coplan, Goetz, et al., 1998).

These experiments marked the end of heightened interest in lactate infusions as a method for elucidating underlying neurobiological mechanisms of biochemically produced panic attacks. But it did not diminish interest in central CO_2 chemoreceptor theory. Interest simply shifted to different methods of provoking panic through stimulating respiration. It is to these methods that I now turn.

RESPIRATION-RELATED PROVOCATION PROCEDURES

Although biochemical provocation of panic received the lion's share of attention prior to 1990, a number of studies provoked intense anxiety and/or panic through procedures directly affecting respiration, or through more psychological methods. These studies assumed more interest with the ascendance of the respiration-related central CO_2 hypersensitivity theory growing out of pharmacological provocation. Although the procedures reviewed have been organized under different headings, we should not lose sight of the fact that all provocation procedures may have similar mechanisms of action—biological, psychological, or (most likely) some combination of the two. Thus one has to rely on operational definitions to categorize procedures. The three procedures grouped in this section—exercise, hyperventilation, and CO_2 inhalation—are superficially quite diverse; however, each technique markedly affects respiration, and alterations in respiration seem heavily implicated in at least some panic attacks.

Exercise

Several years ago a patient, referred to here as "Jack," arrived at our clinic at Albany and presented with a severe case of panic disorder with agoraphobia. Jack was an office manager in his late 40s who had transferred from a higher-paying blue-collar job within his company to his current position. Although industrious and hard-working, he was also impulsive, irritable, and given to angry outbursts. This had led to a stormy relationship with his wife and children, and occasional brief physical altercations with his sons. He reported that in years past his agoraphobia had been so severe that he had spent many days confined to his bed, unable to move for fear of provoking a panic attack. Further questioning revealed that Jack had requested the transfer to the lower-paying desk job, thinking it would be less stressful than his previous job, which had involved a great deal of hard physical labor. Jack had done reasonably well at this desk job for a number of years, but an incident several months ago had precipitated a relapse and resulted in his eventual referral to our clinic.

As Jack described the incident,

> I was feeling pretty good. I really hadn't had any nervous problems to speak of for about a year, and I was able to go places and do things in pretty much of a normal way. [This included taking walks and doing other things around the house.] It was a Saturday morning, and we'd just had a cord of wood delivered for the woodstove. Usually I order the wood cut and split, but this time I was feeling pretty good, so I thought I'd split it myself. Also, I can really use the exercise, since I'm sitting at a desk all day. I got out there fairly early in the morning and started splitting the wood, and worked up a good sweat. Then all of a sudden I felt it coming on. It was the same old problem. I got dizzy and started to tremble, and now the sweat was really

starting to pour off my forehead. My legs were so weak I didn't think I was going to be able to make it to the house. I had the same old feeling that it wasn't really me struggling to get to the house, and that it wasn't really my house, but some kind of nightmare. I managed to crawl into bed and stayed there all weekend. My wife brought me cold towels to put on my forehead, which always seems to help a little bit. Since that time I've been able to struggle in to work, but that's about it.

Jack's story is typical of many patients with panic disorder. In Jack's case, it is interesting that he did not make a tight connection between physical exercise and panic, because, as he put it, "there is nothing scary about chopping wood." But he had managed to arrange his life so that he engaged in as little physical exercise as possible over the years, despite his strength and stature. For example, it seemed that his job transfer was motivated by avoidance of physical exercise rather than by stress or job pressure. Cases like Jack's were undoubtedly responsible for one of the most popular names for panic disorder in the 1940s, "effort syndrome." As noted in Chapter 4, this term, originated by Lewis (1917), came out of World War I to describe soldiers who had great difficulty tolerating the physical exertion connected with army duty. An inability to do hard work, or to engage in strenuous physical exercise or any activity that required an "effort," then became the most prominent sign of what we would now call "panic disorder" during the period between the two World Wars.

At the time, the term "effort syndrome" implied an etiology associated with cardiac problems. However, Jones and Mellersh (1946) reported that during World War II a change occurred. Gradually, effort syndrome came to be considered as more of a psychological than a cardiological problem. As a result, the number of cases diagnosed as "effort syndrome" began to drop, and various diagnoses connected with "anxiety" were utilized instead. Nevertheless, a number of studies continued to examine the response of these patients to exercise in contrast to some comparison group. These studies, it will be recalled, originally suggested the lactate hypothesis (Pitts & McClure, 1967). In 1969, Grosz and Farmer pointed out the very different biological consequences of lactate produced by exercise as opposed to infusions of lactate (exercise produces metabolic acidosis, but lactate infusions produce metabolic alkalosis). After this observation, the early literature on exercise and effort tests was largely ignored. Nevertheless, the fact that increases in blood lactate per se cannot account for panic during exercise (or at any other time) still leaves us with the finding that physical exercise seems capable of provoking anxiety and, occasionally, panic attacks in susceptible patients. For that reason, it is interesting to examine briefly some of these early studies.

Typical of these early experiments are reports by Linko (1950) and Holmgren and Strom (1959). In these reports, it was simply noted that blood lactate levels were somewhat higher in patients with "anxiety" (panic?) during and after exercise, compared to a variety of control groups. Exercise was typically defined as a certain amount of effort on a stationary bicycle. Nothing was mentioned about the psychological responses to exercise in patients with effort syndrome.

In a more complete and sophisticated series of studies carried out by Mandel Cohen and his associates, the response of these patients to exercise was examined more comprehensively (Cohen & White, 1947, 1950). In these studies, walking or running on a treadmill was the exercise. In addition to blood lactate concentration, measures of pulse and respiration, as well as of oxygen consumption during work, were collected. During rest periods, Cohen and White reported that pulse and respiration rates were somewhat higher in patients with "neurocirculatory asthenia" (the term they used), but that measures of oxygen consumption and blood lactate concentration were normal. However, during moderate or exhausting exercise, marked differences emerged between patients and controls. Generally, patients evidenced higher blood lactate concentrations and lower oxygen consumption and ventilatory efficiency. As Cohen and White noted, the more strenuous the exercise, the more clearly these differences emerged. Patients tended to resemble other groups with low work capacity who were in relatively poor physical shape or who exercised infrequently.

Patients in the Cohen and White studies also terminated the treadmill exercise earlier than control subjects and complained of numerous symptoms (e.g., dizziness, weakness, chest pain, trembling, etc.) as reasons for terminating the test. Controls, on the other hand, when they did terminate, almost always stated only that their legs gave out or they ran out of wind.

In fact, these studies of respiration rate and oxygen uptake during exercise showed a very consistent finding: Patients ventilated more rapidly than healthy controls to meet optimal conditions for oxygen assimilation. In other words, patients with "effort syndrome" or "neurocirculatory asthenia" demonstrated a low ventilation efficiency (Cohen & White, 1950; Jones & Mellersh, 1946). Furthermore, both Jones and Mellersh (1946) and Cohen and White (1950) found higher rates of respiration at rest in patients than in controls. Jones and Mellersh reported a very large difference, with patients breathing approximately twice as fast and half as deeply as healthy controls at rest. Cohen and White reported a much smaller difference—a respiratory rate of 15.8 breaths per minute for patients, compared to 13.2 breaths per minute for controls. These differences in patterns of breathing suggest that chronic hyperventilation might be responsible for symptoms. But Jones and Mellersh (1946) reported no evidence of hyperventilatory alkalosis in patients, and also reported adequate oxygen saturation of the blood. Jones and Mellersh concluded that these patients were hyperventilating, but not to the point of markedly altering pH levels.

Low ventilation efficiency does not seem to have been the whole story in these early exercise studies. Cohen and White (1950) also reported that for the same amount of work and at the same rate of ventilation, there was a substantially greater awareness of shortness of breath among patients than among control subjects. Dyspnea, of course, is one of the most prominent and frequent symptoms associated with panic attacks (see Chapter 4). Heightened sensitivity to dyspnea and other somatic events is also a hallmark of patients with panic disorder.

Although the Cohen and White (1947, 1950) studies only hinted at the patients' subjective response to exercise, the earlier study by Jones and Mellersh (1946) provided what may be more useful information. In this study, 10 patients with effort syndrome were compared to 10 patients with "anxiety states" and "somatic anxiety symptoms," but with no evidence of effort syndrome. Both groups of anxious patients were compared with 20 control subjects. The patients with effort syndrome showed symptoms typical of descriptions of this syndrome in the 1940s. In addition to difficulties associated with putting forth "effort," they evidenced excessive emotional response to any excitement. When described in detail, they sound very much like patients with panic disorder. The remaining patients in this study with "anxiety states" seem to have resembled patients with GAD, although there is no way to confirm this.

Response to pedaling a stationary bicycle revealed patterns similar to the studies described previously with effort syndrome patients. But a new finding emerged from this study: Both patients with effort syndrome and patients with anxiety states showed some deficiencies in oxygen uptake. Blood lactate concentrations were also higher, along with pulse rate, for both patient groups at baseline as well as during exercise. Jones and Mellersh concluded that the patients with anxiety states were not really different from those with effort syndrome in their response to these tests on physiological measures. However, they were very different in terms of their subjective response to exercise. As the authors put it,

> In the one group the patient is conscious of this poor exercise response and tends to associate his symptoms with physical effort (in fact develops an effort phobia); in the other group no such awareness is present and the somatic anxiety symptoms are not correlated with exercise. This conforms to the clinical impression that most ES [effort syndrome] patients are indistinguishable from anxiety states, except for the fact that they do have an effort phobia. (Jones & Mellersh, 1946, pp. 185–186)

This is an intriguing hypothesis that was not pursued by these investigators. However, over 50 years later, similar hypotheses have now received increased attention—a topic to which I return below.

Finally, an observation was made in these early studies that would be confirmed repeatedly in the decades to follow. Anxious patients, with or without effort syndrome, evidenced elevated pulse and respiration rates and other indices of chronic hyperarousal *while at rest* (see Chapter 6). In summary, the results of these important early studies suggest an interaction of chronic hyperarousal and a subjective or cognitive sensitivity to these somatic sensations as crucial mechanisms in effort syndrome.

This early work could provide only the barest hints of important relationships. Among the many problems was the necessity of equating old diagnostic categories with new diagnostic categories, as well as the lack of definition of panic in these early experiments. Although these findings are thus of historical interest only, recent studies have replicated these early studies with more up-to-date methodology and assessment procedures. For example, J. M. Stein et al. (1992) exercised 16 patients with panic disorder and 15 normal controls on a stationary bicycle, utilizing procedures similar to those employed by Jones and Mellersh (1946) and Cohen and White (1950). Consistent with observations by Grosz and Farmer (1969), exercise-produced lactate was unrelated to the physical or psychological consequences of exercise. One patient was recorded as experiencing a full-blown panic attack, compared to none in the control group. In addition, 10 of the 16 patients and 5 of the 15 controls stopped the exercise prematurely, but only 4 patients were stopped by the investigators for meeting or exceeding heart rate goals. Patients showed significantly increased levels of epinephrine during the test and reported some increases on cognitive symptoms of panic attacks (going crazy or losing control), compared to no reports whatsoever of these cognitive symptoms among the control group; but these differences did not reach statistical significance. Unfortunately, measures of exercise-related anxiety were not taken.

These results seem consistent with the earlier studies (to the extent that measures were similar), in that patients with panic disorder showed less tolerance of exercise; levels of lactate seem unrelated to this tolerance; and there were some hints of subjective distress to the exercise paradigm, although this was not adequately measured. The authors interpreted the results to suggest that the principal between-group differences lay in physical conditioning. Of course, this difference may have been due to anxiety-related avoidance of exercise on the part of patients, as noted by Jones and Mellersh (1946) and Cohen and White (1950).

Cameron and Hudson (1986) exercised 36 patients with panic attacks and, while noting similar very low rates of panic, observed that as many as 31% of patients experienced marked increases in anxiety during the exercise that was directly related to the intensity of the exercise. This result compared to only 7% of 30 patients with anxiety disorders *without* panic attacks in the picture. Martinsen, Raglin, Hoffart, and Friis (1998) also exercised 35 patients with panic disorder on a stationary bicycle. Consistent with previous studies, only 1 patient evidenced a full-blown panic attack, and exercise-related lactate levels were unrelated to panic or anxiety. Also consistent with previous studies, the patients as a group were less fit than normal subjects were.

Finally, Taylor et al. (1987) compared 40 patients with panic disorder and 40 age-matched controls during exercise on a treadmill. They also reported that patients evidenced higher heart rates, tended to avoid physical activity, and were probably less fit than controls. Only 1 patient experienced a panic attack during exercise. Similarly, Gaffney, Fenton, Lane, and Lake (1988) compared 10 patients with panic disorder to 10 controls on a stationary bicycle exercise test and also found lower fitness levels in patients, but no evidence of panic.

It should also be noted that several studies utilizing ambulatory monitoring have looked for naturalistic associations between exercise and panic attacks (e.g., Freedman, Ianni, Ettedgui, & Puthezhath, 1985; Lint, Taylor, Fried-Behar, & Kenardy, 1995; Margraf, Taylor, Ehlers, Roth, & Agras, 1987; Taylor, Telch, & Haavik, 1983). Many of these studies have been reviewed in Chapter 4. Generally, it seems a rare occasion when clear evidence of physical exertion precedes a panic attack. In one review it was noted that of 91 naturally occurring panic attacks recorded, only 1 seemed related to physical exertion (O'Connor, Smith, & Morgan, 2000).

In summary, the results from these studies dating back to the 1940s are remarkably consistent. Patients with panic disorder (or its historical equivalent) are consistently less fit than matched controls, tend to avoid or escape exercise, and evidence anxiety focused on the somatic consequences of exercise (effort phobia), although few manifest full-blown panic attacks. This is consistent with widespread clinical observations that patients with panic disorder tend to avoid exercise-produced somatic sensations, particularly those that resemble their naturally occurring panic attacks (Asmundson & Stein, 1994a). Of course, none of the above-described experiments directly tested that notion in a satisfactory manner. In addition, as pointed out by Martinsen et al. (1998), the unexpected occurrence of somatic sensations from incidental exercise may well be very different from the very controlled, purposeful exercise-related induction of somatic sensations in the experimental laboratory. That is, incidental exercise of the type not directly examined in ambulatory monitoring studies may be more panicogenic. Early studies also report relatively consistent evidence for low ventilatory efficiency and relatively rapid ventilation (as possible correlates of poor physical fitness), and a greater awareness of these states, in patients with panic disorder. One may conclude, then, that the physical effects of exercise have little or no relation to panic provocation. Rather, the subjective sensitivity to somatic sensations, and perhaps low ventilatory efficiency and awareness of breathlessness, in patients with panic attacks may be what produce any differences observed in exercise provocation studies.

Studies on the effects of exercise are now few and far between. However, despite the lack of evidence that hyperventilation mediates exercise-provoked anxiety (or panic), the intriguing findings on ventilatory inefficiency remained. Interest in the effects of hyperventilation was reinvigorated during the 1980s, when clear evidence that instructions to hyperventilate can provoke panic attacks began to appear.

Hyperventilation

Hyperventilation is a common human experience familiar to many of us, at one time or another. The basis of hyperventilation is very straightforward: Any time one overbreathes or blows off an excess of CO_2, a hyperventilation syndrome may develop. In its more severe form, sustained overbreathing leads to dramatic symptoms, such as unconsciousness or tetany. However, the more common signs and symptoms of hyperventilation include chronic sighing, as well as a variety of physical symptoms such as dizziness, paresthesias, palpitations, and dyspnea (Fried & Grimaldi, 1993; Fried, 1994; Lum, 1975, 1976). These symptoms are also common during panic attacks. For that reason, there was sustained interest during the 1980s in the possibility that hyperventilation under certain circumstances causes panic. A natural step was to attempt provocation of panic attacks through hyperventilation.

The Physiological Basis of Hyperventilation

The physiological basis of hyperventilation is relatively well worked out. The function of respiration is to provide oxygen, which is transported from inhaled air to blood and then to various tissues and organs to meet metabolic needs. The brain takes a disproportionate share of this oxygen. Increased breathing removes CO_2, a by-product of respiration, from the lungs faster than it can be manufactured by the body. This action decreases the partial pressure of arterial CO_2 (pCO_2). A pCO_2 reading below 35 mm/Hg is defined as hypocapnia (normal would be between 35 and 45 mm/Hg). The loss of CO_2 through hyperventilation produces respiratory alkalosis when pH exceeds 7.45. This is caused by a reduction in free hydrogen ions.

Hypocapnic alkalosis is directly related to the symptoms experienced during hyperventilation. This is because oxygenation is somewhat impaired, since oxygen binds more tightly to hemoglobin (the oxygen-transporting protein in red blood cells), during hypocapnia. Hypcapnia also causes vascular constriction. Eventually, as hyperventilation continues, reduced cerebral blood flow and reduced availability of oxygen produce hypoxia. This condition stimulates dilation of the cerebral vasculature as well as several other compensatory mechanisms to attempt to bring the pH level back into balance. The decrease in cerebral blood flow and relative lack of oxygen seem to account for the symptoms of lightheadedness, dizziness, derealization and depersonalization, blurred vision, and other physiological symptoms mentioned above. The extra work of breathing rapidly (or increases in heart rate because of indirect effects of hypocapnia) may produce chest pain in the intercostal muscles and sensations of breathlessness. With chronic hyperventilation, pH and cerebral blood flow may return to nearly normal due to the effects of various compensatory mechanisms, even though pCO_2 and related physiological markers of hyperventilation remain low. It is this state of "chronic hyperventilation" that may be maintained by several deep breaths per hour or several long "sighs," but even slight increases in ventilatory rate while in this state may reestablish the hypocapnic, alkalotic state (McNally, 1994; Papp, Klein, & Gorman, 1993).

Hyperventilation Provocation Studies

Early studies examined individual differences in resting pCO_2 levels that seem to be associated with a greater sensitivity to increased ventilation. In other words, only small increases in rates of breathing trigger the beginnings of hyperventilation symptoms for some people, whereas more rapid breathing is required to produce the same symptoms in others (Lum, 1975, 1976). Some individuals may maintain this lower resting pCO_2 level through a habit of rapid breathing as described above. For example, Huey and West (1983) used a screening questionnaire containing hyperventilation-related symptoms to choose either "likely hyperventilators" or "unlikely hyperventilators" from an otherwise normal student population. They found that "likely hyperventilators" ventilated more rapidly during baseline conditions and developed more somatic symptoms after a period of overbreathing then did "unlikely hyperventilators." This was one of the few experiments on hyperventilation to provide adequate controls for demand characteristics. These early results suggested that individuals who panic may be individuals likely to hyperventilate who have developed a "habit" of rapid breathing.

The next step was to examine the effects of voluntary hyperventilation in patients with panic disorder. In one early experiment testing the relationship of hyperventilation and panic, Garssen, VanVeenendaal, and Bloemink (1983) asked 28 patients with DSM-III agoraphobia with panic attacks to hyperventilate. Specifically, they were asked to breathe as deeply and rapidly as possible until pCO_2 was decreased to approximately half of its resting value and was maintained at this level for a period of at least 90 seconds. After hyperventilating, the patients reported on the similarity of this experience to their panic attacks. In this procedure, 17 (or 61%) of the 28 patients experienced panic symptoms while hyperventilating. However, it is not clear whether any subject reported an actual panic attack, since this was not part of the procedure. The patients simply reported that the somatic symptoms were similar or identical to those experienced during a panic attack.

Rapee (1986) carefully selected 20 patients with panic disorder, as well as 13 subjects with DSM-III GAD who had never experienced a panic attack. In this study, patients with panic disorder evidenced lower resting pCO_2 and higher resting heart rate then those with GAD. Since patients with GAD who had experienced any panic attacks were excluded, it is possible that these patients were less severely anxious than the patients with panic disorder.

After 90 seconds of voluntary hyperventilation, patients were administered a questionnaire on which they indicated the number of symptoms they experienced and the amount of distress caused by each symptom on a rating scale. Patients with panic disorder reported a significantly greater number of symptoms, as well as greater mean distress associated with each symptom, than did patients with GAD. Furthermore, when asked about the similarity of their experience to naturally occurring anxiety, 80% of the group with panic disorder reported a marked similarity of symptoms, while 20% reported no resemblance. This compares to 25% of the patients with GAD who reported the experience to be similar and 75% who said that the hyperventilatory symptoms were quite dissimilar from their (generalized) anxiety. No subject reported an actual panic attack. All patients indicated that they did not "panic" because they knew what was causing the symptoms and felt that they were in a safe environment.

Since that time a number of studies have reported the effects of voluntary hyperventilation in patients with panic disorder, compared with a number of different control groups. The rather consistent finding is that anywhere from 20% to 50% of patients will report a panic attack during these procedures, with the modal percentage in the 20–30% range. Of course, these reports depend greatly on definitions of panic and other experimental procedures that vary from study to study. In one notable early study, Gorman et al. (1984) compared hyperventilation to lactate provocation as well as a maximum of 20 minutes of breathing 5% CO_2. During hyperventilation, 3 out of 12 subjects, or 25%, evidenced a panic attack based on independent ratings of the occurrence of panic attacks developed in this laboratory. This rate was substantially less than that observed under conditions of lactate infusion or CO_2 inhalation—a finding to be repeatedly observed in future studies. Curiously, the panic attacks during hyperventilation as described by these patients were reported as being dissimilar to their naturally occurring panic attacks (or to lactate-induced or CO_2-induced panics).

In any case, subsequent studies have produced similar results (e.g., Gorman, Fyer, Kinney, & Klein, 1988; Holt & Andrews, 1989a, 1989b; Spinhoven, Onstein, Sterk,

& le Haen-Versteijnen, 1992). For example, Gorman et al. (1994) noted that 13% of 23 patients (as defined by independent raters) or 30% of 20 patients (when subjectively reported) evidenced panic attacks during voluntary hyperventilation. Once again, these rates were considerably lower than comparative conditions involving inhalation of CO_2 (to be reviewed below).

Representative of the effects of hyperventilation in these studies, and the largest study of its type yet conducted, is a report by our group (Rapee, Brown, Antony, & Barlow, 1992). In this study, 198 patients with diagnosed anxiety disorders and 25 nonanxious control subjects underwent a 90-second challenge of voluntary hyperventilation. This condition was compared to inhalations of 5.5% CO_2 in air. Between 25 and 40 patients from each of the major anxiety disorder diagnostic categories were evaluated. Reports of both psychological and physical reactions, as well as similarity to naturally occurring panic attacks, were taken on well-established psychometrically sound questionnaires (Rapee, Brown, et al., 1992). Detailed results are presented in Table 5.2. Significant differences among groups were apparent for all of the cognitive symptoms, with patients with panic disorder generally evidencing the highest scores on cognitive symptoms and the nonanxious control group the lowest score. No analyses were done on respiratory rate or pCO_2 levels, since these were intentionally manipulated during the experiment, although mean results are presented in the table. The success of the hyperventilation manipulation is demonstrated by the fact that pCO_2 during hyperventilation is around half that of resting pCO_2.

To examine in a meaningful way the percentage of patients meeting criteria for panic attacks during a hyperventilation challenge, patients were aggregated into four groups: those with panic disorder with or without agoraphobia as a principal diagnosis ("panic disorder primary"); patients with some other anxiety disorder as a principal diagnosis but with panic disorder with or without agoraphobia as an additional (less severe) diagnosis ("panic disorder additional"); patients with anxiety disorders without panic disorder anywhere in the diagnostic picture ("anxiety disorders, no panic"); and nonanxious controls. In addition, panic attacks were defined by both liberal and conservative criteria. In the more liberal criteria, patients had to report four or more DSM-III-R panic symptoms, at least one of which was a cognitive symptom, together with a feeling of fear or panic at an intensity of at least 1 on a 0–8 scale. Because this definition involved a low degree of fear, a more conservative a priori definition was devised that involved the same somatic and cognitive criteria but required a fear intensity rating of 5 or above on a 0–8 scale (more than moderate fear).

The results are presented in Figure 5.2, as are the results from breathing 5.5% CO_2 in air (to be described below). There were significant overall differences in the number of subjects who experienced a panic attack according to both the liberal and conservative criteria in response to both hyperventilation and CO_2. As one can see, 20–46.7% of patients in the "panic disorder primary" group met one set of criteria or another for experiencing a panic attack during hyperventilation. This compared to 6.7–33.3% in the "panic disorder additional" group; 6.5–17.2% in the "anxiety disorders, no panic" group; and 0–8% in the nonanxious control group. Notice that these figures are substantially less than the percentages reported during CO_2 provocation, which is consistent with other studies. In addition, 11 subjects in the "panic disorder primary" group (15.5%) terminated the CO_2 inhalation before the end of the 15-minute challenge. This compared with 3 (10.3%) in the "panic disorder additional" group, 6 (6.5%) in the "anxiety disorders, no panic" group, and 1 (4.0%) in the control group. This was not a significant difference.

Several interesting findings emerged from this experiment. First, all groups actually seemed to evidence peripheral physiological changes to similar degrees. The major differ-

TABLE 5.2. Means and Standard Deviations of Measures Taken after Hyperventilation

Variable	Group						
	PDA	PD	GAD	SOC	SP	OCD	Control
No. physical symptoms							
M	5.4_a	4.9_{ab}	3.9_{bc}	4.2_{bc}	3.6_c	3.3_c	1.9
SD	2.7	2.6	2.3	2.9	2.4	2.2	1.4
No. cognitive symptoms							
M	0.7_a	0.8_a	0.5_{ab}	0.2_{bc}	0.2_{bc}	0.4_{abc}	0.1_c
SD	0.8	1.0	0.8	0.6	0.5	0.9	0.3
Intensity of physical symptoms							
M	3.4_a	3.5_a	2.9_{ab}	3.4_a	2.8_{ab}	2.5_b	2.1_b
SD	1.5	1.4	1.3	1.6	1.8	1.1	1.2
Intensity of cognitive symptoms							
M	2.1_a	1.6_{ab}	1.2_{bc}	0.6_{cd}	0.5_{cd}	0.5_{cd}	0.1_d
SD	2.5	2.1	1.9	1.4	1.2	0.9	0.4
Intensity of fear							
M	3.4_a	2.7_{ab}	1.7_{bc}	1.3_{cd}	1.8_{bc}	1.3_{cd}	0.3_d
SD	2.5	2.2	2.1	1.9	2.3	1.6	0.7
Anxiety immediately after hyperventilation							
M	4.4_a	4.3_a	3.8_{ab}	3.6_{ab}	3.1_b	3.2_b	1.4
SD	1.8	1.6	2.0	1.9	1.9	1.9	1.4
Similarity to usual panic or anxiety							
M	3.1_a	2.4_{ab}	2.0_{bcd}	2.2_{bc}	1.8_{bcd}	1.3_{cd}	1.1_d
SD	2.1	1.9	1.9	2.0	1.5	1.1	1.8
No. catastrophic thoughts							
M	1.7_a	1.8_a	1.6_a	0.7_{bc}	0.6_{bc}	1.1_{ab}	0.1_c
SD	1.3	1.8	1.9	1.0	1.0	1.3	0.3
No. noncatastrophic thoughts							
M	2.3	2.2	2.2	1.8	2.3	1.9	3.0
SD	1.3	1.5	1.7	1.6	1.5	1.5	1.6
Heart rate (beats/min)							
M	97.8	101.9	97.8	104.8	100.6	92.9	100.1
SD	19.6	14.7	16.5	16.6	18.8	16.4	15.7
Respiratory rate (breaths/min)							
M	45.5	41.8	42.6	39.9	45.6	45.2	46.0
SD	19.1	16.7	15.6	12.2	14.3	18.1	17.3
pCO_2 (mm/Hg)							
M	23.0	21.2	20.5	20.6	21.1	21.6	21.1
SD	4.5	3.4	4.2	2.9	3.8	3.4	4.0

Note. PDA, panic disorder with agoraphobia (moderate to severe avoidance); PD, panic disorder (none or mild avoidance); GAD, generalized anxiety disorder; SOC, social phobia: SP, simple phobia; OCD, obsessive–compulsive disorder; Control, nonanxious control. Means with the same subscripts are not significantly different at $p < .05$. From "Response to Hyperventilation and Inhalation of 5.5% Carbon Dioxide-Enriched Air across the DSM-III-R Anxiety Disorders" by R. M. Rapee, T. A. Brown, M. M. Antony, and D. H. Barlow, 1992, *Journal of Abnormal Psychology, 101,* 538–552. Copyright 1992 by the American Psychological Association. Reprinted with permission.

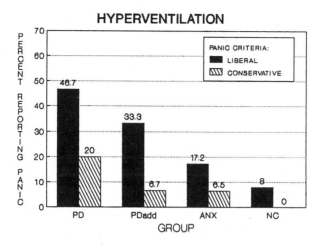

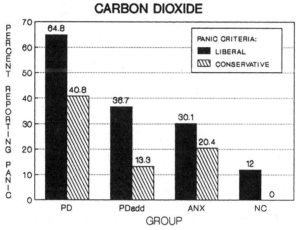

FIGURE 5.2. Proportion of subjects in each comorbid category who reported a panic attack (according to either liberal or conservative criteria) in response to each challenge procedure. (PD, panic disorder as principal diagnosis; PDadd, panic disorder as additional diagnosis; ANX, other anxiety disorder without panic disorder; NC, nonanxious controls.) From "Response to Hyperventilation and Inhalation of 5.5% Carbon Dioxide-Enriched Air across the DSM-III-R Anxiety Disorders" by R. M. Rapee, T. A. Brown, M. M. Antony, and D. H. Barlow, 1992, *Journal of Abnormal Psychology, 101,* 538–552. Copyright 1992 by the American Psychological Association. Reprinted with permission.

ences among groups were on subjective measures, or the response to these somatic changes. It is also interesting to note, consistent with findings reported above, that panic disorder anywhere in the picture seemed to heighten the probability of responding with panic to these provocation procedures. This result underscores the importance of assessing comorbid diagnoses.

Mechanisms of Hyperventilation-Provoked Panic Attacks

Despite clear evidence that hyperventilation challenge can provoke panic attacks in at least some patients, a clear consensus has developed among investigators with many different views that the physiological consequences of hyperventilation are not a direct and unique cause of panic attacks. For example, Gorman et al. (1986) demonstrated that metabolic alkalosis is not the proximate cause of panic during lactate infusions, since patients who went on to panic kept their pH level very close to that of nonpanicking patients. Weiner (1985) also described dissimilarities between physiological effects of anxiety and hyperventilation.

Holt and Andrews (1989a) found that patients with panic disorder showed higher rates of hyperventilatory symptoms than patients with other anxiety disorders or normal subjects, as well as on measures of respiratory rate at rest, but these differences did not correlate with direct measures of expired pCO_2 at rest or of respiratory alkalosis. Furthermore, Holt and Andrews (1989a) found that hyperventilation symptoms increased not only during a hyperventilation challenge, but also during the physiologically converse CO_2 challenge condition. They argued that the greatest differences between groups lay in their perception of the effects of the experimental procedures, rather than in any fundamental physiological consequences of hyperventilation. They conclude that this does not rule out the occasional case where a clear hyperventilation syndrome accompanied by substantial drops in pCO_2 is associated with subsequent panic attacks (e.g., Salkovskis, Warwick, Clark, & Wessels, 1986), but that this could not be the direct and proximate cause of panic in the majority of cases. Similarly, Spinhoven et al. (1992) found no differences in respiratory physiology between patients who rated their symptoms during a hyperventilation challenge as similar to those occurring during panic attacks in daily life, compared to those who did not rate their hyperventilation symptoms similar to their panic symptoms. Patients who experienced a panic attack during hyperventilation challenge also showed no independent changes in respiratory physiology. They concluded, as did Holt and Andrews (1989a), that reports of severe panic and hyperventilation symptoms are more closely related to the level of anxiety than to respiratory physiology.

Garssen, Buikhuisen, and van Dyck (1996) explored the association between transcutaneous pCO_2 levels and panic attacks during long-term ambulatory measurement and found that a decrease in pCO_2 was observed during only 1 of 24 registered panic attacks in a group of 28 patients with panic disorder. Hibbert and Pilsbury (1989) came to similar conclusions.

Thus the overwhelming body of evidence indicates that hyperventilation is not a cause of panic attacks. Rather, hyperventilatory symptoms (but not necessarily hyperventilatory respiratory physiology) may be a function of high levels of anxiety that may in turn be associated with distorted perceptions of bodily sensations. These perceptions are what may trigger full-blown panic attacks. In other words, consistent with data from the Rapee, Brown, et al. (1992) study, the subjective response to hyperventilatory symptoms is more crucial in the production of panic than underlying respiratory physiology.

CO_2 Inhalation

The third provocation procedure in which respiratory symptoms are strongly implicated involves inhaling various amounts of CO_2. It is particularly interesting to compare and contrast the panicogenic qualities of voluntary hyperventilation with those of CO_2 inhalation.

Testifying once again to the long historical tradition of provocation studies, the inhalation of CO_2 was demonstrated very early to provoke panic-like symptoms in susceptible patients. In 1919, Drury found that patients with "irritable heart syndrome" displayed an exquisite sensitivity to the inspiration of even low percentages of CO_2. This sensitivity included symptoms that would now be described as panic.

Cohen and White (1950) reported an experiment in which 43 patients and 27 control subjects first breathed oxygen for 12 minutes, and then inhaled air containing 4% CO_2 for 12 minutes. Of the 43 patients, 47% developed symptoms rated as identical to their anxiety attacks, while another 37% developed symptoms described as similar to their attacks. Thus a substantial proportion of 84% of the patients found that inhaling CO_2 was anxiogenic and possibly panicogenic. These findings were overlooked until the 1980s, although it is not clear why. One possibility is that for a period of years, inhalations of CO_2 were used to reduce anxiety in anxious patients. Beginning with Wolpe (1958), who first popularized the method, a number of clinical reports suggested that inhalations of CO_2 were effective in reducing anxiety in patients with a variety of anxiety problems, including what we would now call panic (Latimer, 1977; Ley & Walker, 1973; van den Hout & Griez, 1982; Wolpe, 1973). In fact, some investigators (e.g., Thyer, Papsdorf, & Wright, 1984) have used the apparent anxiolytic effects of CO_2 inhalation to further support the possibility of a hyperventilatory etiology of panic, where CO_2 is rapidly blown off! van den Hout and Griez (1982), who have both increased and decreased anxiety with CO_2 inhalations, conclude that CO_2-induced sensations are either pleasant or unpleasant, depending upon prior expectations. For example, Ley and Walker (1973) instructed their patients to expect less anxiety, and this is what they found. The issue of expectations and demand in panic provocation studies is taken up again below.

From the point of view of mechanisms of action, 35% CO_2 initially produces respiratory acidosis. This would seem to make it incompatible with hyperventilation and possibly lactate infusion, which produce respiratory (and metabolic) alkalosis. But as van den Hout (1988) pointed out, the intense stimulation of a breath of 35% CO_2 produces a hypocapnic undershoot. This results very quickly in a rebound to a state of alkalosis. Therefore, 35% CO_2 seems to produce the same effects as hyperventilation, despite the process of blowing off CO_2 on the one hand and inhaling it on the other. For this reason, among others, there has been more interest from a theoretical point of view in procedures where (approximately) 5% CO_2 is inhaled. The 5% CO_2 produces a clear acidosis with no rebound. This provides a clear contrast to effects of hyperventilation or lactate. And yet, beginning with the Cohen and White (1950) study described above, the evidence is as firm on the panicogenic effects of inhaling 5% CO_2 as it is for any other provocation procedure, including lactate.

Gorman et al. (1984), in the experiment described earlier, had the same 12 patients who had previously undergone lactate infusions inhale air containing 5% CO_2. Of these 12 patients, 7 panicked and reported the attacks as being very much like both lactate panics and their naturally occurring attacks. These patients reported being particularly uncomfortable with having their respiration increased or "driven" in an out-of-control manner. Cohen and White (1950) also reported that rapid, out-of-control breathing was particularly discomforting to their patients.

Several other well-controlled early studies pointed to the panicogenic effects of 5% CO_2. In one study, 7 out of 10 medication-free patients with agoraphobia and panic attacks who inhaled a 5% CO_2 mixture experienced panic attacks. These 7 (along with another patient who had a strong reaction but did not actually report panic) indicated that the experiences were very similar to naturally occurring panics. This compared to 4 out of 22 control subjects who reported panic (Woods et al., 1986). The investigators specifically tested the hypothesis that patients with panic might have abnormally high central medullary chemoreceptor sensitivity—a hypothesis that became increasingly popular in subsequent years, since CO_2 exerts its primary effects in the respiratory center located in the brain stem (specifically, the reticular substance of the medulla oblongata and the pons). As Coplan and Klein (1996) point out, the diversity of agents capable of provoking panic would seem to imply a low threshold for the triggering of panic pathways by a variety of mechanisms. However, no differences in ventilatory responses to CO_2 emerged between patient and control groups in this particular study. These investigators then conducted a second, more intensive study (Woods, Charney, Goodman, & Heninger, 1987) in which many different physiological, biochemical, and behavioral measures were collected over a period of 3 hours surrounding the provocation procedure. In addition, healthy control subjects breathed two different mixtures of CO_2 (one containing 5% and another containing 7.5%). This study retains importance. Of 14 patients, 8 experienced panic attacks while breathing 5% CO_2, compared to 3 out of 11 control subjects. In an interesting development, 7 out of 8 healthy control subjects experienced panic attacks at the higher 7.5% level of CO_2.

This last study is important for three reasons. First, this study was among the first that was placebo-controlled. Second, it included a substantial majority of normal healthy subjects reporting clear panic attacks defined not only by somatic symptoms but also by cognitive symptoms (marked subjective anxiety, fear of losing control, etc.). In this regard, normal control subjects differed from patients only in requiring a stronger concentration of CO_2 before panicking. Third, no differences emerged on physiological or biological measures between patients and controls at any point in the experiment. This included the 5% CO_2 inhalation comparison, where patients reported significantly more anxiety and panic attacks than did controls. Once again, this raises questions about the basic mechanisms of action of panic.

Another well-done early study yielded similar results. Ehlers, Margraf, and Roth (1987) administered a 5.5% CO_2 mixture to 16 patients with panic and 18 control subjects. These investigators also observed a similar response to the provocation procedure on the part of patients and controls. What made this study interesting at the time was the observation that patients reported significantly more anxiety as well as more panic attacks (depending on the criteria used) as a function of differences in baseline anxiety prior to the CO_2 inhalation. That is, the patients were more anxious to begin with, but there were no differences in absolute increases in subjective or physiological measures of anxiety over and above those demonstrated by control subjects.

These findings do not agree entirely with those of Woods, Charney, Goodman, and Heninger (1987), since the patients in the latter study did show greater increases in anxiety and some phsyiological measures over baseline values, compared to controls. Repeated ratings of anxiety during CO_2 inhalations from the Woods, Charney, Goodman, and Heninger (1987) experiment are presented in Figure 5.3. Physiological measures showed similar patterns.

These early studies produced heightened interest in CO_2 provocation as a valid marker of panic attacks, and perhaps panic disorder. This is because CO_2-induced panic attacks seem to be fairly specific to patients with panic disorder, although not necessarily sensitive (Sanderson & Wetzler, 1990). Also, Papp, Klein, Martinez, et al. (1993) showed in their study that 35% CO_2 was significantly more panicogenic than increased airway resistance that produced similar amounts of respiratory distress and breathlessness, implying a more fundamental neurobiological mechanism.

Two more recent studies directly comparing panic provocation by either CO_2 inhalation or hyperventilation have been mentioned above (Gorman et al., 1994; Rapee, Brown,

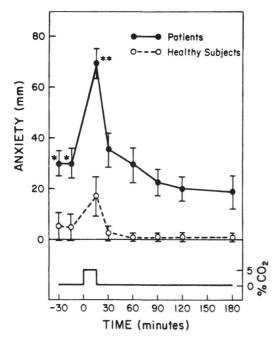

FIGURE 5.3. Anxiety visual analogue scale ratings and inspired CO_2 concentrations on the 5% CO_2 day in patients with panic disorder and healthy subjects. $*p < .001$, baseline values, patients versus healthy subjects, unpaired t test, two-tailed; $**p < .001$, time point versus baseline, paired t test, two-tailed, and $p < .05$, change from baseline, patients versus healthy subjects, unpaired t test, two-tailed. From Woods, Charney, Goodman, and Heninger (1987). Copyright 1987 by the American Medical Association. Reprinted by permission.

et al., 1992). Furthermore, both 5% and 7% CO_2 were administered and compared in the Gorman et al. (1994) study. In this study, only between 13% and 30% of patients panicked (depending on the definition used) during voluntary hyperventilation, whereas between 29% of 21 patients (as defined by independent raters) or 71% of 17 patients (when subjectively reported) evidenced panic attacks during 5% CO_2 inhalation. This compared to 0 out of 17 control subjects when independently rated, and 1 out of 14 control subjects when subjectively reported. During administration of 7% CO_2, 13 (68%) of 19 patients but only 2 (12%) of 17 control subjects panicked as defined by independent raters, and 13 (81%) of 16 patients and 1 (7%) of 14 control subjects reported panicking. Notice that the results for control subjects with 7% CO_2 differed substantially from the results reported by Woods, Charney, Goodman, and Heninger (1987) for control subjects inhaling 7.5% CO_2. The reasons for this discrepancy are not clear, but most likely reside in methodological differences. Measures taken before and after a 20-minute baseline period in the Gorman et al. (1994) this experiment showed that patients with panic scored significantly higher than normal control subjects on all measures of anxiety, and that scores increased during baseline for patients on some measures. Analyses of panic status during provocation as a function of baseline anxiety were not undertaken, but it was noted that no patients experienced a panic attack during baseline.

Some of the results from the Rapee, Brown, et al. (1992) experiment comparing inhalations of 5.5% CO_2 to hyperventilation have been described above. Reports of both psychological and physical reactions, as well as similarity to naturally occurring panic attacks after CO_2 inhalation are presented in Table 5.3 for the different diagnostic groups. Notice that this table parallels the results for hyperventilation provocation in Table 5.2. Once again, the percentage of patients meeting criteria for panic attacks during CO_2 inhalation is represented in Figure 5.2. As one can see, between 40.8% and 64.8% of the patients in the "panic

TABLE 5.3. Means and Standard Deviations of Measures Taken after CO_2 Inhalation

Variable	Group						
	PDA	PD	GAD	SOC	SP	OCD	Control
No. physical symptoms							
M	5.6_{ab}	5.9_a	4.8_{abc}	4.2_c	4.2_{bc}	3.9_{cd}	2.6_d
SD	3.2	2.7	2.9	2.7	2.4	2.6	2.3
No. cognitive symptoms							
M	1.0_a	1.0_a	0.6_{ab}	0.4_{bc}	0.3_{bc}	0.7_{ab}	0.1_c
SD	1.0	0.9	0.9	0.7	0.5	0.9	0.3
Intensity of physical symptoms							
M	3.7_a	4.0_a	3.3_{ab}	3.4_{ab}	3.3_{ab}	3.1_{ab}	2.5_b
SD	2.0	1.7	1.7	1.5	1.6	1.4	1.6
Intensity of cognitive symptoms							
M	2.5_a	2.5_a	1.2_b	1.1_b	0.9_b	1.4_b	0.2_b
SD	2.6	2.4	1.7	2.0	1.5	1.8	0.7
Intensity of fear							
M	3.6_{ab}	4.3_a	2.9_{bc}	2.2_{cd}	3.1_{abc}	2.9_{abc}	1.1_d
SD	2.8	2.7	2.4	2.3	2.7	2.3	2.0
Average anxiety during inhalation							
M	4.2_a	4.3_a	3.7_a	3.3_a	3.5_a	3.9_a	1.9
SD	2.4	1.8	1.9	1.7	2.4	2.2	1.7
Similarity to usual panic or anxiety							
M	3.1_{ab}	3.5_a	2.4_{abc}	2.6_{ab}	2.9_{ab}	2.2_{bc}	1.3_c
SD	2.5	2.3	1.9	2.2	2.4	1.6	1.8
No. catastrophic thoughts							
M	2.2_{ab}	2.6_a	1.7_{bc}	1.1_{cd}	1.0_{cd}	1.5_{bc}	0.5_a
SD	1.9	1.9	1.9	1.2	1.2	1.7	1.1
No. noncatastrophic thoughts							
M	1.9	1.4	2.1	1.4	1.7	1.9	2.2
SD	1.7	1.4	1.8	1.5	1.6	1.3	1.7
Heart rate (beats/min)							
M	80.2	78.4	74.6	77.5	79.6	73.5	77.0
SD	13.5	12.8	9.8	12.5	10.9	8.3	9.4
Respiratory rate (breaths/min)							
M	18.9_a	15.7_a	16.7_{ab}	15.8_a	18.1_{ab}	18.3_b	16.7_{ab}
SD	5.6	4.0	4.0	4.1	5.0	3.7	4.4
pCO$_2$ (mm/Hg)							
M	47.2	46.4	45.8	46.7	45.8	46.6	48.3
SD	3.1	3.9	5.0	3.7	4.7	4.0	3.4
Duration of CO_2 inhalation (in min)							
M	13.3	14.3	14.2	14.9	14.6	14.9	14.5
SD	3.7	2.4	2.5	0.5	1.9	0.4	2.4

Note. PDA, panic disorder with agoraphobia (moderate to severe avoidance); PD, panic disorder (none or mild avoidance); GAD, generalized anxiety disorder; SOC, social phobia: SP, simple phobia; OCD, obsessive-compulsive disorder; and Control, nonanxious control. Means with the same subscripts are not significantly different at $p < .05$. From "Response to Hyperventilation and Inhalation of 5.5% Carbon Dioxide-Enriched Air across the DSM-III-R Anxiety Disorders" by R. M. Rapee, T. A. Brown, M. M. Antony, and D. H. Barlow, 1992, *Journal of Abnormal Psychology, 101,* 538–552. Copyright 1992 by the American Psychological Association. Reprinted with permission.

disorder primary" group met one set of criteria or another for experiencing a panic attack during CO_2 inhalation. Percentages of patients meeting criteria for panic attack were generally higher for CO_2 than for hyperventilation.

As observed in previous experiments, patients evidenced higher scores on measures of anxiety at baseline than controls did, and this seemed to account for many of the differences. However, when similar measures were taken immediately *after* the challenge procedures, a significant group × time interaction emerged, suggesting the specificity of this procedure for patients with panic attacks somewhere in the picture. Interestingly, a predictor analysis showed that one robust predictor of responding to these challenge procedures with panic attacks was anxiety focused on somatic sensations, as reflected in high scores on the Anxiety Sensitivity Index.

During the 1990s, numerous studies have replicated both the robust nature and specificity of CO_2 inhalation as a potential marker of panic disorder or panic attacks. For example, Perna, Bertani, Arancio, Ronchi, and Bellodi (1995) showed this specificity for inhalation of 35% CO_2 in patients with panic disorder compared to patients with obsessive–compulsive disorder alone (without comorbidity), who did not differ from normal controls. Bellodi et al. (1998) even demonstrated a significantly higher concordance for 35% CO_2-induced panic attacks among monozygotic compared to dizygotic twins (55.6% vs. 12.5%) without panic disorder, which the authors interpret as perhaps reflecting a preexisting vulnerability to panic—a conclusion also reached by Goetz et al. (1994). Unfortunately, comparable measures of anxiety sensitivity that could possibly account for the results in the Goetz et al. (1994) study were not taken.

Mechanisms of Panic Provoked by Respiration-Related Procedures

On the whole, studies from respiration-related provocation procedures would seem to reinforce findings from biochemical provocation studies concerning multiple underlying biological processes associated with provocation of panic. The inhalation of 5% CO_2 is incompatible with respiratory alkalosis, which is the physiological consequence of hyperventilation. Similarly, exercise, to the extent that it is panicogenic, would also seem incompatible with respiratory alkalosis, since increased oxygen consumption is necessary to meet increased metabolic demands. What all three procedures have in common, of course, are the discomfort and distress associated with suddenly increased rates of ventilation. This is the out-of-control, "driven" respiration mentioned by Liebowitz, Gorman, Fyer, Levitt, et al. (1985) as a possible panic trigger in lactate infusion. Papp, Klein, Martinez, et al. (1993) observed that respiratory distress alone could not account for all of the effects of CO_2 inhalation, although their procedure involved a very "controllable," temporary, laboratory-created airway impedance that may not have been as anxiogenic as unexpected respiratory distress. In any case, this observation of ventilatory irregularities—first reported in the 1940s (Jones & Mellersh, 1946; Cohen & White, 1950)—and competing biological and psychological explanations for these irregularities have become the principal foci of attention in explanations of panic provocation in the laboratory.

Despite the negative findings from Woods and colleagues (Woods et al., 1986; Woods, Charney, Goodman, & Heninger, 1987), partially replicated in subsequent studies such as Roth et al. (1992), and Asmundson and Stein (1994b) intense interest has continued to focus on data suggesting a neurobiologically based CO_2 hypersensitivity as a possible etiological factor in panic attacks. In earlier studies, Gorman et al. (1988) observed abnormal ventilatory physiology in patients with panic disorder. A number of subsequent studies have observed at least "soft" signs of CO_2 hypersensitivity (Pine et al., 1998; Griez & Verburg,

1999). These "soft" signs (which could be accounted for by other factors), include excessive hyperventilation in room air, variable breathing rates, and of course specific sensitivity to CO_2 provocations.

Another reason for the interest in this hypothesis is the observed high frequency of panic attacks and panic disorder among those patients with chronic respiratory disease, where feelings of "suffocation" are common. For example, Pollack, Kradin, et al. (1996) examined 115 patients referred for pulmonary function testing and found that 17% met criteria for panic disorder, with a total of 41% reporting panic attacks. Out of 9 patients with chronic obstructive pulmonary disease, 6 met criteria for panic disorder. Verburg, Griez, Meijer, and Pols (1995) studied 82 patients with panic disorder compared to 68 patients with other anxiety disorders, and found that the rate of respiratory disorders before the onset of panic disorder was 42.7%, compared to 16.2% before the onset of other anxiety disorders. A summary of these results is presented in Figure 5.4. Griez and Verburg (1999) summarized a number of additional studies confirming this elevated rate of respiratory disorders preceding the development of panic disorder. Since CO_2 physiologically simulates the process of suffocation, these findings are not surprising.

Klein's False-Suffocation-Alarm Theory

In the context of rising interest in the contribution of respiratory factors to panic, and the attractiveness of CO_2 hypersensitivity in particular, Donald Klein (1993) has proposed a false-suffocation-alarm theory of spontaneous panic attacks and related conditions. Klein proposes that spontaneous or unexpected panic attacks are triggered by a hypothetical "monitor" in the brain stem that detects conditions that may lead to suffocation. These would include increased levels of CO_2 that would be detected centrally. Klein notes that during evolution, the experience of breathing excessive CO_2 would occur if individuals were forced to rebreathe their own exhalations, as would happen while trapped in a cave or during asphyxiation for various reasons. Those individuals with a particularly sensitive "suffocation alarm monitor" would be more likely to compensate through increased respiration and accompanying urges to escape the site where the suffocation might take place. Klein speculates that over evolutionary time, environmental cues may have become associated with the suffocation alarm response—including situations where there is no ready exit, or where stuffy, stale air signals that there may be no ready exit. Other situations might include large crowds where it is difficult to move because of the large number of people, or observing someone else who appears to be suffocating. From this point of view,

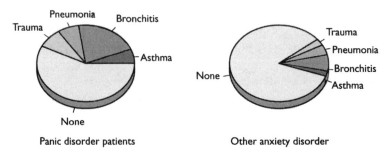

FIGURE 5.4. History of respiratory disorders in patients with panic disorder versus patients with other anxiety disorders. From Verburg, Griez, Meijer, and Pols (1995). Copyright 1995 by Elsevier Science Ltd. Reprinted by permission.

chronic hyperventilation could be understood as a method for keeping levels of CO_2 at manageable levels. Klein cites several interesting anecdotes in support of this notion, including commonly observed "gas hysteria" during World War I, where entire army units would break ranks and run in response to threats of suffocation from gas without any objective provocation.

This theory has attracted much attention and has provided considerable heuristic value (Griez & Verburg, 1999; McNally & Eke, 1996). Klein (1993) makes several assumptions that underlie this theory. First, as noted above, Klein assumes the existence of a "suffocation monitor" existing somewhere in the brain stem. In support of this assumption, he describes an "experiment of nature" called "Ondine's curse." Basically, this congenital condition is characterized by a central hypoventilation syndrome in which an infant may breathe normally while awake, but once asleep can stop breathing, quickly develop an acute oxygen deprivation, and possibly die. Ventilatory support procedures are necessary for such children to survive. But it is one characteristic of these children that attracts Klein's attention: They seem to show no distress or anxiety while in a state of hypoxia, which Klein interprets as "a striking indication of the loss of a specific suffocation detector" (1993, p. 309). Klein also makes the assumption that unexpected and uncued panic attacks are fundamentally different from the basic emotion of fear, mostly due to the predominance of dyspnea in panic attacks, but not in fear. However, as described in Chapter 4, the evidence does not consistently support this differential symptom picture in panic attacks versus fearful episodes. In fact, most observations of dyspnea seem to occur during lactate provocation or other challenge procedures that specifically activate respiratory symptoms (e.g., Goetz, Klein, & Gorman, 1996).

Of course, the most direct observation in support of a hypersensitive suffocation detector would be evidence for CO_2 hypersensitivity. As reviewed above, some studies report evidence for this hypersensitivity (e.g., Gorman et al., 1988; Papp, Klein, & Gorman, 1993; Pine et al., 1998). Other studies find no direct evidence of this hypersensitivity (e.g., Woods et al., 1986; Holt & Andrews, 1989a).

For example, among additional studies reporting evidence supporting possible central CO_2 hypersensitivity, Schwartz, Goetz, Klein, Endicott, and Gorman (1996) compared a group of patients with panic disorder (combined with patients with late-luteal phase dysphoric disorder, who have been shown to be vulnerable to panic attacks) to 15 nonanxious volunteers. They found that the clinical group met a rigorous criteria for sighing more frequently than the control subjects during lactate infusion. Hegel and Ferguson (1997) reported that a group of patients with panic disorder demonstrated significantly lower end-tidal CO_2 levels than either a group of patients with GAD, or a group of normal controls, in spite of the equivalence of the patients with panic disorder to those with GAD on baseline anxiety levels. Evidently, a higher level of respiratory symptoms during panic attacks accounted for the bulk of the observed differences. From another point of view, Coryell (1997) reported that first-degree relatives of patients with panic disorder evidenced a higher rate of panic attacks following inhalation of 35% CO_2 than did similarly composed groups of first-degree relatives of patients with mood disorders or alcoholism. Similar findings were reported by Bellodi et al. (1998).

On the other hand, McNally, Hornig, and Donnell (1995) compared patterns of symptoms during panic attacks reported by patients with panic disorder compared to nonclinical subjects who had experienced unexpected panic attacks, on the assumption that suffocation-type symptoms might discriminate the clinical group from the nonclinical group. The results revealed that three cognitive symptoms—fear of dying, fear of heart attack, and fear of loss of control—best discriminated clinical from nonclinical panic, but not suffocation sensations. Also, Schmidt, Telch, and Jaimez (1996) directly tested the suffocation monitor theory by noting that biological challenges *lowering* pCO_2 levels, as hyperventilation procedures do, should result in lower fear and less likelihood of panic. This is in contrast to increased fear and greater likelihood of panic in response to biological challenges where pCO_2 levels are increased, as with inhalation of CO_2 gas. However, observations of potential indicators of the suffocation monitor, including severity of dyspnea symptoms, frequency of dyspnea symptoms, heightened respiration rate, and lowered pCO_2 levels, did not predict differential emotional responding to hyperventilation versus 35% CO_2 challenge.

Conditional Anxiety and Respiratory Disease

Despite these contradictions, we do observe some irregularities in ventilation—even if not directly related to a centrally based CO_2 hypersensitivity—in studies dating back to the 1940s, as noted above. What could account for these findings? In addition to poor physical fitness due to avoidance of exercise, one alternative hypothesis is the development (learning) of anxiety associated with breathing irregularities (Craske, 1999). For example, Carr, Lehrer, Jackson, and Hochron (1996) assessed airway impedance responses to psychological stressors among 113 individuals: 61 with asthma only, 10 with asthma and panic disorder, 24 with panic disorder only, and 18 controls with neither condition. Interestingly, individuals with asthma displayed higher airway impedance, whereas those individuals with panic disorder with or without asthma displayed lower airway impedance than those without panic disorder. Thus the patients with panic disorder, with or without asthma, had more bronchodilated airways, which the authors note would allow greater ventilation in a potential fight-or-flight situation. Although this result could represent a biological adaptation to the threat of increased levels of CO_2, the authors suggest that a more likely interpretation is a general effect of greater anticipatory anxiety, in that individuals with panic disorder show greater respiratory preparedness for stress (or panic). In other words, the airways of individuals with panic disorder are in a chronic state of preparedness, which may on occasion promote hyperventilation. Since this would be adaptive in the presence of comorbid respiratory disorders (as anxiety and its effects are adaptive in the presence of any potential danger), the development of this association between anxiety and respiratory irregularities would seem reasonable and logical.

On the other hand, Pine et al. (1994) evaluated the presence of anxiety symptoms in 13 children with "Ondine's curse" or central hypoventilation syndrome (described above), in a test of Klein's theory. The authors compared rates of anxiety disorders in three children to a group of community subjects (n = 292) containing a subgroup of children with asthma (n = 15), as well as a subgroup with other chronic medical illnesses (n = 66). The idea was that the children with "Ondine's curse" would be expected to develop anxiety and fear focused on respiration on a par with the asthmatic children, due to their severe respiratory condition and near-death experiences, if fear conditioning were the operative mechanism. Klein's observations, on the other hand, point to little or no conditioned anxiety in these children. Two of the 13 children, or 15%, in the group with congenital central hypoventilation syndrome met criteria for anxiety disorders, compared to 24% of the community group, 32% of the chronically ill comparison subgroup, and 47% (7 of 15) of the group with asthma. Although none of these results were statistically significant according to conventional probability levels, the particularly low rate of anxiety disorders in the central hypoventilation group is remarkable. Of course, this study is only preliminary, since very low numbers of subjects were involved. In addition, subjects in the hypoventilation group were significantly younger than patients in the other two groups, potentially giving them less time to develop full-blown anxiety disorders (although, as the authors point out, the presence of nonpathological anxiety symptoms may be more prevalent in younger children). In addition, Klein's suffocation monitor theory is specific to panic disorder, but the authors chose to evaluate the presence of all anxiety disorders, and rates of panic disorder specifically in the samples are not given.

Although Pine et al. (1994) note these results as antithetical to fear conditioning notions (and supportive of Klein's theory), some clear differences exist between children with respiratory diseases, such as asthma, and children with central hypoventilation syndrome. Children with asthma experience dyspnea and acute respiratory distress, often accompanied directly by feelings of suffocation and associated anxiety. Children with central hypoventilation syndrome, on the other hand, presumably experience none of these aversive cues; their respiration tends to cease only during sleep, and then evidently without distress. The authors note that the considerable medical attention (including frequent hospitalizations, as well as chronic interactions with ventilatory support and/or mechanical ventilation) can be distressing, but one might question whether these are the conditions under which fear conditioning to respiratory cues might occur. Nevertheless, the Pine et al. (1994) study is a fascinating preliminary look at this phenomenon.

Other studies have produced ambiguous results in evaluating central CO_2 sensitivity theories versus more psychological explanations. Taylor and Rachman (1994) found that individuals who, at pretest, were assessed as being particularly fearful of suffocation were also more likely to evidence increased anxiety and even panic while breathing through a narrow straw. Asmundson and Stein (1994c) noted that patients with panic disorder held their breath for significantly shorter durations than patients with generalized social phobia or normal controls. Again, this could be either due to a greater sensitivity to CO_2 or to anxiety focused on somatic sensations produced by this procedure. In addition, McNally and Eke (1996) examined predictors of response to a CO_2 challenge (breathing deeply and rapidly into a paper bag for 5 minutes) among 78 normal college students. Once again, fear of suffocation measured before the test was the only significant predictor of both anxiety and increased bodily sensations during this challenge.

Respiratory Irregularities as Factors in Panic: Conclusions

Debate on the merits of neurobiologically based respiratory irregularities as at least substantial etiological factors in the genesis of panic attacks and panic disorder continues. Nevertheless, since the first edition of this book (Barlow, 1988), the field has advanced substantially, in that there is wide agreement among neurobiological investigators that many hypothetical mechanisms once thought to account for panic have been eliminated. Interest remains in a possible common denominator among at least some substances. Specifically, substances that stimulate preexisting irregularities in ventilation may reflect a hypersensitive central CO_2 mechanism, possibly in the form of a faulty suffocation monitor. However, as noted above, Coplan and Klein (1996) observed that the diversity of substances successful in provoking panic would seem to imply that a low threshold for triggering panic could be associated with a number of different neurobiological pathways. At the same time, evidence supporting the strong contribution of psychological reactions to the variety of provocation procedures as a substantial, and perhaps the predominant, etiological factor in the genesis of panic attacks and panic disorder has continued to grow. The juxtaposition of these two rival theories—biologically based respiratory abnormalities and psychologically based reaction to somatic activation—is now very much the central focus of attention. It is to the latter hypothesis that I now turn.

PSYCHOLOGICAL MECHANISMS IN LABORATORY-PROVOKED PANIC

I have noted that the inability to elucidate common neurobiological pathways to panic from provocation by various biochemical substances left investigators with the assumption that there must be multiple biological pathways to panic in the laboratory, each with its own distinctive mechanism of action (Nutt & Lawson, 1992). This conclusion was particularly compelling to theorists who did not accept the possibility of a unifying psychological account of panic provocation as a response to suddenly occurring, misperceived seemingly dangerous somatic events, in whatever form they might appear.

Prior to 1967, the prevailing view of the data produced from the myriad of infusion studies suggested a complex interaction of biological and psychological processes in the production of anxiety attacks and panic. For example, Breggin (1964), in reviewing the early studies on adrenaline or epinephrine, specified four separate factors interacting to produce panic: (1) the elicitation of physiological sensations; (2) the strength of the subject's previously learned association between physiological sensations and psychological feelings of acute anxiety; (3) the degree of current (baseline) anxiety; and (4) the degree of anxiety elicited by the experimental setting (in other words, the "experimental demand" in the situation). Essentially, Breggin suggested that for patients who have already experienced an anxiety attack, any physiological sensations resembling the attack may further increase anxiety or apprehension. This anxiety is then exacerbated by the experimental demand in the situation. This process is most likely to occur if the patient comes into the situation already anxious. As Breggin put it,

> When the past conditioning of internal cues is taken into account, some differences in the results of various experiments still remain unexplained. Most of these differences can be accounted for by a second variable: the degree to which the experimental environment or external cues reinforce anxiety. This second variable must be separated out by inference since there are very few studies which attempt to control the environment. For example, the presence or absence of a psychiatric interviewer is an important variable which has not been controlled but which seems significant in several studies. (1964, p. 560)

The influences of various psychological procedures on the provocation of panic have been examined, including instructional sets, the presence of safety cues or signals, and the manipulation of a sense of control in these laboratory procedures. Some of these investigations of potential psychological mechanisms have occurred in the context of more traditional biological provocation paradigms. But what is perhaps the most common provocateur of panic is the occasional paradoxical effect of relaxation.

Relaxation

One of the first empirical observations that suggested the presence of substantial psychological factors in the provocation of panic were the observed paradoxical effects of relaxation. In Chapter 4, the panic attacks of Jill and Mary have been described in some detail. Seemingly, these were "spontaneous" or uncued attacks that just happened to occur while these patients were attempting to relax. Another possibility is that the process of relaxation itself is panicogenic for susceptible patients. Early clinical reports abound describing what seems to be a relatively common problem during the early stages of relaxation or meditation. Jacobson and Edinger (1982) observed rapid exacerbation in anxiety during relaxation at a sufficient frequency to term it a "side effect" of relaxation. Kennedy (1976) reported depersonalization occurring as a consequence of some meditational techniques. Others have reported similar problems (Fewtrell, 1984).

One of the leading investigators of the effects of relaxation, Thomas Borkovec, observed this phenomenon frequently; as a result, he began a systematic attempt to examine anxiety and panic provoked by relaxation and meditation techniques (Heide & Borkovec, 1983, 1984). In the preliminary study (Heide & Borkovec, 1983), 14 subjects meeting the DSM-III criteria for GAD were recruited. Each subject experienced one session of training in each of two relaxation methods: progressive relaxation and mantra meditation. Prior to the session, subjects briefly practiced the specific procedure to be used. During this practice period, four subjects reported increases in anxiety, such as restlessness, feeling uptight, and fear of losing control. An additional subject reported what seemed to be a full-blown panic attack, characterized by crying and reports of intense anxiety. She chose to terminate the experience immediately. Posttreatment questionnaires, as well as results from the physiological measures, revealed that 31% of the subjects reported feeling increased tension during progressive relaxation on either subjective or physiological measures of anxiety or both. Moreover, 54% reported increased anxiety during the meditation procedure. From a number of psychological scales, the investigators attempted to determine what factors mediated these increases in anxiety. Generally, fear of losing control and the experience of sensory side effects of relaxation were strongly associated with poor outcome on the relaxation measures. Norton, Rhodes, Hauch, and Kaprowy (1985) reported similar results.

These preliminary experiments would seem to establish the phenomenon of relaxation-induced anxiety. Nevertheless, these studies really say very little about the possibility of relaxation-provoked panics, since panic was not the object of the investigation, nor was it systematically measured. Several years ago, a study from our clinic at Albany examined the panicogenic properties of relaxation in a group of 15 patients with panic disorder with or without agoraphobia (Adler, Craske, & Barlow, 1987). Each patient listened to three 15-minute audiotapes in random order: a relaxation tape, a tape with instructions on muscle tension, and a neutral tape containing a passage from a popular novel. Significant differences emerged among the three tapes on the number of severe DSM-III-R panic symptoms reported. The greatest symptomatology was associated with the relaxation tape, which also elicited reports of a significantly greater similarity to natural panic, and less of a sense of control, than responses to the other tapes. Abrupt, if modest, elevations in heart rate were associated with these symptoms in some patients. Two of the patients reported panicking; both reported that their panics occurred during the relaxation condition.

None of these experiences was nearly as severe as the panics experienced by Jill and Mary and described in Chapter 4, and although this phenomenon is now well accepted clinically (Dattilio, 1994; Schwartz & Schwartz. 1995; Wells, 1990), few studies have followed up on these findings in a systematic empirical manner. In one interesting study of clinical electroencephalographic findings, Knott, Bakish, Lush, and Barkley (1997) noted theta and alpha increments during relaxation procedures in control subjects, but not patients with panic disorder, indicating continued high levels of arousal independent of reports of relaxation.

Relaxation is surely the strangest of panic provocation procedures, since abrupt surges of anxiety (panic) occur without the type of neurobiological "push" associated with pharmacological or respiratory provocators. But a common thread running through all provocation studies is the possibility that panic is provoked by specific sensitivity to certain somatic sensations or events. These somatic sensations may have come to be associated with a sense of loss of control. During relaxation, subjects are often instructed to give up control of specific somatic responses (e.g., "Let go totally of your muscles; make no attempt to control them"), as they were in the relaxation tape in the Adler et al. (1987) study. Both in Borkovec's early work and in the Adler et al. (1987) study, fear of losing control, and a seeming sensitivity to sensory side effects of relaxation, mediated anxiety and panic when these occurred. These findings reinforced a psychological contribution to the provocation of panic, and underscored the importance of determining the contribution of psychological factors to more biological methods of panic provocation in a systematic manner.

Safety Cues

Additional studies have examined the effects of manipulating cues that signal that the anticipated threat or danger will not occur, or "safety" cues. We (Rapee, Telfer, & Barlow, 1991) divided patients with panic disorder into two groups, all of whom inhaled 5.5% CO_2 for 15 minutes. Subjects in the "safe" group experienced the presence of a "doctor" in a white laboratory coat, as well as a professionally dressed graduate assistant. Subjects in the "unsafe" group were told that the doctor had suddenly been called away and that their test would continue anyway, but would be administered by a "student" assistant who was dressed very unprofessionally. Unfortunately, credibility ratings of the manipulation demonstrated that the concept of "safety" was not successfully imparted to the experimental groups. However, a post hoc median split of subjects feeling more or less safe prior to the infusion indicated that subjects feeling safer had a lower intensity of fear, had lower anxiety ratings, and were less likely to report a panic attack than subjects who felt less safe. In a more systematic study, M. M. Carter, Hollon, Shelton, and Carson (1995) utilized more sophisticated procedures by requiring each patient with panic disorder to be accompanied by someone with whom he or she felt safe. These patients then underwent the CO_2 inhalation procedure either in the presence of their safe persons or in their absence, having been previously informed that they might be in either group. A nonanxious control group also experienced the inhalation procedure without safe persons. For several individuals in the panic disorder group, a psychiatrist served as the safe person, but most brought friends or relatives. Patients exposed to CO_2 without their safe persons reported significantly greater distress and more catastrophic cognitions than did patients exposed in the presence of their safe persons. Interestingly, "nonsafe" patients also evidenced a greater level of physiological arousal. The "safe" group did not differ from nonanxious controls on most measures.

Instructional Sets

One of the first studies to directly evaluate the importance of psychological factors was reported by Rapee, Mattick, and Murrell (1986), who arranged for patients with panic disorder (or social phobia without "spontaneous" panic) to inhale a very strong 50% CO_2 mixture. Half of each group received instructions on exactly what somatic symptoms to expect, while routine instructions that did not specify the somatic symptoms were administered to the other half (the no-explanation condition). Subjects with panic disorder who were given no explanation reported significantly more intense somatic symptoms, more catastrophic thoughts, and significantly greater similarity of the experience to naturally occurring panics than did patients with panic disorder who were told what symptoms to expect in some detail. Patients with social phobia, on the other hand, evidenced no difference as a function of the instructions.

Clark, Salkovskis, and Anastasiades (1990), using very similar procedures, reported a nearly identical outcome during lactate infusion of patients with panic disorder. Schmidt and Telch (1994) also reported similar findings with nonpatient anxious volunteers undergoing hyperventilatory procedures.

As noted above, a theme running through all provocation studies is the potential importance of a sense of loss of control. In fact, this is one of the defining features of panic, and it is also the major cognitive symptom in the DSM-IV panic attack symptom list. Experiments manipulating expectancies and demand may be affecting this sense of control. For example, in the Rapee et al. (1986) experiment, a full explanation of symptoms on the part of the experimenter communicated that the experimenter was in control. Several years ago in our laboratory at Albany, we directly manipulated perceptions of control on the part of patients with panic disorder during inhalations of 5.5% CO_2 mixtures.

We (Sanderson, Rapee, & Barlow, 1989) administered 5.5% CO_2 to two groups of 10 patients with panic disorder under two different conditions. Both groups were told that manipulating a dial would regulate the inflow of CO_2 when a light on a panel in front of them was illuminated. For one group, the light was always illuminated during the 15-minute CO_2 administration period. For the other group, the light was never illuminated. In other words, one group assumed they were in control of the CO_2 (illusion-of-control group); in fact, they were not. The second group was not under this illusion of control. The no-illusion group reported a greater number of panic symptoms, rated the symptoms as more intense, reported more subjective anxiety, reported a greater number of catastrophic cognitions, and reported a greater resemblance of the overall inhalation experience to a naturally occurring panic attack (see Table 5.4 for all values). Eight patients in the no-illusion group reported panic attacks compared to two patients in the illusion group. Ratings of DSM-III-R symptoms broken down by group are presented in Table 5.5.

Since that time, several studies have replicated the importance of a sense of control on CO_2 provocations of panic (e.g., Zvolensky, Lejuez, & Eifert, 1998). In a particularly well-done study, Zvolensky, Eifert, Lejuez, and McNeil (1999) administered 20% CO_2-enriched air to 30 nonclinical participants reporting elevated levels of anxiety sensitivity. In the first phase of this experiment, subjects were randomly assigned to either a condition that permitted subjects to turn off the gas if they felt it necessary, or a condition where this was not possible. This manipulation was similar to that in the Sanderson et al. (1989) study. However, in this experiment the conditions were reversed in a second phase, such that individuals who had control no longer had control, and vice versa. Across both phases, lack of control was associated with greater self-reported anxiety compared to the condition in which subjects were able to turn off the gas. This effect was particularly marked for individuals moving from the no-control condition in Phase 1 to the control condition in Phase 2. Since individuals with high anxiety sensitivity are at risk for developing panic attacks and panic disorder, the experimental effects of control in this study may be particularly relevant to treatment and prevention.

At least one significant study only partially replicated the Rapee et al. (1986) and Sanderson et al. (1989) findings. Welkowitz, Papp, Martinez, Browne, and Gorman (1999)

TABLE 5.4. Means of Self-Reported Data for No-Illusion and Illusion-of-Control Groups after the CO_2 Assessment

	Group			
	No-illusion ($n = 10$)	Illusion-of-control ($n = 10$)	F	$p <$
Similarity to naturally occurring panic attacks[a]	4.5 (2.1)	1.8 (1.7)	9.64	.0061
No. of symptoms reported	9.2 (4.1)	4.3 (1.9)	11.76	.0030
Mean intensity rating of symptoms[b]	4.0 (1.5)	2.7 (1.2)	6.01	.0235
No. of catastrophic cognitions[c]	2.4 (2.2)	0.9 (1.0)	3.95	.0624
No. of noncatastrophic cognitions[d]	1.5 (1.3)	2.1 (1.2)	1.18	.2912
Peak subjective anxiety rating[e]	5.9 (1.1)	4.1 (1.7)	4.08	.0830

Note. Standard deviations are in parentheses. From Sanderson, Rapee, and Barlow (1989). Copyright 1989 by the American Medical Association. Reprinted by permission.
[a]Diagnostic Symptom Questionnaire—Form B (DSQ-B) question asking for similarity rating between effects of CO_2 inhalation and a naturally occurring panic attack (9-point scale: 0, "not at all"; 2 "slightly"; 4 "quite"; 6 "very"; and 8, "identical").
[b]Intensity rating of symptoms reported; scale range from 1, "slightly felt," to 8, "very strongly felt."
[c]Number of catastrophic thoughts verified on the DSQ-B (total, six).
[d]Number of noncatastrophic thoughts verified on the DSQ-B (total, four).
[e]Scale range from 0, "not anxious at all," to 8, "as anxious as I can imagine."

randomly assigned 37 patients with panic disorder to one of three instructional set conditions during inhalations of both 5% and 7% CO_2 concentrations in random order. The first condition was similar to the Rapee et al. (1986) instructional set in assuring the patients that there was nothing to fear. The second provided patients with a dial that actually did reduce CO_2 concentration in the canopy, in a manner similar to the Sanderson et al. (1989) manipulation, thus providing a sense of control (which was evidently not illusory, since the dial actually worked). The number of patients who actually reached for the dial was not reported. A third group evidently received only standard instructions about the laboratory procedures. A manipulation check indicated that subjects in the reassurance group felt (significantly) more reassured than the basic-instruction group, although values on this scale were not reported. Since manipulation checks were not reported for the sense-of-control group, this manipulation was evidently ineffective.

Results revealed that the reassurance group scored significantly lower on the Borg scale of respiratory exertion during 5% CO_2 but not 7% CO_2 inhalations, compared to the basic-instruction group. However, scores on scales assessing anxiety or panic symptoms did not differ significantly among groups. Percentages of subjects in the various groups who panicked were not reported. The numerous methodological differences and differences in assessment devices among the above-described studies, and the seeming failure to instill a valid and credible instructional set in at least the sense-of-control group, makes it difficult to compare the Welkowitz et al. (1999) data with the Sanderson et al. (1989) and Rapee et al. (1986) data. Nevertheless, the report of basically no differences on measures of anxi-

TABLE 5.5. Percentage of Patients in Each Group Who Reported Experiencing DSM-III-Revised Panic Symptoms during the CO_2 Inhalation

| | Group, % | | |
| | No Illusion ($n = 10$) | Illusion of Control ($n = 10$) | |
Symptom			p^a
Physical			
Numbness or tingling in face or extremities	60	20	.1698
Trembling or shaking	50	30	.6499
Dizziness, light-headedness, unsteadiness	90	80	.9999
Pounding or racing heart	70	60	.9999
Breathlessness or smothering sensation	80	80	.9999
Faintness	80	30	.0697
Chest tightness or pain	70	10	.0197
Choking	60	20	.1698
Sweating	40	30	.9999
Hot flushes or cold chills	50	10	.1408
Feeling unreal or in a dream	70	10	.0197
Nausea or abdominal distress	40	30	.9999
Cognitive			
Fear of dying	50	0	.0325
Fear of going crazy	40	0	.0866
Fear of losing control	70	20	.0697

Note. From Sanderson, Rapee, and Barlow (1989). Copyright 1989 by the American Medical Association. Reprinted by permission.
[a]Fisher's exact test, two-tailed probability.

ety during CO_2 provocation from this reputable laboratory underscores the need to examine these findings more closely.

Now an important report from the leading group of biological investigators would seem to confirm the basic tenets of Breggin's ideas. Gorman et al. (2001) examined differences in respiratory responses to CO_2 in four distinct groups, in an attempt to pinpoint functional anxiogenic mechanisms related to this procedure. The four groups consisted of patients with panic disorder, patients with premenstrual dysphoric disorder (PMDD), patients with major depression without panic, and normal controls. Subjects from these four groups were asked to breathe 5% and 7% CO_2 for up to 20 minutes each.

The breathing produced the expected increases in relevant respiratory variables. Nevertheless, although CO_2 did cause a higher rate of panic attacks in the patients with panic disorder (and those with PMDD) compared to the other groups, physiological features of the attacks appeared similar across groups. The authors conclude from this sophisticated study that there seems to be no primary abnormality in respiratory physiology in individuals with panic disorder. Rather, these individuals seem overly sensitive to somatic sensations, such as breathlessness, produced by inhalations of CO_2. However, if a panic attack is triggered in these groups, measures of respiration (including minute ventilation and respiratory rate) increase substantially, whether an individual carries a diagnosis of panic disorder or not. In many ways, this study represents definitive work from a group predisposed to entertain alternative biological hypotheses. As such, it represents the best of our science.

CONCLUSIONS

It seems safe to say that a number of widely varying procedures are capable of provoking panic attacks in the laboratory. In fact, the variety of methods used to provoke panic forms a long and rich experimental tradition that has been limited only by the imaginations of clinical investigators, or, more accurately, by their ability to take advantage of serendipitous observations. It also seems safe to say at this time that there is no single underlying biological mechanism of action that can account for these diverse provocation procedures. For example, flumazenil produces panic seemingly without respiratory distress. Lactate seemingly does not activate a central CO_2 sensitivity, but other substances do. Thus there is direct evidence of the incompatibility of hypothetical biological mediating factors in many of these procedures (Coplan & Klein, 1996).

Thus far, several factors emerge as common across all panic provocation procedures. First, a high level of apprehension or high baseline anxiety seems a consistent predictor of panic in the laboratory across different procedures (e.g., Coplan, Goetz, et al., 1998; Ehlers et al., 1986; Liebowitz et al., 1984). For example, Liebowitz et al. (1984) reported that patients who panicked had a greater sense of anxiety prior to infusion than patients who did not panic. Also, heart rate, as reported in Liebowitz, Gorman, Fyer, Levitt, et al. (1985), averaged 83.98 beats per minute (BPM) during baseline for patients who went on to panic, as opposed to 75.30 BPM during baseline for patients who did not panic. Heart rate in control subjects was 62.79 BPM. This finding of greater subjective reports of anxiety, as well as of higher baseline autonomic levels in patients who go on to panic, is fully consistent with most reports (Coplan, Goetz, et al., 1998). Baseline differences in the levels of anxiety between patients and controls before panic provocation have been reported in almost all studies dating back to the 1940s (e.g., Cohen & White, 1950).

The second factor common across most provocation studies is the elicitation of a specific somatic response that is associated with anxiety or a sense of loss of control. Procedures with very different physiological consequences, such as exercise, hyperventilation, CO_2 inhalations, and lactate infusions, have in common somatic signs and symptoms such as rapid breathing, which are often perceived by vulnerable patients as indications of being "out of control." This sense of loss of control is vividly illustrated in the case report at the beginning of this chapter and plays an important role in the conceptions of emotion reviewed in Chapter 2.

Of course, it is not clear from these studies what causes a sense of loss of control, since it could be a by-product of the alarm reaction itself. But the fact that manipulations of a sense of control (Sanderson et al., 1989; Rapee et al., 1986; Zvolensky et al., 1999) dramatically affect whether provocation challenges are reported as panic or not highlights psychological contributions to provocations, although at least one study did not replicate this result (Welkowitz et al., 1999). But it would seem that the elicitation of intense somatic symptoms, particularly respiratory symptoms, may be an important but not sufficient cause of panic in the laboratory. These somatic symptoms may have to interact with psychological factors to result in panic.

This interaction differs in one important respect from the "nonspecific" stress mechanism of action mentioned by some early investigators (e.g., Levin, Liebowitz, Fyer, Gorman, & Klein, 1984) as one possible unifying explanation for the genesis of panic in provocation studies. The implication of the nonspecific stress hypothesis is that any "stressor" (somatic disruption) will be panicogenic. But we see time and again that only very specific stimuli are panicogenic in the laboratory, and that these vary from individual to individual. This has never been better illustrated than in the study reported long ago by Lindemann and

Finesinger (1938), where individual patients responded differently to adrenaline or acetyl-choline. But it is also evident in numerous recent studies reviewed above that individuals are specifically sensitive to widely varying and dissimilar provocation procedures. This implies that individuals may have learned a specific association between panic and certain discrete somatic sensations, possibly associated with an earlier major alarm reaction. This explanation is more parsimonious at the present time than postulating an entirely different set of causal mechanisms for each individual pattern of panic would be. Of course, if somatic sensations are sufficiently intense, such as the feelings of suffocation induced by 7.5% CO_2 in the Woods, Charney, Goodman, and Heninger (1987) study, even normal subjects may panic if psychological conditions are appropriate (i.e., if the sensations are unexpected). This may be the purest example of the innate emotion of fear. This reaction in normals also suggests that patients with panic and normal controls respond in a similar fashion (at least to CO_2), but that the patients are far more sensitive and respond to less intense levels of the stimulus, perhaps because they have "learned" to associate the physical symptoms with loss-of-control sensations. On the other hand, inhalation of 7% CO_2 was not panicogenic for normal subjects in the Gorman et al. (1994) study.

In any case, these are not new ideas. Breggin's (1964) suggested four factors that seem to interact to produce panic in the laboratory are worth reiterating: (1) the elicitation of physiological sensations; (2) the strength of the subject's previously learned association between physiological sensations and fear; (3) the degree of current (baseline) anxiety; and (4) the degree of anxiety elicited by the experimental setting (demands, a sense of control, etc.). Of course, we know much more about panic now than we did when Breggin wrote his review. Therefore, Breggin's model is accurate in only a general sense, and is incomplete as far as it goes. In addition, any model of panic provocation in the laboratory cannot account for the appearance of an initial panic or the development of panic disorder (see Chapters 7 and 8). But this psychobiological model, now well over 35 years old, would seem to accommodate the laboratory provocation data to a degree that no unidimensional psychological or biological model can attain.

CHAPTER 6

Biological Aspects
of Anxiety and Panic

As our science becomes more complex and more specific, the overriding relationship between biology and behavior is often forgotten. For centuries scientists, approaching behavior from an evolutionary point of view, have argued persuasively that biology serves behavior. In this view, all biological processes have a purpose or a function in behavioral or emotional expression that enhances adaptation and survival. Anxiety in its various manifestations is no exception.

Anxiety has been thought to serve several functions, as noted in Chapter 1. The most usual and common function of anxiety or "stress" is to prepare the organism both biologically and psychologically to meet the challenges and conflicts of day-to-day life. Contemporary human challenges are numerous and include such usual and customary activities as meeting a deadline, taking an examination, or introducing oneself to new people. As noted in previous chapters, as long ago as 1908, Yerkes and Dodson demonstrated that "anxiety" does in fact facilitate performance up to a point, usually termed "moderate" anxiety. Beyond this point, further increases lead to deterioration of performance.

Another important function long subsumed under the term "anxiety" is the massive alarm reaction experienced in response to imminent threat or danger. This is the well-known "fight-or-flight" response first described by Cannon (1929) and mentioned in all theories of emotion since that time.

Traditionally these two functions of anxiety, preparation and alarm, have been assumed to be on a continuum, with the alarm reaction clearly at one extreme. The alternative suggestion addressed in previous chapters is that these functions are distinct to a certain extent. That is, although a degree of overlap obviously exists both behaviorally and biologically, some system characteristics are not shared. My suggestion in the first edition of this book (Barlow, 1988) was that the biological and behavioral dimensions of the alarm reaction gone awry represent panic, while the pathological expression of the organizing function of anxiety is more "generalized" anxiety or anxious apprehension. My suggestion also implies different biological underpinnings—an assumption that has received increasing support, as outlined briefly in Chapter 1 and described in more detail below.

In Chapter 5, evidence relating to neurobiological (and other) correlates of panic attacks provoked in the laboratory has been reviewed. But this is a very narrow perspective, fraught with a number of conceptual and methodological difficulties, as outlined in that chapter. The purpose of this chapter is to examine biological aspects of panic and anxiety within a more comprehensive biopsychosocial framework. Information from genetic, psychophysiological, endocrinological, and neurobiological studies is reviewed and integrated. This information plays a necessary and important role in the theory of panic and anxiety initially described in the first edition of this book, and updated and elaborated in Chapters 7 and 8.

The biological basis of anxiety and panic can be examined from a number of different perspectives. One of the more intriguing perspectives addresses the strong evidence concerning a genetic basis for anxiety and panic. This field has been very active during the past decade and, with increasing data to examine, has organized itself around two competing propositions. The first proposition is that individual anxiety disorders such as panic disorder or specific phobia have differential heritabilities (or "breed true"). The second proposition is that the genetic contribution to anxiety disorders (and closely related disorders such as depression) is nonspecific. At the present time, as reviewed below, the best evidence supports the existence of a nonspecific genetic contribution to anxiety and related disorders, although room certainly exists for alternative interpretations. In addition, there is reasonably good evidence that major features of the anxiety disorders, such as panic attacks and more generalized anxiety, may have somewhat different (albeit overlapping) genetic bases.

FAMILY AND GENETIC STUDIES

Genetic Contributions to Specific Anxiety Disorders

In the difficult field of genetic determinants of behavior and emotion in humans, we are quite confident that being "high-strung," "nervous," or "emotional" runs in families and has a genetic component. This conclusion is supported by several different lines of evidence (Eysenck, 1967; Gray & McNaughton, 1996). For example, animal behaviorists have demonstrated that it is possible to breed emotionality in rats and dogs (Bignami, 1965; Broadhurst, 1975; Fuller & Thompson, 1978; Gray, 1971, 1982). Most notable in this regard is the work of Stephen Suomi (1986, 1991, 1999; Suomi, Kraemer, Baysinger, & DeLizio, 1981). By all estimates, this "emotionality" is the analogue of anxiety in humans.

In addition, studies of normal personality or normal emotional experience almost always isolate a factor that is termed "anxiety," "neuroticism," "negative affect," or "behavioral inhibition." The nature and structure of these personality dimensions have been reviewed in some detail in Chapter 2. There is strong evidence that this personality dimension is heritable (L. A. Clark, Watson, & Mineka, 1994; Shields, 1962; Eaves & Eysenck, 1976; Young, Fenton, & Lader, 1971; Jardine, Martin, & Henderson, 1984). Eysenck (1967) estimated, based on research with personality questionnaires, that approximately 50% of variance in the trait of neuroticism is attributable to genetic factors—a figure that is remarkably consistent with estimates of heritability of other major personality traits (Plomin, DeFries, McClearn, & Rutter, 1997). Similar personality traits or temperaments, such as behavioral inhibition, also evidence relatively robust genetic contributions (DiLalla, Kagan, & Reznick, 1994). As reviewed elsewhere in this book (see Chapter 2), the relationships among the closely related traits of neuroticism, negative affect, and behavioral inhibition have yet to be fully worked out. But it is very likely that each represents variations on a theme underlying a biological vulnerability to develop emotional disorders generally.

Although published reports estimating genetic contributions to anxiety disorders were relatively few at the time of the publication of the first edition of this book, numerous studies utilizing a variety of methods (family studies, twin studies) have appeared since that time.

Most of these studies have been organized around specific disorders, and I briefly review these reports, highlighting two disorders that have accumulated the most data: panic disorder (with and without agoraphobia) and specific phobia.

Panic Disorder with and without Agoraphobia

Various early studies (e.g., Raskin, Peeke, Dickman, & Pinkster, 1982; Terhune, 1949; Webster, 1953) looked at anxious patients' reports of developmental antecedents to their anxiety, such as parenting characteristics, using questionnaires or brief interviews. Many of these studies were conducted on patients with panic disorder with or without agoraphobia. On occasion, control groups were included, and some brief questions referred to the existence of panic or other symptomatology in relatives. Some of these studies on developmental antecedents are reviewed in Chapters 7 and 8 in the context of discussions of etiology.

But the difficulty with trying to determine in this manner whether differences exist among families of different patient groups is that such reports are subject to considerable distortion. The person who is asked must know the information about a specific family member; he or she must also remember it. For this reason, ascertaining relevant factors about psychological problems in the families of patients by asking the patients usually requires lengthy, carefully constructed interviews. This strategy is called the "family history method."

An even better method is to interview the family members of patients directly. Although the personnel and effort required by such interviews are considerable, there are many reasons to undertake them. For example, if a disorder aggregates in families, then it is possible that some genetic contribution to the disorder exists. Of course, the fact that a problem aggregates in families is neither a necessary nor a sufficient proof that a genetic link exists. In specific phobia, for example, we know that social influence or modeling is sufficient to instill severe fears in some cases (see Chapter 11). However, a lack of familial aggregation for a specific disorder would all but rule out any genetic link. For this reason, family studies are very important from the point of view of etiology.

FAMILY STUDIES. A series of studies on the incidence of panic disorder in families of patients with panic disorder, compared to families of patients with other types of anxiety, during the past two decades is summarized in Table 6.1. As one can see, the lifetime prevalence of panic disorder in relatives of patients with PDA ranges between 7.9% and 41%. The rate for controls is never above 8%. Two notable family studies in this series are reviewed briefly here.

In 1983, Crowe, Noyes, Pauls, and Slymen reported data collected from 278 first-degree relatives of 41 hospitalized patients with panic disorder. In addition, they collected data on 262 first-degree relatives of a group of control subjects who were either surgical patients or employees of the hospital. Over 60% of these relatives were interviewed directly. Data from the remainder were collected by interviewing the patients using the family history method. Members of the control group were matched with the patient group for age and sex, and did not have panic disorder, according to the diagnostic interview.

After completing the large amount of work involved in interviewing these first-degree relatives over a number of years, the investigators established diagnoses in a "blind" fashion. The diagnoses in which they were particularly interested were panic disorder (including "probable panic disorder," which refers to the presence of limited-symptom attacks or very mild panic attacks) and generalized anxiety disorder (GAD). Because these patients were

TABLE 6.1. Family Studies of Panic Disorder

Authors and references	Method	Lifetime prevalence (%) for first-degree relatives		
		Probands	Controls	Relative risk
Crowe, Pauls, Slymen, & Noyes (1980)	History	31	4	7.8
(all relatives interviewed only)	Direct	41	8	5.1
Crowe, Noyes, Pauls, & Slymen (1983)	Direct	17.3	1.8	9.6
Moran and Andrews (1985)	History	12.5	—	—
Noyes, Crowe, & Harris (1986)	Direct	14.9	3.5	4.3
Hopper, Judd, Derrick, & Burrows (1986)	History	11.6	—	—
Weissman (1993)	Direct	14.2	0.8	17.7
Mendlewicz, Papadimitriou, & Wilmotte (1993)	Direct	13.2	0.9	14.6
Maier, Lichtermann, Minges, Örlein, & Franke (1993)	Direct	7.9	2.3	3.4
Fyer, Mannuzza, Chapman, Martin, & Klein (1995) (panic disorder with agoraphobia)	Direct	10	3	3.3

Note. "Direct" indicates direct interview of relatives; "History" indicates the family history method. From Lépine and Pélissolo (1999). Copyright 1999 by Martin Dunitz Ltd. Reprinted by permission.

diagnosed before *Diagnostic and Statistical Manual of Mental Disorders* (DSM) criteria were available, the 41 patients with panic disorder were not distinguished into subtypes. Retrospectively, the authors reported that 11 of the 41 patients could be diagnosed as having DSM-III agoraphobia with panic attacks (DSM-IV panic disorder with moderate to severe agoraphobia), while an additional 11 had limited but distinct avoidance behavior, which would probably classify them in DSM-IV as having panic disorder with mild agoraphobia. This left 19 subjects who had panic attacks with no appreciable avoidance.

Based on these data, the risk of a relative in the patient group having panic characterized by either major attacks or limited-symptom attacks or both was 24.7%, as opposed to a risk of 2.3% for a relative in the control group. These data are presented in Table 6.2. To put it another way, 20 of the 41 families of patients had at least one member with a definite panic disorder, and 13 families had one member with "probable panic disorder" (limited-symptom attacks). Altogether, 25 of the 41 families (51%) had a relative with either diagnosis.

Importantly, there was no difference in the incidence of GAD among first-degree relatives of the two groups. That is, a family member of a patient with panic disorder did not stand a greater risk of having GAD than did a family member of a control subject. The finding of no differences in incidence seemed, on the face of it, to suggest a lack of association between the syndromes of GAD and panic disorder.

In another particularly well-done early study, Moran and Andrews (1985) concentrated on panic disorder with moderate to severe agoraphobia. Using the family history method, they interviewed 60 patients, and observed a lifetime prevalence of panic disorder with at least moderate agoraphobia (conservatively diagnosed) in 12.5% of first-degree relatives. They noted that 12.5% is considerably above the estimates of the prevalence of agoraphobia in the population (4.14%), based on the Epidemiologic Catchment Area data (Robins et al., 1984). Although a prevalence of 12.5% is not as high as fig-

TABLE 6.2. Anxiety Disorders in Patients' and Control Families

	Patients' families	Control families
Morbidity risk (%)[a]		
Definite panic disorder	17.3 ± 2.5	1.8 ± 0.9
Probable panic disorder	7.4 ± 1.7	0.5 ± 0.5
Generalized anxiety disorder (definite and probable)	4.8 ± 1.4	3.6 ± 1.4
Families with familial disorder (no.)[b]		
Definite panic disorder	20	4**
Probable panic disorder	13	1*
Generalized anxiety disorder (definite and probable)	10	8

Note. From Crowe, Noyes, Pauls, and Slymen (1983). Copyright 1983 by the American Medical Association. Reprinted by permission.
[a]Risks are given as means ± SEs.
[b]These families had the specified disorder diagnosed in one or more of the proband's first-degree relatives.
*p = .0007 (Fisher's exact test).
**p = .0002 (Fisher's exact test).

ures obtained in studies reviewed above, only patients and family members with agoraphobia were included.

Moran and Andrews (1985), in analyzing the possible modes of transmission, came to a somewhat different conclusion than Crowe et al. (1983), and echoed a theme on which the evidence is converging: Both simple genetic transmission and purely cultural transmission are ruled out. Their conclusion was that a nonspecific diathesis or vulnerability for panic (and agoraphobia) may be inherited, but that the expression of the disorder is a function of environmental factors (e.g., stress).

TWIN STUDIES. Of course, even family studies with the strongest results provide only suggestive evidence of genetic transmission. An equally likely interpretation is that something in the environment facilitates the acquisition of various emotional disorders or disordered behaviors in families. To explore a possible genetic link, it is necessary to find individuals who have identical gene pools but who do not necessarily share the same environmental influences. Only the study of twins fulfills this qualification. For this reason, twin study methodology is at the heart of human behavioral genetics, and we are fortunate to have several studies of this type dealing with panic disorder.

In a well-done early study, Torgersen (1983a) was able to locate 32 monozygotic and 53 dizygotic adult, same-sex twins, at least one of whom had an anxiety disorder. As anyone familiar with research in genetics knows, this is a difficult type of study to complete, because of the problems in locating a large number of twin pairs in which one member has a certain diagnosis. Most of these studies come from Scandinavia, where excellent demographic records are available. For this reason, along with the fact that the Scandinavian countries are relatively small, it becomes easier to locate and keep track of twins. Torgersen completed his study in his native Norway.

Even with the relatively large number of twins in Torgerson's study, in which at least one member was found to have an anxiety disorder, the numbers were quite small and many comparisons did not reach statistical significance. However, for our purposes, one analysis is very important. Torgersen created a category termed "anxiety disorder with panic attack." Into this category fell twins who met the diagnoses of DSM-III panic disorder, and agoraphobia with panic attacks, as well as a diagnosis termed "possible panic disorder." (Rather than the limited symptom attacks discussed above, "possible panic disorder" referred only to frequency of panic attacks, and included twins having between one and four panic attacks a month.) The minimum criterion for inclusion in the "anxiety disorder with panic attack" category was one panic attack in a 1-month period at any time during a patient's life. This is a very liberal criterion, but it is tempered somewhat by the fact that all of these probands (the identified twins with the anxiety disorder) sought treatment for their problem at some point. Thus the anxiety problem was severe enough to motivate a visit to a therapist.

When this group was compared with a group of probands diagnosed as having DSM-III GAD, some significant differences emerged (Torgersen, 1983a). If the probands (patients) had either panic disorder or agoraphobia with panic, then the frequency of Torgersen's category of "anxiety disorder with panic attack" was 31% in monozygotic twins but 0% in dizygotic twins. The 31% figure represented 4 out of 13 possible monozygotic twins, while the 0% figure was based on 16 dizygotic twins (admittedly, small numbers). This difference was statistically significant. On the other hand, only two dizygotic and no monozygotic cotwins of probands with GAD had "anxiety disorder with panic attack." This suggests a genetic component for panic. In fact, when all panic-related anxiety disorders with the exception of GAD were lumped together, the concordance for anxiety disorders in the proband group was 45% in monozygotic pairs against 15% in dizygotic pairs. This difference was also statistically significant.

It is possible that identical twins raised in the same family are treated more nearly alike and experience more similar environmental influences then fraternal twins. Therefore, the difference could be explained by environmental rather than genetic factors. In fact, Torgersen concluded that this was unlikely, since he found no relationship between similarity in environment and the likelihood of a cotwin's having an anxiety disorder or not. Therefore, this study supported the family studies demonstrating familial aggregation of panic disorder (and agoraphobia), but it took the evidence a step further by indicating a genetic basis for this aggregation. It also raised once again the puzzling finding of a lack of heritability for GAD.

The report by Torgersen is one of several studies suggesting a specific genetic contribution to panic disorder. For example, Carey (1982; Carey & Gottesman, 1981) followed a number of twins with phobias, where most of the probands met criteria for DSM-III agoraphobia with panic attacks. Fully 88% (i.e., 7) of 8 monozygotic cotwins had at least mild phobic features, but only 38% of 13 dizygotic cotwins presented with these features. Of course, these latter two studies did not separate out panic disorder specifically.

More recently, Skre, Onstad, Torgersen, Lygren, and Kringlen (1993) studied concordance rates for panic disorder in 20 monozygotic twin pairs compared to 29 dizygotic twin pairs and found concordance rates of 42% versus 17%, respectively. On the other hand, examining a large Australian twin registry containing 446 twin pairs, Andrews, Stewart, Allen, and Henderson (1990) found no differences in concordance between monozygotic and dizygotic twins for patients with panic disorder.

More recent studies have attempted to link panic disorder to certain specific genes, or at least certain specifically defined areas on chromosomes—mostly without success, for reasons reviewed below. For example, Crowe, Noyes, Wilson, Elston, and Ward (1987) studied 26 families in which a proband was diagnosed with panic disorder and reported some preliminary evidence for a linkage with an area on chromosome 16. However, as is often the case in this line of research, a subsequent study (Crowe, Noyes, Samuelson, Wesner, & Wilson, 1990) could not replicate these findings. Subsequent studies have also excluded candidate genes for adrenergic and gamma-aminobutyric acid (GABA) receptors, and other closely related genes in panic disorder pedigrees (Mutchler, Crowe, Noyes, & Wesner, 1990; Wang, Crowe, & Noyes, 1992; Schmidt, Zoega, & Crowe, 1993; Crowe et al., 1997). As noted below, most investigators now favor polygenic models, with numerous genes from a variety of different chromosomal areas making small contributions to panic and anxiety.

GAD and "Anxiety Neurosis": Differential Heritability from Panic Disorder?

Many of the studies reviewed above attempted to analyze familial aggregation of, and genetic contributions to, panic and panic disorder specifically, but most early studies did not distinguish between panic and generalized anxiety. These studies usually looked at clinical anxiety under a broad term, such as "anxiety neurosis." It is possible that some of those with "anxiety neurosis" also suffered from panic attacks, but since persons experiencing frequent panics often ended up in the offices of cardiologists with diagnostic labels such as "neurocirculatory asthenia" or "effort syndrome," it is not clear how many individuals with "anxiety neurosis" might have suffered from panic disorder. It is clear from the criteria for "anxiety neurosis" that the diagnosis encompasses what is now referred to as "GAD," by various DSM definitions. This section briefly examines the evidence from these early studies bearing on the heritability of generalized anxiety and possible differences from the heritability of panic.

Whether investigators have used the family history method or have interviewed family members directly, a consistent finding has been that "anxiety neurosis" aggregates in families. For example. Cohen, Badal, Kilpatrick, Reed, and White (1951) found that approximately 15% of first-degree relatives also manifested an anxiety disorder. Other early studies (e.g., Brown, 1942) found a similar percentage affected. For example, Wheeler, White, Reed, and Cohen (1948) found that 49% of the children of parents with anxiety neurosis also presented with clinical anxiety, compared to only 6% of a group of control children whose parents were not anxious. The rather higher figures in this study may be accounted for by the fact that only children, not parents, were surveyed concerning anxiety in the children. Also, the children were directly interviewed, as opposed to the more indirect method of asking the parents about anxiety in their children. The Crowe et al. (1983) study described above, with a larger number of subjects, showed that the percentage of relatives who had definite or probable panic disorder was 24.7%; however, if GAD was added, the percentage rose to approximately 30%. Therefore, studies in which relatives have actually been interviewed have yielded consistently higher percentages with clinical anxiety. Early twin studies also suggested a genetic contribution to the development of anxiety disorders in general. The most famous study was the Slater and Shields (1969) investigation. Slater and Shields found that 41% of monozygotic cotwins also could be diagnosed as having an anxiety disorder, while 4% of dizygotic twins carried this diagnosis.

But several early studies reviewed above (e.g., Torgersen, 1983a; Crowe et al., 1983) produced the surprising finding that any genetic contribution to the anxiety disorders might be accounted for entirely by the heritability of panic disorder, since GAD did not aggregate differently in "anxious" families compared to control families, or in monozygotic twins compared to dizygotic twins. There were several problems with this conclusion. First, a diagnostic convention in DSM-III introduced an artifact into these data. According to DSM-III, GAD was a residual category to be diagnosed only in the absence of any other anxiety-based symptoms, such as panic, phobic avoidance, or obsessive thoughts. In fact, almost all patients with panic disorder also present with marked "generalized anxiety" (Barlow, Blanchard, Vermilyea, Vermilyea, & Di Nardo, 1986). Most of these patients are severely anxious, whether they have panicked recently or not. But the only patients included in the DSM-III category of GAD in the Crowe et al. (1983) study were those who were not panicking at all. It is likely that these patients were less severely anxious than the patients with panic. Similar confounds affected the Torgersen (1983a) study. In addition, Torgersen (1983b) found a higher concordance for monozygotic twins only among inpatient "neurotic" probands compared to outpatients, and only among male twins rather than female twins. In other words, if Torgersen had restricted the sample in this study to females (who in fact present with the majority of anxiety disorders) or to outpatient clinics (where most anxiety disorders are found), he would have found no genetic contribution to neurotic disorders! These results differ substantially from those of earlier studies; Torgersen attributed this difference to sampling variation.

It is important to review these early studies since conclusions on differential heritability of panic disorder and GAD still find their way into current interpretations of genetic contributions to anxiety disorders (e.g., Lépine & Pélissolo, 1999). More recent studies present a different picture. For example, Kendler, Neale, Kessler, Heath, and Eaves (1992a) looked at the heritabilitiy of GAD among 1,033 female twin pairs. In this study, the unaffected monozygotic twins of probands with GAD were more than twice as likely to be diagnosed with GAD as unaffected dizygotic cotwins were. Notably, Kendler et al. (1992a) used DSM-III-R criteria (where the confound of severity did not exist, since comorbid diagnoses were allowed). In fact, when Kendler et al. reanalyzed the data, eliminating some comorbid cases, evidence for heritability of GAD disappeared, most likely because the more severe cases were eliminated. (Comorbidity is associated with higher overall levels of severity.) Skre et al. (1993) also found a marked difference in affected monozygotic versus dizygotic cotwins of 60% versus 14%, respectively, for GAD if cases with comorbid diagnoses were included.

Specific Fears and Phobias

TWIN STUDIES. There is also some evidence for a genetic contribution to specific fears and phobias. For example, Torgersen (1979) studied specific fears in a large groups of twins. Eleven pairs of twins were specifically selected because one of the twins in each pair had been hospitalized for a neurotic disorder; the remaining pairs consisted of a relatively unselected sample. Scores on a fear questionnaire indicated that monozygotic twins were more strongly concordant than dizygotic twins for specific fears of animals, mutilation, and social situations (but, interestingly, not for separation fears). Nevertheless, Torgersen pointed out that the most likely reasons for this discrepancy between monozygotic twins and dizygotic twins were differences in personality development (e.g., learning) due largely to psychosocial, not genetic, influences. Using a similar approach, Rose and Ditto (1983) found greater concordance among monozygotic than among dizygotic twins for a variety of fears, such as fears of small animals and social fears. Similar findings were observed for fear of the unknown, fear of injury and small animals, fear of danger, and total fear score in a genetic analysis of twin data derived from the Fear Survey Schedule for Children— Revised (Stevenson, Batten, & Cherner, 1992). In an important study described below, Kendler, Neale, Kessler, Heath, and Eaves (1992b) also found greater concordance for animal phobias in monozygotic versus dizygotic twins (25.9% vs. 11%), but no differential concordance for situational specific phobias or blood–injection–injury phobia. In an extension of this study correcting for measurement error, Kendler, Karkowski, and Prescott (1999) also found differential concordance for situational and blood–injection–injury phobias. Kendler et al. concluded that phobias are moderately heritable, but individual specific environmental experiences play an important role. However, all of these data, with the exception of Kendler et al. (1992b, 1999), describe "normal" fears rather than clinical phobias. On the other hand, Skre et al. (1993) found no significant difference between monozygotic and dizygotic twins in concordance rates of specific phobia, and Page and Martin (1998) reported that unique environmental events accounted for the majority of the variance in blood–injection–injury fear in a nonclinical sample of twins, although the tendency to faint in general evidenced a genetic contribution.

FAMILY STUDIES. Several important family studies on specific phobia have been conducted by Abby Fyer and her colleagues. In the first preliminary report (Fyer et al., 1990), 49 first-degree relatives of probands with specific phobia were directly interviewed by evaluators unaware of the study's hypotheses, and their results were compared to interview results from 119 relatives of controls who had never been mentally ill. Relatives of probands with specific phobia evidenced a significantly higher risk for specific phobia themselves compared to control relatives (31% vs. 11%; relative risk = 3.3). Female relatives were more likely to be affected than male relatives (48% vs. 13%). Fredrikson, Annas, and Wik (1997) also found an increased risk for phobias among relatives of subjects with phobias as compared to relatives of controls. Carey (1982; Carey & Gottesman, 1981) also demonstrated that phobias of all types aggregated in families of volunteer probands with agoraphobic symptoms, but specific types of fears did not seem connected.

In a subsequent study, Fyer, Mannuzza, Chapman, Martin, and Klein (1995) compared 15 probands with specific phobia and 79 of their relatives to similarly composed groups with panic disorder with agoraphobia and social phobia, as well as never-ill controls. Findings suggested that relatives of each proband group were at risk for developing the same phobia as the proband (e.g., showing social phobia), but not other phobias, although there was a trend for a risk for specific phobias, but not other phobias, to be spread across all groups of relatives except the not ill controls.

In a follow-up collaborative study between our center at Boston University and Fyer's group at the New York State Psychiatric Institute, we are attempting to replicate previous findings of familial aggregation of specific phobias to determine whether specific phobia aggregates by subtype. In other words, do relatives of individuals with each phobia subtype have an increased risk for the proband's phobia, but not for other phobia subtypes, as compared to relatives of not-ill controls? If this were the case, it might support a distinction between these syndromes, as well as the validity of the DSM-IV specific phobia subtypes (i.e., animal, situational, blood–injection–injury, and natural environment). Preliminary data from 105 probands (75 with specific phobias and 30 not-ill controls) as well as 203 relatives (143 relatives of probands with specific phobias and 60 of not-ill controls) recruited at both sites replicate the finding that specific phobia is familial. Furthermore, the preliminary evidence suggests that subtypes of specific phobia also aggregate. More precisely, specific phobias were diagnosed in 28% of relatives of probands with specific phobias, as compared to 10% of relatives of controls. Rates of other anxiety disorders, or of other psychiatric disorders, did not differ significantly between these two sets of relatives.

Subdivided by DSM-IV subtypes, the 75 probands with specific phobias included 12 (61%) with animal phobias; 16 (21%) with blood–injection–injury; 18 (24%) with situational; 9 (12%) with natural environment; 4 (5%) with other; and 16 (21%) with mixed (more than one subtype). Relatives of probands with animal and blood–injection–injury phobias each had higher rates of these type of phobias than controls. For those with animal phobias, the difference was specific (no excess of other phobia subtypes) and reached the .05 level of significance (4/23 versus 3/60, Fisher's exact test, two-tailed, $p = .047$). Rates of situational phobias did not differ between the relatives of those with situational phobias versus controls (11% vs. 8%). The current sample size for natural environment phobias is too small for meaningful interpretation of family data.

Confirmation of these preliminary findings will have to await analysis of the full sample, but the initial conclusion is that specific phobias aggregate in families by subtype (at least for animal and blood–injection–injury phobias) and may be associated with a specific genetic contribution. Of course, psychological transmission via modeling or some other mechanism is an equally strong hypothesis in any family study. But a genetic contribution would be consistent with the data from Kendall et al. (1999) and with the potential genetic influence on the development of specific fears proposed by Seligman (1971) and others, who suggest that evolution has favored some fears, and that we are more "prepared" to learn these fears because of specific genetic contributions. Over the course of our evolution, these objects or situations threatened the survival of our ancestors, although this may no longer be the case in our civilized world. Thus, based on this theory, many of us still fear spiders, heights, and snakes, but not guns, hammers, and other more dangerous modern inventions. A related idea is that some fears are innate; that is, they do not require conditioning or learning experiences to find expression and are "nonassociative" (Gray, 1982; Menzies & Clarke, 1995c). However, there is little evidence to support this idea, since almost all models of the etiology of phobia require the activating effect of unique experience (Bouton, Mineka, & Barlow, 2001; Kendler et al., 1999). The notion of preparedness to learn fears (or phobias) and associated issues are examined in the discussion of the etiology of phobias in Chapter 7.

Evidence for a Nonspecific Genetic Contribution to Anxiety and Related Disorders

In addition to the studies reviewed above providing some evidence for separate heritabilities for specific anxiety disorders, particularly specific phobias, a relatively large body of evidence has accumulated over the last decade supporting a more nonspecific genetic contribution to a biological vulnerability for anxiety and related disorders in general. Much of these data have been produced by one of the leading behavioral geneticists in the world, Kenneth Kendler, and his colleagues.

In two important series of studies, Kendler and his colleagues reported that anxiety and depression have a common genetic basis, and that specific differences in these two disorders are best accounted for by environmental factors. In the first of these reports (Kendler, Heath, Martin, & Eaves, 1987), a number of anxious and depressive symptoms evidenced heritability. Genetic factors accounted for approximately 27% of the total variance, based on questionnaire responses from over 3,700 pairs of twins from an Australian twin registry. In the second of these reports (Kendler, Neale, Kessler, Heath, & Eaves, 1992c), as well as a follow-up study (Kendler, 1996), the investigators found that a common genetic contribution to GAD and major depressive disorder best accounted for the findings. Specifically, utilizing bivariate twin analyses on direct personal interview data from 1,033 pairs of female twins, Kendler and colleagues determined that whether a vulnerable woman develops major depression or GAD is a result of her unique environmental experiences, but that the liability to develop either disorder is influenced by the same genetic factors. The direct interview data, of course, lend increased credibility to this report. Kendler et al. (1995) expanded their analysis to include not only GAD but also panic disorder, phobias, and major depression, as well as two nonanxiety disorders, bulimia nervosa and alcoholism; they continued to find evidence, for the most part, for a nonspecific genetic contribution, with differentiation among these disorders due to individual life experiences.

The one important caveat is a tendency, based on preliminary analyses, for disorders characterized by what Kendler and colleagues refer to as acute, short-lived, or "paroxysmal" clinical manifestations to have a somewhat separate heritability (Kendler et al., 1995). These reactions would seem to subsume panic-related phenomena (referred to below), and also additional episodic emotional reactions, such as binge eating in bulimia nervosa.

This evidence is further buttressed by growing support for polygenic models of heritability. That is, as with almost all psychological disorders (and unlike hair or eye color), no single gene seems to cause anxiety. Instead, weak contributions from many genes in several different areas on chromosomes collectively make us vulnerable to anxiety (Kendler et al., 1995; Lesch et al., 1996; Plomin et al., 1997). This is not to say that investigators may not ultimately narrow down areas on chromosomes that may differentially contribute to a nonspecific vulnerability to become anxious. For example, recent studies using quantitative methods have identified relevant areas on a number of chromosomes in animals, including 1, 12, and 15. Numerous genes in these areas seem to create a tendency to be "uptight," overemotional, or anxious (Flint et al., 1995).

Separate Heritabilities for Panic Attacks?

Although a growing consensus supports a nonspecific genetic contribution to anxiety and related disorders, there is some evidence for the differential heritability of the fundamental emotions of anxiety on the one hand and fear (panic) on the other, as mentioned in Chapter 2. This differential heritability may also show up in Kendler et al.'s (1995) "paroxysmal" clinical manifestations, as noted above. Chapter 1 has discussed the ancient, seemingly innate defensive reactions of freezing when under attack by a predator and fainting at signs of blood and injury. Although remnants of the freezing or tonic immobility (TI) response seem to occur seldom if ever in humans, fainting at the sight of blood is fairly common (see Chapter 11). The interesting fact is that both of these reactions seem to have a marked genetic contribution. For example, Gallup (1974) reported that extreme TI reactions could be bred quickly in chickens. Though this has not been observed in humans, a phobic reaction to blood seems to aggregate more strongly in families than does any specific anxiety disorder (Marks, 1986). For example, fully 67% of individuals with blood phobias reported biological relatives with the same reaction (Öst, Lindahl, Sterner, & Jerremalm, 1984). Individuals with blood phobias experience a very specific and unusual response at the sight of blood. As noted above, they develop extreme bradycardia and hypotension, and occasionally faint. As Marks (1986) suggests, it is most likely this reaction that is genetically transmitted. The phobia develops over the possibility of having another reaction (see Chapter 7). Data from Page and Martin (1998) would seem to confirm that fainting is mostly heritable, whereas fear is learned.

But what about panic? It has been suggested in Chapter 2 that panic may also be a manifestation of an ancient, hard-wired alarm reaction. It is possible that this mode of responding to stressful situations has a strong genetic component, much as fainting and freezing are strongly genetically determined responses in certain similar situations. In this manner one may inherit a tendency to be "nervous" or "emotional"—or, more precisely, to be very reactive biologically to environmental changes. One may also be disposed to experience an alarm (panic), much as people are more or less disposed to faint at the sight of blood. This may reflect a differential, biologically based threshold for specific emotions, as posited by some emotion theorists. In each case the response (alarm or fainting) is unexpected, at least at first, and may lead to the development of a phobia concerning possible recurrences of the response in the future. This process is described more fully in Chapters 7 and 8. Thus tendencies to be "nervous" and to panic may both be genetically trans-mitted independently. In fact, a variety of evidence now exists supporting differential heri-tabilities of anxiety and panic (Craske, 1999). For example, Kendler, Heath, Martin, and Eaves (1986) ascertained unique sources of genetic variance for symptoms of anxiety ver-sus symptoms of panic. Martin, Jardine, Andrews, and Heath (1988), presenting data from 2,903 same-sex twin pairs, also determined that symptoms of panic (such as breathless-ness and rapidly accelerating heart rate) were related to different genetic factors than those affecting the more general trait of neuroticism. Specifically, "the common genetic factor that accounts for 51% of the total variance in neuroticism only accounts for 5% in heart pounding and 13% in feelings of panic" (p. 703). Martin et al. (1988) concluded that the existence of a differential genetic contribution to the physical symptoms of panic suggest "that this response has been subject to intense natural selection during the course of human evolution" (p. 705), and that "symptoms of panic seem to be shaped, in part by unique genetic influences which do not affect other anxiety symptoms" (p. 698). Also, Kendler et al. (1995) reinforced observations of separate heritabilities for panic and anxiety, as noted above.

Alternatively, when activated by stress, genetically determined emotional reactivity may lower the threshold for the expression of a specific emotion such as fear, and for its strong escapist action tendencies through a psychological process. This explanation receives some support from evidence in Chapter 5 that successful panic provocation can be pre-dicted by high levels of anxiety prior to the provocation. In this way, anxiety may serve as a "platform" for panic. What is inherited may be a proneness to anxiety associated with a biologically labile response to stress, but this anxiety proneness may interact with specific psychological and environmental triggers (internal and external) in a complex way to deter-mine expression of fear and panic.

Summary of Family and Genetic Studies

It seems safe to conclude that some aspects of anxiety run in families and are almost cer-tainly heritable. However, the safest bet is that what seems to be inherited is a "vulnerability" to develop an anxiety disorder, rather than a specific clinical syndrome itself (e.g., Kendler et al., 1995). But what exactly is this vulnerability?

Early on, Eysenck (1967) made a strong case for a labile or "overly responsive" auto-nomic nervous system as the underlying biological vulnerability predisposing the develop-ment of a clinical anxiety syndrome under the right combination of environmental or psychological conditions. Early supportive evidence for this proposition was provided by twin studies on the heritability of specific autonomic nervous system traits. For example, Hume (1973) and Lader and Wing (1964) both showed that habituation of the galvanic skin response (GSR), as well as pulse rate and number of spontaneous fluctuations in GSR, seems to be genetically determined. As McGuffin and Reich (1984) suggested, these psycho-physiological characteristics may well reflect the substrate on which both the personality trait of "emotionality" and the clinical anxiety disorders are based. Large twin studies also point to the centrality of this anxiety substrate as opposed to categorical disorders when data on heritability are analyzed (e.g., Andrews, Stewart, Morris-Yates, Holt, & Henderson, 1990; Kendler, 1996). What is this substrate? Evidence reviewed in the next section points to overactivity in various brain-regulated systems during interactions with specific envi-ronmental events or "stressors." Smoller and Tsuang (1998) also surmise that the search for genetic underpinnings may be more fruitful if a general "anxiety diathesis" rather than narrowly defined diagnostic categories is specified.

Furthermore, this vulnerability in and of itself may not be "anxiety." This same vulnerability may also underlie stress disorders such as essential hypertension, where little or no "anxiety" is present. Evidence now exists supporting the heritability of stress reactions of this type (Rose & Chesney, 1986; Brannon & Feist, 1997). The subsequent development of anxiety, stress, anger, or even depression may depend on psychological elaboration (see Chapter 8).

Now an important report has suggested that behavioral and endocrine responses to stress may be transmitted across generations *without* direct genetic contributions. Francis, Diorio, Liu, and Meany (1999) carried out a series of "cross-fostering" studies in rats, and discovered that maternal behaviors associated with increased responsiveness to stress in infants were transmitted across generations through modeling or other nongenomic methods. They conclude:

> These findings suggest that individual differences in the expression of genes in brain regions that regulate stress reactivity can be transmitted from one generation to the next through behavior. . . . In humans, social, emotional and economic contexts influence the quality of the relationship between parent and child, and can show continuity across generations. (p. 1158)

An analysis of the nature of these early interactions appears below and in Chapter 8.

One exception to a nonspecific vulnerability may be the tendency to learn some specific "prepared" fears easily (Kendall et al., 1999; Fyer et al., 1995). A second exception to this nonspecific vulnerability may occur in strong alarm reactions or in specific action tendencies or defensive behaviors, such as fainting or freezing. That is, specific emotional reactions, such as fear and its associated action tendencies, may be independently transmitted as suggested above. There is good, if selective, evidence for the heritability of these behavioral action tendencies and their associated physiology in both animals and humans. Indeed, the intensity of the first expression of a coherent fear response, stranger distress, seems to have a genetic component (as reviewed in Chapter 2).

Even if these processes are independently transmitted, they may be related. Genetically determined stress-produced biological reactivity, possibly elaborated psychologically into anxiety (see Chapter 8), may in turn trigger off basic emotions or defensive reactions as a function of differential inherited thresholds for these action tendencies. This model depicts a dual genetic vulnerability, which nevertheless would still not account for the full expression of a clinical disorder. Alternatively, and perhaps more parsimoniously, a nonspecific biological vulnerability may simply lower the threshold for the expression of specific emotions and associated defensive action tendencies, the form of which may be determined, for the most part, by psychological and environmental factors. In this way, panic (or other emotions—e.g., depression, anger; see Chapter 8) may "spike off" a baseline of stress-related reactivity or "anxiety." Lang describes a similar arrangement referred to as "emotional priming" (Lang, Bradley, Fitzsimmons, et al., 1998). That is, activation of various neurobiological systems may present a sufficient number of response or stimulus propositions to trigger specific emotional action tendencies stored deep in memory. Increased arousal itself may provide sufficient stimulus and response propositions under the right circumstances. In this way, a specific action tendency associated with a discrete emotion may occasionally "fire" out of situational context. In other words, under stress-produced biological reactivity, perhaps elaborated into anxiety, or activation of Lang's primitive motivational circuitry (Lang, Bradley, & Cuthbert, 1997; see Chapter 8), one may experience specific action tendencies such as panic in the absence of any external danger. This hypothetical organization is depicted in Figure 7.2 and is described further in Chapter 7.

Thus, with our present knowledge, it would be difficult to assume that a specific clinical anxiety disorder—even a specific phobia—can be directly inherited as one intact behavioral and emotional response set in some sort of simple Mendelian mode, much as hair and eye color are inherited. The demonstrated psychosocial influence on the formation of these behavioral and emotional patterns almost surely points to a complex, interactive, biopsychosocial model of the development of anxiety disorders.

At present, in fact, there is no behavioral or emotional disorder for which a classical Mendelian model of single-gene heredity seems applicable. Even for the major psychotic disorders, where genetic links have long been suspected, almost all investigators (including geneticists) believe that an underlying vulnerability interacts with a variety of psychological and social factors to produce the disorder (Plomin et al., 1997; Gottesman, 1991). At most, geneticists suggest that a polygenic–multifactorial model may be appropriate, in which the underlying genetically determined vulnerability is normally distributed across the population through the additive effect of many genes ("polygenic"), but environmental factors also account for a necessary contribution ("multifactorial") (Kendler, 1995). This view of the role of the genetic contributions to anxiety disorders is in keeping with the biopsychosocial approach advocated here. In conclusion, the evidence is clear that genetic factors are implicated in anxiety. Discovering the precise nature of this inherited vulnerability, as well as the specific operations of the interaction of this generalized vulnerability with specific emotional alarm reactions and action tendencies, is a task that still lies ahead of us. But hints of promising future directions may be found in other areas of the biological investigation of anxiety.

PSYCHOPHYSIOLOGICAL ASPECTS OF ANXIETY

If a nonspecific genetic vulnerability to experience anxiety can be detected, where is it most likely to be manifested? One logical place to look is in psychophysiological functioning of anxious patients compared to nonanxious subjects, both at rest and under conditions of stress. The psychophysiological measurement and assessment of anxiety has a long and distinguished tradition but is fraught with methodological difficulties. Nevertheless, the last decade has witnessed a developing consensus on two findings. First, additional research has supported the idea, presented in some detail in the first edition of this book (Barlow, 1988), that chronically anxious individuals seem to evidence a persistant preparatory set as evidenced by elevated sympathetic functioning. A more recent development is the finding of relative autonomic inflexibility in chronically anxious and stressed individuals. Finally, a fascinating web of evidence has emerged highlighting asymmetrical patterns of brain activation associated with anxiety and panic. I briefly review each of these three areas.

Elevated Sympathetic Activity

One of the most robust findings to emerge from the study of anxiety is that anxious subjects from both nonclinical and clinical populations are highly aroused and alert, and generally in a state of "overpreparedness" as indicated by physiological measures. Hyperarousal has been demonstrated in normal subjects made anxious in the laboratory by means of such procedures as the threat of painful electric shock while performing a task. With anxious patients, we have long known that an anxiety-producing situation is not necessary to produce hyperarousal; rather, it seems to be chronic (Lader, 1975, 1980a, 1980b).

An early experiment of ours illustrates this nicely (Holden & Barlow, 1986). In this study 10 women with panic disorder with at least moderate agoraphobia and 10 control subjects were carefully matched on age, physical condition, and other factors that might influence physiological responding. They were then tested in a variety of ways. The major assessment was a behavioral test in which the subjects would walk a specified course away from the clinic toward a downtown area, making it increasingly anxiety-provoking (Agras, Leitenberg, & Barlow, 1968). The patients carried a small map of the mile-long course, which was divided into 20 approximately equidistant stations. When they reached a station, they were instructed to tell us how anxious they felt at that station on a self-report scale of 0–100 (subjective units of disturbance). Each subject made this report into a lapel microphone connected to a small tape recorder carried in a purse or pocket. Each subject was also fitted with a portable and rather unobtrusive device for measuring heart rate directly as she walked.

In this study, patients participated in this assessment before treatment, halfway through treatment, and immediately following treatment. For purposes of this experiment, however, both patients and control subjects actually walked this course three times before the patients began treatment. The walks were separated by at least several days and occurred over approximately 2 weeks. Whenever a patient took the walk, her matched control subject was also ready to take the walk within the hour. This helped control for the myriad factors that could influence heart rate, such as temperature, time of day, and traffic conditions on the course. Our patients then received 12 weeks of treatment, taking the walk once again halfway through, or after 6 sessions. The control subjects also walked at this time. After treatment was over, the patients again took three walks over approximately a 2-week interval, and the control subjects continued to walk at nearly identical times. Thus each subject took a total of seven walks.

We also administered baseline measures of heart rate after each walk. In one baseline condition, the patients and control subjects rested comfortably in a chair in a quiet room. This was termed a "resting" baseline. In another baseline condition, they walked the hallways of the clinic for approximately 6 minutes, but did not leave the safety of the clinic. Thus patients experienced the same type of "exercise" as they did during the behavioral test, but were not anxious. This was termed a "walking" baseline. Both of these baseline procedures were administered after the patients had taken their walks around town, in order to insure that the patients were not experiencing anticipatory anxiety about the upcoming walk.

Heart rate was calculated in five different ways to control for various factors, such as how far patients walked. But the primary data of interest are presented in Figure 6.1. As one can see, the mean heart rate for the patients with agoraphobia was consistently higher at each walk than that of the control subjects. However, much to our surprise, heart rate decreased or habituated in both groups over the seven walks. The only difference in the slope of this change was in the very last walk, when our patients with agoraphobia showed a marked increase in heart rate that was significantly different from the continuing habituation showed by the control subjects. Perhaps the patients knew it was the last walk and reacted with what Grey, Sartory, and Rachman (1979) have termed a "final exam" effect.

When one subtracts baseline heart rate from heart rate during the walk, another interesting finding emerges. This measure, which we termed "heart rate response" (Holden & Barlow, 1986), is presented in Figure 6.2. The data indicate no difference between the two groups in their heart rate during the supposedly frightening (for the patients) walk, relative to what their heart rate happened to be on that day as measured during resting baseline procedures. This indicates that higher heart rate during the walk for the patients

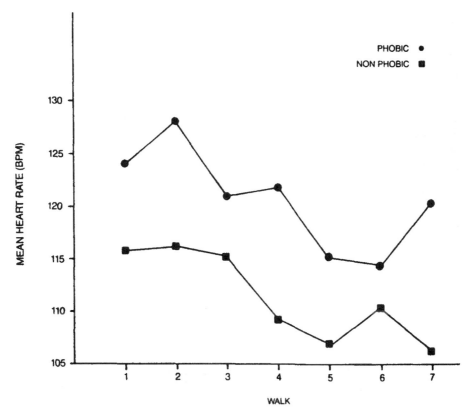

FIGURE 6.1. Mean heart rate of both groups during the seven walks. From Holden and Barlow (1986). Copyright 1986 by the Association for Advancement of Behavior Therapy. Reprinted by permission.

was due entirely to the fact that they came in that day with higher heart rate, as reflected in their baseline measures. In other words, the test does not seem to be specific for changes in anxiety associated with panic disorder with agoraphobia, as measured by a physiological response. Rather, it seems to reflect simply the finding that patients are chronically over aroused.

In summary, then, the clinical sample presented with a chronically high and labile heart rate compared to controls, whether they were engaged in a fear-provoking task or not. These findings echo a well-done but seldom cited early study by White and Gildea (1937), who also reported that heart rate was higher and more variable in patients with "anxiety states" than in normal controls, both at rest (baseline) and during the cold pressor test (a common stress test in which subjects submerge their hands in a bucket of cold water for as long as they can tolerate it).

Our experiment (Holden & Barlow, 1986) was separated from that of White and Gildea (1937) by almost 50 years; yet the common finding, still evident, is that patients with anxiety disorders are more aroused than nonanxious subjects, and that this arousal carries over into various experimental tasks, whether these tasks are stressful or not (Roth et al., 1992). The central finding of chronic overarousal has been demonstrated many times in the intervening 50 years, and since then has been obtained with a variety of psycho-physiological measures, both peripheral and central. For example, in studies reviewed in

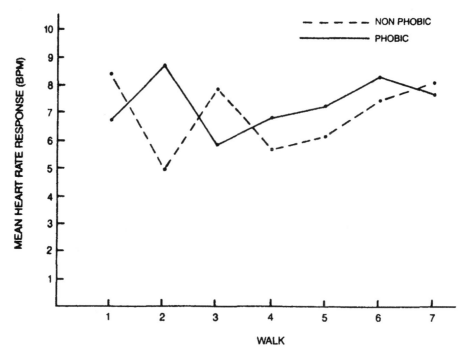

FIGURE 6.2. Mean heart rate response (increase over baseline) of both groups during the seven walks. From Holden and Barlow (1986). Copyright 1986 by the Association for Advancement of Behavior Therapy. Reprinted by permission.

Chapter 5, Cohen and White (1947, 1950) reported chronic overarousal in patients with "effort syndrome" or "neurocirculatory asthenia" as compared to controls. Excellent reviews of this work were published periodically by Malcolm Lader (e.g., Lader, 1975, 1980a, 1980b). Among various physiological measures showing resting differences between anxious patients and controls, in addition to heart rate, are forearm blood flow (Kelly, 1966), electromyographic (EMG) activity (Goldstein, 1964; Hazlett, McLeod, & Hoehn-Saric, 1994; Hoehn-Saric, McLeod, & Zimmerli, 1989), and GSR (Lader & Wing, 1966; Raskin, 1975). Differences in GSR are evident, whether measured as levels of conductance or as spontaneous fluctuations. Robust differences in colonic motility, a process thought to underlie irritable bowel syndrome, are also found in anxious patients when compared to controls (Neff & Blanchard, 1987). Findings of chronic overarousal are not limited to humans. Monkeys bred for anxiety-like behavior also demonstrate chronic hyperarousal and greater physiological reactions to stress than non-"anxious" monkeys exhibit (Kalin, Shelton, & Davidson, 2000; Suomi, 1986, 1991).

Equally interesting are comparisons made between patients and controls using more central physiological measures. For example, studies using electroencephalographic (EEG) procedures have consistently shown less alpha and more beta activity in anxious patients than in controls (Lindsley, 1951). This type of activity, of course, is correlated with subjective reports of tension or relaxation, and indicates that anxious patients are less relaxed. Other central measures that differentiate anxious patients from controls include various aspects of the contingent negative variation (McCallum & Walter, 1968; Walter, 1964), as well as harmonic driving in EEG induced by photic stimulation. "Harmonic driving" refers to alpha responses that mimic certain frequencies of a rapidly flickering light in a laboratory procedure. Shagass (1955) demonstrated that harmonic driving was much higher in anxious patients than in nonanxious controls or depressed patients. Ulett, Gleser, Winokur, and Lawler (1953) illustrated how this response increased with increasing anxiety in patients. As Lader (1980a) points out, these results fit in with the findings of elevated beta activity in the resting EEG of anxious patients.

In recent years, 24–hour ambulatory recordings of physiology have provided another opportunity to compare patients with anxiety disorders to nonanxious controls. In this methodologically difficult area, the results are mixed. Consistent with studies above, some ambulatory monitoring studies have found clear physiological indices of elevated arousal during ambulatory monitoring in patients compared to controls (Anastasiades et al., 1990; Bystritsky, Craske, Maidenberg, Vapnik, & Shapiro, 1995). Other studies, however, have not found markedly different levels of arousal (e.g., Shear et al., 1992).

Ambulatory monitoring, though technically challenging, remains a very promising area of study. Physiological indices of arousal such as heart rate and blood pressure obviously reflect a plethora of bodily functions other than anxiety, and somehow these must be factored out if we are to gain a more precise appreciation of the chronic effects of anxiety on physiological responsiveness. In addition, it may be that chronically elevated arousal over days or weeks may be a function of severity of the disorder, or frequency of contact with internal or external anxiety-provoking cues.

Another important paradigm for studying physiological responses involves examining the rate at which subjects habituate to various stimuli, which may simply provide another reflection of high tonic arousal (Craske, 1999). For example, in a classic experiment, Lader and Wing (1964) devised a paradigm in which, following a 10–minute rest period, 20 identical auditory stimuli of 100-dB intensity and 1-second duration were administered at intervals varying randomly between 45 and 80 seconds. GSRs to the stimuli, as well as spontaneous fluctuations, were calculated. Lader and Wing (1964) demonstrated that habituation of GSR was much slower in patients than in controls. Patients also had a higher frequency of spontaneous skin conductance fluctuations and heart rates 15 beats per minute higher than those of controls. Furthermore, the more anxious the patient (according to ratings and direct observations), the slower the habituation and the more rapid the fluctuations. Whereas all control subjects had fully habituated after 20 repetitions of the auditory stimuli, only 6 of the anxious patients had done so at that time. This finding of slower habituation has been repeated often (Johnstone et al., 1981; Maple, Bradshaw, & Szabadi, 1981), and has also been replicated using other physiological measures, both peripheral and central, (e.g., contingent negative variation; Walter, 1964).

Of course, there are difficulties with these studies that make interpretation problematic under certain circumstances. Most of these difficulties are due to the fact that many date back 30 years or more, when diagnostic standards were different (or, more often, nonexistent). Most usually, the diagnoses of patients in these studies were lumped together under the general heading of "anxiety neuroses." However, in a landmark study that changed thinking on the classification of anxiety disorders, Lader (1967) examined physiological responsiveness among a number of well-defined groups of patients. Lader applied the habituation procedure to the following groups of subjects: (1) patients with both anxiety and depression; (2) patients whose main complaint was pervasive anxiety; (3) patients with agoraphobia; (4) patients with social phobia; (5) patients with specific phobias; and (6) normal subjects. These groups are arrayed on the basis of habituation rate and spontaneous skin conductance fluctuations in Figure 6.3 (Lader, 1980b).

In this study, normal controls and patients with specific phobias were indistinguishable, in that they both habituated quickly and had fewer spontaneous fluctuations. They

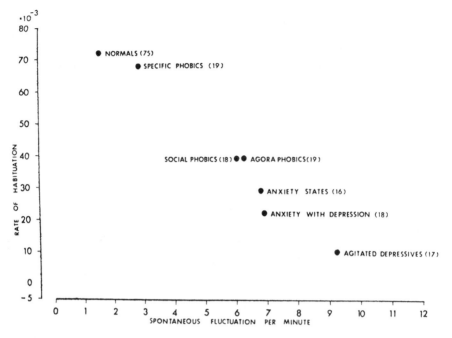

FIGURE 6.3. Relationship between habituation rate and spontaneous skin conductance fluctuations in various groups of subjects. The figures in parentheses are the numbers in each group. From Lader (1980b). Copyright 1980 by Marcel Dekker, Inc. Reprinted by permission.

were also rated clinically as less overtly anxious. On a discriminant-function analysis, all other patients with anxiety disorders clustered together and were quite different from the normal subjects and the patients with specific phobias (Lader, 1967). Only 3 out of 19 patients with specific phobias and 8 out of 71 other patients were misclassified using the author's cutoff score.

This study demonstrated that patients with specific phobias are not in the same state of overarousal or overpreparedness that characterizes the other anxiety disorders. Nevertheless, the anxiety states, as well as social phobia and agoraphobia, clearly demonstrate chronic overarousal. This finding has been demonstrated repeatedly in studies of anxiety disorders, including obsessive–compulsive disorder, which was not one of the groups in the Lader (1967) study (Turner, Beidel, & Nathan, 1985).

Comparisons of Anxious Patients and Nonanxious Controls during Stressful Tasks

The finding that anxious patients are generally overaroused and overalert is robust when measures are taken at rest or during baseline procedures. But the finding is surprisingly less robust, and often disappears, when patients are compared to nonanxious controls while performing a mildly to moderately stressful laboratory task. This discrepancy has been overlooked by most investigators, but may have marked implications for studies into the nature of anxiety. For example, in the Holden and Barlow (1986) study, the supposedly difficult test of walking away from the safe clinic was reported as frightening by the patients with agoraphobia, but provoked an equally strong heart rate response from the normal control subjects, despite the fact that this was not a bit frightening for the controls (according to their reports). Differences in heart rate, once again, were accounted for totally by levels of heart rate at rest.

A careful examination of studies in which patients and controls were compared during a variety of contrived "stressful" situations reveals similar findings (Kelly, 1966; Malmo, Shagass, & Heslam, 1951; McCallum & Walter, 1968; Wilkinson et al., 1998).

How can we account for the lack of differences between anxious and control subjects during performance? There are several possibilities. First, one must consider the nature of the task. The tasks used in psychophysiological studies most often involve mild stress or conflict. In fact, Malmo et al. (1948) stipulated that the requirements of an anxiety-provoking task should include its being relatively mild, as well as being uniform and controllable. The number of tasks meeting these criteria have been limited only by the ingenuity of investigators. The task most widely adopted for humans has involved anticipating painful but harmless electric shock. However, other tasks include anticipating or actually undergoing thermal pain, as in the cold pressor task; watching stressful movies (e.g., a movie in which a victim is about to be attacked by a chainsaw); or threatening subjects with a variety of negative evaluations if they do not perform some task at a certain level. Although some of these tasks may have face validity as "anxiety"-producing, many of the tasks simply require performance of some kind under time limits or some other "stress."

What all of these test situations have in common is their novelty. Very few experiments of this type repeatedly test subjects over time. In addition, investigators often present the subjects with the necessity of meeting a challenge, such as performing under pressure. These tasks elicit the increased alertness and preparation for responding that most people bring to any new task they undertake. Although there may be some minor individual differences, the primary responses common to both anxious patients and nonanxious controls include increased vigilance, muscle tension, and autonomic and central nervous system activity, as well as a variety of endocrinological responses. These tasks (no matter how carefully devised) are not tapping a clinically significant anxiety response, but rather the general response of preparation or mobilization for a task.

One factor that seems to differentiate patients from controls, at least on a physiological level, is that the patients come to these tasks with a higher state of arousal and habituate more slowly from levels of arousal reached during the task itself. These differences, of course, could be due to any number of factors. For example, it is possible that anxious patients are chronically "ready" or prepared to meet life's challenges. This "vigilance" in turn could be due to chronic, exaggerated, negative cognitive activity regarding upcoming challenges or tasks; to basic biological hyperreactivity; or, most likely, to a combination of the two, as suggested in Chapter 3.

Toughening Up

But chronically high arousal does not seem to be the whole story. To return to animal models once again, there is a fascinating phenomenon, reviewed in the first edition of this book, referred to as "toughening up." Originally this concept was proffered as a biochemical explanation for the phenomenon of learned helplessness (Weiss, Glazer, & Poherecky, 1976). Based on original observations by Neil Miller (1980), Weiss et al. (1982) speculated, with some evidence, that the mechanism of "toughening up" or increasing resistance to the effects of stressful life events is one in which repeated experiences with early stressful events in animals results in a down-regulation of noradrenergic receptors in the locus ceruleus, and therefore a drop in noradrenergic transmission to the forebrain. What seems important in the animal laboratories is that these early experiences with stress be both brief and controllable or predictable (Dienstbier, 1989). In the first edition of this book, I specu-lated that some successful drug treatments for anxiety may involve roughly similar mecha-nisms of receptor down-regulation and resulting alteration of levels of norepinephrine or serotonin (Charney & Heninger, 1985). This effect may be observed with administration of tricyclic antidepressants and also, more recently, selective serotonin reuptake inhibitors (SSRIs). That is, exposure-based procedures and certain anxiolytic drugs may have in com-mon a mechanism involving enhanced monoaminergic activity, followed by receptor down-regulation.

But this mechanism does not seem to hold for all pharmacological agents. For example, Gray (1985) reviewed a number of early studies showing that the administration of benzo-diazepines to animals interfered with the process of toughening up. Essentially, animals were more sensitive to anxiety-producing situations after the removal of arousal-reducing drugs (such as benzodiazepines) then they would have been had they never received the drugs at all, despite similar amounts of exposure to these situations.

In any case, Dienstbier (1989) described how intermittent stressors activate catechola-mine responding, but how, in predictable and controllable stressful situations that allow adequate coping, animals evidence a minimal cortisol response mediated by the hypotha-lamic–pituitary–adrenocortical (HPA) axis. Thus individuals with this type of positive learn-ing history may actually evidence increased catecholamine responding potential when faced with stressful events, which has been associated with enhanced performance (O'Hanlon & Beatty, 1976) and lower neuroticism scores (Forsman, 1981). Early expo-sure to stressors with minimal predictability and controllability, on the other hand, seems to result in heightened cortisol responding and, possibly catecholamine depletion. Thus early exposure to controllable and predictable stressful manipulations such as shock and rough handling can actually lead to less fear or reactivity when animals are exposed to subsequent threats (Denenberg, 1964; Levine, 1960). In other words, this early experience may actually immunize animals to later excessive emotional responding when confronted with these threats (Hannum, Rosellini, & Seligman, 1976).

The healthy organism, then, demonstrating resilience or "toughness" in the face of threats, will present with low resting arousal and strong, responsive challenge- or stress-induced arousal. This "healthy" arousal is associated with lower resting levels of cortisol, and perhaps more flexible autonomic (sympathetic) nervous system responding to actual threats and stressors, which may be mediated by low parasympathetic tone. A discussion of this topic follows. These findings anticipate the fuller discussion of the crucial role of the corticotropin-releasing factor (CRF) system in anxiety found later in this chapter and in Chapter 8.

Autonomic Inflexibility

The second distinctive psychophysiological finding in the study of patients with anxiety disorders that has emerged robustly over the past several years is the observation of auto-nomic inflexibility. As Craske (1999) points out, this particular finding has renewed interest in the psychophysiology of anxiety. Initial findings in this area can be traced to the work of Thomas Borkovec (e.g., Borkovec, 1994a) and Rudolph Hoehn-Saric (Hoehn-Saric et al., 1989). The key to this work is a close study of the parasympathetic nervous system (PNS). For example, several studies reviewed by Hoehn-Saric and McLeod (1988) suggest that anxious patients show a weaker skin conductance response and less variability in skin conductance and heart rate in response to challenge or stress. Moreover, as noted above, anxious patients appear to take longer to return to baseline than normal subjects. Reductions in variability of EMG activity have also been found among anxious patients, suggesting that low variability of response may apply to muscle tension as well (Hazlett et al., 1994). It is these results that led Borkovec and Hoehn-Saric to postulate that anxiety, particularly chronic anxiety, may be characterized by a degree of sympathetic restriction and a resulting "autonomic inflexibility" (Thayer, Friedman, & Borkovec, 1996). In Chapter 3, I have reviewed evidence that autonomic inflexibility seems specifically associated with the worry process, and may actually represent a coping response that emerges when anxiety becomes chronic, rather than a biological marker of anxiety itself.

Other recent studies have elaborated on findings of autonomic restriction by examining the role of the PNS in autonomic arousal of anxious patients. As Thayer et al. (1996) have highlighted, previous studies of autonomic activity in anxiety have generally been assessed via sympathetic nervous system (SNS) indices. This approach neglects the role of the PNS, as well as its relationship to the SNS—factors that may play a particularly important role in heart rate regulation. Lyonfields, Borkovec, and Thayer (1995) compared subjects who met criteria for GAD except for the severity criterion ("GAD analogue" subjects) and nonanxious controls during baseline, a period of aversive imagery related to a topic of great concern, and a period of worrying about that topic. Throughout the experiment, cardiovascular variability was measured by the mean successive difference of heart rate interbeat interval. Cardiovascular variability assesses the degree of vagal (parasympathetic) control of heart rate activity. In general, low parasympathetic activity (low vagal tone) is associated with a high and stable heart rate and has been linked with decreased heart rate reactivity (Thayer et al., 1996).

Results indicated that the "GAD analogue" subjects evidenced very little heart rate variability throughout the experiment, and significantly less variability than the control group at baseline. In contrast, the control subjects displayed more variability during baseline, but significant reductions in variability from baseline to aversive imagery and to worrisome thinking. These findings led the authors to conclude that "GAD analogue" participants experienced chronically low parasympathetic tone as a result of their perpetual negative thinking, even while at rest.

In a related experiment, Thayer et al. (1996) examined the autonomic characteristics of GAD and worry in patients meeting full criteria for GAD (as opposed to "GAD analogue" subjects) and nonanxious controls during baseline, relaxation, and worry periods. Similar to the study above, cardiovascular responses were measured using parasympathetic indices of heart rate variability. Patients with GAD showed increased heart rate and less vagally mediated heart rate variability across all conditions. In addition, relative to baseline and relaxation periods, worry was characterized by decreased cardiac parasympathetic activity (and decreased variability) in both patients with GAD and controls. The authors interpreted this finding to suggest that the worry process is directly associated with lowered parasympathetic control of cardiovascular functioning, which accounts for the autonomic inflexibility seen in patients with GAD. Innovative pilot work in connection with this study suggests that a sample of the patients with GAD displayed significant increases in heart rate variability and parasympathetic tone following successful intervention with cognitive-behavioral therapy (Friedman, Thayer, Borkovec, & Lyonfields, 1993). Thayer et al. (1996) conclude that anxiety, and particularly the worry process, may be associated with rigid and unresponsive autonomic nervous system activity that is associated with decreased parasympathetic tone, but that this situation can be modified with successful treatment.

As Thayer et al. (1996) highlight, a relationship between anxiety (worry) and autonomic inflexibility has been noted by several researchers. In particular, the behaviorally inhibited children studied by Kagan and colleagues (Kagan, Reznick, & Snidman, 1988;

Kagan, Gibbons, Johnson, Reznick, & Snidman, 1990; Kagan & Snidman, 1999), typically manifest higher resting heart rates and stability compared with behaviorally uninhibited children. Indeed, inflexibility and reductions in variability of various biological systems in response to environmental demands may be indicative of a generic response associated with psychological and physiological dysfunction (Thayer et al., 1996). Borkovec (1994a) suggests that the autonomic inflexibility found in anxious patients is related to the fact that the stimuli feared by these patients are not produced by external environmental stressors, but are (chronically present) internally generated thoughts about potential future threats.

Furthermore, autonomic inflexibility seems to be a characteristic of anxiety disorders in general, rather than a psychophysiological feature associated with just one disorder. For example, this inflexibility has been noted in patients with panic disorder (Hoehn-Saric, McLeod, & Zimmerli, 1991) and obsessive–compulsive disorder (Hoehn-Saric, McLeod, & Hipsley, 1995), as well as GAD. Also, M. B. Stein, Tancer, and Uhde (1992) observed differential autonomic responding, presumably due to low vagal tone, in a group of patients with anxiety disorders who were subjected to orthostatic challenge.

Sophisticated electrocardiographic recordings, from which an energy ratio index can be calculated, confirm decreased heart rate variability in patients with anxiety disorders (Klein, Cnaani, Harel, Braun, & Ben-Haim, 1995). Finally, 24–hour ambulatory monitoring also revealed decreased heart rate variability measures in patients with anxiety disorders, specifically panic disorder, compared to control subjects (Sloan et al., 1999). As noted in Chapter 1, reduced heart rate variability has been associated with increased risk of cardiovascular morbidity (Kawachi, Sparrow, Vokonas, & Weiss, 1995).

Asymmetrical Patterns of Brain Activation

A very new and promising area of psychophysiological investigation focuses on characteristics of brain waves in depressed and anxious individuals. Richard Davidson and his colleagues (e.g., Davidson & Tomarken, 1989) have pioneered much of this work. Basically, this line of research has strongly suggested that increased EEG activation of left-hemisphere anterior regions is associated with heightened positive affect and decreased negative affect, whereas increased relative right-hemisphere anterior EEG activation has been linked to heightened negative affect and decreased positive affect. Interestingly, these responses are evident in most studies both during emotionally confrontive tasks and at rest; this suggests that these differences may be biological markers to differentially experience negative affect, particularly negative affect with a strong negative emotional valence (Tomarken, Davidson, Wheeler, & Doss, 1992). Kalin, Shelton, Rickman, and Davidson (1998) and Kalin et al. (2000) have demonstrated relatively higher right frontal lobe activity in abnormally fearful rhesus macaques, further suggesting the robustness of this phenomenon across species.

Extending these findings to psychopathological states, a number of investigators (e.g., Davidson, 1993b; Heller & Nitschke, 1997) have noted differential alpha activity in the two hemispheres of the brain in depressed individuals. That is, depressed individuals exhibit more right-sided and less left-sided EEG activation than nondepressed individuals do. Furthermore, right-sided anterior EEG activation is also found in patients who are no longer depressed in some studies (Gotlib, Ranginath, & Rosenfeld, 1998), suggesting that this brain function may possibly reflect a vulnerability to depression. Now several studies have demonstrated that this frontal brain asymmetry is also a characteristic of patients with anxiety disorders. For example, Wiedemann et al. (1999) assessed 23 patients with panic disorder without a diagnosis of depression, and compared the results to those for 25 healthy control participants during a variety of conditions. These included while at rest and during exposure to several stimuli/situations, including an emotionally neutral stimulus (a picture of a mushroom), a neutral panic-relevant situation (emergency situations), an anxiety-relevant but panic-irrelevant stimulus (a picture of a spider), an anxiety-irrelevant but emotionally relevant context (erotic pictures), and finally performance of a motor task. The motor task required subjects to trace a line on a sheet of paper, to control for level of concentration associated with focusing on the pictures.

In patients with panic disorder, asymmetries were noted during resting phases, and also when the patients were confronted with anxiety and panic-relevant stimuli. Once again, the expected pattern of right frontal activation as indicated by reduced frontal alpha amplitude was observed relative to controls. However, these observations were only apparent while the subjects were at rest and when confronted with anxiety and panic-relevant stimuli. They were not evident when subjects were otherwise "distracted" by examining an emotionally neutral picture or performing a motor task. Several other recent studies have made similar observations of right frontal activation in anxious patients (Bruder et al., 1997).

Heller, Nitschke, Etienne, and Miller (1997) have now provided the first data articulating these asymmetric brain patterns more specifically in anxiety, depression, and panic (anxious arousal). As mentioned in Chapter 4, Heller et al. (1997) observed right parieto-temporal activation for anxious arousal (panic-like symptoms) but not anxious apprehension. However, instead of right frontal activation for anxious apprehension, in their paradigm they observed left frontal activation (or, more accurately, right frontal inhibition). In a cogent discussion, Heller et al. (1997) observed that the anterior regions of the brain are uniquely involved with pleasant or unpleasant valence dimensions of the emotional state. Pleasant affect is clearly associated with greater left anterior activity, as noted above, and unpleasant affect is associated with greater right activity. But the subjects used in Heller et al. (1997) were undergraduates who were specifically screened to match the control group on measures indexing affective valence, including the Positive and Negative Affect Scales—Expanded Form (Watson & Clark, 1991). In this study, then, students with "anxious apprehension" differed from controls only on state anxiety, but not on negative affect, and the procedure involved listening to several distinctive narratives. Thus it is possible that this component of anxious apprehension was what accounted for the relative decrease in right-hemisphere activity in this study. Heller et al. (1997) point out that more sophisticated and specific measurement of patterns of brain activity may serve not only to distinguish panic (anxious arousal) from anxious apprehension, but also to distinguish anxiety from depression.

What make this latter finding particularly interesting are earlier reports of left frontal EEG activation in anxious patients and nonanxious controls during periods of worry (Carter, Johnson, & Borkovec, 1986). As Craske (1999) points out, and as Roemer and Borkovec (1993) have suggested, worry may well restrict strong autonomic activity, particularly autonomic activity reflecting negative affect; it thus may serve as a coping mechanism that is negatively reinforced by the temporary avoidance of negative affect. In Chapter 3, I review why this process may well account for the "chronic" nature of worry in clinically anxious individuals, particularly (but not exclusively), those with GAD. As also noted in Chapter 4, Heller et al. (1997) observed right parieto-temporal activation for anxious arousal (panic-like symptoms) but not anxious apprehension, where left frontal activation was observed (or, more accurately, relative right frontal inhibition). In any case, the results from Heller et al. (1997) are consistent with Borkovec's findings, in that Borkovec and colleagues may have observed relative right frontal inhibition, rather than left frontal activation reflecting worry and anxious apprehension. Furthermore, to the extent that it is right frontal inhibition we are observing rather than left frontal activation, this process may be related to autonomic restriction as described above.

Evidence also exists for an additional important relationship between prefrontal cortical activation and the amygdala (Abercrombie et al., 1996; Dolski et al., 1996). Specifically, as Wiedemann et al. (1999) point out, frontal cortical activity may regulate and restrain subcortical structures related to affect. Conversely, weakening of these influences may facilitate activity of the amygdala, thereby releasing uncontrolled bursts of emotion, including anxiety and panic. Although this is highly speculative for the moment, here once again we see a more intuitively appealing systemic account of brain systems possibly underlying anxiety and panic.

These three rather robust psychophysiological characteristics—elevated tonic sympathetic arousal or "physiological readiness," autonomic inflexibility, and patterns of brain asymmetry—bear a fascinating relationship to recent discoveries pertaining to neuro-endocrine functioning (particularly in the HPA axis) and to other neurobiological functions. It is to this subject that I now turn.

THE NEUROBIOLOGY OF ANXIETY AND PANIC

The last decade has produced a veritable explosion of knowledge on neurocircuitry and brain systems underlying anxiety and panic. It is instructive to review very briefly some of the origins of current neurobiological research dating from as early as the 1970s, if only to see how far we have come. These early studies, while laying the foundation for research described below, tended to focus on small segments of brain functioning using animal models, and often on single neurotransmitter systems. More recently, interest has centered on neuromodulators of the HPA axis as crucial neurobiological processes underlying anxiety and related emotional states. It is this brain system that is at the core of more integrative neurobiological accounts described below. Before focusing on this important work, I review its origins.

The Noradrenergic System

In the late 1970s, Eugene Redmond and his colleagues highlighted a noradrenergic connection for anxiety and panic. They began an interesting series of experiments in which they electrically or pharmacologically stimulated noradrenergic neurons in stump-tailed monkeys. A major nucleus in this noradrenergic system is an area of the brain called the locus ceruleus. The locus ceruleus is situated in the pons with projections to the cerebral cortex and limbic system, as well as the brain stem, the reticular system, and the pain-sensitive neurons in the dorsal horn of the spinal cord (Redmond, 1977, 1979; Redmond & Huang, 1979). Redmond and his colleagues noted that the reaction induced by stimulation appeared very similar in these monkeys to what happens in the wild when the animals are exposed to an overwhelming natural threat. The implication is that this reaction may be analogous to intense fear or panic. This observation led to a series of studies on the effects of yohimbine (an alpha-2-adrenergic receptor antagonist that increases locus ceruleus activity) and clonidine (an alpha-2-adrenergic receptor agonist that inhibits locus ceruleus activity). Some of these experiments have been reviewed in Chapter 5. Although promising, the evidence from these studies was inconclusive, since it seemed on occasion that panic attacks could occur in the absence of heightened noradrenergic activity (Woods, Charney, McPherson, Gradman, & Heninger, 1987). Other studies focusing on specific markers of central noradrenergic activity, such as 3-methoxy-4-hydroxyphenylglycol (MHPG, a norepinephrine metabolite), also proved inconclusive (Ko et al., 1983; Charney, Heninger, & Breier, 1984).

Another line of research over the last several decades has produced the consistent observation that catecholamines are reliably increased in nonanxious individuals in response to stress. The types of "stress" that produce these normal increases are wide-ranging and include exercise, concentration, temperature changes, and even postural changes (Dimsdale & Moss, 1980; Kopin, 1984). In fact, almost any change in stimulation seems to increase catecholamine secretion (Weiner, 1985). We have also known for years that this reaction to stimulation seems to be true not only for epinephrine and norepinephrine, but for their major metabolites (Uhde, Siever, & Post, 1984; Uhde et al., 1982). In view of this evidence, it has been assumed that catecholamine levels may be chronically higher in anxious patients than in controls. Nevertheless, the evidence for this in early studies was mixed, with some studies finding some differences in catecholamine levels between patients and control subjects, and other studies finding none (Mathew, Ho, Kralik, Taylor, & Claghorn, 1981; Mathew, Ho, Francis, Taylor, & Weinman, 1982; Lader, 1980a; Liebowitz, Gorman, Fyer, Levitt, et al., 1985; Ballenger et al., 1984; Stokes, 1985). Notably, in one well-done study, Nesse, Cameron, Curtis, McCann, and Huber-Smith (1984) reported elevated epinephrine and norepinephrine levels in patients with panic disorder and agoraphobia, compared to controls. These differences seemed "chronic" in that they were present at baseline and maintained throughout a series of tasks, recalling the findings on chronic overarousal described above.

Despite the mixed results, Redmond's interesting theorizing isolated noradrenergic activity and the area of the locus ceruleus in particular as very likely implicated in anxiety and panic, and these ideas were picked up by other investigators (e.g., Gray, 1985; Charney & Heninger, 1986a; Nutt, 1986). Although inconclusive in its early stages, this early work on the noradrenergic system paved the way to a deeper understanding of what has come to be called the locus ceruleus–norepinephrine (LC-NE) system (Chrousos & Gold, 1992). More recent research suggests that neurons active in the production and regulation of norepinephrine (or noradrenaline) originate in the locus ceruleus as well as other nuclei in the brain stem, and project throughout the brain. This system also has effects outside the central nervous system, most notably through activation and regulation of the autonomic nervous system.

The Serotonergic System

At about this time, investigators were also becoming interested in serotonergic models of anxiety and panic. In the first edition of this book, I suggested that panic is the discrete emotion of fear; echoing Lang (1985, 1994a), I also suggested that emotions are fundamentally behavioral action tendencies—a proposition now more widely accepted. In Chapter 1 and above, I have referred to the closely related action tendency of TI in animals. TI (a state resembling freezing but characterized by waxy flexibility) is interesting here because it seems also to be associated with the emotion of fear in animals, but may be programmed to occur only after the primary action tendency (escape) has failed, and then only under the specific stimulus condition of contact with a predator. Between attempts to escape, and the response of TI, are aggressive action tendencies directed at the predator (see also Craske, 1999). TI has obvious survival value in animals, since movement cues often trigger predation.

It would seem that panic in humans has little to do with TI, since we seldom see people who panic "freezing," although there are occasional reports of people being "scared stiff" or "frozen with fear." People experiencing panic attacks are seldom aggressive, either. But it is possible that we may see vestiges of this response in humans on the far edge of terror during rape and on the battlefield. The personally tragic but theoretically intriguing phenomenon of rape-induced paralysis has been described in Chapter 1.

In view of this potential connection, the neurobiology of TI and other parameters affecting the response became of interest during the 1980s. For example, hyperventilation occurs during TI, and the duration of the response of TI in animals is greatly influenced by baseline anxiety levels. Any manipulations that increase anxiety prior to TI, such as conditioned aversive stimuli, loud noises, injections of adrenaline, or suspension over a visual cliff, will prolong the response. On the other hand, most procedures that reduce baseline anxiety, such as safety signals and handling, antagonize the reaction. These findings are similar to data from the laboratory provocation studies of panic reviewed in Chapter 5.

The neurobiological process that underlies TI is reasonably well worked out and heavily involves the serotonergic system, among other systems (Boren, Gallup, Suarez, Wallnau, & Gagliardi, 1979; Wallnau & Gallup, 1977). The evidence for this comes from several sources. Manipulations of tryptophan, the essential amino acid precursor to serotonin, results in the expected increases or decreases in the duration of TI. Also, drugs that systematically affect serotonin concentration in turn systematically affect TI (Boren et al., 1979). Among the more interesting of these drugs is imipramine, which, when administered peripherally, clearly blocks TI in animals (Maser & Gallup, 1974). On the other hand, early investigations of serotonergic activity as a possible basis for panic and anxiety also proved inconclusive (Cloninger, 1986; Evans et al., 1986; Charney & Heninger, 1986b). In any case the advent of the SSRIs and their proven effectiveness, not only for depression but for anxiety disorders (e.g., Stein et al., 1998), has energized interest in this system in the context of more comprehensive integrative models described below.

The Benzodiazepine–GABA System

If early speculation centered on noradrenergic (and serotonergic) neurotransmitter systems as neurobiological substrates of panic, equally interesting speculations in the 1970s and 1980s suggested that the benzodiazepine system may be a specific neurobiological substrate for more generalized anxiety. In 1977 the discovery of the benzodiazepine receptor was reported (Mohler & Okada, 1977; Squires & Braestrup, 1977). Subsequent work showed that the inhibitory neurotransmitter GABA potentiates the binding of benzodiazepines to the receptor sites (e.g., Skolnick & Paul, 1982). One interesting consequence of these discoveries is the realization that there must be naturally occurring clinical substances in the brain that are specific for benzodiazepine receptors. These substances, which may be anxiolytic, have yet to be isolated.

Evidence supporting the benzodiazepine model has come largely from investigating the effects of anxiolytic drugs, specifically the benzodiazepines, on various paradigms for provoking "anxiety" in animals. Many such paradigms exist, most of which have been utilized for almost a century to produce what some have termed "experimental neuroses." The nature of experimental neuroses is explored more thoroughly in Chapter 8. For now, suffice it to say that these situations typically produce mild anxiety through threat of shock, the omission of expected reward ("frustrative nonreward"), or the punishment of previously reinforced behavior. The prototypical paradigm is the Geller–Seifter conflict test (Geller & Seifter, 1960), where liquid reinforcers are paired with foot shock, setting up a conflict over pressing the bar for the liquid. These paradigms are thought to be analogous to anxiety rather than panic, since there is little evidence of an overwhelming alarm response. Rather, a state of relatively "chronic" anxiety is assumed, since an animal's behavior is characterized by increased attention and vigilance, arousal, and the interruption of ongoing behavior.

Evidence for the involvement of the benzodiazepine system in anxiety came from several sources. First, several GABA antagonists seem to be anxiogenic. That is, anxiety in the context of various animal models is increased by GABA antagonists (Gray, 1985; Insel, 1986). Conversely, the benzodiazepines seem to exert anxiolytic effects by virtue of the enhanced GABA-ergic inhibition they produce, although the benzodiazepines have other well-known actions, including sedation, anticonvulsant effects, and muscle relaxation. This diversity of functions continues to make it difficult to conclude that the GABA system is specifically anxiolytic.

Particularly interesting were early experiments showing acute modification in number of benzodiazepine receptors as a function of stress or anxiety. For example, exposing animals to stress, such as immersion in ice water or convulsions, can increase cortical benzodiazepine receptors by 20% within 15 minutes. This level returns to normal after 60 minutes (Paul & Skolnick, 1978, 1981). This work presaged the exciting explication of the effects of environmental and psychological variables on brain function reviewed below.

Even this evidence, however, did not identify the GABA system as specifically anxiolytic. Investigation concluded that the reduction in generalized arousal associated with sedative and anticonvulsant effects could also be the mechanism of action for any anxiolytic effects observed, although arousal reduction need not be as great as for sedative effects. This in fact was the assumption of a leading psychopharmacologist, Malcolm Lader (1985). In addtion to sedative and muscle relaxant effects, Bond and Lader (1979) found that benzodiazepines reduce anger, hostility, and aggression. Even more interesting was the finding of reduction in reports of positive emotional states, such as "eager anticipation" and pleasure (Lader, 1975). Thus Lader (1985) concluded that benzodiazepines may act to reduce emotion in general, or, more likely, the arousal associated with many emotional or affective states.

More recent research indicates that the benzodiazepine–GABA system is more complex and more intimately interrelated to other systems than previously supposed. For example, activation of central benzodiazepine–GABA receptor complexes also suppresses HPA axis activity, and consequently cortisol levels, which becomes important when HPA function is discussed below (Spiegel & Barlow, 2000c). In addition to these central receptor complexes, benzodiazepine recognition sites of different type are present widely in cells outside the central nervous system. These so-called peripheral benzodiazepine receptors are believed to be instrumental in controlling the syntheses of regulatory steroids. Their role in the anxiolytic actions of benzodiazepines is unknown. For example, although they bind some benzodiazepines (e.g., diazepam), they have low affinity for others (e.g., clonazepam). Interestingly, peripheral benzodiazepine receptors are decreased in blood cells of individuals with untreated GAD, but return to normal levels after successful treatment with benzodiazepines. Their numbers also vary in response to stress, being elevated following acute stressors and reduced during chronic stress (Spiegel & Barlow, 2000c).

A possible explanation for those changes has been suggested by Rocca et al. (1998). These investigators note that peripheral benzodiazepine receptors in brain glial cells control the production of neurosteroids that act as modulators of GABA-A receptor sensitivity.

Their effect on GABA functioning appears to be opposite to that of clinically effective benzodiazepines; that is, they *decrease* rather than increase the inhibitory effects of GABA. It is hypothesized that an endogenous ligand of these glial cell receptors (possible diazepam binding inhibitor) is released during stress, initiating the cycle of events depicted in Figure 6.4. The immediate effect of these events would be to enhance the stress-induced release of cortisol. However, prolonged cortisol excess is hypothesized to down-regulate peripheral benzodiazepine receptors, resulting in the reduced receptor densities found in patients with GAD. Administration of a clinically effective benzodiazepine drug would interrupt the proposed pathway at the point of the central GABA receptor, lowering cortisol levels and restoring synthesis of peripheral benzodiazepine receptors (Speigel & Barlow, 2000c). Once again, these latter findings become important in more integrative accounts of anxiety described below implicating the CRF system.

Adrenocortical Function

In an interesting series of studies, George Curtis, Randolph Nesse, and their colleagues provoked panic in patients with specific phobia by confronting them with their feared object (usually a small animal), while examining adrenocortical functioning. They noted, much to their surprise, no response in the adrenocortical system as reflected in measures of pro-

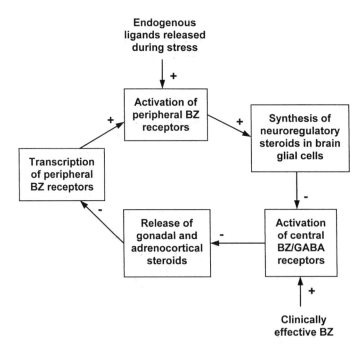

FIGURE 6.4. Possible involvement of peripheral benzodiazepine receptors in acute and chronic stress reactions (based on descriptions by Rocca et al.). BZ, benzodiazepine; GABA, gamma-aminobutyric acid. From Spiegel, D. A., and Barlow, D. H. (2000c). Generalized anxiety disorders. In M. G. Gelder, J. J. Lopez-Ibor, and N. C. Andreasen (Eds.), *The new Oxford textbook of psychiatry*. New York: Oxford University Press. Copyright 2000 by the Oxford University Press. Reprinted by permission.

lactin, thyroid-stimulating hormone, and plasma cortisol (Curtis, Buxton, Lippman, Nesse, & Wright, 1976). This lack of response occurred despite the fact that by all other criteria, the subjects seemed clearly tõ be panicking. On the other hand, there were slight increases in growth hormone response. Stokes (1985) points out that, contrary to most studies with normal subjects, there was no uncertainty or novelty in this situation. That is, these patients were clearly informed of what was to occur and experienced repeated flooding sessions with the phobic object. Furthermore, Curtis et al. (1976) did report some increase in adrenocortical responding at the first session, when patients came in for initial measurements, perhaps again reflecting novelty or anticipation. This, of course, would be consistent with other physiological responses.

In a particularly well-done study from the same laboratory utilizing this paradigm, Nesse et al. (1985) were able to observe weak and inconsistent increases in cortisol, growth hormone, and insulin in response to phobic (expected) panic. However, even this weak response decreased by the second trial. Of course, all physiological and catecholamine responses (with the exception of blood pressure), as well as subjective anxiety, also decreased at the second trial; this raised the possibility that the results reflected therapeutic changes rather than just habituation to novelty. On the other hand, these results with patients were certainly puzzling, since substantial increases in HPA axis functioning and resulting hypercortisolemia would be expected. Nesse et al. (1985) reversed their earlier lack of results only by exercising extreme care in the timing of their measurements, as well as other experimental control procedures.

In fact, several more recent studies have also observed the puzzling finding of normal or decreased adrenocortical activity in patients with anxiety disorders. Most of these observations have been made in patients with posttraumatic stress disorder, but more recent reports suggest that patients with panic disorder and social phobia also evidence this phenomenon (e.g., Yehuda, 1997; Yehuda, Lowy, Southwick, Shaffer, & Giller, 1991; Yehuda, Boisoneau, Lowy, & Giller, 1995; Yehuda, Teicher, Trestman, Levengood, & Siever, 1996; Roy-Byrne, Geraci, & Uhde, 1986; Goldstein, Halbreich, Asnis, Endicott, & Alvir, 1987; Tancer, 1993). These findings, of course, are consistent with the studies by Curtis et al. (1976) and Nesse et al. (1985) described above, but are inconsistent with results in patients suffering from depression (Heim & Nemeroff, 1999). And yet other studies seem to clearly indicate increased CRF secretion in patients with anxiety disorders, which should produce the same type of hypercortisolemia noted in depressed patients (Yehuda, Levengood, et al., 1996; Bremner, Licinio, et al., 1997). The best interpretation of these findings is that there is a pronounced increase in CRF secretion in these anxious patients (consistent with that observed in depressed patients, but that negative feedback systems inhibiting activity of the HPA axis are particularly pronounced in patients with anxiety disorders, due perhaps to some form of peripheral adaptation. It is this increase in negative feedback systems that seems to result in normal, or perhaps even decreased, adrenocorticol activity. This hypothesis is consistent with the findings of Rocca et al. (1998), who noted the down-regulation of peripheral benzodiazepine receptors as a function of prolonged excesses of cortisol.

In view of these disappointing results, the study of neuroendocrine function languished for a time during the late 1980s and early 1990s. But other investigators with different points of view were originating new and exciting inquiries into neuroendocrinological correlates of anxiety and stress. Prominent among these efforts is the programmatic research of Charles Nemeroff and his colleagues on HPA axis functioning in rats. I take up their findings below and in Chapter 8.

Toward an Integrative Brain System Account of Anxiety and Fear

By the 1990s it was clear that understanding the neurobiology of any one isolated system would provide only a small contribution to the complex biopsychosocial construct of anxiety. As early as 1986, Insel pointed out that lesioning pathways in the forebrain in one system (such as noradrenergic pathways) would lead to substantial reductions in other systems (such as benzodiazepine receptors). At that time, Uhde, Boulenger, et al. (1984) also pointed out that anxiety and panic are most likely multiply loaded in the brain because of their important survival value. Both the noradrenergic system and the serotonergic system—organized with cell bodies in the brain stem, and having diffuse projections throughout the brain—are capable of the global function of alerting and alarming the organism.

The Septo-Hippocampal System (Behavioral Inhibition System)

Perhaps the first investigator to attempt a true description of an integrated whole-brain system was Jeffrey Gray (1982, 1985). For example, Gray noted:

> [Cortical areas] afford a route by which language functions of the neocortex can control the activities of the limbic structures which are the chief neural substrate of anxiety. In turn, limbic structures, via subicular and hippocampal projections to the entorhinal cortex, are able to scan verbally coded stores of information when performing the functions allotted to them in the theory outlined above. In this way, it is possible for human anxiety to be triggered by verbal stimuli (relatively independently of ascending monoaminergic influences) and to utilize verbally coded strategies to cope with perceived threats. It is for this reason, if the theory is correct, that lesions to the prefrontal and cingulate cortices are effective in cases of anxiety that are resistant to drug therapy (Powell, 1979). (Gray, 1985, p. 10)

As noted earlier, Gray (1982) hypothesized that the septo-hippocampal system, together with the Papez circuit (a neural loop connecting the subicular area in the hippocampal formation to the mammillary bodies, anterior thalamus, cingulate cortex, and back to the subiculum), is responsible for mediating the emotion of anxiety as well as the major effects of anxiolytic drugs. In Chapter 2, I have noted that Gray called this network the behavioral inhibition system (BIS), because he believed that when it is activated, it interrupts ongoing behavior and redirects the organism's attention to signs of possible danger.

According to Gray's model (Gray & McNaughton, 1996; Gray, 1982), and as briefly described in Chapter 2, the BIS receives information about the environment from the sensory cortex via the temporal lobe and hippocampal formation. The system checks the information for consistency with predictions, which are updated continuously by the Papez circuit based on preceding information and stored patterns, as well as for consistency with the immediate goals of the organism. When a mismatch is found, or if a predicted event is aversive, the outputs of the BIS are activated, resulting in a constellation of emotional and behavioral effects consistent with anxiety (see Figure 6.5).

The activation of the BIS appears to be moderated by ascending noradrenergic and serotonergic projections to the septo-hippocampal complex, providing a possible mechanism for the anxiolytic actions of some drugs. The amygdala also provides inputs to the BIS and may relay its outputs to the hypothalamus and autonomic nervous system, thereby mediating anxious arousal. Sustained activation of the BIS may therefore account for many of the features of anxiety. Although this model has its critics (e.g., Davis, 1998; Lang, Davis, & Öhman, in press), it was this kind of thinking that led the way to current integrated work on the neurobiology of anxiety and panic.

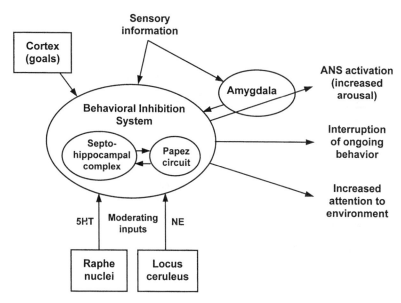

FIGURE 6.5. The behavioral inhibition system (based on descriptions by Gray & McNaughton). ANS, autonomic nervous system; 5HT, serotonin; NE, norepinephrine. From Spiegel, D. A., and Barlow, D. H. (2000c). Generalized anxiety disorders. In M. G. Gelder, J. J. Lopez-Ibor, and N. C. Andreasen (Eds.), *The new Oxford textbook of psychiatry*. New York: Oxford University Press. Copyright 2000 by the Oxford University Press. Reprinted by permission.

The Amygdala and the Bed Nucleus of the Stria Terminalis

Some of the most exciting research on the neurobiology of anxiety and fear (and, in my view, its clinical manifestation of panic) has centered on the central role played by the amygdala in the mediation of fear reactions, and, more recently, on the functions of the bed nucleus of the stria terminalis (BNST). For example, it is now clear that the BNST is an important link in the larger septo-hippocampal system (Spiegel & Barlow, 2000c).

The amygdala is thought to be responsible for the detection of potential threats to the organism and the mobilization of a range of defensive responses (LeDoux, 1996, 1998). A representation of fear pathways based on theorizing by LeDoux (1996) and Michael Davis (1998) is presented in Figure 6.6. Through connections with the hypothalamus, it can activate the SNS and the HPA axis. Through efferent fibers to the central gray area of the midbrain, it can mediate behavioral defense responses such as the fight-or-flight response and behavioral "freezing." And through connections to the nucleus reticularis pontis caudalis, it can enhance the defensive startle reflex.

Interestingly, and at least in the case of fear conditioning using auditory cues, information concerning a possible dangerous situation seems to be relayed to the amygdala following two different parallel pathways, both of which lead to the lateral nucleus of the amygdala. The first pathway, proceeding rapidly from the thalamus to the amygdala, provides information, unprocessed by higher cortical regions and seems to enable immediate action. This is LeDoux's "low road" to emotional activation, unfettered by cortically based cognitive processing. A second pathway, proceeding from the thalamus through the cortex (the "high road") to the amygdala, allows more considered action, probably by calling

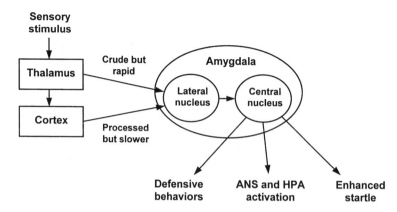

FIGURE 6.6. Fear pathways (based on descriptions by LeDoux and Davis). ANS, autonomic nervous system; HPA, hypothalamic–pituitary–adrenocortical axis. From Spiegel, D. A., and Barlow, D. H. (2000c). Generalized anxiety disorders. In M. G. Gelder, J. J. Lopez-Ibor, and N. C. Andreasen (Eds.), *The new Oxford textbook of psychiatry.* New York: Oxford University Press. Copyright 2000 by the Oxford University Press. Reprinted by permission.

on stored memories of past experience with the potential threat. The central nucleus of the amygdala is the region most critical for the expression of what LeDoux (1996) terms a conditioned "fear" response. This nucleus has multiple projections throughout the brain. For example, projections to the periaqueductal gray seems to activate a variety of anxiety-related behaviors, including freezing (hypervigilance). Projections to the BNST (described below) activate the HPA axis. Further projections to the ventral tegmental area, the locus ceruleus, and the raphe nuclei connect it with other key monoaminergic systems, including dopaminergic, noradrenergic, and serotonergic systems (Sullivan, Kent, & Coplan, 2000).

The extent to which these pathways are involved in the neurobiology of anxiety (as opposed to fear) is unclear. However, a structure closely related to the amgdala, the BNST, may well make a more substantial contribution to the emotion of anxiety. The BNST resembles the amygdala in its neurotransmitter content, cell morphology, and hypothalamic and brain stem connections; like the amygdala, it also exerts a modulating effect on the startle reflex (Davis, 1998). Administration of CRF into the cerebral ventricles of rats produces a state of generalized arousal resembling anxiety. Under those conditions, the startle reflex also is enhanced. Exposing rats to bright light for 5 to 20 minutes has similar effects. These effects are not blocked by damage to amygdala, but are blocked by lesions to the BNST and by treatment with benzodiazepines or buspirone. Conversely, infusion of CRF directly into the BNST, but not the amygdala, produces a rapid increase in startle. Based on these observations, Davis (1998) has suggested that the BNST may play a role in anxiety analogous to that of the amygdala in fear reactions, and, furthermore, that prolonged or repeated stimulation of the BNST by CRF during periods of stress may lead to sustained activation and thus to persistent anxiety.

More recent integrative models build on early theorizing as well as new findings, particularly those findings reviewed above involving the HPA axis. For example, building on the work of Chrousos and Gold (1992), Sullivan et al. (2000) specify two brain systems as particularly relevant underpinnings of anxiety and fear: the LC-NE system, mentioned above, and the CRF system.

The CRF System

The CRF system is assuming center stage in recent neurobiological theorizing on the underpinnings of anxiety, since CRF has emerged as a neurotransmitter that may play a very central role in anxiety and depression. At least partly because of the findings reported above exploring adrenocortical correlates of anxiety and depression, other groups of investigators have turned their attention to the operations of the HPA axis—and in particular to the role of the CRF system—in psychopathological states, especially depression and anxiety. Notable among these investigations is the work of Charles Nemeroff and his associates (e.g., Heim & Nemeroff, 1999; Heit, Owens, Plotsky, & Nemeroff, 1997; Ladd et al., 2000). These investigators have gone beyond simply characterizing the HPA axis and the role of CRF. Rather, these investigators have characterized whole-brain systems implicated in stress, anxiety, and depression, in which CRF plays a central role. They have also outlined the potential implications of these alterations for the development of anxiety and depression. Before these interesting findings are discussed, it is important to review briefly the structure and function of the HPA axis. A schematic of these operations is presented in Figure 6.7.

Various stressful or threatening cues may activate input from several regions of the brain, including the brain stem (particularly the locus ceruleus), the limbic system (particularly the hippocampus and the amygdala), and the prefrontal cortex. These inputs then activate CRF, which is stored predominantly in the hypothalamic paraventricular nuclei (PVN). CRF neurons are found not only in the PVN of the hypothalamus, but also in the central nucleus of the amygdala and the lateral BNST (Sullivan et al., 2000). CRF also acts synergistically with another hormone emanating from the PVN of the hypothalamus, known as arginine vasopressin (AVP); CRF and AVP are what directly result in increased pituitary–adrenal activity (Chrousos, 1995). CRF and related substances such as AVP, in turn, stimulate the synthesis and release of adrenocorticotropic hormone (ACTH) from the anterior pituitary gland. ACTH then stimulates the production and release of glucocorticoids. The glucocorticoids (cortisol in primates) then combine with catecholamines released from the adrenal medulla and sympathetic nerve terminals to raise circulating glucose levels, and to increase heart rate and blood pressure. As noted above, this system is controlled and regulated by a glucocorticoid-mediated negative feedback system located primarily in the hippocampus and septum, but with receptors found in other parts of the brain also (Ladd et al., 2000).

It now seems clear that CRF mediates not only endocrine responses to stress, but also wide-ranging brain and behavioral responses, including autonomic nervous system and immune system responses. A representation of these wide-ranging effects is presented in Figure 6.8. Particularly important is the relatively recent finding that a number of classical neurotransmitter systems are believed to stimulate hypothalamic CRF release. These include the benzodiazepine–GABA system, as well as monoamines such as serotonin and norepinephrine, which have long been implicated in the pathophysiology of anxiety and depression. Furthermore, as noted above, two critical brain structures—the locus ceruleus and the central nucleus of the amygdala—are innervated by a particularly dense set of CRF nerve terminals. Of course, the locus ceruleus has long been implicated in the pathophysiology of both mood and anxiety disorders, and is the main source of noradrenergic neurons innervating the forebrain. Both acute and chronic stressors elevate CRF concentrations in the locus ceruleus (Chappell et al., 1986). Furthermore, infusions of CRF into the locus ceruleus produce anxiety-like behavior in animal studies (Butler et al., 1990).

Similarly, infusions of CRF into the central nucleus of the amygdala produce anxiety and fear-like behavior (Wiersma, Baauw, Bohus, & Koolhaas, 1995), and other findings suggest that CRF neurons in the amygdala may regulate serotonergic transmission (Boadle-

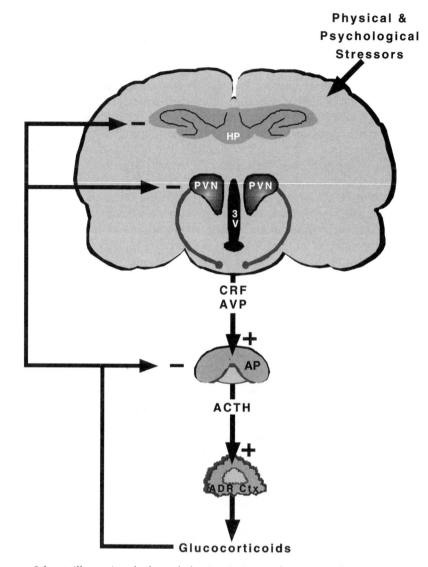

FIGURE 6.7. Scheme illustrating the hypothalamic–pituitary–adrenocortical (HPA) axis. Viscerosensory and emotional stimuli are encoded within the central nervous system and funnel to the hypothalamic paraventricular nuclei (PVN), adjacent to the third ventricle (3V), where they activate secretion of corticotropin-releasing factor (CRF) and arginine vasopressin (AVP) from nerve terminals in the external zone of the median eminence (ME) ending in the perivascular spaces of the primary portal capillary plexus. These peptides enter the hypophysial portal vascular system via fenestrations in the walls of these capillaries and are carried by the long portal vessels to the anterior pituitary gland, where they diffuse from capillaries of the secondary portal plexus to act at corticotropes. CRF stimulates transcription of the propiomelanocortin (POMC) gene, providing the precursor peptide for adrenocorticotropin (ACTH). Both CRF and AVP facilitate the secretion of stored ACTH into the systemic circulation. ACTH binds to its membrane receptor on adrenocortical cells, resulting in the de novo biosynthesis and release of glucocorticoids (corticosterone in the rat, cortisol in primates), which then act throughout the organism via cytoplasmic receptors. The circulating glucocorticoids also complete a negative feedback loop to damp ongoing and subsequent activity of the HPA axis through actions at cytoplasmic glucocorticoid receptors (GR) distributed in pituitary corticotropes, the hypothalamic PVN, the hippocampus (HP), and numerous other regions within the central nervous system. Input from regions such as the brain stem and cortico-limbic regions modulates HPA axis activity. From Ladd et al. (2000). Copyright 2000 by Elsevier Science Ltd. Reprinted by permission.

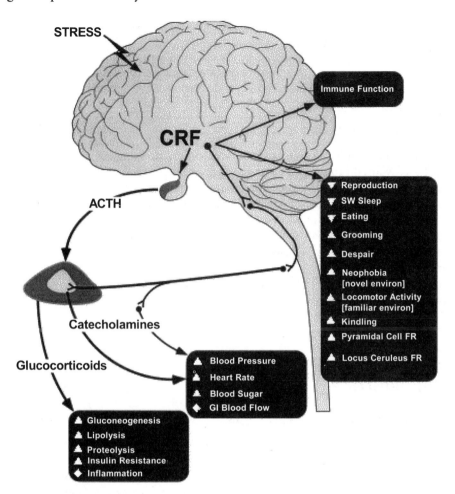

FIGURE 6.8. Representation of the ability of central CRF neurons to integrate endocrine, behavioral, autonomic, and immunological responses to stress. From Heit, Owens, Plotsky, and Nemeroff (1997). Copyright 1997 by Williams & Wilkins. Reprinted by permission.

Biber, Singh, Corley, Phan, & Dilts, 1993). Numerous studies in animals link the administration of CRF to behavioral indices of anxiety and depression (Heit et al., 1997; Ladd et al., 2000; Nemeroff, 1996; Coplan, Goetz, et al., 1998; Sullivan et al., 2000). As Sullivan et al. (2000) point out, CRF has emerged as a key neurotransmitter in terms of its role in the expression of stress, anxiety, and depression, because of its wide distribution throughout key anatomical regions in the brain.

As summarized above, it is now clear that CRF neurons and LC-NE neurons in the brain stem are linked (Chrousos, 1998). Also, dopaminergic pathways, including those from the ventral tegmentum to the prefrontal cortex, are linked to both brain systems (Sullivan et al., 2000). It is very possible that these dopaminergic pathways are involved in anxious anticipation and vigilance (major components of anxiety)—a suggestion that has recently received some support from Shively (1998) in work with cynomolgus monkeys. Other monoaminergic pathways are also connected to both brain systems, including serotonergic pathways originating in the raphi nuclei, which seem to activiate CRF and LC-NE neurons and to have complex effects on the functioning of the amygdala (Graeff, Guimaraes, DeAndrade, & Deakin, 1996; Sullivan et al., 2000). Finally, Kalin et al. (2000) have recently reported that rhesus monkeys with extreme right frontal brain activity had increased CRF concentrations in cerebrospinal fluid for a period spanning 5 years, suggesting a strong link between these manifestations of chronic anxiety.

Neurobiological Findings: Conclusions

It is clear that our thinking on the neurobiological underpinnings of anxiety, depression, and fear has advanced rapidly during the past few years. From narrowly focused investigations of single monoaminergic systems, research has led us to appreciate the complex interplay of a variety of brain systems (particularly the CRF system) acting both centrally and peripherally to support fundamental important emotions such as anxiety and fear. It also seems clear that what we now know will also be substantially dated in a relatively short period of time. However, research by leading neuroscientists has been made even more intellectually satisfying by a clear recognition that we must go beyond the brain to fully understand the workings of the brain. In fact, it is from these leading neuroscientists that we are coming to appreciate more fully the influence of psychological and environmental factors on brain functioning—a topic to which I now turn.

THE RECIPROCAL RELATIONSHIP OF NEUROBIOLOGY AND PSYCHOLOGY

Early Findings from Animal Paradigms

When strong evidence began to appear that neurotransmitter system functions in isolation are insufficient to account for anxiety even in animal models, leading investigators began to theorize that they must superimpose psychological constructs, such as meaning and interpretations or attributions, as well as conditioning and learned coping responses. For example, Segal and Bloom (1976) stimulated the locus ceruleus in awake rats. They found that electrical activity or firing rate of hippocampal neurons was either increased or decreased, depending on prior learned associations the animals had made with specific stimuli. It also became clear that noradrenergic functioning was strongly influenced by the adequacy of coping responses, as in a learned helplessness paradigm (Anisman, 1984). This was demonstrated for serotonergic functioning as well (Maser & Gallup, 1974). Similar observations were made concerning animal paradigms involving conflict, which may underlie more generalized anxiety. For example, Cassens, Roffman, Kuruc, Orsulak, and Schildkraut (1980) demonstrated clear increases in MHPG, a metabolite of norepinephrine, in rats after exposure to previously neutral stimuli that had been paired with stress (conditioned stimuli). Bandura, Taylor, Williams, Mefford, and Barchas (1985), in a particularly well-done experiment, demonstrated that changes in perceived self-efficacy alter catecholamine secretion.

From another perspective, scientists such as Kandel (1983) were working out the molecular and neurobiological basis of the development of anxiety in organisms low on the phylogenetic scale, such as sea snails (*Aplysia*). Using classical fear conditioning paradigms, Kandel observed profound changes in synaptic strength and number of receptors as a function of learning and experience. These results recalled the work on alteration of the number of benzodiazepine receptors as a function of learning and experience (Paul & Skolnick, 1978, 1981).

Although chronic arousal seems to be a biological marker for most anxiety disorders, it was not entirely clear in the early1980s whether chronic overarousal is directly inherited, or whether it is the product of a complex psychobiological interaction. The work of Kandel (1983) and others on the biology of learning indicated that at the level of individual cells, increases in both receptors and neurotransmitters involved in fear conditioning seem to be permanent as a result of learning. Kandel (1983) speculated that the very genetic structure of cells within the central nervous system is changed as a result of learning. Specific inactivated genes become active during learning, leading to such changes in structure as the increase in receptors. If the behavior is extinguished, the change is reversed. These preliminary observations on the fundamental effects of experience and psychological factors on brain function and structure were clearly confirmed during the 1990s (Kandel, Jessell, & Schacter, 1991; Owens, Mulchahey, Stout, Plotsky, 1997; Wallace, Kilman, Withers, & Greenough, 1992). For this work, Kandel was awarded the Nobel Prize in 2000. To take just one interesting example, some scientists have begun to pin down the complex interaction among psychosocial factors, brain structure, and brain function, as reflected in neurotransmitter activity. Yeh, Fricke, and Edwards (1996) studied two male crayfish that were battling to establish dominance in their social group. When one of the crayfish won the battle and established dominance, the scientists found that serotonin made a specific set of neurons in that animal more likely to fire; however, in the animal that lost the battle, serotonin made the same neurons less likely to fire. Thus Yeh et al. (1996) discovered that naturally occurring neurotransmitters have different effects depending on the previous psychosocial experience of the organism. Furthermore, this experience directly affects the structure of neurons at the synapse by altering the sensitivity of serotonin receptors. These investigators also discovered that the effects of serotonin are reversible if the losers once again become dominant.

Emerging Evidence for the Influence of Adverse Early Life Events on Brain Function

Now there is dramatic evidence that early stressful life events may effect rather permanent alterations in brain function (particularly in CRF-containing neurons and receptors), that may mediate the neurobiological vulnerability to develop chronic anxiety and depression later in life. As noted above, much work in this area has emerged from the laboratories of Charles Nemeroff and his colleagues at Emory University (e.g., Heit et al., 1997; Ladd et al., 2000; Heim & Nemeroff, 1999). Building on pioneering work on the effects of early stress on later behavior by scientists such as Ader and Grota (1969), Denenberg (1964), Miller (1979), and Weiss et al. (1982), reviewed briefly above, Nemeroff and his colleagues have studied more systematically the effects of stressful early separation on later behavior in rats. As such, this group has provided the clearest articulation to date of the diathesis–stress model of the etiology of anxiety and related emotional states such as depression. This animal model is particularly useful, since maternal separation during crucial periods just after birth is a particularly stressful occurrence.

In a typical paradigm, maternal separation would occur for 2 weeks immediately after birth for either 180 minutes a day (HMS180, the stressful condition), compared to removal for 15 minutes a day (HMS15, a nonstressful condition), or a normal animal facility rearing (AFR) condition with no separation. In one experiment, levels of circulating ACTH and corticosterone were normal in adults of all rearing conditions, but response to psychological or physical stressors were very different. For example, a psychological stressor such as an airpuff startle elicited clear hyperreactivity in the HPA axis, as indicated by marked elevations in ACTH and corticosterone in HMS180 animals (see Figure 6.9). The authors point

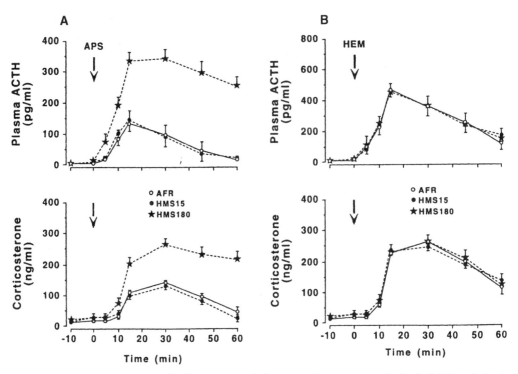

FIGURE 6.9. Rearing-associated differences in adult responsiveness to psychological (A) and physical (B) stressors. In the maternally separated adults (HMS180), the ACTH and corticosterone responses to the psychological stressor of airpuff startle (APS) was enhanced relative to the responses in animal facility reared (AFR) colony controls or handling controls (HMS15). In contrast, no difference in responsiveness was evident among the groups in response to the physical stressor of 15% hemorrhage (HEM). Data are shown as mean ± *SEM*. From Ladd et al. (2000). Copyright 2000 by Elsevier Science Ltd. Reprinted by permission.

out that other psychological stressors, such as exposure to a novel environment and restraint, produced similar responses in animals stressed early in life; however, comparable physical stressors (e.g., hemorrhage) did not produce this activation. The suggestion from these and other data (e.g., Ladd et al., 2000), is that early environmental factors exert a significant impact on the developing HPA axis, resulting in persistent alterations in the adult organism's responsiveness to psychological stressors. As a mechanism, these investigators suggest that sensitivity of the hippocampus and frontal cortex to circulating glucocorticoids is attenuated, thereby decreasing the efficacy of negative feedback inhibition over HPA axis activity. This in turn would increase CRF and AVP synthesis in the hypothalamic PVN, and, perhaps, increased expression of CRF in the central nucleus of the amygdala (Ladd et al., 2000). This latter finding is supported by observation of elevated levels of CRF in a variety of sites, including the central nucleus of the amygdala and the BNST, in adult rats who had been subjected to separation immediately after birth. What is important about these findings is that a psychological variable, early separation seems to result in a chronic alteration of neurobiological function that may underlie chronic emotionality and perhaps neuroticism. These experiments lead directly to models of the etiology of anxiety and anxiety disorders articulated in Chapter 8. In the context of the neurobiological underpinnings reviewed in this chapter, it is now possible to outline in more detail models of the etiology of panic, anxiety, and the anxiety disorders.

True Alarms, False Alarms, and Learned (Conditioned) Anxiety

The Origins of Panic and Phobia

Only in the mid-1980s did we begin to collect information on the nature of panic. Much of what is known has been presented in the preceding chapters. But the accumulating evidence points to a complex biopsychosocial process. This process involves the interaction of an ancient alarm system, crucial for survival, with inappropriate and maladaptive learning and subsequent cognitive and affective complications. Some of the thinking on the origins of pathological panic presented in theoretical form below remains speculative, but there should be enough coherence within the theory to enable investigators to design research protocols that result in confirmation or disconfirmation. This chapter begins with a brief analysis of the alarm system most commonly known as fear.

TRUE ALARMS

There is general agreement that fear occurs when we are directly threatened with a dangerous, perhaps life-threatening, event. An impending attack from wild animals is something few of us experience today, but our ancestors knew this threat well in millennia past. This history may account for our somewhat greater susceptibility to becoming "alarmed" in the presence of snakes and mountain lions (Cook, Hodes, & Lang, 1986; Öhman, 1999; Öhman, Flykt, & Lundqvist, 2000; Seligman, 1971). Relevant threats today include speeding vehicles, guns, drowning, or seeing the safety of our children threatened. Under these conditions, the emotion of fear mobilizes us physically and cognitively for quick action and sometimes "superhuman" efforts. Most typically, running away or escaping is the behavioral manifestation of fear. Occasionally, directed action to counter the threat is apparent, such as attacking a predator or single-handedly lifting an automobile so that a child trapped underneath can escape. These reactions represent Cannon's emergency reaction characterized by the compelling action tendencies of "fight or flight." Sometimes these actions are counterproductive, as in the case of a drowning victim's vainly struggling when the rational response would be to lie still and attempt to float. The ancient response of "freezing" (tonic immobility) may be called forth if other action tendencies, such as escape or aggression, are ineffective or not available and one is under direct attack by a predator, as mentioned in Chapters 1 and 6. Most theorists would agree that these basic responses are primitive alarm reactions observed far down the phylogenetic scale. As such, they have profound evolutionary significance.

FALSE ALARMS

In the first edition (Barlow, 1988), I described the phenomenon of false alarms. That is, "spontaneous" or "uncued" panic seems nearly identical in all respects to fear phenomenologically, except for the ability of the individual to specify an antecedent (Carter & Barlow, 1995; Forsyth & Eifert, 1996). The evidence for this has been reviewed in Chapter 4. The very definition of panic, specifying as it does sudden feelings of marked apprehension and impending doom that are associated with a wide range of distressing physical sensations, would certainly qualify as a definition of fear in other contexts. Although few would disagree that panic seems to be intense fear, a continuing goal for future research is to compare directly the expressive-behavioral, neurobiological, and cognitive aspects of intense fear and uncued panic. In any case, if fear is an alarm, then we are faced with the phenomenon of false alarms, where marked fear or panic occurs in the absence of any life-threatening stimulus, learned or unlearned. How common are false alarms, and why do they occur?

False alarms or panic attacks seem to be far more prevalent in the general population than was assumed previously. In fact, studies from around the world are converging to suggest that occasional panic attacks occur relatively frequently in the general population. Detailed evidence on the frequency of panic has been reviewed in Chapter 4. For example, data from the clinic at Albany (Rapee, Sanderson, & Barlow, 1987) and from epidemiological surveys (e.g., Wittchen & Essau, 1991) suggest that between 10% and 14% of the population has experienced an unexpected, uncued panic attack. Typically, attacks are less intense and less frequent in individuals with nonclinical panic than in patients. Panic attacks also occur during sleep in those with nonclinical panic and aggregate more strongly in the families of these individuals than in families of subjects who have not experienced panic (Craske, 1999; Norton, Dorward, & Cox, 1986). The frequency of panic in the general population plays an important role in models of anxiety disorders outlined below.

Although false alarms seem remarkably prevalent, relatively few people seek treatment for this problem—an issue that is also discussed further below. Nevertheless, it is important to determine the "causes" of false alarms, since they may represent the beginning of panic disorder, although false alarms alone clearly are not sufficient to account for panic disorder (Bouton, Mineka, & Barlow, 2001). We have made progress in our search for the causes of false alarms, particularly initial false alarms, during the past decade. Ongoing lines of investigation are targeting a complex web of preexisting biological and psychological vulnerabilities interacting with contemporaneous events (e.g., life stress) in the genesis of initial false alarms (panic).

Causes of False Alarms

Genetic Contributions

In Chapter 6, I have reviewed evidence for specific genetic contributions to innate defensive reactions such as freezing, or experiencing a vasovagal reaction to the sight of blood. Conceptualizing false alarms as yet another defensive reaction, I have also reviewed a variety of evidence supporting the differential heritability of false alarms (panic) from anxiety. To quote Martin, Jardine, Andrews, and Heath (1988) once again, "this response has been subject to intense natural selection during the course of human evolution" (p. 705), and "symptoms of panic seems to be shaped in part by unique genetic influences which do not affect other anxiety symptoms" (p. 698). I have then described a hypothetical arrangement in which more generalized stress-produced neurobiological hyperreactivity (possibly elaborated psychologically into anxiety) may trigger basic emotions or defensive reactions such as panic attacks, as a function of differential inherited thresholds for these action tendencies. In other words, panic attacks may "spike off" a baseline of stress-related reactivity or possibly "anxiety." In this way, the action tendencies associated with discrete emotions such as fear (panic) may occasionally "fire" out of situational context. That is, one may experience a false alarm. One implication of considering a specific genetic contribution to experiencing false alarms is that there may be an associated biological dysregulation.

Biological Dysregulation

It would certainly seem logical that a biological dysregulation may underlie false alarms. After all, the very nature of false alarms specifies that there is no readily identifiable external or internal antecedent or cue. For this reason, investigators have attempted to identify a biological marker in patients with panic disorder that would be associated with an underlying biological dysregulation, or that at least would point in the direction of a biological dysregulation. This research has been reviewed in Chapters 5 and 6. As I conclude in those chapters, at the present time there is no evidence for any specific biological marker; nor, for that matter, is there evidence for any important functional neurobiological differences between patients with panic disorder and individuals without panic. The exception, of course, is chronic hyperarousal, which seems a biological and/or psychological marker of sorts. But in Chapter 6 I have reviewed evidence that preexisting chronic hyperarousal and its biological underpinnings characterize almost all anxiety disorders, and thus should not constitute a specific biological marker for panic. However, hyperarousal may interact with other variables and contribute to the genesis of false alarms in a manner suggested below.

As noted in Chapter 4, there is always the possibility that we are looking in the wrong place. Patients with panic disorder present with a number of emotional complications. It may be that their panic attacks are no longer purely false alarms, but rather learned (or conditioned) alarms that are contaminated by substantial emotional interference in the form of generalized anxiety and depression, and that therefore present somewhat differently than do "pure" false alarms (e.g., Taylor et al., 1986; Bouton et al., 2001). If this is so, investigators in their search for crucial biological markers may be better off studying people with infrequent panic attacks who have not yet presented for treatment (e.g., Kenardy & Taylor, 1999).

Separation Anxiety

An early hypothesis focused on the relationship of separation anxiety in children to the later development of false alarms (and, subsequently, panic disorder with agoraphobia). Separation anxiety has occupied a prominent place in many theories of child development and psychopathology (Bowlby, 1973, 1982). Bowlby's influential writings on attachment theory, taken up in more detail in Chapter 8, purports that attachment to others is a powerful evolutionarily favored drive with early attachment to a mother figure as the prototype. Separation from an attachment figure thus produces an intense affective response called "separation anxiety." Early separation has also become the principal paradigm for studying the effect of intense early stress on later emotional functioning in animal models (e.g., Heim & Nemeroff, 1999; see Chapter 6). Since agoraphobia often represents the experience of fear when one is away from familiar surroundings, or alone, Bowlby (1973) viewed agoraphobia as a function of insecure attachments in adulthood.

Early clinical reports (Klein & Fink, 1962) also suggested that the panic attacks seen in patients with agoraphobia could be a "mature" expression of the type of distress and panic some children evidence upon separation, particularly from their mothers. Klein (1981), drawing on Bowlby's ideas, theorized that "spontaneous" panic attacks might be an expression of a "protest–despair" mechanism contingent on threats of separation in those with a biologically determined lowered threshold for this response. Several years ago, Rachel Gittelman-Klein evaluated evidence, both pro and con, concerning the relationship of separation anxiety to the development of panic attacks, panic disorder, and agoraphobia (e.g., Gittelman & Klein, 1985). Generally, there were three lines of evidence supporting this relationship: similarity of drug treatment effects for separation anxiety and adult agoraphobia; family concordance for separation anxiety and agoraphobia; and history of childhood separation anxiety in adults with agoraphobia.

Gittelman-Klein and Klein (1973) treated 44 children who had severe school phobia with imipramine; they found that, when compared to a group receiving placebo, most of the children reported feeling better, had fewer complaints on school days, and showed less distress at separation as reported by the mothers. Since studies indicate that imipramine is effective for panic disorder (see Chapter 10), these investigators suggest that panic and separation anxiety may be similar.

Weissman, Leckman, Merikangas, Gammon, and Prusoff (1984), in a well-designed study, examined the family concordance of separation anxiety and adult anxiety. They determined the prevalence of separation anxiety in the 6- to 18-year-old children of depressed and nondepressed adults identified in community surveys. These adult patients, diagnosed by direct structured clinical interview, were classified into four groups: (1) depressed with no anxiety disorder, (2) depressed with agoraphobia, (3) depressed with panic disorder, and (4) depressed with generalized anxiety disorder at any time in their adult lives. Separation anxiety was diagnosed in 24% of the children whose parents had a diagnosis of both depression and agoraphobia or panic. In contrast, none of the children of adults with pure depression, and only 6% of the children of parents with depression and generalized anxiety disorder reported separation anxiety. This study suggested a connection between separation anxiety and panic disorder, with or without agoraphobic avoidance.

Gittelman and Klein (1985) reported on the incidence of separation anxiety in adults with agoraphobia. These data were collected from clinical interviews with adults with agoraphobia who were asked to recall separation anxiety in their childhoods. This method suffers from the weaknesses of any retrospective study, but it remains one of the few studies of its type to employ a control group consisting of individuals with specific phobias. Nevertheless, in both childhood and adolescence (the periods examined), patients with agoraphobia recalled significantly more separation anxiety than the comparison group of patients with specific phobias who were also asked about these recollections. Intriguingly, this group difference was due entirely to a high prevalence of separation anxiety disorder in females with agoraphobia. No differences were found between males with agoraphobia and males with specific phobias. Fully 48% of females with agoraphobia reported separation anxiety, compared to only 20% of females with specific phobias. More recently, Biederman et al. (1993) reported in a prospective study that behaviorally inhibited children diagnosed with separation anxiety disorder were more likely to develop agoraphobia 3 years later than were inhibited children without separation anxiety disorder.

Unfortunately for the separation anxiety hypothesis, considerable evidence exists contradicting these positive results. For example, Thyer, Nesse, Curtis, and Cameron (1986) administered carefully structured questionnaires to 23 patients with panic disorder and 28 patients with small-animal phobias, and found essentially no differences in reports of childhood separation anxiety. This research group (Thyer, Nesse, Cameron, & Curtis, 1985) also found no differences in reports of separation anxiety when comparing individuals with agoraphobia to individuals with specific phobias. Other studies have also failed to find an increased incidence of reports of separation anxiety during the childhood of patients with agoraphobia (Buglass, Clarke, Henderson, Dreitman, & Presley, 1977; Parker, 1979). For example, Lipsitz et al. (1994) found no differences in the prevalence of separation anxiety in the childhood of patients with panic disorder versus patients with other anxiety disorders. van der Molen, van den Hout, van Deren, and Griez (1989) also found this nonspecificity, with nonanxious controls reporting as much or more past separation anxiety as patients with panic disorder. Shear (1996) similarly concluded that there is no specific association between separation anxiety and the onset of panic attack or panic disorder. Examining the issue from another perspective, Tennant, Hurry, and Bebbington (1982) found no association between forced childhood separations due to illnesses or other family circumstances, and the later development of anxiety and depression. Similarly, Gittelman-Klein (1975) failed to find any incidence of agoraphobia or panic disorder in the parents of 45 children with school phobia. In fact, Gittelman-Klein (1995), in reviewing five studies that examined self-reported retrospective ratings of adults with panic disorder (based on self-report), found a higher frequency of separation anxiety compared to other anxiety disorders in only one study.

The specific connection between separation anxiety and panic disorder, to the extent that it exists, is not convincing and is subject to alternative explanations. For example, Gittelman and Klein (1985) reported a history of separation anxiety only in women with current agoraphobia. Chambless and Mason (1986) found that sex role inventory measures of masculinity were inversely related to severity of avoidance behavior in agoraphobia. That is, the less "masculine" the scores on these inventories, the more the subjects tended to use avoidance as a coping mechanism, regardless of biological sex. Numerous studies have since noted that the proportion of females increases as agoraphobic avoidance becomes more severe (e.g., Craske, 1999; Thyer, Himle, Curtis, Cameron, & Nesse, 1985). What these data suggest (the suggestion is taken up in detail in Chapter 10) is that the incidence of panic in men and women is actually nearly equal, but that women cope with panic by avoiding, whereas men tend to cope with panic in other ways, such as consuming alcohol. This difference in coping strategies may account for the high percentage of individuals with agoraphobia who are females. What Gittelman and Klein may have discovered is that separation anxiety reflects an early expression of a greater tendency toward avoidance, which in females is culturally acceptable in our society. Therefore, reports of separation anxiety in the history of females with agoraphobia may simply reflect the early expression of a generalized gender-specific method of coping with stress and anxiety. If this is true, then the relationship between separation anxiety and subsequent panic may be only incidental to the stronger relationship between separation anxiety and the use of avoidance as a coping mechanism for stress or anxiety in general. In other words, if one sees children, particularly females, avoiding (and/or refusing to separate) in childhood, one can predict that they will continue to cope with any stress or anxiety as adults by avoiding. While interesting, this observation tells us very little about the causes of false alarms.

It is also possible that females are more inclined to report separation anxiety as children than are males because of the same cultural factors that seem to determine the use of avoidance as a method of coping with panic. That is, any differences may be an artifact of selective reporting. It is difficult to get around these issues in retrospective studies.

In addition, it is not entirely clear how the phenomenon of separation distress, as studied intensively by the developmentalists and reviewed in Chapter 2, relates to clinical manifestations of childhood separation anxiety on the one hand, or to the occurrence of forced separations during childhood as studied by Tennant et al. (1982) on the other. Evidence reviewed in Chapter 2 indicates that separation distress may begin as early as 4 months, reaching a peak at 13–18 months, and thereafter diminishing in the third year of life (Emde, Gaensbauer, & Harmon, 1976). Shiller, Izard, and Hembree (1986) suggest that separation distress in infants more closely reflects the basic emotion of anger rather than fear, as noted in Chapter 2. These investigators (Emde et al., 1976; Shiller et al., 1986) consider stranger distress rather than separation distress to be the innate precursor of a fear or panic response in humans, and the first sign of the emergence of a coherent fear system. As concluded in Chapter 2, variations in the intensity of stranger distress may have a stronger relationship to the later adult phenomenon of false alarms than separation distress may have.

The relationship of forced separations as studied by Tennant et al. (1982) in later childhood to separation distress during this early crucial period is also not clear. It would seem from this research that many children undergo forced separations of one type or another during childhood after the age of 3, and during adolescence, without any ill effects whatsoever.

To enable us to determine that the clinical presentation of separation anxiety is an important precursor to panic rather than a learned method of coping with stress or anxiety, several lines of evidence would have to converge. First, a relationship would need to be established between separation distress during the crucial biological period peaking at about 18 months and later separation anxiety in childhood or adolescence. With this evidence, we might begin to talk of a specific connection linking the seemingly hard-wired response of separation distress to the clinical syndrome of separation anxiety and the subsequent development of panic. Without this evidence, there would be little reason to assume that separation anxiety (or avoidance) is anything more than a learned and culturally acceptable method for coping with stress and anxiety in families that are anxiety-prone—a trait for which we already have good evidence of familial aggregation and perhaps genetic transmission (see Chapter 6). In other words, the behavior of avoiding separation in children would have no direct connection with later false alarms. Rather, both would be consequences of the underlying temperament of behavioral inhibition or neuroticism.

Evidence supporting this assertion comes from Goldsmith and Gottesman (1981), who found that monozygotic twins were more concordant for separation distress at age 7 than dizygotic twins were. Similarly, Silove, Manicavasagar, O'Connell, and Morris-Yates (1995) found that genetic factors contributed 41% of the variance to female adult twins' recollections of separation anxiety experiences. Since behavioral inhibition relates strongly to fundamental traits of neuroticism or introversion, as discussed in Chapter 2 (and may well be a consequence of these traits), it is likely that the relationship of separation anxiety to agoraphobic avoidance can be best accounted for by biological contributions to personality, combined with cultural influences favoring the utilization of avoidance as a coping mechanism.

Now a large prospective study would seem to confirm this conclusion. Hayward, Killen, Kraemer, and Taylor (2000), in a study to be reported more fully below, evaluated 2,365 students enrolled in four northern California high schools. Students were evaluated initially as they entered high school, and then prospectively for up to 4 years following the initial evaluation. The presence of separation anxiety disorder, as assessed by earlier structured interviews of these students at age of primary school entry, did not relate to the subsequent development of later initial panic attacks or the onset of panic disorder.

Dangers from Within: Unpredictable Bodily Sensations and Anxiety Sensitivity

Among the many things we learn to fear in childhood, including monsters, strangers, darkness, and separation, it seems that a substantial proportion of us are taught that our own bodies may be the source of some of the greatest threats to our integrity and well-being. One of the most persuasive demonstrations of the existence of this acquired apprehension is evident in an experiment by Anke Ehlers (1993). Ehlers (1993) assessed 121 patients with panic disorder, as well as several other comparison groups of subjects. These included 86 individuals who experienced infrequent unexpected, uncued panic attacks (at least one lifetime) but did not meet criteria for panic disorder; 38 patients with other anxiety disorders (mostly specific phobias, but including social phobia and generalized anxiety disorder) who had never experienced an unexpected, uncued attack; and 61 control subjects with no prior history of panic attacks or mental disorders. All individuals in the study were asked about general parental encouragement of sick role behavior when, for example, they were sick with colds or the flu, as well as about the incidence of chronic illness of at least 6 months' duration in their family members. In addition to questions concerning sickness in general, all subjects were also asked about their own panic symptoms (racing heart, dizziness, etc.) while growing up, and their parents' reactions to these symptoms that they now realized were the beginnings of panic attacks. Subjects also reported on their parents' panic symptoms and how their parents handled these symptoms if they experienced them. Finally, subjects were also asked about the occurrence of temper tantrums or other uncontrollable emotional responses while under the influence of substances on the part of parents and other members of their household, on the premise that patients with panic disorder frequently report that members of their household have abused substances. A descriptive summary of the major results is presented in Table 7.1.

The first finding reported by Ehlers (1993) was that patients with panic disorder, individuals with infrequent panic attacks, and patients with other anxiety disorders, when compared to the control group, all reported that their parents encouraged greater sick role behavior in response to panic-like symptoms by communicating to them to take special care of themselves when these symptoms occurred. They were also encouraged to avoid strenuous activities or social engagements if they experienced anxiety or panic-like symptoms significantly more than the control group was encouraged. In addition, all anxious groups reported more "uncontrollable emotional responses" on the part of parents than the control group did. In contrast, no differences emerged among groups, including the control group, in the parental encouragement of sick role behavior in the event of colds or flu.

Importantly, individuals experiencing panic attacks (those with infrequent panic and patients with panic disorder) reported observing more panic symptoms in their parents than the group with other anxiety disorders or the control group did (although they did not necessarily observe their parents react with more distress and anxiety to the experience of these symptoms than the group with other anxiety disorders). The two groups experiencing panic attacks also reported a significantly higher number of chronic illnesses in their households while they were growing up, as compared to those with other anxiety disorders or controls.

TABLE 7.1. Results of the Learning History Questionnaire

	Panic disorder (n = 121)	Infrequent panic (n = 86)	Other anxiety disorders (n = 38)	Normal controls (n = 61)
Subject's sick role experiences/ panic symptoms (scale 0–9)	Mdn: 0.0 M: 1.1 SD: 1.8	0.0 1.0 1.6	0.0 0.8 1.4	0.0 0.1 0.3
Measure combining:				
Frequency of subject's panic symptoms (scale 0–3)	Mdn: 1.0 M: 1.1 SD: 1.2	0.0 0.9 1.1	0.0 0.8 1.2	0.0 0.3 0.7
Encouragement of sick role/panic (scale 0–3) (only Ss with symptoms)	M: 1.0 SD: 0.8	0.9 0.8	1.1 0.5	0.5 0.6
Observation of parental sick role/panic symptoms (scale 0–9)	Mdn: 2.2 M: 2.8 SD: 2.9	2.4 2.8 2.9	0.0 1.8 2.3	0.0 0.9 1.6
Measure combining:				
Frequency of parental panic symptoms (scale 0–3)	Mdn: 2.0 M: 1.6 SD: 1.3	2.0 1.6 1.2	0.0 1.0 1.2	0.0 0.6 0.9
Modeling of sick role/panic (scale 0–3) (only parents with symptoms)	M: 1.6 SD: 0.9	1.6 0.9	1.7 0.7	1.3 0.7
Encouragement of sick role/colds (scale 0–3)	M: 1.4 SD: 0.9	1.3 0.9	1.5 0.7	1.1 0.7
Frequency of uncontrolled behavior (scale 0–3)	Mdn: 2.0 M: 1.4 SD: 1.3	1.0 1.3 1.2	1.0 1.2 1.2	0.0 0.5 0.9
Number of chronically ill [family members] (scale 0–3)	Mdn: 1.0 M: 0.8 SD: 1.0	1.0 0.8 0.9	0.0 0.4 0.6	0.0 0.5 0.8

Note. The table shows medians (Mdn), means (M), and standard deviations (SD) if the scale was not normally distributed. Otherwise, means and standard deviations are given. From Ehlers (1993). Copyright 1993 by Pergamon Press. Reprinted by permission.

This study suffers from all the weaknesses of retrospective reports, and we cannot be confident about the findings until appropriate prospective studies are completed. But it seems that caregivers can model the "dangers" of somatic symptoms such as panic attacks, and that this modeling may confer a risk for reacting to attacks with distress and anxiety in all individuals with anxiety disorders. In addition, the specific experience of individuals with panic disorder or panic attacks seems to be that observing physical suffering in general, in the form of chronic illness, can contribute to a belief that bodily sensations (signifying, perhaps, the beginnings of illness) are dangerous and need attention. The fact that unexplained somatic events, such as the autonomic symptoms characterizing a panic attack, are perceived as occurring more frequently in parents may simply reflect the differential heritability and familial aggregation of panic attacks.

Other studies also report that early experiences may lead to anxiety focused on specific somatic symptoms as adults.. For example, Whitehead, Winget, Fedoravicius, Wooley, and Blackwell (1982), in a retrospective study of over 800 subjects, found that adults who more often sought medical help and missed work or school because of perceived illnesses reported that when they were children, their parents attended much more closely to similar symptoms and reinforced them (with toys or special food, etc.) when ill. In a follow-up study with 351 women, Whitehead, Bush, Heller, and Costa (1986) found a more direct relationship between the types of illness-related symptoms to which parents paid special attention and help-seeking behavior when the women became adults. This study was particularly well done, since subjects' retrospective reports were independently corroborated by their parents. For example, if parents of these women expressed substantial concern focused on the physical consequences of menstruation during adolescence, the women as adults would seek medical attention more often, and miss work or school more frequently, because of menstrual symptoms. Similarly, if these females were taught to be very careful of colds as children, they would seek medical help and miss work/school with these symptoms as adults. Finally, Turkat (1982) found in another retrospective study that a group of 27 individuals with diabetes tended to display greater sick role behavior, including avoiding work, if their parents had engaged in illness-related avoidance behavior themselves.

The consequence of these early learning experiences seems to be a tendency to focus anxiety on bodily sensations, particularly unexplained bodily sensations, and to develop beliefs about the dangers of these symptoms or sensations. A number of questionnaires have been developed to capture this network of beliefs. Some of these questionnaires, such as the Body Sensations Questionnaire (Chambless, Caputo, Bright, & Gallagher, 1984), have been designed to assess specifically anxiety focused on bodily sensations in panic disorder and have proved useful for this purpose. A questionnaire that has attracted somewhat more interest is the Anxiety Sensitivity Index (ASI; Reiss, Peterson, Gursky, & McNally, 1986), mentioned briefly in previous chapters. This questionnaire purports to measure a set of beliefs that anxiety and its associated symptoms, (particularly somatic symptoms) may cause deleterious physical, psychological, or social consequences that go beyond any immediate physical discomfort. Generally, anxiety sensitivity has been found to be normally distributed in the population, suggesting that it is a dimensional construct.

Research has begun to appear examining the utility of the ASI in predicting later anxiety-related problems, particularly panic attacks. Schmidt, Lerew, and Jackson (1997) administered the ASI to military recruits and found that higher initial scores on the scale predicted greater anxiety and depression after a stressful course of basic military training, as well as a greater number of panic attacks during the training. These results are presented in Figure 7.1. In a second study, Schmidt, Lerew, and Jackson (1999) replicated these results, finding a somewhat stronger relationship with later anxiety and panic than with later depression. These are the first studies to successfully predict the occurrence of an initial panic attack in individuals who had heretofore not experienced panic attacks; therefore, the finding is relevant to an analysis of factors contributing to the origins of panic. However, Schmidt and colleagues caution that the results were relatively weak in this sample of well-adjusted military recruits and accounted for a rather small percentage of the variance—for example, 2% of the variance in predicting unexpected panic attacks in the Schmidt et al. (1999) study. Furthermore, it seems that anxiety sensitivity does not bear a unique relationship to the etiology of panic attacks, since high ASI scores also predicted later anxiety and depression more generally. Nevertheless, the evidence now seems clear that early experiences sensitizing individuals to the potential dangers of physical symptoms and sensations may well contribute to a specific vulnerability to develop panic attacks and panic disorder.

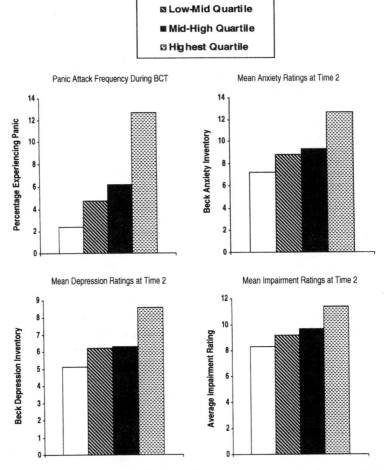

FIGURE 7.1. Panic attacks, symptomatology, and impairment across anxiety sensitivity groups on the basis of quartile cutoffs from Anxiety Sensitivity Index (ASI) scores. Means are adjusted for Time 1 scores. Impairment ratings are based on an average score of four questions assessing impairment. There were significant group effects for all indices (p's < .001). Post hoc group comparisons indicated that the highest-quarter ASI group was significantly higher than all other groups on all indices (p's < .05). BCT, basic cadet training. From Schmidt, Lerew, and Jackson (1997). Copyright 1997 by American Psychological Association. Reprinted by permission.

The prospective study reported by Hayward et al. (2000) and mentioned above sheds more light on the role of anxiety sensitivity as a risk factor for initial false alarms. In this study of 2,365 high school students, the investigators evaluated the risk of negative affectivity, separation anxiety, anxiety sensitivity, and female gender in predicting the initial onset of panic attacks consisting of the four or more symptoms required by the *Diagnostic and Statistical Manual of Mental Disorders*, fourth edition (DSM-IV). Although separation anxiety disorder and female sex were not predictive of initial panic attacks, as noted above, both negative affectivity and anxiety sensitivity predicted the onset of panic attacks, based on univariate analyses. These data are presented in Table 7.2. Multivariate analysis revealed that negative affectivity more robustly predicted initial panic attacks, with anxiety sensitivity manifesting a trend relationship. The authors conclude that negative affectivity is a risk factor for "internalizing" symptoms and disorders, and that panic attacks may be a nonspecific sign of distress that does not necessarily relate to the subsequent onset of emotional disorders. Thus anxiety sensitivity does not contribute to the predictive power of negative affect in multivariate analyses assessing vulnerabilities for initial panic attacks, but may mediate the development of panic disorder in those adolescents who report initial panic attacks. Since anxiety sensitivity is most usually conceptualized as a second-order factor within the structure of anxiety, with negative affect as a higher-order factor (Brown, Chorpita, & Barlow, 1998; Craske, 1999), and since higher anxiety sensitivity discriminates panic disorder from other anxiety disorders, it is likely that negative affect is a more fundamental vulnerability. In this arrangement, anxiety sensitivity may be a more specific vulnerability for panic disorder to develop, given negative affect and the occurrence of panic attacks. Thus this topic is taken up once again in Chapter 8, where I discuss the development of specific psychological vulnerabilities placing individuals at risk for panic disorder. In the context of these developments, the question remains: What triggers initial panic attacks in those individuals with negative affect and anxiety sensitivity?

Stress as a Precipitant

A remarkably consistent retrospective observation of biological and psychological clinicians and investigators has been the report of negative life events preceding the first panic attack in patients who later present with panic disorder. What makes this observation interesting is that few of these patients can identify a precipitating event when asked a question such as "What caused your first panic attack?" As noted above, the defining characteristic of false alarms is that, at least initially, they are uncued and unexpected (out of the blue). However, systematic questioning about life events reveals that approximately 80% of these patients describe clearly one or more negative life events preceding their first panic (Buglass et al., 1977; Doctor, 1982; Finlay-Jones & Brown, 1981; Mathews, Gelder, & Johnston, 1981; Roth, 1959; Snaith, 1968; Solyom, Beck, Solyom, & Hugel, 1974; Uhde, Boulenger, Roy-Byrne, et al., 1985). In one large series of 404 patients who had panic dis-

Table 7.2. Hazard Ratios (95% Confidence Intervals) for Onset of Panic Attacks by Risk Factors

Risk factor	Four-symptom panic attack ($n = 32$)
Negative affectivity	2.39 (1.27–4.50)**
Female sex	1.28 (0.89–1.82)
Anxiety sensitivity	1.04 (1.01–1.07)*
Childhood separation anxiety disorders	1.37 (0.85–2.22)

Note: Hazard ratio for panic adjusted for the effects of past or concurrent major depression. Adapted from Hayward, Killen, Kraemer, and Taylor (2000). Copyright 2000 by the American Academy of Child and Adolescent Psychiatry. Adapted by permission.
$^*p < .05$; $^{**}p < .01$.

order with agoraphobia (Doctor, 1982), separation and loss (31%), relationship problems (30%), and new responsibility (20%) were the most common precipitants of the initial panic attack.

Typical of these studies and the types of negative life events reported are results from an early series of 58 individuals with agoraphobia (53 females and 5 males) from our clinic at Albany (Last, Barlow, & O'Brien, 1984). The occurrence of negative life events was assessed by a structured clinical interview. Categories of life events and the frequencies with which they were reported are presented in Table 7.3. Of the 58 individuals with agoraphobia, 81% reported one or more of these stressful life events, while 19% reported no significant life events prior to the development of agoraphobia. For heuristic purposes, we collapsed life events reported by our patients into conflict events versus endocrine/physiological reactions, and the results are presented in Table 7.3. These two major categories accounted for approximately 91% of the life events reported. Liebowitz and Klein (1979) also reported a large proportion of individuals developing panic attacks after experiencing endocrinological changes, and Klein (1964), in an early survey, noted "endocrine fluctuations" (e.g., those associated with birth, menopause, and gynecological surgery) as events immediately preceding panic in a subgroup of patients.

Perhaps the best among these early studies was also one of the first to examine these issues. Roth (1959) found that 96% of a sample of 135 individuals with agoraphobia reported some type of background stress preceding the development of their disorder. The stressors of 83% of these patients were categorized as follows: bereavement or a suddenly developing serious illness in a close relative or friend (37%); illness or acute danger to the patient (31%); and severance of family ties or acute domestic stress (15%). In an additional 13% of the women, panic began during pregnancy or after childbirth, and was characterized by an abrupt onset shortly after delivery. What makes this study important is that Roth was the first investigator to employ a control group. He found that the incidence of identifiable stressors in his patients with agoraphobia was significantly greater than that found in 50 control patients suffering from some other form of "neurosis," as well as in 50 additional individuals who had recently recovered from a physical illness but had never

TABLE 7.3. Life Events Occurring Prior to Onset of Agoraphobia

Precipitating events	Frequency (n = 58)	%
Interpersonal conflict situations		
Marital/familial	20	34.5
Death/illness of significant other	9	15.5
Total	29	50.0
Endocrine/physiological reactions		
Birth/miscarriage/hysterectomy	17	29.3
Drug reaction	7	12.1
Total	24	41.4
Other		
Major surgery/illness (other than gynecological)	2	3.4
Stress at work/school	2	3.4
Move	2	3.4

Note. Frequencies exceed the number of patients interviewed because many patients reported more than one significant life event occurring prior to their first panic attack. From Last, Barlow, and O'Brien (1984). Copyright 1984 by *Psychological Reports*. Reprinted by permission.

suffered a psychiatric disorder. Pollard, Pollard, and Corn (1989) and Roy-Byrne, Geraci, and Uhde (1986) also found a greater occurrence of negative and more impactful life events in patients with panic compared to healthy controls in the year prior to the first panic, whereas Faravelli (1985) and Faravelli and Pallanti (1989) reported similar results for the 2-month period preceding the first panic attack. However, we (Rapee, Litwin, & Barlow, 1990) asked patients with panic disorder to recall stressful events occurring during the period of 6 months prior to the beginning of their disorder (approximately 2 years before the study), but also asked a yoked control group to list stressful life events occurring at a similar time approximately 2 years before the study. Results suggested no differences in number of events, but patients reported experiencing the events as more uncontrollable, undesirable, and distressing than did control subjects.

Although the majority of these studies point to a relationship between stressful life events and the onset of initial panic attacks, controlled retrospective reports have produced mixed results: Some studies have found excessive stressful life events preceding the initial panic attack compared to comparison groups, while other studies have not found excessive numbers of stressful life events (Rapee, Litwin, & Barlow, 1990). Of course, we now know that one major difficulty is in the retrospective nature of these reports. If one inquires of individuals who are currently anxious and perhaps suffering from panic attacks, "What happened when you first began panicking years ago?," one may get different answers from those they would give if they were not currently anxious and panicking. Because anxiety and other moods tend to distort memories, most investigators have concluded that the only useful way to study stressful life events is to follow people prospectively, to determine more accurately the precise nature of events and their relation to subsequent psychopathology. Furthermore, it is obviously insufficient simply to count stressful events and assume that they have a somewhat similar impact on different individuals. Far more important is to examine the context and the individual meaning of the events in a given person's life, as clearly articulated several years ago by George Brown and his associates (e.g., Brown & Harris, 1989; Kessler, 1997). For example, losing a job would count in most inventories as a stressful life event, but might be a blessing to some individuals who disliked their job in the first place, had adequate financial and social support to compensate for lost income, and took the opportunity to initiate an exciting new career.

Nevertheless, it seems likely from the studies reviewed above that stress (particularly in the form of negative life events) is related to the onset of initial panic attacks, or at the very least has a greater emotional impact on individuals who go on to experience a panic attack. Indeed, a growing body of evidence, some of it from prospective studies that consider context and meaning, has begun to demonstrate a robust relationship between stress and the onset of syndromal mood and anxiety disorders (Kessler, 1997; Brown, 1993). Thus, by inference, it is likely that a similar relationship will emerge between stress and initial panic attacks when more appropriate studies are conducted.

Setting the Stage: The Functional Relationship of Panic Attacks to Stress

Previously (Barlow, 1991a; Barlow, Chorpita, & Turovsky, 1996; see Chapters 5 and 6), I have outlined the functional relationship of panic attacks to stress or anxiety. That is, an individual possessing the biological (genetic) and psychological vulnerabilities to develop anxious apprehension (see Chapter 8) may experience an initial panic attack in at least one of two distinct ways. First, heightened neurobiological reactivity to stress ("neuroticism") may trigger discrete emotions or defensive reactions as a function of differentially inherited thresholds for these action tendencies, or perhaps, shared neurotransmitter functions. In other words, prolonged stress and its neurochemical consequences, combined with a low threshold for experiencing panic attacks (and/or other stress-related responses, such as headaches), may trigger an initial false alarm. Rosen and Schulken (1998) propose something similar when they note that stressful life events may sensitize fear circuits in the limbic system, resulting in a state of "hyperexcitability" that would lower the threshold for a false alarm. Interaction of the corticotropin-releasing factor system with the locus ceruleus–norepinephrine system (described in Chapter 6) would be a logical neurobiological mechanism.

I have also suggested an alternative, albeit related, explanation in Chapter 6 that would be predicted by Lang's (1985, 1994a) bioinformational emotion theory. In this model, stressful life events and the resulting activation of various neurobiological and cognitive–affective systems best described as negative affect or perhaps "anxiety" (see Chapter 3) may present a sufficient number of response, stimulus, and meaning propositions (threatening negative cognitions, negative valence, high arousal, etc.) to trigger specific emotional action tendencies stored deep in memory. In this way, a specific action tendency associated with a coherent, tightly organized emotional response may occasionally "fire" out of context. The analogy to neuronal discharge is intentional. There is still room within this Langian perspective for a differential heritability of the tendency to experience a panic attack, or other output from a defensive motivational system. while under stress. Once again, this would be consistent with the notion that a variety of specific stress-related responses (e.g., headaches, hypertension, and irritable bowel syndrome) tend to be strongly familial reactions to stress and are probably heritable in some way (Barlow et al., 1996). In this view, the tendency to experience an initial panic attack may simply be another stress-related response that runs in families, particularly families prone to experiencing negative affect and/or anxiety.

Baseline Anxiety

In Chapter 5, I have reviewed the robust finding that the most powerful predictor of whether panic attacks will occur in the laboratory in response to CO_2 provocation, for example, is high "baseline" anxiety. This observation may also elucidate the relationship between stress and panic noticed in survey research described below. Specifically, baseline differences in levels of anxiety between patients and controls before specific panic provocation trials have been reported in almost all studies dating back to the 1940s (e.g., Cohen & White, 1950). Once again, as summarized in Chapter 5, these "baseline" differences seem to increase the likelihood of a full-blown panic attack that is often construed by the individual as "unexpected" or "out of the blue." This caused Breggin (1964) to suggest that degree of current "baseline" anxiety is one of the major determinants of laboratory provocation of panic attacks.

To take one example, the studies by Liebowitz et al. (1984) and Liebowitz, Gorman, Fyer, Levitt, et al. (1985) summarized in Chapter 5 reported that patients who went on to panic had a greater sense of anxiety prior to the infusions with lactate than patients who did not evidence panic attacks, and that heart rate was higher for patients who went on to evidence panic attacks during baseline than for patients who did not panic in response to the infusion. Coplan, Goetz, et al. (1998) reported similar results. Basoglu, Marks, and Sengun (1992) examined the issue in a different way: They asked 39 patients who had panic disorder with agoraphobia to monitor the duration and intensity of panic attacks and anxiety episodes over three 24-hour periods, using an event-sampling technique. Of the

32 patients who reported at least one panic attack, 69% reported that their attacks occurred in the context of heightened anxiety. Only 13% reported no awareness of increased anxiety preceding their panic attacks. Kenardy, Fried, Kraemer, and Taylor (1992), using prospective 24-hour ambulatory monitoring procedures, determined that patients who went on to panic reported elevated apprehension in the hour preceding the panic attack or concern about having an attack, which the authors concluded supported the position that "an underlying apprehension is a precursor to the panic" (Kenardy et al., 1992, p. 672). Similar results were reported with 10 patients by Kenardy and Taylor (1999). Of course, some of these latter studies involved individuals with existing panic disorder, which confounds a clean analysis of the contribution of anxiety to the origins of initial or nonclinical panic attacks. However, combined with other data, the best evidence is that preexisting anxiety does potentiate panic attacks. As noted in Chapter 6, this arrangement would make sense from an ethological point of view, since these emotional defensive reactions seem to be arranged hierarchically along a dimension of imminence of threat, where the hypervigilant state of anxious apprehension is followed by a flight-or-fight response when the threat becomes imminent. It is therefore reasonable to assume that on occasion, and in the context of other predisposing factors, a preexisting state of anxiety will provide the setting for a false alarm, and may mediate the observed relationship between stressful life events and initial panic attacks as described above.

Conclusions about False Alarms

The circumstantial evidence supporting a crucial role for stress—not only in the genesis of false alarms, but also in the etiology of all anxiety and mood disorders—is strong. This requires detailed examination of the nature of stress and why some vulnerable individuals become either anxious or depressed or both when subjected to negative life events. This evidence in turn leads to an exploration of the essential differences between anxiety and depression, and the place of panic in this broader perspective. These complex issues are addressed in Chapter 8.

Suffice it for now to suggest that a variety of evidence indicates that certain individuals are susceptible to stress produced by negative life events because of constitutional factors, relatively low social support, and/or some combination of personality and cognitive dispositions. In the case of individuals who experience initial false alarms (panic attacks), I have suggested individual-specific genetic contributions to the development of broad characteristics of personality, such as neuroticism or negative affect, to be relevant dispositions. A heritable lowered threshold for experiencing the defensive action tendencies of fear may also be operative. The tendency to focus on somatic sensations as threatening may contribute a small amount of variance, but is probably not a major factor in the occurrence of initial false alarms (although this tendency seems to play a more substantial role in the possible subsequent development of panic disorder). These individuals then react to negative life events in much the same way they might react to physical threats from wild animals or snakes. That is, they evidence a fear response much as they would when confronted with any other threat to their well-being. As suggested above, these alarms are mediated initially by neurobiological responses to stress. In any case, because the fear response is not temporally associated (within hours) with the negative life event, the individual is unable to specify an antecedent to or a "cause" of the fear. Indeed, there is no antecedent that would require an immediate alarm reaction, with all of its associated action tendencies of fight or flight. For that reason, the alarm is false. A depiction of this model can be found in Figure 7.2.

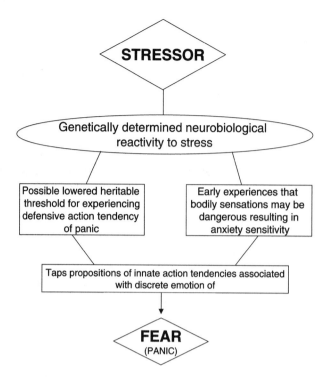

FIGURE 7.2. Hypothetical model of the role of genetic vulnerability in producing panic.

If the stress–diathesis model of false alarms (panic) is correct, then one would predict that individuals with infrequent, nonclinical panic will continue having occasional false alarms of varying severity, depending on the intensity and frequency of experienced negative life events, their neurobiological disposition, and possibly their threshold for action tendencies associated with alarms. In addition, the presence of moderating variables such as anxiety sensitivity may affect the propensity for experiencing alarms. But even when circumstances line up correctly, the relationship does not stay as simple as this. The overwhelming experience of panic in some individuals seems to insure that learning will take place that markedly affects the subsequent course of false alarms.

LEARNED (CONDITIONED) ANXIETY

Before the critical issue of learned (conditioned) anxiety is discussed, it is necessary to consider briefly what we now know about how one learns to be afraid. Although many emotion theorists consider fear to be innate and universally present across cultures and species, none would suggest that all objects or situations that elicit fear or anxiety are also innate. Indeed, it is crucial for the survival of any species to be flexible. "Flexibility," in this context, implies a capacity to learn quickly to be anxious in the presence of new threatening objects or situations. Although this is a far more complex issue than previously assumed, one of the fundamental laws of learning, discovered and elaborated in the laboratories of experimental psychology, is that anxiety can be learned by a process of association. In fact, this universally acknowledged process is central to many theoretical approaches to anxiety and psychopathology. For example, both psychoanalytic and behavioral approaches posit that anxiety can be associated with neutral objects (signal anxiety) or conditioned stimuli (CSs), although there are some disagreements on the source of the original anxiety and the degree to which symbolic processes may be involved. The importance of this associational process, whether one is "aware" of it or not, cannot be underestimated. Although it is a very normal psychological process, it also seems a crucial step in the development of psychopathology under certain conditions. Echoing the discussion of fundamental ancient emotions in Chapter 2, this form of learning is also primitive, heavily biological, and subject to evolutionary pressures. It occurs across cultures and species, and far down the phylogenetic scale. Researchers have isolated the process underlying the learning of anxiety at the level of the single cell in the sea snail, as described in Chapter 6 (Kandel, 1983). Although this is not the only way one learns to be afraid, it is important, in the context of the present discussion, to describe this process (most commonly called "classical" or "Pavlovian" conditioning) in some detail. It is also important to note at the outset that this process cannot account for either panic attacks or the subsequent development of anxiety disorders; however, conditioning plays a role in a more comprehensive theory of panic and the origins of anxiety disorders, outlined below. Finally, the learned (conditioned) response has been described traditionally as "fear" in the experimental literature; but, consistent with the terminology described in Chapter 2, and for reason's outlined in detail below, it seems clear that what is learned is "anxiety" (see also Boutin et al., 2001). Thus, in the next section, I will describe the experimental work consistent with the original literature, but the term "fear" will appear in quotes.

"Fear" Conditioning

The paradigm (or operation) of classical "fear" conditioning, familar to everyone who has read elementary psychology, is that neutral stimuli that are present during a fear-arousing experience acquire the capacity to elicit "fear." This "fear" is termed "conditional" or "conditioned," because only under certain conditions (the symbolic or actual reappearance of the neutral stimulus) will "fear" (the conditioned response, or CR) occur. Typically, the strength of the "fear" response depends on a number of factors. These factors include, but are not limited to, the number of pairings of the new CS with the unconditioned stimulus (UCS—the original source of the fear) and the intensity of fear evoked by the UCS. Stimuli that are similar to the CS also come to elicit "fear" as a direct function of their similarity; the more similarity, the more "fear." This relationship between the CR and similarity of the evoking stimulus to the CS is called a "generalization gradient." Watson and Raynor (1920) conducted some of the earliest research demonstrating these principles in humans. In this well-known study, a young child, Albert, was exposed to a loud noise (the UCS) while viewing a rat (the CS) on several occasions. Albert subsequently developed a conditioned "fear" of rats that spread or "generalized" to other creatures that resembled rats, such as rabbits and other furry animals. Most of the principles of classical "fear" conditioning have been well worked out in the laboratories of experimental psychology over the ensuing decades (cf. Eysenck, 1979; Bouton et al., 2001). In fact, this is one of the most widely researched forms of affective learning.

Conditioning is also well established as a method of learning emotional responses in humans. One of the most dramatic examples, occurring daily in our major hospitals, involves the widespread acquisition of conditioned nausea in patients with cancer who are undergoing chemotherapy (e.g., Jacobsen et al., 1993, 1995; Redd & Andrykowski, 1982). Typically, these patients develop moderate to severe nausea reactions to any "neutral" stimuli associated with the administration of chemotherapy. Most usually, the stimuli are associated with nursing staff administering the therapy and can include sights, sounds, and often smells, such as a particular perfume or cologne. This effect is very strong. For example, 60–80% of an early series of patients with Hodgkin's disease clearly evidenced conditioning (Cella, Pratt, & Holland, 1986). Estimates from a review of a larger series of studies suggest that a variable but somewhat lower percentage of patients undergoing chemotherapy develop this response (Burish & Carey, 1986; Morrow & Dobkin, 1988). Among factors that seem to account for conditionability (or lack of it) in these patients is the strength of the nausea-producing properties of the drug (the UCS) and the intensity of the initial nausea reaction. To deal with this problem therapeutically, oncologists and psychologists working in cancer units have come up with a number of methods to counter and minimize the effects of classical conditioning. These methods are also derived from basic knowledge of classical conditioning elaborated in the animal laboratories (e.g., Cella et al., 1986).

What is particularly interesting for our purposes is that this type of conditioning can be very rapid in both humans and animals. For example, in a theoretically interesting experiment that may have some bearing on the discussion of etiology below, Campbell, Sanderson, and Laverty (1964) produced an intense "fear" CR to neutral tones in just one trial. Ordinarily, this would be very unusual during classical "fear" conditioning, since a number of trials are usually required to condition "fear" successfully. However, one variable accounting for the speed of this response clearly stands out: Campbell et al. used succinylcholine as the UCS. This drug, once injected, produces respiratory paralysis in a matter of seconds. As a result, subjects cannot breathe and feel that they are suffocating and dying.

The results are seldom as dramatic in terms of clear conditioning effects as those reported in the experiments above, or those seen daily on the oncology ward (Barlow, 1978). One probable reason is that seldom is a UCS as powerful as succinylcholine or chemotherapy ever used in these paradigms. But there are other reasons as well.

Modifications to Conditioning Theory

In the 1950s and 1960s, with the rise of behavior therapy, it was widely assumed that all phobias are learned through simple traumatic conditioning (e.g., Wolpe, 1958; Marks, 1969) and that therapy should involve extinction of these traumatically learned fears. The success of behavior therapy with phobias strengthened this assumption about etiology. By the late 1960s, however, it was becoming clear that traumatic conditioning alone cannot account for the genesis of phobic reactions, since conditioning cannot accommodate several facts about clinical phobias. Among other objections, it was noted that conditioning theory cannot explain the selectivity of phobias (Marks, 1969). Specifically, why do people learn to "fear" some objects or situations more than other? Another objection specified the failure of phobias to extinguish despite repeated exposure to the CS—a phenomenon that is almost always seen in the animal laboratories (Rachman, 1977, 1991). Finally, it became clear that fears and phobias can be acquired through simple provision of information (instructions), as well as vicariously (Bandura, 1969; Rachman, 1977, 1978). The clinical implications of observational or instructional acquisition of phobias are discussed below and in subsequent chapters. At this point, it is important to turn our attention to recent developments in our knowledge of classical "fear" conditioning itself.

An early modification to classical "fear" conditioning theory was the avoidance learning model (Mowrer, 1947), which hypothesizes that fears or phobias will fail to extinguish if one successfully learns to avoid the feared stimulus. The idea here was that substantial avoidance prevents the individual from "reality testing" or learning that there is no longer any reason to be afraid. This notion, known as the "two-factor theory," was popular for decades, since it seemed to explain why phobias do not extinguish: "Fear" is originally learned through classical conditioning and is subsequently maintained due to avoidance.

But various difficulties also arose with a strict transfer of this paradigm from animal laboratories to clinical phobias. Among these difficulties were obvious differences between the amount of "fear" or distress produced by avoidance conditioning paradigms and that observed in clinical phobias. Animals seem to display no subjective distress after they learn to avoid the "feared" stimulus successfully, presumably because they do not encounter it. But the avoidance response itself is highly resistant to extinction. Humans with clinical phobias, on the other hand, can often overcome their avoidance behavior, but they continue to experience marked distress in the "feared" situation. This "distress" does not always seem to extinguish. In fact, enduring these situations with dread is a defining characteristic of clinical phobias in DSM-IV. This failure to extinguish is part of the "neurotic paradox" referred to in Chapter 1. Modifications to this theory, specifying the importance of "cognitive" variables, seemed necessary to account for the data (Mineka & Zinbarg, 1996; Rescorla & Wagner, 1972; Seligman & Johnston, 1973; Wagner, 1981). In fact, modern learning theorists have long since abandoned a mechanistic behavioral framework in studying animals. The more integrative approach employs a wide range of cognitive concepts—including, but not limited to, concepts of probability learning, information processing, attention, surprise, short-term memory, and the like—to explain even simple conditioning (e.g., Martin, 1983; Martin & Levey, 1985; Mackintosh, 1975; Mineka & Zinbarg, 1996; Pearce & Hall, 1980).

Nevertheless, the evidence is now very strong that the process of emotional learning is a fundamentally distinct process to which the principles of conditioning are particularly applicable (Bouton et al., 2001). This is in contrast to the more usual conscious, cognitive acquisition of what has been described as propositional declarative knowledge dependent on verbal input. There is much evidence to support this contention. For example, classically conditioned emotional responses are not necessarily influenced by verbal instruction (Hamm & Vaitl, 1996). More importantly, emotional conditioning in general, and "fear" conditioning specifically, do not depend on conscious awareness (LeDoux, 1996; Öhman, 1997; Morris, Öhman, & Dolan, 1998). One particularly elegant experiment illustrates this important principle. Bechara et al. (1995) demonstrated a dissociation between emotional learning (conditioning) and verbal declarative knowledge. One individual with a damaged amygdala (the locus of "fear" conditioning, as described in Chapter 6) did not acquire classical autonomic conditioning after a standard classical conditioning experience, but he was able to verbally report the probability that a CS would predict a UCS. On the other hand, a second patient with a damaged hippocampus (the area of the brain implicated in short-term memory) was able to acquire the classical autonomic conditioning response reflective of emotional learning, but could not report the relationship between the CS and the UCS. As we (Bouton et al., 2001) point out, findings such as these suggest that "conscious declarative or propositional knowledge about conditioning contingencies is not necessary or sufficient for emotional conditioning" (p. 9). Thus the evidence supports the notion that emotional learning occurs in largely subcortical emotional networks connected to defensive motivational systems, as described in Chapter 2.

This is not to say that conditioning and propositional systems do not sometimes overlap and interact. Human classical conditioning may modify certain rational cognitive processes, such as expectancies about the occurrence of the UCS (Davey, 1992), and it seems possible to influence conditioned responding with verbal information or cognitive processes (Lovibond, 1993). But, as we have noted (Bouton et al., 2001), it would seem that this sort of verbal influence on basic subcortical emotional learning does not necessarily happen; it will depend on the type of conditioning, the brain systems involved, and a variety of other factors. In fact, this interaction and occasional conflict between rational and emotional (sometimes irrational) processes become the battleground on which emotional disorders are played out. Although this notion will not be new to many clinicians (Freud, 1926/1959), the scientific developments specifying these interactions are new.

One important modification to conditioning theory is the question of why humans seem to learn "fears" and phobias selectively (Mineka, 1985b; Seligman, 1971). One possibility is that certain types of objects or situations have become highly prepared for learning over the course of evolution, because this learning facilitates survival of the species. This explanation is the theory of evolutionary "preparedness," which integrates biological points of view with classical conditioning. (Cook & Mineka, 1991). Öhman and his colleagues performed the initial important work in this area (e.g., Öhman, Erixon, & Lofburg, 1975). Although this notion still has weaknesses (see McNally, 1987, for a review), it has received increasing support over the decades (Cook et al., 1986; Mineka, 1985b; Öhman, Dimberg, & Öst, 1985a; Öhman, 1993; Öhman, Flykt, & Lundqvist, 2000; Öhman & Mineka, 2001). Öhman et al. (1985a) outline two important evolutionarily derived behavioral fear systems: a system for defense against predators such as attacking animals, and a system that facilitates yielding to members of the group who are dominant or higher in the social hierarchy. As Öhman et al. (2000) point out, there is a premium on speed in these particular response systems, since it will be adaptive to avoid dangerous individuals or predators before any damage can be done, and the fact that angry faces are more quickly recognized than neutral or happy faces has been demonstrated. Öhman et al. (2000) have documented that emotional activation of these systems can bypass the cortex and activate circuits directly in the emotional brain that would be out of awareness; this may account for lower reaction times. For example, Morris et al. (1998) showed subjects slides of two angry faces, one of which had been previously conditioned to a burst of noise. In half of the trials, the slide with the angry face that had been conditioned (the target face) was presented for a very brief period of time that was too short to allow conscious perception, and was immediately followed by a slide with a neutral face (the masked condition). In the other half of the trials, the target was shown for a sufficient period of time to allow conscious perception. The investigators examined neural activity in the amygdala during the experiment, using brain imaging procedures. In a landmark finding, the results suggested that emotional responses that were out of awareness, as opposed to conscious, activated different pathways. The unmasked target faces that were consciously perceived elicited neural response in the left nucleus of the amygdala, whereas the masked targets that were not consciously perceived produced substantial neural activity in the right nuclei of the amygdala.

To return to the evolutionary perspective once again, the implication (as noted in Chapter 2) is that some aspect of what individuals learn to fear, in addition to the "fear" response itself, may be innate. Furthermore, these prepared stimuli are often out of awareness.

Along similar lines, Pitman and Orr (1986) also demonstrated that both patients with anxiety disorders and matched controls developed an emotional CR to pictures of angry faces, but not to pictures of neutral faces. But the next finding in this study is particularly important for our perspective on the origins of clinical phobias: The CR in patients failed to extinguish, even though the electrodes were removed and they were told that no further mild shocks (the UCS) would occur. The control subjects, on the other hand, demonstrated CR extinction. This difference in the process of extinction reflects the common finding, reviewed in Chapter 2, that individuals with anxiety or "neuroticism" condition more easily and extinguish more slowly. But this apparent biological vulnerability interacts with the type of object or situation with which one is faced. As noted above, it is not hard to imagine how survival might be associated with a propensity to respond fearfully to angry faces, much in the same way that it seems selectively associated with snakes and spiders. Of course, other explanations of these preliminary findings are still possible.

Another development was the demonstration by Cook et al. (1986) that certain UCSs "belong" with certain CSs in humans. These findings hark back to the work of Garcia and his colleagues, who observed very rapid (one-trial) development of aversion in animals to the taste of certain foods that had previously resulted in nausea or illness (e.g., Garcia, McGowan, & Green, 1972). It is easy to see how survival might be associated with the capacity to learn quickly to avoid noxious food. Pairing another UCS, such as shock, with food would not produce learning as quickly or intensely, since this association is presumably not as important from an evolutionary point of view. Tomarken, Mineka, and Cook (1989) illustrated this phenomenon by showing that humans tend to overestimate the likelihood that fear-relevant stimuli, in contrast to neutral stimuli, will be associated with an aversive outcome. This "covariation bias" has been demonstrated in small animals such as snakes and spiders (Tomarken et al., 1989), angry faces (Mineka, Sutton, Luten, & Roener, 1996), and blood–injection–injury stimuli (Pury & Mineka, 1997). This covariation bias seems to reflect biological preparedness, and may facilitate more rapid fear conditioning (and delayed extinction) to these objects and situations.

Another selective association to account for the prevalence of certain CSs in phobic disorders is proposed below. Specifically, situations or circumstances that prevent strong action tendencies of some emotional responses, such as alarms, are more likely to become CSs (phobic situations). Thus situations that prevent, even partially, the powerful action tendency of escape during a false alarm (the unconditioned response, or UCR) most likely intensify the alarm further, resulting in strong emotional learning. This may account for the prevalent feelings of being "trapped" in many phobias. More is said about this below.

In addition to the recognition of evolutionary pressures on the origins of fears and phobias, and the establishment of the importance of a myriad of cognitive variables in the process of "fear" conditioning, other developments have occurred in this active area that are not well known outside of a small group of specialists (Bouton et al., 2001). Nevertheless, a full understanding of the complexity of the relationship between CRs and UCRs, and of the various stimuli and contexts that modulate this arrangement, provides a particularly rich and nuanced view on the development of fear across species. An in-depth review of this area, particularly as it applies to panic disorder, has recently appeared (Bouton et al., 2001).

THE ETIOLOGY OF PHOBIAS

With this in mind, we can now consider ways in which false alarms may be learned, and implications of these for the etiology of phobias. For years, investigators have searched the histories of individuals with phobias for signs of traumatic conditioning. This line of inquiry has all of the weaknesses inherent in asking any patient with any disorder to recall situations or facts that may have occurred many years ago. Nevertheless, the research has produced interesting information. The primary finding is that most of these individuals cannot recall a traumatic conditioning event to account for the development of their fears or phobias (e.g., Ehlers, Hofmann, Herda, & Roth, 1994; Menzies & Clarke, 1993c, 1995b). For example, Rimm, Janda, Lancaster, Nahl, and Dittmar (1977) found that 36% of their subjects with phobias could not account for their "fears" in terms of past learning experiences of any kind. This finding is even more apparent for minor fears. For example, Murray and Foote (1979) found that most college students who were afraid of snakes could not recall a bad experience with snakes. Rather, they had acquired their "fears" through verbal or vicarious means. Usually they reported hearing about the dangers of snakes from a parent or observing a parent behave fearfully in the presence of snakes. In fact, casting further doubt on the importance of traumatic conditioning, Murray and Foote reported that three individuals in their large sample had actually been bitten by snakes but reported no fear whatsoever!

One of the strongest demonstrations of vicarious learning of "fear" as opposed to direct traumatic conditioning has been reported, paradoxically, with laboratory monkeys. Mineka and her colleagues (e.g., Cook, Mineka, Wolkenstein, & Laitsch, 1985; Cook & Mineka, 1989; Mineka & Cook, 1993; Mineka, Davidson, Cook, & Keir, 1984) introduced laboratory-reared adolescent monkeys to their wild-reared parents. Prior to the reunion, the lab-reared animals had displayed no avoidance behavior to snakes whatsoever. They observed their parents reacting fearfully in the presence of real, toy, and model snakes for short periods of time. After only brief periods of observation, Mineka and colleagues found that the offspring demonstrated behavioral avoidance and disturbances that were not significantly different from the parents' behaviors. The intensity of these "fear" responses did not change at a period extending up to 3 months.

The overwhelming evidence is that many phobias and the majority of fears are not learned through a traumatic experience. (More is said about the phenomenon below.) On the other hand, Öst and Hugdahl (1981, 1983) reported that a large number of their patients with specific phobias and agoraphobia recalled a traumatic conditioning experience, and that few remembered acquiring their "fear" through vicarious means. For example, Öst and Hugdahl (1983) found that 48% of patients with animal phobias, 58% of those with social phobias, 61% of those with blood and dental phobias, 69% of those with claustrophobias, and 91% of those with agoraphobias identified direct conditioning histories. The remainder identified vicarious or informational transmission as crucial events responsible for the acquisition of their "fears." Between 10% and 20% of all groups could not remember any incident that might account for their fears.

The Öst and Hugdahl (1983) findings seemed, at the time, totally at odds with our clinical understanding of the etiology of panic and agoraphobia. Clearly, individuals with agoraphobia are very seldom (if ever) run down by a car in the parking lot of a shopping mall. Nor are they assaulted in church, or a movie theater, or some other crowded location. What is the traumatic experience Öst and Hugdahl are talking about that leads to "conditioning"? Before the answer to this is considered, it is interesting and useful to refer to other retrospective information concerning patients with specific phobias.

McNally and Steketee (1985) interviewed 22 outpatients presenting for treatment with animal phobias. When questioned about etiology, the majority (15) of these patients could not remember what had happened. Of the remaining 7 cases, 5 had had a frightening encounter with an animal, whereas 2 seemed to have acquired their "fear" through instructional or vicarious modes. Nevertheless, what they all dreaded now was not attack from their feared animal; rather, they were afraid they would panic and suffer the consequences of panic following an unavoidable encounter with the animal. Munjack (1984), in an interesting retrospective analysis, questioned individuals with a more common type of specific phobia about the etiology of their "fear" of driving. Of his 30 subjects, a few (20%) reported some traumatic incident while driving that seemed to lead to their fears, such as a collision. Almost half (40%) reported no such incident. Rather, they noted that suddenly, for no apparent reason, they had "panicked" while driving and since then had been unable to drive on freeways. Although these patients presented with a fear of driving, what actually seemed to make them anxious, much as with McNally and Steketee's patients, was the possibility of having unexpected panic attacks. It also seems possible that in cases where the etiology was less clear, experiences similar to panic or possibly limited symptom attacks played a role.

Clinicians are familiar with one of the most common types of specific phobias, "fear" of flying. It is the rare individual who reports developing a "fear" of flying after crashing in an airplane, or even after reading about a crash in the newspaper. The more common situation is that an individual who may have flown successfully for years suddenly develops an incapacitating "fear" of flying. The example of John Madden, a well-known sports announcer in the United States, has been described in some detail in Chapter 1. Often such people will report, when pressed, that they are afraid some catastrophe will occur or that the plane will crash. What they really seem to "fear" is the possibility of having another panic attack.

In this context, the Öst and Hugdahl findings mentioned above become clear. The majority of these individuals with specific phobias, social phobia, and agoraphobia, reported experiencing an intense, overwhelming false alarm in situations or contexts that subsequently became "phobic" for these individuals. It was the false alarm, rather than a realistic traumatic event, that seemed implicated in their "conditioning."

It is entirely possible that some individuals with specific phobias experience an alarm reaction in response to a realistic threat to their well-being, which then becomes associated with the same or similar objects or situations. Being attacked by a dog may be an example. A larger number of persons with specific phobias experience a false alarm, which is of such intensity that learning occurs. Specifically, false alarms become strongly associated with the object or situation that set the occasion for the first false alarm. In this model, the individual who develops a phobia evidences anxiety in the presence of the object or situation (or similar objects or situations) that have set the occasion for the first false alarm, but anxiety occurs primarily over the possibility of having another (unpredictable) false alarm in the presence of the cues that signal the possibility of this alarm.

As noted above, this association is not a random event. Conditioning is more likely to occur to some evolutionarily prepared stimuli than to others. Similarly, some CSs and UCSs are more likely to "belong" to each other, as in taste and illness reactions surrounding food. But another possible association may account for much of the nonrandom quality of phobic reactions. A common theme is the danger of being trapped. This theme is obvious in individuals with agoraphobia. Fears of sitting too far from the door in a church, synagogue, or movie theater, or of being trapped in a crowded mall, are prototypic agoraphobic situations. One early name for agoraphobia, the "barber's chair syndrome," reflects the difficulty that many of these individuals have with confinement to dentists' or beauticians' chairs. But the feeling of being "trapped" is also strongly present in phobias of driving, flying, or other forms of transportation. It is also present in fears of crossing bridges. What these situations have in common is that the context prevents easy escape in the event of a false alarm. That is, the overwhelmingly powerful and ethologically ancient action tendency of escape is blocked. At the very least, this intensifies and prolongs the alarms and potentiates learning. Interference or conflict with this survival-based behavior is probably the most important factor in "convincing" the organism not to let this happen again at any cost. And the cost is often high. If emotions are fundamentally behavioral acts (Lang, 1985), or evolutionary process responses to make us do what our ancestors had to do to pass genes on to coming generations (Öhman, 1993), anything that interferes with the execution of this most important of all emotional acts (escape) should have profound significance.

The implications of this model for the development of a specific phobia is clear. An actual traumatic event (true alarm) involving the phobic object or situation may not be necessary. Only a false alarm may be required in the presence of a previously benign object or situation, particularly where escape is difficult, or where the context is "prepared" in some other way. These conditions may insure that a learned alarm or conditioned anxiety occurs the next time the object or situation is encountered. These ideas concerning the etiology of specific phobias are elaborated in Chapter 11.

As noted in the first edition of this book, the occurrence of a false alarm may be one of the "missing links" in a traumatic conditioning etiology of some phobias. This missing link—identifying as it does an intense UCS, capable of providing strong emotional learning in as little as one trial—fulfills a theoretical prediction made years ago by Wolpe (1952, 1954). In "vicarious" learning, a similar phenomenon is present (Mineka & Cook, 1993; Mineka & Zinbarg, 1996). Mineka (1987) has demonstrated in monkeys that what is crucial for vicarious acquisition of a phobic response is the intensity of the fear reaction of the model. Fear intensity correlates almost perfectly with the intensity of the alarm from the subject and with the subsequent strength of the phobic reaction. Thus the well-known principle of "emotion contagion" from the emotion theory literature may underlie observational etiology of phobia. Emotion contagion in turn reflects the social communication function of emotional behavior.

Thus the occurrence of a false alarm may be one crucial element heretofore overlooked in etiological accounts of phobias. But there is another link (described below) that, in my view, is required for a satisfactory etiological account.

False Alarms and Panic Disorder: Interoceptive Conditioning

What of patients with panic disorder, with or without agoraphobia? The majority of these individuals are unable to report a clearly demarcated cue for their alarms, although individuals with agoraphobia often report a series of diffuse situations of which they are wary, many of which revolve around being "trapped" away from a safe place. But agoraphobic avoidance is sometimes limited in panic disorder. It is possible that the major difference between panic disorder and other phobic disorders may be in the association (or lack thereof) between a false alarm and a specific cue, as suggested in Chapter 4. What is learned then in this case? To understand this more fully, let us consider an important but little-known line of research conducted by Russian investigators.

For years Russian investigators conducted a series of experiments demonstrating that fear could be conditioned to internal physiological stimuli. These stimuli came to be known as "interoceptive" (Razran, 1961). To take a typical example, the colon of a dog was slightly stimulated (the CS) at the same time that an electric shock was administered. As a result of this procedure, the dog began to evidence signs of intense conditioned anxiety during the natural passage of feces. The Russians demonstrated that this type of learning was particularly resistant to extinction. That is, it would persist indefinitely, despite repeated physiological sensations in the absence of the original UCS (shock). These findings are robust (e.g., Dworkin, 1993; Martin, 1983). The clear implication is that it is possible to learn an association between internal cues and false alarms, and that these internal cues serve the same function for patients with panic disorder (with or without agoraphobia) that external cues do for individuals with specific phobias. That is, they signal the possibility of another false alarm. Of course, there is no clear demarcation between specific phobias and panic disorder in regard to external versus internal cues for false alarms. Although panic disorder seems to be characterized by a predominance of internal cues (see Chapter 10), external cues for false alarms can also be identified. Similarly, for specific phobias, internal somatic cues may make a substantial contribution to the generation of anxiety and, on occasion, false alarms (Chosak, 2000; Craske, Mohlman, Yie, Glover, & Valeri, 1995; Davey, Menzies, & Gallardo, 1997).

The evolution of knowledge concerning interoceptive conditioning in the ensuing years has been outlined in some detail recently (Bouton et al., 2001). One particularly interesting type of interoceptive conditioning, reviewed in more detail in Bouton et al. (2001), involves the case in which a low dose of a drug signals a higher dose of the same drug. For example, a typical UCR to a drug of any kind in organisms is a compensatory response; that is, if the drug is a stimulant, a compensatory response will involve suppression. Kim, Siegel, and Patenall (1999) found evidence of this kind of learning with single administrations of morphine in rats. After an injection, followed by a long exposure to morphine (which suppresses arousal), rats were given a short "probe" injection that mimicked the internal physical early-onset properties of the longer injection. The rats' response to the short probe resembled their response to the longer probe, but only if the shorter probe had been paired with a longer probe. Thus interoceptive cues to the onset of a long interoceptive stimulus became associated with the remainder of the stimulus. Dworkin (1993) has termed this type of conditioning, in which early onset is associated with an event's later aspects, a "homoreflex." This is in contrast to the more usual textbook description of classical conditioning, where the CS and UCS are different. The applicability to panic disorder, where early signs of a false alarm signal the remainder of the full-blown panic episode, is evident. As we (Bouton et al., 2001) point out, "since early onset cues are presumably similar to the U[C]S's later effects, they may be especially easy to condition; theoretically they might therefore overshadow learning about other perfectly valid predictors of the U[C]S—such as other predictive external cues. This scenario suggests that interoceptive conditioning may be a major contributor to the development of panic disorder" (p. 12). Evidence is not limited to the animal laboratory, but is present in numerous case examples from the clinic. To take an example, Hegel and Ahles (1992) describe the successful treatment of a case where urges to void urine triggered a gagging and vomiting reflex established some years earlier in the context of severe alcohol abuse and heavy smoking.

Over the years, various commentators have criticized this conception of classical conditioning on a variety of counts. Some have supposed that this conditioning approach lacks conceptual clarity when applied to panic disorder (e.g., McNally, 1994, 1999; Reiss, 1987). For example, the point is made that there is confusion about what constitutes the CS, UCS, CR, and UCR, and that the distinction between the CS and the CR is blurred, since they seem to be two arbitrary points on a continuum of arousal. Others have argued, reasonably, that this theory would lead to an overprediction of panic attacks, since every somatic sensation that had been associated with panic should lead to a new attack (Clark, 1988). A third criticism of the role of interoceptive conditioning in the etiology of panic disorder is the notion that interoceptive conditioning should extinguish when a bodily sensation that has become a CS is not followed by a panic attack (van den Hout, 1988; Rachman, 1991). As we have detailed (Bouton et al., 2001), a more contemporary perspective on the properties of classical conditioning and learning theory in general obviates these criticisms. In fact, the "homoreflex" described above, in which early properties of a physiological response signal the full response, may be one of the most powerful forms of classical conditioning. The critique noting an overprediction of panic fails to consider the variety of modulating stimuli found in the background of the occurrence of any CS. Finally, it has become clear that the process of extinction depends heavily on contextual factors (Bouton, 1991, 1993) that would preclude simple extinction's occurring by nonreinforced pairing.

Learned (Conditioned) Anxiety

Thus the association of false alarms with internal or external cues results in *learned* (conditioned) anxiety. A characteristic of any learned response is that it need not fully replicate its unlearned counterpart. Contrary to textbook illustrations of classical conditioning (which focus on one small part of a response, such as salivation), the constellation of responses to a particular CS, both internal and external, are actually far more complex (Bouton et al., 2001). For example, in defensive conditioning in animals, the CR may include freezing and other natural defensive behaviors, as well as various physiological changes: increases in blood pressure and heart rate, changes in respiration, and the release of endogenous opiates that reduce pain (e.g., Bolles & Fanselow, 1980). The principal purpose of conditioned defensive behavior is to prepare the organism to deal with upcoming threat (Hollis, 1997). Once again the analogy to phobia or panic disorder seems clear, in that the complex CR to interoceptive cues would serve to prepare the individual for an upcoming false alarm by facilitating vigilance and possible escape or avoidance behavior.

As noted above, one clear consequence of this learning in individuals who become phobic is the rapid development of acute sensitivity and vigilance concerning the newly acquired phobic cues. Someone recently bitten by a dog will quickly become acutely sensitive to any sign of dogs. This vigilance will extend to unfamiliar areas where dogs may be roaming free. Someone experiencing a false alarm in an elevator will become acutely aware of any plans in the immediate future that may require entry into an elevator. And someone who has learned to associate interoceptive cues with false alarms will become acutely sensitive to, and vigilant for, specific somatic cues that may signal the beginning of another alarm.

To reiterate, the response described above that becomes conditioned to interoceptive (or exteroceptive) cues is *anxiety* and not panic (Bouton et al., 2001), albeit a brief burst of discrete conditioned anxiety. The function of anxiety is to prepare the organism for the next false alarm or panic attack, or other threat to the organism's integrity. That is, in the presence of both interoceptive and exteroceptive cues, anxiety now occurs; this also makes it possible for new operant behaviors that serve to avoid or reduce the anxiety to be reinforced. This emphasis is fully consistent with the literature on conditioning of defensive responses in animals. In this paradigm, the CRs, such as endogenous analgesia or freezing, are not the same as the UCR to a noxious UCS, which often involves bursts of activity and pain. In this view, the UCR would be equivalent to a false alarm or panic attack, whereas the CR is a forward-looking set of responses that prepares the organism for the upcoming threat.

As we (Bouton et al., 2001) point out, it is also possible under certain conditions that panic itself can be conditioned to certain interoceptive or exteroceptive cues associated with panic attacks. To follow a distinction made throughout this book, a panic attack, unlike anxiety, represents an emergency reaction designed to deal with imminent or ongoing threat or danger. Animal and human studies that have arranged conditions so that cues that are particularly close in time to the onset of panic, such as some of its proximal interoceptive correlates, may be more likely than other kinds of stimuli to evoke this particular CR (Cook et al., 1986; Domjan, Huber-McDonald, & Holloway, 1992; Forsyth & Eifert, 1996, 1998; Stegen, de Bruyne, Rasschaert, van de Woestijne, & van den Bergh, 1999). But this is most likely the exception rather than the rule. The most usual response to internal and external cues would be (anticipatory) anxiety.

Recently, Forsyth and colleagues (e.g., Forsyth & Eifert, 1996) have developed the notion of interoceptive conditioning as a process underlying the development of phobias and panic disorder, elaborating on ideas presented in the first edition of this book and outlined above. Furthermore, data have begun to appear articulating the nature of this process in humans; these data demonstrate the importance of the intensity of the UCR (false alarm), as opposed to the nature of the UCS (e.g., Forsyth, Eifert, & Thompson, 1996; Forsyth & Eifert, 1998; Stegen et al., 1999). For example, Forsyth et al. (1996) evaluated as CSs fear-relevant and fear-irrelevant video stimuli depicting either internal bodily processes or external environmental situations. The internal fear-relevant stimulus was a close-up of a human heart beating arrhythmically. The internal fear-irrelevant stimulus was a magnified view of human sperm swimming. (This stimulus was chosen because it was easily discriminable and produced an animated stimulus.) The environmental stimuli included a fear-relevant view of a poisonous snake moving toward the viewer, whereas the fear-irrelevant stimulus depicted a field of daisies swaying in the wind. The UCS paired with these stimuli was 20-second inhalations of a premixed 20% CO_2-enriched air mixture. Both physiological and self-report measures were collected. Participants were randomly assigned to either the internal or external stimulus condition. Within each of these groups, participants were also randomly assigned to pairings of either the fear-relevant or fear-irrelevant stimulus with the CO_2 inhalations. For example, subjects in the internal fear-relevant group viewed both the arrhythmically beating heart and the sperm, but only the arrhythmically beating heart was paired with the CO_2. Thus the beating heart segment was designated as CS+. For subjects in the internal fear-irrelevant group, the same film segments were presented, but the sperm served as the CS+ in that it was paired with CO_2 inhalations. Subjects in the external groups viewed the snake and flower segments with either the snake, which was the fear-relevant stimulus, or the flower, which was the fear-irrelevant stimulus, designated as the CS+.

Results for skin conductance, presented as first-interval anticipatory responses (FARs), are presented in Figure 7.3. Both acquisition and extinction data for FARs are shown. As one can see, responses to fear-relevant stimuli were more easily acquired, were of higher magnitude, and showed greater resistance to extinction than did responses to fear-irrelevant stimuli. This was true whether the stimuli were representations of internal or external context, although conditioning was more pronounced to external (snake) than to internal (heart) phobic stimuli. Parallel results on subjective measures (subjective units of disturbance, or SUDs) are presented in Figure 7.4.

Forsyth and Eifert (1998) expanded on this important line of research by looking at different intensities of CO_2 inhalation paired with either fear-relevant stimuli (snakes or heart beating arrhythmically) or fear-irrelevant flowers. Specifically, 20% versus 13% mixtures of CO_2-enriched air were compared across the three stimuli in three independent groups of subjects. Results for FAR responses are presented in Figure 7.5. Subjective distress ratings (SUDs) are presented in Figure 7.6. Once again, it is clear that for fear relevant stimuli, the intensity of the internal UCS is very relevant in the acquisition of conditioned fear responses and in their resistance to extinction. The analogy to unexpected uncued panic attacks (false alarms) seems clear.

Finally, Stegen et al. (1999) paired images of fear-relevant (being stuck in an elevator or a sauna) and fear-irrelevant (reading a book overlooking the sea) contexts with inhalations of 5.5% CO_2-enriched air. Once again, participants exposed to the fear-relevant images showed significant conditioning both physiologically and subjectively. That is, subjects showed altered respiratory behavior and cardiac/warmth symptoms to the fear-relevant images, as well as subjective symptoms of anxiety. The authors note that "a little stress induced hyperventilation in association with a phobia-relevant place or an image thereof may evoke the experience of similar symptoms of anxiety on next confrontations, even without apparent hyperventilation" (p. 150).

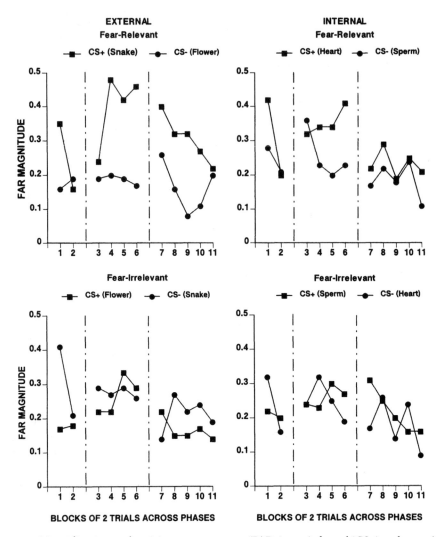

FIGURE 7.3. Mean first-interval anticipatory responses (FARs) to reinforced (CS+) and nonreinforced (CS–) stimuli across trial blocks for each phase of the experiment. FARs were recorded in microsiemens and corrected for individual differences in range. Trial block numbers correspond to the following phases: habituation (1–2), acquisition (3–6), and extinction (7–11). From Forsyth, J. P., Eifert, G. H., and Thompson, R. N. (1996). Systematic alarms in fear conditioning: II. An experimental methodology using 20% carbon dioxide inhalation as an unconditioned stimulus. *Behavior Therapy, 27,* 391–415. Copyright 1996 by the Association for Advancement of Behavior Therapy. Reprinted by permission of the publisher.

A variety of additional evidence supports the contention that in patients with panic disorder and phobias, interoceptive cues trigger anxiety. Chapter 5 has reviewed the substantial body of evidence, dating back 60 years, on the provocation of panic via both pharmacological and behavioral methods. As suggested there, the weight of the evidence indicates that anxiety can be a learned response to a variety of somatic cues, particularly respiratory, cardiovascular, and vestibular. Evidence reviewed in Chapter 5 (e.g., Linde-

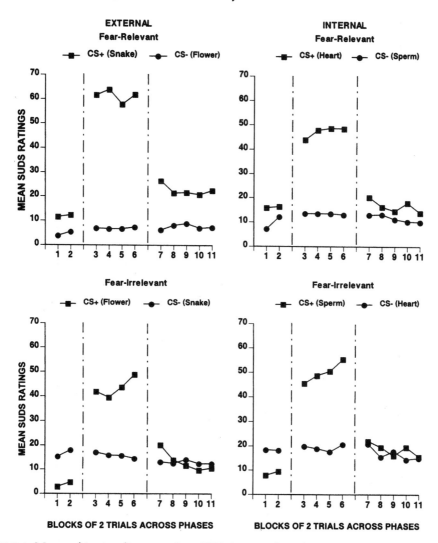

FIGURE 7.4. Mean subjective distress ratings (SUDs) to reinforced (CS+) and nonreinforced (CS–) CS types for each phase of the experiment. Trial block numbers correspond to the following phases: habituation (1–2), acquisition (3–6), and extinction (7–11). From Forsyth, J. P., Eifert, G. H., and Thompson, R. N. (1996). Systematic alarms in fear conditioning: II. An experimental methodology using 20% carbon dioxide inhalation as an unconditioned stimulus. *Behavior Therapy, 27,* 391–415. Copyright 1996 by the Association for Advancement of Behavior Therapy. Reprinted by permission of the publisher.

mann & Finesinger, 1938) also suggests that anxiety becomes associated with specific interoceptive cues rather than with the general physiological activation of nonspecific stress.

The interesting phenomenon of nocturnal panic, reviewed in Chapter 4, suggests that conditioned anxiety may be associated with sudden changes in physiological homeostasis, even when these changes are ordinarily anxiolytic. A case in point involves relaxation and the closely associated state that occurs during the beginning of slow wave-sleep.

From this perspective, it is tempting to speculate on the origins of seemingly vastly different "anxiety" disorders found in other cultures, as reviewed in Chapter 1. Could *koro*

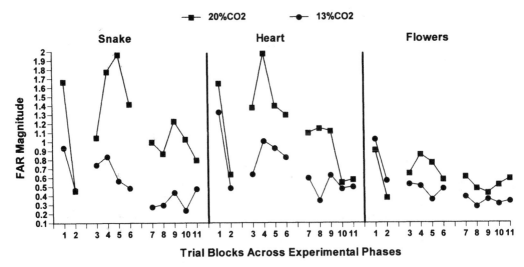

FIGURE 7.5. Mean first-interval anticipatory response (FAR), recorded in microsiemens, across trial blocks for each experimental phase. Trial blocks for each phase are designated as follows: habituation (1–2), acquisition (3–6), and extinction (7–11). From "Response Intensity in Content-Specific Fear Conditioning Comparing 20% versus 13% CO_2-Enriched Air as Unconditioned Stimuli" by J. P. Forsyth and G. H. Eifert, 1998, *Journal of Abnormal Psychology, 107,* 291–304. Copyright 1998 by the American Psychological Association. Reprinted with permission.

result from a false alarm that is then attributed to a culturally popular cue or cause? Is "heart distress" in Iran similar to what was called "irritable heart syndrome" in the early part of the century in the United States? If so, perhaps both "heart distress" and "irritable heart syndrome" are precipitated by a false alarm attributed to a cardiovascular disease process.

Internal versus External Cues

If this account is correct, what accounts (1) for the development of more chronic anxiety associated with external or internal cues, and (2) for the variety of anxious propositions (including types of causal attributions) present during the episode? One factor would seem to involve the particular situation in which the individual finds him- or herself during an initial false alarm. In the case of a true alarm, where one's welfare is threatened, the location of the first alarm is not an issue (at least initially), since all attention is focused on the source of the threat (e.g., a car careening out of control). When one experiences a false alarm, however, attention may be allocated in many different ways, since there is no obvious cause for alarm. If one is "trapped" in a situation where no exit is possible while experiencing the full effects of a false alarm, with its associated sense of death, dying, and loss of control, then it is intuitively likely that the largest share of attention will be directed to the "trapped" situation, which prevents the powerful action tendency of escape. Common examples mentioned above include planes or other means of public transportation; dentists' or hairdressers' chairs, where it is difficult to suddenly get up and leave; or public places such as churches or synagogues, where a quick exit may prove embarrassing.

When one is alone at home, one's attention may be focused more fully on internal cues associated with the false alarm. Evidence from our clinic at Albany indicates that the location of the individual during the first panic is important in this respect, since

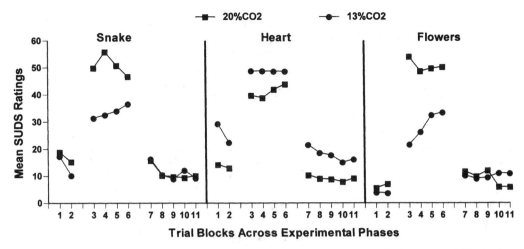

FIGURE 7.6. Mean subjective distress ratings (SUDs) across experimental phases. Trial blocks for each phase are designated as follows: habituation (1–2), acquisition (3–6), and extinction (7–11). From "Response Intensity in Content-Specific Fear Conditioning Comparing 20% versus 13% CO_2-Enriched Air as Unconditioned Stimuli" by J. P. Forsyth and G. H. Eifert, 1998, *Journal of Abnormal Psychology, 107*, 291–304. Copyright 1998 by the American Psychological Association. Reprinted with permission.

patients who have panic disorder without agoraphobic avoidance tend to have more of their first panics at home while accompanied; patients who have panic disorder with agoraphobia tend to have their first panic attacks out of the house, alone (Craske & Barlow, 1988).

It is unlikely, however, that one's attention will be as neatly divided in the event of a false alarm as is implied by this description. Clinical experience indicates that patients present with a varying mixture of apprehension to internal and external cues, with only a minority fearing one or the other exclusively. Examples in the latter category include a person with a airplane phobia who experiences a false alarm while flying but has associated this alarm exclusively with planes, or a patient who has panic disorder with no avoidance whatsoever (a very rare occurrence indeed; see Chapter 10) whose concern is focused exclusively on somatic sensations. But most patients who have experienced false alarms fall somewhere in between and are apprehensive about a varying mixture of internal and external cues.

It is also interesting to consider the minority (approximately 30%) of patients with panic disorder who can clearly cite an unfavorable experience with drugs such as anesthesia, cocaine, or marijuana as the setting event for their first panic (Aronson & Craig, 1986). Here the "cause" in terms of a temporally associated event seems clear, and the anesthesia or the recreational drug is subsequently avoided. But a full panic disorder syndrome also develops, including marked sensitivity to a variety of somatic cues and repeated panic attacks in the absence of external cues. This division of attention between internal and external cues may be more typical of a clinical phobia. But whether a drug is involved in the etiology or not, aversive unexplained arousal clearly becomes the major focus of concern and the stimulus component of the anxious propositions. Internal or external cues that happen to be associated with an initial false alarm, even if prepotent in some way (as in "trapped" situations), cannot fully account for the development of all anxiety disorders. In the subsequent chapters of this book devoted to each clinical disorder, we suggest factors in addition to the location of the first alarm that determine the focus of anxious apprehension.

Finally, the avoidance behavior that develops (whether the initial reaction is a true or a false alarm) in specific or social phobia seems to differ somewhat from the avoidance behavior that develops subsequent to a false alarm in panic disorder with agoraphobia. As described in more detail in Chapter 10, much of the extensive avoidance behavior sometimes seen in panic disorder with agoraphobia, resulting in eventual housebound status, seems secondary to a false alarm. For example, if these people are home alone during the first false alarm and then begin experiencing an increasing number of panic attacks associated with various internal cues, they will come to avoid a variety of situations where they do not feel "safe" in the event of an unexpected panic attack (if cultural, social, and environmental contingencies allow such avoidance). This type of secondary avoidance then becomes a method of coping with false alarms and is more readily understood from the point of view of a safety signal analysis (e.g., Rachman, 1984). That is, where and with whom is it safe to be if one has a panic attack? For this reason, the avoidance in agoraphobia is more diffuse and variable than that in specific or social phobias. It is also more clearly related to the presence or absence of a "safe" person (Craske, 1999; Salkovskis, Clark, & Gelder, 1996). The development of expectancies regarding the likelihood of future attack also plays a substantial role in determining the extent of agoraphobic avoidance (Craske & Barlow, 1988). This issue is discussed further in Chapter 10.

ALARMS AND CLINICAL ANXIETY DISORDERS

Thus far, I have highlighted the role of stress and associated neurobiological reactions in the genesis of an initial false alarm. The fact that at least some of these alarms are associated with a variety of internal and external cues also receives substantial support. One final link in the etiological chain derives from the fascinating issue of who develops clinical disorders associated with false alarms and who does not. As noted earlier (e.g., Norton et al., 1986; Wittchen & Essau, 1991), many more people seem to experience alarms (true and false) than those who actually present with clinical disorders. In fact, individuals with nonclinical panic form a substantial minority of the population. At present, the difference between those who develop full-blown clinical syndromes and those who do not is largely speculative, since we know so little about those with infrequent panic. For example, persons with nonclinical panic who have occasional alarms seem to experience them less frequently, although a small minority may be experiencing as many as those with clinical disorders and yet have evidently not considered seeking help. These subjects also seem to experience their alarms less intensely.

It is possible, of course, particularly among those who are experiencing more frequent panics, that full-blown panic disorder will develop. But another possibility is that they simply do not "fear" these alarms, or, more accurately, that they do not become chronically apprehensively anxious about them. Some may even evidence conditional anxiety to specific situations that have become associated with alarms and develop normal "fears" that cause occasional avoidance, or at least temporary increased vigilance (nonclinical panic), but that do not interfere with functioning. What could account for individuals who do not develop a clinical disorder? One possibility is that the alarms simply are not of sufficient intensity to result in clinical complication. But a more likely possibility is that people who develop full-blown panic or phobic disorders are specifically susceptible to developing more intense, chronic anxiety and negative affect over aversive uncomfortable events perceived as aversive, unpredictable, and uncontrollable, such as recurring false alarms, because of a combination of individual biological and psychological vulnerabilities. Among these vulnerabilities may be biologically based stress reactivity, perceptions of unpredictability and uncontrollability of the alarms or other negative events, and poor coping skills or social support (as described in Chapter 3). In other words, if an alarm calls forth a variety of anxious propositions (in Lang's sense) characterized by perceptions of unpredictability–uncontrollability, and a shift of attention to internal self-evaluative modes, then it is possible that the conditions will be ripe for the development of an emotional disorder. If, on the other hand, one does not experience unpredictability or loss of control as a result of this event, one may find it disconcerting, but simply attribute it to benign events of the moment ("something I ate," "a fight with my boss"). In this case, one will not experience an internal self-evaluative shift in attention (see below), and the false alarm will be just that. Life will then go on as before, with perhaps an occasional rather mild false alarm reappearing from time to time under stressful conditions.

In any case, the lack of chronic distress or anxiety over the possibility of having another alarm, found in a large percentage of the general population and perhaps in a few nonpsychiatric medical patients, suggests a fundamental distinction between these individuals and patients with anxiety disorders. To develop an anxiety disorder, one must be susceptible to developing chronic anxiety or apprehension over the possibility of subsequent alarms or other negative events. What determines this susceptibility? What are the factors that lead to the development of chronic anxiety? It is to this topic that I now turn.

CHAPTER 8

The Origins of Anxious Apprehension, Anxiety Disorders, and Related Emotional Disorders

Triple Vulnerabilities

The experience of the last decade has strengthened speculations offered in the first edition of this book (Barlow, 1988) on an interacting set of vulnerabilities or diatheses relevant to the development of anxiety, anxiety disorders, and related emotional disorders. Evidence reviewed in preceding chapters now becomes relevant to a full integrative discussion of etiology. I begin with a brief review of genetic contributions to the development of anxiety and negative affect that constitute a generalized biological vulnerability. This is followed by a detailed explication of the contributions of early life experience to the later development of anxiety and related emotional states. Evidence now suggests that these early life experiences, under certain conditions, contribute to a psychological vulnerability or diathesis to experience anxiety and related negative affective states generally (a generalized psychological vulnerability). Although the unfortunate co-occurrence of generalized biological and psychological vulnerabilities may be sufficient to produce anxiety and related states, a third set of vulnerabilities seems necessary to account for the development of at least some specific anxiety disorders. In this regard I refer to certain learning experiences that seem to *focus* anxiety on certain life circumstances; that is, these circumstances or events become imbued with a heightened sense of threat and danger. It is this specific psychological vulnerability that, when coordinated with the generalized biological and psychological vulnerabilities mentioned above, seems to contribute to the development of discrete anxiety disorders such as social phobia (social anxiety disorder), obsessive–compulsive disorder (OCD), panic disorder, and specific phobias.

A full discussion of these three sets of vulnerabilities then makes possible a description of a model of the development of anxiety disorders. A description of this model is followed by an extension of this theory to other related emotional disorders, including anger and stress, depression, and mania. Emerging evidence since the first edition of this book, where many of these ideas were initially proposed, has strengthened the conception of the commonalities among these emotional disorders, and the resulting implications for etiology and treatment.

GENERALIZED BIOLOGICAL VULNERABILITY: GENETIC CONTRIBUTIONS

In Chapters 2 and 6, I have reviewed in some detail evidence pertaining to genetic contributions to personality traits or temperaments related to anxiety and its disorders. Evidence reviewed there suggests that the fundamental trait of being "high-strung," "nervous," or "emotional" runs in families and has a genetic component. More formal studies of temperaments such as "anxiety," "neuroticism," "negative affect," or "behavioral inhibition" also evidence a substantial genetic component (L. A. Clark, Watson, & Mineka, 1994). As noted earlier, the relationships among these closely related traits and temperaments have yet to be fully worked out, but it is likely that each represents variations on a theme underlying a biological vulnerability to develop emotional disorders generally. Genetic contributions to the expression of these generalized traits are most usually estimated to run in the range of 30–50% of the variance. More importantly, it has now been established that traits of neuroticism or negative affectivity are strongly related to anxiety and anxiety disorders (Trull & Sher, 1994; L. A. Clark et al., 1994; Zinbarg & Barlow, 1996; Brown, Chorpita, & Barlow, 1998). Of course, many of these early studies are correlational, but more satisfactory prospective designs detailing the relationship between neurotic temperaments and the later development of anxiety are now appearing. For example, Gershuny and Sher (1998) evaluated the extent to which personality dimensions of neuroticism (as well as extraversion and psychoticism) predicted global anxiety ratings in over 400 young adults. They found that an interaction of neuroticism and extraversion predicted both global anxiety and depression 3 years after initial assessment. They conclude that personality variables, particularly the combination of high neuroticism and low extraversion, constitute an important vulnerability for the later development of anxiety and its disorders (although the purpose of this study was not to predict the occurrence of specific anxiety disorders). Furthermore, Gershuny and Sher (1998) found a lack of specificity for predicting anxiety versus depression, in that the personality variables measured seemed to provide a common diathesis—a subject to which I return below.

Although some tantalizing evidence exists on more circumscribed genetic contributions to some disorders, particularly specific phobia (e.g., Fyer, Mannuzza, Chapman, Martin, & Klein, 1995; Kendler, Karkowski, & Prescott, 1999; Page & Martin, 1998), the strong consensus is that anxiety and related emotional disorders (such as depression) have a common genetic basis, and that specific differences in these disorders are best accounted for by environmental factors (e.g., Kendler 1996; Andrews, Stewart, Allen, & Henderson, 1990; Martin, Jardine, Andrews, & Heath, 1988). Furthermore, as noted in Chapter 6, there is no reasonable evidence to date confirming the existence of a specific "anxious gene." Instead, weak contributions from many genes in several different areas on chromosomes (i.e., a polygenic model) seem to contribute to a generalized biological vulnerability to become anxious (e.g., Plomin, DeFries, McClearn, & Rutter, 1997).

The one deviation from the consensual conclusion regarding nonspecific genetic contributions to emotionality is the evidence reviewed in Chapter 6 for a differential, if overlapping, heritability for panic and perhaps related defensive reactions. That is, certain defensive reactions, such as responding to stressful situations with panic attacks, may have a separate genetic component, much as fainting and freezing in response to certain specific stimulus situations seem to evidence a strong heritable tendency (Marks, 1986; Page & Martin, 1998; Kendler et al., 1995).

Thus, as noted in Chapter 6, one may inherit a tendency to be "nervous" or "emotional"—or, more precisely, to be very reactive biologically to environmental changes. This reactivity constitutes a generalized biological vulnerability to develop anxiety *only* if appropriate psychological vulnerabilities are properly coordinated. My own view is that this genetic contribution is nonspecific to the point that it underlies labile emotionality more generally, including positive affective states. But it is entirely possible that it is restricted to more negative affective states. In any case, as noted already, one may also be disposed genetically to experience an alarm reaction or some other defensive response. Thus the tendencies to be generally "anxious" or "nervous" on the one hand, and to experience an alarm response or panic attack on the other, may have separate if overlapping genetic components. I have outlined in Chapter 7 how a heritable proneness to anxiety may interact with the somewhat separable heritability to experience panic attacks in a manner that "sets the stage" for a more frequent experience of panic attacks (see Figure 7.2). This makes sense from an ethological point of view, since "being ready" for danger (anxiety) should lower the threshold for a flight-or-fight reaction when danger occurs (panic). Nevertheless, in the absence of concurrent psychological diatheses discussed below, the individual with this nonspecific biological vulnerability will presumably not develop anxiety or other negative emotional states later in life, but rather will manifest tendencies to emotionality or exaggerated responsiveness to stress that are within "normal" limits. To activate the specter of anxiety and related negative affectivity, this normative personality trait must incubate in the fertile ground of early experience. This nonspecific genetic vulnerability may also influence the propensity to develop conditioned emotional responses when one is experiencing panic and anxiety, since it has been established that temperamental variables with known genetic contributions influence other forms of conditioning (Bouton, Mineka, & Barlow, 2001; Mineka & Zinbarg, 1996).

GENERALIZED PSYCHOLOGICAL VULNERABILITY: A DIMINISHED SENSE OF CONTROL

Experimental Neurosis and the Centrality of a Sense of Control: Animal Models and Their Implications

In Chapter 3, I have noted that individuals suffering from anxiety and related disorders evidence a marked sense of uncontrollability when faced with certain tasks or challenges that may be in some way threatening. For these individuals, failures or perceived deficiencies are indications of a chronic inability to cope with unpredictable uncontrollable negative events, and this sense of uncontrollability is associated with negatively valenced emotional responding. Functional or "normal" individuals, on the other hand, seem to manifest what has been described as an "illusion of control," in which response deficiencies are attributed to passing external causes or to trivial and temporary internal states. But it is not possible from the evidence presented in Chapter 3 to ascribe causal status to these perceptions of controllability.

In the difficult area of etiology, the isolation of potentially important variables contributing to a disorder is often limited to a retrospective search of the patient's history. Short of longitudinal studies conducted over the course of decades to examine children at risk for the development of certain disorders, there are few methods available to help answer this most essential of all questions. For this reason, the ability to produce an emotional disorder in the laboratory is an enormously important step. Experimentally induced anxiety permits systematic exploration of the factors contributing to the disorder. Thus one chapter of this book (Chapter 5) has been devoted to the fascinating area of the laboratory provocation of panic in patients, with all of its problems and promises.

The Production of Experimental Neurosis in Animals

Although it would seem that there is no adequate laboratory analogue of anxious apprehension, the evidence actually suggests that we can produce severe anxious apprehension in the laboratory, and that we have been doing so for over 50 years. In experiment after experiment, most of them now classic, investigators have produced behavior characterized by extreme agitation, restlessness, distractibility, hypersensitivity, increased autonomic responding, muscle tension, and interference with ongoing performance. The names of the investigators associated with these experiments occupy a prominent place in every textbook of introductory psychology: Pavlov, Masserman, Liddell, and Gantt. The phenomenon they produced was commonly termed "experimental neurosis."

Why has this work been largely ignored by clinical researchers? Probably because the subjects were animals rather than people, and these early investigators made few systematic attempts to match the phenomena they were producing in the laboratory with human clinical conditions. In addition, many different paradigms were used to produce what came to be called "experimental neurosis," and each was accompanied by sometimes radically different theoretical explanations, based on the biological, psychodynamic, or behavioral predilections of the investigator. For this reason, animal models of psychopathology in general were not popular for a number of years.

Now interest has been rekindled in possible animal models of anxious apprehension, because of the striking similarity of these emotional states produced in the laboratory to clinical anxious apprehension. Particularly notable is the persistence or chronicity of these learned emotional states. Establishing a persistent, self-defeating emotional state begins to address the issue of Mowrer's "neurotic paradox" (see Chapter 1).

Anyone observing species closely related to humans, such as nonhuman primates, has realized that in addition to displaying all of the behavioral and physiological signs of anxiety, these animals "look" extremely anxious in a number of more qualitative nonquantifiable ways (e.g., Suomi, Kraemer, Baysinger, & DeLizio, 1981; Suomi, 1986, 1999, 2000). Of course, one must be cautious about generalizing too readily from animal models. Nevertheless, experimental neurosis would seem to be one of the best animal analogues of human psychopathology (Mineka, 1985a; Mineka & Zinbarg, 1996). Therefore, it is important to determine possible causes of this laboratory phenomenon.

Experimental neurosis in animals has been produced by a number of different procedures: the punishment of appetitive responses: the presentation of insoluble problems, accompanied by the punishment of mistakes; long periods of restraint and monotony; and the introduction of extremely difficult discriminations that are required to obtain food. Some of these models, such as the punishment of appetitive responses in the Geller–Seifter paradigm described in Chapter 6, are often used for testing the effects of anxiolytic drugs.

At first glance, it would seem very difficult to abstract common themes from the variety of paradigms used to produce experimental neurosis. Mineka and Kihlstrom (1978), in an important review, made a compelling case for the specification of one causal factor running through all paradigms. They suggested that the cause of anxiety in these animals is that "environmental events of vital importance to the organism become unpredictable, uncontrollable, or both" (p. 257).

A body of basic experimental work has demonstrated the markedly different consequences of exposing organisms to exactly the same stimuli in a predictable and controllable versus an unpredictable and uncontrollable way. For example, Weiss (1971a, 1971b) exposed rats to the same amount and intensity of electric shock, and then examined their stomachs. He found greatly increased ulceration in rats whose shock was unpredictable, whether or not shock occurrence or its absence was signaled. Similarly, providing rats with some control over the shocks (the capability of terminating the shock by pressing a bar) produced significantly less ulceration than in rats that received the same amount of shock without any control. Much of this early work was conducted by Seligman (1968) and his colleagues (see also Maier & Seligman, 1976; Seligman, 1975). In the classic experiment in this series (Overmier & Seligman, 1967), a dog was exposed to a continuing regimen of inescapable shock. Later, when actively escaping the shock became possible, the dog, appearing emotionally distressed, failed to take advantage of this opportunity.

The mention of Seligman's name will quickly recall to any student of psychopathology the concepts of learned helplessness and depression. But conceptions of helplessness and lack of control have long been thought to underlie anxiety. For example, Mandler (1966) suggested that perceptions of lack of control (caused by aversive interruptions) are central to all views of anxiety. Early experiments with both animals and humans similar to those carried out by Weiss (1971a, 1971b) have repeatedly demonstrated the strong and crucial relationship between anxiety and perceptions of lack of control over events, particularly "stressful" events (Geer, Davison, & Gatchel, 1970; Haggard, 1943; Mowrer & Viek, 1948; Neale & Katahn, 1968; Pervin, 1963; Staub, Tursky, & Schwartz, 1971; see also Miller, 1979, for a review). In a particularly cogent experiment, Rodin and Langer (1977) informed one group of nursing home residents that they would exercise control and responsibility over the arrangement of items in their room, as well as the scheduling of their time. After 18 months, residents receiving this message evidenced a significantly better mortality rate than did residents who did not have control and responsibility. Miller (1979) was one of the first to suggest that it is not even control per se, but rather the "illusion of control," that is important. Organisms may then "predict" that future danger will be held to a minimum. Geer et al. (1970) demonstrated this phenomenon with college students. Studies supporting the importance of an illusion of control have been reviewed in Chapter 3. Seligman's important and influential observations on helplessness and depression have overshadowed the relationship of uncontrollability and anxiety.

In fact, experience with unpredictable and/or uncontrollable events consistently produces emotional disturbance in animals, but the form of the emotional disturbance varies considerably from animal to animal. In addition, the threshold for appearance of the emotional disturbance is different. In other words, some animals tolerate significantly more frequent or more intense unpredictable or uncontrollable events before showing signs of emotional disturbance. Many animals, under conditions of unpredictability–uncontrollability, first appear extremely anxious; this is followed by severe depression, as indicated by passive, retarded, and apparently helpless behaviors. Some animals seem to develop depression as an initial response to stressful experiences. As Mineka and Kihlstrom (1978) pointed out, "Some [animals] become very agitated with increases in general activity level and signs of high autonomic arousal (increased breathing rate, piloerection, struggling, howling, etc.). Others showed decreased activity levels and generally looked passive and withdrawn, sometimes becoming socially isolated from their conspecifics" (p. 260). Reasons for these individual differences are not clear, but they have a marked parallel in human clinical psychopathology, as indicated below.

Seligman (1975) suggested early that there may be differences between unpredictability and uncontrollability. Specifically, unpredictability may lead to anxiety, whereas excessive amounts of uncontrollability may lead to depression. Mineka (1985a; Mineka & Zinbarg, 1996) in turn suggested that these concepts necessarily overlap. Indeed, she argued that many if not all of the effects commonly attributed to the uncontrollability of the aversive event may be more appropriately attributed to the unpredictability of the event. This is true because animals who have control over shock termination are able to predict shock absence. This view is based on the observation that although controllable shock results in less fear conditioning than does equivalent exposure to uncontrollable shock, this difference can be removed by providing the animal with a "feedback" stimulus, which will predict shock absence, during the uncontrollable experience (Mineka, Cook, & Miller, 1984). This feedback stimulus is also called a "safety signal"—a term that appears subsequently in this book. However, Rosellini, Warren, and DeCola (1987) demonstrated in animals that the effects of controllability and predictability are separable and do exert an independent influence. They found that (1) the acquisition of fear follows a different pattern in animals having control than it follows in those having only prediction of shock absence; and (2) controllability of shock results in lower levels of fear conditioning under conditions where these effects cannot be mediated by predictability. Miller (1979) also concluded that the majority of human studies on this issue suggest that having control reduces emotional arousal after a stressful event, even when predictability is held constant. Investigators are continuing to untangle these effects and their relative importance in the generation of "anxiety."

In summary, it seems crucial that events important to the organism, such as the acquisition of food and escape from pain, occur in a predictable and/or controllable manner. Even aversive events of substantial intensity or duration will be better tolerated (with marked individual differences) if they occur predictably, and if the organism at least perceives that some control over these events is possible. Lack of predictability or controllability of these "stressful" events seems to lead to chronic anxiety and/or depression.

The Development of "Anxiety" in Primates

Although experiments on uncontrollability and unpredictability have been carried out with a variety of laboratory animals, some of the most compelling evidence comes from experiments with our close relatives, the primates—particularly rhesus monkeys and baboons. For example, Suomi and his colleagues have been studying "anxiety" in rhesus monkeys for years (e.g., Suomi, 1986, 1999, 2000). In particular, they have been interested in chronic displays of anxiety in the absence of specific fear stimuli, and factors that increase or decrease the intensity of this anxiety. Monkeys display all of the signs and symptoms of anxiety: tension, agitation, vigilance, and autonomic hyperactivity. Additional evidence that these behaviors and reactions represent anxiety comes from observations of similar or identical behaviors on the part of the monkeys when faced with cues or signals of danger. Of course, rhesus monkeys have species-specific expressions of anxiety, in addition to more general manifestations that seem to be shared by several species. Nevertheless, work by these investigators and others examining causes of chronic anxiety in monkeys provides useful, suggestive evidence to guide a search for causes of anxiety in humans.

What these investigators have found (e.g., Suomi et al., 1981; Suomi, 1999, 2000; Sapolsky, 1990, 1992; Coplan et al., 1996; Coplan, Trost, et al., 1998) is that unpredictable and uncontrollable stressful negative life events during development produce long-term increases in anxiety levels. These events are characterized as potentially life-threatening, such as separation from a primary caregiver or introduction to a group of strangers. In each case a "panic-like" reaction in the young monkey occurs, followed by long-term chronic anxiety that may last several years. Anxious behavior over the long term is likely to occur in novel or stressful situations to which the monkey is subsequently exposed. Introduction to strangers is a particularly interesting event, in terms of the evidence reviewed in Chapter 2 on the seemingly innate (if short-lived) fear of strangers that develops in human infants at approximately 8 months of age. Fear of strangers in rhesus monkeys is an adaptive response, since a young monkey attempting to join a new group in the wild is often severely beaten or killed by these "strangers" if the newcomer does not display the appropriate submissive behaviors. In any case, this sequence seems to be an example of a stressful event leading to an alarm reaction (panic?), which is followed by chronic anxiety.

There are also marked individual differences in responses among primates, which can be traced to a combination of experiential and neurobiological/genetic factors. For example, rhesus monkeys seem to inherit varying levels of autonomic hyperactivity in response to stress (e.g., Suomi, 1986, 1999, 2000). High reactivity predisposes them to more severe anxiety. Again, this reactivity in and of itself would seem to be nonspecific in regard to emotional expression. In addition, experiencing stress of various sorts (which increases generalized arousal and reactivity) prior to the experience of an unpredictable life-threatening experience also seems to produce more intense anxiety subsequently.

THE CAUSES OF PRIMATE ANXIETY IN THE LABORATORY. Some fascinating research from Mineka, Insel, and their colleagues in the 1980s began to illustrate not only the seeming importance of negative life events in the production of anxiety in rhesus monkeys, but also their interaction with uncontrollability or unpredictability in what would seem to be a very unlikely context. For example, Insel, Scanlan, Champoux, and Suomi (1988) reared two groups of rhesus monkeys identically except for their control over nonaversive stimuli. One group (the control group) had free access to toys and food treats, but identical items were presented to a yoked group only when they were first selected by an animal in the control group. When these two groups were exposed to a traumatic social separation in their third year of life, the yoked group exhibited more anxiety.

In an interesting twist, these investigators then administered a benzodiazepine inverse agonist (see Chapter 6) in order to examine responses to this pharmacological anxiogenic substance in the two groups of monkeys. This drug seems to produce a severe burst of negative affect. Once again, the yoked group displayed anxiety, and an increase in cortisol secretion. The monkeys that had control over their environment, on the other hand, made more aggressive threats under these conditions, with significantly less cortisol secretion. The authors conclude that these anxiogenic compounds have differential behavioral effects, depending on rearing history. Specifically, experiences of control and mastery early in life may have long-term consequences for the development of anxiety and coping behavior.

Mineka, Gunnar, and Champoux (1986) conducted a similar but even more sophisticated experiment with similarly defined groups, as well as a group receiving no reinforcers (toys or treats). Infant monkeys were assigned to one of three groups: master, yoked, and standard-reared. Monkeys in the master group had control over the delivery of food, drink, and other appetitive stimuli. Monkeys in the yoked group received equal amounts of these reinforcers, but did not have control over their delivery. Monkeys in the standard-reared group were treated according to standard laboratory procedures. Testing began when the monkeys were approximately 7 months of age. Results showed that master monkeys engaged in significantly more exploring behavior and less clinging than did the yoked monkeys. Master monkeys also showed reduced fear to a toy robot compared with yoked monkeys. Finally, when separated from peers, master monkeys used coping strategies more effectively to reduce distress. These findings are significant in that they demonstrate the negative influence of experiences with uncontrollability in the early environment. In addition, whereas experimental neurosis paradigms suggest the importance of control over aversive stimuli, this study suggests that control over appetitive stimuli may be equally important.

Several features of these experiments are particularly interesting. First, exposure to traumatic negative experiences (social separation, threatening objects) resulted in the predictable alarm response, followed by long-term (chronic) anxious apprehension. This result seems to replicate previous animal work on exposure to uncontrollable aversive events in a dramatic fashion. But prior experiences with controllability of nonaversive events (toys and treats) also predicted response to subsequent aversive events. This differential response was even more clearly evident during the experience of a noxious, stressful event: the administration of a drug causing anxiety. In fact, the animals in the group that learned control over an aspect of their environment dealt with this anxiogenic compound by becoming more aggressive—certainly one way of coping with difficult situations or experiences. Now an important extension of these findings has emerged from a bellwether program of research conducted by a prominent neuroscientist, Robert M. Sapolsky, who studies free-ranging baboons in a national reserve in Kenya.

THE DEVELOPMENT OF PRIMATE ANXIETY IN THE WILD: SAPOLSKY'S BABOONS. Like most primates, baboons arrange themselves in a social hierarchy with dominant members at the top and more submissive members at the bottom. And life at the bottom of a social hierarchy is difficult indeed! Among baboons, these subordinate animals undergo continual attack from dominant animals; they also have less access to food, preferred resting places, and sexual partners. Sapolsky (1990; Sapolsky, Alberts, & Altman, 1997; Sapolsky & Ray, 1989) has examined levels of cortisol in these animals as a function of their social rank and discovered that dominant males have lower resting levels of cortisol than subordinate males. However, when some "emergency" occurs, levels of cortisol rise more quickly in the dominant males than in the subordinate males. These findings recall an earlier independent conclusion by Dienstbier (1989), described in Chapter 6, on what constitutes "physiological toughness" or healthy resilience. The combination of low resting arousal and strong and responsive challenge, or stress-induced arousal, according to Dienstbier, is correlated with enhanced performance in complex tasks, emotional stability, and healthy responsiveness of the immune system.

Cortisol, of course, is the final step in a cascade of hormone secretion that begins with the limbic system in the brain during periods of stress or anxiety, as described in some detail in Chapter 6. As noted there, the hippocampus is very responsive to corticosteroids. When stimulated by these hormones during hypothalamic–pituitary–adrenocortical (HPA) axis activity, the hippocampus contributes to a down-regulation of the stress response, thus articulating the close link between the limbic system and various parts of the HPA axis. When produced chronically, cortisol can have damaging effects on a variety of physiological systems, ultimately causing damage to the hippocampus and the immune system. This damage to the hippocampus after a period of chronic stress may then lead to reduced negative feedback sensitivity, to chronic secretion of stress hormones, and ultimately to physical disease and death. I discuss the phenomenon of hippocampal degeneration in more detail below.

Sapolsky and his colleagues searched out the causes of these differences between dominant and subordinate animals by working backward up the HPA axis. They found that the most likely explanation was excess secretion of corticotropin-releasing factor (CRF) by the hypothalamus in subordinate animals, combined with a diminished sensitivity of the pituitary gland (which is stimulated by CRF). Therefore subordinate animals, unlike dominant animals, are continually secreting the hormone cortisol, probably because their lives are so stressful. In addition, they have an HPA system that is less sensitive to the effects of cortisol, making the system less efficient in turning off the stress response (this is probably related to hippocampal atrophy).

But Sapolsky's careful observations suggest that it is more than simply being at the top or bottom of a social hierarchy that is crucial in this regard. For example, he observed baboons during years when several males were sitting at the top of the hierarchy with no clear "winner." Although these males dominated the rest of the group, they were continually attacking and stressing each other. Under these conditions, they displayed hormonal profiles more like those seen in subordinate males than in dominant males. Thus Sapolsky concluded that the most important factor in regulating stress physiology seems to be a psychological factor—a sense of control (Sapolsky, 1992; Sapolsky et al., 1997; Sapolsky & Ray, 1989). Those animals that are in control of social situations and are able to cope with any tension that arises can go a long way toward blunting the long-term effects of stress or anxiety. Although Sapolsky characterizes his work as research on "stress," and the neuroendocrine responses in the HPA system are typically called "stress hormones," the experience of these baboons—with their profound sense of uncontrollability over future threat, and their continual physiological "readiness" for danger—would certainly fit almost any definition of anxiety, including my own. Of course, the processes in patients with anxiety seem more complex, in that (as noted above) increased CRF in patients seems to be accompanied by enhanced feedback inhibition of HPA functioning.

In any case, what makes this work even more interesting is that another prominent psychophysiological characteristic, autonomic inflexibility, can be linked to Sapolsky's work. Specifically, Sapolsky (1990, 1992) and Dienstbier (1989) both note that the process of anxiety, as it becomes chronic, results in physiological responses characterized by low vagal tone that are not optimal for the organism, and are opposite to the responses one would observe in an organism that has acquired "physiological toughness" (Dienstbier, 1989).

Thus it seems that Sapolsky's subordinate baboons are caught in a perpetual state of scanning for danger, probably as a function of perceived lack of control over their condition, resulting in chronic arousal and reduced reactivity (autonomic restriction) to actual stressors. These findings may reflect a psychological and neurobiological link between Sapolsky's "stressed" baboons and patients suffering from chronic anxiety (Mathews, 1990). As reviewed above, the finding of low vagal tone in anxious patients is very robust and has been observed in many studies utilizing very different paradigms. The work of Sapolsky and others has led to more complex interactive accounts of the role of CRF and the HPA axis in anxiety and fear, as detailed in Chapter 6.

Interestingly, early and chronic stress seems to result in more than anxiety. In fact, the "personalities" of these baboons are radically altered. Personality characteristics that reflect a sense of control, or a lack of it, are shown in Figure 8.1. Dominant males with a sense of control manifest certain personality traits, and have lower base levels of cortisol, than baboons without these traits. These dominant males can more easily distinguish between threatening and neutral actions of a rival, are more likely to start a fight with a threatening rival instead of waiting to be attacked; know which fights to pick, and thus are likely to win the fights they initiate; and can distinguish between having won and lost the fights (Sapolsky & Ray, 1989).

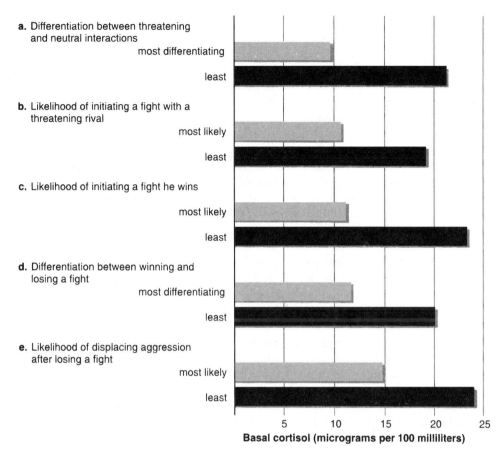

FIGURE 8.1. Personality characteristics in baboons that reflect a sense of control. Dominant baboons with certain personality traits (lighter bars) have lower base levels of cortisol than do other dominant males (darker bars), which suggests that attitude is a more important mediator of physiology than is rank alone. Dominant males that can distinguish between the threatening and neutral actions of a rival have cortisol levels that are about half as high as those of other dominant males (a). Similarly, low cortisol levels are found in males that start a fight with a threatening rival instead of waiting to be attacked (b); that know which fights to pick, and so are likely to win fights they initiate (c); that distinguish between having won and lost a fight (d); and that, when they do lose, take out their frustration on subordinates (e). From Sapolsky and Ray (1989). Copyright 1989 by Wiley-Liss Inc. Reprinted by permission.

EARLY EXPERIENCE AND CRF IN MACAQUES. In another pivotal experiment, Coplan et al. (1996) and Coplan, Trost, et al. (1998) evaluated a similar model of the development of anxiety in infant bonnet macaques. In this model, nursing mothers of infant monkeys were subjected to three different conditions involving foraging for food, which led to differential interactions with their infants. In the first condition, mothers were exposed to a context of low foraging demand (LFD), where food was readily available. In the second condition, consistently high (but predictable) foraging demand (HFD) was in effect. In the third condition, the monkeys were subjected to variable (and unpredictable) foraging demand (VFD). Interestingly, infants that were subjected to mothers exposed to the VFD condition exhibited heightened anxiety-like behavior during development, as well as substantially increased behavioral inhibition to a variety of novel and anxiety-producing contexts (Coplan, Rosenblum, & Gorman, 1995). Of more importance, CRF levels of these monkeys in cerebrospinal fluid were persistently elevated, and cortisol levels depressed (Coplan et al., 1996). CRF levels were also correlated with heightened cerebrospinal fluid levels of serotonin and dopamine metabolites (Coplan, Trost, et al., 1998). Some of these findings are displayed in Figure 8.2.

Coplan, Trost, et al. (1998) concludes that increasing adversity during early childhood results in enhanced CRF activity, which in turn causes alteration in other systems underlying the adult expression of stress and anxiety. Behaviors associated with the VFD condition included inconsistent, erratic, and dismissive behaviors on the part of the mothers—behaviors likely to result in diminished maternal attachment. Furthermore, the results seemed due to the unpredictability of the VFD condition, since adult mothers engaged in the predictable HFD condition did not exhibit the elevated CRF concentrations. Thus Coplan, Trost, et al. (1998) suppose, as do Nemeroff and his colleagues (e.g., Ladd et al., 2000) that adverse early experience—in combination, of course, with a genetic predisposition—creates a neurobiological diathesis. This diathesis becomes activated in later life by the experience of additional stressful life events or other triggers, completing the diathesis–stress model of the development of anxiety. As Sullivan, Kent, and Coplan (2000) note, "The combination of a 'jumpy' CRF and LC-NE [locus ceruleus–norepinephrine] system due to early environmental sculpting and increased amygdala-mediated cue and contextual fear memories due to past adversity, may make future responses much less specific such that anxious and/or avoidant behavior predominates" (p. 21).

The finding of *suppressed* cortisol levels in these animals is particularly interesting, in light of recent findings from patients who meet criteria for posttraumatic stress disorder (PTSD). Coplan et al. (1996) also noted that the reduced cortisol concentrations in these animals is precisely what is observed in patients with PTSD but that this observation seems

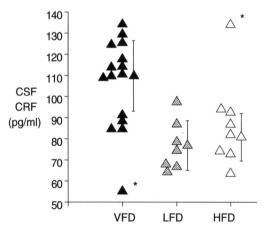

FIGURE 8.2. Cerebrospinal fluid CRF concentrations in differentially reared primates. Scatterplot showing cerebrospinal fluid CRF concentrations in grown bonnet macaques whose mothers were exposed to low, high, and variable foraging demands as infants. Pooled data are expressed as means ± *SD*. *Not used for the determination of mean group concentrations. From Coplan et al. (1996). Copyright 1996 by the National Academy of Sciences. Reprinted by permission.

at odds, on the face of it, with Sapolsky's findings of *heightened* levels of cortisol. Differences in negative feedback mechanisms may be implicated.

THE INFLUENCE OF PARENTING STYLES ON EMOTIONALITY IN PRIMATES. Finally, some recent findings from cross-fostering studies in rhesus monkeys have important implications for a discussion of the contribution of parenting styles to a generalized psychological vulnerability to develop anxiety in humans. In these studies with rhesus monkeys, Suomi and colleagues (Suomi, 1999, 2000) experimented with a particularly emotional and stress-reactive group of young monkeys by cross-fostering them to nonreactive mothers. Reactive young animals who were raised by calm mothers for the first 6 months of their lives were able to overcome their biological vulnerability to be reactive. These animals developed normally, demonstrating the kinds of social competence characteristic of nonreactive animals. Furthermore, these changes in their "temperaments" seemed to be permanent, in that they raised their own offspring in a nonreactive and calm manner, much to the benefit of their offspring. On the other hand, infants with the same biological vulnerability raised by emotional and stress-reactive mothers retained their emotionality, perhaps because they developed a synergistic psychological vulnerability. These findings, of course, have implications for the prevention of anxiety (and depression), although we are still a long way from understanding how this process might work in humans. A discussion of the effects of parenting styles on the development of anxiety in humans is provided later in this chapter.

Hippocampal Degeneration and Regeneration in Primates and Patients

The findings on hippocampal alterations as a function of prolonged stress in Sapolsky's baboons are of particular concern, since hippocampal lesions, or changes in hippocampal volume, could potentially predict additional deficits in functioning. Now results suggesting decreased hippocampal volume have been replicated in a number of studies of patients with anxiety disorders, particularly PTSD. For example, Bremner, Randall, Scott, et al.(1995) measured hippocampal volume in 26 Vietnam combat veterans who met diagnostic criteria for PTSD, as well as 22 noncombat, nonanxious control subjects matched on a number of demographic and physical variables. Results indicated an 8% decrease in hippocampal volume for patients with PTSD relative to control subjects. Stein, Koverola, Hanna, Torchia, and McClarty (1997) found very similar results in women who were survivors of childhood sexual abuse, compared to women who had not been thus abused. Gurvits, Shenton, Hokama, and Ohta (1996) also compared Vietnam veterans with PTSD to well-constructed control groups, and confirmed decreased hippocampal volume in patients with PTSD (compared to combat veterans without PTSD, as well as nonanxious nonveterans). Furthermore, there were no statistically significant group differences in the intracranial cavity, the whole brain, the ventricles, the ventricle–brain ratio, or the amygdala among these groups. In an interesting and important finding, hippocampal volume was directly correlated with amount of combat exposure, which further strengthens the link between hippocampal damage and stress. Similarly, Bremner, Vermetten, Southwick, Krystal, and Charney (1998) did not find a difference in volume of the amygdala between patients with combat-related PTSD and control subjects. Bremner, Randall, et al. (1997) also examined hippocampal volume in 17 male and female adults with a history of severe childhood physical and/or sexual abuse who met current criteria for PTSD. When these patients were compared to 17 healthy control subjects, a 12% reduction in hippocampal volume was found. More recently, hippocampal atrophy has also been found in patients with either current or past major depressive disorder (Sheline, Wang, Gado, Csernansky, & Vannier, 1996; Bremner, 1999).

Of course, it is well known that the hippocampus plays an important role in new learning and memory (Zola-Morgan & Squire, 1990; Bremner, 1999). As Bremner (1999) points out, patients with PTSD *do* present with a variety of cognitive deficits—including deficits in declarative memory, as well as commonly observed fragmentation of memories, particularly concerning trauma-related material. For example, decreases in immediate and delayed recall, as well as short-term memory, have been demonstrated in patients with PTSD (Sass et al., 1992; Bremner, Randall, Capelli, et al., 1995). Deficits in implicit memory have also been noted (see Brewin, Dalgleish, & Joseph, 1996). These memory deficits are in evidence in Desert Storm veterans as well (Vasterling, Brailey, Constans, & Sotker, 1998). Interestingly, Bremner, Randall, Capelli, et al. (1995) suggest that this fragmentation of memory reported clinically in patients suffering from past trauma is what may account for difficulty in recalling at least some aspects of the trauma, thereby providing a possible anatomical basis for some aspects of this controversial clinical phenomenon. Of course, fragmentation of memory would be quite different from total inability to recall any details of the trauma, and then later recovering that memory some years after that trauma occurred.

Fortunately, as Bremner (1999) points out, there is suggestive evidence that hippocampal atrophy may be reversible. Thus Gould, Tanapat, McEwen, Flugge, and Fuchs (1998) have demonstrated in monkeys that the hippocampus is unique in its capacity to regenerate neurons even after neuronal death. Now Starkman et al. (1999) report results from 22 patients with hippocampal atrophy due to Cushing's disease (which causes chronic hypercortisolemia) and found increases of up to 10% in hippocampal volume following successful treatment.

Summary of Findings from Animal Studies

Findings from the animal laboratories have important implications for the relationship of experiences with unpredictability and uncontrollability to fear and panic. For example, Mineka's monkeys evidenced more extreme fear (alarm, panic) when confronted with a potentially life-threatening situation if they had experienced unpredictability or uncontrollability over important life events. During development, presumably, they were already in a cycle of anxious apprehension. We also know from evidence reviewed in Chapter 5 that among the best predictors of successful panic provocation in the laboratory are the high baseline anxiety and arousal characteristic of "chronically" anxious individuals. It is possible that the results described above constitute an animal analogue of the common clinical observation that panic attacks tend to "spike off" a platform of high baseline anxiety, leading to a classic vicious spiral of anxious apprehension and panic. More precisely, chronic anxious apprehension lowers the threshold for panic. It is also possible that panic attacks represent learned alarms to the arousal cues associated with the catecholamine surges and HPA axis activity characteristic of anxiety, as detailed in Chapters 6 and 7.

Taken together, this evidence indicates that in animals at least, early stress—particularly uncontrollable and/or unpredictable life events—leads to increased HPA axis responding, negative emotionality (chronic anxious apprehension), and alarm reactions. Instillation of a sense of mastery or control during development seems to protect against the likelihood of an anxious response. Other evidence indicates that monkeys receiving social support from a monkey peer group will have fewer anxiety reactions than will monkeys reared in isolation (Mineka, 1985a, 1985b). The results from cross-fostering studies of positive partnering remained above (Suomi, 1999) also seem to produce marked reductions in stress reactivity and anxiety, and suggest the possibility of preventive strategies. The development of coping responses that imply a sense of control (whether real or apparent) buffers anxiety as well (Suomi, 1986; Coplan et al., 1996; Heim & Nemeroff, 1999). With this suggestive evidence in mind, it becomes possible to examine findings on the etiology of human anxious apprehension.

The Development of Anxiety in Humans

Locus of Control and Attributional Style

Efforts to examine directly the role of control in humans actually date back to the work of Julian Rotter (1954). Rotter theorized that one's "locus of control" could be rated along a dimension of internal to external causality, and developed an instrument to measure perception of control (Rotter, 1966). He suggested that the extent to which a person attributes a response–stimulus relationship as internally or personally controlled mediates the extent to which an event is reinforcing. Rotter's ideas sparked a new generation of research on cognitive manifestations of a sense of control in humans, including "locus of control," "attributional style," and psychometrically sound questionnaires to measure these constructs. After several unsuccessful attempts by other investigators, Nowicki and Strickland (1973) developed the first psychometrically sound measure of locus of control in children, the Nowicki–Strickland Locus of Control Scale (Barlow, Charpita, & Turovsky, 1996). Using this scale, investigators found that an external locus of control was significantly positively correlated with both anxiety (Nunn, 1988) and depression (McCauley, Mitchell, Burke, & Moss, 1988; Siegel & Griffin, 1984) in clinical samples of children. These studies suggested once again that a sense of being unable to control one's environment is associated with higher levels of anxiety.

Of course, definitional issues become prominent when these constructs are applied to humans. For example, locus of control may be a somewhat different construct from perceptions of control related to anxiety, in that locus of control is rather general, and therefore perhaps less relevant to the development of negative emotions (e.g., Rapee, Craske, Brown, & Barlow, 1996; Chorpita & Barlow, 1998). For example, we (Rapee et al., 1996) demonstrated in an adult sample that a more specific measure of perceived control over threat and one's reactions to threat (the Anxiety Control Questionnaire) was more highly correlated with measures of anxiety in adult clinical samples than was Rotter's more general measure. In any case, it appears that the measurement of perceived control as a vulnerability to negative emotional states requires more development in both adults and children (e.g., Skinner, Chapman, & Baltes, 1988; Weisz & Stipek, 1982).

Research on control-related cognitions has also emerged from the multidimensional construct of attributional style, although, as noted above, much of the initial focus of this work was on depression. As stated earlier, Seligman (1975) hypothesized that when repeatedly faced with negative life events, people develop a belief that they do not have control over their environment. Feeling helpless, they cease to act on the environment (or cease attempting to cope), and depression ensues. Abramson, Seligman, and Teasdale (1978) reformulated this theory. They suggested that the relationship between negative life events and learned helplessness is moderated by one's attributional style. That is, the experience of negative events is not sufficient to develop helplessness. Rather, negative life events are most likely to lead to learned helplessness when a person makes internal, global, and stable attributions regarding the negative events. Abramson, Metalsky, and Alloy (1989) modified this theory further and emphasized the role of hopelessness rather than helplessness as more specific to depression. They suggested that for many forms of depression, attributions play a causal role only when they contribute to a sense of hopelessness in which individuals despair of ever attaining any influence over important events in their world. Helplessness, in their view, is more relevant to anxiety.

The most rigorous attempts to examine the role of attributional style in the development of anxiety and depression have involved prospective methodology. For example, Nolen-Hoeksema, Girgus, and Seligman (1986) examined attributional style in a sample of 168 schoolchildren in a 1-year longitudinal investigation. A composite score from the six scales of the Children's Attributional Style Questionnaire (CASQ; Seligman et al., 1984) was used to assess attributional style. Composite scores were found to be correlated with concurrent depression as measured by the Children's Depression Inventory (CDI; Seligman et al., 1984). More noteworthy, however, the composite CASQ scores were found to be predictive of increases in CDI scores over time. The relationship held in the other direction as well: CDI scores were found to predict changes in CASQ style over time.

Nolen-Hoeksema, Girgus, and Seligman (1992) extended the investigation, and in so doing provided fascinating information regarding the development and subsequent effects of cognitive response styles in childhood and early adolescence. They conducted a 5-year longitudinal study that aimed to identify predictors of depression in childhood. Children were recruited from third-grade classes in suburban elementary schools. At nine assessment points over the 5-year period, children and teachers completed self-report questionnaires. The authors found that in early childhood, negative life events rather than control cognitions or explanatory style were the best predictors of depression. But they also found that the presence of depression in early childhood led to a deterioration of explanatory style. Specifically, children who experienced depression at a young age developed an increased tendency to make internal, stable, and global attributions for negative life events, and to make external, unstable, and specific attributions for positive events. This pessimistic explanatory style was found to predict a recurrence of depression in later childhood, with negative life events predicting the specific time at which relapse occurred. In other words, there is a suggestion that cognitive style comes to *mediate* negative life events and depression in older children. I return to a discussion of structural models of etiology below.

The results of this study suggest that adult models of depression (e.g., Abramson et al., 1978) may apply only to older children. The data indicate that by early adolescence, certain cognitive response styles develop. Maladaptive cognitive response styles (which may result from childhood depression, early negative life events, or a combination) serve as a psychological vulnerability or diathesis. Thus, when faced with negative life events, adolescents with such cognitive styles seem to be at a greater risk of developing depression.

Some important new findings suggest that the focus on the relationship of control cognitions to depression has been misleading, and that anxiety is the first consequence of this negative cognitive style. For example, Cole, Peeke, Martin, Truglio, and Seroczynski (1998) have conducted what may be the most informative study to date of the temporal relationship between the development of anxiety and depression in children. A total of 330 elementary school students and their parents participated in this 3-year longitudinal study. Data were collected from both children and parents on the presence of anxiety and depressive symptoms every 6 months during the 3-year period. After prior levels of depressive symptoms were controlled for, the findings clearly indicated that high levels of anxiety symptoms at one point in time predicted high levels of depressive symptoms at subsequent points in time. These results were consistent across self-reports and parent reports. Results from this prospective longitudinal study clearly supported the temporal hypothesis that anxiety leads to depression in children and adolescents. In fact, this finding had been repeatedly obtained in prior studies, albeit with less satisfactory methodologies (Hershberg, Carlson, Cantwell, & Strober, 1982; Kovacs, Gatsonis, Paulauskas, & Richards, 1989; Orvaschel, Lewinsohn, & Seeley, 1995; Lewinsohn, Gotlib, & Seeley, 1995).

In a similar vein, Lutin, Ralph, and Mineka (1997) reported that a pessimistic attributional style was related more strongly to underlying negative affect than to anxiety or depression specifically. They also suggest that a generalized psychological vulnerability—as represented by a pessimistic attributional style reflecting a sense of uncontrollability—may lead initially to anxiety, followed by depression.

Gender Differences in Cognitive Styles

I have argued elsewhere (along with several of my colleagues, particularly Susan Nolen-Hoeksema) that the effects of negative life events, uncontrollability, and attributional style account in part for the preponderance of women among those with anxiety or depressive disorders (Barlow, 1988, 1991a; Mineka, 1985a; Nolen-Hoeksema, 1987, 1990; Nolen-Hoeksema & Girgus, 1994). The notion behind this argument is that, compared with boys, girls may be subjected to a larger number of negative life events during childhood and adolescence. In addition, girls may learn that their behaviors have less impact on their environment. Both of these factors are thought to contribute to a sense of uncontrollability in girls and foster the development of pessimistic attributional styles. Maladaptive cognitive responses, then, may place girls at higher risk for emotional disorders. In support of this argument, there are data suggesting that girls may be more likely to experience negative life events (e.g., childhood sexual abuse) that lead to a sense of helplessness (Cutler & Nolen-Hoeksema, 1991; Nolen-Hoeksema & Girgus, 1994). Furthermore, results from a number of studies suggest that both parents and teachers respond more to the actions (positive and negative) of boys than to those of girls (see Nolen-Hoeksema, 1990, for a review). As a result, females may be more likely than males to learn from interactions with others that their behavior does not have an impact on the environment (Barlow et al., 1996; Nolen-Hoeksema, 1987).

Of course, studies on cognitive style are correlational for the most part, and provide only limited insight into the development of a sense of uncontrollability (manifested, perhaps, in a specific pattern of control cognitions or attributional style). These studies do not answer the question concerning the origins of these control-related cognitions, although hints of these origins are present in the negative life events experienced by young children who later became depressed in the Nolen-Hoeksema et al. (1992) study. But what were these events? More relevant information has emerged only recently through a series of studies on early environment and the role of parenting styles.

The Influence of Parenting Styles

In discussing how a sense of control might develop, Shear (1991) draws a specific connection between the psychological dimension of control and a child's early experience with parenting when she states,

> It is certain that interpersonal relationships influence importantly the development of an individual's sense of control. As already noted, the human infant is almost completely helpless. Its only route to controlling the environment is via its effects on caretakers. In this sense, the infant and small child experience the world much as the yoked control in . . . animal experi-

ments . . . (Mineka et al., 1986). The adults exert control and the child is the passive recipient. (p. 90)

When parents are insensitive to their child's expressive, exploratory, and independent behaviors, the child is at risk of developing inhibition and a sense of uncontrollability over his or her world, which may contribute to anxiety. This notion is similar to Bowlby's (1980) view of parents as attachment objects (see below); however, Shear (1991) states that lack of perceived control need not necessarily be instilled by separation or loss experiences, or by a high frequency of stressful experiences. Rather, a "malfunctioning relationship" involving an intrusive, overprotective, or controlling parenting style could be expected to make a strong contribution to a cognitive vulnerability for anxiety.

At present, there is some evidence supporting two related propositions: first, that a particular set of family characteristics is associated with the development of a sense of control, most often manifested as control-related cognitions in children (e.g., Schneewind, 1995); and, second, that a particular set of family characteristics is associated with the development of anxiety and its disorders (e.g., Turner, Beidel, & Costello, 1987), as well as with depression. After selected evidence is reviewed for each of these two propositions, it becomes possible to propose that family characteristics, a sense of control, and anxiety are linked in a mediational structure in early development.

PARENTING STYLES AND THE DEVELOPMENT OF A SENSE OF CONTROL. Some evidence has appeared on the relation of family structure to the development of a sense of control. One might predict that children who have access to undivided attention from parents, and who need not compete with siblings for attention or other reinforcers, should be more likely to develop a sense of control over events. A number of studies have documented this relationship, demonstrating, for example, that first-born children display a more internal locus of control than later-born children (Crandall, Katkovsky, & Crandall, 1965; Hoffman & Teyber, 1979; Krampen, 1982). In addition, some hints have appeared that family size is related to a sense of control, such that beliefs about external locus of control increase in later-born children as family size increases (Walter & Ziegler, 1980). But what are the specific parental behaviors within these family structures that facilitate or inhibit the development of a sense of control?

A consensus has developed that two dimensions should be most important (Chorpita & Barlow, 1998). First, parents who are more contingently responsive should provide children with more opportunities to exercise control over their environment by influencing their parents' behavior (particularly the provision of attention, food, etc.) early in life in a consistent, predictable manner. Second, parents who are less intrusive and protective should provide children with more occasions to explore their world and develop new skills to cope with unexpected environmental occurrences. Manipulating their environment in this way should help cultivate an enhanced sense of control over events. These parenting dimensions can be abbreviated as follows: (1) warmth or sensitivity, consistency, and contingency; and (2) encouragement of autonomy and absence of intrusion or of an overcontrolling style (Chorpita & Barlow, 1998).

The relation of both dimensions of parenting to the development of a sense of control have received empirical support, and this evidence has been thoroughly reviewed elsewhere (Chorpita & Barlow, 1998). First, the children of parents who are consistently and contingently responsive evidence a more internalized locus of control (Diethelm, 1991; Schneewind & Pfeiffer, 1978). For example, Davis and Phares (1969) documented an association between inconsistent parental behavior during a family decision-making task and children's external locus of control. Similarly, Skinner (1986) used observational methodology to assess parental contingent responsiveness and found a tendency for high parental responsiveness to be positively associated with children's internal locus of control.

Second, parents who provide more opportunity for autonomy and independence, and who encourage the development of new skills, are more likely to foster beliefs about internal locus of control in their children (Chandler, Wolf, Cook, & Dugovics, 1980; Gordon, Nowicki, & Wichern, 1981). Parents of children with a more highly developed sense of control are more likely to reward, value, or encourage independence (e.g., Gordon et al., 1981). Conversely, Carton and Nowicki (1994) reviewed several studies documenting the association between high external locus of control in children and parental dimensions of overprotectiveness (e.g., Biocca, 1985) and intrusive governing (e.g., Washington, 1974). Thus it appears that both parental dimensions (warmth, consistency, and contingency on the one hand, and encouraging autonomy on the other) provide opportunities for a child to experience control over reinforcing events in early development, through social contingency and mastery of the environment. Over time, such experiences can become part of the child's stored (learned) information and contribute to a generalized sense of control (e.g., Bryant & Trockel, 1976; Carton & Nowicki, 1994).

Nolen-Hoeksema, Wolfson, Mumme, and Guskin (1995) examined the influence of these dimensions of parenting in a particularly elegant manner. Two groups of 5- to 7-year-old children were compared with respect to their ability to demonstrate mastery versus helplessness in a puzzle task, completed jointly with their mothers. But one group of mothers suffered from major depressive disorder. Mothers in the other group did not. Interestingly, a maternal diagnosis of major depression did not account for differences in children's display of helplessness; rather, the degree to which mothers were responsive and able to encourage active problem solving was the important factor. This highlights the importance of a specific link between parental behavior and a sense of control in children. That is, it does not seem to be maternal depressed affect per se that influences children's development of a sense of diminished control, but specific parental behaviors that provide and encourage opportunities for control over events. Of course, the studies described above do not establish that a diminished sense of control ultimately leads to anxiety or depression.

PARENTING STYLES AND THE DEVELOPMENT OF ANXIETY AND DEPRESSION. Studies relating parenting style to the later development of anxiety and depression in children implicate the same two dimensions of parenting behavior reviewed above as influential. For example, Stark, Humphrey, Crook, and Lewis (1990) assessed families in which a child was diagnosed with a mood disorder, an anxiety disorder, both a mood disorder and an anxiety disorder, or neither a mood nor an anxiety disorder. Fifty-one children and their mothers completed a self-report measure assessing their perception of their family interactions. Mothers of anxious children did not differ significantly from mothers of controls in their perceptions of the family. However, children with emotional disorders (an anxiety disorder, a mood disorder, or both) rated their parents as significantly less supportive, less socially engaged, more enmeshed, and less willing to involve them in decisions being made about them and their families. Of course, the emotional disorders may have influenced the children's reports. But this study at least suggests that children who are less likely to develop a sense of autonomy, and who feel they are not involved in making decisions that affect them, may experience a sense of uncontrollability that then leads to an emotional disorder. This study is also limited by its reliance on self-report measures, and the fact that children were assessed only for mood and anxiety disorders, not for other forms of psychopathology.

Siqueland, Kendall, and Steinberg (1966) examined a similar question with improved methodology. They assessed families with and without children who had an anxiety disorder to examine differences in family interactions. Participants were 17 families with a child who met *Diagnostic and Statistical Manual of Mental Disorders*, Fourth edition (DSM-IV) criteria for an anxiety disorder, and 27 families that served as nonclinic controls. The Anxiety Disorders Interview Schedule for Children (Silverman & Nelles, 1988) was administered to children and parents in the clinical group. Each family completed self-report measures and participated in four videotaped interaction tasks in which the child, and one or both parents, were asked to discuss a topic about which they disagreed. Ratings by independent observers indicated that parents of children with anxiety disorders gave their children less psychological autonomy than did nonclinic parents. In addition, children with anxiety disorders rated their parents as less accepting than did nonclinic children.

In a study that yielded similar results, Dumas, LaFreniere, and Serketich (1995) evaluated the nature of interpersonal exchanges in mother–child dyads. A total of 126 children were recruited from preschools and were classified as socially competent, aggressive, or anxious. The children were asked to complete a task while mothers observed and assisted. Mother–child interactions were videotaped and rated for the presence of control, coercion, and positive and aversive behavior and affect. Positive interactions included use of laughter, assistance, and affection. Aversive interactions included use of critical punishment, disapproval, or sarcasm. The authors found that, compared with mothers of aggressive or socially competent children, mothers of anxious children were more controlling and more likely to exercise control through aversive behavior or affect. In addition, mothers of anxious children were more likely to use coercive behaviors, and were less likely to comply with children's efforts to assert control. Finally, anxious children complied with their mothers less often than did their aggressive and socially competent counterparts. Taken together, these studies provide evidence that overcontrolling, intrusive parenting styles are associated with anxiety disorders in children. This conclusion is also consistent with findings from a series of studies by Parker and colleagues (Parker, 1983; Silove, Parker, Hadzi-Pavlovic, Manicavasagar, & Blaszczynski, 1991). Parker developed an instrument for adults that retrospectively measures their perception of their mothers' and fathers' parenting styles. The Parental Bonding Instrument is a self-report scale that measures the two dimensions Parker saw as underlying parental attitudes and behaviors: care and protection (Parker, Tupling, & Brown, 1979). Protection is measured along a dimension ranging from affection, emotional warmth, and empathy to indifference, emotional coldness, and rejection. Parker (1983) hypothesized that the parenting style most often associated with anxiety in children is a combination of high protection and low care. He referred to this parenting style as "affectionless control."

Silove et al. (1991) administered the Parental Bonding Instrument to 80 patients seeking treatment for panic disorder or generalized anxiety disorder. This information was compared with data obtained from a matched control sample. The authors found that, overall, patients reported receiving less parental care and greater parental overprotection as children. Results of logistical regression indicated that patients with panic disorder tended to rate their parents as affectionate and overprotective, whereas patients with generalized anxiety disorder tended to rate their parents as affectionless and overprotective.

It is clear that there is evidence for a relation between high levels of anxiety in children and overcontrolling, intrusive family environments. However, at this point the relationship must be described as correlational. Longitudinal studies focusing on very young children are needed to determine whether these overcontrolling, intrusive parenting styles predate the onset of anxiety disorders, or whether this parenting style is a response to anxious behavior in children. Thus far, however, the data are at least consistent with the notion that a low sense of control related to specific parenting styles contributes to high levels of anxiety.

Well-done studies have also examined the effects of parenting styles on the development of later depression. Reiss et al. (1995) conducted a cross-sectional evaluation of the effects of various dimensions of parenting on symptoms of depression in adolescents from 708 families. In a structural equation analysis, multiple indicators of parenting variables were examined in terms of their relation to self- or parent-reported symptoms of depression in the adolescent. Parenting was measured by observing coded videotaped interactions of parents with their adolescents, as well as through self-report. Parental behavior was classified into domains of conflict–negativity, warmth–support, and monitoring–control. The results suggested that paternal and maternal warmth-support (cf. Parker's dimension of care) had significant path coefficients (–0.26 and –0.37) to adolescent depressive symptoms, suggesting that low warmth was related to increased depressive symptoms in the offspring. In a second analysis, monitoring–control was not found to be related to depressive symptoms; however, one of this domain's lower-order factors, parental "attempts at control" over an adolescent, was found to have an observable influence on depressive symptoms in that adolescent. Of course, it is not clear that constructs such as "attempts at control" in the Reiss et al. (1995) study are directly related to the parenting styles defined above. But the data support, in general terms, the findings reviewed thus far from studies focusing on the development of anxiety (Chorpita & Barlow, 1998).

Finally, it is important to recognize that although studies of the relation of parenting style to the development of anxiety or depression implicate high protection and intrusiveness and low warmth as significant influences, few studies have examined the role of the purported mediating variable of a diminished sense of control (e.g., attributional style, locus of control). The exception is a study that obtained some preliminary findings in the context of attribution and childhood depression (Nolen-Hoeksema et al., 1992). Similarly, studies reviewed earlier suggesting a link between parenting styles and a sense of uncontrollability did not explore the consequences of this link in terms of subsequent anxiety or depression. Because findings from biological, cognitive, and emotion theory research support the hypothesis that early experiences with control may contribute to the origin of a generalized psychological vulnerability, it is important to continue to examine the structural relationship of parenting styles, a diminished sense of control, and the development of anxiety.

RELATION TO ATTACHMENT THEORY. Before more sophisticated attempts to model the causes of anxiety and depression are examined, it is useful to consider briefly the links between early childhood experience and a diminished sense of control with propositions from attachment theory alluded to above (Bowlby, 1969, 1973, 1980, 1982). These links have been described in some detail in Chorpita and Barlow (1998) but are reviewed briefly here, because early experiences with attachment figures have also been implicated in the existence of long-standing psychological vulnerabilities to develop emotional disorders.

The fundamental notion in attachment theory is that the parent provides a protective and secure base (attachment object) from which the child operates. Thus a secure and predictable relationship with the caregiver (parent) is critical to healthy development. Of interest to us here is the notion that the quality of the relationship with the caregiver is an important antecedent to the development of a possible generalized psychological vulnerability to develop anxiety and depression (Thompson, 1998). For example, Thompson states, "Another kind of expectation emerging from . . . early interactive experiences concerns the infant's emerging sense of agency or effectance," and further, "An awareness that [infants'] signals and actions can have predictable effects on others is fostered by the contingency inherent in the adult's responsiveness" (1998, p. 29). From this observation, one can make a connection between the mutual social influences inherent in secure attachment, and the ideas of consistency and autonomy highlighted in the literature on the development of control cognitions (e.g., Carton & Nowicki, 1994).

Both Rutter (1980) and Sroufe (1990) have detailed the importance of specific parent–child interactions in which the parent is sensitive and empathic to the infant, and allows the infant to communicate his or her needs more clearly, resulting in effective action by the parent to achieve the child's ends. Sroufe (1990), in particular, hypothesizes that a parent's failure to modulate his or her behavior based on perceived desires of the infant may result in the child's internalizing a diminished sense of control over the environment. This process in which internal working models of the earlier attachment relationship are carried forward into adulthood has been referred to as "attachment representations." These representations may reflect one possible method for the development of a generalized psychological vulnerability (Fonagy et al., 1996). It is of some interest that conceptual models and data from attachment theory are closely concordant with independently conceived notions on the development of a sense of controllability and its relation to later emotional disorders (Chorpita & Barlow, 1998).

Advances in Modeling Causes of Anxiety and Depression

A number of researchers have promoted diathesis–stress models of anxiety and depression in adults (see Barlow et al., 1996; Chorpita & Barlow, 1998). In such models, negative life events interact with preexisting vulnerabilities, resulting in emotional disorders. The work of Nolen-Hoeksema et al. (1992) provides preliminary support for this general notion. Before I proceed, it becomes important to delineate two somewhat different structural relations that reflect variations on a stress–diathesis model of the development of emotional disorders (Chorpita & Barlow, 1998). In a "mediational" model, the effects of negative or stressful life events activate the hypothesized generalized psychological vulnerability reflecting a diminished sense of control, which in turn contributes to the development of anxiety or depression. In contrast, a "moderational" model describes a direct relationship between the negative life event and the development of anxiety or depression, which is enhanced or strengthened by the influence of the generalized psychological vulnerability. A depiction of these two models is presented in Figure 8.3 (Chorpita & Barlow, 1998). What Nolen-Hoeksema et al. (1992) have suggested is that moderational models may apply to depression in adults and older children, but may not be applicable for younger children.

Cole and Turner (1993) used structural equation modeling to explore these alternative models. Participants were nonclinical fourth-grade ($n = 123$), sixth-grade ($n = 118$), and eighth-grade ($n = 115$) boys and girls from elementary and middle schools. The children completed self-report instruments designed to measure depressive symptoms, attributional style, and the frequency and valence of positive and negative events; peers' impressions of children's competency were also collected. With use of structural equation modeling, the data were applied to both mediational and moderational models of depression. The results indicated that negative peer competency evaluations and negative life events influenced attributional style, which in turn influenced depressive symptoms. These results also support a mediational model of depression in childhood. Limited support for a moderational model of childhood depression emerged, in contrast to adult depression, where moderational models seem better supported.

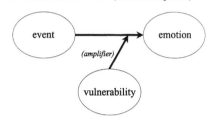

A Mediational Model (early development)

B Moderational Model (later development)

FIGURE 8.3. Mediational and moderational models of the influence of psychological factors on the expression of emotion. From "The Development of Anxiety" by B. F. Chorpita and D. H. Barlow, 1998, *Psychological Bulletin, 124,* 3–21. Copyright 1998 by the American Psychological Association. Reprinted with permission.

As the authors themselves admonish, the results of this study are correlational and must be interpreted with caution. Nevertheless, this study points the way to a better theoretical understanding of childhood depression and possibly other emotional disorders. Once again, the results support the notion that the moderational model often applied to adult depression may not accurately reflect the development of depression in children. It suggests, instead, the potential fit of a mediational model, in which the influence of life events and peer competency evaluations on depressive symptoms is mediated by attributional style and control cognitions.

In a subsequent study, Turner and Cole (1994) once again administered self-report instruments to fourth-grade (*n* = 149), sixth-grade (*n* = 131), and eighth-grade (*n* = 129) children. The self-report instruments were designed to measure attributional style, cognitive errors, and depressive symptoms. A modified version of the Children's Activity Inventory (Shelton & Garber, 1987) was used to measure the occurrence of pleasant and unpleasant events in three domains: sports, academics, and social. In this study, the authors specifically tested for the effects of grade, the domain of events (sports, academic, social), and cognitions associated with each domain. The results of regression analyses indicated a significant interaction of grade (or age), event, and cognitive style for the academic and social domains (but not sports). The authors suggest that such an interaction may be specific to areas in which children deem success more important. Furthermore, results indicated that the interaction between cognitive style and events was significant for eighth graders, but not for fourth and sixth graders, and that cognitive style *moderated* the effects of events in producing depression in these older children. The authors concluded that a moderational diathesis–stress model of depression may apply to older but not to younger children.

We (Chorpita, Brown, & Barlow, 1998b) utilized a cross-sectional design to evaluate these hypotheses in the context of anxiety. Ninety-three families with children between the ages of 6 and 15 years were studied. Sixty-two families were selected from referrals to the Child and Adolescent Fear and Anxiety Treatment Program at Albany; each child had received a principal or co-principal diagnosis of an anxiety or mood disorder. Thirty-one additional families whose children did not meet criteria for any DSM-IV Axis I diagnosis were also recruited as a nonclinical control group. Before hypothetical structural models were evaluated, an initial measurement model allowing all latent variables to be freely intercorrelated was tested. The measurement model and a depiction of the latent variables are presented in Figure 8.4. Model indicators are also presented in this figure. The major hypothesis was that an overcontrolling family environment that fosters diminished personal control should in fact produce a sense of uncontrollability, as reflected in a more external locus of control. This external locus of control should in turn contribute to increased negative affect, and ultimately to clinical symptoms. We also evaluated the possibility, based on evidence from childhood depression studies, that attributional style should function as a mediator in the model.

Compared to a number of alternative models, the model depicting a diminished sense of personal control (external locus of control) functioning as a mediator between a family environment fostering less autonomy, and subsequent negative affect and clinical symptoms, was the best fit for the data. The results are reflected in Figure 8.5 (as the revised hypothesized model). These findings once again suggest that a family environment characterized by limited opportunity for personal control is associated with later anxiety and

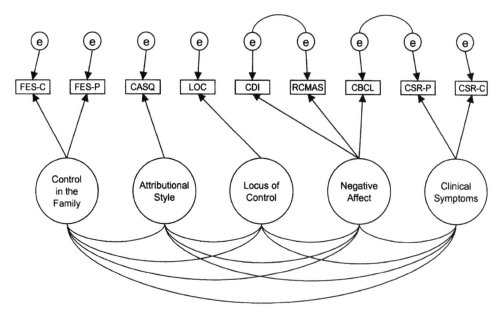

FIGURE 8.4. Measurement model. FES-C, Family Environment Control Scale, child report; FES-P, Family Environment Control Scale, parent report; CASQ, Children's Attributional Style Questionnaire, Stable Negative Scale; LOC, Nowicki–Strickland Locus of Control Scale; RCMAS, Revised Children's Manifest Anxiety Scale; CDI, Children's Depression Inventory; CBCL, Child Behavior Checklist, Internalizing Scale; CSR-C, clinical severity rating, child interview; CSR-P, clinical severity rating, parent interview. From Chorpita, Brown, and Barlow (1998b). Copyright 1998 by the Association for Advancement of Behavior Therapy. Reprinted by permission.

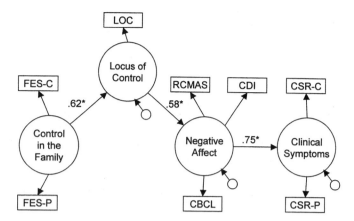

FIGURE 8.5. A structural model of the relation of perceived control to family environment, negative affect, and clinical symptoms. Abbreviations as in Figure 8.4. *$p < .05$. Adapted from Chorpita, Brown, and Barlow (1998b). Copyright 1998 by the Association for Advancement of Behavior Therapy. Adapted by permission.

negative affect. This relationship is mediated by low perceived control in the children, which appears to be a more robust mediator than attributional style.

In summary, the literature on child attributional style has begun to outline a model of the development of anxiety and depression characterized by a generalized psychological vulnerability (or sense of relative uncontrollability) as a mediator between events and anxiety or depression early in development. The general contrast between evidence for a mediational model in early childhood and a moderational model for late childhood and adulthood (Chorpita, Brown, & Barlow, 1998b; Cole & Turner, 1993; Hammen, Adrian, & Hiroto, 1988; Nolen-Hoeksema et al., 1992) suggests an important developmental progression in the formation of this vulnerability. That is, the environment may help to foster a (cognitive) template, with early experience contributing to the formation of a vulnerability (i.e., mediational model). Later in development, this vulnerability may then begin to operate as an amplifier for environmental events (i.e., moderational model). This developmental structure seems to be consistent across models of anxiety and depression.

Family Influences on Neuroendocrine Responding

Earlier in this chapter I have reviewed animal models of anxiety, noting the profound effect of early stressful exposure on neuroendocrine functioning (specifically, HPA axis and CRF activity). As mentioned in that discussion, a common neuroendocrine correlate of anxiety (and depression) is elevated basal cortisol level. As also noted above, Kagan, Reznick, and Snidman (1987) found that children classified as behaviorally inhibited evidenced elevated levels of cortisol. Kagan's temperament of inhibition has been found to be associated with the increased likelihood for the development of anxiety disorders (Hirshfeld et al., 1992). I have also reviewed cross-fostering studies with primates, which demonstrate the buffering effect of positive parenting by calm, emotionally nonreactive mothers on young rhesus monkeys with heightened HPA axis activity and elevated reactivity to stress (e.g., Suomi, 1999). An emerging area of research in humans involves family influences on neuroendocrine responding.

Several studies illustrate this theme. In one study, Nachmias, Gunnar, Mangelsdorf, Parritz, and Buss (1996) examined cortisol responding in 77 infants exposed to novel stimuli (e.g., clowns, puppets). As expected, only inhibited children showed elevations in salivary cortisol. However, examing parenting behavior among the inhibited children revealed a more interesting finding: salivary cortisol change scores were noted only for those with insecure attachment (avoidant or resistant). The responding of the securely attached inhibited children looked like that of the uninhibited children. These findings suggest that inferences about the developmental elaboration of inhibited temperament may need to consider the influence of parenting. The connection between attachment quality and perceptions of control suggests that a sense of control exerts a potentially important influence on temperament.

Gunnar, Larson, Hertsgaard, Harris, and Broderson (1992) examined the influence of control cognitions by examining caretakers' ability to influence HPA axis activity (specifically, cortisol responding). In this study, Gunnar (1994) conceptualized separation from parents as involving loss of control: "Not only is the child blocked from access to the mother (loss of control over proximity), but the child also loses the mother's help in controlling the internal and external environment" (p. 182). Gunnar et al. (1992) demonstrated that 9-month-old infants showed an elevated cortisol response when separated from their mothers, but that this effect was eliminated when an infant was accompanied by a highly responsive caretaker versus a less responsive caretaker. These results suggest that contingent access (control) over positive (appetitive) stimulation may play an important role in reducing HPA axis responding, recalling the findings of Mineka et al. (1986) with primates. Along with the findings of Nachmias et al. (1996), these results highlight the potential importance of the reciprocal influence between parent–child interaction and temperamental factors related to anxiety.

Finally, Granger, Weisz, and Kauneckis (1994) specifically examined the effects of a sense of control, as well as of current behavioral and emotional problems, on cortisol levels in children as a function of a parent–child conflict task. They assessed 102 clinic-referred children and adolescents aged 7–17. Patients presented with a variety of difficulties. The task involved prompting parent–child conflict in the session through discussion of current issues, such as chores or homework, that both the parent and child agreed were conflictual. The dependent variables were cortisol levels (based on salivary samples). They found that children with higher neuroendocrine activation were more socially withdrawn and socially anxious, had more social problems, and perceived themselves as having less personal control over the outcomes of their lives. They also tended to perceive social outcomes as being less contingent on their actions in general than did low reactors. Although the findings are correlational, they suggest that children with a lower sense of control during parent–child conflict may evidence exaggerated HPA axis reactivity in the face of stressors.

These studies, then, create an important link between the effects of early stressful experiences (particularly those associated with intrusive, controlling parenting styles) and the development of a generalized psychological vulnerability (manifested as diminished control cognitions). This vulnerability in turn directly influences the expression of clinical and neurobiological correlates of anxiety and depression in both humans and animals.

Protective Factors

Of course, nonoptimal parenting and related early experiences are not the only factors influencing the development of a sense of control. A number of alternative experiences seem to contribute in a constructive fashion to an adaptive sense of control. In Chapter 6, I have reviewed evidence summarized by Dienstbier (1989) that early exposure to stressful manipulations in rats, such as shock or rough handling, can actually lead to a healthy psychological profile characterized by low resting levels of cortisol and autonomic flexibility when the rats are confronted with stress or challenges. To produce the desirable psychophysiological profile that becomes adaptive in the face of stressful experiences later in life, these early experiences must be brief, predictable, and controllable. Dienstbier refers to this adaptive psychophysiological profile as "toughening," extending Neal Miller's (1980) conception of "toughening up."

Parallel investigations examining the varied effects of stress on children have been carried out by Garmezy and colleagues (Garmezy, 1986; Garmezy & Rutter, 1983; Masten, Best, & Garmezy, 1991). Garmezy has referred to the effects of these protective factors as the "steeling effect" (Garmezy, 1986), in which certain stressors may actually immunize or enhance subsequent functioning of the individual. The parallel to Dienstbier's "toughening" is clear. Rachman's (1979) notion of "required helpfulness" describes a related phenomenon. Specifically, Rachman describes a number of studies in which children from high-risk environments were called on to contribute to efforts of the larger group, such as a family or a community, to deal with substantial short-term or long-term adversity. The efforts of these children at coping with adversity as best they could, and therefore helping those around them, seems to have produced a similar "steeling effect" or "toughening effect" when faced with their own adversity later in life (e.g., Elder, 1974).

Masten et al. (1991) specify four factors that could contribute to this "steeling effect." In addition to responsive parenting (reviewed at length above) in both primates and humans, intellectual skill and social-cognitive ability seem to make separate contributions to later adaptive functioning. Masten et al. cite Bandura's (1986) notion of self-efficacy as a fourth factor, and this notion is very close to the construct of controllability referred to throughout this chapter. Thus much of the important body of research produced during the past 20 years on self-efficacy becomes somewhat relevant. However, as noted in the first edition of this book, there are also some subtle differences in definition between self-efficacy and a sense of control. In the present model, control is related to the degree to which an organism has the possibility to influence opportunities for positive or negative reinforcement, and is not specific to the organism's actual performance. Self-efficacy, on the other hand, has traditionally been tied more closely to performance. But the constructs do overlap somewhat, and undoubtedly research findings from each tradition have relevance to the other.

Generalized Psychological Vulnerability: Conclusions

It is important to note that acquisition of a generalized psychological vulnerability, in isolation, is unlikely to lead to a clinical disorder. The expected outcome in the absence of a synergistic biological (heritable) vulnerability would be a personality style characterized by pessimism, low self-confidence and self-esteem, and lack of initiative. Of course, these dimensions of personality associated with biological and psychological vulnerabilities rarely occur in isolation from one another, and my purpose here is to outline a model of the development of anxious apprehension based on generalized biological (genetic) and generalized psychological (early experience) dimensions.

As detailed elsewhere (Chorpita & Barlow, 1998) and discussed above, genetic contributions to the development of anxious apprehension seem to account for approximately 30–50% of the variance. But the neurobiological processes underlying anxious apprehension that may emerge from this biological (genetic) diathesis seem to be influenced substantially by early psychological processes, contributing to a generalized psychological vulnerability. In this sense, early experiences with controllability and predictability, based in large part (but not exclusively) on interactions with caregivers,

> ... contributes to something of a psychological template, which at some point becomes relatively fixed and diathetic. Stated another way, this psychological dimension of a sense of control is possibly a mediator between stressful experience and anxiety, and over time this sense becomes a somewhat stable moderator of the expression of anxiety.... (Chorpita & Barlow, 1998, p. 16)

A preliminary conceptual model outlining these operations is presented in Figure 8.6.

Once again, early experiences with uncontrollable or unpredictable events lead to low perceptions of control and increased neurobiological activity, perhaps best reflected as increased activity in Gray's behavioral inhibition system or BIS ("Gray's anxiety") with heavy involvement of the CRF system. This is followed by a variety of undifferentiated somatic outputs, as described early by Kagan and colleagues (e.g., Kagan et al., 1987). At a later developmental period, this diminished sense of controllability then acts as a diathesis in the context of stressful life events. The resulting long-term effects of chronic activation of the BIS and CRF systems may lead to hypercortisolism and glucocorticoid feedback insensitivity, which in turn may result in further BIS activation. This generalized psychological vulnerability also accounts for the chronic cognitive biases seen in anxiety and related disorders. Thus a "neurotic temperament" is formed.

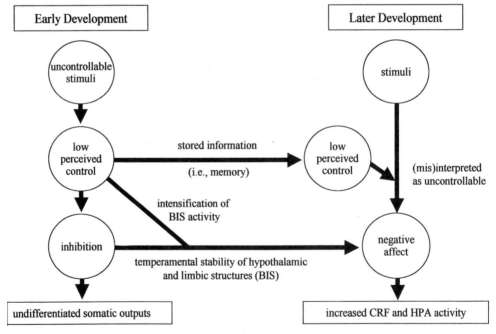

FIGURE 8.6. Model of the development of vulnerability for anxiety and depression. BIS, behavioral inhibition system; CRF, corticotropin-releasing factor; HPA, hypothalamic–pituitary--adrenocortical. From "The Development of Anxiety" by B. F. Chorpita and D. H. Barlow, 1998, *Psychological Bulletin, 124*, 3–21. Copyright 1998 by the American Psychological Association. Reprinted by permission.

In summary, a synergism of generalized biological (genetic) and generalized psychological (early experience) vulnerabilities is likely to lead to the clinical syndromes of generalized anxiety disorder and the depressive disorders, as outlined in Figure 8.7. Notice that false alarms (panic attacks) may occur as a function of stressful life events, facilitated by high levels of baseline anxiety, emerging as a function of these synergistic generalized vulnerabilities. But these false alarms are not in themselves implicated in a clinical disorder. For that to occur, an additional layer of more specific psychological vulnerabilities must be considered.

SPECIFIC PSYCHOLOGICAL VULNERABILITIES: LEARNING WHAT IS DANGEROUS

In the first edition, I alluded to a third set of psychological vulnerabilities that predisposes an individual to focus anxiety on some specific object or event. This particular set of vulnerabilities, also a function of early learning experiences, becomes relevant for certain anxiety disorders where anxious apprehension is focused on potentially dangerous key features. In panic disorder, these are somatic (interoceptive) and other cues signaling the possible occurrence of the next panic attack. In specific phobia, this set of vulnerabilities contributes substantially to determining the particular object or situation that becomes the focus of fear. In social phobia, there is evidence that individuals developing this problem have been differentially subjected to early experiences in which the potential danger of social evaluation was clearly communicated by parents or other important caregivers or friends. In OCD, where obsessional thoughts, images, or urges themselves become the focus of anxiety, there is some evidence that at least some of these individuals have previously learned to equate dangerous thoughts with dangerous actions ("Thinking it is as bad as doing it," or thought–action fusion).

Learning what is threatening, and its later contribution to the development of a disorder, seems to extend beyond the anxiety disorders to closely related somatoform and eating disorders, to take just two additional examples from the "neurotic spectrum." For example, considerable evidence exists that individuals (particularly adolescent girls) who engage in activities where the "dangers" of being overweight are frequently conveyed are

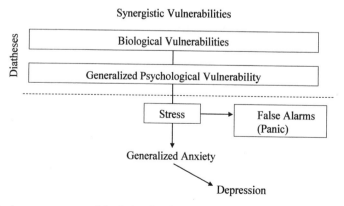

FIGURE 8.7. Diatheses–stress model of the development of generalized anxiety and depression.

at somewhat greater risk for developing an eating disorder than if they are not exposed to those experiences (Barlow & Durand, 1999). Similarly, individuals developing hypochondriasis or body dysmorphic disorder undergo similar experiences relating to the potential dangers of becoming sick or being evaluated on the basis of physical appearance, respectively (Barlow & Durand, 1999). But our focus here is on anxiety disorders. It is also important to note that, much as with other, more generalized biological and psychological vulnerabilities, the presence of this specific vulnerability set seems insufficient in isolation to lead to the development of an emotional disorder. Rather, there must be a synergy among generalized biological and psychological vulnerabilities and more specific psychological vulnerabilities to set the occasion for the development of one emotional disorder versus another, as outlined in Figure 8.8.

To take the example of panic disorder, as noted in the first edition of this book,

> A substantial determinant [of the focus of anxiety on future panic attacks] may be a pre-existing disposition to focus anxiety specifically on somatic events . . . [which] may be the reason why so many patients with panic disorder end up in the offices of cardiologists and other non-psychiatric physicians . . . while patients with other anxiety disorders (often with equal frequencies of panic [attacks]) do not. It is for this reason also that a large overlap exists between panic disorder and somatization disorders . . . (Barlow, 1988, pp. 367–368)

We (Bouton et al., 2001) review evidence for the acquisition of this specific psychological vulnerability in some detail. Many of these studies have been reviewed in Chapter 7, where I conclude that this predisposition contributes a small amount of the variance to the development of panic attacks (both clinical and nonclinical), but is far more relevant as a vulnerability to developing panic disorder. Thus it is important to recap the evidence briefly. For example, Turkat (1982) and Whitehead, Winget, Fedoravicius, Wooley, and Blackwell (1982) found that individuals as adults were more likely to engage in sick role behavior (not going to work, canceling activities, seeking medical help, etc.) if they had been differentially attended to or reinforced when they were ill as children. This information often seems transmitted via the well-known psychological mechanism of modeling, in which parental reactions to somatic symptoms, illness, and disease are transmitted to their offspring—particularly if these reactions involve fear, anxiety, or perceived danger.

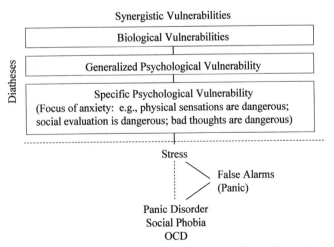

FIGURE 8.8. Triple vulnerabilities in the development of certain anxiety disorders.

In one of the most comprehensive studies addressing the development of these specific vulnerabilities for panic disorder, Ehlers (1993) analyzed early learning experiences encouraging sick role behavior and/or negative evaluations of somatic symptoms in patients with panic disorder, individuals with infrequent panic, patients with anxiety disorders other than panic disorder (mostly specific phobias), and normal controls (see Chapter 7 for details). Support was found for the notion that patients with panic disorder, as well as individuals with infrequent panic, reported experiencing a greater frequency of chronic illness in their households while growing up than patients with other anxiety disorders or control subjects reported. Ehlers noted, "Observing physical suffering can also contribute to the evaluation that somatic symptoms are dangerous and that special care is needed" (1993, p. 276). Patients with panic disorder and persons with infrequent panic attacks also reported observing their parents experience more panic-like somatic symptoms than did subjects in the other groups, and all three groups with anxiety received more parental encouragement for sick role behavior during their own experience of panic-like symptoms ("Take care of yourself and avoid strenuous activities," etc.) than did the nonanxious controls. Remarkably, there were no reported differences in the encouragement of sick role behavior among groups in the event of common colds or other physical illnesses. Thus the focus on the potential danger of somatic symptoms, and the increased frequency of observing these symptoms, seem specific to those who go on to develop anxiety or anxiety disorders.

There is even evidence that preexisting and previously learned sensitivity to specific somatic sensations, such as suffocation cues, differentially predicts panic attacks to respiratory challenges that provoke this specific sensation, such as breathing into a paper bag (e.g., Taylor & Rachman, 1994; McNally & Eke, 1996). That is, those individuals with specific dispositions focusing on the potential danger of one physical symptom will focus anxiety on the possible future occurrence of that symptom, even if it occurs in the context of a web of additional somatic symptoms of equal or greater intensity. More recently, Craske, Poulton, Tsao, and Plotkin (2001) noted the same effect among individuals who had experienced chronic obstructive pulmonary disease among their relatives while growing up. That is, a specific sensitivity to respiratory symptoms as potentially dangerous later developed.

In the context of the development of social phobia, Barrett, Rapee, Dadds, and Ryan (1996) noted that the parents of socially anxious children spent a great deal of time discussing the potential threatening nature of social situations with their children when given the opportunity, and reinforced among their children the tendency to avoid these situations. Earlier work from our center at Albany (Bruch, Heimberg, Berger, & Collins, 1987; Bruch & Heimberg, 1994) suggested that parents of individuals with social phobia are significantly more socially fearful and concerned with evaluative opinions of others than the parents of individuals with panic disorder with agoraphobia. More comprehensive discussions of evidence pertaining to the development of specific psychological vulnerabilities that tend to focus anxiety on one specific key feature or another are provided in the chapters of this book devoted to specific anxiety disorders (Chapters 10–15).

In summary, vicarious learning of anxiety as focused on a variety of key features or situations seems to serve as a specific type of psychological vulnerability for the development of individual anxiety disorders. Once again, these experiences in isolation are not sufficient to produce a clinical disorder. For example, individuals who vicariously learn that physical sensations are potentially dangerous may well develop hypochondriacal tendencies as adults, or differentially attend to illness-related behaviors in their children, but are unlikely themselves to develop a clinical disorder such as panic disorder or hypochondriasis in the absence of more generalized biological and psychological vulnerabilities, as detailed in Figure 8.8.

A MODEL OF CLINICAL ANXIETY DISORDERS

Having presented a model of the development of anxiety, I now discuss in more detail the origins of anxiety disorders. Research reviewed in earlier chapters supporting a clear distinction between the emotional states of panic and anxiety leads directly to a model of the development of clinical anxiety disorders. Specifically, the experience of unexpected panic attacks seems to be a rather common feature in the population at large, as detailed in Chapter 7 (Norton, Harrison, Hauch, & Rhodes, 1985; Norton, Dorwood, & Cox, 1986; Salge, Beck, & Logan, 1988; Telch, Lucas, & Nelson, 1989; Wittchen, 1986; Wittchen & Essau, 1991). But very few of these individuals who experience panic attacks go on to develop a clinical anxiety disorder, such as panic disorder. The difference between these individuals with "nonclinical" panic and those who develop panic disorder is quite striking. Individuals with nonclinical panic show little or no concern over the attacks or the possibility of experiencing another one. Rather, they dismiss the attacks as associated with some passing event or episode, such as something they ate or a difficult day at work. They seem to put the experience behind them quickly. The distinguishing characteristic of individuals with panic disorder is the development of anxious apprehension focused on the next potential unexpected panic attack. Thus individuals with panic disorder apprehensively anticipate the next attack, perceive the attacks as uncontrollable, and are extremely vigilant for somatic symptoms that might signal the beginning of the next attack. The criteria for panic disorder in DSM-IV specify that unexpected panic attacks must be accompanied by anxiety or concern over future attacks (or a change in behavior reflecting this concern) (American Psychiatric Association, 1994). Notice also that nonclinical panickers seem to display a kind of "illusion of control" or a resistance to developing a dysfunctional cognition response set, as mentioned earlier. The illusion of control may well reflect the lack of a generalized psychological vulnerability to develop anxiety focused on what for others would be traumatic events, and/or well-developed emotion regulation skills (Gross & Munoz, 1995; see Chapter 3). Thus, experiencing a false alarm (panic attack) must then be followed by the development of anxious apprehension over the next panic attack in order to meet the criteria for panic disorder, based, of course, on the presence of specific psychological vulnerabilities to focus anxiety on potentially dangerous somatic symptoms, as discussed above. This arrangement is displayed in Figure 8.9 (Barlow et al., 1996).

It should also be noted that one may experience a "true alarm"—that is, a legitimate traumatic experience—and yet follow the same course on the way to developing a clinical disorder. But the disorder in this case should be PTSD rather than panic disorder. Evidence has been developed elsewhere that these two disorders seem to have much in common (Jones & Barlow, 1990). In a similar vein, other anxiety disorders, such as OCD, social phobia, and specific phobia, may also reflect a combination of the occurrence of alarms or panic attacks and the development of anxious apprehension in the context of the triple vulnerabilities described above. For example, social phobia is often characterized by false alarms occurring in social and evaluative situations following a stressful event. The individual then focuses anxiety on upcoming social and evaluative situations (based on having learned that these contacts are potentially threatening) where he or she might experience undue anxiety and possibly a panic attack, resulting in social failure and ridicule. Anxiety focused on intrusive, unacceptable thoughts that may themselves trigger panic attacks often characterizes OCD. Specific phobia reflects alarms learned to specific cues, as well as anxious apprehension in the presence of a specific object or situation.

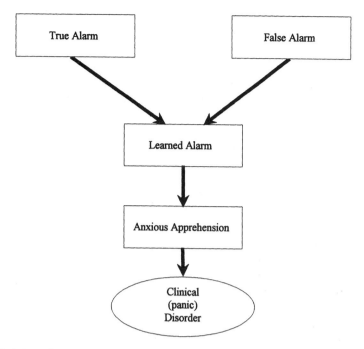

FIGURE 8.9. Origins of panic-related disorders. From Barlow, Chorpita, and Turovsky (1996). Copyright 1996 by University of Nebraska Press. Reprinted by permission.

It would also seem that these conceptualizations of fear, panic, anxiety, and their functional relationship in the context of clinical anxiety disorders have implications for the structure of other emotional disorders such as stress and mood disorders, and for the nature of anger and depression.

THE RELATION OF ANXIETY DISORDERS TO OTHER EMOTIONAL DISORDERS

Anger and Stress

Throughout this book, I have referred to the fight-or-flight reaction. In fact, this is the term that Gray (1987) chooses to describe a single brain system underlining these behavioral action tendencies. Furthermore, on any circumplex of emotion (utilized by theorists to describe hypothetical relations of one emotional state to another), anger and fear are very closely related (see Chapter 2).

But it is "flight" that is the hypothetical behavioral action tendency of fear. The "fight" side of the reaction, reflecting as it does resistance to a dangerous threat and/or attack, is most closely associated with the emotion of anger. The one differentiating characteristic between anger and fear arising out of factor-analytic studies is that anger is characterized by a sense of control and mastery (e.g., Lang, 1994a). This may reflect the notion that angry individuals are directing their attention outward toward the source of threat and attempting to cope actively with the situation. Individuals experiencing fear, on the other hand, do not share this sense of actively coping with the threat.

What determines whether one experiences anger or fear? Once again, there is evidence that early experiences with mastery and control over one's environment may have a substantial influence. In one very relevant experiment, described earlier and summarized here once again for clarity, Insel et al. (1988) reared two groups of rhesus monkeys identically, except for their experiences with nonaversive stimuli in their cages. One group was given free access to toys and food treats. This group served as the control group. For a second group, identical toys and food treats were presented only when they were selected by a matched animal in the control group. Thus this "yoked" group had the same exposure to the toys and food treats, but did not experience *control* over accessing these items. Later in life when these groups were exposed to a traumatic social separation, it was the "yoked" group that exhibited more anxiety. But the more relevant experimental manipulation occurred next. Insel et al. (1986) administered a benzodiazepine inverse agonist to both groups of monkeys. This drug produces a very severe burst of negative affect. Once again, the yoked group displayed significantly more anxiety as indicated by social withdrawal and distress vocalizations. But the monkeys that had experienced control over positive aspects of their environment while growing up had a very different response. They evidenced extreme hostility and aggression, often attacking other monkeys that happened to be nearby.

It is tempting to conclude that reactions expressed by the Insel et al. (1988) animals reflected either flight or fight, and that this varying reaction, at least in this experimental situation, was a function of early experience with mastery and control. Of course, based on the ethological work reviewed above, it seems that all animals will experience either flight reactions or aggressive or resistive responses under some conditions, such as decreasing distance from a predator. But, perhaps, the threshold for one reaction or another differs as a function of early experience. In any case, individuals experiencing anger or fear may share the same biological vulnerability to be overly responsive to stress or challenge. Similarly, they may also experience "false alarms" in response to negative life events, much as do individuals with panic disorder. But individuals experiencing anger, with their momentary mastery and sense of control, have quite a different emotional experience from that of those experiencing fear.

In fact, it seems that many individuals with clinical disorders, including some entering the treatment system, experience repeated "anger attacks." In many cases these anger attacks seem to occur in the context of other emotional disorders, such as panic disorder or major depressive disorder. One patient of ours reported experiencing his first "attack" as an inappropriate angry outburst. This event occurred during a business meeting where the individual felt threatened and stressed. The anger he felt was so overwhelming that he found himself temporarily unable to speak in a coherent manner. At that point, he very consciously experienced a lack of control (over his inability to speak or behave appropriately) and found that his anger attack was quickly transformed into a classic panic attack. This immediately led to the development of social phobia accompanied by anxiety and marked vigilance for somatic symptoms that might signal the beginning of the next attack, particularly during business meetings where some participation was expected.

Similar cases of "anger attacks" appearing in clinics have been reported in other centers (Fava, Anderson, & Rosenbaum, 1990; Rosenbaum et al., 1993). Thus "anger disorder" may bear marked similarities to anxiety and mood disorders and may represent yet another emotional disorder. There is also evidence that anger outbursts occur relatively frequently in the population, with at least one study (Deffenbacher, 1992) reporting that 4–7% of college samples experience anger attacks—a frequency similar to the population frequency of nonclinical panics. As with anxiety and mood disorders, the close relationship between stress and anxiety insures that individuals may present with considerable overlap between the two. For example, Lee and Cameron (1986) reported that almost 75% of a group of patients with anxiety disorders had presented with Type A behavior (based upon a questionnaire), which of course is characterized by frequent angry outbursts. It is also noteworthy that some investigators have noted the importance of distinguishing brief periods of anger or anger attacks from more enduring trait characteristics of anger (Spielberger et al., 1985; Spielberger, Krasner, & Solomon, 1988). Finally, excessive anger is treated in a very similar fashion to anxiety, both psychologically (e.g., Biaggio, 1987; Novaco, 1975, 1994; Robins & Novaco, 2000) and pharmacologically (Fava et al., 1990; Fava & Rosenbaum, 1998; Rosenbaum et al., 1993). Interestingly, in the latter cases, tricyclic antidepressants were often successfully used to treat anger attacks. Thus, experiencing out-of-control attacks of anger to a clinically significant degree may represent another emotional disorder closely paralleling panic disorder. That is, individuals with anger disorder and those with panic disorder may share some of the same biological vulnerabilities, as well as the experience of false alarms. However, people experiencing anger attacks exclusively should be relatively unlikely to focus anxiety on the next upcoming attack, and therefore should present for treatment less often. In describing their patients with anger disorder, Fava et al. (1990; Fava & Rosenbaum, 1998) note that the presence of anger attacks was characterized by episodes of anger that were of short duration and grossly out of proportion to precipitating psychosocial stressors. Somatic symptoms associated with these attacks included sudden surges of autonomic arousal, including symptoms such as increased heartbeat, sweating, and flushing, as well as a feeling that the anger was out of control. None of the patients described anxious, panicky, or fearful emotions. The perception that the attack was out of control may well have come after the fact. Nevertheless, it might have ultimately motivated these particular patients to come for help.

Research suggests that experiencing repeated anger attacks is dangerous. For example, Ironson et al. (1992) instructed individuals with heart disease to imagine situations or events in their own lives that made them angry, compared to imagining other situations (such as exercise) that also increased heart rate. They found that the emotion of anger actually impaired the pumping efficiency of the heart, putting these individuals at risk for arrhythmias. When the same subjects were asked to imagine getting into situations producing performance anxiety (such as having to give a speech or take a difficult test), these experiences did *not* have the same effect on their hearts as the emotion of anger, at least not in those individuals with preexisting coronary heart disease. This raises the interesting possibility of a differential physiological consequence of experiencing anger versus fear or perhaps anxiety. But the finding of impaired pumping efficiency, or lack of it, would have to be first established in individuals *without* coronary heart disease, and then in individuals in the midst of a panic attack, to confirm this differential physiological consequence. On the other hand, new epidemiological facts presented in Chapter 1 suggest that at least in men, chronic anxiety leads to cardiac arrhythmias and increased mortality (Kawachi, Sparrow, Vokonas, & Weiss, 1995).

Finally, I have suggested that both anxious and stressed individuals may share the same biological vulnerability to be overresponsive to stress or challenge. But individuals presenting with classic "stress disorders" such as hypertension or the loosely defined "Type A syndrome" display little or no anxiety over the stress they experience. In fact, the process of anxious apprehension never seems to begin, since their focus of attention remains external and task-oriented. As in the caricature of the hard-driving executive, the coping methods of these individuals seem characterized by hard work, continual attention to achievement, and remarkable confidence in their abilities to deal with problems. The exaggerated sense of mastery and control seems to lead to an almost exclusively external focus of attention on the task at hand (Scheier, Carver, & Matthews, 1983), often at the expense of physical well-being. Evidence suggests that these individuals ignore the warning signs of physical malfunctioning associated with stress disorders. As Scheier et al. (1983) point out, this external focus of attention results in a marked decrease in the amount of attention available for internal focus, and a subsequent lack of sensitivity to internal bodily events. Suls and Fletcher (1985a) confirmed that individuals lower in self-consciousness become ill more often, probably as a result of internal insensitivity. Thus patients with anxiety versus stress disorders may differ not only in terms of perceptions of controllability, but also in self-directed versus externally directed focus of attention. These individuals, with the same biological vulnerabilities reflected in a hyperresponsivity to stress, seem to experience this stress in very different ways—with the subsequent "alarm" response representing flight on the one hand and fight on the other.

Depression

Considerable attention has been focused during the last decade on the relation of anxiety to depression (e.g., Barlow, 1991b; Clark & Watson, 1991; Kendall & Watson, 1989), and this relationship is taken up in some detail in Chapter 9. But an emerging consensus, some of which has been detailed in Chapters 2 and 6 and alluded to earlier in this chapter, suggests that anxiety and depression are variable manifestations of similar (or identical) neurobiological processes (Barlow, 1991a; Brown et al., 1998; Gray & McNaughton, 1996) producing similar symptom profiles. When groups of patients with anxiety disorders can be differentiated from those with depressive disorders, depressive signs and symptoms, not anxious signs and symptoms, are what best discriminate these groups. Specifically, almost all depressed patients are anxious, but not all anxious patients are depressed. This is a robust finding reflected in analyses of self-rating scales, patterns of comorbidity in clinical studies (Brown et al., 1998; Moras, Di Nardo, Brown, & Barlow, 1995; Sanderson, Di Nardo, Rapee, & Barlow, 1990), and examination of broad mood factors of negative and positive affect as originally isolated by Auke Tellegen (e.g., Tellegen, 1985). Specific symptoms that do seem to discriminate individuals with depression from those with anxiety can be characterized as loss of pleasurable engagement, or "anhedonia," along with cognitive and motor retardation, or "slowing." These symptoms constitute the classic "melancholic" cluster (Rush & Weissenburger, 1998). Broadly speaking, these symptoms have been characterized as "low positive affect" in Tellegen's terms; however, the most recent information suggests that social phobia may share this feature with depression (Brown et al., 1998), further obscuring the boundaries. This information, along with the often observed finding that anxiety tends to precede the occurrence of depression, suggests that at least certain types of depression seem to grow out of anxiety, or are complications of anxiety occurring in some people under some conditions. Arriving at a similar conclusion, Alloy, Kelly, Mineka, and Clements (1990) refer to depression emerging out of a state of anxiety as "hopelessness depression." The findings of Cole et al. (1998), reviewed above, confirm the robustness of this finding. Thus the origins of depression may be similar (if not identical) to the origins of anxiety, in that both states may arise out of common biological vulnerabilities, as well as very similar generalized psychological vulnerabilities emerging from early experiences with (lack of) control. When these biological and psychological vulnerabilities line up correctly, the trigger of a stressful negative life event should lead to clinical anxiety and, possibly some time later, to depression. In this view, then, depression simply reflects an extreme psychological vulnerability to experiences of unpredictability and uncontrollability, based on early experiences with controllability and coping. To put it another way, the determination of whether one becomes anxious and stays that way, or also becomes depressed, depends on the extent of one's psychological vulnerability, the severity of the current stressor, and the coping mechanisms at one's disposal.

But the model suggested above for panic disorder, and possibly anger disorder, also suggests the occurrence of a discrete alarm response (fight or flight) that is elaborated into panic or possibly anger attacks. In the case of panic disorder, there is good evidence that individuals focus apprehensive anxiety onto the possibility of a future panic attack, and that this state of affairs is what accounts for the development of a clinical disorder. In other words, the occurrence of a stress-produced isolated panic attack, with its very short duration, should not lead to a clinical disorder if one does not become anxious about its happening again. Similarly, very few people with angry, hostile outbursts come for treatment of their own accord, since they do not usually experience disruptions in their sense of control over their emotional responding. Does something similar happen in depressive disorders? In other words, can one experience a basic and rather acute loss of positive affect with the resulting anhedonia and slowing, much as one might experience the basic emotion of fear or panic? That is, could this reaction occur for no discernible reason (unexpected and uncued) and be experienced by certain individuals as unpredictable and/or uncontrollable?

Clinically, this seems to happen. John Teasdale (1985) may have best captured the essence of this phenomenon:

> It is not uncommon for depressed patients to misinterpret symptoms of depression as signs of irremediable personal inadequacy: for example, the lack of energy, irritability or loss of interest and affection that characterizes depression are seen as signs of selfishness, weakness, or as evidence that a person is a poor wife or mother. Such interpretations, as well as making the symptoms more aversive, imply that they are going to be very difficult to control. (p. 160)

What this observation reflects is that the basic experience of the symptoms of sudden low positive affect in the form of a major depressive episode is in itself perceived as uncontrollable in these patients. There is also evidence from nonclinical populations that fear of experiencing episodes of sadness is a distinct factor in factor-analytic studies of the Fear Survey Schedule (Taylor & Rachman, 1991, 1992).

There are two implications of this model of depression. The first is that these major depressive episodes should be time-limited, and should occur in relative isolation without the emotional complications attendant on perceptions of uncontrollability and hopelessness. In fact, it is very clear that discrete depressive episodes are time-limited; the probability of full remission of an episode approaches 90% even without intervention (Thase, 1990), although the minimum time one must experience the symptoms to qualify for a major depressive episode is 2 weeks (American Psychiatric Association, 1994). In fact, the average length of time of a major depressive episode is 6–9 months (Tollefson, 1993). Although major depressive episodes are defined by a heterogeneous mix of symptoms, research suggests that the somatic or vegetative symptoms, as reflected in low positive affect, are most central to these episodes (Buchwald & Rudick-Davis, 1993).

I have noted above that panic attacks—representing, as I think they do, the basic emotion of fear—may serve an adaptive value by promoting the immediate escape from danger (when danger is present). In this case, what is the purpose of major depressive episodes? Some have speculated (e.g., Beck, 1972) that the shutdown accompanying major depressive episodes may accomplish an important conservation of energies and resources, which might be necessary in the event of the loss of important and loved providers. Another possibility is that a depressive episode—if it is appropriate, such as upon the death of a loved one (see below)—may marshal social support, empathy, and the reestablishment of new social networks (Barnett, King, & Howard, 1979; Izard, 1992). Thus this emotional reaction may also be normal and adaptive in its original purpose, but inappropriate and untimely in its pathological expression. Therefore, the extension of the present model of emotional disorders to mood disorders posits two fundamentally different kinds of "depression." These are (1) the discrete depressive reaction with its accompanying cognitive and motoric shutdown, which I refer to as "endogenous depression"; and (2) the more chronic neurotic or "hopelessness" type of depression, which I, along with Alloy et al. (1990), posit as being an extension of anxious apprehension.

It is also important to consider the usual course of a strong but "normal" major depressive episode in the form of a grief reaction. Although the severe manifestations of most depressive grief reactions resolve within 2 months, it is not uncommon for some individuals to grieve for a year or longer (Jacobs, Hansen, Berkman, Kasi, & Ostfield, 1989). It is also common for grieving people to experience increases in their grief at significant anniversaries, such as births, holidays, and other meaningful occasions (including the 1-year anniversary of the death), where symbolic psychosocial representations of the loss become evident. In approximately 20% of bereaved individuals, what we consider a "normal" major depressive reaction will develop into a pathological grief reaction or impacted grief reaction (Jacobs, 1993; Horowitz et al., 1997). This happens when severe incapacitating grief lasts beyond 2 months, or even 1 year, and substantial impairment in functioning remains. Interestingly, many of the same psychological and social factors that seem to contribute to the onset of mood disorders in general also predict the development of a "normal" grief response into a formal mood disorder (Jacobs et al., 1989; Horowitz et al., 1997). Thus the major depressive episode most often occurring during the process of grief may be the best representation of a "nonclinical" depressive episode, despite the fact that the suffering can be intense and the impairment in functioning readily evident. The only clear distinction between this reaction and one meriting a formal diagnosis of major depressive disorder, single episode, is the presence of a clear and socially acceptable cue or trigger and the resulting attributions for the episode on the part of the patient.

But remember that the more chronic negative affective states of anxious apprehension and "hopelessness" depression (which may also map closely onto the clinical state of dysthymia) may really be more similar than different, as I have suggested above. That is, both may reflect the profound sense of uncontrollability over life events that make one vulnerable to subsequent stressors, particularly when combined with certain biological vulnerabilities. In this view, both panic attacks and discrete major depressive episodes may occur anywhere along the continuum of perceptions of uncontrollability that characterize anxiety and more "chronic" hopelessness depression. For that matter, panic and major depressive episodes may occur outside the context of these negative affective states. Of course, if one experiences a major depressive episode for any reason, the fact that it may last several weeks or months rather than a few minutes insures that the episode will be associated with substantial impairment in functioning, and therefore may need intervention even if it is not part of a recurring pattern against the background of more chronic negative affect. Only when clear precipitants are available, as in the case of the death of a loved one, does society provide the kind of social support and make the necessary allowances (at least for several months) that may obviate the need for more formal intervention.

Mania (Excitement Disorder)

In addition to major depressive episodes, a second fundamental experience contributing to mood disorders is a period of abnormally marked elation, joy, or euphoria referred to as "mania." As any clinician knows, this state often seems to resemble a pure emotional experience of elation or excitement. It is also important to note that the average duration of a manic episode without treatment is approximately 6 months, with full remission most usually occurring even without the treatment. But recent discoveries provide some interesting parallels with the model of anxiety, stress, and depressive disorders outlined above. It has become apparent over the last decade that a substantial number of patients studied at the peak severity of a manic phase, present with marked degrees of anxiety and negative affect (e.g., Post et al., 1989). In DSM-IV, this type of episode is referred to as a dysphoric manic, or "mixed episode" (American Psychiatric Association, 1994; see also McElroy et al., 1992). Patients with mixed episodes are generally more severely impaired than those with "pure" manic episodes without negative affect, in that they tend to experience a significantly greater number of previous hospitalizations and respond less well to treatment. It also seems clear that manic reactions (excitement), much like other emotions, can be conditioned to a variety of internal and external events or stimuli (Post, Rubinow, & Ballenger, 1986). Clinically, patients experiencing mixed episodes report distress over their manic behaviors and feelings, which they experience as out of their control. What this suggests is that much as with fear, depressive episodes, and anger, a time-limited basic emotion of excitement can emerge frequently and inappropriately in that it can be perceived as unpredictable and out of one's control, resulting in the emergence of negative affect (anxiety, dysphoria) focused on the mania itself. The phenomenon of mixed episodes completes the better part of a circumplex of emotions associated with emotional disorders. What is common to each of these disorders is a discrete emotion occurring unexpectedly or inappropriately in a manner that is experienced as at least somewhat out of control. This model of emotional disorders is depicted in Figure 8.10.

Finally, preliminary data now exist directly testing the extension of the present model of panic disorder to the emotions of anger, depression/sadness, and excitement in the nonclinical population (Craske, Brown, Meadows, & Barlow, 1995). Specifically, over 300 undergraduates were surveyed with a carefully constructed questionnaire to determine the

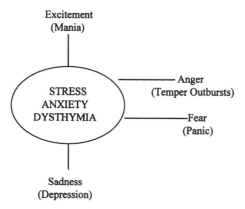

FIGURE 8.10. A model of the development of sadness (depression), fear (panic), anger (temper outbursts), and excitement (mania in a "mixed episode" as defined by DSM-IV). From Barlow (1991a). Copyright 1991 by Lawrence Erlbaum Associates. Reprinted by permission.

prevalence of both cued and uncued panic attacks, anger outbursts, episodes of sadness, and surges of excitement, as well as the degree of worry or distress over the recurrence of each type of emotional experience. The numbers and percentages of the sample who answered affirmatively to having experienced either cued or uncued emotions ever, and in the past 3 months, are shown in Table 8.1.

It is noteworthy that 32% of the sample reported no uncued emotional experiences. Overall, significantly more of the sample reported experiencing uncued surges of excitement than uncued panic attacks and uncued anger attacks. Ratings of worry about the recurrence of specific emotional episodes and the degree to which they interfered with daily functioning are shown in Table 8.2. Uncued depressive episodes were more anxiety-provoking than were uncued panic episodes, uncued anger episodes, or uncued surges of excitement. Uncued anger attacks and panic attacks were in turn, significantly more anxiety-provoking than surges of uncued excitement.

It seems clear, based on these data (and pending replication), that uncued surges of various types of emotion occur in a substantial minority of the population. Although one should expect inflationary reports with this type of study, the proportions are still surprisingly high, with at least 68% of the sample experiencing at least one uncued emotion in the previous 3-month interval. The estimate of 10% of the population experiencing uncued panic is consistent with estimates obtained from earlier questionnaire-based studies (e.g., Telch, Lucas, & Nelson, 1989). However, it is noteworthy that surges of other emotions were evident in much higher proportions, with 34% of the sample reporting depressive episodes. Furthermore, depressive episodes were associated with the most distress. Nevertheless, in this population, distress ratings were mild on average, with a very small percentage of the sample "moderately or more so" worried about the recurrence of specific emotions. The percentages meeting this criteria were less than 1% for uncued panic, 4.4% for uncued anger, 14.5% for uncued depression, and almost 0% for uncued excitement.

More recently, Williams, Chambless, and Ahrens (1997) constructed a questionnaire, the Affective Control Scale, to directly assess anxiety focused on loss of control of discrete emotions, including sadness, excitement or positive emotions, and anger. Data from college students in this and a subsequent study (Berg, Shapiro, Chambless, & Ahrens, 1998) confirmed the validity of this concept, and suggested that anxiety focused on these differing emotions shares common components. Utilizing this instrument with clinical populations will be an important next step.

TABLE 8.1. Lifetime and 3-Month Prevalence of Cued and Uncued Panic Anger, Depressive Episodes, and Excitement ($n = 317$)

	Panic attack	Anger outburst	Depressive episode	Excitement surge
Lifetime				
Cued	191 (60%)	244 (77%)	250 (79%)	298 (94%)
Uncued	43 (14%)	59 (19%)	122 (40%)	137 (44%)
Past 3 months				
Cued	132 (42%)	204 (64%)	217 (69%)	282 (89%)
Uncued	32 (10%)	55 (17%)	109 (34%)	130 (41%)

Note. Percentages are rounded. From Craske, Brown, Meadows, and Barlow (1995). Copyright 1995 by Elsevier Science Ltd. Reprinted by permission.

TABLE 8.2. Means (and Standard Deviations) for Ratings of Worry about Recurrence and Interference Caused by Cued and Uncued Panic, Anger, Depressive Episodes, and Excitement over the Past 3 Months

	Panic attack	Anger outburst	Depressive episode	Excitement surge
Worry about recurrence (0–8)				
Cued	1.64 (1.6)	1.53 (1.6)	2.65 (2.0)	0.29 (0.9)
Uncued	1.07 (1.1)	1.89 (1.9)	2.90 (2.0)	0.33 (0.9)
Interference with functioning (0–8)				
Cued	1.78 (1.7)	1.92 (1.8)	3.30 (1.9)	1.47 (1.7)
Uncued	1.19 (1.5)	2.33 (1.8)	3.13 (1.9)	1.09 (1.4)

Note. From Craske, Brown, Meadows, and Bartlow (1995). Copyright 1995 by Elsevier Science Ltd. Reprinted by permission.

The convergence of findings from basic and clinical research is only beginning. Findings from cognitive science and emotion theory have only become truly applicable to clinical disorders in the past several years. Additional research integrating findings from basic scientific explorations of affect and cognition should further enhance our knowledge of the nature and treatment of emotional disorders.

Classification of Anxiety and Mood Disorders

TIMOTHY A. BROWN

DAVID H. BARLOW

Classification is at the heart of any science. Without some objective ordering and labeling of objects or experiences, investigators would be unable to communicate with each other, and knowledge would not advance. Each individual would then have to develop his or her own personal science, which could not be applicable beyond his or her own subjective experience. In dealing with rocks or insects, these ideas are fundamental. But when the subject matter is human behavior, particularly emotional or behavioral disorders, controversy surrounds all aspects of the endeavor—including the basic issue of whether classification should even be attempted. For example, major controversies have arisen surrounding what is "normal" or "abnormal" in emotional expression; the boundaries among the various proposed categories; and/or which features of the anxiety disorders should be dimensionalized or scaled to provide a more complete picture (Blashfield, 1990; Brown, in press; Clark, Watson, & Reynolds, 1995; Frances, Widiger, & Fyer, 1990). Because diverse phenomena such as the somatic manifestations of panic, the percept of derealization, intrusive thoughts, and massive agoraphobic avoidance behavior are all subsumed under the broad heading of "anxiety disorders," deciding on logical and useful groupings is difficult, to say the least. Problems are not limited to the practical issue of what features to be grouped together. The organization or classification of emotional disorders involves issues fundamental to the conceptualization of human behavior.

The classification of anxiety disorders, as the old adage goes, has a long past but a very recent history. Although observations of phobic, obsessive–compulsive, and other anxiety-based phenomena stretch back to the earliest recorded observations of human behavior, only recently have these problems been defined and included in nosological systems. For example, as late as 1959, only three out of nine systems for classifying psychiatric disorders in various countries listed "phobic disorder" as an independent diagnosis (Marks, 1969). Even the term "anxiety" did not appear in the *International Classification of Diseases* (ICD) until the seventh revision, published in 1955. At that time, the listing was "anxiety reaction without mention of somatic symptoms" under the general heading of "psychoneurotic disorders" (Jablensky, 1985).

Any reasonable system of classification, whether dimensional or categorical, should accomplish several important goals. First, it should describe specific subgroups of symptoms or dimensions of behavior that are readily identifiable by independent observers on the basis of operational definitions ("reliability"). Second, there should be some usefulness or value in identifying these subgroups or dimensions. Within the area of emotional and behavioral disorders, this usefulness ("validity") usually refers to predicting specific response to treatment, course of the disorder, and possibly etiology. For example, someone with social phobia not only should differ from someone with specific phobia by definition, but should also present with a different etiological picture, require somewhat different psychological or pharmacological treatment, and follow a somewhat different course over the years in regard to fluctuations and the possibility of spontaneous recovery. If the major features of all the anxiety disorders alluded to above are classified dimensionally rather than categorically, then these distinctions should apply to individuals whose symptoms are more severe on some dimensions and less severe on others. In summary, diagnostic categories should include defining features that permit differentiation among the categories and preferably show some differences in etiology, course, prognosis, choice of treatment, or all of the above. Investigators working in the area refer to successful categorization of natural objects or events as "cutting nature at the joints" (e.g., Kendell, 1975).

As with everything else in the study of anxiety disorders, this is easier said than done. Currently, we are not at an advanced state in this area of investigation. One reason is the recency of this effort. Formal classification systems for most anxiety disorders did not begin to appear until close to 1950, as noted above; at that time, they were deeply influenced by prevailing theoretical conceptions of anxiety disorders. Therefore, full attention to the presenting descriptive characteristics of anxiety disorders, as well as empirical data on the validity of these disorders, received little attention.

This chapter reviews and integrates current knowledge on the organization and classification of anxiety disorders and associated phenomena. This knowledge is related to the models of panic and anxiety developed in earlier chapters. This information is a prelude to a detailed description of the nature, etiology, assessment, and treatment of each of the anxiety disorders in Chapters 10–15, based on the theoretical conceptions developed in this book and on current evidence.

CRITERIA FOR EVALUATING A NOSOLOGICAL SYSTEM

This book is organized around the categories found in the fourth edition of the *Diagnostic and Statistical Manual of Mental Disorders* (DSM-IV; American Psychiatric Association, 1994), for convenience. But clinicians and investigators should not assume complacently that this system represents reality, or even the best thinking available in the world today on classification. In fact, as one travels from country to country, numerous differences emerge in categorizing the major features of anxiety disorders. As the cultural gaps become broader, these differences are accentuated to the point where the presenting disorder itself may seem to have little or no parallel in another culture. Essential questions regarding marked cross-cultural differences in presentation, as described in Chapter 1, go to the heart of basic controversies concerning the nature of anxiety.

Do such differences matter? Personal preferences aside, there are really only two ways to answer this question, as suggested above. First, is the system reliable? Second, is the system useful? One would think that answers to these questions would have been established decades ago. In fact, investigators are only beginning to establish answers to these questions, and most of the data are in a very preliminary form indeed. In this regard, the DSM descriptions of anxiety disorders have provided a substantial advantage to those studying the classification of these disorders.

THE REVISIONS OF DSM

The DSM of the American Psychiatric Association has undergone four revisions over the decades, but the third edition (American Psychiatric Association, 1980) departed the most radically from its predecessors. Though controversial, DSM-III was widely used because of several advantages over alternative systems—notably, its relatively atheoretical approach and its specificity. Many clinicians objected to the implementation of a nosological system that not only departed radically from accepted customs (including the custom of not diagnosing at all), but also introduced new categories without full empirical support. Their objections are understandable. Nevertheless, DSM-III proved to have enormous heuristic value for clinical investigators. For the first time, diagnostic criteria within the anxiety disorders were specified in sufficient detail to allow studies of reliability and validity. In addition, investigators could communicate with each other more accurately on the subject matter of their investigations, in areas of both psychopathology and treatment outcome, thereby advancing the clinical science.

DSM-III-R was published in 1987, and DSM-IV, the most recent edition, was published in 1994. More recently, a text revision of DSM-IV has been published that does not entail changes to the diagnostic criteria of disorders, but provides updated empirical reviews for each diagnostic category regarding associated features, cultural, age, and gender features, prevalence, course, familial patterns, and differential diagnosis (DSM-IV: Text Revision; American Psychiatric Association, 2000). Although specific features of each DSM-IV anxiety disorder category are reviewed in subsequent chapters, it is informative to have an overview of the development of these criteria from DSM-II to DSM-IV. The major categories presented in each of these four versions of DSM are presented in Table 9.1.

The major shift in DSM-III, of course, was conceptual: The time-honored term "neurosis" was deleted. For most of the previous 75 years or so, it had been enough to say that anxiety was a major part of the neurotic condition. Automatically, this had shifted the focus from the observable features of anxiety disorders to hypothetical, underlying, unconscious conflicts maintaining the anxiety. Several developments led to deletion of the term "neurosis." First, new theories regarding etiological and maintaining factors for anxiety disorders were suggested, as detailed in earlier chapters. Some of these were biological, while others were based on psychological and social learning concepts that departed from specific theoretical conceptions underlying the term "neurosis." Second, many pointed out that the term "neurosis" did not facilitate research in classification. "Neurosis" was too general a term and one that could not be defined reliably. This generality also made it difficult to answer questions concerning the usefulness or validity of the concept. DSM-III encouraged clinicians and investigators to look at anxiety more descriptively. This in turn highlighted a number of specific problems or major features deemphasized within the neuroses. These features became the basis for DSM-III categories.

The neuroses were based on hypothetical etiological constructs. These constructs were associated not only with observable symptoms of anxiety, such as obsessions or phobic avoidance, but also with anxiety that was controlled unconsciously and automatically by conversion, displacement, and various other psychological mechanisms. Many disorders

TABLE 9.1. The Classification of Anxiety Disorders in DSM-II, DSM-III, DSM-III-R, and DSM-IV

DSM-II	DSM-III	DSM-III-R	DSM-IV
Phobic neurosis	Phobic disorders (or phobic neuroses) Agoraphobia with panic attacks Agoraphobia without panic attacks Social phobia Simple phobia	Phobic disorders Social phobia Simple phobia Agoraphobia without history of panic disorder	Anxiety disorders Panic disorder with agoraphobia Panic disorder without agoraphobia Agoraphobia without history of panic disorder Social phobia (social anxiety disorder) Specific phobia Generalized anxiety disorder Obsessive–compulsive disorder Posttraumatic stress disorder Acute stress disorder Anxiety disorder due to a general medical condition Substance-induced anxiety disorder Anxiety disorder not otherwise specified
Anxiety neurosis	Anxiety states (or anxiety neuroses) Panic disorder Generalized anxiety disorder	Anxiety states Panic disorder with agoraphobia Panic disorder without agoraphobia Generalized anxiety disorder Obsessive–compulsive disorder	
Obsessive–compulsive neurosis	Obsessive–compulsive disorder (or obsessive–compulsive neurosis)		
	Posttraumatic stress disorder Acute Chronic or delayed	Posttraumatic stress disorder	
	Atypical anxiety disorder	Anxiety disorder not otherwise specified	
Neuroses not classified as anxiety disorders in DSM-III (and above) Hysterical neurosis			
Depressive neurosis Neurasthenic neurosis	Somatoform disorders Dissociative disorders Affective disorders [Eliminated]		

were subsumed under this broad heading, and therefore the listing of DSM-II "neurotic disorders" in DSM-III ranged far and wide. Only those neurotic disorders in which anxiety is experienced directly were grouped together in the new class of DSM-III anxiety disorders. The remaining DSM-II neurotic disorders were distributed among other classes, such as somatoform disorders, dissociative disorders, and affective disorders. Greater specificity was achieved in DSM-III anxiety disorders through the provision of precise descriptions of narrower, more manageable categories. Panic disorder and posttraumatic stress disorder (PTSD) were new to DSM-III.

The revisions in DSM-III-R were limited to clarifications, with the exception of panic disorder, agoraphobia with panic attacks, and generalized anxiety disorder (GAD). In these categories, more substantial revisions were introduced. Specifically, agoraphobia with panic attacks was subsumed under panic disorder. Agoraphobic avoidance within the new cate-

296 ANXIETY AND ITS DISORDERS

gory of panic disorder with agoraphobia was rated on the basis of severity, from mild to severe (see Chapter 10). The definition of GAD was specified to a much greater extent. This allowed the identification of GAD in addition to other anxiety disorders; previously, it had been a residual category diagnosed only when no other anxiety disorders were identifiable. In addition, chronic worry (defined as unrealistic or excessive worry about two or more life circumstances) was designated as the essential feature of this disorder.

Another major revision introduced in DSM-III-R was the elimination of almost all hierarchical exclusionary rules. In DSM-III, hierarchical conventions dictated that a patient could not receive an anxiety disorder diagnosis if he or she was depressed. Similarly, a more pervasive anxiety disorder, such as obsessive–compulsive disorder (OCD), would automatically exclude a less pervasive anxiety disorder, such as simple phobia (renamed "specific phobia" in DSM-IV). These hierarchical exclusionary systems, which are characteristic of most classification systems, greatly distorted the presenting clinical picture in a manner discussed below.

With the publication of the DSM-IV in 1994, 12 anxiety disorder categories now exist in the formal nomenclature: panic disorder, panic disorder with agoraphobia, agoraphobia without a history of panic disorder, social phobia, specific phobia, GAD, OCD, PTSD, acute stress disorder, anxiety disorder due to a general medical condition, substance-induced anxiety disorder, and anxiety disorder not otherwise specified (NOS) (see Table 9.1). A 13th category, mixed anxiety–depressive disorder, was considered for inclusion in DSM-IV but currently resides in the appendix of disorders in need of further study as a possible addition to the fifth edition of the DSM (cf. Zinbarg et al., 1994, 1998). In addition to the creation of three new categories (acute stress disorder, anxiety disorder due to a general medical condition, and substance-induced anxiety disorder), numerous revisions to the definitions of existing categories were made in DSM-IV. Table 9.2 summarizes these revisions and provides an overview of key diagnostic features for major anxiety disorder categories. These changes, as well as clarification in the definitions of other disorders, are discussed in some detail in the subsequent chapters on these specific disorders.

DSM-IV perpetuates the steady increase in the number of categories across its preceding editions. For instance, whereas 12 anxiety disorders reside in DSM-IV, only three categories existed in DSM-II. This increase could be viewed as corresponding to expanding cumulative knowledge of the nature of psychopathology and in the classification of disorders. However, many researchers (e.g., Andrews, 1996; Tyrer, 1989) have expressed concern that the expansion of our nosologies has come at the expense of less empirical consideration of shared or overlapping features of emotional disorders that, relative to "unique" features of specific disorders, may have far greater significance for our understanding of the prevention, etiology, and course of disorders, and for predicting their response to treatment.

Moreover, this expansion has led to questions of compromised discriminant validity—namely, whether our current classification systems are erroneously distinguishing symptoms and disorders that, in reality, are inconsequential variations of broader syndromes. For instance, many anxiety disorders share constituent *processes* (e.g., apprehension of situations or objects, protective or anxiety-reducing actions), and differ primarily (or solely) at the descriptive level in *content* or *focus* of apprehension (e.g., worry about rejection or embarrassment in social phobia; worry about contamination in OCD; worry about a number of daily matters in GAD) or in the *form* of protective action (e.g., situational avoidance in agoraphobia, specific phobia, and social phobia; compulsions in OCD; safety behaviors in all anxiety disorders). Similarly, virtually all current cognitive-behavioral treatments of anxiety disorders contain the elements of exposure (situational, imaginal, intero-

TABLE 9.2. Overview of Key Features and Changes to the Definitions of Majo Disorders Introduced in DSM-IV

Disorder	Key feature(s)	Changes in DSM
Panic disorder	Recurrent, unexpected panic attacks Persistent worry/concern about additional attacks or their consequences	Elimination of p specifiers (mild, moderate, severe) Introduction of a panic typology (unexpected, situationally bound, situationally predisposed) "Recurrent" replaces requirement of history of at least four panic attacks in a 1-month period Increased emphasis on cognitive features (e.g., worry about panic, cognitive misappraisals) Criterion of "significant change in behavior related to the attacks" for coverage of "nonfearful panic disorder"
Panic disorder with agoraphobia	Meets criteria for panic disorder Agoraphobia: Fear/avoidance of situations where panic attacks might occur	See panic disorder Elimination of agoraphobia severity specifiers (mild, moderate, severe)
Social phobia	Marked fear/avoidance of social situations due to possibility of embarrassment or humiliation	Diagnosis permitted in presence of unexpected panic attacks, if attacks confined to social situations (i.e., situationally predisposed attacks)
Specific phobia	Fear/avoidance of circumscribed objects or situations (e.g., heights, enclosed places, receiving injections)	Introduction of phobia types (animal, natural environment, situational, blood–injury–injection, other) Diagnosis permitted in presence of unexpected panic attacks, if attacks confined to phobic situation/object Previously named "simple phobia"
Generalized anxiety disorder	Chronic excessive, uncontrollable worry about a number of events or activities (e.g., job performance, finances)	Criterion of uncontrollable worry "A number of events/activities" replaces requirement of two or more worry spheres List of associated symptoms reduced from 18 to 6, primarily via elimination of autonomic symptoms

(cont.)

TABLE 9.2. (*cont.*)

Disorder	Key feature(s)	Changes in DSM-IV
		Replaces category of "overanxious disorder" as a child/adolescent diagnosis
Obsessive–compulsive disorder	Recurrent, intrusive thoughts, images, or impulses (e.g., excessive doubting, thoughts of contamination) Repetitive behaviors or mental acts aimed at reducing distress or to "neutralize" an obsession	Recognition of mental/covert compulsions Inclusion of differential diagnostic criterion involving boundary of obsessions and chronic worry Introduction of "with poor insight" specifier for cases where obsessions and compulsions not recognized as excessive or unreasonable
Posttraumatic stress disorder	Persistent reexperiencing (e.g., dreams, flashbacks), distress, and avoidance of stimuli associated with prior exposure to extreme stress (e.g., rape, combat)	Traumatic event criterion revised to require subjective response (intense fear, horror, helplessness) Introduction of course specifier (acute, chronic) Introduction of a new category, acute stress disorder, for coverage of short-term extreme stress responses emphasizing dissociative symptoms

Note. DSM-IV, *Diagnostic and Statistical Manual of Mental Disorders*, fourth edition (American Psychiatric Association, 1994). From Brown (in press). Copyright by the American Psychiatric Association. Reprinted by permission.

ceptive) and cognitive restructuring. Although differentiation may be helpful in conveying information about the nature of the disturbance, the empirical question exists as to whether these manifestations are sufficiently distinct (e.g., beyond variations in content) to warrant separation. This issue can be addressed by the cumulative evidence on the reliability and validity of the various anxiety and mood disorder categories and the symptoms that constitute these syndromes.

RELIABILITY

From DSM-III on, when the specificity and complexity of diagnostic criteria became increasingly evident, the use of standardized interview protocols became more and more important. These protocols are necessary to test fairly the reliability of these categories, as well as to sample the broad range of phenomenology present even in the most discrete categories, such as specific phobia. Examples of these instruments include the Structured Clinical Interview for DSM-IV Axis I Disorders (SCID-I; First, Spitzer, Gibbon, & Williams, 1997), the Schedule for Affective Disorders and Schizophrenia—Lifetime Anxiety Version

(SADS-LA; Fyer, Endicott, Mannuzza, & Klein, 1985), and the Composite International Diagnostic Interview (CIDI; World Health Organization, 1990). Unfortunately, neither these nor other newly developed structured interviews cover sufficient information to permit differential diagnoses among all of the anxiety disorders. For example, the CIDI was designed for quite a different purpose (epidemiological research) and was designed for administration by a layperson. Whereas interviews such as the SCID-I and SADS-LA are very useful instruments for general screening purposes, to make them manageable it is necessary to collect the minimum amount of information on each of the major DSM-IV disorders. This makes it particularly valuable for screening in a general outpatient clinic, but less valuable for detailed inquiry into any one set of disorders, such as the anxiety disorders.

Anxiety Disorders Interview Schedule

In order to proceed more effectively with our own research in 1981, we began developing a detailed structured interview specifically for the anxiety disorders, which we termed the Anxiety Disorders Interview Schedule (ADIS; Di Nardo, O'Brien, Barlow, Waddell, & Blanchard, 1983). Because much of the information on classification presented in this chapter involves data collected with various versions of the ADIS, this instrument is described in some detail here, along with guidelines governing its use. The original ADIS was designed not only to permit differential diagnoses among the DSM-III anxiety disorder categories (American Psychiatric Association, 1980), but to provide data beyond the basic information required for establishing the diagnostic criteria. To this end, information regarding history of the problem, situational and cognitive factors influencing anxiety, and detailed symptom ratings provided a data base for clinical investigation and important information for differential diagnosis and treatment planning. Because depression is often associated with anxiety, a fairly detailed examination of depressive symptoms as well as their relationship to symptoms of anxiety disorders was included in this interview. Screening questions for addictive, psychotic, and relevant organic disorders were included as well.

Although many of the items in the original ADIS were developed by our own staff, some items were adapted from the SADS and the Present State Examination (Wing, Cooper, & Sartorius, 1974). Also embedded in all versions of the interview are the Hamilton Anxiety Rating Scale (Hamilton, 1959) and the Hamilton Rating Scale for Depression (Hamilton, 1960). To ensure the continuity of the interview, the items of the Hamilton scales are grouped according to content so that similar items can be rated simultaneously.

The ADIS was revised several times in subsequent years, according to our experience and to revisions across editions of the DSM. In 1988, the Anxiety Disorders Interview Schedule—Revised (ADIS-R) was published to be fully compatible with DSM-III-R, and to provide expanded coverage for all mood disorders and selected somatoform disorders such as hypochondriasis and somatization disorder (Di Nardo & Barlow, 1988). During its tenure, the ADIS-R was translated into over six languages and was used in over 150 clinical and clinical research settings around the world.

The Anxiety Disorders Interview Schedule for DSM-IV: Lifetime Version (ADIS-IV-L) was published in 1994 (Di Nardo, Brown, & Barlow, 1994). The revisions in the ADIS-IV-L go well beyond updating the ADIS-R to be consistent with DSM-IV criteria. Unlike the ADIS-R, the ADIS-IV-L provides assessment of both current and *lifetime* disorders, as well as a diagnostic timeline that fosters accurate determination of the onset, remission, and temporal sequence of these conditions. (In addition, a nonlifetime version of the ADIS-IV was developed that focuses on current diagnoses only; Brown, Di Nardo, & Barlow, 1994.) Moreover, the ADIS-IV-L provides diagnostic assessment of a broader range of conditions (e.g., substance use disorders) and dimensional assessment of the key and associated features of disorders, regardless of whether a formal DSM-IV diagnosis is under consideration (e.g., even when the DSM-IV diagnosis of social phobia does not appear warranted, interviewers inquire about and assign 0–8 ratings on the patient's fear and avoidance of a variety of social situations; cf. Brown, Di Nardo, Lehman, & Campbell, 2001). The latter revision is based on the position that many features of emotional disorders operate on a continuum rather than in a categorical, "presence–absence" fashion as in DSM diagnosis (cf. Brown, 1996; Brown, Chorpita, & Barlow, 1998; Brown et al., 2001; Costello, 1992). Dimensional assessment of the key and associated features of emotional disorders fosters many important clinical and diagnostic endeavors, such as determination of the severity of the disorder or presence of subthreshold manifestations (e.g., a pronounced fear of snakes that does not satisfy the interference–distress criterion for DSM-IV specific phobia). These data also serve important empirical functions such as measures of outcome in clinical trials (e.g., Borkovec & Costello, 1993; Brown & Barlow, 1995) and dimensional indicators in studies of latent structure and taxometric analysis (e.g., Brown et al., 1998; Waller & Meehl, 1997).

From DSM-III-R on, most diagnostic hierarchy rules were eliminated, allowing for the assignment of multiple Axis I and II diagnoses in the same individual (comorbidity). For example, we now know that anxiety and mood disorders rarely present in isolation from co-occurring Axis I diagnoses (e.g., Brown & Barlow, 1992; Brown, Campbell, Lehman, Grisham, & Mancill, 2001; Kessler et al., 1996, 1997, 1998; Kessler, Stang, Wittchen, Stein, & Walters, 1999; Magee, Eaton, Wittchen, McGonagle, & Kessler, 1996; Sanderson, Di Nardo, Rapee, & Barlow, 1990; Wittchen, Zhao, Kessler, & Eaton, 1994). When two or more diagnoses are present, the clinician makes a distinction between a principal and an additional disorder, based on severity, distress, and interference with life functioning. The temporal relationship between or among the disorders is noted and often helps to establish their independence, but does not in and of itself determine the principal versus additional status of the disorders. We do not assume that the more long-standing disorder is necessarily the principal problem, unless the information indicates that the more recent problem can be subsumed under the long-standing one. Indeed, if symptoms that would meet the criteria for one disorder are clearly part of another disorder, no separate diagnosis is given. For example, many persons with panic disorder with agoraphobia report fears of heights or enclosed places, because such situations represent the unavailability of an escape route in case of panic. A diagnosis of specific phobia is not assigned in this case. In another example, persons with specific phobia or OCD may "panic" when confronted with a circumscribed phobic object or an intrusive thought, respectively; however, panic attacks are not diagnosed as panic disorder even if the criteria are otherwise met. Thus the ADIS-IV-L is not designed for administration by a layperson, but requires clinical judgments and some experience with the emotional disorders and DSM-IV.

Accordingly, for each current and lifetime diagnosis, ADIS-IV-L interviewers assign 0–8 clinical severity ratings (CSRs) to indicate the degree of distress and interference in functioning associated with the disorder (0 = "none" to 8 = "very severely disturbing/disabling"). In instances where patients meet criteria for two or more current diagnoses, the "principal" diagnosis is the one receiving the highest CSR. Occasionally a patient presents with two distinct emotional disorders, both of which are of equal severity and associated with the same levels of interference with functioning. In these cases, "coprincipal" diagnoses are given. Other current and lifetime disorders that meet or surpass the threshold for a formal DSM-IV diagnosis are assigned CSRs of 4 ("definitely disturbing/disabling") or higher ("clinical" diagnoses). Current clinical diagnoses that are not deemed to be the principal diagnosis are referred to as "additional" diagnoses. When the key features of a current or lifetime disorder are present but are not judged to be extensive or severe enough to warrant a formal DSM-IV diagnosis (or for DSM-IV disorders in partial remission), CSRs of 1–3 are assigned ("subclinical" diagnoses). When no features of a disorder were present, CSRs of 0 are given.

To summarize, if one disorder can be clearly subsumed under another, the subsumed disorder is neither diagnosed nor assigned as an additional diagnosis. But if two disorders are judged to be independent, principal status is determined on the basis of relative severity and interference with functioning, rather than on the basis of temporal relationships or other hierarchical assumptions.

Reliability Studies

"Diagnostic reliability" refers to the extent to which two (or more) independent raters or interviewers agree on the presence or absence of a given diagnosis. Studies examining the diagnostic reliability of anxiety and mood disorders are very important to the endeavor of evaluating and revising the diagnostic categories in the extant nosology (e.g., DSM-IV). In addition to determining overall rates of diagnostic agreement, it is important to examine the sources of unreliability when diagnostic disagreements occur (cf. Brown, Di Nardo, et al., 2001; Chorpita, Brown, & Barlow, 1998a; Di Nardo, Moras, Barlow, Rapee, & Brown, 1993; Mannuzza et al., 1989). For instance, if a diagnostic category is associated with a high proportion of disagreements due to one rater's subsuming its features under a comorbid disorder, this result should raise concerns about the discriminant validity of the disorder. On the other hand, if unreliable diagnosis is largely due to disagreements on whether the condition should be assigned as a clinical or subclinical disorder, this outcome may reflect a poor operational definition of the DSM-IV distress–interference criterion and may perhaps signify the difficulties associated with imposing a categorical classification (i.e., presence–absence of DSM-IV diagnosis) on symptom expression that is largely dimensional (e.g., individual differences in the number, frequency, and severity of symptoms; Brown, in press; Brown et al., 2001).

The approach to studying diagnostic reliability of the emotional disorders has usually taken one of two methods, both involving use of structured clinical interviews such as the ADIS-IV-L or SCID-I. The first approach is "test–retest": On two separate occasions, the patient is interviewed by different independent evaluators (e.g., Brown et al., 2001; Di Nardo et al., 1993). The second method is "simultaneous": A diagnostic interview is video- or audiotaped and rated by an independent evaluator (e.g., Riskind, Beck, Berchick, Brown, & Steer, 1987; Skre, Onstad, Torgersen, & Kringlen, 1991). In both approaches, the most widely used index of interrater agreement is the kappa coefficient (κ; Fleiss, Nee, & Landis, 1979), which ranges in values from 0 (chance agreement) to 1.00 (perfect agreement). The conventional standard in reliability studies of DSM emotional disorders (e.g., Di Nardo et al., 1993; Mannuzza et al., 1989; cf. Shrout, Spitzer, & Fleiss, 1987) has been to interpret κ coefficients as follows: excellent agreement ($\kappa \geq .75$), good agreement (κ between .60 and .74), fair agreement (κ between .40 and .59), and poor agreement ($\kappa < .40$).

The strategy of interviewing patients on separate occasions is the more stringent approach to estimating diagnostic reliability, given that it introduces several potential sources of disagreement not found in the single-interview method (e.g., variation in patient report, change in clinical status). Whereas these issues could be viewed as limitations of this approach, the single-interview method has also been criticized for its potential to provide an overly optimistic estimation of diagnostic reliability. For example, the independent evaluator's judgments may be strongly influenced by the nature and extent of follow-up questions asked by the initial interviewer, or the interview may fail to address the short-term stability in symptoms or in patient report—factors that may bear on confidence in judgments of the presence/absence of a DSM diagnosis (cf. Segal, Hersen, & Van Hesselt, 1994).

Reliability studies (using the test–retest method) based on DSM-III-R and DSM-IV definitions of anxiety and mood disorders indicate that these categories are associated with differential levels of agreement (Brown et al., 2001; Di Nardo et al., 1993; Mannuzza et al., 1989; Williams et al., 1992). For instance, results have shown that categories such as panic disorder with agoraphobia, OCD, social phobia, and specific phobia have good to excellent reliability, whereas certain categories such as dysthymia are associated with fair agreement at best.

Interrater agreement for current diagnoses (i.e., principal diagnoses; any current diagnosis collapsing across principal and additional diagnostic status) from our large-scale DSM-III-R ($N = 267$; Di Nardo et al., 1993) and DSM-IV ($N = 362$; Brown et al., 2001) reliability studies are presented in Table 9.3. In both studies, the reliability sample was randomly selected from the normal flow of our intake assessments to receive two independent ADIS-R or ADIS-IV-L interviews. In the majority of cases (e.g., 79% in Brown et al., 2001), the second interview occurred within 2 weeks of the first interview. After both interviews had been completed and the interviewers had independently recorded their diagnostic judgments, cases were presented in weekly staff meetings that entailed the presentation of interviewers' diagnoses, discussion of factors contributing to any diagnostic disagreements, and establishment of consensus diagnoses.

As seen in Table 9.3, all DSM-IV principal diagnostic categories evidenced good to excellent reliability, with the exception of dysthymia (the n for PTSD was insufficient to calculate κ). In comparison to the reliability study of DSM-III-R disorders (Di Nardo et al., 1993), improved reliability was noted for the vast majority of DSM-IV categories, and no DSM-IV category was associated with a markedly lower reliability estimate. Diagnoses showing the most improvement were panic disorder and GAD. The improvement in GAD was particularly encouraging, because this category was in jeopardy of being removed from DSM-IV, in part due to evidence of poor to fair reliability of its DSM-III-R definition (Brown, Barlow, & Liebowitz, 1994; see Chapter 14). Although not shown in Table 9.3, good to excellent reliability was also found for the majority of lifetime DSM-IV anxiety and mood disorders; excellent interrater agreement was also obtained for lifetime alcohol and other substance use disorders (κ's = .83 and .82, respectively), indicating the potential utility of the ADIS-IV-L to provide reliable DSM-IV diagnosis of these conditions.

A similar pattern of results was noted when we examined *any* current clinical disorder, collapsing across principal and additional diagnoses (see Table 9.3). For example, excellent reliability was obtained in the DSM-IV study for panic disorder with agoraphobia, OCD, social phobia, and panic disorder, collapsing across the presence–absence of agoraphobia. The categories associated with good reliability were specific phobia, GAD, and any mood disorder (major depression or dysthymia). Fair reliability was found for panic disorder, major depression, and PTSD; dysthymia continued to be associated with poor reliability. As was the case for principal diagnoses only, higher κ's were obtained for all DSM-IV categories relative to DSM-III-R with the exception of dysthymia, which went from .35 to .31, and OCD, which did not change (κ = .75 in both Brown, Di Nardo, et al., 2001, and Di Nardo et al., 1993).

TABLE 9.3. Diagnostic Reliability of Current DSM-IV Diagnoses (*N* = 362) and Current DSM-III-R Diagnoses (*N* = 267)

	Principal diagnosis				Principal or additional diagnosis			
	DSM-IV[a]		DSM-III-R[b]		DSM-IV[a]		DSM-III-R[b]	
	κ	*n*	κ	*n*	κ	*n*	κ	*n*
PD	.72	14	.43	38	.56	22	.39	44
PDA	.77	83	.72	131	.81	102	.71	142
PD & PDA	.79	94	.79	152	.79	120	.75	168
Specific phobia	.86	56	.82	21	.71	100	.63	47
Social phobia	.77	80	.79	45	.77	152	.66	84
GAD	.67	76	.57	38	.65	113	.53	108
OCD	.85	33	.80	19	.75	60	.75	24
PTSD	—	—	.46	3	.59	14	.55	8
MDD	.67	53	.65	8	.59	111	.55	46
DYS	.22	15	−.05	5	.31	53	.35	25
MDD & DYS	.72	61	.46	13	.63	138	.56	64

Note. κ, kappa; *n*, number of cases in which diagnosis was assigned by either or both raters; —, insufficient *n* to calculate kappa; PD, panic disorder; PDA, panic disorder with agoraphobia; GAD, generalized anxiety disorder; OCD, obsessive–compulsive disorder; MDD, major depressive disorder; DYS, dysthymia; PTSD, posttraumatic stress disorder. From "Reliability of DSM-IV Anxiety and Mood Disorders: Implications for the Classification of Emotional Disorders" by T. A. Brown, P. A. Di Nardo, C. L. Lehman, and L. A. Campbell, 2001, *Journal of Abnormal Psychology.* Copyright by the American Psychological Association. Reprinted with permission.
[a]The data are from Brown, Di Nardo, Lehman, and Campbell (2001).
[b]The data are from Di Nardo, Moras, Barlow, Rapee, and Brown (1993).

Another important aspect of these studies was the examination of the sources of diagnostic unreliability. In the DSM-IV study (Brown, Di Nardo, et al., 2001), the primary source of unreliability for each diagnostic disagreement was recorded via the following rating system:

1. Difference in patient report—patient gives different information to the two interviewers (e.g., variability in responses to inquiry about the presence, severity, or duration of key symptoms).
2. Threshold—consistent symptom report is provided across interviews, but interviewers disagree on whether these symptoms cause sufficient interference and distress to satisfy the DSM-IV threshold for a clinical disorder.
3. Change in clinical status—there is a clear change in the severity or presence of symptoms between interviews.
4. Interviewer error—interviewer improperly applies DSM-IV diagnostic or exclusion rules or fails to obtain necessary diagnostic information during ADIS-IV-L administration (e.g., skips out of an ADIS-IV-L diagnostic section prematurely).
5. Diagnosis subsumed under another condition—there is disagreement on whether symptoms are attributable to, or better accounted for by, a co-occurring disorder.
6. DSM-IV inclarity—disagreement stems from limitations of the DSM-IV criteria in providing clear direction for differential diagnosis.

Table 9.4 presents the results on the sources of unreliability for each current DSM-IV anxiety and mood disorder (collapsing across principal and additional diagnoses). The prevailing sources of unreliability differed substantially across the anxiety and mood disorders. For instance, the majority of disagreements involving social phobia, specific phobia, and OCD (62% to 67%) entailed cases where one interviewer assigned the diagnosis at a clinical level, and the other rated the diagnosis as subclinical; for other categories (e.g., panic disorder with agoraphobia, GAD, major depression, dysthymia), this was a relatively rare source of unreliability. Indeed, the "threshold" issue was the most common source of disagreements for the diagnoses of specific phobia and social phobia. This unreliability source also accounted for the observed decline in the interrater agreement of panic disorder, OCD, and specific phobia as diagnoses anywhere in the clinical picture (collapsing principal and additional diagnoses), relative to their estimates as principal diagnoses only (this decline also occurred for social phobia in the DSM-III-R study; see Table 9.3). By definition, a "principal" diagnosis is the disorder associated with the highest degree of distress–interference, and thus would be less susceptible than an additional diagnosis to disagreements involving the DSM-IV threshold.

"Difference in patient report" was otherwise the most prevalent source of unreliability, although with wide-ranging frequency across the anxiety and mood disorders (i.e., from 22% in specific phobia to 100% in PTSD; cf. Mannuzza et al., 1989, who found that "information variance" across interviews accounted for over half of the diagnostic disagreements in their DSM-III-R reliability study). Considerable variability was also evident across categories for the frequency with which other disorders were involved in diagnostic disagreements. Whereas disagreements with other disorders were relatively uncommon for social phobia, OCD, and PTSD (8% to 13%), another clinical diagnosis was involved in over half of the disagreements with dysthymia, panic disorder with agoraphobia, major depression, and GAD (54% to 74%). As can be seen in Table 9.4, disagreements entailing another clinical diagnosis quite often involved disorders with overlapping definitional features, and that differed mainly in the duration or severity of symptoms (e.g., panic disorder vs. panic disorder with agoraphobia; specific phobia vs. agoraphobia without a history of panic disorder; major depression vs. dysthymia). Consistent with prior evidence that mood disorders may pose the greatest boundary problem for GAD (T. A. Brown, Marten, & Barlow, 1995; Clark & Watson, 1991; Starcevic, 1995), 22 of the 35 GAD disagreements (63%) involving another diagnosis were with mood disorders (dysthymia = 10, major depression = 9, depressive disorder NOS = 2, bipolar disorder = 1). In addition, this overlap was evident in disagreements involving anxiety disorder NOS and depressive disorder NOS diagnoses. For example, a category frequently involved in disagreements with GAD was anxiety disorder NOS (GAD) ($n = 10$), where one interviewer noted clinically significant features of GAD (i.e., CSR $\geq$ 4) but judged that all criteria for a formal DSM-IV GAD diagnosis had not been met (e.g., number or duration of worries or associated symptoms). This was also the case for the NOS diagnoses associated with disagreements in other disorders; for example, in the two OCD disagreements involving another disorder, both were with anxiety NOS (OCD).

In addition to the preponderance of disagreements stemming from DSM-IV threshold issues (i.e., both interviewers recorded key features of the disorder, but disagreed as to whether or not these symptoms met or surpassed the threshold for a formal DSM-IV diagnosis), the high rate of disagreements involving NOS diagnoses illustrates the problem of measurement error introduced by imposing categorical cutoffs (i.e., DSM-IV criteria for the presence–absence of a disorder) on diagnostic features that operate largely in a continuous fashion (e.g., number, severity, and duration of symptoms; degree of distress). A similar result was noted when the reliability of DSM-IV categorical speci- fiers (e.g., "mild," "moderate," or "severe" depressive episode in major depression) was compared to the interrater stability of these ratings in dimensional form (e.g., ADIS-IV-L 0–8 ratings of the seven symptoms that accompany depressed mood and diminished interest/pleasure in activities to form the key criterion for a major depressive episode). For example, whereas dimensional ratings of the severity of major depression features were quite reliable ($r = .74$), the DSM-IV categorical specifiers of major depression severity evidenced poor reliability ($\kappa = .36$). Because of the measurement error, loss of information, and validity problems associated with the purely categorical approach to diagnostic classification in DSM-IV, researchers have called for incorporation of dimen- sional components in future nosological systems (e.g., Blashfield, 1990; Brown, in press; Frances et al., 1990)—an issue to which we return at various points throughout this chapter.

VALIDITY

Overview

Historically, studies of the validity of anxiety and mood disorders have been greatly hindered by the lack of reliable definitions. With more precise definitions in place since DSM-III for most disorders, these studies have proceeded. Although questions on the validity of diag- nostic categories can be addressed in many different ways, much of the extant research has addressed issues bearing on convergent and discriminant validity. As noted earlier in this chapter, this inquiry has centered on the question of whether the anxiety and mood disorders represent distinct entities, or whether the increase in the number of diagnostic categories across editions of the DSM reflects compromised discriminant validity to the point that the classification system is erroneously distinguishing categories that are minor variations of broader underlying syndrome(s) (Andrews, 1990; Andrews, Stewart, Morris- Yates, Holt, & Henderson, 1990; Brown, in press; Brown et al., 1998).

The classification scheme currently in place in DSM-IV corresponds to one side of this argument, which asserts the merit of extensive categorical differentiation of the symp- toms comprising the anxiety and mood disorder constructs (i.e., 12 anxiety disorder cate- gories, 9 mood disorder categories). On the other side of this issue is the argument for a "general neurotic syndrome," which contends poor discriminant validity of DSM-IV, and which collapses the spectrum of anxiety and mood disorder symptoms under a single entity akin to the construct of "neurosis" in DSM-II (Andrews, 1990, 1996; Tyrer, 1989). Under this conceptualization, heterogeneity in the expression of emotional disorder symptoms (e.g., individual differences in the prominence of social anxiety, panic attacks, anhedonia, etc.) is regarded as trivial variations in the manifestation of a broader syndrome (i.e., this variability is of little clinical importance and does not warrant diagnostic differentiation). Intermediate to these two stances are positions that acknowledge the considerable overlap among the anxiety and mood disorder categories (e.g., shared symptom features and etio- logical factors), but that contend that the differentiation reflected in DSM-IV is important because it has important implications for treatment planning and prognosis, prediction of course and complicating factors, and so on (e.g., Barlow, Chorpita, & Turovsky, 1996; Brown et al., 1998; L. A. Clark, Watson, & Mineka, 1994). Similar to the theoretical model put forward in this book (see Chapter 8), these conceptualizations draw from the empirical evidence that anxiety and mood disorders emerge from shared psychosocial and biological/

TABLE 9.4. Factors Contributing to Diagnostic Disagreements for Current DSM-IV Anxiety and Mood Disorders

Diagnosis:	PD	PDA	SPEC	SOC	GAD	OCD	PTSD	MDD	DYS
Total disagreements (n):	13	26	37	39	47	21	8	53	41
Proportion (and n) of:									
Disagreements involving another clinical diagnosis	.38 (5)	.54 (14)	.27 (10)	.08 (3)	.74 (35)	.10 (2)	.13 (1)	.64 (34)	.71 (29)
Disorders involved in the disagreement:									
PD		.15 (4)	—	—	.02 (1)	—	—	—	—
PDA	.31 (4)		.08 (3)	—	—	—	—	—	—
SPEC	—	.19 (5)		—	—	—	—	—	—
SOC	—	—	—		—	—	—	—	—
GAD	—	.04 (1)	.03 (1)	—		—	—	.04 (2)	.15 (6)
OCD	—	—	—	—	—		—	—	—
PTSD	—	.04 (1)	—	—	.02 (1)	—	—	—	—
MDD	—	—	—	—	.19 (9)	—	—		.39 (16)
DYS	—	—	—	—	.21 (10)	—	—	.39 (16)	
Depression NOS	—	—	—	—	.04 (2)	—	—	.23 (12)	—
Anxiety NOS	.08 (1)	.08 (2)	—	.05 (2)	.21 (10)	.10 (2)	.13 (1)	.28 (15)	.12 (5)
AGw/oPD	—	.04 (1)	.14 (5)	.03 (1)	—	—	—	.02 (1)	—
Adjustment disorder	—	—	—	—	.02 (1)	—	—	—	—
Other	—	—	HYPO^c	—	BIP	—	—	.06 (3) PAIN	.02 (1) SOM

306

Clinical vs. subclinical disagreements[a]

.46 (6)	.12 (3)	.62 (23)	.67 (26)	.13 (6)	.62 (13)	.25 (2)	.17 (9)	—

Sources of unreliability									
Threshold[b]	.46 (6)	.12 (3)	.46 (17)	.41 (16)	.09 (4)	.29 (6)	—	.15 (8)	.05 (2)[d]
Difference in patient report	.31 (4)	.50 (13)	.22 (8)	.36 (14)	.55 (26)	.48 (10)	1.00 (8)	.55 (29)	.66 (27)
Interviewer error	.23 (3)	.19 (5)	.14 (5)	.10 (4)	.19 (9)	.14 (3)	—	.11 (6)	.15 (6)
Diagnosis subsumed under comorbid disorder	—	.15 (4)	.08 (3)	.10 (4)	.15 (7)	.10 (2)	—	—	.15 (6)
Change in clinical status	—	.04 (1)	.03 (1)	—	.02 (1)	—	—	.17 (9)	—
DSM-IV inclarity	—	—	.05 (2)	.03 (1)	—	—	—	—	—
Missing	—	—	.03 (1)	—	—	—	—	.02 (1)	—

Note. PD, panic disorder; PDA, panic disorder with agoraphobia; SPEC, specific phobia; SOC, social phobia; GAD, generalized anxiety disorder; OCD, obsessive–compulsive disorder; PTSD, posttraumatic stress disorder; MDD, major depressive disorder; DYS, dysthymia; Depression NOS, depressive disorder not otherwise specified; Anxiety NOS, anxiety disorder not otherwise specified; AGw/oPD, agoraphobia without a history of panic disorder; HYPO, hypochondriasis; BIP, bipolar disorder; PAIN, pain disorder; SOM, somatization disorder. From "Reliability of DSM-IV Anxiety and Mood Disorders: Implications for the Classification of Emotional Disorders" by T. A. Brown, P. A. Di Nardo, C. L. Lehman, and L. A. Campbell, 2001, *Journal of Abnormal Psychology.* Copyright by the American Psychological Association. Reprinted with permission.

[a]Cases where both raters recorded the diagnosis, but disagreed on whether it should be assigned at the clinical level.

[b]Note that for SPEC and other diagnoses, the frequency of cases where "Threshold" was the primary source of unreliability does not necessarily equal the number of disagreements entailing assignment of the disorder at clinical and subclinical levels. This is because each of the other unreliability sources (e.g., change in clinical status, variability in patient report regarding number or severity of symptoms) could also result in clinical vs. subclinical disagreements.

[c]This disagreement pertained to a boundary issue between specific phobia, other type (contracting an illness) and hypochondriasis.

[d]In these 2 cases, disagreements stemmed from a threshold issue of MDD (chronic) versus DYS—that is, whether the features were sufficiently severe to be classified as a chronic major depressive episode.

307

genetic diatheses (which account in part for the communality of symptom dimensions such as negative affect), but differ on many salient dimensions (disorder-specific features) that arise from environmental determinants (e.g., Kendler, Neale, Kessler, Heath, & Eaves, 1992a, 1992c; Watson, Clark, & Harkness, 1994).

Over the past decade, much research has accrued that bears on the convergent and discriminant validity of the anxiety disorders. In the remainder of this chapter, these issues are addressed by a review of recent studies on diagnostic comorbidity, treatment specificity, and latent structure of dimensional features of the emotional disorders. This review also considers the distinctiveness of anxiety and depression, in view of evidence that mood disorders (major depression, dysthymia) may pose serious boundary problems for some anxiety disorders such as GAD.

Diagnostic Comorbidity

Hierarchical Exclusionary Systems

In order to achieve the acceptable levels of diagnostic reliability now possible for most disorders, as described above, disorders are defined in a specific and rather narrow fashion. Although the old category of "neurosis" in DSM-II was so heterogeneous that the label communicated very little, the categories within the DSM-IV anxiety disorders describe the nature of a presenting problem precisely. However, clinicians have known for years that patients seldom present with just one problem, and that trying to "force" patients into one and only one category is not a good way to represent the reality of clinical presentation. Nonetheless, the hierarchical exclusionary systems present in most systems of classification often require one and only one diagnosis.

Explicit or implicit hierarchies of disorders are introduced into classification systems to assist choosing among related diagnoses when decisions are difficult. Associated with these hierarchies are often complex exclusionary rules reflecting the assumptions of the hierarchies. For some disorders in DSM-III, a diagnosis was excluded if, in the clinician's judgment, its symptoms were "due to" a coexisting disorder that occupied a higher position in the hierarchy. Thus a diagnosis of specific phobia may have been excluded by a number of disorders, including major depression and OCD. GAD may have been excluded by any other anxiety disorder, as well as by major depression. More generally, any of the anxiety disorders could be excluded by major depression. The primary difficulty in establishing these hierarchical relationships among various disorders for any given patient was that DSM-III provided no guidelines for determining when a particular disorder was "due to" another. Excellent discussions of the origin and nature of hierarchical exclusionary systems within diagnostic categories are provided by Kendell (1975), Surtees and Kendell (1979), Sturt (1981), and Boyd et al. (1984).

Below the level of organic disorders, few of these exclusionary systems in their totality have any empirical support (Surtees & Kendell, 1979). Their most important function is to allow clinicians to assign only one diagnosis. However, Sturt (1981) made the convincing argument that even exclusionary systems with some face validity may simply reflect the tendency of every symptom to show a highly significant association with the total symptom score. A study by Boyd et al. (1984) indicated that when diagnoses are applied without exclusionary restrictions, individuals who meet the basic criteria for any one DSM-III disorder are likely to meet the criteria for one or more additional diagnoses. Such findings suggest that arbitrary exclusionary systems may obscure true relationships among disorders or syndromes.

On the other hand, the results of Boyd et al. also indicated that the practice of simply listing all diagnoses for which a patient meets the basic criteria also obscures existing relationships among syndromes, because such a procedure makes no provision for recording these relationships. That is, in some cases, symptoms fitting the criteria for two different diagnoses either may be part of the same problem or may not be. For example, in a case of severe OCD with washing rituals, fear of dirt is not a separate specific phobia. But a fear of heights may be, particularly if it had a different time of onset or otherwise has nothing to do with feelings of contamination, which are an integral part of many presentations of obsessive–compulsive syndromes. Automatically including every "specific phobia" that happens to be present in a person with OCD would be as misleading as automatically excluding every specific phobia. Thus the issue becomes one of carefully delineating the exclusionary guidelines used in a diagnostic system, rather than eliminating hierarchical or exclusionary assumptions altogether.

Recognizing these difficulties, Spitzer and Williams (1985) critically evaluated some of the assumptions underlying the hierarchical organization of DSM-III anxiety disorders. For example, they noted that DSM-III excluded a diagnosis of agoraphobia in the presence of OCD, because individuals with the latter disorder are often fearful of going out of the house alone. This exclusionary rule fails to recognize that a person with agoraphobia and a person with OCD may be housebound for different reasons. In agoraphobia, fear of leaving the house is mediated by anticipation of panic attack or sudden incapacitation; such fears are not a part of the picture in OCD.

The Functional Relationship among Disorders

These issues, along with empirical data, led to the deletion of most aspects of the hierarchical exclusionary system in DSM-III-R and DSM-IV (although a few diagnostic hierarchy rules still exist for some disorders, such as the guideline that DSM-IV GAD cannot be diagnosed if its features occur exclusively during the course of a mood disorder). But it has not been replaced with the practice of simply listing all diagnoses, for reasons mentioned above. Rather, clinicians must examine the functional relationship of problems or disorders. A central element is the distinction between "associated features" of a disorder and "coexisting complications" of a disorder. An "associated feature" refers to a symptom that is a typical aspect of the clinical picture of a more pervasive disorder. In the presence of the more pervasive disorder, the associated symptoms do not warrant a separate diagnosis. For example, as noted earlier, phobic avoidance of dirt is a typical feature in patients with obsessive thoughts about contamination, so a separate diagnosis of specific phobia is not warranted. Similarly, fear and avoidance of enclosed places such as elevators, sufficient to meet the criteria for specific phobia, are often reported by persons with panic disorder with agoraphobia. These symptoms usually prove to be an associated part of the agoraphobia, because the feared situations represent the unavailability of an escape route in the event of panic. That is, a fear of heights is "functionally related" to or "better accounted for" by the agoraphobic syndrome.

"Coexisting complications," on the other hand, are additional disorders that are also present but cannot be subsumed under another disorder. These additional diagnostic entities may have implications for etiology, treatment, or prognosis. For example, research has routinely shown higher rates of mood disorder comorbidity in patients who have panic disorder with extensive agoraphobia than in patients who have panic disorder with no or minimal agoraphobic avoidance (e.g., Brown & Barlow, 1992; Brown, Campbell, et al., 2001). That is, marked agoraphobia is not an integral part of depression, but if it is present it seems to be associated with coexisting complications, with different implications for treatment. In fact, any time two or more distinct diagnoses are present, treatment approaches may be different than they would be for one disorder. In such cases, it is important to be able to assign joint diagnoses.

Rates and Patterns of Comorbidity

Consistent evidence of high comorbidity among anxiety and mood disorders is frequently cited in support of skepticism about the distinguishability of the emotional disorders (Andrews, 1990; Tyrer, 1989). Comorbidity studies based on DSM-III-R criteria routinely indicated that at least 50% of patients with a principal anxiety disorder have one or more additional diagnoses at the time of assessment (e.g., Brawman-Mintzer et al., 1993; Brown & Barlow, 1992; Sanderson et al., 1990). Similar findings were obtained in a large-scale study that we recently completed for the DSM-IV anxiety and mood disorders (Brown et al., in press). These data were derived from a large sample ($n = 1,127$) of patients carefully diagnosed with the ADIS-IV-L. It is important to note that this study (like others) probably yielded conservative estimates of diagnostic co-occurrence, due to limits in generalizability such as the nature of inclusion–exclusion criteria used (e.g., active substance use disorders and presence of suicidality were exclusion criteria), its outpatient setting, and so forth. Nevertheless, comorbidity rates for many categories were quite high. Results indicated that 55% of patients with a principal anxiety or mood disorder had at least one additional anxiety or depressive disorder at the time of the assessment (Table 9.5); this rate increased to 76% when lifetime diagnoses were considered (Table 9.6). The principal diagnostic categories of PTSD, major depression, dysthymia, and GAD had the highest comorbidity rates, and specific phobia had the lowest. Although 65% of patients with principal GAD had at least one additional current diagnosis, this comorbidity rate was significantly lower than the estimate (82%) in our previous study using DSM-III-R definitions (Brown & Barlow, 1992). This finding is noteworthy, because the high comorbidity rate associated with DSM-III-R GAD was viewed by some researchers as evidence of its poor discriminant validity and questionable utility as a formal DSM diagnosis (Brown, Barlow, & Liebowitz, 1994). However, as shown in Table 9.5, several diagnostic categories had comparable or higher levels of comorbidity to GAD in the DSM-IV study. By far the most common additional diagnosis was major depression (20% and 50% for current and lifetime, respectively), followed by social phobia (22% for current).

Analyses examining patterns of covariation among current and lifetime disorders (collapsing across principal and additional diagnostic status) also yielded many interesting findings (Brown, Campbell, et al., 2001). For example, in both current and lifetime analyses, significant odds ratios were obtained for the associations between social phobia and the mood disorders (major depression, dysthymia). Although PTSD had a higher rate of comorbidity overall, the presence of this disorder was associated with significantly increased risk of panic disorder with agoraphobia, mood disorders, and substance use disorders. Other categories associated with increased risk of substance use disorders were panic disorder with agoraphobia and major depression.

Nevertheless, several aspects of the Brown, Campbell, et al. (2001) study indicated where comorbidity data based on the DSM-IV diagnostic level produce misleading findings regarding the overlap among disorders. For example, the presence of social phobia and specific phobia was associated with decreased likelihood of panic disorder with agoraphobia (and vice versa), which would suggest that although these conditions possess overlapping features (e.g., situational avoidance, panic attacks), they co-occur relatively infrequently. However, it is likely that findings of significantly decreased odds ratios were artifacts of the issues discussed earlier regarding DSM-IV differential diagnosis and hierarchy rules (e.g., features of social phobia were judged to be better accounted for by panic disorder with agoraphobia). A clear instance of this phenomenon is evident in findings on the comorbidity of GAD and mood disorders. For instance, when adhering strictly to DSM-IV diagnostic rules, the comorbidity between GAD and dysthymia was 5%. However, when the hierarchy rule that GAD should not be assigned when it occurs exclusively during a course of a mood disorder was ignored, this comorbidity estimate increased to 90% (see Table 9.5). Such findings reflect how investigation focused solely at the diagnostic level provides limited information about the discriminant validity of emotional disorders (e.g., diagnostic-level studies are bound to the diagnostic system being evaluated, are at increased risk for measurement error associated with categorical thresholds of the dimensional frequency and severity of symptoms, etc.).

Another noteworthy finding from the Brown, Campbell, et al. (2001) study is the high rate in which anxiety disorder NOS and depressive disorder NOS diagnoses were current and lifetime comorbid conditions (in Tables 9.5 and 9.6, disorders under the headings "Other anxiety" and "Other mood" were almost exclusively NOS diagnoses, except for the rare anxiety or mood disorder due to a general medical condition). For instance, in analyses collapsing across principal anxiety and mood disorders, the lifetime prevalence of such diagnoses was 5%—a rate greater than or equal to the rates as additional diagnoses of nonresidual categories such as panic disorder and PTSD (2% and 5%, respectively; see Table 9.6). Recall, too, that NOS diagnoses were frequently involved in diagnostic disagreements with GAD, OCD, major depression, and dysthymia in Brown et al. (2001) (see Table 9.4). In addition to the problem of measurement error discussed earlier (imposing a categorical threshold on individual differences in the expression of symptoms), the high rate of these unclassifiable boundary cases (NOS diagnoses) is indicative of poor diagnostic coverage of the current nosology (Clark et al., 1995).

Explanations for Descriptive Comorbidity Findings

In addition, the multiple conceptual explanations for diagnostic comorbidity are sufficiently wide-ranging either to support or to invalidate current nosologies of emotional disorders (cf. Blashfield, 1990; Frances et al., 1990). Accounts for comorbidity that challenge current classification systems include the possibility that disorders co-occur because (1) they share overlapping definitional criteria; or (2) they represent inconsequential variations of a broader underlying syndrome that has been erroneously separated by the classification system (i.e., the "general neurotic syndrome" discussed earlier in this chapter). In regard to the first explanation, for example, as currently defined by DSM-IV the associated symptom criteria for GAD overlap almost entirely with defining features of major depression and dysthymia (e.g., sleep disturbance, fatigability, concentration difficulties, restlessness). This overlap could contribute to findings of a differentially high comorbidity rate of GAD and mood disorders (e.g., Brawman-Mintzer et al., 1993; Brown & Barlow, 1992; Brown, Campbell, et al., 2001), although DSM-IV attempts to adjust for this with a hierarchy rule stating that GAD should not be assigned if its features occur exclusively during the course of a mood disorder. The second explanation aligns with arguments for a "general neurotic syndrome" discussed earlier in this chapter.

On the other hand, explanations for comorbidity that do not imply problems in the classification system include the possibility that the co-occurrence of disorders is due to the following: (1) Artifacts exist, such as their base rates of occurrence in the study set-

TABLE 9.5. Percentages (and Odds Ratios) of Current Additional Diagnoses in Patients with Current Principal Anxiety and Mood Disorders (N = 968)

Current additional diagnosis	DSM-IV principal diagnosis (n)											
	PD (36)	PDA (324)	PD/A (360)	SOC (186)	GAD (120)	OCD (77)	SPEC (110)	PTSD (13)	MDD (81)	DYS (21)	MDD/DYS (102)	Overall[a]
Any Axis I	42 (.73)	62 (1.14*)	60 (1.09)	46 (.78*)	68 (1.24*)	57 (1.01)	34 (.56*)	92 (1.64*)	69 (1.25*)	76 (1.36*)	71 (1.28*)	57
Any anxiety/mood	42 (.75)	60 (1.16*)	59 (1.12)	45 (.79*)	65 (1.21*)	53 (.96)	33 (.56*)	92 (1.69*)	68 (1.26*)	76 (1.40*)	70 (1.30*)	55
Any anxiety disorder	36 (.84)	47 (1.17*)	46 (1.14)	28 (.61*)	52 (1.25*)	39 (.91)	27 (.61*)	62 (1.45)	64 (1.58*)	57 (1.35)	63 (1.56*)	43
Any mood disorder	17 (.58)	33 (1.28)	31 (1.19)	29 (1.04)	36 (1.32*)	32 (1.17)	10 (.34*)	77 (2.79*)	11 (.37)	38 (1.36)	17 (.56)	28
Anxiety Disorders												
PD	—	—	—	01 (.28)	03 (3.25)	01 (.86)	00 (—)	00 (—)	04 (3.25)	00 (—)	03 (2.48)	01
PDA	—	—	—	03 (.24*)	15 (2.09*)	08 (.88)	05 (.58)	23 (2.75)	15 (1.90*)	14 (1.68)	15 (1.96*)	
PD or PDA	—	—	—	03 (.24*)	18 (2.24*)	09 (.88)	05 (.49)	23 (2.33)	19 (2.08*)	14 (1.42)	18 (2.03*)	10
SOC	08 (.37)	15 (.58*)	15 (.53*)	—	36 (2.33*)	26 (1.21)	09 (.38*)	15 (.70)	41 (2.07*)	48 (2.25*)	42 (2.24*)	22
GAD	19 (1.59)	16 (1.50*)	16 (1.64*)	13 (1.10)	—	12 (.93)	05 (.40*)	23 (1.87)	05 (.37*)	05 (.38)	05 (.36*)	13
GAD: no hierarchy	22 (.87)	22 (.79)	22 (.78*)	21 (.78)	—	16 (.59)	07 (.26*)	38 (1.52)	67 (3.16)	90 (3.80*)	72 (3.73*)	25
OCD	06 (.83)	07 (1.12)	07 (1,08)	08 (1.29)	04 (.59)	—	03 (.38)	23 (3.62)	09 (1.35)	05 (.71)	08 (1.21)	07

312

SPEC	08 (.65)	15 (1.36)	15 (1.28)	08 (.58)	12 (.91)	12 (.91)	15[b] (1.17)	15 (1.21)	15 (1.18)	10 (.75)	14 (1.09)	13
PTSD	00 (—)	04 (2.30*)	04 (1.95)	03 (1.09)	01 (.30)	00 (—)	00 (—)	—	06 (2.84*)	00 (—)	05 (2.20)	03
Other anxiety	03 (.92)	04 (1.86)	04 (1.81)	03 (1.10)	01 (.25)	03 (.86)	03 (.90)	00 (—)	02 (.81)	00 (—)	02 (.63)	03
Mood Disorders												
MDD	08 (.41)	24 (1.41*)	23 (1.28)	14 (.66*)	26 (1.39)	22 (1.14)	03 (.12*)	69 (3.67*)	—	33 (1.73)	—	20
DYS	08 (.99)	07 (.73)	07 (.74)	13 (1.75*)	06 (.66)	10 (1.26)	04 (.40)	23 (2.80*)	11 (1.36)	—	—	08
Other mood	03 (.74)	03 (.87)	03 (.84)	05 (1.40)	06 (1.71)	04 (1.05)	04 (.98)	00 (—)	00 (—)	05 (1.29)	01 (.24)	04
Other Disorders												
Somatoform	00 (—)	02 (.99)	01 (.84)	01 (.65)	04 (3.53)	01 (.83)	00 (—)	00 (—)	02 (1.68)	00 (—)	02 (1.31)	02
Other Axis I	03 (.92)	02 (.63)	02 (.64)	01 (.31)	06 (2.25)	06 (2.41)	02 (.58)	00 (—)	06 (2.28)	00 (—)	05 (1.77)	03

Note. PD, panic disorder; PDA, panic disorder with agoraphobia; PD/A, panic disorder with or without agoraphobia; SOC, social phobia; GAD, generalized anxiety disorder; GAD: no hierarchy, generalized anxiety disorder ignoring DSM-IV hierarchy rule with mood disorders; OCD, obsessive-compulsive disorder; SPEC, specific phobia; PTSD, posttraumatic stress disorder; MDD, major depressive disorder; DYS, dysthymia; MDD/DYS, major depressive disorder or dysthymia. From Brown, Campbell, et al. (2001). Copyright 2001 by American Psychological Association. Reprinted by permission.

[a]Overall frequency category was assigned as an additional diagnosis.

[b]Indicates that 15% of patients with principal specific phobia had additional specific phobias of another type.

*Significantly increased or decreased risk of co-occurring disorder (95% confidence interval).

TABLE 9.6. Percentages (and Odds Ratios) of Additional Lifetime Diagnoses in Patients with Current Principal Anxiety and Mood Disorders (N = 968)

Lifetime additional diagnosis	DSM-IV principal diagnosis (n)											Overall[a]
	PD (36)	PDA (324)	PD/A (360)	SOC (186)	GAD (120)	OCD (77)	SPEC (110)	PTSD (13)	MDD (81)	DYS (21)	MDD/DYS (102)	
Any Axis I	75 (.93)	82 (1.03)	81 (1.01)	72 (.86*)	92 (1.16*)	86 (1.07)	65 (.78*)	100 (1.24*)	91 (1.15*)	100 (1.25*)	93 (1.18*)	81
Any anxiety/mood	69 (.91)	77 (1.01)	76 (1.00)	67 (.86)	88 (1.19*)	83 (1.10)	56 (.72*)	100 (1.32*)	90 (1.20*)	100 (1.32*)	92 (1.24*)	76
Any anxiety disorder	53 (.98)	56 (1.07)	56 (1.07)	37 (.63*)	71 (1.38*)	45 (.84)	45 (.81)	69 (1.30)	73 (1.40*)	62 (1.16)	71 (1.37*)	54
Any mood disorder	44 (.74)	60 (1.03)	59 (.99)	57 (.95)	73 (1.28*)	71 (1.23*)	36 (.58*)	85 (1.44*)	57 (.95)	76 (1.29*)	61 (1.03)	59
Anxiety disorders												
PD	03	01 (.50)	01 (.56)	01 (.22)	08 (5.78*)	01 (.61)	00 (—)	00 (—)	05 (2.74)	00 (—)	04 (2.12)	02
PDA	11 (.92)	11	11	04 (.31*)	20 (1.82*)	10 (.85)	11 (.89)	23 (1.93)	22 (1.99*)	14 (1.19)	21 (1.86*)	12
PD or PDA	14 (1.00)	12 (.84)	13	05 (.30*)	27 (2.20*)	12 (.83)	11 (.76)	23 (1.67)	27 (2.13*)	14 (1.02)	25 (1.93*)	14
SOC	08 (.39)	19 (.87)	18 (.79)	01	39 (2.17*)	27 (1.36)	16 (.77)	15 (.74)	43 (2.32*)	52 (2.62*)	45 (2.54*)	21
GAD	19 (1.63)	17 (1.80*)	18 (1.93*)	14 (1.19)	03	12 (.96)	06 (.42*)	23 (1.92)	09 (.69)	05 (.39)	08 (.62)	12
GAD: no hierarchy	22 (.95)	23 (1.01)	23 (1.00)	22 (.91)		16 (.65)	07 (.29*)	38 (1.67)	67 (3.45)	90 (4.15*)	72 (4.07*)	23
OCD	08 (.92)	10 (1.16)	10 (1.14)	10 (1.17)	08 (.92)	04	04 (.38)	31 (3.54*)	14 (1.58)	05 (.52)	12 (1.36)	09
SPEC	14 (.89)	18 (1.23)	18 (1.20)	10 (.59*)	17 (1.05)	13 (.80)	20 (1.23)	23 (1.46)	19 (1.18)	10 (.59)	17 (1.05)	16

PTSD	03 (.50)	08 (1.91*)	08 (1.75)	04 (.64)	07 (1.26)	01 (.22)	02 (.31)	00 (—)	10 (1.95)	00 (—)	08 (1.51)	05
Other anxiety	08 (1.73)	06 (1.55)	07 (1.69)	04 (.84)	04 (.82)	04 (.77)	05 (1.11)	00 (—)	02 (.48)	00 (—)	02 (.37)	05
Mood disorders												
MDD	36 (.71)	52 (1.04)	50 (1.00)	44 (.87)	64 (1.33*)	61 (1.24*)	27 (.51*)	77 (1.55*)	52	76 (1.54*)	57	50
DYS	11 (.99)	09 (.69)	04 (.70)	17 (1.67)	13 (1.13)	12 (1.04)	07 (.62)	23 (2.08)	12 (1.11)	05	11	11
Other mood	06 (.74)	06 (.82)	06 (.79)	11 (1.62)	09 (1.27)	10 (1.44)	06 (.84)	08 (1.03)	01 (.15)	05 (.64)	02 (.24)	07
Other disorders												
Alcohol	17 (1.14)	17 (1.29)	17 (1.31)	15 (1.03)	12 (.77)	09 (.60)	07 (.47*)	31 (2.13)	16 (1.10)	29 (1.99)	19 (1.31)	15
Drug	06 (.55)	11 (1.17)	11 (1.09)	11 (1.16)	10 (1.00)	05 (.50)	09 (.90)	23 (2.34)	07 (.72)	14 (1.44)	09 (.87)	10
Alcohol or drug	19 (1.05)	23 (1.36*)	22 (1.35*)	17 (.94)	18 (.93)	10 (.54)	12 (.61)	38 (2.10*)	17 (.92)	29 (1.56)	20 (1.06)	19
Somatoform	00 (—)	02 (.82)	02 (.70)	02 (.60)	06 (2.91*)	04 (1.65)	02 (.71)	00 (—)	02 (1.00)	00 (—)	02 (.77)	02
Other Axis I	11 (1.48)	06 (.79)	07 (.86)	05 (.73)	08 (1.10)	10 (1.40)	11 (1.51)	00 (—)	10 (1.33)	00 (—)	08 (1.03)	08

Note. PD, panic disorder; PDA, panic disorder with agoraphobia; PD/ A, panic disorder with or without agoraphobia; SOC, social phobia; GAD, generalized anxiety disorder; GAD: no hierarchy, generalized anxiety disorder ignoring DSM-IV hierarchy rule with mood disorders; OCD, obsessive-compulsive disorder; SPEC, specific phobia; PTSD, posttraumatic stress disorder; MDD, major depressive disorder; DYS, dysthymia; MDD/DYS, major depressive disorder or dysthymia. From Brown, Campbell, et al. (2001). Copyright 2001 by American Psychological Association. Reprinted by permission.

[a] Overall frequency category was assigned as an additional diagnosis.

*Significantly increased or decreased risk of co-occurring disorder (95% confidence interval).

ting; (2) the features of one disorder act as risk factors for another disorder (e.g., severe agoraphobia leads to mood disturbance due to hopelessness, restricted mobility, etc.); and (3) they emerge from the same diatheses. As an illustration of the first explanation, major depression was found to be the most frequently assigned lifetime additional diagnosis in the Brown, Campbell, et al. study (2001) (50%). This result may have been more a reflection of the fact that major depression is a highly prevalent diagnosis in our research setting and general population (Kessler et al., 1994) than indicative of a boundary problem with other emotional disorders. In regard to the second explanation, findings from the Brown, Campbell, et al. (2001) study indicated that the presence of PTSD was associated with a significantly elevated risk of panic disorder with agoraphobia, and that in the majority of comorbid cases, PTSD preceded panic disorder. These descriptive findings could be interpreted to suggest that the high autonomic arousability and low perceptions of personal control associated with PTSD may have served as precipitants to panic disorder. The third explanation is intriguing in terms of its alignment with theories discussed earlier, which posit that anxiety and mood disorders emanate from shared genetic, biological, and psychosocial vulnerabilities (Barlow et al., 1996). By this account, a certain amount of co-occurrence among disorders would be presumed due to their shared etiological roots.

Effects of Psychosocial Treatment on Comorbid Disorders

Nevertheless, other aspects of extant comorbidity findings perpetuate questions about the discriminant validity of the anxiety and mood disorders. Findings indicate that psychosocial treatment for a given anxiety disorder produces a significant decline in other anxiety or mood diagnoses that are not addressed in treatment (Borkovec, Abel, & Newman, 1995; T. A. Brown, Antony, & Barlow, 1995). For instance, we (T. A. Brown, Antony, & Barlow, 1995) examined the course of additional diagnoses in a sample of 126 patients who were enrolled in a short-term (11-session) psychosocial treatment program for DSM-III-R panic disorder with minimal agoraphobic avoidance. At pretreatment, 26% of patients had an additional diagnosis of GAD. However, the rate of comorbid GAD declined significantly at posttreatment to 9%, and remained at this rate at a 2-year follow-up (see Figure 9.1). Whereas it might be tempting to attribute this decline to treatment generalization (e.g., elements of the treatment, such as cognitive restructuring, were sufficiently powerful to reduce symptoms of both panic disorder and GAD), evidence of the resistance of GAD to current psychosocial and drug treatments mitigates the plausibility of this explanation (cf. Brown, Barlow, & Liebowitz, 1994). Rather, other factors such as a lack of independence between disorders, random measurement error (e.g., diagnostic unreliability), or systematic measurement error (e.g., demand characteristics to overreport symptoms at pretreatment or underreport them at posttreatment; Brown & Barlow, 1992) might be more compelling explanations for the sharp decline in GAD.

However, an interesting pattern of results was obtained when overall comorbidity was examined (i.e., collapsing across all additional diagnoses). In this analysis, a significant pre- to posttreatment decline was still evident—from 40% to 17%. At the 2-year follow-up, however, the rate of comorbidity had increased to a level (30%) that was no longer significantly different from that at pretreatment. This was despite the fact that in the aggregate, patients maintained or improved upon gains for panic disorder across the follow-up interval, indicating considerable independence between panic disorder symptoms and overall comorbidity. Although highly speculative, these findings could be interpreted in accord with the explanation for comorbidity and theoretical models stating that disorders emerge

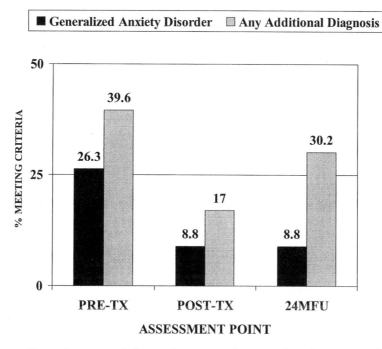

FIGURE 9.1. Effects of cognitive-behavioral treatment for panic disorder on comorbid diagnoses. PRE-TX, pretreatment; POST-TX, posttreatment; 24MFU, 24-month follow-up). Adapted from "Diagnostic Comorbidity in Panic Disorder: Effect on Treatment Outcome and Course of Comorbid Diagnoses Following Treatment" by T. A. Brown, M. M. Antony, and D. H. Barlow, 1995, *Journal of Consulting and Clinical Psychology, 63,* 408–418. Copyright 1995 by the American Psychological Association. Adapted with permission.

from shared vulnerabilities. Specifically, it could be argued that cognitive-behavioral treatment was generally effective at ameliorating the symptoms and maintaining processes of panic disorder, but did not result in substantial reductions in the general predispositional features (e.g., trait negative affect) that left patients vulnerable to the emergence or continuation of other disorders.

Nonspecificity of Treatment Response

The fact that numerous disorders respond similarly to the same psychosocial or drug treatment has also been cited as evidence of their overlap and poor discriminant validity (Hudson & Pope, 1990; Tyrer et al., 1988). Findings that a wide range of emotional disorders (e.g., major depression, dysthymia, OCD, panic disorder) respond equivalently to antidepressant medications has been interpreted as indicating overlap or a shared pathophysiology among these syndromes (e.g., Hudson & Pope, 1990).

In one of the largest studies bearing on this issue to date, Tyrer et al. (1988) treated 210 outpatients with GAD, panic disorder, or dysthymia with one of the following five interventions: diazepam, dothiepin, placebo, cognitive-behavioral therapy, or a self-help program. Although some treatment condition differences were noted at posttreatment (e.g., diazepam was less effective than dothiepin, cognitive-behavioral therapy, and self-help), no diagnostic group differences were obtained. In view of the lack of diagnostic group treatment response differences, Tyrer et al. concluded that differential diagnosis of anxiety and mood disorders does not provide a sound basis for treatment prescription. However, these conclusions are limited by several issues, such as the absence of long-term outcome data and the use of nonspecific psychosocial treatments rather than more recent interventions designed specifically to target the key and maintaining features of the disorders in question (cf. Brown, O'Leary, & Barlow, 2001; Craske & Barlow, 2001; Young, Weinberger, & Beck, 2001).

Latent Structure of Dimensional Features of Emotional Disorders

Reliability and comorbidity studies conducted at the diagnostic level are limited in their ability to make strong and compelling contributions to the validation of current nosologies of emotional disorders. As we have discussed at length elsewhere (Brown, 1996, in press; Brown et al., 1998), the categorical approach to analysis has many limitations (cf. Costello, 1992; Livesley, Schroeder, Jackson, & Jang, 1994). For instance, studies conducted at the diagnostic level (e.g., comorbidity, genetic or familial aggregation, across-diagnosis comparisons) are restricted by their adherence to the disorders defined by the classification system. That is, by using diagnoses as the units of analysis, researchers are implicitly accepting or are bound to the nosology they are evaluating. Moreover, analyses at the diagnostic level rely largely on data that do not reflect the dimensional nature of psychopathological phenomena. Categorization of dimensional variables usually forfeits meaningful information by artificially (and often erroneously) collapsing variability above and below an arbitrary threshold (e.g., presence–absence of a DSM-IV disorder). In addition to reducing statistical power and limiting the ability to detect more complex uni- or multivariate relationships, this categorization often unnecessarily introduces additional measurement error. In the Brown et al. (2001) study reviewed earlier in this chapter, a common source of unreliability consisted of interviewer disagreements on whether or not the features of a disorder met or surpassed the DSM threshold. Moreover, dimensional ratings of the constituent features of major depression were found to be far more reliable than the DSM-IV categorical severity descriptors (mild, moderate, severe). Thus, whereas considerable concordance was observed at the dimensional level, error was inflated when a qualitative system was imposed on these ratings. In contrast, when evaluation is conducted at the dimensional level, the interrelationships among symptoms and syndromes can be examined, as can the extent to which the latent structure of these features corresponds to that specified by major classification systems such as DSM-IV.

In addition, many studies bearing on the classification of emotional disorders are limited because specific disorders are often evaluated in isolation from other disorders (Watson et al., 1994). For example, the associated symptom criterion for DSM-IV GAD was revised (i.e., autonomic arousal symptoms were eliminated) without empirical consideration of how this might further obfuscate its boundary with the mood disorders (Brown, Barlow, & Liebowitz, 1994; T. A. Brown, Marten, & Barlow, 1995; Marten et al., 1993). The decision to emphasize the parameter of the uncontrollability of worry in DSM-IV was based largely on its ability to distinguish GAD from nonpathological worry, rather than from other anxiety and mood disorders (Abel & Borkovec, 1995; Borkovec, 1994a; Starcevic, 1995). Ideally, evaluations of the structure and construct validity of emotional disorders should entail features of the full range of anxiety and mood disorders, given the strong relationship and potential overlap of these domains (Clark & Watson, 1991; Kendall & Watson, 1989; Watson et al., 1994).

Initial Studies of Latent Structure

Large-scale studies that evaluate the latent structure of the dimensional features of emotional disorders are beginning to appear in the literature (e.g., Brown et al., 1998; Spence, 1997; Zinbarg & Barlow, 1996). For example, Spence (1997) examined the structure of anxiety symptoms in 698 children (8–12 years of age), using confirmatory factor analysis of a questionnaire of the frequency of symptoms from six DSM-IV constructs: panic disorder, separation anxiety disorder, social phobia, specific fears, OCD, and GAD. Compared to competing models in which disorders were collapsed or factors were constrained to be orthogonal, the six-factor model provided a superior fit to the data. Although factorially distinct, the six disorder factors were highly intercorrelated (range of r's = .67 to .88). However, the considerable covariance in these latent factors was satisfactorily accounted for by a higher-order model in which the six disorder factors loaded significantly onto a single second-order factor. This higher-order model is consistent with the DSM-IV nosology, which asserts that panic disorder, separation anxiety disorder, social phobia, specific phobia, OCD, and GAD, albeit distinct, belong to a common family of disorders. This higher-order model was replicated in a second cohort and was found to be consistent across sexes and age groups. Although this research was limited to some degree by its use of a single self-report measure and a nonclinical sample, as well as its failure to include a depression factor (i.e., mood disorders may be highly overlapping with some anxiety disorders such as GAD), the results are encouraging with regard to the correspondence of the obtained latent structure with the nosology outlined in DSM-IV.

In another study (Zinbarg & Barlow, 1996), the symptoms of DSM-III-R anxiety disorders were assessed dimensionally by questionnaire and clinical ratings in 432 adult patients and 32 normal controls. Exploratory factor analyses produced a six-factor solution consisting of the following factors: Social Anxiety, Generalized Anxiety, Agoraphobia, Panic, Obsessions and Compulsions, and Simple Fears. Confirmatory factor analysis indicated that a hierarchical model consisting of one higher-order factor (on which each of the six primary factors loaded significantly) provided a significantly better fit than a model in which the six primary factors were constrained as orthogonal. In line with recent conceptual models (e.g., L. A. Clark et al., 1994; Watson et al., 1994), this higher-order factor was labeled Negative Affect. Using factor scores for the first- and higher-order factors, the extent to which the different anxiety disorder groups (determined by the ADIS-R) displayed characteristic factor score profiles was examined. A discriminant-function analysis yielded six statistically significant functions. One function, defined primarily by the Negative Affect factor, discriminated each of the patient groups from the normal controls with no significant differences among patient groups. The second function, defined by the Panic factor, discriminated the patients with a DSM-III-R principal diagnosis of panic disorder with or without agoraphobia from each of the other groups. The third function, defined by the Agoraphobia factor, discriminated patients with panic disorder with agoraphobia from the other groups. The fourth function, defined by the Social Anxiety factor, discriminated patients with social phobia from the other groups. The fifth function, defined by the Obsessions and Compulsions factor, discriminated patients with OCD from each of the other groups. The sixth function, defined by the Generalized Anxiety factor, discriminated patients with specific phobia and normal controls from the other groups.

Thus the results indicated a reasonably good match between the discriminant function classification and the DSM-defined anxiety disorder diagnoses. In addition, the results of the exploratory factor analyses and discriminant-function analyses provided some empirical support for the construct validity of these diagnostic classifications. As in the study by Spence (1997), the emergence of the higher-order factor and its corresponding discriminant function indicated that the various anxiety disorders are related and belong in a common family or group of disorders (yet, this conclusion was limited by the fact that the higher-order factor was theoretical in nature and was not quantified by observed measures). However, the primary factors and their corresponding discriminant functions indicated that it is possible to differentiate reliably among the members of this family. Although encouraging, these findings were limited by such factors as the preponderant use of self-report measures (e.g., method variance could account in part for the structure observed) and the fact that mood disorders were poorly represented (i.e., depressive symptoms were assessed by a single measure, which was a scale under psychometric development). This latter limitation is quite noteworthy in view of evidence that mood disorders (i.e., major depression, dysthymia) show greater overlap with certain anxiety disorders than do other anxiety disorders (cf. T. A. Brown, Marten, & Barlow, 1995; Brown et al., 1998; D. A. Clark, Steer, & Beck, 1994; Starcevic, 1995).

Distinguishability of Anxiety Disorders and Mood Disorders

Indeed, we now know that evaluation of the discriminant validity of the anxiety disorders cannot be accomplished without consideration of boundary issues with depression. Many of the studies discussed thus far in this chapter underscore the overlap between anxiety and depression. For example, in our large-scale diagnostic reliability study of the DSM-IV anxiety and mood disorders (Brown, Di Nardo, et al., 2001), in the 35 diagnostic disagreements with GAD that involved another clinical disorder, the majority (19, or 54%) entailed major depression or dysthymia. In our recent study of the comorbidity among DSM-IV anxiety and mood disorders (Brown, Campbell, et al., 2001), major depression was by far the most common lifetime additional diagnosis in patients with a principal anxiety disorder. Findings from this study also strongly supported prior evidence of the relative infrequency of cases of "pure" depression (i.e., patients who present with mood disorders without current or past anxiety disorders; cf. Alloy, Kelly, Mineka, & Clements, 1990; Mineka, Watson, & Clark, 1998). Specifically, of the 670 patients who had lifetime major depression or dysthymia, only 33 (5%) did not have a current or past anxiety disorder. In the majority of cases of comorbid anxiety and depression, anxiety disorders were more likely to precede than to follow the onset of mood disorders, although this temporal sequence was more evident for major depression than for dysthymia.

Historically, psychometric studies of anxiety and depression have also noted considerable overlap in these constructs (Kendall & Watson, 1989). For instance, intercorrelations among widely used self-report measures (e.g., the State–Trait Anxiety Inventory, the Beck Depression Inventory) and clinical rating scales (e.g., the Hamilton Anxiety and Depression Rating Scales) of anxiety and depression have typically exceeded .70 (Clark & Watson, 1991). These findings, in tandem with studies conducted at the diagnostic level, led investigators to question whether clinical anxiety and depression are in fact empirically distinct phenomena. Based on a comprehensive review of this literature, Clark and Watson (1991) concluded that although anxiety and depression share a significant nonspecific component encompassing general affective distress and other common symptoms, the two constructs can be distinguished by certain unique features. Accordingly, these authors proposed a tripartite structure of anxiety and depression, consisting of (1) negative affect (symptoms of general distress such as worry, irritability, tension); (2) positive affect (defined as the level of pleasurable engagement with the environment and characterized by features such as cheerfulness, sociability, energy, and enthusiasm); and (3) autonomic arousal (characterized by symptoms such as rapid heart rate, shortness of breath, and trembling). As originally proposed, the tripartite model asserts that negative affect is a shared feature of anxiety and mood disorders (i.e., symptoms of tension, worry, irritability, etc., are present in both anxiety and depression). However, autonomic arousal is seen as specific to anxiety, whereas an absence of positive affect (anhedonia) is viewed as differentiating mood disorders from anxiety disorders.

Sophisticated studies have emerged in support of the tripartite structure in adult and child samples (e.g., Chorpita, Albano, & Barlow, 1998; Joiner, Catanzaro, & Laurent, 1996; Watson, Clark, et al., 1995; Watson, Weber, et al., 1995). Although the primary intent of the tripartite model was the delineation of the shared and unique features of anxiety and mood disorders, subsequent research has suggested that this model may have considerable relevance to the understanding of the pathogenesis of these conditions. Findings suggest that negative affect and perhaps positive affect represent trait vulnerability factors for the development of emotional disorders. Negative affect evidences considerable temporal stability: It has 12-year test–retest correlations > .70; is strongly heritable; and, as a higher-order factor, accounts for covariance or communality in lower-order symptom dimensions (e.g., Costa & McCrae, 1988; Tellegen et al., 1988; Watson & Clark, 1984; see Watson et al., 1994, for a review). Although developed independently, the constructs of negative affect and positive affect coincide closely with trait vulnerability constructs of other leading theories, such as Gray's (1987), Eysenck's (1981), and our own (Barlow et al., 1996). For instance, negative affect is a construct similar to behavioral inhibition, neuroticism, and anxious apprehension in the Gray, Eysenck, and Barlow et al. models, respectively. The construct of positive affect is analogous to behavioral activation and extraversion in the Gray and Eysenck models, respectively.

Conceptualizations emphasizing the construct of negative affect as a higher-order, pathogenic factor that is shared by anxiety and depression have strong bearing on the classification of emotional disorders (L. A. Clark et al., 1994; Watson et al., 1994). For instance, these models align with a theoretical explanation that the high co-occurrence of anxiety and mood disorders is due in part to the fact that these conditions emerge from the same etiological sources. Recent genetic evidence is consistent with this position. As reviewed in Chapter 6, in a study of 1,033 "blindly" assessed female twin pairs, Kendler et al. (1992a) found that GAD is a moderately familial disorder, with a heritability estimated at about 30%. Subsequent research in both all-female (Kendler et al., 1992c) and mixed-sex twin samples (Roy, Neale, Pedersen, Mathé, & Kendler, 1995) has indicated that whereas a clear genetic influence exists in GAD, the genetic factors in GAD are completely shared with major depression. Whereas this shared genetic basis could be viewed as further indication of the poor boundaries of these conditions, other empirical evidence suggests that this may not be the case. Although the disorders share genetic factors, the environmental determinants of GAD and major depression were found in Kendler et al. (1992c) to be largely distinct.

These findings are consistent with the aforementioned conceptual models of emotional disorders (e.g., Barlow et al., 1996; see Chapter 8), which view the anxiety and mood disorders as sharing vulnerabilities but differing on important dimensions (e.g., focus of attention, degree of psychosocial vulnerability arising from environmental experiences), to the extent that differentiation of these psychopathological phenomena is warranted. Whereas biologically or genetically based traits such as negative affect and behavioral inhibition may underlie social phobia and panic disorder, whether or not one or both conditions become manifest could depend on environmental determinants (specific psychological vulnerabilities) such as direct experiences with social humiliation or scrutiny, vicarious exposure (e.g., parental modeling) to shyness/introversion or hypochondriacal behavior, and so on. Predictions based on the tripartite model (Watson et al., 1994) would further assert that though anxiety and depression possess common vulnerability dimensions, it is possible that unique diatheses exist as well (e.g., low positive affect in depression; cf. Brown et al., 1998; L. A. Clark et al., 1994).

Structural Relationships of Dimensions of Emotional Disorders and Dimensions of the Tripartite Model

We recently published a study that examined the latent structure of the dimensional features of major emotional disorders (panic disorder with/without agoraphobia, social phobia, OCD, GAD, unipolar mood disorders) and the constructs composing the tripartite model of anxiety and depression (negative affect, positive affect, autonomic arousal) (Brown et al., 1998). This study extended prior investigations (e.g., Spence, 1997; Zinbarg & Barlow, 1996) of the latent structure of emotional disorders in a number of ways: (1) multimethod measurement (use of self-report measures and clinical ratings derived from the ADIS-IV-L); (2) inclusion of indicators of mood disorders; and (3) specification of higher-order factors defined by observed measures (i.e., in Spence, 1997, and Zinbarg & Barlow, 1996, the common higher-order factor was hypothetical in nature and did not entail indicators of negative affect, positive affect, etc.).

Using a sample of 350 patients with DSM-IV anxiety and mood disorders, we (Brown et al., 1998) found that a confirmatory factor analysis of the latent structure of dimensions of key features of the DSM-IV disorders supported the discriminant validity of DSM-IV for the five constructs examined, consistent with the earlier findings of Spence (1997) and Zinbarg and Barlow (1996). Specifically, four models were fitted to the data: (1) a five-factor model consistent with the DSM-IV typology distinguishing mood disorders, panic disorder with/without agoraphobia, social phobia, OCD, and GAD; (2) a one-factor model in accord with a "general neurotic syndrome" (cf. Andrews, 1990; Tyrer, 1989), asserting that the features of a broader underlying syndrome have been erroneously distinguished as separate disorders; (3) a two-factor model consisting of anxiety versus mood disorders; and (4) a four-factor model in which the features of GAD and mood disorders were collapsed to load on a single factor. Relative to the other models, the five-factor model (i.e., mood disorders, panic disorder with/without agoraphobia, social phobia, OCD, GAD) provided the best fit for the data. Notably, model fit was degraded significantly when indicators of GAD and mood disorders were collapsed into a single factor, thereby lending support for the differentiation of these features.

While upholding the discriminant validity of these domains, inspection of the zero-order correlations among latent factors highlighted areas of overlap. For instance, the GAD latent factor was most strongly correlated with the mood disorder latent factor ($r = .63$), supporting contentions that the features of GAD have the most overlap with the mood disorders. Moreover, the OCD latent factor had its strongest correlation with the GAD factor ($r = .52$), consistent with the position that the closest "neighbor" to OCD among the various anxiety and mood disorders is GAD (perhaps due to the overlap in chronic worry and obsessions; Abramowitz & Foa, 1998; Brown, Moras, Zinbarg, & Barlow, 1993; Turner, Beidel, & Stanley, 1992). Whereas the distinction of GAD from other anxiety and mood disorders was supported by the superiority of the five-factor model, these data also indicated that GAD had the highest degree of overlap with the other DSM-IV disorder factors (i.e., the latent factor DSM-IV GAD consistently had the strongest zero-order correlations with other DSM-IV factors). Moreover, the GAD latent factor evidenced a strong association with the nonspecific trait dimension of negative affect ($r = .74$).

In addition to examining the latent structure of anxiety and mood disorders, we (Brown et al., 1998) comparatively evaluated several structural models of the interrelationships among the five DSM-IV disorder latent factors and three latent factors corresponding to the tripartite model of anxiety and depression (i.e., negative affect, positive affect, autonomic arousal). Consistent with the theoretical predictions, superior data fit was associated with a model that specified Negative Affect and Positive Affect as higher-order factors to the DSM-IV disorder factors (with significant paths from Negative Affect to each of the five DSM-IV factors, and significant paths from Positive Affect to the Mood Disorder and Social Phobia factors only), and that specified Autonomic Arousal as a lower-order factor (with significant paths from Panic Disorder/Agoraphobia and Generalized Anxiety Disorder to Autonomic Arousal). This model is presented in Figure 9.2. Notably, although all paths were statistically significant, the strongest paths from the higher-order factor of negative affect to the various DSM-IV factors were to GAD and mood disorder. These results are consistent with predictions of the tripartite model that negative affect is a shared dispositional (vulnerability) trait of anxiety and mood disorders, but that GAD and mood disorders are associated with the highest levels of this dimension (although these interpretations require verification in longitudinal research).

Of further interest was the finding that although the Generalized Anxiety Disorder and Autonomic Arousal factors were positively correlated at the zero-order level ($r = .48$), in the structural model the path from Generalized Anxiety Disorder to Autonomic Arousal was negative ($-.22$, $p < .001$). Thus a suppressor effect was operative in this portion of the model, which was attributed to the findings that at the zero-order level, both Generalized Anxiety Disorder and Autonomic Arousal were strongly correlated with Negative Affect (both r's = .74). In other words, when variance in Negative Affect was removed (which occurred in the structural model when Negative Affect was specified as a higher-order factor), the true relationship between Generalized Anxiety Disorder and Autonomic Arousal

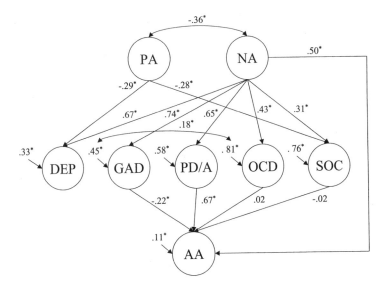

FIGURE 9.2. Structural Model of the Interrelationships of DSM-IV Disorder Constructs and Negative Affect, Positive Affect, and Autonomic Arousal. PA, positive affect; NA, negative affect; DEP, mood disorders; GAD, generalized anxiety disorder; PD/A, panic disorder with/without agoraphobia; OCD, obsessive–compulsive disorder; SOC, social phobia; AA, autonomic arousal. *$p < .01$. From "Structural Relationships among Dimensions of the DSM-IV Anxiety and Mood Disorders and Dimensions of Negative Affect, Positive Affect, and Autonomic Arousal" by T. A. Brown, B. F. Chorpita, and D. H. Barlow, 1998, *Journal of Abnormal Psychology, 107,* 179–192. Copyright 1998 by the American Psychological Association. Reprinted with permission.

was explicated (i.e., the direction of their association was reversed). Therefore, the presence of autonomic symptoms in Generalized Anxiety Disorder may be due to the high levels of negative affect associated with this disorder. However, in accounting for variance in Autonomic Arousal due to negative affect, the true direct influence of the disorder-specific features of Generalized Anxiety Disorder on Autonomic Arousal (i.e., autonomic suppression) may have been illuminated. This finding is noteworthy in view of its concordance with laboratory studies indicating that GAD and chronic worry are associated with the suppression of autonomic responsivity (e.g., Borkovec, Lyonfields, Wiser, & Diehl, 1993; Hoehn-Saric, McLeod, & Zimmerli, 1989). Moreover, modification indices from the structural model indicated that data fit would not be improved with the addition of a path from DSM-IV Mood Disorders to Autonomic Arousal, thereby highlighting another possible point of distinction between generalized anxiety disorder and the mood disorders (i.e., generalized anxiety disorder, but not the disorder-specific features of clinical depression, is associated with autonomic inflexibility).

However, counter to predictions of the tripartite model, paths from the DSM disorder factors Obsessive-Compulsive Disorder and Social Phobia to Autonomic Arousal were nonsignificant (see Figure 9.2). These results suggest that, although generally unrelated to mood disorders, autonomic arousal symptoms may be weakly related or of less discriminant value for certain anxiety disorders (e.g., discrete social phobias). Accordingly, these findings contributed to a refinement of the tripartite model with regard to autonomic arousal. Although autonomic arousal was initially posited to be a discriminating feature for the entire range of anxiety disorders, these data suggest that the relevance of autonomic arousal may be limited primarily to panic disorder with or without agoraphobia. This interpretation is reflected in the most recent iteration of the tripartite model (Mineka et al., 1998).

As was true for Negative Affect, results involving the higher-order factor of Positive Affect were generally consistent with prediction. Support for the tripartite model was obtained by findings of a significant path from (low) Positive Affect to Mood Disorders and small modification indices indicating that model fit would not improve (i.e., the paths would be nonsignificant) if paths were added from Positive Affect to Generalized Anxiety Disorder, Panic Disorder/Agoraphobia, or Obsessive-Compulsive Disorder. Thus, such findings support the contention that low positive affect is more specifically linked to depression. However, somewhat counter to expectations, an equally strong association was obtained between positive affect and social phobia (cf. Amies, Gelder, & Shaw, 1983; Watson, Clark, & Carey, 1988). In addition, the social phobia latent factor had a significantly stronger zero-order relationship with positive affect than did the other anxiety disorder factors. The relationship of social phobia to positive affect has been interpreted as being based on the interpersonal character of low positive affect (e.g., low confidence, unassertiveness; L. A. Clark et al., 1994). Moreover, such findings could be interpreted as suggesting diagnostic overlap between the social phobia and mood disorder constructs, or perhaps as indicating that these disorders share a vulnerability dimension (low positive affect) that is not found in other emotional disorders.

Along these lines, it is interesting to note the findings from our DSM-IV comorbidity study of the strong and statistically significant aggregation of the mood disorders and social phobia (Brown, Campbell, et al., 2001). By far the most frequent additional current or lifetime diagnosis in principal major depression and dysthymia was social phobia (excluding other mood disorders). These associations were confirmed by odds ratio findings: For both current and lifetime diagnoses, the presence of social phobia was associated with a significantly increased risk of major depression and dysthymia (and vice versa). In fact, social phobia was the only DSM-IV anxiety disorder to be associated with increased risk of both current and lifetime dysthymia.

SUMMARY AND CONCLUSIONS

Shortcomings and Usefulness of the DSM System

Much of the evidence reviewed in this chapter has underscored the shortcomings of a purely categorical approach to classifying the anxiety and mood disorders. To name just a few of these problems, the purely categorical system of the DSM has been associated with (1) measurement error (diagnostic unreliability) arising from threshold disagreements (i.e., whether the features of a given disorder are sufficient in number, duration, or severity to warrant a DSM-IV diagnosis; Brown, Di Nardo, et al., 2001); (2) high prevalence of and diagnostic unreliability involving NOS categories (Brown, Campbell, et al., 2001; Brown, Di Nardo, et al., 2001); (3) artifactual rates of comorbidity due to the differential diagnosis and diagnostic hierarchy rules (e.g., lower rate of current and lifetime comorbidity between mood disorders and GAD because of the DSM-IV hierarchy rule; Brown, Campbell, et al., 2001); and (4) loss of important information regarding the severity and associated features of disorders (e.g., a DSM-IV diagnosis of panic disorder with agoraphobia conveys no information about frequency and intensity of panic attacks and the severity of agoraphobic avoidance). Moreover, the disjunctive approach to categorical classification embedded in DSM (e.g., DSM-IV major depression can be assigned in the context of any five symptoms from a list of nine) promotes a high level of within-diagnosis heterogeneity that further mitigates the validity and utility of the diagnostic system (Clark et al., 1995). For instance, the inability to empirically establish a relationship between comorbid major depression and treatment response for anxiety disorders (cf. Brown & Barlow, 1995) could be due partially to the fact that only certain symptom clusters within the category of major depression (e.g., psychomotor retardation, hopelessness, anhedonia) are poor prognostic indicators; the presence and heterogeneity of these constituent symptoms is largely ignored by DSM, which emphasizes the presence or absence of diagnosis. However, DSM-IV has attempted to address this issue to some extent by the introduction of specifiers and subtypes for some categories (e.g., the various types of DSM-IV specific phobia).

In addition, the extant literature points to considerable overlap among the various anxiety and mood disorders. At the diagnostic level, this lack of independence is evidenced by high rates of current and lifetime comorbidity (Brown & Barlow, 1992; Brown, Campbell, et al., 2001; Kessler et al., 1996, 1997, 1998; Kessler, Stang, et al., 1999; Magee et al., 1996; Wittchen et al., 1994), nonspecificity of treatment response (e.g., Tyrer et al., 1989), and the remission of comorbid conditions following psychosocial treatment of the principal disorder (Borkovec et al., 1995; T. A. Brown, Antony, & Barlow, 1995). An even stronger degree of overlap is found at the symptom level, supported by the wide-ranging and consistent evidence that important definitional features such as worry, social anxiety, negative affect, and panic attacks are found to varying degrees in all emotional disorders and in persons not meeting formal diagnostic criteria for a mental disorder (e.g., Borkovec, 1994a; Brown et al., 1998; Craske, Rapee, Jackel, & Barlow, 1989; Norton, Cox, & Malan, 1992; Rapee, Sanderson, & Barlow, 1988).

On the other hand, initial evidence indicates that the dimensional key features of the DSM anxiety and mood disorders, though overlapping to various degrees, display a high level of discriminant validity (e.g., Brown et al., 1998; Spence, 1997; Zinbarg & Barlow, 1996). Moreover, most of the shared variance of these emotional disorder constructs can be accounted for by a higher-order dimension of general distress/negative affect, and in the case of mood disorders and social phobia, low positive affect as well (Brown et al., 1998). Such findings would seem to argue against the utility of a "general neurotic syndrome" where the various emotional disorder features are collapsed into one broad entity. Instead, these data suggest a *family* of constructs that are interrelated in part because of their common relationship to higher-order traits (i.e., negative affect) associated with a genetic basis, high temporal stability, and strong predictive value for etiology, course, and treatment response of psychopathological conditions (L. A. Clark et al., 1994; Watson et al., 1994).

On a more basic level, there remains the issue of whether classification should be categorical or dimensional (Brown, 1996; Clark et al., 1995; Frances et al., 1990). With marked overlap in symptoms, it is tempting to turn to purely dimensional analyses for anxiety and mood disorders. On the other hand, there seems to be evidence of the importance of identifying at least some of the clusters of symptoms specified in the DSM-IV anxiety and mood disorder categories. If one can forgo the notion that these are distinct entities with single causes and no particular relation to other descriptive psychopathology, then identifying certain disorders seems more useful than does a strictly dimensional analysis. For example, there is growing evidence for the importance of identifying anxiety focused on panic in panic disorder (see Chapter 10). Anxiety focused on negative evaluation and other performance anxieties currently grouped under the category of social phobia seem to be processes that define a boundary in relation to other anxiety and mood disorders (see Chapter 13). Blood–injection–injury phobia is characterized by a physiological response distinct from that of other specific fears (Öst, Sterner, & Lindahl, 1984)—a finding that is reflected in the specific phobia subtypes introduced in DSM-IV (see Chapter 11). Moreover, although considerable consensus exists for the conclusion that measures of psychopathological symptoms operate dimensionally, expression of symptoms on a continuum cannot be taken alone to confirm or refute the absence of underlying taxa (e.g., quantitative indicators can have dichotomous latent influences, such as presence–absence of a gene; cf. Meehl, 1995; Waller & Meehl, 1997).

Thus diagnostic categories such as those specified in DSM-IV, though not qualifying in any sense as real entities (Kendall & Butcher, 1982; Kendell, 1975), seem to be useful concepts or constructs that emerge as "blips" on a general background of a varying mixture of anxious and depressed symptoms. Researchers (e.g., Tyrer, 1984) have described the somewhat confused state of the classification of emotional disorders and have called for longitudinal studies to determine the patterns and relationships of these symptoms over time. This will be an important step. In the meantime, in view of the relatively good reliability of most DSM-IV anxiety and mood disorder categories, a full description of these problems as they exist in each individual—a description based on functional relationships, but without regard to arbitrary hierarchical exclusionary systems—seems an important step in both clinical and research settings.

Future Classification Systems

One issue in the area of classification on which everyone can agree is that DSM-IV does not represent the last word on classifying anxiety and mood disorders. We have concluded that at present, a combination of categorical and dimensional classification best represents reality and should be most helpful in clinical planning. Potential advantages of including dimensional elements within the classification system include (1) reduced measurement error associated with categorical cutoffs; (2) enhanced diagnostic coverage and reconciliation of the problem of frequent NOS diagnoses; (3) better parsimony through the identification of a smaller set of basic dimensions (compared to the 300+ categories that exist in DSM-IV); and (4) recognition of the severity and heterogeneity of symptom expression, as well as other important clinical information that is largely ignored by a purely categorical approach. As stated earlier in this chapter, studying the nature of psychopathological phenomena at the dimensional level will accelerate the advances in the clinical science, because this inquiry is relatively independent of the classification system in place at the time (e.g., the results from studies of diagnostic comorbidity are influenced strongly by existing definitional criteria and are subject to problems associated with categorical assessment, such as elevated measurement error).

On the other hand, much work must be done before a dimensional system can be seriously considered for incorporation in the formal nosology. Investigators involved in the preparation of DSM-IV considered and rejected the adoption of a dimensional classification, in part because "there is as yet no agreement on the choice of the optimal dimensions to be used for classification purposes" (American Psychiatric Association, 1994, p. xxii). Indeed, whereas many researchers have acknowledged the potential utility of such systems, an enormous amount of empirical and conceptual groundwork is needed on the identification, measurement, and validation of the core dimensional elements. As succinctly stated by Clark et al. (1995), "it is time to halt the general call for dimensional systems and to begin the hard work of developing specific dimensional proposals in targeted domains" (p. 147).

In the meantime, it is hoped that a dimensional assessment of psychopathology will gain greater prominence in research on classification and pathogenesis, such as in familial/genetic and longitudinal studies. In twin studies, greater emphasis on dimensional assessment (e.g., latent disorder constructs), in tandem with a structural equation modeling approach to analysis (cf. Boomsma, Martin, & Neale, 1989) could lead to important advances beyond evidence on the heritability and familial aggregation of disorders focused at the diagnostic (categorical) level (i.e., estimates of genetic liability are limited by heightened measurement error and lower statistical power when dimensional symptom variability and severity are collapsed above and below the DSM threshold). Genetic studies of this nature have begun to appear in the literature (e.g., Kendler, Heath, Martin, & Eaves, 1987).

At least two important avenues for longitudinal research exist. One avenue involves the study of at-risk or large nonclinical samples to determine the predictive validity of dimensions implicated as generalized vulnerability factors (e.g., negative affect) to emotional disorders, and to establish whether these "higher-order" traits are more explanatory than vulnerability constructs suggested to be disorder-specific (e.g., anxiety sensitivity, thought–action fusion, autonomy–sociotropy; Ingram, Miranda, & Segal, 1998; Salkovskis, 1996; Taylor, 1999; Watson et al., 1994). Some preliminary results from studies of this nature have been reviewed in Chapter 8. A second avenue entails large-scale clinical studies that examine the temporal stability and covariation of latent factors corresponding to the emotional disorders and their underlying vulnerability constructs. This methodology is crucial to the better understanding of the direction of the relationships among disorders and potential vulnerability constructs (e.g., theory-driven tests of selected conceptual accounts for comorbidity such as the features of a disorder that serve as risk factors to another disorder). For instance, whereas the findings of the Brown et al. (1998) study were consistent with the position that negative affect operates as a higher-order trait, the cross-sectional nature of this study precluded conclusions about the direction and the possible reciprocal nature of these relationships. This and other important questions regarding the classification of emotional disorders await longitudinal study. With this perspective in mind, it is now possible to focus on a detailed description of the presenting characteristics, etiology, assessment, and treatment of each of the anxiety disorders—a task that occupies the remainder of this book.

Panic Disorder and Agoraphobia

KAMILA S. WHITE
DAVID H. BARLOW

The evolution of our understanding of panic disorder with agoraphobia (PDA) and its treatments over the last two decades has been rapid and exciting. Since it was formally recognized as a discrete disorder in the revised third edition of the *Diagnostic and Statistical Manual of Mental Disorders* (DSM-III-R; American Psychiatric Association [APA], 1987), PDA has become the most investigated of the anxiety disorders. Conceptualizations of PDA in the first edition of this book (Barlow, 1988)—panic disorder as anxiety focused on somatic sensations associated with panic attacks, and agoraphobia as a strategy for coping with panic attacks by avoiding unsafe situations where attacks might occur—are increasingly supported today. In addition, evidence continues to accumulate supporting the efficacy of cognitive-behavioral and drug treatments for PDA. In this chapter we review the modern developments in the conceptualization, assessment, and treatment of PDA. The chapter begins with an overview of the clinical presentation and diagnostic classification of PDA, followed by our model of etiology and development. After a discussion of effective methods for diagnosis and assessment, we review the empirically supported psychological and drug treatments for PDA—including the cognitive-behavioral treatment (CBT) protocol developed in our clinic, "panic control treatment" (PCT). We conclude by highlighting our recent efforts to improve long-term outcome for patients with PDA, and by discussing areas in need of further research.

A HISTORICAL CONTEXT

Westphal (1871) coined the term "agoraphobia" in the late 1800s; however, the condition known as agoraphobia only became well known during the late 1970s and the 1980s. Since that time, PDA has become one of the most widely recognized and publicized anxiety disorders. The earlier views of agoraphobia as a fear of venturing into crowded areas are inconsistent with the model alluded to in previous chapters, which highlights the centrality of panic in generating agoraphobia. In fact, the term "agoraphobia" is somewhat misleading, based on our current model of PDA. Were it not for an accident of history, this seeming misdirection might not have occurred. In 1870, a year before Westphal, Benedikt (1870) suggested another name for what was certainly the same condition. The German term *platzschwindel*, referring to the sensation of dizziness in public places, conveys what now seems to be a more accurate conception of the disorder. We now know that individuals with this disorder focus on and attempt to avoid internal physical sensations associated with panic, and dizziness is indeed one of the primary symptoms of panic. Over the years, clinicians have suggested alternative labels to capture this essential feature of PDA, as did Roth (1960) when he referred to agoraphobia as the "phobic anxiety–depersonalization syndrome." In any case, what these clinicians were communicating was that the central problem in PDA is anxiety focused on the symptoms of panic; hence the well-known and commonly accepted characterization of agoraphobia as "fear of fear."

Since that time, evidence has indeed accumulated (reviewed below) supporting our basic assumption that agoraphobic avoidance behavior is a secondary but associated feature of unexpected panic. This avoidance behavior is multiply determined and maintained, and it is closely associated (at least initially) with the escapist action tendencies of the basic emotion of fear (i.e., panic). Over time, agoraphobic avoidance may become one way of coping with anxiety over the possibility of additional unexpected panics.

DIAGNOSTIC CLASSIFICATION AND CLINICAL OVERVIEW

Panic Disorder and the Nature of Panic Attacks

As detailed in DSM-IV (APA, 1994) and in Chapter 4, a "panic attack" is an intense, discrete episode of fear or discomfort accompanied by various somatic and cognitive symptoms; these may include palpitations, chest pain, sweating, trembling, shortness of breath, and paresthesias (i.e., numbness or tingling), as well as fears of dying, losing control, or going crazy. Although panic attacks can occur as a part of all anxiety disorders, panic disorder is distinguished by the occurrence of unexpected, often seemingly uncued or "out-of-the-blue" panic attacks. The DSM-IV diagnostic criteria for panic disorder require recurrent panic attacks (operationalized as a minimum of two unexpected attacks). The attacks must peak in severity within 10 minutes and must be followed by 1 month or more of persistent worry about future attacks, worry about the consequences of the attacks (e.g., dying, having a heart attack, going crazy, losing bowel control), or a behavioral change because of the attacks (e.g., cutting back on work, more frequent medical check ups, placing the phone next to the bed at night). This "behavioral change" criterion covers "nonfearful" panic attacks in which the individual does not report anxiety about future attacks, but seems to manifest this anxiety through changes in behavior (see Chapter 4). And, as with the other anxiety disorders, the symptoms cannot be the direct result of the effects of a substance (e.g., caffeine) or a general medical condition (e.g., hyperthyroidism, hypoglycemia). This is usually determined by noting whether the onset and offset of symptoms is directly related to the onset and offset of the medical condition.

Agoraphobia

Panic disorder may occur with or without the presence of agoraphobia, although at least mild agoraphobia is almost always present (see Chapter 9). "Agoraphobia" refers to the avoidance or endurance with distress of situations that might be difficult to escape or in which help is unavailable in the event of a panic attack or panic-like symptoms. As a result of anxiety concerning panic-like sensations, the individual with agoraphobia may avoid travel outside the home or may require the accompaniment of a companion when away from home. The experience of agoraphobia can range from mild to severe restriction in lifestyle, and a severe case may result in the individual's being completely housebound or unable to leave home unaccompanied. Avoided activities may include driving (locally or long distance); traveling over bridges; going to grocery stores, malls, theaters, churches, or temples; being in crowds; going to restaurants; using public transportation; going to the barber or hairdresser; or being in enclosed or being in wide-open spaces. It is not uncommon for patients with agoraphobia to define a "safe zone" around their homes, and to be unable to venture outside this radius.

In addition to these situational clusters of avoidance, the patient may manifest avoidance of substances (e.g., caffeine, alcohol, taking medication) or physical activities (e.g., exercise, sexual activity) that produce somatic sensations resembling the symptoms associated with panic. We have referred to this cluster of responses as "interoceptive avoidance" (Rapee, Craske, & Barlow, 1995; Shear et al., 1997), and it seems clear that it is every bit as important as more classical agoraphobic avoidance. Examples of interoceptive activities typically avoided by individuals with agoraphobia are presented in Table 10.1. These persons may also engage in "safety behaviors" (e.g., carrying a bottle of water, mints, or anxiolytic medications) that they believe may prevent or protect them in some way in the event of a panic.

Although most persons with panic disorder also have agoraphobia, when agoraphobia is not accompanied by panic attacks, it is diagnosed as agoraphobia without history of panic disorder (AWOPD; APA, 1994). Individuals suffering from AWOPD typically present with panic-like sensations or other embarrassing symptoms (e.g., vomiting, loss of bladder control), but have never met criteria for panic disorder (e.g., never experienced a full-blown panic attack, panic attacks have not peaked within 10 minutes, no recurrent unexpected panic attacks). Occurrences of "limited-symptom attacks" that do not meet full diagnostic criteria for panic attacks (i.e., fewer than four panic symptoms) are usually what distinguish patients with AWOPD from patients with PDA. Indeed, 57% of patients with AWOPD report limited-symptom attacks (Goisman, Warshaw, et al., 1995). Because the

---

TABLE 10.1. Common Interoceptive Activities Avoided by People with Agoraphobia

Running up flights of stairs	Eating heavy meals
Walking outside in intense heat	Watching exciting movies or sports events
Hot, stuffy rooms	Getting involved in "heated" debates
Hot, stuffy cars	Taking showers with the doors and windows closed
Hot, stuffy stores or shopping malls	Taking a sauna
Walking outside in very cold weather	Hiking
Aerobics	Sports
Lifting heavy objects	Drinking coffee or any caffeinated beverage
Dancing	Eating chocolate
Sexual relations	Standing quickly from a sitting position
Watching horror movies	Getting angry

Note. Adapted from Barlow and Craske (2000). Copyright 1994 by Graywind Publications Inc. Adapted by permission.

pattern of agoraphobia in AWOPD is quite similar to that of PDA, some have posited that this condition occurs on a continuum with PDA rather than as a distinct disorder (Goisman, Warshaw, et al., 1995).

The Connection between Panic Attacks and Agoraphobia

The long-standing controversy regarding the nature of the relationship between agoraphobic avoidance and panic attacks continues today. As late as 1980, when DSM-III was published, agoraphobia was considered a separate phobic disorder that may or may not be accompanied by panic attacks (APA, 1980). However, due in large part to Klein's (1981) argument, agoraphobia came to be viewed as a conditioned avoidance response to the aversive stimulus of spontaneous attacks, and the diagnostic view of agoraphobia changed considerably. By the time DSM-III-R (APA, 1987) was published, panic disorder was viewed as diagnostically primary with or without the existence of agoraphobia (secondary), based largely on clinical research. An important factor in this change was the early observation by Klein and others (Craske & Barlow, 1988; Turner, Williams, Beidel, & Mezzich, 1986) that agoraphobia rarely develops without being preceded by panic attacks or limited-symptom attacks in clinical samples. Although some have found otherwise (Fava, Grandi, & Canestrari, 1988; Marks, 1987), most clinical research supports Klein's contention that the occurrence of panic attacks generally precedes agoraphobia (Katerndahl & Realini, 1997; Swinson, 1986; Thyer & Himle, 1985), and that patients with panic disorder are more likely to develop agoraphobic avoidance of situations or locations that were associated with the first panic attack (Faravelli, Pallanti, Biondi, Paterniti, & Scarpato, 1992). Several explanations have been put forward for the temporal sequence of panic and agoraphobia. First, the expectation of a panic attack while in a particular situation predicts the development of agoraphobic avoidance (Craske, Rapee, & Barlow, 1988; Kenardy & Taylor, 1999; Telch, Brouillard, Telch, Agras, & Taylor, 1989). This expectation appears to be more critical in predicting agoraphobia than the severity, frequency, or duration of the panic attack (Craske, Sanderson, & Barlow, 1987). With few exceptions (Turner et al., 1986), this finding has been supported by others (Cox, Endler, & Swinson, 1995; Telch, Brouillard, et al., 1989). Similarly, Cox et al. (1995) found no relationship between anxiety sensitivity and the presence of catastrophic cognitions across levels of agoraphobia, contradicting findings of such associations by others (Norton, Pidlubny, & Norton, 1999). Second, factors such as social embarrassment resulting from the panic attack (Amering et al., 1997) and occupational status at panic attack onset (de Jong & Bouman, 1995) have also predicted the development of agoraphobia. Such findings are consistent with earlier theorizing in this area (Craske & Barlow, 1988) that secondary gain (positive or negative reinforcement) may contribute to development of agoraphobia.

Prevalence

Contributing to the enduring controversy over the relationship between panic attacks and agoraphobia are the large differences between clinical and community study estimates of prevalence of PDA and AWOPD, and the changes in these estimates over time. The prevalence of agoraphobia was formerly estimated at approximately 0.5% on the basis of probability samples of the population as late as the 1960s (Agras, Sylvester, & Oliveau, 1969); however, more recent epidemiological studies have documented significantly higher prevalence rates of panic disorder, PDA, and AWOPD. Lifetime prevalence of PDA is estimated to be between 1.5% and 3.5%, with 1-year prevalence rates estimated between 1% and

2% (APA, 1994; see Chapter 1). This increase in population prevalence probably does not reflect an actual increase in prevalence, but is likely due to variability in definitions of agoraphobia, assessment techniques, and/or the geographic areas and age ranges sampled. In addition, research design differences may affect the results (e.g., cross-sectional vs. longitudinal). The National Comorbidity Survey conducted in the United States reported a 3.5% lifetime prevalence for PDA or panic disorder without agoraphobia, and a 5.3% lifetime prevalence of AWOPD (Kessler et al., 1994).

The diagnosis of AWOPD is a controversial category about which we know very little. Years ago, when DSM-III-R was being compiled, a difference of opinion arose between the clinicians on the one hand and the epidemiologists on the other. Whereas clinicians reported almost never seeing a case of agoraphobia without panic (Barlow, 1988; Swinson, 1986; Thyer, Himle, Curtis, Cameron, & Nesse, 1985), epidemiologists reported a substantial percentage of people with extensive avoidance who did not present with panic attacks (Weissman, 1985; Weissman, Leaf, Blazer, Boyd, & Florio, 1986). This discrepancy continues to date. Whereas epidemiological studies report high rates of agoraphobia without panic (2.8% last 6 months, 5.3% lifetime; Kessler et al., 1994), clinical samples show that individuals with agoraphobia who seek treatment almost always have a precipitating history of panic (Craske, Miller, Rotunda, & Barlow, 1990; Noyes et al., 1986; Pollard, Bronson, & Kenney, 1989). For example, in the Harvard–Brown Anxiety Disorder Research Program (mentioned briefly in Chapter 1)—a naturalistic, longitudinal study of anxiety disorders that included 562 patients with panic disorder—Goisman, Warshaw, et al., (1995) found that only 6% of patients with agoraphobia met criteria for AWOPD. Community studies, however, have found that a substantial proportion of subjects with agoraphobia do not report a history of panic attacks (Thompson, Bland, & Orn, 1989; Faravelli, Degl' Innocenti, & Giardinelli, 1989; Joyce, Bushnell, Oakley-Brown, Wells, & Hornblow, 1989). The Epidemiologic Catchment Area (ECA) study conducted with more than 18,000 Americans (and based on DSM-III criteria) found that the majority of individuals with agoraphobia did not report panic attacks (Eaton, Dryman, & Weissman, 1991). Recent research by Wittchen, Reed, and Kessler (1998) also showed AWOPD to be more prevalent than PDA. Attempts to reconcile these discrepant findings have led researchers to conclude that (1) individuals with panic are more likely to seek treatment (Boyd, 1986); (2) clinical samples have higher rates of comorbidity than samples of untreated individuals (Berkson, 1946); and/or (3) epidemiological studies may have overestimated prevalence due to misdiagnosis, particularly misdiagnosis of specific phobia (Horwath, Lish, Johnson, Hornig, & Weissman, 1993). For example, it seems that lay interviewers in the ECA study mistook fear of venturing out in an unsafe area among people living in a poor neighborhood for AWOPD. Nevertheless, it is clear that not all patients with panic develop agoraphobia, and that the magnitude of agoraphobic avoidance is quite variable (Craske & Barlow, 1988).

Age of Onset

Panic disorder is generally a disorder of adulthood. The disorder has a median age of onset of 24 years (Burke, Burke, Regier, & Rae, 1990). The ECA study found a bimodal distribution in age of onset occurring between ages 15–24 years and 45–54 years (Eaton, Kessler, Wittchen, & Magee, 1994). The average age at which people seek treatment for panic is 34 years (Breier, Charney, & Heninger, 1986; Craske et al., 1990). Prepubescent children are known to experience panic attacks and occasionally PDA, although this is rare (Albano, Chorpita, & Barlow, 1996; Kearney, Albano, Eisen, Allen, & Barlow, 1997; Moreau &

Weissman, 1992). The interesting observation has been made that most unexpected panic attacks begin during or after puberty. In fact, puberty seems a better predictor of unexpected panic attacks than age, since higher rates of panic attacks are found in physically mature girls (Hayward et al., 1992). In addition, many prepubertal children seen by pediatricians present with symptoms of hyperventilation that may well be unrecognized panic attacks. It may be that these children do not report fears of dying or losing control (which might look more like panic to pediatricians), since they are not at a stage of their cognitive development where they can make these attributions (Nelles & Barlow, 1988). In general, PDA seems less pervasive among the elderly, but estimates are not yet firm (e.g., Beck & Stanley, 1997). Lindesay (1991) studied 60 cases of phobic disorders in the elderly, mostly PDA; they found that PDA had a late onset (after age 50) and was often related to a particularly severe stressful life event, usually an illness or injury.

Clinical Course and Correlates

Several noteworthy naturalistic longitudinal investigations have revealed the clinical course of PDA to be chronic and disabling. Rate of remission for PDA or panic disorder without agoraphobia at 5 years has been reported to be 39% and is equivalent in men and women; however, recurrence of panic symptoms is higher in women (82%) than men (51%; Yonkers et al., 1998). The Harvard–Brown project found 1-year remission rates of 37% for panic disorder and 17% for PDA. Perhaps more important, however, was the finding that among patients who attained remission, relapse was common (Keller et al., 1994). At the 3-year follow-up, the cumulative probability of symptom recurrence was very high: For panic disorder the probability was .65 for women and .39 for men, and for PDA the probability was .75 for women and .47 for men (Keller et al., 1994). Findings like these demonstrate the importance of longitudinal studies for adequately and most accurately capturing the course of PDA. With the Harvard–Brown study as a model, longitudinal investigations of clinical course may actually show increased prevalence estimates, because they capture relapse and/or symptom recurrence (unlike more limited cross-sectional evaluations). Nevertheless, inferences about the true natural course of the disorder must be drawn with prudence, because of the inherent limitation of examining course in a clinical sample where events may in fact be influenced by participating in the study.

Stress has been identified as a clinical correlate of panic onset, most likely due to its strong relationship with the initial unexpected panic attack. The large majority (70%) of individuals describe identifiable stressors at panic attack onset, particularly relating to interpersonal difficulties or physical well-being; stressors of the latter type include frightening experiences with drugs (either legitimate, such as anesthesia, or illegitimate, such as marijuana). But the triggering role of stress seems similar across all anxiety disorders, and is not unique to panic disorder (Craske, Miller, Rotunda, & Barlow; 1990, see Chapter 8 for an extended discussion).

Gender and Cultural Factors

One of the most fascinating mysteries about PDA is the marked gender difference in presentation: Women report more than two times greater incidence than men (Katerndahl & Realini, 1993). This 2:1 sex ratio has been consistently found in both community and clinical studies around the world (Wittchen, Essau, Von Zerssen, Krieg, & Zaudig, 1992; Bland, Orn, & Newman, 1988), and it appears to hold up whether patients are presenting for treatment (Mathews, Gelder, & Johnson, 1981) or are participating in random samples of the population (Myers et al., 1984; Thorpe & Burns, 1983). In fact, one meta-analysis found three-fourths of treatment research participants to be women (Gould, Otto, & Pollack, 1995). Similarly, other reports (Myers et al., 1984; Thorpe & Burns, 1983), including the National Comorbidity Study (Kessler et al., 1994), found lifetime prevalence of panic disorder and AWOPD to be almost twice as high among women (5% and 7%, respectively) as among men (2.0% and 3.5%, respectively). Increasing severity of agoraphobia is also associated with a higher proportion of women. At the most severe level of agoraphobia in our clinic at Boston University, fully 89% are women.

Various reasons have been offered to explain this gender discrepancy, including greater cultural acceptability of avoidance for women and/or a difference in coping strategies between men and women. The cultural acceptability explanation is based on the assumption that in most cultures around the world, it is generally more culturally acceptable for women to report fear and to act by avoiding a large number of situations because of it, whereas men are expected to minimize fears and to overcome them through avoidance. Chambless and Mason (1986) found that the tendency to avoid situations while alone for individuals with agoraphobia, whether male or female, was significantly correlated with masculinity scores on a sex role scale. That is, the less "masculine" one's scores on a sex role scale, the more agoraphobic avoidance, regardless of gender. Pierce and Kirkpatrick (1992) and Ginsburg and Silverman (2000) reported similar findings in which males (in samples of college students) and children (with anxiety disorders) underreported fear, respectively. This supports the notion that agoraphobic avoidance behavior is in large part culturally determined, and it highlights the potential importance of associated personality characteristics described below.

In addition, many more men than women cope with anxiety and panic by self-medicating with alcohol or other substances, as reviewed in some detail in Chapter 1 (e.g., Kushner, Abrams, & Borchardt, 2000). Essentially, men may self-medicate (e.g., with alcohol or nicotine) more than women in an attempt to endure rather than avoid the feared situations. Recent research has indeed found substantially higher prevalence of nicotine use among patients with panic disorder, although gender differences were not found (Amering et al., 1999). In addition, panic symptoms may be influenced by certain phases of the female reproductive cycle, and symptoms may worsen during the premenstrual and/or the postpartum period, due to increased unexplained somatic symptoms.

Consideration of the social and cultural context of anxiety and panic can have important implications for assessment and treatment of panic. Although population-based studies have not found any differences in PDA prevalence among African American, Hispanic American, and European American groups (Eaton et al., 1991; Horwath, Johnson, & Hornig, 1993), African Americans are largely underrepresented in treatment outcome programs (Paradis, Hatch, & Friedman, 1994). Additional clinical characteristics for African Americans with PDA include a later age of onset and different modes of coping relative to European Americans; specifically, African Americans tend to use coping strategies like counting one's blessings and religiosity more often than European Americans do. However, they show less self-blame (L. C. Smith, Friedman, & Nevid, 1999). Friedman, Paradis, and Hatch (1994) found similar characteristic panic symptoms among European American and African American individuals with anxiety in general, but African Americans had more health care utilization (i.e., psychiatric hospitalizations, emergency department visits) and life stress (i.e., childhood trauma). Furthermore, higher rates of fears of dying have been reported among African American patients than among majority group patients (L. C. Smith et al., 1999). To date, it is unclear to what extent potential confounds such as socioeconomic status or social support factors may be operating in this discrepancy, and future research conducted to examine these cross-cultural differences is needed. As noted in Chapters 1 and 4, the occurrence of panic-like isolated sleep paralysis is also significantly higher in African Americans with PDA, with rates as high as 59.6%, compared to European Americans or other groups with PDA (see Figure 10.1).

Not surprisingly, the characterization of PDA differs across the cultural landscape; societal and cultural variables (e.g., ethnic identity, gender roles within the family, communication styles, and level of acculturation) play significant roles in clinical presentation, assessment, and treatment, as described in Chapter 1 (Friedman, 1997). Two examples illustrate this differential clinical presentation of panic disorder. First, *ataque de nervios* is a syndrome commonly reported in Hispanic populations, including those from Caribbean and Latin American areas (Guarnaccia, Canino, Rubio-Stipec, & Bravo, 1993; Liebowitz et al., 1994). This condition includes somatic symptoms similar to panic, including trembling, numbness, palpitations, as well as heat mounting in the head; also, the individual may respond with cursing, falling to the ground, and/or memory loss following the attack. Like panic disorder, *ataque de nervios* generally occurs concurrent with stressful circumstances (e.g., death of a loved one, familial conflict) and is considered to be a culturally acceptable response to difficult circumstances (Guarnaccia, Rubio-Stipec, & Canino, 1989).

Second, a common panic-like experience reported in Cambodian populations involves what is generally referred to as "sore neck syndrome." This syndrome is characterized by panic-like attacks consisting of headache, dizziness, disturbed vision, and other forms of somatic arousal (e.g., increased heart rate, trembling). In a study of 89 Khmer patients, 60% were diagnosed with panic disorder (Hinton, Ba, Peou, & Um, in press-a), and although most did not endorse panic attacks per se, patients reported common triggers for

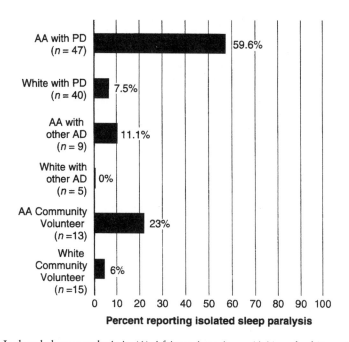

FIGURE 10.1. Isolated sleep paralysis in (1) African Americans (AA) and whites with panic disorder (PD), (2) other anxiety disorders (AD) but not panic disorder, and (3) community volunteers with no disorder. From Paradis, Friedman, and Hatch (1997). Copyright 1997 by John Wiley & Sons, Ltd. Reprinted by permission.

the attacks that included orthostatically induced olfactory stimuli, hunger, and dizziness. Most of these patients identified a fear of dying during the attack from a rupture of blood vessels in the neck resulting from increased wind pressure and blood flow. This fear reflects the cultural belief in "wind overload" (*kyol goeu*) as a cause of somatic symptoms that could signal a blockage of an important vessel in the neck carrying wind and blood to the body. In spite of some differences, it seems clear that these attacks resemble Western concepts of panic attacks.

Functional Impairment and Costs

Patients with panic disorder, especially those with PDA, suffer high levels of social, occupational, and physical disability (Klerman, Weissman, Ouellette, Johnson, & Greenwald, 1991; Leon, Portera, & Weissman, 1995; Markowitz, Weissman, Ouellette, Lish, & Klerman, 1989; Siegel, Jones, & Wilson, 1990). Moreover, numerous studies have shown that panic disorder is associated with persistent general medical health consequences as well as poor perceived physical health (Antony, Roth, Swinson, Huta, & Devins, 1998; Barsky, Delamater, & Orav, 1999; Klerman et al., 1991; Markowitz et al., 1989; Sherbourne, Wells, & Judd, 1996). Individuals with panic are among the highest utilizers of ambulatory medical services, including emergency departments, and are more likely than other psychiatric patient groups to be hospitalized for physical problems (Klerman et al., 1991). In comparison to people with other psychological disorders, individuals with panic disorder have the highest use of emergency services for problems with an emotional basis (Rees, Richards, & Smith, 1998; Weissman, 1991). Siegel et al. (1990) found that their patients with panic disorder had up to seven times the number of medical visits expected for the general population, and missed up to twice as many work days. Antony et al. (1998) found that individuals with panic disorder reported more subjective impairment than individuals with chronic medical conditions such as end-stage renal disease or multiple sclerosis. On the other hand, in comparison to those with other anxiety disorders (e.g., social phobia, obsessive–compulsive disorder), research has generally found that individuals with panic disorder do not report higher levels of impairment (Antony et al., 1998), although there are some exceptions to this finding (e.g., Rees et al., 1998).

The costs of panic disorder extend beyond individuals' suffering to include tremendous direct (e.g., hospitalizations, medications) and indirect (e.g., work productivity) costs to the health care system (Salvador-Carulla, Segui, Fernandez-Cano, & Canet, 1995). As detailed in Chapter 1, the estimated cost of anxiety disorders as a group was estimated to be in excess of $46 billion, of which panic disorder accounted for a substantial part (Katon, 1996). In light of these striking findings, it is not surprising that efforts to improve identification and treatment of patients with panic disorder in medical settings have attracted much recent attention and are increasingly becoming goals of investigation (Mostofsky & Barlow, 2000; Roy-Byrne & Katon, 2000).

Diagnostic Comorbidity

The diagnosis of panic disorder rarely occurs in isolation. As noted in Chapter 9 (see Table 9.5), over half of individuals with PDA present with comorbid psychological disorders (60%, Brown, Campbell, Lehman, Grisham, & Mancill, 2001; 51%, T. A. Brown, Antony, & Barlow, 1995), and this has been a consistent finding. Common psychological disorders comorbid with panic disorder include other anxiety disorders (Goisman, Goldenberg, Vasile, & Keller, 1995; Sanderson, Di Nardo, Rapee, & Barlow, 1990), mood disorders (Chen & Dilsaver, 1995; Lesser et al., 1988), substance use disorders (Cox, Norton, Swinson, & Endler, 1990), and personality disorders (Chambless, Renneberg, Goldstein, & Gracely, 1992; Diaferia et al., 1993). The large study described in Chapter 9 (Brown et al., in press) obtained patterns of comorbidity for 360 patients carefully diagnosed with PDA according to the Anxiety Disorders Interview Schedule for DSM-IV: Lifetime (ADIS-IV-L), and found 59% with a comorbid anxiety or mood disorder and 46% with a comorbid anxiety disorder alone. Among specific disorders, 23% presented with a comorbid major depressive disorder, 16% with generalized anxiety disorder, and 15% each with social phobia or specific phobia. Other studies have found similar high rates of comorbidity (First, Spitzer, Gibbon, & Williams, 1996). Several studies have reported that most nonpanic psychological conditions usually precede panic disorder in individuals with multiple psychological disorders (Katerndahl & Realini, 1997; Starcevic, Uhlenhuth, Kellner, & Pathak, 1993).

It has been estimated that from 25% to 65% of individuals with PDA also meet criteria for an Axis II personality disorder, usually dependent, avoidant, or histrionic personality disorder (Brooks, Baltazar, & Munjack, 1989; Chambless, Goldstein, Gallagher, & Bright, 1986; Chambless et al., 1992; Diaferia et al., 1993; Reich, Noyes, & Troughton, 1987). Estimates of comorbidity and the nature of the association between PDA and the personality disorders are imprecise and remain to be fully investigated. Indeed, the validity of the "personality disorder" diagnoses is disputed in light of findings by some investigators(e.g., Black, Monahan, Wesner, Gabel, & Bowers, 1996; Mavissakalian & Hamman, 1987), who found that abnormal personality traits improved and some "personality disorders" even remitted following successful treatment of PDA.

Suicide Risk

Issues of diagnostic comorbidity have complicated past investigations of suicide risk in panic disorder and PDA. Indeed, a high occurrence of suicidal attempts and ideation has been reported in individuals with panic disorder (Cox, Direnfeld, Swinson, & Norton, 1994), and the presence of panic attacks is reportedly predictive of suicide risk (Clayton, 1993). However, the original report that 20% of individuals with panic disorder had attempted suicide (Johnson, Weissman, & Klerman, 1990; Weissman, Klerman, Markowitz, & Ouellette, 1989) was reanalyzed with statistical controls for comorbidity. This reanalysis failed to find this connection (Hornig & McNally, 1995). In a retrospective review of patients with panic disorder, where it was observed that 25% of patients with panic disorder and comorbid borderline personality disorder reported a past suicide attempt, only 2% of individuals with panic disorder alone reported past attempts (Friedman, Jones, Chernen, & Barlow, 1992). Thus, among individuals with panic disorder, suicide attempts tend to occur more often when a comorbid condition is present (e.g., depressive disorders, borderline personality disorder, substance use disorders; Cox et al., 1994; Friedman et al., 1992; Warshaw, Massion, Peterson, Pratt, & Keller, 1995). In fact, among individuals who commit suicide, a diagnosis of panic disorder is rare (Henriksson et al., 1996), but among those with panic disorder who have attempted suicide, the attempt generally preceded the panic disorder onset (Mannuzza, Aronowitz, Chapman, Klein, & Fyer, 1992).

What is the cause of this discrepancy? Among several possibilities, the method of assessment and the type of interview used in the various studies differed considerably. The epidemiological studies reported by Weissman et al. (1989) were conducted by lay interviewers who were not necessarily trained in determining suicidal risk. Also, the lay interviewers were interviewing a random sample of the population rather than a sample drawn from clinic outpatients. In addition, the lay interviewers did not necessarily identify other disorders individuals with panic disorder might have had in the past that could have accounted for suicidal ideation. But there are other possibilities. The epidemiological studies may have included individuals who were unaware that treatment existed. As a result, they might have become particularly hopeless and begun to think about suicide. All of the patients at the outpatient clinics, on the other hand, were about to receive treatment, and therefore had some hope of recovering. Although Hornig and McNally's (1995) analysis does not support this interpretation, it is important to collect further data to clarify the true relationship between panic disorder and suicide.

Controversy exists regarding the treatment of individuals with panic disorder or PDA who have comorbid personality disorders. Research has found that individuals with PDA and personality disorders may improve more slowly (Marchand, Goyer, Dupuis, & Mainguy, 1998), and presence of a comorbid personality disorder has been found to be a negative predictor of outcome, whereas absence of a personality disorder is a positive predictor of recovery (Black, Wesner, Gabel, Bowers, & Monahan, 1994). In contrast to these findings, some of our research (Hofmann et al., 1998) on the effects of treatment of PDA (i.e., CBT or imipramine) on personality disorder characteristics in patients with PDA, found not only a marked reduction in panic symptomatology, but also a favorable effect on most personality disorder characteristics as described below. Contrary to previous research, we found that personality disorder characteristics did not predict treatment outcome for either treatment. In addition, case research conducted at our Boston center has provided preliminary evidence for use of a modification of our treatment, PCT, with a patient with comorbid schizophrenia (e.g., Bufka & Hofmann, 1999).

A MODEL OF PANIC DISORDER AND PDA

In Chapters 7 and 8, independent models for the development of panic attacks and anxiety have been presented that integrate neurobiological and psychological vulnerabilities and experiences. These chapters have reviewed the necessity of a generalized biological (heritable) vulnerability that seems to account for between 30% and 50% of the variance in developing anxious apprehension. They have also noted that this nonspecific biological vulnerability may be expressed as undifferentiated somatic outputs, heightened stress-responsive arousal, and labile emotionality, but that this vulnerability may well lie dormant unless activated by early psychological experiences. Specifically, early experiences with uncontrollability and unpredictability (based in large part, but not exclusively, on interactions with caregivers) may lead to low perceptions of control. This sense of uncontrollability then acts as a diathesis in the context of stressful life events, creating a generalized psychological vulnerability to experience anxious apprehension. The synergism of these two generalized vulnerabilities is essential for the development of anxiety disorders, as outlined in Figure 8.7.

An extensive review of data on the heritability of panic disorder is presented in Chapter 6. Whereas early family and twin studies suggested an independent genetic contribution to panic disorder (see Table 6.2), more comprehensive analyses (e.g., Kendler et al., 1995) support a nonspecific genetic contribution to emotionality or negative affect generally, as noted above, with environmental factors determining whether panic disorder develops specifically. The exception to this formulation is evidence for differential heritability for panic attacks and other defensive reactions relative to anxiety (e.g., Martin, Jardine, Andrews, & Heath, 1988). Thus one may possess a heritable tendency to react to stress with panic attacks (versus some other reaction such as headaches), which, in the context of a generalized biological vulnerability to experience emotionality or negative affect, creates a neurobiological diathesis for the development of panic disorder. The hypothetical relationship of these two separate heritabilities, in which heightened negative affect lowers the threshold in those vulnerable to stress-related attacks, is presented in Figure 7.2.

Chapter 7 has reviewed in some detail the origins of false alarms, which may occur as a function of stressful life events in biologically vulnerable individuals and may be facilitated by high levels of negative affect. But these false alarms in and of themselves are not implicated in a clinical disorder unless a more specific layer of psychological vulnerabilities exists. In other words, individuals must be taught early what specific objects or events in life are dangerous. As reviewed in some detail in Chapter 8 and in Bouton, Mineka, and Barlow (2001), individuals who go on to develop panic disorder manifest a clear tendency to focus anxiety on somatic events that are perceived to be unpredictable and dangerous. It is for this reason that many patients with panic disorder end up in the emergency department, or in the offices of cardiologists or other nonpsychiatric physicians, whereas individuals with other anxiety disorders do not. That is, individuals who go on to develop panic disorder seem to be exposed early in life to adults who evaluate physical symptoms as dangerous and perhaps encourage sick role behavior. Ehlers (1993) found that observing physical suffering can also contribute to the idea that somatic symptoms are dangerous and require one's full attention.

In this fertile context, the association of an initial false alarm with interoceptive or somatic cues seems particularly crucial in the development of panic disorder. In the case of PDA in particular, two principal types of avoidance behavior then develop to these feared cues: classical agoraphobic avoidance, and a cluster of behaviors with the purpose of avoiding activity that produces somatic cues, termed "interoceptive avoidance." Subsequently, the degree and extent of avoidance behavior seem to be functions of particular coping skills employed by the individual to cope with unexpected panic. The development of avoidance behavior to deal with panic is determined at least partly by experiential and cultural factors as outlined above. Fluctuation in agoraphobic and interoceptive avoidance behavior is largely a function of perceptions of safety on the part of the individual. That is, does a place exist where it is relatively safe to have a panic attack, or does an individual exist with whom it is relatively safe to have a panic attack (Rachman, 1984; Craske, 1999)?

Thus patients with panic disorder or PDA are biologically predisposed to react to negative life events with emotionality, negative affect, and perhaps false alarms (panic attacks). They are psychologically predisposed to develop anxiety with its sense that events are proceeding out of control, and they are predisposed specifically to focus this anxiety on internal somatic events associated with a false alarm. The arrangement of these triple vulnerabilities in the context of panic disorder in general and PDA in particular is illustrated in Figure 10.2.

ASSESSMENT

A comprehensive multimodal approach to the assessment of PDA includes a clinical interview, functional behavioral analysis, medical evaluation, self-monitoring, self-report measures, and behavioral tests. Each of these techniques examines specific aspects of PDA, and the different instruments often tap unique aspects of the disorder that are important for treatment planning and evaluation.

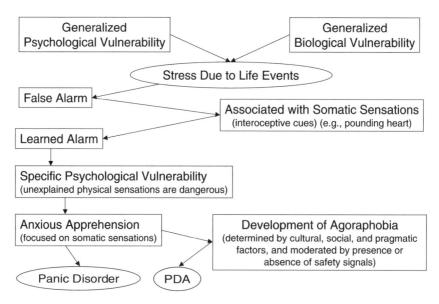

FIGURE 10.2. A model of the etiology of panic disorder and PDA.

Semistructured Diagnostic Interviews

The value of semistructured interviews lies in their contribution to reliable differential diagnosis and systematic assessment of issues important to consider in any functional analysis of a disorder. Such structured interviews are especially important in assessing PDA, because panic attacks can occur across the full range of anxiety disorders. Use of structured clinical interviews is highly recommended in both clinical and research settings, because they insure that the clinician follows systematic assessment procedures to obtain critical information. Previous research has shown that approximately one-third of diagnostic disagreements are related to inconsistencies on the part of the diagnostician rather than in the diagnostic criteria (cf. Blanchard & Brown, 1998). Moreover, in a National Institute of Mental Health consensus development conference on the treatment of panic disorder, it was recommended that all research on the treatment of this disorder include a semistructured diagnostic interview (Shear & Maser, 1994).

A commonly used and empirically supported semistructured interview developed in our Clinic is the ADIS-IV (Brown, Di Nardo, & Barlow, 1994; for the Lifetime Version [ADIS-IV-L],) see also Di Nardo, Brown, & Barlow, 1994; see Chapter 9 for a full description). As detailed in Chapter 9, the ADIS-IV assesses the full range of anxiety disorders as well as mood, substance use, and other commonly comorbid disorders (e.g., hypochondriasis). The interview includes a medical history as well as brief screens for the presence of psychotic disorders. The ADIS-IV-L is particularly useful for understanding the nature, course, and manifestations of the disorders that may influence treatment response.

The ADIS-IV is a clinician-administered interview that follows a hierarchical structure in which those symptoms central to a disorder are queried first, followed by additional inquiry if the basic, defining criteria for that disorder are met. Among the data obtained are the frequency, intensity, and duration of panic attacks; their antecedents; and patterns of avoidance behavior or other coping responses. Variability across time in the pattern of panic and avoidance behavior is also examined. Since many patients with PDA often (initially) identify many of the attacks they experience as triggered and predictable, and deny unexpected or spontaneous panic attacks, utilizing the ADIS assists in identifying unexpected panic attacks.

Psychometric qualities of the ADIS-IV are good. A recent study using the ADIS-IV-L to examine diagnostic agreement on 362 individuals with anxiety disorders reported a strong kappa coefficient of .79 for panic disorder and PDA (Brown, Di Nardo, Lehman, & Campbell, 2001). Moreover, the interrater reliability of the ADIS-IV-L dimensional ratings for number of panic attacks, anxiety focused on future panic attacks, agoraphobic avoidance, and clinical severity rating were very good at .58, .53, .86, and .83, respectively. The full ADIS-IV or ADIS-IV-L is used mostly in clinical research settings. Since it is impractical in many nonresearch settings due to the length of administration (usually 2–4 hours), clinicians often systematically administer sections of interest to arrive at diagnoses and to obtain necessary information. Other commonly used semistructured interviews with promising diagnostic reliability are the Schedule for Affective Disorders and Schizophrenia—Lifetime version modified for anxiety disorders (Fyer, 1995) and the Structured Clinical Interview for DSM-IV Axis I Disorders (First et al., 1996).

Functional Analysis

An initial diagnostic classification of PDA will point the clinician in the proper directions for further assessment. A functional analysis is commonly used to elaborate on the characteristic and idiosyncratic responses of each individual patient. Although diagnostic classification provides the clinician with good clues about which problematic behaviors to assess, the functional analysis allows the clinician to assesses each patient individually to determine the manner in which the disorder presents itself. For example, two people who meet diagnostic criteria for PDA may present with very different clinical pictures, depending on their age, social support system, gender, and socioeconomic status, as well as on the presence or absence of other associated problems.

The most important part of a behavioral assessment of PDA is to determine the functional relationship among panic, avoidance, and cognitive patterns, as well as their relationship to internal and external cues. In a functional analysis, the clinician will assess how maladaptive behaviors and feelings are related to specific events that result in an individual pattern of responding. For example, one patient may have health-related concerns (such as apprehension over possible heart attacks) that may be cued directly by unexpected panic attacks and result in immediate increases in avoidance behavior. In another patient, health concerns and avoidance behavior may be more independent of unexpected panic, resulting in a more functionally autonomous pattern of responses. It is this determination, over and above the initial diagnostic classification, that is necessary if the clinician is to tailor a standardized set of therapy principles to the individual patient.

It can be helpful to organize a comprehensive assessment according to the three major response systems of anxiety and panic: behavioral or motoric, cognitive or subjective, and physiological or somatic (Barlow, 1981; Lang, 1968, 1977b). Within the behavioral response system, avoidance and or other behavioral attempts at coping with panic are assessed. Cognitive aspects requiring assessment include reports of subjective disturbance or intensity of the various symptoms and feared consequences of panic. Physiological or somatic assessment often involves monitoring and report of autonomic nervous system reactivity accompanying anxiety and panic, such as increased heart rate, respiration, and other physiological signs of arousal that may underlie action tendencies associated with these emotions or affective states. The principal goal of behavioral assessment in PDA is to examine the three components of anxiety and panic as they relate to each other and to the individual's environment—with the ultimate goal being to arrive at an appropriately tailored treatment strategy for that individual patient. For example, an elderly woman residing in a fourth-floor walk-up apartment in an urban area will inevitably present with different problems and goals for treatment than will a young male living with a large family in a rural area who must drive 35 miles to work each day.

Cognitive Components

The cognitive components of PDA relate to the patient's thoughts and beliefs about the presumed deleterious nature of panic attacks. Panic-related cognitions can vary considerably among individuals. Common attributions that may develop include fears of having a heart attack, a seizure, or a stroke; suffocating, fainting, or losing control (e.g., unable to drive a car, unable to make a decision); going crazy (e.g., attacking someone, running around screaming); or dying as a result of a panic attack. These appraisals often emerge from attacks that appear to be uncued or apparently from "out of the blue." Thus, because an external trigger does not readily explain the symptoms, patients are likely to turn inward and develop such erroneous beliefs based on preexisting vulnerabilities (see Chapter 8). In addition to assisting the clinician in making an accurate diagnosis, understanding the nature of cognitions related to panic attacks is an important aid in treatment (as discussed later in this chapter).

Behavioral Components

Behavioral components of PDA relate to those behaviors a patient may engage in or refrain from doing that are believed to "protect" him or her from experiencing panic attacks. These "protective" behaviors fall into four categories: agoraphobic avoidance, interoceptive avoidance, distraction, and safety behaviors.

AGORAPHOBIC AVOIDANCE. Agoraphobic avoidance can include avoiding public transportation, driving, theaters, crowds, and sporting events. The general theme involves being unable to reach a safe place or safe person quickly and without embarrassment; feeling trapped is also particularly difficult (see "Agoraphobia" section above).

INTEROCEPTIVE AVOIDANCE. "Interoceptive avoidance" refers to a strong sensitivity to physical sensations associated with anxiety and panic. Anxiety about experiencing these sensations may lead patients to avoid activities that naturally elicit sensations similar to panic attacks. For example, exercising, drinking caffeine, and having sexual relations are commonly avoided activities. Assessing the various feared physical sensations and resulting avoidance is particularly important, since, as discussed in detail later, this assessment provides the foundation for designing interoceptive exposure exercises—a fundamental treatment component for decreasing a patient's anxiety and sensitivity to physical sensations. Similarly, those activities that are avoided because of the sensations they create are often added to the patient's situational fear and avoidance hierarchy in the treatment program.

DISTRACTION. Distraction involves subtle forms of avoidance that are often insidious. For example, patients with PDA may attempt to thwart a panic attack by distracting themselves away from the anxiety—often by turning up the radio, engaging in conversations, watching television, or reading a newspaper. These behaviors can undermine treatment if not identified and eliminated, as we discuss later.

SAFETY BEHAVIORS.   Safety behaviors are those actions that a patient engages in to help him or her feel more secure or protected in the event that a panic attack should occur. Safety behaviors often represent long-standing habits. Thus the clinician will want to pay particular attention to the degree of reliance on safety signals, such as a "safe" place, person, or thing (Rachman, 1984). Examples of common safety behaviors include going places only with a safe person or carrying a cell phone, a water bottle, a lucky charm, or a bottle of medication. A safe person is commonly a significant other whose company enables the patient to feel more comfortable going places than he or she can be either alone or with other people. Usually, this person is considered "safe" because he or she knows about the panic attacks. Notably, even if the safe person does not approve of the panics (as is the case with some spouses), the patient feels that this person would take him or her to the hospital or help in other ways if the patient became incapacitated by panic. A summary of safety signals (excluding safe people) used by 125 consecutive patients with PDA seen in our Boston clinic is presented in Table 10.2. Although other safety behaviors have more substantial "safety" value, the most common talisman is the medication bottle, often unused or even empty. A thorough assessment of safety behaviors is integral to successful treatment as patients are gradually weaned from these ritualistic props, and an ongoing assessment of these behaviors may be beneficial to insure that no new safety behaviors are picked up as old ones are eliminated.

Physiological Components

Research studies on PDA have often examined psychophysiological responding. A number of different psychophysiological functions can be measured (e.g., electrodermal response,

TABLE 10.2. Safety Signals (Excluding Safe People) of Consecutive Patients with PDA ($n = 125$)

Safety signal	Frequency	Percentage
Anxiety medication	60	48
Food/drink	17	14
Bags, bracelets, objects	8	6
Smelling salts/antacid	5	4
Paper bag	5	4
Religious symbols	5	4
Flashlight/money/CB radio	4	3
Reading material	3	2
Cigarettes	3	2
Alcohol	3	2
Relaxation tapes/coping statements/ therapist's phone number	2	2
Pets	0	0
No safety signals (excluding a safe person)	32	26
One safety signal	58	46
Two safety signals	29	24
Three safety signals	6	4

respiration rate, blood pressure, heart rate), and such an assessment can be effectively combined with a behavioral avoidance test (BAT) or other components of treatment. Also, the psychophysiological techniques can be used to confirm a complex differential diagnosis or to observe a patient's anxiety response. Such techniques are generally difficult to administer and interpret, because multiple factors affect arousal; moreover, the various psychophysiological indicators often do not correlate, since they target different bodily response systems. Nevertheless, such approaches can serve a unique function in the assessment and treatment of panic disorder.

Behavioral Assessment Strategies

Behavioral assessment approaches can be used to individually tailor treatments, to systematically track progress in treatment, and to continually evaluate the success of the treatment.

Symptom Induction Tests

Perhaps the most compelling behavioral tests for PDA are symptom induction tests. The primary goal of these tests is to work with the patient to identify sensations that have become triggers of anxiety or fear, even when provoked deliberately in the safe context of a clinician's office. Symptom induction tests involve having the patient purposefully engage in exercises that elicit physical sensations mimicking a patient's naturally occurring panic attacks. Figure 10.3 presents a therapist's record of in-session symptom induction tests. Exercises are performed for a fixed duration (usually 30 seconds to 2 minutes) and are ordered in such a way as to reduce the amount of carryover symptoms from one exercise to the next. Patients are encouraged to bring on the sensations as strongly as they can tolerate, but are also told that they may discontinue the test at any time. Common induction tests include breathing through a coffee straw for 2 minutes, spinning in a chair for 1 minute, and running in place for 2 minutes. Exercises can be tailored to imitate a patient's attacks more closely (e.g., tying a scarf around the patient's neck to induce feelings of choking sensations). Anxiety is rated before, during, and after the exercise, and the intensity of the sensations of panic and their similarity to natural panics are rated. These tests serve a twofold purpose for assessment: They objectively confirm the presence of the anxiety and panic response, and they help to identify the specific physical sensations that elicit anxiety and panic. Moreover, these symptom induction tests are the foundation on which interoceptive exposure practices are based in treatment.

Although highly specialized, additional panic provocation procedures described in some detail in Chapter 4, such as inhalation of a mixture of CO_2 and air or lactate infusions, can be used to profile panic symptoms and track responses to treatment on a pre–post basis (Biber & Alkin, 1999; Coplan, Goetz, et al., 1998; Forsyth, Lejuez, & Finlay, 2000; Fyer et al., 1989; Sanderson, Rapee, & Barlow, 1989; Schmidt, Trakowski, & Staab, 1997).

Behavioral Avoidance Tests

A behavioral assessment technique that assesses the classic behavioral markers of agoraphobia is a BAT (Craske, Barlow, & Meadows, 2000). The BAT affords many advantages to the clinician; perhaps most importantly, it provides a solid foundation on which to build and tailor the treatment program. Advantages of the individualized BAT for assessment purposes include (1) a direct observation of the patient's anxiety response system; (2) an

For each test you do in session, have the patient rate (0 = none, 8 = extreme) the overall intensity of the sensations, how anxious or afraid the patient felt during the procedure, and the similarity of the sensations to those the patient experiences during naturally occurring panic attacks.

Procedure	Sensations experienced	Intensity	Anxiety/Fear	Similarity
Shake head from side to side, 30 sec.				
Head between knees (30 sec.), then lift quickly				
Run in place, 1 min.				
Hold breath, 30 sec.				
Complete body muscle tension, 1 min.				
Breathe through a thin straw, 2 min.				
Spin in a chair or twirl in place, 1 min.				
Hyperventilate, 1 min.				
Stare at a light (<40 watt bulb) for 1 min., then read a paragraph				
Other:				

FIGURE 10.3. Therapist's record of in-session symptom induction tests. Reprinted by permission of the Center for Anxiety and Related Disorders, Boston University.

objective indication of the degree of distress, anxiety, and avoidance of certain situations; (3) an identification of any safety behaviors or other idiosyncratic behaviors; and (4) a more objective and perhaps more accurate measurement of agoraphobic avoidance than self-report. The BAT is also particularly useful in evaluating treatment outcome, because the tests are quite sensitive to treatment effects and are broadly generalizable to other situations. To objectively assess the degree or severity of agoraphobia, BATs are often used systematically in a variety of naturalistic situations and are often individually tailored to assess more personally relevant behaviors or situations. BATs range from those conducted in the home for the most personal relevance (Barlow, O'Brien, & Last, 1984; Mathews et al., 1981; Mathews, Teasdale, Munby, Johnston, & Shaw, 1977) to those tasks contrived to take place at the clinic (Mavissakalian & Michelson, 1983).

A typical BAT entails the selection of about five items from the patient's hierarchy of feared situations, chosen to cover a range of difficulty levels. As recommended by Williams (1985), items should be chosen to reach a high ceiling to account for potential demand characteristics (i.e., the tendency of patients to "push" themselves for a clinician), and to be sensitive to any treatment-produced change. Examples of items may include driving to a local market or riding a subway for 10 minutes. The assessment generally takes place over a time period of 1–2 hours. Patients are asked to rate their anticipatory anxiety concerning the upcoming test on a 0–8 scale (with 0 indicating little or no anxiety and 8 indicating the most anxiety they have ever experienced). All situational tests are structured for a specified duration, and patients are strongly encouraged to persevere as long as possible; however, they are also instructed that they may discontinue the task at any time. A caveat: To eliminate the confound between behavioral and subjective components of anxiety, patients should be instructed to stay in the situation as long as they possibly can. Throughout the task, patients report their anxiety ratings approximately every 30 seconds. A patient is instructed to attempt all five items in the order of difficulty, and each item is scored on a 3-point scale as follows: 0, "refused item (complete avoidance)"; 1, "partial completion of item (partial avoidance)"; and 2, "successful completion of item (no avoidance)."

Some additional caveats: First, it is ideal that the patient complete the BAT independently of the clinician. As discussed above, individuals with agoraphobia are often able to perform certain behaviors quite successfully when accompanied by someone they perceive as "safe" (cf. Baker, Patterson, & Barlow, in press; Barlow & Waddell, 1985; Rachman, 1984). Thus, if at all possible, the assessor should not accompany the patient on the test itself. The patient's behavior can be unobtrusively monitored by clinic personnel or verified by other means, including odometer readings (e.g., Williams & Rappoport, 1983) or sales receipts. Second, as noted above, it has been observed that patients will "push" themselves under the implicit demands of the situation to accomplish tasks they would not even attempt ordinarily. Although this may be true, a clinician can be confident that a BAT reflects a patient's true behavioral capacity. Likewise, the clinician/assessor should insure that the BAT samples the maximally difficult items for a given patient, to provide a true indication of the patient's behavioral capacity.

Although the individualized BAT is often the most clinically relevant assessment for agoraphobia, standardized BATs have been used in agoraphobia research for years (Agras, Leitenberg, & Barlow, 1968; Bandura, Adams, Hardy, & Howells, 1980; Barlow, O'Brien, & Last 1984; Emmelkamp & Wessels, 1975; Vermilyea, Boice, & Barlow, 1984; Williams & Rappoport, 1983), often as a component to evaluate treatment outcome. Common standardized BATs include the behavioral walk (Vermilyea et al., 1984), driving on a progressively difficult route (Williams & Rappoport, 1983), and other behavioral assessments across multiple areas of functioning (Bandura et al., 1980; Craske et al., 2000). Importantly, one common use of the BAT at our Boston center is to pair it with a symptom induction exercise (i.e., an interoceptive exposure exercise). It is not uncommon for patients to report minimal anxiety related to symptom induction exercises—largely because of the purposeful, planned nature of bringing on the symptoms themselves, as well as because they feel safe in the clinician's office. This paired approach has the distinct advantage of inducing anxiety symptoms in a naturalistic setting that affords the opportunity to assess avoidance of both situations and symptoms. The anxiety ratings on these tests can then be used to track the patient's progress in treatment and to identify sensations and situations for exposure therapy.

Fear and Avoidance Hierarchy

Although it is not a psychometrically established assessment, a fear and avoidance hierarchy (FAH) can be a useful clinical tool for assessment, for guiding treatment, and for evaluating progress in treatment. The FAH is one of the most convenient and convincing indicators of assessing treatment progress from the patient's point of view. The clinician and the patient collaboratively develop a FAH, and its structure is organized around the patient's specific agoraphobic fears (cf. Craske et al., 2000). Figure 10.4 presents an example of an individualized FAH for one patient. Broadly speaking, constructing a FAH involves compiling a rank-ordered list of the patient's feared situations, covering the range of lower or easier situations to higher or more difficult situations. The clinician should utilize information from the initial structured interview and assessment, as well as any additional information provided by the patient during the initial appointment. Although the FAH plays a prominent role in treatment, patients are not specifically informed about this beforehand, as it may compel them to withhold reporting difficult items in their environments for fear of being "forced" to deal with the situations before they are ready. Once the list is compiled, the patient is instructed to rate both his or her fear of and avoidance of each situation on a 0–8 scale, where 0 represents no anxiety, panic, and/or avoidance, and 8 represents extreme anxiety, panic, and/or avoidance. It is important to develop a FAH that encompasses a full range of anxiety and avoidance; therefore, particularly difficult situations may need to be broken down into components early in the assessment process, to enhance the patient's willingness to engage in exposure to the items later in the treatment process. It is also critical to include the most difficult or severe situations on the hierarchy, as these constitute some of the most important goals for therapy. All FAH items also include liberal reference to interoceptive cues, such as dyspnea and palpitations. If the patient denies any avoidance behavior, the list should be made up of situations that may provoke panic attacks. By providing a guide to treatment, the FAH is a useful, and perhaps essential, tool for developing a systematic plan for confronting feared situations.

Standardized Self-Report and Clinician-Rated Measures

Other instruments designed to assess PDA and its components are valuable in understanding individual aspects of a patient's clinical presentation. Measures that tap unique aspects of the disorder and its key features from both the patient's and the clinician's perspective are equally useful to confirm the initial diagnosis, but are also used to gauge severity of the disorder and to design a tailored treatment plan. Below is a review of several measures with good psychometric properties that have been designed to assess the key features of PDA and may be used to track the disorder over time. For an exhaustive description of all extant measures, see Baker et al. (in press).

Measures of the Severity of Panic and Avoidance

Because PDA often follows a variable course and consists of loosely related components that may vary independently of one another (e.g., severity of panic attacks, agoraphobic avoidance), it is important to assess comprehensively the components of PDA over time. Several clinician-rated and self-report scales have been developed for this purpose. Among these are the Panic Disorder Severity Scale (PDSS; Shear et al., 1997) and the Panic and Agoraphobia Scale (PAS; Bandelow, 1995).

PANIC DISORDER SEVERITY SCALE. The PDSS (Shear et al., 1997) assesses seven key dimensions of PDA during the past month, including frequency of panic attacks, anxiety focused on future panic, distress during panic, interoceptive avoidance, situational avoidance, and interference related to social realms and work. It can be clinician-administered

Activity	Anxiety Rating*	Avoidance Rating*	Conditions That Would Make My Anxiety Worse	Conditions That Would Make My Anxiety Less
Flying	8	8	Longer flight, esp. overseas, smaller plane, over water or mountains	Short flight, larger plane, not over water
Being out of the city	8	8	Farther from home, unfamiliar city, overnight	Closer to home, familiar city, back home the same day
Driving on the highway	7	5	In traffic, fewer exits, unfamiliar area, certain stretches of road, bridges, tunnels, narrow berms	Less traffic, more exits, driving more slowly, familiar area, wide berms, no bridges or tunnels
Taking a bus	7	8	Crowded, standing, certain routes	Not many people, sitting, other routes
Being in a shopping mall	7	3	Bigger mall, more people, being farther from an exit, phones, and restrooms, in a crowded store	Smaller mall, closer to home, familiar, fewer people, being in center or near exit or restroom
Being at home alone	6	4	At night, without a car, lights out, radio and TV off	Daytime, car available, radio and TV on
Eating in a restaurant	6	6	More formal and expensive, with people who don't know about my panic, drinking coffee	Smaller, more casual, quicker, no coffee, eating alone, sitting at counter
Going to a movie	5	4	Scary movie, farther from home, unfamiliar theater, at night	Funny movie, familiar theater, closer to home, during the day
Doing something physically strenuous	5	3	Outside on a hot day or at the health club with my clothes in a locker, more strenuous, tired	At home, cool day, less strenuous, less tired
Going for a walk	4	3	Farther from home or in a busy downtown area, in open spaces like parks, hot day, no houses nearby	Near home, near houses, cool day, familiar area

*The 0–8 rating of anxiety or avoidance when activity is done *alone and without any other safety behavior.*

FIGURE 10.4. Individualized fear and avoidance hierarchy (FAH) for one patient. Reprinted by permission of the Center for Anxiety and Related Disorders, Boston University.

in about 10–15 minutes, and the seven items are rated on 5-point Likert scales that can be totaled for an overall score. Psychometrically, the PDSS has demonstrated excellent interrater reliability (kappa = .87) and promising internal consistency (alpha = .65), and the total score has been found to correlate with the clinical severity ratings for PDA on the ADIS (r = .55; Shear et al., 1997). Furthermore, in a recently reported large multicenter clinical trial described later, the PDSS proved to be the one comprehensive outcome measure with the most sensitivity to change. Given these promising findings, the PDSS appears to have considerable utility for efficiently assessing the major components of PDA and its treatment. A self-report version of the PDSS has been developed and is currently under evaluation.

PANIC AND AGORAPHOBIA SCALE.   Much like the PDSS, the PAS (Bandelow, 1995) was designed to assess the severity of PDA as well as the frequency and duration of panic attacks, panic-related avoidance, functional impairment, and anticipatory anxiety. The scale has two versions, patient report and clinician-rated, and consists of 13 items. The self-report version of the scale has demonstrated good internal consistency (alpha = .88), and the clinician-rated scale has demonstrated satisfactory interrater reliability (kappa = .78). The scale has been found to correlate with other measures of similar constructs (e.g., $r = .82$ with the Panic-Associated Symptom Scale; Argyle et al., 1991). Other scales with similar goals, but more limited objectives or less developed psychometrics, include the Panic-Associated Symptoms Scale (Argyle et al., 1991), the Panic Attack Symptoms Questionnaire (Clum, Broyles, Borden, & Watkins, 1990), and the Panic–Agoraphobia Spectrum Questionnaire (Cassano et al., 1997).

Measures of Panic-Related Cognitions

A number of questionnaires exist for assessing cognitions associated with PDA and the extent to which the patient believes them. Cognitions include maladaptive thoughts about the causes and consequences of panic as well as perceived ability to cope with panic. Among measures addressing various cognitive components of PDA are the Agoraphobic Cognitions Questionnaire (AgCQ; Chambless, Caputo, Bright, & Gallagher, 1984) and the Panic Appraisal Inventory (PAI; Feske & de Beurs, 1997).

AGORAPHOBIC COGNITIONS QUESTIONNAIRE.   The AgCQ (Chambless et al., 1984) is perhaps the best-known measure of its type. The ACQ assesses the frequency of frightening or maladaptive thoughts about the consequences of panic and anxiety. The ACQ is a 14-item self-report scale that contains 6 behavioral–social and 8 physiological items (e.g., "I am going to pass out"), rated on a 5-point Likert format. The ACQ has good internal consistency (alpha = .80) and good test–retest reliability ($r = .86$), and it is correlated with other related constructs, including the Body Sensations Questionnaire (BSQ) ($r = .67$).

PANIC APPRAISAL INVENTORY.   The PAI (Feske & de Beurs, 1997) is designed to measure three domains of panic appraisal: anticipation of panic, consequences of panic, and perceived ability to cope with panic. Patients rate the perceived likelihood that they will have a panic attack in 15 different situations that would be confronted alone and without the use of any safety signals. Ratings are also obtained on the perceived distress and the perceived ability to cope in each of the situations. Feske and de Beurs (1997) report that the scale has five subscales that comprise the three domains identified; the Consequences of Panic subscale is further divided into three subscales, including Physical Consequences, Social Consequences, and Loss of Control. Internal consistency ranges from .86 to .90 for the subscales, and the PAI was found to correlate with physiological concerns on the AgCQ ($r = .80$) and with the BSQ ($r = .44$).

Other instruments with similar goals include the Agoraphobic Cognitions Scale (Hoffart, Friis, & Martinsen, 1992), the Cognition Checklist (Taylor, Koch, Woody, & McLean, 1997), the Catastrophic Cognitions Questionnaire—Modified (Khawaja & Oei, 1992), the Panic Attack Cognitions Questionnaire (Clum et al., 1990), and the Panic Belief Questionnaire (Greenberg, 1988).

Measures of Anxiety Focused on Emotions or Physical Sensations

ANXIETY CONTROL QUESTIONNAIRE. The Anxiety Control Questionnaire (AnxCQ; Rapee, Craske, Brown, & Barlow, 1996) assesses perceived control of reactions in emotional situations (e.g., "When I am put under stress, I am likely to lose control," "Whether I can successfully escape a frightening situation is always a matter of chance with me"). The scale contains 30 items rated on a 6-point Likert scale ranging from "strongly disagree" to "strongly agree." The AnxCQ has shown considerable promise psychometrically in clinical samples: It has demonstrated good internal consistency (alpha = .87), good convergent and discriminant validity, and adequate sensitivity to change following CBT.

ANXIETY SENSITIVITY INDEX. "Anxiety sensitivity" refers to the belief that beyond any immediate physical discomfort, anxiety and its accompanying symptoms may cause deleterious physical, psychological, or social consequences (McNally & Lorenz, 1987; Reiss, Peterson, Gursky, & McNally, 1986; Taylor, Koch, McNally, & Crockett, 1992). The Anxiety Sensitivity Index (ASI; Reiss et al., 1986), the most widely used scale of its type, consists of 16 items rated on a 5-point Likert scale. The ASI has good internal consistency (Cronbach's alpha = .88; Peterson & Heilbroner, 1987) and promising discriminant validity for distinguishing patients with PDA from patients with other anxiety disorders (Telch, Shermis, & Lucas, 1989). The construct of anxiety sensitivity appears to be multidimensional (Cox, Parker, & Swinson, 1996), and recent research supports the hierarchical structure of the ASI as containing three lower-order factors loading onto a single higher-order factor (Zinbarg, Barlow, & Brown, 1997). The three lower-order factors include physical concerns, mental incapacitation, and social concerns. Notably, although anxiety sensitivity is most often associated with PDA and plays a small role in predicting onset of initial panic attacks (see Chapter 7), it has also proven to be an important construct in several other clinical disorders (i.e., depression, chronic pain, substance abuse) (Asmundson, 1999; Cox, Borger, & Enns, 1999; Stewart, Samoluk, & MacDonald, 1999). Thus the ASI may tap a trait-like construct reflecting a specific psychological vulnerability—namely, the belief that unexplained somatic sensations are dangerous (see Chapter 8). Taylor and Cox (1998) recently expanded the ASI to include 20 additional items; however, this revised version awaits further psychometric evaluation. Using the expanded version of the ASI, these researchers (Taylor & Cox, 1998) found the ASI—Revised to distinguish patients with panic disorder from patients with other anxiety or nonanxiety psychological disorders.

BODY SENSATIONS QUESTIONNAIRE. The BSQ (Chambless et al., 1984) is the oldest scale to assess anxiety focused on bodily sensations. Seventeen items are rated on a 5-point scale; patients are asked to rate the degree to which they experience anxiety related to specific bodily sensations (e.g., heart palpitations, pressure in chest, numbness in arms). The scale has been shown to correlate with the ASI ($r = .66$; McNally & Lorenz, 1987) and the AgCQ, as noted above. Test–retest reliability is fair (.67), and the scale has good internal consistency (.87).

BODY VIGILANCE SCALE. The 4-item, Body Vigilance Scale (BVS; Schmidt, Lerew, & Trakowski, 1997), asks individuals to rate how closely they pay attention to bodily symptoms, how sensitive they are to those sensations, how much time they spend checking for symptoms, and how much attention they pay to a range of panic sensations (e.g., chest pain, numbing, palpitations). Published data support the internal consistency of the BVS (alpha = .82); it has adequate test–retest reliability ($r = .58$); and some promising findings support the discriminant validity of the scale, with patients with panic disorder showing significantly higher levels of body vigilance than nonclinical samples.

Measures of Avoidance

ALBANY PANIC AND PHOBIA QUESTIONNAIRE. The Albany Panic and Phobia Questionnaire (APPQ; Rapee et al., 1995) is designed to measure anxiety and avoidance focused on interoceptive or more traditional agoraphobic situations. Using a 9-point Likert scale, patients rate their fear in a variety of situations (e.g., running up stairs, playing a vigorous sport on a hot day). Three subscales are derived from the 27 items: Interoceptive Avoidance (alpha = .87), Situational Agoraphobia (alpha = .90), and Social Phobia (alpha = .91). The APPQ has shown promising psychometric properties.

MOBILITY INVENTORY. The Mobility Inventory (MI; Chambless, Caputo, Gracely, Jasin, & Williams, 1985) is a 27-item questionnaire designed to assess agoraphobic avoidance behavior. The scale is made up of 26 situations commonly avoided by patients with agoraphobia (e.g., driving, restaurants). The instructions include ratings of the severity of avoidance when alone and when accompanied—two related but often very different aspects of avoidance behavior. Ratings of panic frequency during the past week are also obtained. Adequate reliability and validity data are reported for this inventory, which has been shown to discriminate between patients with agoraphobia and patients with other anxiety disorders (Craske, Rachman, & Tallman, 1986). The two subscales, Avoidance Alone and Avoidance Accompanied, have shown excellent internal consistency (Cronbach's alpha = .90 and .96 respectively).

FEAR QUESTIONNAIRE. The Fear Questionnaire (FQ; Marks & Matthews, 1979) is commonly used to monitor changes in phobic avoidance. It yields three subscales (Agoraphobia, Blood Injury Phobia, and Social Phobia) derived by Marks (1981), as well as a total score. The 15-item scale requires patients to rate their avoidance of a variety of situations on a 9-point scale, where 0 indicates "no avoidance" and 8 indicates "total avoidance." The FQ has been shown to have adequate reliability and validity with patients with agoraphobia (Cox, Swinson, Parker, Kuch, & Reichman, 1993), and the results of a confirmatory factor analysis of the scale with data from patients with PDA provide further empirical support for the three factors of the scale (Cox et al., 1993). Normative data have also been published on this scale (Gillis, Haaga, & Ford, 1995), and these may be useful for comparison.

Self-Monitoring

Self-monitoring involves continuous monitoring of behavioral and emotional events related to anxiety and panic, and is an important component of behavioral assessment (Barlow & Craske, 2000). Adequate self-monitoring includes a daily record of the frequency, intensity, and duration of panic and general anxiety. Because self-monitoring does not rely on extensive memory recall of events, it is considered more accurate and reliable than other modes of self-report assessment. Retrospective reports of anxiety (e.g., answers to the question "How many panic attacks have you had in the past week?") have been shown to be characterized by marked distortion and exaggeration (Turner, Beidel, & Jacob, 1988), and simple frequency data on the number of panic attacks are experienced are inadequate and potentially misleading (Chambless et al., 1986). For example, after becoming educated and sensitive to the components of anxiety, patients often record transient, less intense "bursts" of anxiety as full-blown panic attacks. Alternatively, a patient may record only the most severe episodes of prolonged panic, thereby recording a misleading clinical picture. Because self-monitoring is used both as a treatment outcome measure and as a measure of ongoing progress in treatment, it is most important to use measures that capture the true clinical picture of each patient at a particular time.

Years of research in this area have led to the development and refinement of the Daily Panic Attack and Anxiety Record (DPAAR; see Figure 10.5, modified from Craske & Barlow, 2000). As illustrated, this self-monitoring form assesses the time of onset, frequency, intensity, and duration of panic attacks, as well as the average and peak levels of general anxiety each day. In addition, the patient indicates medication use (i.e., dosages, if appropriate) and whether the panic attack was "unexpected" or "cued" (i.e., expected). Importantly, we retain use of the distinction between "unexpected" and "cued" panic attacks. A panic attack, whether it occurs within the context of panic disorder or a specific phobia, may be expected or unexpected (Barlow, Brown, & Craske, 1994); however, in specific phobia, all panics are cued by definition. In PDA multiple cues can often be identified, including interoceptive cues as well as situational cues (e.g., crowds, shopping malls), and the latter may be more properly considered as discriminative stimuli or "learned settings" where safety signals are not present (Rachman, 1984). In the early stages, panic may not be associated with obvious cues (which is the origin of the often-used term "spontaneous"). Thus the "expected" and "cued" nature of panic attacks may vary independently, and both factors should be noted and recorded (see Chapter 4 for an extended discussion).

Patient compliance with self-monitoring presents a common practical challenge. Many suggestions have been offered to improve compliance and the reliability of the data obtained (cf. Barlow, Hayes, & Nelson, 1984). Among these, we recommend the following to clinicians in regard to self-monitoring: (1) Educate the patient on the importance of maintaining accurate daily records throughout the course of treatment; (2) train the patient in the monitoring procedure; (3) encourage the patient to complete monitoring records for several weeks prior to treatment, for training and practice; and (4) systematically review, reinforce, and provide corrective feedback to the patient on the accuracy and completeness of the records at each treatment session.

Psychophysiological Assessment Techniques

Uses of Psychophysiological Assessment

Although research in past decades on the importance of physiological assessment in PDA suggested that physiological assessments are generally unreliable measures of change, as noted above (Arena, Blanchard, Andrasik, Cotch, & Myers, 1983; Holden & Barlow, 1986), and are not necessarily valid indicators of treatment response (Michelson & Mavissakalian, 1985), there are several reasons to assess the physiological component of anxiety and panic (Agras & Jacob, 1981; Barlow & Wolfe, 1981; Hofmann & Barlow, 1996; Jansson & Öst, 1982). The panic attack, with its surge of physiological activity, is the defining characteristic of panic disorder; important results from physiological monitoring of panic attacks have been presented in Chapter 4. Physiological responding may well underlie the all-important action tendencies associated with any emotional or affective state (Barlow et al., 1994). Physiological assessment can also be used to provide objective evidence of physiological responding to the patient and improve interoception. Finally, demonstration of habituation may be indicative of therapeutic change and serve to reassure the patient (Hofmann & Barlow, 1996).

Initials: _____ ID: _____ Date: ____/____/_____

Part 1. Did you have any panic or limited symptom attacks on this day?
[ ] Yes (Please complete a column for each attack.)
[ ] No (Please skip to Part 2.)

Attack Number	1	2	3	4	5	6	7	8	9	10
About the attack										
Time it began	:	:	:	:	:	:	:	:	:	:
A.M./P.M.	A P	A P	A P	A P	A P	A P	A P	A P	A P	A P
Time to peak (minutes)										
Unexpected/situational	U S	U S	U S	U S	U S	U S	U S	U S	U S	U S
Maximum anxiety (0–8)										
Check which symptoms you experienced during the attack										
Pounding heart										
Chest tightness or pain										
Short of breath										
Dizzy										
Trembling										
Sweating										
Choking										
Nausea										
Feeling of unreality										
Numbness or tingling										
Hot or cold flash										
Fear of dying										
Fear of going crazy										
Fear of losing control										

Part 2. On this day (circle a number):

What was your average anxiety?	0	1	2	3	4	5	6	7	8
What was your maximum anxiety?	0	1	2	3	4	5	6	7	8
How much did you fear a panic attack?	0	1	2	3	4	5	6	7	8

Part 3. Please list any medications you took on this day that were prescribed for your panic disorder or that you took because of panic or anxiety symptoms, muscle tension, or difficulty sleeping:

FIGURE 10.5. Daily Panic Attack and Anxiety Record (DPAAR). From Craske and Barlow (2000). Reprinted by permission of the Center for Anxiety and Related Disorders, Boston University.

A Clinical Application

We used ambulatory psychophysical monitoring in the treatment of a patient with PDA (see Hofmann & Barlow, 1996, for a fuller account). Following successful treatment, the patient relapsed after a stressful life event and again became concerned that the panic attacks might reflect heart problems. Ambulatory physiological monitoring served two purposes. First, it demonstrated to the patient that she was in fact overestimating her actual heart rate. Second, because the increase in heart rate and respiration followed anxious thoughts, the patient was able to recognize that rather than coming from "out of the blue" as she had initially thought, the attacks were indeed precipitated by anxious thoughts and were therefore manageable. Although historically, ambulatory monitoring of heart rate and finger temperature have been most often used to corroborate self-reported panic attacks, this case example suggests the beneficial uses of psychophysiological assessment in the treatment of PDA. Although the costs associated with ambulatory monitoring are dropping, its utility in assessment and treatment planning needs to be balanced against the costs. Nevertheless, such physiological monitoring devices appear to hold promise for the future.

Issues of Medical Comorbidity and Evaluation

Whereas panic attacks are typically associated with anxiety disorders, similar attacks can be a sign of an underlying medical condition. Thus a key component of a diagnostic assessment includes obtaining a thorough medical history to ensure that potential medical causes for the panic symptoms are ruled out. Medical conditions may have a direct impact on the patient's somatic presentation or may actually be causally related to the incidence of panic attacks. As Zaubler and Katon (1996) have pointed out, it can be difficult to identify whether a medical condition is a cause, a correlate, or a complicating factor in panic disorder. Because the physical manifestations of panic attacks can mimic cardiorespiratory, gastrointestinal, and otoneurological illness, a large percentage of patients with panic disorder or PDA may initially seek care in the medical setting (cf. Zaubler & Katon, 1996). As we review below, a number of major physical disorders can be responsible for anxiety and panic-like symptoms; however, a medical etiology for the physical disorder does not necessarily rule out the coexistence of panic disorder or PDA, and thus the necessity of treating panic attacks directly.

Medical Conditions That May Mimic Panic Attacks

Specific disorders that may show panic-like symptoms and should be ruled out include endocrine disorders (e.g., hypoglycemia, hyperthyroidism, Cushing's syndrome, menopause, premenstrual dysphoric disorder, pheochromocytoma); cardiovascular disorders (e.g., mitral valve prolapse [MVP], cardiac arrhythmias, congestive heart failure, hypertension, myocardial infarction); respiratory disorders (e.g., chronic obstructive pulmonary disease, asthma); neurological disorders (e.g., epilepsy, Huntington's disease, vestibular disorders, multiple sclerosis); and substance-related anxiety following intoxication with drugs such as caffeine, cocaine, amphetamines, or withdrawal from drugs such as alcohol, barbiturates, or opiates. The effects of caffeine in provoking panic have been reviewed in Chapter 5. To illustrate the clinical overlap in symptomatology, hyperthyroidism results from excessive thyroid gland activity, and 95% of patients with this disorder report nervousness and episodic anxiety as their primary complaint. More than two-thirds of this group also report palpitations, tachycardia, and dyspnea (difficulty breathing)—all common panic attack symptoms. As for PDA, the age of onset for hyperthyroidism is between 20 and 40 years, and the disorder is more common among females. Importantly, any of the above-mentioned physical conditions may coexist with panic attacks and interact with psychological factors to exacerbate the effects of the panic attacks. Therefore, the diagnosis of a comorbid physical disorder should not rule out the potential necessity of treating the panic attacks directly.

The medical condition that has unquestionably received the greatest attention in relation to possible organic etiologies of panic is MVP. MVP is the most commonly occurring cardiac condition and results from an alteration (sagging) in the connective tissue of the mitral valve of the heart. It is characterized in its extreme form by chest pain, palpitations, dyspnea, tachycardia, lightheadedness, fatigue, and anxiety, and is accompanied by an unusual and difficult-to-characterize systolic murmur. The early excitement concerning the relation of PDA to MVP was caused by the fact that a series of early studies reported a high percentage of patients with recurrent panic attacks who also presented with MVP (Crowe, Pauls, Slymen, & Noyes, 1980; Grunhaus, Gloger, Rein, & Lewis, 1982; Kantor, Zitrin, & Zeldis, 1980). These early data provoked a flurry of speculation that MVP might be a biological marker for panic in a substantial number of patients. However, more sophisticated examinations using echocardiogram procedures failed to confirm the earlier-reported high prevalence of MVP, and to date there is no firm evidence for a common genetic factor linking panic disorder and MVP (Rosenman & Swan, 1988). Researchers have generally concluded that the high prevalence of MVP in anxiety disorders found in earlier studies was due to biased screening, and sophisticated studies point to bias and erroneous classification of differences as reasons for early positive findings (cf. Shear, Devereux, & Kramer-Fox, 1991). Indeed, as pointed out by Dager, Comess, Saal, and Dunner (1986), even expert cardiologists cannot agree on the presence or absence of MVP, as reflected in kappa coefficients below .20. Follow-up studies have failed to find an association between MVP and panic disorder (e.g., Bowen, D'Arcy, & Orchard, 1991; Hamada, Koshino, Misawa, Isaki, & Gejyo, 1998; Toren et al., 1999).

MVP has a benign prognosis (Bouknight & O'Rourke, 2000), and current consensus on MVP and panic disorder holds that there is little if any clinical significance in distinguishing patients with both disorders from those with only panic disorder (Singh, 1996). There appears to be no increased risk for MVP in patients with PDA, based on studies from around the United States that have found the prevalence of MVP in patients with PDA to be no greater than that found in the normal population (e.g., Mazza, Martin, Spacavento, Jacobsen, & Gibbs, 1986; Toren et al., 1999). Current rates of MVP prevalence are quite variable, due to different diagnostic criteria. Conservative estimates range from 4% to 7%, and prevalence is higher among women and appears to be a function of age, peaking during the 30s. Panic attacks do not appear to exert any effect on MVP (Yang, Tsai, Hou, Chen, & Sim, 1997). Interestingly, Kearney and colleagues (1996) found that children with MVP who were aware of their medical diagnosis reported significantly more anxiety than children with other cardiac conditions and higher than normative values reported in the literature. Nevertheless, the presence of MVP comorbid with PDA does not appear to affect clinical course or response to treatment (Singh, 1996), and there appears to be no clinical reason to alter clinical strategies in patients with PDA who also have MVP.

Medical Comorbidity

In addition to anxiety disorders' mimicking physical complaints, anxiety disorders often coexist with genuine medical illness. Patients with PDA have an increased rate of medical illnesses, including migraine (Stewart, Linet, & Centenano, 1989), hypertension, coronary artery disease, ulcer, and asthma (Katon et al., 1986; Rogers et al., 1994). The rate of panic disorder in patients with cardiac ailments is higher than the general population (9%, Goldberg et al., 1990; 23%, Katon et al., 1988; 16%, Yinglin, Wulsin, Arnold, & Rouan, 1993). In addition, patients with PDA have an increased rate of respiratory illnesses such as asthma (Carr, Lehrer, Rausch, & Hochron, 1994; Perna, Caldirola, Arancio, Bellodi, 1997) and chronic obstructive pulmonary disease (Karajgi, Rifkin, Dodd, & Kolli, 1990; Smoller, Pollack, Otto, Rosenbaum, & Kradin, 1996), as well as an increased rate of disability related to vestibular disease (Stein, Asmundson, Ireland, & Walker, 1994).

The presence of PDA may function to alter a medical disorder's presentation, course, and treatment outcome. PDA can worsen cardiac disease (Katon et al., 1990), and, as reviewed in Chapter 1, longitudinal studies have shown phobic anxiety to be associated with sudden cardiac death (Kawachi, Sparrow, Vokonas, & Weiss, 1994, 1995). Similarly, some medical conditions have been identified as risk factors for panic disorder. For instance, the development and severity of asthma may put an individual at risk for panic (Carr, 1998, 1999; Feldman, Giardino, & Lehrer, 2000). Substance use is also frequently considered a risk factor for development of panic (Cox et al., 1990), and caffeine, marijuana, and cocaine use have been associated with panic onset (e.g., Aronson & Craig, 1986; Geracioti & Post, 1991; Louie, Lannon, & Ketter, 1989; Schnoll & Daghestani, 1986; Szuster, Pontius, & Campos, 1988).

Recognition of PDA in Medical Settings

Nearly 85% of patients with PDA initially seek medical attention for their symptoms (Katerndahl & Realini, 1995); however, PDA is poorly recognized in medical settings. Indeed, past studies have shown that the majority of patients with PDA (70%) saw an average of 10 physicians before finally being diagnosed (Sheehan, 1982). This finding is consistent with more recent studies describing high rates of physician nonrecognition of PDA (61% in primary care, Spitzer, Williams, Kroenke, et al., 1994; 98% in emergency departments, Fleet et al., 1996; and 80% in general medical patients referred for psychiatric evaluation, Roy-Byrne & Katon, 2000). Thus it is quite common for patients presenting to mental health clinics with PDA to have had a thorough battery of medical evaluations to rule out a medical etiology. Nevertheless, clinicians should be aware of the various physical disorders that can mimic panic attacks.

Roy-Byrne and Katon (2000) have cited several reasons for the nonrecognition of anxiety in medical settings, including patient barriers (e.g., stigma of mental illness, lack of knowledge of mind–body connection, cultural differences in clinical presentation), physician barriers (e.g., tendency to look for physical causes of somatic symptoms, overemphasis on not missing medical disorders in our litigious society, tendency to see anxious patients as "difficult") (Hahn et al., 1996), and system and process-of-medical-care barriers (e.g., lack of adequate time for primary care physician diagnosis, overwhelmed medical system, need for health care reform). Compounding the lack of recognition of PDA in medical settings, a number of studies have shown that even when recognized, anxiety disorders are inadequately treated (Fifer et al., 1994; Mathias et al., 1994; Yelin et al., 1996). As Higgins (1994) suggests, improved recognition alone is inadequate to increase identification and treatment of anxiety disorders in medical settings.

Several researchers (e.g., Ballenger, 1997; Roy-Byrne & Katon, 2000) have proposed solutions to improve identification of PDA in medical settings. Roy-Byrne and Katon (2000) cite interventions that strengthen and support self-management by promoting physician–

patient collaboration focused on patient education and activation, development and implementation of expert systems, and process-of-care changes (i.e., increased integration of mental health professionals into primary care). To improve diagnostic screening of PDA, Ballenger (1997) has recommended a thorough workup, including (1) evaluation of medical, psychiatric, and social history; (2) physical and neurological examination; (3) family history assessment; (4) medication and drug use history; (5) an electrocardiogram (in patients over 40 years of age); and (6) laboratory tests (i.e., blood chemistry panel, thyroid function test).

In summary, there is little question that the various physical disorders described above can produce symptoms that mimic panic attacks, and as we have seen, it is not uncommon for a medical disorder to coexist with PDA. The complicating factor is that it is clear that individuals with PDA are overly sensitive to and vigilant for patterns of internal physical changes. Patients who develop learned alarms to these somatic events through the process of interoceptive conditioning are more likely to experience anxiety and panic than if the sensations produced by the physical disorder are not present. Similarly, those patients without PDA who present with one or more of these physical problems generally do not experience anxiety or panic once the underlying reasons for the physiological sensations have been thoroughly explained by a health care professional. The ultimate test is whether the symptoms of panic disorder diminish or disappear once the disorder is properly diagnosed and treated. If not, the panic disorder requires treatment in its own right.

OVERVIEW OF TREATMENT COMPONENTS

Treatments for PDA generally fall into one of two categories: (1) techniques targeting agoraphobia and related avoidance behaviors; and (2) techniques targeting panic attacks (i.e., frequency, intensity, and duration of panic attacks) and anxiety focused on panic attacks.

Treating Agoraphobia and Related Avoidance Behaviors

The Discovery of Exposure

As late as the 1960s, there were no proven effective treatments for agoraphobia or panic. Donald Klein had begun his work with imipramine, but only preliminary results were available. At about the same time, pioneering behavioral investigators were experimenting with possible behavior therapy approaches to agoraphobia. For example, Meyer and Gelder (1963) began encouraging patients with agoraphobia to venture away from their homes or the clinic along routes that were very difficult for them. However, they cautioned their patients to avoid experiencing any anxiety and to turn back if this occurred. This resulted in very limited improvement in a few patients, at an excruciatingly slow rate of progress (Mathews et al., 1981). This procedure was soon given up in favor of the predominant behavioral treatment for phobia in those days, systematic desensitization in imagination. Evidence began to accumulate at that time that systematic desensitization was effective with patients with specific and mixed phobias, at least some of whom also had agoraphobia, when compared to psychotherapy (Gelder & Marks, 1968; Gelder, Marks, & Wolff, 1967). Nevertheless, in studies confined to patients with severe agoraphobia, systematic desensitization did not provide a significant advantage over psychotherapy, and overall improvements were small with both treatments (Emmelkamp, 1982; Gelder & Marks, 1966; Marks, 1971).

In the late 1960s, we experimented with the possibility of strongly encouraging patients with agoraphobia to expose themselves to real-life frightening situations (e.g., Agras et al, 1968). A course was set up that led from the clinic to an increasingly busy downtown area about 1 mile away. As patients walked further along this course (and therefore began to experience and tolerate greater anticipatory anxiety and panic), the value of this exercise was discussed with them, and they were effusively praised. If they were unable to make progress on a given trial, very little was said, although they were encouraged to try harder next time. Although these patients were told to return if they experienced what was vaguely defined as "undue anxiety," in fact the demands of the situation produced Herculean efforts on the part of many of these patients.

According to behavioral observations of distance walked along this course, the initial three patients in this series did extremely well in a relatively short period of time (Agras et al., 1968). But a surprising finding began to emerge, which we were to isolate experimentally only in later years. Although we were betting on the therapeutic value of praise and encouragement from a therapist with whom a patient had a good relationship, many of these patients began improving in a "baseline" phase before this encouragement was even introduced. That is, the opportunity to practice by walking further along this difficult course seemed therapeutic in and of itself. These results are graphically demonstrated in Figure 10.6 for one of the patients in this early series. As one can see, this patient was already improving in terms of distance walked and time away from a safe place during baseline. The slope of this improvement was not substantially affected by the introduction of social reinforcement, although removal of this reinforcement in a systematic way at a later date did exert some control over agoraphobic behavior. In fact, later studies in this series indicated quite clearly that the opportunity to practice in a systematic way by exposing oneself to feared situations accounted for the largest part of therapeutic benefit (e.g., Leitenberg, Agras, Edwards, Thompson, & Wincze, 1970; Mavissakalian & Barlow, 1981).

By the mid-1980s, positive outcomes for of exposure-based treatments were found fairly consistently over a number of different studies conducted by clinicians in various parts of the world. If dropouts were excluded, the best estimates of outcome indicated that from 60% to 70% of those individuals with agoraphobia completing treatment showed some clinical benefit. Follow-up studies revealed that these effects were maintained, on the average, for periods of 4 years or more (Burns, Thorpe, & Cavallaro, 1986; Cohen, Monteiro, & Marks, 1984; Emmelkamp & Kuipers, 1979; Jansson, Jerremalm, & Öst, 1986; Jansson & Öst, 1982; McPherson, Brougham, & McLaren, 1980; Munby & Johnston, 1980). The effectiveness of this approach was demonstrated repeatedly in controlled experimentation when exposure was compared to no treatment or some good placebo (e.g., Mathews, 1978; Mavissakalian & Barlow, 1981; O'Brien & Barlow, 1984).

The Administration of Exposure-Based Procedures: A Current Perspective

In vivo exposure involves systematic, repeated contact with the avoided situation. The approach to exposure can vary from graded or hierarchical to intense exposure, from therapist-directed to self-directed exposure, from massed to spaced exposure, from endurance to controlled-escape exposure, and from attention-based to distraction-based exposure. Choice of strategy generally depends on the patient's motivation and willingness to engage in exposures, and these may be strongly influenced by a patient's degree of avoidance.

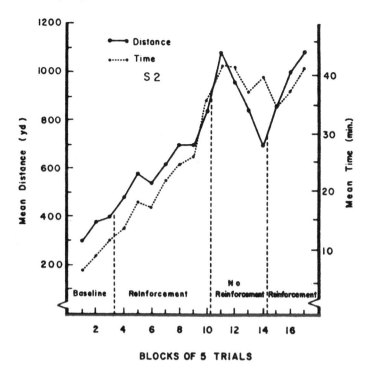

FIGURE 10.6. The effect of reinforcement and nonreinforcement upon the performance of a patient with agoraphobia (Subject 2). From Agras, Leitenberg, and Barlow (1968). Copyright 1968 by the American Medical Association. Reprinted by permission.

MASSED VERSUS SPACED EXPOSURE AND THE NEW THEORY OF DISUSE. Long, continuous exposure sessions would seem generally more effective than shorter, interrupted sessions on the face of it (Chaplin & Levine, 1981; Marshall, 1985; Stern & Marks, 1973), but the optimal rate for repeated exposure is not clear. For many years we thought that spaced exposures were generally preferable, because dropout rates (Emmelkamp & Ultee, 1974; Emmelkamp & Wessels, 1975) and relapse rates (Hafner, 1976; Jansson & Öst, 1982) were higher following massed exposure. Also, it seemed that rapid changes resulting from massed exposure made family adjustments to the change more difficult (Barlow, O'Brien, & Last, 1984). In contrast, Chambless (1990) did not find such detrimental outcomes, and in fact found massed exposure to be equal in effectiveness to graded exposure after treatment and at a 6-month follow-up with no differential relapse rates. However, a selection bias was operating in the massed-exposure group, since a number of potential patients were unwilling to participate (as is often the case to some extent, if the proposed schedule for exposure is too intense).

It may be that we have been attending to the wrong segment of treatment in deciding between massed and spaced sessions. In 1992, Bjork and Bjork proposed that an expanding-spaced schedule, once initial learning has occurred, is the most beneficial for long-term retention (Lang, Craske, & Bjork, 1999). As applied to PDA and other phobias treated with exposure, sessions could be relatively massed initially, since the theory predicts that some difficulty in learning results in better retention (Schmidt & Bjork, 1992). But as progress is made, and perhaps fear and anxiety have diminished considerably, sessions should be scheduled at increasingly spaced intervals to prevent return of fear. Bjork and

Bjork (1992) refer to this notion as the "new thoery of disuse." Craske and her colleagues have begun to test this notion with volunteers with nonclinical fears, as well as some patients with specific phobias, with promising results (e.g., Lang & Craske, 2000; Rowe & Craske, 1998a; Tsao & Craske, 2000). To date, studies have not examined this arrangement with PDA, but its success with specific phobias and its grounding in solid principles of learning should make this evaluation a priority.

GRADUATED VERSUS INTENSE EXPOSURE. In a related procedural strategy, exposure can be conducted in a graduated format, progressing from least to most difficult situations, or in an intensive format, beginning with most feared items on a hierarchy. An impressive series of studies examining a particularly aggressive and intensive form of exposure therapy with patients with PDA has been reported by Wolfgang Feigenbaum and his associates in Germany (Ehlers, Feigenbaum, Florin, & Margraf, 1995; Feigenbaum, 1988). This strategy involves intense, therapist-accompanied, ungraded, massed exposure. For example, in a comparison study of graduated ($n = 23$) versus intensive exposure ($n = 25$) in patients with severe agoraphobia, Feigenbaum (1988) found both treatment conditions to be equally effective at posttreatment and 8-month follow-up, but ungraded (intensive) exposure was clearly superior at 5-year follow-up (76% patients receiving intensive exposure vs. 35% from the graded condition were symptom-free). Interestingly, the patients receiving graded exposure reported the treatment to be more distressing than those in the intensive condition reported! After this finding, the next 104 subjects were treated with the intensive strategy. Results remained promising, with 78% remaining of the entire group symptom-free at 5-year follow-up. Moreover, these authors (Ehlers et al., 1995) found low attrition rates and comparable response rates to other studies at 2-year follow-up (e.g., Fava, Zielezny, Savron, & Grandi, 1995).

LEVEL OF ANXIETY REDUCTION DURING EXPOSURE. Based on extinction models of fear reduction, it has long been assumed that exposure should continue until anxiety decreases substantially (Marks, 1978). Newer emotional processing models of fear reduction also assume that long-term fear reduction is generally dependent on activation of fear arousal during the session, as well as on within-session and between-session habituation or fear reduction (Foa & Kozak, 1986; Rachman, 1980). But research in this area has produced inconsistent results, and it is far from clear whether high levels of fear arousal followed by substantial reductions in fear and anxiety during exposure sessions are prerequisites for long-term fear reduction. For example, we found benefits of exposure without endurance of high levels of anxiety when we instructed patients to terminate the exposure session when they experienced "undue levels of anxiety" (Agras et al., 1968; see also Emmelkamp, 1982). On the other hand, Marshall (1985) observed substantial benefit from longer periods of exposure with time allowed for complete anxiety reduction. Others have found equally effective results, whether escape or endurance paradigms were used (de Silva & Rachman, 1984; Rachman, Craske, Tallman, & Solyom, 1986). Interestingly, Rachman et al. (1986) found patients in the escape condition to report more perceived control and less fear during the exposure than patients in the endurance condition, suggesting that maximal fear elicitation and subsequent habituation are not essential for therapeutic benefit. As suggested in previous chapters and in the first edition of this book (Barlow, 1988), reinforcing a sense of control, and preventing emotionally driven escapist action tendencies (also perceived to be out of volitional control by the patient), more accurately represent the process of emotional change and fear reduction—an idea that has similarities to Bandura's self-efficacy model (Bandura, 1977, 1988).

DISTRACTION DURING EXPOSURE. It seems common sense that distraction procedures during exposure exercises are basically avoidant strategies and should be counterproductive (e.g., counting to 100, saying a prayer, snapping a rubber band on a wrist, etc.). Thus it is standard procedure to make all attempts to eliminate distraction strategies during exposure. However, we are aware of only one study that has investigated this assumption with patients with PDA (Craske, Street, & Barlow, 1989). In this study, we administered therapist-directed and self-directed exposure in small groups for 11 sessions. In one condition ($n = 16$), patients were instructed to monitor bodily sensations and thoughts objectively throughout *in vivo* exposure and to use thought stopping and focusing self-statements to interrupt distraction; patients in the other condition ($n = 14$) were taught to use specific distraction tasks during *in vivo* exposures (e.g., word rhymes, spelling, etc.), and to use thought stopping and distracting self-statements to interrupt focusing attention on feared bodily sensations and images. Treatment groups did not differ at posttreatment; however, consistent with previous research in obsessive–compulsive disorder (Grayson, Foa, & Steketee, 1982), the focused-exposure group improved significantly from posttreatment to follow-up, in contrast to slight deterioration in the distracted-exposure group.

ELIMINATING SAFETY SIGNALS. An often overlooked treatment target is the elimination of safety signals—the "talismans" that are such prominent features in the lives of patients with PDA, as described earlier (Craske et al., 2000; Rachman, 1983, 1984). Although few therapists would ignore the necessity of attending to the functional impairment that results from requiring the presence of a safe person such as a spouse on ventures out, other safety signals receive less attention. As noted in Table 10.2, more subtle safety behaviors (e.g., empty pill bottles, sheets of paper containing coping self-statements, or even pets) may be unobtrusive companions. Therefore, an individual cannot be considered "recovered" with a continuing dependence on these items—a dependence that is readily acknowledged to be irrational.

The difficulty with ignoring this residue of extensive avoidance lies in the danger of the individual's misplacing or otherwise forgetting the item after treatment is over. This of course may result in anxiety, a return of avoidance, or even relapse. At the very least, it will bring the patient to a realization that he or she has not recovered and that loss of control and panic may be just around the corner, depending on the presence or absence of a small piece of paper or an empty pill bottle. Since it is a rather small matter, in our experience, to wean patients from the variety of safety signals as part of their structured exposure exercises, there seems little reason not to do it. We consistently and carefully examine for the presence of safety signals, which on occasion have become so integrated with patients' routines that they may not report their presence. Once identified, all safety signals are removed prior to the beginning of exposure exercises.

PARTNER-ASSISTED EXPOSURE. Agoraphobia is a problem that invariably impinges on the social system of the patient. For this reason, family members are important possible sources of support for patients with PDA. Over the years, several groups of investigators have included significant others or partners in the treatment of PDA, with the notion that involving a motivated partner would initially support a patient during exposure practices in the home environment, which is the social system in which a patient exists on a day-to-day basis. The first investigators to examine this issue were Hand, Lamontagne, and Marks (1974). They noted that patients with agoraphobia who were treated in what became a cohesive group stayed in touch with one another and supported each other after treatment, and this evidently resulted in further improvement after completion of treatment. Mathews et al. (1977), in an uncontrolled clinical trial, included spouses of patients with agoraphobia as cotherapists and noted that over 90% of these patients were much improved at the end of treatment, with improvement continuing at follow-up. Munby and Johnston (1980) followed up a series of studies carried out by the same group of investigators. They concluded that the treatment in which spouses were directly included produced continuing improvement. The results were superior at a 4- to 9-year follow-up to the results of treatments where patients with agoraphobia were treated in separate clinical trials, but more intensively and without spouses. Sinnott, Jones, Scott-Fordham, and Woodward (1981) noted that patients with agoraphobia selected from the same neighborhood and treated as a group had superior outcomes on many measures to those of patients from diverse geographical regions (who presumably did not meet, socialize, or generally support each other during or after therapy). It seems likely that the reason for greater improvement in these experiments lay in support and motivation for continued "practice" in facing feared situations between sessions and after treatment was over.

We have also found that attending to a patient's social support system may enhance the effects of exposure. Specifically, we tested the feasibility and benefit of including patients' spouses directly in treatment (Barlow, O'Brien, & Last, 1984; Barlow, O'Brien, Last, & Holden, 1983). Results indicated an advantage for the spouse-assisted group compared with the nonassisted group. These posttest differences actually increased in favor of the spouse-assisted group at 1- and 2-year follow-ups (Cerny, Barlow, Craske, & Himadi, 1987). On the other hand, evidence from one of our studies (Barlow, O'Brien, & Last, 1984) indicated that in a well-adjusted marriage, the formal inclusion of the spouse in the treatment process made little difference. However, in a more poorly adjusted marriage, inclusion of the spouse seemed to override the influence of a poor relationship. Indeed, Arnow, Taylor, Agras, and Telch (1985) found that in marriages that were well adjusted at baseline, communication training further improved the effectiveness of treatment. These experiments underline the importance of considering the social system that provides the context for the treatment of agoraphobia, and highlights the role families may play in treatment. Moreover, as discussed above, educating family members on subtle reinforcement of agoraphobic behaviors (e.g., their role as potential safe persons) and the importance of modifying their behavior in response to the patients as they progress in treatment would seem to be important in maintaining success. Of course, the best "partner" may not always be a patient's spouse. We have often utilized adult children or even close friends and neighbors to assist with treatment.

This literature has been updated over the years (Carter, Turovsky, & Barlow, 1994; Daiuto, Baucom, Epstein, & Dutton, 1998; Marten & Barlow, 1993). Although some investigators have not found support for the importance of including significant others in treatment (e.g., Emmelkamp et al., 1992), the majority of studies generally support attending to a patient's social system and enlisting that social system in a supportive manner while treating agoraphobia. Unfortunately, there has been little systematic research on this as it relates to long-term improvement. Daiuto et al. (1998) point to the need for considerably more effort in this area, and the importance of targeting both agoraphobic behavior and the structure of relationships with significant others, particularly the spouse.

Recent Results of Exposure-Based Treatment

Since the 1980s and the development of psychological treatments for PDA, fewer studies have appeared evaluating exposure-based procedures in isolation from a CBT package. One notable exception is a study by Fava et al. (1995), who reported on long-term follow-up of 90 patients who had received 12 sessions of graduated self-paced exposure-based treatment. These treatments were administered biweekly over a 6-month period, approximating the kind of expanding-spaced schedule derived from the new theory of disuse described above (Lang et al., 1999). At the end of treatment, 87% were free of panic and were considered much improved. More importantly, using survival analysis to estimate the probability that responders to treatment would successfully remain in remission, Fava et al. (1995) reported that 96% remained in remission for the first 2 years, 77% throughout the first 5 years following treatment, and 67% after the first 7 years. The most important predictors of relapse were the presence of residual agoraphobia (suggesting the need to continue with treatment until agoraphobia is eliminated) and the presence of a personality disorder.

Exposure Combined with Drug Treatments

During the 1980s and early 1990s, prior to the new emphasis on CBT for panic, research on the efficacy of combined treatments focused on adding drugs to exposure-based treatments for patients with agoraphobia. Most of these studies examined the benefits of tricyclic antidepressants (TCAs) such as imipramine, with Matig Mavissakalian the leading investigator in this area. These studies, for the most part, reported evidence for superior results for combined treatment at the conclusion of therapy (Mavissakalian, 1996a; Mavissakalian & Perel, 1989; Telch, Agras, Taylor, Roth, & Gallen, 1985). However, the benefits generally disappeared at follow-up, after discontinuation of the drug (e.g., Mavissakalian, 1993; Mavissakalian & Michelson, 1986; Telch & Lucas, 1994). Marks et al. (1993) also found that a combined treatment consisting of alprazolam, a high-potency benzodiazepine, and *in vivo* exposure was similar in its efficacy to either alprazolam or exposure administered alone. But patients receiving combination treatment also experienced a high relapse rate 6 months after discontinuation of the alprazolam, to the point that overall therapeutic gains were less than with exposure alone. In other studies combining antidepressants with exposure, de Beurs, van Balkom, Lange, Koele, and van Dyke (1995) found that the addition of fluvoxamine to exposure was superior to exposure alone in reducing avoidance. Long-term naturalistic follow-up of this study 2 years later, however, showed that the effects in the two groups were equivalent (i.e., the fluvoxamine-plus-exposure group was no longer superior to the other treatment groups) (de Beurs, van Dyke, Lange, & van Balkom, 1999). Cottraux et al. (1995) found that the combination of CBT and buspirone was superior in the short term (16 weeks), but that the addition of the medication provided no advantage over the CBT condition alone at 1 year posttreatment.

Briefer Cost-Effective Modifications to Exposure-Based Procedures

Investigators have examined the effectiveness of more self-directed treatments for agoraphobic avoidance. First, Ghosh and Marks (1987) examined three combinations of self-directed exposure treatment over 10 weeks (i.e., therapist-instructed, computer-instructed, and text-instructed). These researchers found support for all three conditions, with no significant differences between conditions. As such, this study provides sound support for clinically effective and cost-effective treatment for agoraphobic avoidance. Second, in a similar study with patients suffering from moderate or severe agoraphobia, Swinson, Fergus, Cox, and Wickwire (1995) found support for a telephone-administered exposure treatment compared to a wait-list control group—and follow-up assessments at 3 and 6 months showed continued gains. Moreover, the gains made were reportedly comparable to those for traditional in-person treatment sessions. It is important to note, however, that some of our past research did not find support for bibliotherapy with patients who had more severe agoraphobia (Holden, O'Brien, Barlow, Stetson, & Infantino, 1983). Third, Côté, Gauthier, Laberge, Cormier, and Plamondon (1994) examined standard CBT with standard therapist contact (approx. 20 hours) compared with reduced therapist contact (approx. 10 hours). They found comparable results for both treatment conditions, and fully 73% of patients reported panic-free status and clinical improvement at 6-month follow-up. Finally, Lidren et al. (1994) found self-directed bibliotherapy to be as effective as group CBT when both were compared with a wait-list control condition, and gains were maintained at 3- and 6-month follow-ups.

Treating Panic and Associated Anxiety

Pharmacological Treatments and Their Effectiveness

Pharmacological approaches to the treatment of PDA have been the focus of an increasing number of controlled clinical trials during the last decade. The recent explosion of public marketing campaigns and research attention devoted to evaluating these drug treatments has led to an array of available medicinal agents with varying efficacy data. These medications are associated with a host of individual advantages and disadvantages for each patient, and appropriate treatment is often complicated by patients seeking treatment from multiple caregivers (Sanderson & Wetzler, 1993) and combination treatments for the same problems (Rapaport et al., 1996; Waikar, Bystritsky, Crasker, & Murphy, 1994–1995). Below we review the pharmacological management of PDA. We begin with a brief discussion of the historical evolution of pharmacological therapies, followed by a review of meta-analyses and efficacy data documented in recent clinical trials.

Following some historic clinical observations by Donald Klein (discussed at some length in Chapter 3; Klein, 1964; Klein & Fink, 1962), early pharmacological management of PDA emphasized the suppression of panic attacks. The expectation was that control of panic attacks would naturally result in reduced anticipatory anxiety and agoraphobic avoidance. In this way, Klein "pharmacologically dissected" panic attacks from more generalized anticipatory anxiety—an observation that had a profound impact on our conception of the nature of anxiety and panic, and led to the creation of the diagnosis of panic disorder. Pharmacotherapies and their efficacy in the treatment of PDA have evolved considerably over the past several decades (Spiegel, Wiegel, Baker, & Greene, 2000). The drug discovered by Klein as potentially effective was a TCA, imipramine. Beginning at that time and into the 1970s, TCAs, monoamine oxidase inhibitors (MAOIs), and barbiturates established the foundation of pharmacological treatments for PDA. In the 1980s, high-potency benzodiazepines were introduced as a safer and better-tolerated alternative to barbiturates. More recent pharmacological treatments include the use of selective serotonin reuptake inhibitors (SSRIs) and related agents. In Table 10.3 we present a list of medications with empirically established efficacy for PDA and their recommended dosages for healthy adults.

TRICYCLIC ANTIDEPRESSANTS. Since the early reports from Klein, over 15 controlled clinical trials have demonstrated the efficacy of the TCAs with panic disorder (APA, 1998), and the TCAs are still considered by many to be the "gold standard" for pharmacotherapeutic efficacy with this disorder (Spiegel et al., 2000). The TCAs have demonstrated both short-term and long-term effectiveness (Mavissakalian, 1996b; Mavissakalian & Perel, 1989, 1992a, 1992b, 1995, 1999); as such, they are the most studied of the medications

TABLE 10.3. Typical Doses for Medications with Empirically Supported Efficacy for the Treatment of PDA in Healthy Adults with No Concurrent Medications

Medication	Usual starting dose (mg/day)	Initial target dose (mg/day)	Maximum rec'd dose (mg/day)
Benzodiazepines			
Alprazolam[a] (++)	0.75	2–3	10
Clonazepam[b] (++)	0.25–0.50	1	4
Lorazepam[b] (+)	0.50	1–3	10
TCAs			
Imipramine[c] (++)	10	100–150	300
Clomipramine (++)	25	50–100	250
SSRIs[d]			
Paroxetine (++)	10	40	60
Sertraline (++)	25	50	200
Fluoxetine (+)	5–10	20	80
Fluvoxamine (+)	25	100	300
Citalopram (+)	10	20	60

Note. Combine medication with exposure instructions for patients with significant agoraphobia. ++, probably effective (efficacy demonstrated in at least one large, well-designed, double-blind trial or in several uncontrolled trials by different investigators). +, effective (efficacy demonstrated in at least two large, well-designed, double-blind trials conducted at multiple sites or by different investigators comparing the drug with placebo or to another drug with established efficacy). TCA, tricyclic antidepressants; SSRI, selective serotonin reuptake inhibitors. Adapted from Spiegel, Wiegel, Baker, and Greene (2000). Copyright 2000 by Allyn & Bacon. Adapted by permission.
[a] Alprazolam is usually taken in divided doses 3–4 times daily to avoid between-dose symptoms.
[b] This medication . . . is usually taken in divided doses 2–3 times daily.
[c] There may be a therapeutic window for imipramine for overall response.
[d] Low starting doses may be required to avoid initial hyperstimulation. If one SSRI is effective, others are likely to be as well.

used in the treatment of panic disorder and PDA. One large clinical trial (Cross-National Collaborative Panic Study, 1992; Klerman, 1992) found that imipramine was superior to placebo and comparable to the high-potency benzodiazepine alprazolam, although alprazolam exerted its effects sooner. In addition, in the large multicenter clinical trial investigating the treatment of panic disorder reported below (Barlow, Gorman, Shear, & Woods, 2000), imipramine was clearly superior to placebo after acute treatment (3 months after the beginning of the study), with drug–placebo differences even larger at the end of maintenance treatment (9 months after the beginning of the study). Although less well studied, other TCAs have shown similar efficacy, including clomipramine (Cassano et al., 1988; Modigh, Westburg, & Ericksson, 1992), desipramine (Lydiard, Morton, et al., 1993), and nortriptyline (Roy-Byrne, Wingerson, Cowley, & Dager, 1993). Pharmacologically, the TCAs are thought to exhibit their effects through the inhibition of the postrelease reuptake of norepinephrine or serotonin into presynaptic nerve terminals. A notable study by Mavissakalian and Perel (1995) found that imipramine may have an optimal therapeutic window for phobic anxiety, with preferred dosages at approximately 130 mg/day. As noted above, a far less specific dose–response relationship was found for panic. The evidence suggests that TCAs, particularly imipramine, are as effective as the newer SSRIs even after attrition is considered, clinical impressions notwithstanding.

Despite their effectiveness, the TCAs are often accompanied by troublesome side effects (e.g., blurred vision, weight gain, constipation) that are difficult for many patients to tolerate (Papp et al., 1997). Perhaps more importantly, the TCAs have been shown to cause central nervous system (CNS) activation and a side effect called "jitteriness syndrome" characterized by anxiety, panic, shakiness, insomnia, and irritability (Pohl, Wolkow, & Clary, 1998). This effect is reported in a substantial minority of patients with panic disorder. Generally, this side effect is time-limited; it often occurs at the outset of treatment; and it can be minimized by starting at low doses with slow titration. Nevertheless, it is a common case of treatment discontinuation. Similar to the benzodiazepines, termination of TCA use is linked with high relapse rates (D. M. Clark et al., 1994; Katschnig et al., 1995; Wiborg & Dahl, 1996). One nonrandomized comparison, however, suggested that *relapse* was significantly lower in patients treated with imipramine for 18 months versus only 6 months (Mavissakalian & Perel, 1992a).

It is interesting to note that imipramine does potentiate exposure-based treatments, but, despite Klein's (1964) provocative hypotheses, very little evidence has accumulated over the last decades that imipramine directly affects panic attacks. Despite a few suggestions to the contrary (Uhlenhuth, Matuzas, Warner, & Thompson, 1997), the weight of the evidence strongly suggests that imipramine has its effects on more generalized (or anticipatory) anxiety. This conclusion is buttressed by general findings that imipramine potentiates exposure treatments in which the focus is not on reducing anxiety and panic, but rather on increasing anxiety in the service of changing behavior, at least in the short term. On the other hand, imipramine does not seem to potentiate CBT for panic and associated anxiety. This may be because CBT focuses directly on anxiety and panic, via perhaps a different mechanism than imipramine and other antidepressants. Thus imipramine and related anxiolytics, such as the high-potency benzodiazepines (see below), not only do not potentiate therapeutic effects of CBT; they may well interfere with their effects by dampening the provocation of anxiety under controlled circumstances, which is an integral part of all forms of CBT (Barlow et al., 2000; Spiegel & Bruce, 1997; Spiegel et al., 2000).

Evidence on the anxiolytic versus panicolytic effects of antidepressants such as imipramine can also be found in the seeming lack of dose–response relationships in the Mavissakalian and Perel (1995) study reported above. In fact, this replicates important earlier studies by Mavissakalian and colleagues showing dose–response relationships for imipramine in the overall outcome of treatment for PDA, but no relationship whatsoever between drug dosage or plasma concentrations of drug on the one hand, and reductions in panic on the other. That is, PDA responded equally well to all dosages of imipramine in several important studies in the 1980s (Mavissakalian & Michelson, 1986; Marks et al., 1983). Drug relationships were found only for global response to treatment, and then only at posttreatment. The most likely possibility, in our view, is that imipramine may contribute to exposure-based procedures by directly reducing anxious apprehension (rather than panic). Thus the somatic sensations associated with anxiety that seem to serve as cues for panic would decrease, as well as levels of anxious self-preoccupation (self-focused attention). A sense of control would increase. Panic attacks would then decrease because the platform of anxious apprehension from which panic attacks emerge would be removed (see Chapters 5 and 7). Direct evidence for the anxiolytic effects of imipramine was obtained in other studies in the 1980s (e.g., Kahn et al., 1986). In the Kahn et al. study, imipramine produced substantial anxiolytic effects that were superior to those of a standard benzodiazepine on most measures. Furthermore, this effect was observed despite the exclusion of patients with clear panic and phobic components to their anxiety.

In addition, some evidence exists that drugs for panic disorder do not block naturally occurring alarms or fear. In one study, patients reported that "alarming" events such as near-accidents in automobiles provoked the same response as they did when the patients were not on drugs (Nesse, Cameron, Curtis, & Lee, 1986). In fact, we suggest elsewhere (Barlow, 1988; Barlow, Chorpita, & Turovsky, 1996) that the development of a sense of control, along with changes in action tendencies and alterations in focus of attention, is what may ultimately be the target of all drug and behavioral treatments (see Chapter 3). All drug and behavioral treatments may be effective only to the extent that they reduce anxiety or anxious apprehension.

BENZODIAZEPINES. The first medication approved by the U.S. Food and Drug Administration (FDA) for the treatment of PDA was alprazolam. This approval was based on several pivotal multicenter studies (Ballenger et al., 1988; Cross-National Collaborative Panic Study, 1992; Lesser et al., 1988; Noyes et al., 1988) showing that alprazolam (at an average dose of 6 mg/day) was superior to placebo on critical clinical outcome measures (e.g., disability, panic attacks, panic-related phobias, and global improvement). Subsequent fixed-dose trials have found that patients may benefit from substantially smaller doses (i.e., 2 mg/day; Lydiard et al., 1992; Uhlenhuth, 1998). Additional studies have shown that the acute treatment improvements were maintained at 6-month follow-up with no demonstrable tolerance to the medication (Schweizer, Rickels, Weiss, & Zavodnick, 1993).

Benzodiazepines are generally considered to be safe and quick-acting, with fewer side effects than other drugs used to treat anxiety disorders (Spiegel et al., 2000). Pharmacologically, benzodiazepines are thought to enhance the natural effect of gamma-aminobutyric acid (GABA) on chloride conductance through cell membranes inhibiting cellular excitability (cf. Stahl, 1996). Other anxiolytics have shown similar results in the treatment of panic disorder and PDA, including clonazepam (Beauclair, Fontaine, Annable, Holobow, & Chouinard, 1994; Davidson & Moroz, 1998; Moroz & Rosenbaum, 1999), lorazepam (Schweizer et al., 1990), diazepam (Dunner, Ishiki, Avery, Wilson, & Hyde, 1986; Noyes et al., 1996), lorazepam (Charney & Woods, 1989; Schweizer et al., 1990), and adinazolam (C. S. Carter et al., 1995).

Common concerns about these agents focus on tolerance, abuse, and dependence (cf. Shader & Greenblatt, 1993). Although tolerance develops to the sedative side effects of benzodiazepines, few studies have found tolerance to the anxiolytic effects (Hayward, Wardle, & Higgitt, 1989; Romach et al., 1992). In fact, abuse of benzodiazepines is rare and usually occurs in a pattern of polysubstance abuse (APA, 1998). Several longitudinal studies have found that treatment gains are maintained with no evidence of abuse or dose escalation over time (over 4 years' use of alprazolam, Nagy, Krystal, Woods, & Charney, 1989; over 2 years' use of clonazepam, Worthington et al., 1998).

The difficulty is that with prolonged use, most patients develop physiological dependence that results in withdrawal symptoms (e.g., nervousness, sleep disturbance, dizziness) when the drug is discontinued (Pecknold, Swinson, Kuch, & Lewis, 1988; Schweizer et al., 1990). For example, alprazolam has been shown to increase anxiety during discontinuation (O'Sullivan et al., 1996; Pecknold et al., 1988), particularly if the drug is tapered rapidly; as such, this effect renders the medication particularly addictive. Benzodiazepine discontinuation has been related to high rates of relapse (50–75%), even after 8 months of treatment (Ballenger, 1994; Spiegel, 1998a), and another study found increased rates of return to drug after prolonged use (Wardle et al., 1994). The withdrawal symptoms from medication can overlap considerably with panic attacks and anticipatory anxiety, and may be interpreted by patients as a return of the disorder, leading them to request additional medication. However, Spiegel and Bruce (1997) report that this "rebound" effect can be avoided by a very slow, flexible drug taper. A series of systematic studies investigating the use of psychological strategies to overcome dependence on benzodiazepines is described below.

SELECTIVE SEROTONIN REUPTAKE INHIBITORS. SSRIs are currently considered by many to be the state-of-the-art choice in medications for panic disorder and PDA. Numerous studies have demonstrated the efficacy of the SSRIs, including paroxetine (Ballenger, Wheadon, Steiner, Bushnell, & Gergel, 1998; Oehrberg et al., 1995), citalopram (Lydiard, Pollack, Judge, Michelson, & Tamura, 1997; Wade, Lepola, Koponen, Pedersen, & Pedersen, 1997), fluoxetine (Michelson et al., 1998), fluvoxamine (Bakish et al., 1996; Black, Wesner, Bowers, Gabel, 1993), and sertraline (Pohl, Wolkow, & Clary, 1998; Pollack, Otto, Worthington, Manfro, & Wolkow, 1998). Paroxetine was the first FDA-approved SSRI in the treatment of PDA, and its efficacy has been shown in several multicenter clinical trials (Ballenger et al., 1998; Lecrubier et al., 1997; Oehrberg et al., 1995).

Comparative studies of SSRIs with each other, or with TCAs or benzodiazepines, have been generally inconclusive, with all treatments yielding similarly equivalent results in most analyses (van Balkom et al., 1997; Wilkinson, Balestrieri, Ruggeri, & Bellantuono, 1991). Whereas one meta-analysis by Boyer (1994) found the SSRIs to be superior to imipramine, others have concluded these medications to be equally effective (Bakish et al., 1996). In fact, in four different randomized studies, none found significant differences at the end of the study in intent-to-treat analyses, which included consideration of dropouts (Lecrubier et al., 1997; Bystritsky et al., 1994–1995; Nair et al., 1996; Wade et al., 1997). Although Lecrubier et al. (1997) did find evidence for a more rapid response for the SSRI, Nair et al. (1996) actually found that the TCA, but not the SSRI, was more effective than placebo. Although SSRIs tend to have a longer duration to response than TCAs, the optimal duration of treatment is not known. Ballenger et al. (1998), in an extension of a earlier trial of a fixed dose of paroxetine, crossed half of the responders to 22 weeks of placebo, resulting in a 30% relapse rate for the patients on placebo within 12 weeks. To date, rates of relapse following long-term treatment with paroxetine have not been reported.

Despite these inconclusive findings, the SSRIs are often preferred because they are better tolerated than the TCAs, are easier to dose than the TCAs and the MAOIs, lack the abuse and dependence potentials of benzodiazepines, and are considered safer. Moreover, the SSRIs have a broad band of therapeutic activity that may be especially helpful with comorbid disorders. Pharmacologically, SSRIs exert their action by inhibiting the postrelease reuptake of serotonin into presynaptic nerve terminals (similar to TCAs), but they have less affinity for the postsynaptic receptors associated with many of the adverse side effects of the TCAs. However, the SSRIs may cause side effects that include sexual impairment (in as many as 50–75% of patients), gastrointestinal symptoms, and CNS activation (including the jitteriness syndrome discussed above). As such, the SSRIs may require more informational support, slower titration, lower start doses, and possibly the time-limited use of a sleep medication early in treatment. Despite their advantages, some SSRIs have a varied profile with significant differences in drug interactions, functional half-lives, and use in older populations (Tollefson & Rosenbaum, 1998), all of which require special caution in their use.

OTHER PRESCRIPTION MEDICATIONS. Several less studied agents have demonstrated provisional but promising findings in the treatment of panic disorder, including the MAOIs (Bakish, Saxena, Bowden, & D'Souza, 1993; Buigues & Vallejo, 1987; Roy-Byrne et al., 1993) as well as other antidepressants. The latter include venlafaxine (Papp et al., 1998;

Pollack, Worthington, et al., 1996) and nefazodone, a related agent that has shown efficacy in depressed patients with panic attacks (DeMartinis, Schweizer, & Rickels, 1996; Zajecka, 1996). Because of their side effects and the strict dietary restrictions they necessitate, MAOIs are rarely prescribed.

Psychological Treatments and Their Effectiveness

THE DEVELOPMENT OF INTEROCEPTIVE EXPOSURE AND "PANIC CONTROL TREATMENT." At the heart of the psychological treatment of panic are reproduction of and exposure to the somatic symptoms of panic. The reproduction–exposure process has been accomplished in a variety of different ways, accompanied by different explanations for its effectiveness. Nevertheless, all psychological treatments for panic with any demonstrated success have this process as a core ingredient.

As with all new discoveries, some interesting early examples of this approach were either misinterpreted or ignored. In Wolpe's classic early work, CO_2 inhalations were a common but largely overlooked component of his anxiety reduction procedures. Generally, inhaling CO_2 was conceptualized as facilitating relaxation, and therefore promoting the reciprocal inhibition of anxiety. In fact, this may have been a very effective procedure for systematically exposing panic-ridden patients to their feared cues in the benign setting of the therapist's office (Wolpe, 1958). Other early reports can also be similarly interpreted. Orwin (1973) treated eight patients who had agoraphobia with "the running treatment." In his procedure, patients were instructed to sprint until breathless, and then to approach or enter a feared situation. Running, of course, produced many of the somatic signs of panic, resulting in systematic exposure to these cues. This recalls some of the early panic provocation work using exercise (e.g., Cohen & White, 1950; see Chapter 5). Watson and Marks (1971), in a study with patients with agoraphobia, reported the then-puzzling finding that imaginal flooding to relevant phobic cues (imagining an intensely vivid scene depicting phobic cues) was no more effective than irrelevant flooding (visualizing being eaten by tigers). In fact, irrelevant flooding produced significantly greater therapeutic effects on patients' subjective anxiety while imagining a phobic scene! This is understandable if one considers that arousal cues produced by irrelevant flooding are the primary phobic cues.

One of the most interesting early reports along these lines was that of Bonn, Harrison, and Rees (1971). Following up on the origins of provoking panic in the laboratory with lactate (see Chapter 5), Bonn et al. (1971) carried this procedure to its logical conclusion from the point of view of treatment by administering it repeatedly to 33 patients. Although panic was not directly measured, this procedure seemed quite successful. Interestingly, this result was totally ignored. In another early series, Haslam (1974) treated 16 subjects, 10 of whom panicked following a sodium lactate challenge with repeated CO_2 inhalation. Of the 10 patients who panicked with lactate, 9 demonstrated marked improvement after 6 weeks of CO_2 inhalation treatment. Other early case reports or clinical series by Latimer (1977) and Lum (1976) reported on diverse procedures such as CO_2 inhalation or voluntary hyperventilation, which seemed to result in substantial improvement in cases of what we would now call panic disorder.

Independent of other treatment techniques, fear reduction via interoceptively induced physical sensations has found support in the research. Several classic studies have supported the role of interoceptive exposure in fear reduction—by utilizing repeated infusions of sodium lactate (a drug that produces panic-like bodily sensations; Bonn, Harrison, & Rees, 1971; Haslam, 1974), and still others have found graduated carbon dioxide inhalations to be superior to propranolol (a Beta blocker that suppresses panic-like sensations) in reducing fear of sensations (Griez & van den Hout, 1986). More recently, several studies have replicated this finding, that fear is reduced through repeated exposure to carbon dioxide inhalations (Beck & Shipherd, 1997) and that panic attacks and panic-related fears are significantly reduced following six sessions of CO_2 inhalation (Beck, Shipherd, & Zebb, 1997). Similarly, some recent research examining physical exercise, a type of interoceptive exposure, in comparsion to medication (clomipramine) and pill placebo, found exercise to be superior to the pill placebo but inferior to the drug in the treatment of panic disorder (Broocks et al., 1998).

Cognizant of this early work, in the mid-1980s we developed a CBT approach to treating panic attacks and related anxiety called "panic control treatment" (PCT; Barlow, Cohen, et al., 1984; Barlow, Craske, Cerny, & Klosko, 1989), which has achieved wide acceptance (Barlow & Craske, 2000). Contemporaneously and independently, David M. Clark and colleagues were developing an approach similar in practice, but with greater theoretical emphasis on cognitive changes (Clark, 1986; D. M. Clark et al., 1994). PCT begins with a focus on the panic attacks themselves and anxiety focused on panic, which is then followed by techniques that target agoraphobic avoidance. Specifically, the goals of PCT are to directly influence catastrophic misappraisal of panic and anxiety, hyperventilatory response, and conditioned fear reactions to physical cues.

The first step in this process is psychoeducation to impart knowledge to the patient on the nature of the fight-or-flight response and the physiology of the anxiety system. Via this information, patients are taught that they experience "sensations" rather than "panics," and that these sensations are normal and harmless. See Barlow and Craske (2000) for detailed and verbatim instructions provided to the patient. The second aim of treatment is to identify and challenge anxious thoughts and beliefs through cognitive restructuring. Next, specific information concerning the effects of hyperventilation and its role in panic attacks is provided. This information is commonly combined with extensive practice of breathing retraining—a somewhat controversial technique (see below). Historically, breathing retraining has played a key role in treatments for panic disorder because patients often describe symptoms of hyperventilation as similar to panic attack symptoms, and this procedure is still included in our protocols. Interoceptive exposure exercises are the last component; in these exercises, patients are instructed to repeatedly expose themselves to anxiety-provoking internal cues and sensations to lessen fear, and to provide an occasion to practice cognitive restructuring strategies. Manuals describing the treatment in some detail are available for the patient (Barlow & Craske, 2000; Craske et al., 2000).

RECONCEPTUALIZATION OF BREATHING RETRAINING. Breathing retraining seems to provide some symptomatic relief for patients with PDA (Clark, Salkovskis, & Chalkley, 1985; Bonn, Readhead, & Timmons, 1984). But treatment studies have generally examined breathing retraining as one component of multicomponent treatments, so it is difficult to attribute positive findings solely to breathing retraining. Garssen, de Ruiter, and van Dyck (1992) concluded from a review of its mechanisms of action and efficacy that breathing retraining probably effects change through distraction or imparting a sense of control, rather than through modulation of breathing per se. As such, breathing retraining has been the focus of recent controversy; investigators have questioned its theoretical compatibility and its incremental benefit over other cognitive and behavioral components of treatment (Schmidt et al., 2000; de Ruiter, Rijken, Garssen, & Kraaimaat, 1989). Using a dismantling design, Schmidt et al. (2000) concluded that breathing retraining did not add any clear benefits to a treatment package consisting of education, cognitive restructuring, and exposure-based techniques (both *in vivo* and interoceptive). In addition, although this study was subject to low power, their data showed a trend that patients who received breathing retraining showed lower end-state functioning on both self-report and clinician-rated measures (Schmidt et al., 2000). Thus these authors speculated that breathing retraining may put a patient at greater risk for relapse or decrease the chances for complete recovery. An important limitation of this study, however, is the lack of assessment of each patient's true use of each treatment component—an important question that needs to be examined. Such an evaluation would benefit from a thorough assessment that identifies what treatment techniques were used or not used by the patients, and what nonstudy techniques may have been used. Nevertheless, the Schmidt et al. (2000) study is the only one of which we are aware that has directly evaluated the addition of breathing retraining to the other main components of CBT interventions.

In our view, any behavior that minimizes panic symptoms or enables avoidance of or distraction from the panic sensations is maladaptive. Such avoidance is considered a safety behavior because it is an attempt to keep a patient "safe" from a false threat (i.e., panic symptoms, high anxiety). As such, teaching the skill of breathing retraining in this context could be conceptualized as teaching avoidance as a coping technique—a concept antithetical to the goals of treatment! Thus we instruct patients that use of breathing retraining during exposure practices is discouraged and is maladaptive.

In light of this potential theoretical incompatibility, we are currently experimenting with using breathing retraining in a very different way. In this new approach, controlled breathing is conceptualized as a means of testing whether some of the anxiety symptoms the patient experiences may be due to overbreathing; thus it is used as an experimental procedure in the PCT protocol. The rationale is presented that if the patient is able to reduce the anxiety sensations simply by changing the way he or she breathes, then this is strong evidence that the sensations are the result of overbreathing—and are therefore understandable, predictable, manageable, and harmless. Once the patient correctly draws this conclusion, controlled breathing is faded out, and the emphasis is shifted to using this information to counter anxious thoughts about the sensations. Thus controlled breathing is not encouraged as a means to reduce physical sensations; its use in this way could maintain anxiety focused on panic attacks, because the patient never learns that even strong sensations of overbreathing, though uncomfortable, are not dangerous.

EFFICACY OF PSYCHOLOGICAL TREATMENTS. The efficacy of various forms of CBT for panic disorder and PDA is strongly supported by more than 25 independently conducted controlled clinical trials. Table 10.4 summarizes results from several of the major clinical trials evaluating the efficacy of different versions of CBT, compared to credible alternative treatments. In most studies patients suffered from no more than mild to moderate agoraphobia, although interoceptive avoidance was substantial in some studies. Table 10.5 presents results from a comprehensive meta-analysis of treatment outcome for PDA with all levels of agoraphobic avoidance (Gould et al., 1995). Included in the meta-analysis were 43 controlled studies. As is evident in Table 10.5, CBT was associated with the largest effect sizes and the smallest rate of patient attrition when compared to drug treatments or to approaches that combined psychological and drug treatments. Importantly, treatments utilizing interoceptive exposure were associated with the largest effect sizes, although many of these studies included patients with no more than mild agoraphobic avoidance. It is also important to note that these versions of CBT produce a incremental increase in quality of life for patients (Telch, Schmidt, Jaimez, Jacquin, & Harrington, 1995).

TABLE 10.4. Clinical Trials of Cognitive-Behavioral Treatments for Panic Disorder: Intent-to-Treat Analysis

Clinical trial	Length of follow-up (months)	Treatment (% panic-free)	Treatment comparisons (% panic-free)[a]
Barlow et al. (2000)	12	PCT ($n = 77$), 41%[e]	Yes: PCT + PL ($n = 63$), 31.9% Yes: PL ($n = 24$), 13% Yes: IMI ($n = 83$), 19.7% Yes: PCT + IMI ($n = 65$), 26.3%
Black, Wesner, et al. (1993)	PT	CT ($n = 25$), 32%	Yes: FL = 68% Yes: PL = 20%
Beck et al. (1992)	PT	CT ($n = 17$), 94%	Yes: ST = 25%[d]
Craske et al. (1991)[b]	24	PCT ($n = 15$), 81%	Yes: AR = 36% Yes: PCT & AR = 43%
Craske, Maidenberg, & Bystritsky(1995)	PT	CBT ($n = 16$), 53%	Yes: NPT = 8%
D. M. Clark et al. (1994)	12	CT ($n = 17$), 76%	Yes: AR = 43%[c] Yes: IMI = 48%[c]
Côté et al. (1994)	12	CBTM ($n = 13$), 92% CBTNM ($n = 8$), 100%	—
Klosko et al. (1990)	PT	PCT ($n = 15$), 87%	No: AL = 50% Yes: PL = 36% Yes: WL = 33%
Margraf & Schneider (1991)	1	CT ($n = 22$), 91%	Yes: WL = 5%
Newman et al. (1990)	12	CTM ($n = 24$), 87% CTNM ($n = 19$), 87%	—
Öst et al. (1993)	12	CT ($n = 19$), 89%[c]	No: AR = 74%[c]
Shear et al. (1994)	6	CBT ($n = 23$), 45%	No: NPT = 45%
Telch et al. (1993)	PT	PCT ($n = 34$), 85%	Yes: WL = 30%

Note. Abbreviations: AL, alprazolam; AR, applied relaxation; CBT, cognitive-behavioral therapy; CBTM, cognitive-behavioral therapy and medication; CBTNM, cognitive-behavioral therapy without medication; CT, cognitive therapy; CTM, cognitive therapy and medication; CTNM, cognitive therapy without medication; FL, fluvoxamine; IMI, imipramine; NPT, nonprescriptive treatment; PL, pill placebo; PCT, panic control treatment (exposure and cognitive restructuring); PT, posttreatment; ST, supportive therapy; WL, wait list. Adapted from Barlow and Lehman (1996). Copyright 1996 by the American Medical Association Adapted by permission.
[a]Yes, comparison was significant; No, comparison was not significant;—, comparison was not made.
[b]Follow-up study of Barlow et al. (1989).
[c]Percentage of patients who were panic-free at follow-up and who had received no additional treatment during the follow-up period.
[d]At 8 weeks (the end of supportive therapy), 71% of patients receiving CT were panic-free.
[e]Patients meeting criteria for "responder" status.

A noteworthy finding from the above-described studies is that forms of CBT for panic disorder have consistently proven more efficacious than credible alternative psychosocial treatments, largely eliminating interpretations related to nonspecific factors (expectancy, therapist relationship issues, etc.). This finding is best illustrated in a program of research first reported by Katherine Shear and colleagues (Shear, Pilkonis, Cloitre, & Leon, 1994), who developed a new approach to panic disorder called "emotion-focused therapy" (EFT). This approach focuses on explicating and treating interpersonal triggers for panic attacks

TABLE 10.5. Findings from a Meta-Analysis of 43 Controlled Studies of Treatment of PDA

Study	Effect size	Dropouts
Cognitive-behavioral therapy	0.68	5.6%
Cognitive therapy and interoceptive exposure	0.88	NR
Pharmacological treatment	0.47	19.8%
Combination treatment	0.56	22.0%

Note. NR, not reported. Data source: Gould, Otto, and Pollack (1995).

rather than interoceptive cues. Attrition was high in the first study, but preliminary results were promising. Further evaluation by Shear, Houck, Greeno, and Masters (in press) is now complete. In this study, patients were randomly assigned to receive either EFT, CBT, imipramine, or placebo. Since EFT was evaluated in parallel to the multicenter study reported below, these comparison conditions were drawn from that study. EFT was less effective than either CBT or imipramine. In fact, results of EFT at the end of treatment, and 6 months later after maintenance treatment, were no different from those for placebo. At follow-up, after all treatments were discontinued, EFT fared better than placebo, but was significantly less effective than CBT or imipramine (see Figure 10.7). The fact that this study was carried out by an investigator with allegiance to EFT illustrates the strength of the study, the power of new psychosocial treatments designed for specific patterns of psychopathology, and the growing sophistication of psychotherapy research in elucidating these differences.

THE MULTICENTER STUDY. We have recently reported results from a multicenter clinical trial for panic disorder, the largest combined treatment study to date (Barlow et al., 2000). In this study, we compared the combination of PCT (Barlow & Craske, 2000) and imipramine to each treatment alone, a pill placebo, and PCT plus placebo in 312 patients with mild to moderate agoraphobia. Patients were seen at four different sites: the Departments of Psychiatry at Yale University, Columbia University/Hillside Hospital, and University of Pittsburgh/Western Psychiatric Institute and Clinic, and the Center for Anxiety and Related Disorders at Boston University. All patients were treated weekly for 3 months (12 sessions for the acute phase), and "responders" were then seen monthly for 6 months (maintenance phase). All patients were followed up 6 months after treatment ended; thus the overall duration of the study was 15 months.

Results indicated that both imipramine and PCT were significantly superior to placebo after the acute phase of treatment, as were the two combined treatments in terms of total number of patients meeting a response criterion based on scores on the PDSS. However, the PCT–imipramine combination was not significantly better than the PCT–placebo combination or either of the individual treatments. Notably, among those who responded to treatment (for the moment, excluding those who didn't respond or dropped out), imipramine evidenced a somewhat broader therapeutic effect, since patients were also less depressed and had slightly better results on some self-report measures (see Figure 10.8). At the end of the maintenance phase, all treatments remained significantly better than placebo; most remaining patients in the placebo condition who had done well initially had deteriorated substantially, resulting in even more dramatic treatment-placebo differences. Also, the PCT–imipramine combined treatment proved to be slightly better at this 9-month follow-up data

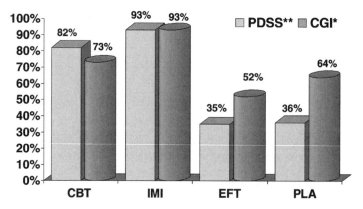

FIGURE 10.7. Response rates among acute treatment completers for cognitive-behavioral therapy (CBT), imipramine (IMI), emotion-focused therapy (EFT), and placebo (PLA). PDSS, Panic Disorder Severity Scale; CGI, Clinical Global Improvement. $*p = .02$. $**p = .001$. From Shear, Houck, Greeno, and Masters (in press). Reprinted by permission of the authors.

point than even PCT plus placebo, although probably not to the point of clinical significance, particularly considering the extra cost associated with this combined treatment. No other differences among treatments were noted at this point (see Figure 10.8). At the 15-month point in the study, 6 months after all treatments were discontinued, patients who had responded to imipramine (either as a single treatment or in combination with PCT) lost any gains they had made, making PCT (either alone or in combination with placebo) significantly more effective than the other conditions (see Figure 10.8). The results suggest that both individual treatments are clearly effective; that there appears to be no worth-

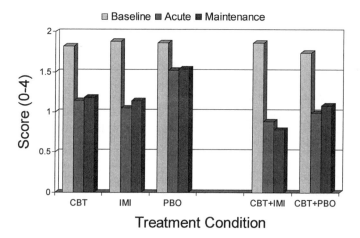

FIGURE 10.8. Comparison of baseline, acute, and maintenance treatment follow-up analyses for intent-to-treat (ITT) sample based on PDSS average item score (n = 312). CBT, cognitive behavioral treatment; IMI, imiprimine; PBO, placebo. From Barlow Gorman, Shear, and Woods (2000). Copyright 2000 by American Medical Association. Reprinted by permission.

while advantage to combining treatments; and that the psychological treatment (i.e., PCT) appears to be more durable in its effects. Indeed, data comparisons of the 6-month post-treatment relapse rate based on the Clinical Global Improvement Scale for intent-to-follow and patients who completed treatment provide some support for the durability of psychological treatment (i.e., PCT) (see Figure 10.9).

Although the study was conducted at two sites known for expertise in psychological treatments (Boston and Pittsburgh) and two sites known for expertise in pharmacological treatments (Yale and Columbia), no site differences were observed in outcome. Thus any "allegiance" effects (in which treatments do better at sites where therapists are adherents to a particular approach) did not seem to contribute to outcome. Attrition analyses from the study indicated that life stressors and lower education level (as a function of household income) were most strongly related to attrition (Grilo et al., 1998). These results are undergoing further analyses.

THE COMBINATION OF CBT AND BENZODIAZEPINES. Most evidence suggests that benzodiazepines do not combine well with CBT or other psychosocial treatments. We have reviewed earlier the study by Marks et al. (1993) in which concurrent administration of alprazolam seemed to detract from long-term effects of exposure, paralleling the effects noted in our multicenter study with PCT and imipramine. But others have noted *synergistic effects* of imipramine and exposure-based treatments under certain conditions (e.g., Mavissakalian, 1996a). Reports that high-potency benzodiazepines may interfere with and detract from CBT are more consistent (Brown & Barlow, 1995; Otto, Pollack, & Sabatino, 1996).

Some innovative research provides insight into the future of combined treatment approaches and possible success of sequential treatment strategies. First, Otto et al. (1993) found that a modified PCT protocol conducted in combination with a slow alprazolam taper over 10 weeks resulted in excellent outcomes. Fully 75% of the patients in the PCT–taper condition discontinued medication, compared with only 25% of those in the taper-only condition. A similar study (Spiegel, Bruce, Gregg, & Nuzzarello, 1994) found that nearly all patients were able to discontinue alprazolam use (80% of those receiving supportive medical management plus taper, and 90% of those receiving PCT plus taper). Importantly, however, at the 6-month follow-up, half of the patients receiving support-

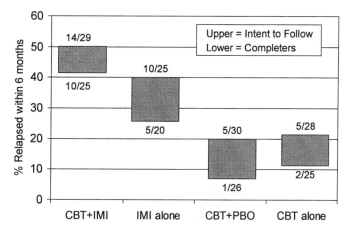

FIGURE 10.9. Posttreatment relapse rate based on Clinical Global Improvement Scale (CGI) for intent-to-follow and completer patients (*N* = 312).

ive medical management plus taper had relapsed, compared to none receiving PCT plus taper. A 3-year follow-up found that one-third of those receiving PCT plus taper had suffered a relapse in the 6–18 months following treatment, compared with 70% in the supportive condition (Spiegel et al., 1994). Taken together, these findings provide support for the potential use of combination treatments that include benzodiazepines (initially to provide immediate relief and/or to treat those who desire medication) followed by or used in conjunction with CBT protocols. The future of these sequential treatment approaches as opposed to comparative or simultaneous approaches awaits further investigation.

Similarly, the effectiveness of psychosocial treatments for those patients who do not show full response to pharmacotherapies has begun to receive attention. Pollack et al. (1994) examined the addition of 12 weeks of CBT for patients who were "medication nonresponders" (i.e., patients who had previously exhibited an incomplete response to pharmacotherapy). Compared to a prior nonresponse to medication, these patients showed marked improvement following the CBT—both improved global functioning and reduced panic attack frequency. It is possible that these patients may represent a unique sample who were nonresponsive to medication and who showed improvement from psychosocial treatments. It is also possible that providing medication for patients who do not resond to CBT (i.e., the reverse sequence) may have comparable outcomes.

EFFECTS OF TREATMENT ON COMORBID CONDITIONS. Effective treatments for panic disorder have been shown to have a positive impact on comorbid conditions of anxiety and depression (T. A. Brown, Antony, & Barlow, 1995; Laberge, Gauthier, Côté, Plamondon, & Cormier, 1993; Tsao, Lewin, & Craske, 1998). That is, following CBT of panic disorder, co-occurring symptoms of depression and other anxiety disorders also show improvement. Moreover, in a recent exploratory single-case design with three patients who reported current alcohol abuse, the alcohol abuse subsided in all three patients after successful treatment with PCT (although one patient later relapsed; Lehman, Brown, & Barlow, 1998). This result is very preliminary and requires extensive investigation before clinicians begin reversing the usual order of treating substance abuse before comorbid anxiety disorders. But it may be a useful strategy, since the onset of anxiety often precedes substance abuse, as described in some detail in Chapter 1. Still other research has found that some personality traits may subside following CBT for panic (Hoffart, 1997; Hoffart & Hedley, 1997; Hofmann et al., 1998; Rathus, Sanderson, Miller, & Wetzler, 1995).

In a recent study (Hofmann et al., 1998), we examined the comparative effects of CBT and pharmacotherapy for panic disorder on personality disorder characteristics in a sample of 93 patients with panic disorder with mild or no agoraphobia. Results of this study showed that both treatments had a positive impact on nearly all personality disorder characteristics, independent of type of treatment and response to the particular treatment. In fact, with some exceptions (i.e., scores on the Schizoid Personality Disorder Scale), all personality disorder characteristics showed significant change from baseline to posttreatment for both treatment groups. Notably, however, personality disorder characteristics did not predict treatment outcome with either CBT or imipramine—a finding consistent with other studies (Dreessen, Arntz, Luttels, & Sallaerts, 1994). A study examining benefits of CBT (T. A. Brown, Antony, & Barlow, 1995) found that the beneficial effects of CBT for panic disorder on comorbid conditions may lessen over time. As such, if the comorbid condition is not completely remitted, both the comorbid condition and the panic disorder may return to pretreatment levels by follow-up. However, other researchers (Woody, McLean,

Taylor, & Koch, 1999) found that reductions in co-occurring diagnoses of depression were no greater after treatment for panic than after a wait-list period. Indeed, these findings raise important questions regarding the mechanisms of action of the treatments and the overlap in treatment components for related anxiety and mood disorders, as well as the nature of psychopathology in anxiety and mood disorders.

SEVERAL CAVEATS. Despite the positive findings reviewed above, research on CBT for panic disorder must be interpreted with only cautious optimism and with several caveats in mind. First, and as noted above, many studies of CBT for panic have excluded patients with severe agoraphobia, and thus findings may overestimate the effectiveness of CBT. Controlled studies including patients with the full range of agoraphobic avoidance have found more attrition and fewer patients showing clinical improvement at posttreatment and follow-up.

Second, methodological rigor and outcome measures are often quite variable across studies and may account for inconsistent outcome findings. Such methodological differences may misrepresent true longitudinal outcome. For example, using very stringent criteria (e.g., recurrence of panic attacks, help-seeking behavior), we (Brown & Barlow, 1995) found that more than one-third of patients with panic who were classified as "panic-free" at 24 months posttreatment had experienced a panic attack in the preceding year. Moreover, we found that a large minority (27%) of this sample had obtained further treatment for panic during the follow-up interval. Such findings highlight the importance of obtaining consistent, longitudinal follow-up on patients, in order to evaluate their clinical status most reliably and validly.

The third caveat concerns the generality of findings from studies reviewed above to clinical settings. Whereas most treatment outcome studies are conducted in highly controlled clinical research settings with thoroughly trained therapists, and are thus designed to maximize both internal validity and the specificity of causal mechanisms of treatment, such controlled conditions are rarely found in the real-world settings to which the treatment is ultimately transported. Researchers have only recently begun to demonstrate the transportability of empirically supported treatments. Fortunately, the early results are encouraging. Wade, Treat, and Stuart (1998), using a benchmarking strategy to compare results from a large community mental health center (CMHC) with those of clinical trial results, found that panic-free status and the percentage of patients achieving normative levels of functioning were comparable across the two settings. These researchers examined 110 patients with PDA or panic disorder without agoraphobia—and patients were *not* excluded on the bases of age, medication use or medication instability, severity of panic, or the presence or absence of agoraphobia. Patients who completed a 15-session CBT protocol in the CMHC were compared with patients from two controlled clinical trials. This transportability study involved extensively trained therapists (both psychologists and master's-level clinicians) and included patients who used concomitant pharmacotherapy when appropriate. Over half (56%) of the CMHC sample reported using anxiolytic medication, compared with somewhat lower percentages in the controlled clinical trial samples (40%, Barlow et al., 1989; 47%, Telch et al., 1993). Moreover, and importantly, the CMHC sample reported having significantly fewer years of education than the clinical trial samples, and a large percentage of the CMHC sample was described as suffering moderate to severe agoraphobia (47%). Findings for the CMHC treatment completers indicated that 87% were panic-free at the end of treatment, and that these patients also exhibited less anticipatory anxiety, less agoraphobic avoidance, less general anxiety, and fewer symptoms of depression. At a 1-year follow-up, these results were maintained with 89% of the CMHC treatment completers free of panic and with a substantial proportion having discontinued any prior benzodiazepine use (Stuart, Treat, & Wade, 2000). The findings from this transportability study are promising indeed and await replication.

Despite these optimistic findings, naturalistic studies examining the likelihood of patients' actually receiving empirically supported treatments outside research settings have had disappointing results (Barlow, Levitt, & Bufka, 1999), For example, Goisman et al. (1993) and Goisman, Warshaw, and Keller (1999) studied patients, many with PDA, presenting to leading clinical centers in New England as part of the Harvard–Brown study. Specifically, 362 patients were interviewed in 1991, and then again in 1995–1996. Only 22% of patients were receiving an empirically supported treatment, and this percentage had not increased over the follow-up period.

Briefer Cost-Effective Treatments for Panic and Associated Anxiety

With their efficacy established, investigations have begun to examine briefer and more cost-effective alternatives to CBT for panic disorder and PDA. Efforts to examine the efficacy of intensive, briefer, or self-directed formats have shown promise. Côté et al. (1994) conducted a study in which patients were randomly assigned to receive CBT with either a standard amount of therapist contact (weekly hour-long sessions) or reduced therapist contact (bimonthly hour-long sessions with bimonthly 10-minute telephone contacts). Results of this study demonstrated that both treatment modalities were equally effective; over 73% of the patients in both groups were both panic-free and clinically improved at the 6-month follow-up assessment. It should be noted that therapist time in the reduced therapist contact condition was still considerable, amounting to approximately 10 hours of contact, as compared with approximately 20 hours of contact in the standard condition.

Several others have examined the efficacy of briefer alternatives. First, Lidren et al. (1994) examined the effectiveness of self-directed treatment utilizing a manual (bibliotherapy) for panic attacks. They found bibliotherapy to be as effective as CBT administered in a group therapy setting. Patients in both conditions were treated for 8 weeks and were compared with patients in a wait-list control condition. The patients in both of the active treatment conditions showed evidence of significant clinical improvement at posttreatment assessments, while the patients in the wait-list control did not. Moreover, patients in the bibliotherapy and group therapy conditions maintained their treatment gains at the 3- and 6-month follow-up assessments. In addition, an attrition rate of 0 was reported for this study, pointing to the desirability of these interventions for patients suffering from panic attacks. In another study, Craske, Maidenberg, and Bystritsky (1995) examined the effectiveness of a brief form of CBT: A four-session PCT protocol was compared to a four-session nondirective supportive therapy protocol. The brief PCT was found to be significantly more effective than the nondirective supportive therapy; the patients' clinical statuses were assessed by noting the frequency of their panic attacks, their degree of worry about panic attacks, and their level of phobic fear. Finally, Clark et al. (1999) randomly assigned 43 patients with panic disorder to either standard cognitive therapy (consisting of up to 12 sessions lasting 1 hour each in the first 3 months) or brief cognitive therapy (where patients attended 5 sessions in addition to using between-session self-study modules). Both treatments produced significantly better results than a wait-list control group.

New Developments: Integrating Treatment for Panic and Avoidance in an Intensive Treatment Format

A promising treatment approach we have been developing and investigating is an intensive treatment program for PDA that combines treatments for panic and avoidance, called "sensation-focused intensive treatment" (SFIT). For a full description of this program and protocol, see Heinrichs, Spiegel, and Hofmann (in press). Inspired by the work of Feigenbaum (1988), this program differs from PCT in several ways. First, the program was designed for patients with PDA whose agoraphobia is moderate to severe. Second, it is conducted intensively in a CBT self-study format (with therapist review) over 8 consecutive days. Third, rather than a hierarchically based exposure plan, treatment involves interoceptive and situational exposures conducted in ungraded massed fashion. That is, patients are exposed to their most feared agoraphobic situations while simultaneously inducing feared somatic sensations. This aspect of the SFIT approach is unique, in that it emphasizes the deliberate provocation and maximal intensification of anxious symptoms without teaching any arousal reduction procedures. Although therapists often accompany patients during the initial exposure trials to insure that the patients conduct the exposure effectively, the therapists are then rapidly removed from the exposure practices. Despite these differences, the program has a number of similarities to our PCT protocol, including education, cognitive restructuring, symptom inductions, and interoceptive and situational exposure practices.

Initial findings for this program appear promising, and long-term outcome evaluations are ongoing. To date (winter 2001), 23 patients with PDA whose agoraphobia is moderate to severe have completed the SFIT protocol, and follow-up data are available on 15 patients (see Spiegel & Barlow, 2000a, 2000b). Following treatment, patients were significantly improved on nearly all self-reported and clinician-rated measures, and the gains have been maintained at follow-up (mean follow-up = 5 months). At posttreatment, the majority (87%) were much or very much improved at posttreatment. Notably, 2 patients evidenced worsening symptoms at follow-up (compared with posttreatment). Of course these results are preliminary, but they are promising enough to warrant replication and comparison with "gold standard" PCT and/or pharmacotherapy.

CHAPTER 11

Specific Phobias

MARTIN M. ANTONY
DAVID H. BARLOW

The diagnosis of specific phobia presents an interesting paradox. In some respects, specific phobia is one of the most significant psychological disorders. It occurs frequently in the general population, with lifetime prevalence estimates of about 11%, based on the largest epidemiological surveys conducted in the United States (Eaton, Dryman, & Weissman, 1991; Kessler et al., 1994). Subclinical fears are even more common (Birchall, 1996). More than half of various population samples report fears of animals, heights, needles, flying, or other specific objects and situations, although these fears often do not meet full criteria for a diagnosis of specific phobia (Agras, Sylvester, & Oliveau, 1969; Curtis, Magee, Eaton, Wittchen, & Kessler, 1998).

In addition, specific phobia is one of the best-understood psychological disorders. Much of what we know about the nature of fear and methods of fear reduction is based on studies of individuals suffering from specific fears and phobias (Antony & Swinson, 2000). Specific phobias are also the most treatable of the anxiety disorders. For certain phobias, up to 90% of individuals achieve clinically significant, long-lasting improvement in as little as one session of behavioral treatment (e.g., Gitin, Herbert, & Schmidt, 1996; Öst, 1989; Öst, Brandberg, & Alm, 1997; Öst, Salkovskis, & Hellström, 1991).

Here is the paradox: Despite the fact that specific phobia is a common, treatable, and well-understood condition, people with specific phobias rarely present for treatment. For example, a recent sample of 522 patients with anxiety disorders referred to a Canadian anxiety disorders center (Antony, 2000), only 6% received a principal diagnosis of specific phobia following a semistructured diagnostic interview. In contrast, other anxiety disorders—such as panic disorder, obsessive–compulsive disorder (OCD), and social phobia (social anxiety disorder)—occurred frequently in this sample. Interestingly, specific phobia frequently occurred as an additional diagnosis (in 23% of patients), although it was rarely the focus of treatment. These findings are consistent with previous findings from our center in Albany, New York, in which only about 5% of patients with anxiety disorders received a principal diagnosis of specific phobia, even though specific phobias occurred frequently as a less severe, additional diagnosis (Antony, Moras, et al., 1994).

Data from epidemiological samples have confirmed that people with specific phobias rarely seek treatment. Among participants in the National Comorbidity Survey (NCS), only

12.5% of those with specific phobia had used specialty services for mental health or addictions in the previous year (Kessler, Zhao, et al., 1999). This percentage was lower than for any other mood or anxiety disorder, except social phobia (11.3%).

It is difficult to know for sure why people tend not to seek treatment for their specific phobias. More than likely, it is because this condition is typically less impairing than are other psychological problems. Because of the circumscribed nature of the disorder, people can often avoid the feared object or situation quite easily. Still, specific phobias should not be thought of as trivial. We have seen numerous individuals who were quite impaired by specific phobias. Some examples include the following:

- A patient who put off surgery to remove a pituitary tumor because of a fear of having necessary blood work before the surgery.
- An individual with a spider phobia who opened her car door and left the car after seeing a spider on her dashboard—while the car was moving.
- A patient with a spider phobia who moved out of her home for several weeks after seeing several spiders over a period of a few days.
- A construction worker who avoided taking certain jobs because of his fear of heights.
- A student who almost dropped out of medical school because of her fear of blood and surgery.
- An individual who would not leave her home on cloudy or rainy days because of an intense storm phobia.
- An individual whose driving phobia prevented her from commuting to work when her company changed locations.
- An executive with a flying phobia who turned down a promotion because his new job required air travel.

DIAGNOSTIC CONSIDERATIONS

In the *Diagnostic and Statistical Manual of Mental Disorders*, fourth edition (DSM-IV), specific phobia is described as a "marked and persistent fear that is excessive or unreasonable, cued by the presence or anticipation of a specific object or situation" (American Psychiatric Association, 1994, p. 410). In addition, the individual must (1) experience the fear nearly every time he or she encounters the phobic stimulus (this may take the form of a panic attack or of crying, tantrums, or freezing in children); (2) recognize that the fear is unreasonable or excessive (in children, this criterion is not needed for the diagnosis); (3) avoid the situation or endure exposure to it with extreme distress; (4) experience significant impairment in functioning or clinically significant distress about having the phobia; (5) have had the problem for at least 6 months (only a requirement for individuals who are under 18 years of age); and (6) not have another DSM-IV disorder that better accounts for the specific phobia symptoms.

These criteria are similar to those that were published in DSM-III-R (American Psychiatric Association, 1987), with several important changes. First, in DSM-III-R this condition was known as "simple phobia."[1] It was renamed in DSM-IV to more accurately reflect the scope of the disorder, which encompasses fears of *specific* objects and situations. In addition, DSM-IV added the requirement that specific phobias be classified into

---

[1]To be consistent with current nomenclature, we use the term "specific phobia" throughout this chapter, even when referring to studies based on earlier versions of DSM, when "simple phobia" was the correct term.

one of five types, each of which is described in the next section. Finally, the criteria used to help the clinician distinguish between specific phobias and other related conditions were widened. Whereas DSM-III-R specified that the fear must not be secondary to symptoms of panic disorder, social phobia, OCD, or posttraumatic stress disorder, DSM-IV took a broader approach, specifying that the fear must not be better accounted for by another mental disorder.

In determining whether a particular fear is better thought of as a specific phobia than as another problem, the clinician must consider the situational content of the fear as well as other features, such as the presence of compulsions or apprehension about experiencing uncued panic attacks. For example, a person with panic disorder who avoids flying only for fear of having an unexpected panic attack on an airplane would not receive a diagnosis of specific phobia. However, an individual with panic disorder who avoids flying because of a fear of crashing in the plane might be diagnosed with both specific phobia and panic disorder, in light of the fact that the fear of flying appears to be unrelated to the person's panic disorder (Craske, 1991; McNally & Louro, 1992).

Recent studies have called into question the usefulness of the criterion specifying that the individual must have insight into the excessiveness and unreasonableness of his or her fear. Originally, this criterion was included to help the clinician distinguish between phobias and delusional fears, in which there is no insight. However, it appears that there are a significant number of people who otherwise meet diagnostic criteria for specific phobia, but who have relatively little insight into the excessiveness of their own fear and distress, even though their beliefs are not delusional in intensity (Jones & Menzies, 2000; Jones, Whitmont, & Menzies, 1996; Menzies & Clarke, 1995a; Menzies, Harris, & Jones, 1998). These findings suggest that some individuals for whom a specific phobia diagnosis is appropriate could be excluded from receiving such a diagnosis because they usually believe that their fears are appropriate.

Specific Phobia Types

Over the years, hundreds of different fears and phobias have been described, most of which are identified by Greek and Latin names. Table 11.1 provides a list of 25 phobias beginning with the letter "A," which was part of a larger compilation taken from a number of different sources, including three medical dictionaries (Maser, 1985). A more recent list posted on the Internet by Fredd Culbertson included more than 500 phobia names and their definitions (about 70 names beginning with the letter "A" alone), all apparently found in various published sources (www.phobialist.com).

The fact that so many phobias have been identified has been a source of fascination to some writers, the mass media, and the public at large. However, lists such as these have had little practical utility for researchers and clinicians who have an interest in phobias. For the most part, the number of different phobias typically seen in clinical settings is relatively small. In fact, DSM-IV defines four main types of phobias (animal type, natural environment type, blood–injection–injury [BII] type, and situational type), as well as a residual "other type." Examples of each of these types are provided in Table 11.2.

The decision to include these specific phobia types in DSM-IV was based on a series of studies and reports suggesting that these types differ in important ways (Craske & Sipsas, 1992; Curtis, Hill, & Lewis, 1990; Curtis, Himle, Lewis, & Lee, 1989; Himle, McPhee, Cameron, & Curtis, 1989; Hugdahl & Öst, 1985). These papers highlighted evidence that specific phobia types could be distinguished on the basis of onset age, sex ratio, patterns of comorbidity among specific phobia types and with other anxiety disorders, focus of

TABLE 11.1. Phobias Beginning with "A"

Term	Fear of:
Acarophobia	Insects, mites
Achluophobia	Darkness, night
Acousticophobia	Sounds
Acrophobia	Heights
Aerophobia	Air currents, drafts, wind
Agoraphobia	Open spaces
Agyiophobia	Crossing the street
Aichmophobia	Sharp, pointed objects; knives; being touched by a finger
Ailurophobia	Cats
Algophobia	Pain
Amathophobia	Dust
Amychophobia	Laceration; being clawed, scratched
Androphobia	Men (and sex with men)
Anemophobia	Air currents, wind, drafts
Anginophobia	Angina pectoris
Anthropophobia	Human society
Antlophobia	Floods
Apeirophobia	Infinity
Aphenphobia	Physical contact, being touched
Apiphobia	Bees, bee stings
Astraphobia	Thunderstorms, lightning
Ataxiophobia	Disorder
Atephobia	Ruin
Auroraphobia	Northern lights
Autophobia	Being alone; solitude; oneself; being egotistical

Note. The definition provided for "agoraphobia" is considerably different from the definition in DSM-IV. From Maser (1985). Copyright 1985 by Lawrence Erlbaum Associates. Reprinted by permission.

apprehension (e.g., fear of internal physical sensations versus external aspects of the object or situation), and physiological response (e.g., panic attacks, fainting).

An impetus for separating situational specific phobias from the other types was a series of reports by George Curtis and colleagues (Curtis et al., 1989, 1990) suggesting that, unlike other specific phobias, situational specific phobias may constitute a variant of agoraphobia. This suggestion is not surprising, given that the situations feared by people with agoraphobia (e.g., enclosed places, driving, flying) overlap considerably with those feared in the situational specific phobias. There is also evidence that situational specific phobias are sometimes difficult to distinguish from agoraphobia (Horwath, Lish, Johnson, Hornig, & Weissman, 1993). Finally, as reviewed later in this chapter, situational specific phobias may share other features with panic disorder and agoraphobia, including stronger fear of panic-related sensations and a greater response to panic induction challenges.

BII phobias were included in DSM-IV as a separate type primarily because of the unique physiological response to the phobic stimulus. As reviewed later in this chapter, BII phobias are the only phobias associated with a tendency to faint in the phobic situation. The decision to include separate types for animal phobias and natural environment phobias was also based on evidence that these phobias differ from other types. First, there is evidence that phobias within these types tend to co-occur. For example, people with one animal phobia are more likely to have another animal phobia than a phobia of a different type. These types also differ from other phobia types on certain demographic features, such as onset age. Findings regarding these features are reviewed later in this chapter.

TABLE 11.2. Specific Phobia Types in DSM-IV

Phobia type	Examples
Animal type	Spiders, *insects*, worms, snakes, dogs, cats, rodents, frogs, birds, fish
Natural environment type	*Heights*, *being near water*, *storms*, wind, sunshine, darkness
Blood–injection–injury (BII) type	*Seeing blood*, *receiving an injection or other invasive medical procedure*, watching surgery, talking about surgical procedures, having a blood test
Situational type	*Public transportation*, *tunnels*, *bridges*, *elevators*, *flying*, *driving*, *enclosed places*
Other type	*Situations that might lead to choking*, *vomiting*, *or illness*, *space phobia*, *loud sounds*, *costumed characters*, clowns, certain flowers or plants

Note. Items printed in italics are listed as examples in DSM-IV. Other examples are based on our own patients who were diagnosed with specific phobias.

Despite some evidence supporting the DSM-IV specific phobia types, we have argued elsewhere (Antony, Brown, & Barlow, 1997a) that assigning specific phobias to types may not be particularly useful diagnostically. First, as we review shortly, there are methodological problems and inconsistencies in the research supporting these types. In addition, practical problems arise in assigning phobias to types. For example, some phobias are not easily classified according to the DSM-IV types. Is a fear of bridges a natural environment phobia (i.e., heights) or a situational phobia (as specified in DSM-IV)? Is a phobia of dentists an example of a BII phobia or a phobia of the "other" type? Does a phobia of the dark belong in the natural environment type or the situational type (in Table 11.2 we have listed it with the natural environment phobias, but one could argue that it belongs with the situational fears)?

A final argument against classifying specific phobias by type is that the types are less informative than simply naming the phobias. Clinically, it would be much more meaningful to give a diagnosis of "specific phobia, heights" or "specific phobia, storms" than a diagnosis of "specific phobia, natural environment type." Naming a phobia communicates more about a patient's condition and is more likely to lead to effective treatment planning.

COMORBIDITY

Comorbidity with Other Psychological Disorders

In a recent study based on data from the NCS (Kessler et al., 1994), Curtis et al. (1998) examined the prevalence and co-occurrence of various specific phobias (i.e., heights, flying, closed places, being alone, storms, animals, blood, water) in the general population. The norm was for specific phobias to co-occur with other specific phobias. In fact, of the 915 individuals with a lifetime history of specific phobias, only 24.4% had a single phobia. The remaining cases had two (26.4%), three (23.5%), four (10.4%), or more than four (17.3%) phobias. These results are consistent with a finding that individuals with specific phobias often endorse multiple fears when completing a fear survey (Hofmann, Lehman, & Barlow, 1997).

In contrast, Fredrikson, Annas, Fischer, and Wik (1996) found multiple phobias to be relatively rare. In their study of 704 participants from Stockholm, Sweden, only 18.1% of individuals with a specific phobia had multiple phobias, even though the point prevalence estimate for specific phobias was relatively high (19.9%) in this study overall.

Note that the numbers of individuals with multiple phobias in the Curtis et al. (1998) and Fredrikson et al. (1996) studies may be inflated, because the interviews and questionnaires used in these studies did not discriminate between multiple *phobias* and fears of multiple *situations* that are due to a single phobia. For example, an individual with claustrophobia who avoids flying exclusively due to claustrophobic fears (e.g., the lack of space and fresh air on the plane) would be diagnosed (according to DSM-IV) with a specific phobia of enclosed places, but not of flying. However, based on the assessment methods used in these studies, such an individual would probably have been diagnosed with specific phobias of both enclosed places and flying.

In addition to finding that multiple specific phobias often co-occur, Curtis et al. (1998) found that the greater the number of specific phobias an individual had, the more likely the person was also to receive other anxiety disorder diagnoses, such as panic disorder, agoraphobia, generalized anxiety disorder, and social phobia. This is noteworthy in light of previous research showing that specific phobias often co-occur with other anxiety disorders (e.g., Sanderson, Di Nardo, Rapee, & Barlow, 1990). However, as reviewed below, the relationship between specific phobias and other anxiety disorders is not symmetrical. When specific phobias co-occur with another anxiety disorder, the phobia is usually of a lesser severity than the comorbid condition.

When a specific phobia is the principal diagnosis (i.e., the diagnosis causing the greatest amount of distress and impairment), it is typically not associated with many other conditions. For example, in a sample of 17 people with specific phobias, Sanderson et al. (1990) found that 47% of individuals did not have any other diagnoses and 53% had only one additional diagnosis (usually social phobia). In comparison, the percentage of individuals with other principal diagnoses who had at least one comorbid condition was 69% for panic disorder with agoraphobia, 58% for social phobia, 91% for generalized anxiety disorder, and 83% for OCD. Furthermore, although no individuals in the specific phobia group had more than one comorbid diagnosis, individuals in the other groups frequently had a greater number of additional diagnoses.

In the large study reported in Chapter 9 (Brown, Campbell, Lehman, Grisham, & Mancill, 2001), 34% of 110 carefully diagnosed patients presenting with a principal diagnosis of specific phobia met criteria for an additional Axis I disorder (see Table 9.5). More specifically, 33% met criteria for either an anxiety or mood disorder, 27% for an anxiety disorder alone, and 10% for a mood disorder alone (major depressive disorder or dysthymia). Interestingly, 15% of patients with a principal diagnosis of one specific phobia also met criteria for another type of specific phobia.

Whereas specific phobias are rarely the *principal* diagnosis when they occur with other anxiety disorders, they often occur as an *additional* diagnosis in the context of other disorders. In fact, Sanderson et al. (1990) found that specific phobias were more likely to be diagnosed as an additional diagnosis (when the principal diagnosis was another anxiety disorder) than were any other anxiety or mood disorders. Thirty-two percent of patients with an anxiety disorder met criteria for an additional diagnosis of specific phobia. Subsequent studies have confirmed that specific phobia occurs frequently as an additional diagnosis (e.g., Curtis et al., 1998; Goisman, Goldenberg, Vasile, & Keller, 1995; Moras, Di Nardo, Brown, & Barlow, 1995).

Despite the high comorbidity rates for specific phobias and other anxiety disorders, it appears that specific phobias may be less frequently diagnosed in the context of certain other psychological disorders. Schwalberg, Barlow, Alger, and Howard (1992) found a lifetime prevalence of 10% for specific phobias in a group of individuals with bulimia nervosa. This rate is close to the lifetime prevalence of specific phobias in the general population (Kessler et al., 1994). Similarly, in a sample of depressed patients, the prevalence of specific phobias was comparatively low, at only 5% (Schatzberg, Samson, Rothschild, Bond, & Regier, 1998). Finally, Lehman, Patterson, Brown, and Barlow (1998) found that specific phobia was less likely to be associated with a lifetime history of alcohol use disorders than any other anxiety or mood disorder except OCD. The relative lack of comorbidity between specific phobias and alcohol use disorders is interesting, in light of previous research showing that alcohol intoxication does not reduce fear and avoidance (more than placebo) during exposure to feared animals (Thyer & Curtis, 1984).

Covariation among Specific Phobias

A large number of studies have examined the ways in which specific phobias and fears group together, using statistical procedures such as factor analysis and cluster analysis. Studies based on statistical covariation among phobias were used to support the initial proposal to include the DSM-IV specific phobia types (Curtis et al., 1989, 1990). However, although some studies have provided evidence that certain specific fears covary according to the DSM-IV types, others have found different factors and clusters (especially in the case of natural environment phobias). For example, in a reanalysis of the data from the Epidemiologic Catchment Area (ECA) study (Eaton et al., 1991), Curtis et al. (1990) found that fears of harmless animals, storms, and being in water were best grouped together in the same clusters. Also, based on a factor analysis of data from the NCS, Curtis et al. (1998) were unable to identify any interpretable factors, lending little support for the DSM-IV specific phobia types.

Even the older studies on which the DSM-IV specific phobia types were in part based have not completely supported these types. For example, a number of studies have found that natural environment phobias (especially heights) most often load on the same factors as situational phobias (Arrindell, 1980; Fredrikson et al., 1996; Landy & Gaupp, 1971; Liddell, Locker, & Burman, 1991; Muris, Schmidt, & Merckelbach, 1999; Wilson & Priest, 1968). Also, findings regarding situational phobias have been somewhat inconsistent across studies. Whereas some studies (e.g., Arrindell, 1980) have found a single factor representing situational fears (plus heights), other studies (e.g., Landy & Gaupp, 1971) have found several situational factors containing mixtures of fears from different DSM-IV types.

To summarize across other studies of statistical covariation, animal phobias often group together, although some studies have found more than one animal factor (Wilson & Priest, 1968). Similarly, fears of blood, injections, and injury-related stimuli typically go together, confirming findings from clinical samples of patients with BII phobias (e.g., Öst, 1992).

Factor-analytic studies should be interpreted cautiously, because they are typically based on nonclinical samples. Therefore, any observed covariation among fears may not be relevant to the covariation of fears in people with specific phobias. It is possible that fears covary differently in the general population than they do among people with specific phobias. For example, covariation among situational fears in the general population may have as much to do with the ways in which these fears covary in people with agoraphobia as the ways in which they covary in people with specific phobias.

DEMOGRAPHIC FEATURES AND EPIDEMIOLOGY

This section summarizes the research literature on the prevalence of specific phobias as well as research on demographic features such as sex, age, and culture. Data on the prevalence of specific phobia in the context of anxiety and related disorders in general are presented in Chapter 1. As you read this section, you should note certain methodological limitations that exist in many of the studies reviewed. For example, findings from large epidemiological studies have often failed to adequately discriminate between specific phobias and other psychological problems, such as agoraphobia. The ECA study defined specific phobias as including fears of animals, heights, bugs, closed places, and water. Agoraphobia was defined as including fears of tunnels, bridges, crowds, public transportation (including flying), going out of the house alone, and being alone (Eaton et al., 1991). In other words, an individual with a specific phobia of flying according to DSM-IV would have received a diagnosis of agoraphobia in the ECA study. Similarly, an individual with panic disorder with agoraphobia (according to DSM-IV) who was fearful of enclosed places as part of his or her agoraphobia would have received a diagnosis of specific phobia in the ECA study.

In addition, several of the studies reviewed in this section are based on findings from comprehensive fear surveys in which participants rated their fear of particular objects and situations. These surveys are commonly used in psychological research, although their validity has been questioned (e.g., Klieger & Franklin, 1993). Also, in addition to including items that are related to common specific phobias (e.g., injections, airplanes), fear survey schedules also tend to include a large number of questions about other types of phobic fears (e.g., public speaking, crowds) and about situations that are not typically associated with fear in people with phobic disorders (e.g., noise of vacuum cleaners, sirens, ugly people, nude men and women, parting from friends).

Finally, most of the older studies reviewed in this section (and throughout this chapter) have not adequately insured that participants met full diagnostic criteria for specific phobia. Therefore, samples from many of these studies may have included individuals with other phobic disorders (especially agoraphobia).

Prevalence

Both the ECA study (Eaton et al., 1991) and the NCS (Kessler et al., 1994) reported lifetime prevalence rates of about 11% for specific phobias. The 30-day prevalence estimate for specific phobias was 5.5% in the NCS (Magee, Eaton, Wittchen, McGonagle, & Kessler, 1996). In both of these studies, diagnoses were determined by structured interviews conducted by trained lay interviewers. Table 11.3 lists lifetime prevalence rates for particular specific fears and phobias, based on findings from the NCS (Curtis et al., 1998). Phobias of animals and heights were the most frequently diagnosed specific phobias, confirming previous findings from the ECA study (Bourdon et al., 1988).

Although the NCS and the ECA study are the two largest epidemiological surveys published (with more than 18,000 and over 8,000 participants, respectively), numerous smaller prevalence studies have been conducted throughout the world. Fredrikson et al. (1996) found that 19.9% of their sample of 704 individuals from Stockholm, Sweden currently met criteria for specific phobias, based on responses to a self-report questionnaire. However, most other international studies have found prevalence rates lower than those in the ECA study and the NCS. In a sample of 3,021 individuals in Munich (ages 14 to 24), Wittchen, Nelson, and Lachner (1998) found lifetime and 12-month specific phobia prevalence estimates of 2.3% and 1.8%, respectively. Prevalence estimates were consider-

TABLE 11.3. Lifetime Prevalence of Specific Fears with and without Specific Phobia

Specific fear	Lifetime fears[a]		Lifetime phobia given fear[b]		Lifetime phobia with specific fear in total sample[c]	
	%	SE	%	SE	%	SE
Height	20.4	0.7	26.2	1.8	5.3	0.5
Flying	13.2	0.7	26.9	2.4	3.5	0.3
Closed spaces	11.9	0.6	35.1	2.5	4.2	0.4
Being alone	7.3	0.6	40.7	3.3	3.1	0.4
Storms	8.7	0.5	33.1	3.4	2.9	0.4
Animals	22.2	1.1	25.8	1.2	5.7	0.4
Blood	13.9	0.7	32.8	2.1	4.5	0.3
Water	9.4	0.6	35.8	2.8	3.4	0.3
Any	49.5	1.2	22.7	1.1	11.3	0.6

Note. From Curtis, Magee, Eaton, Wittchen, and Kessler (1998). Copyright 1998 by Royal College of Psychiatrists. Reprinted by permission.
[a]Prevalence of lifetime fears in the total sample.
[b]Probability of specific phobia diagnosis in people endorsing each fear.
[c]Percentage of people in total sample with specific phobia and each lifetime fear (i.e., 5.3% of total sample had lifetime specific phobia and a height fear).

ably higher (16.0% and 10.7%, respectively) when subthreshold fears were included. Lifetime and point prevalence rates were only 0.63% and 0.45% in an Italian study of 1,110 individuals (Faravelli, Degl'Innocenti, & Giardinelli, 1989).[2] In Iceland, the lifetime prevalence of specific phobias was found to be 8.8% in a sample of 1,087 participants (Líndal & Stefánsson, 1993). Finally, in a Canadian study of 3,258 individuals living in Edmonton, the lifetime prevalence of specific phobia was 7.2% (Bland, Orn, & Newman, 1988).

When the findings across studies are examined, it seems clear that specific phobias are prevalent in the general population. The precise number of sufferers is difficult to estimate, because prevalence studies have tended to vary with respect to assessment methods, sampling methods, populations studied, and diagnostic nomenclature (e.g., DSM-III vs. DSM-III-R or DSM-IV).

Age of Onset

In a group of 152 outpatients with various specific phobias, Thyer, Parrish, Curtis, Nesse, and Cameron (1985) found a mean onset age of 16.1 years. This age is close to the median onset age of 15 years found for specific phobias in the NCS (Magee et al., 1996).

Table 11.4 summarizes the findings from studies that reported age of onset for particular specific phobias, based on individuals from clinical samples. Summarizing from these studies, animal and BII phobias tend to begin in childhood, whereas situational phobias

---

[2]Note that this study used a hierarchical diagnostic decision tree (similar to that from DSM-III), such that participants could receive no more than one diagnosis. Specific phobias were low on this hierarchy and therefore less likely to be diagnosed than other disorders. This procedure would be expected to yield much lower prevalence estimates for specific phobias, compared to studies that allowed for comorbidity.

TABLE 11.4. Mean Age of Onset for Specific Phobias and Agoraphobia in Individuals Presenting for Treatment

Study	Phobia type	n	Age of onset[a]	
Antony et al. (1997a)	Panic disorder with agoraphobia	15	29.07 (P)	28.14 (F)
	Heights	15	34.13 (P)	20.47 (F)
	Animal	15	20.00 (P)	10.80 (F)
	Blood–injection–injury	15	14.50 (P)	7.93 (F)
	Driving	15	32.20 (P)	25.67 (F)
Öst (1987a)	Agoraphobia	100	27.74	
	Animal	50	6.86	
	Blood	40	8.83	
	Dental	60	11.73	
	Claustrophobia	40	20.18	
Marks & Gelder (1966)	Agoraphobia	84	23.9	
	Animal	18	4.4	
	Situational (i.e., any situation, including heights, dark, storms)	12	22.7	
Himle et al. (1989)	Animal	25	14.9	
	Blood	9	12.4	
	Choking/vomiting	8	20.6	
	Situational (i.e., agoraphobia-like situations, including driving, crowds, etc.)	46	27.3	
Craske, Burton, et al. (1989)	Animal	18	17.1	
	Heights	12	15.3	
	Flying	21	22.3	
	Driving	14	29.1	
	Claustrophobia	11	26.5	
	Blood–injection–injury	18	17.1	

[a]P, the age at which full criteria for specific phobia were met; F, = age at which fear first began.

and phobias of heights tend to begin later, in adolescence or adulthood, closer to the onset age for agoraphobia (onset ages for agoraphobia are included in Table 11.4 where available). Studies based on epidemiological samples (e.g., Curtis et al., 1990) have yielded similar results, although the differences across specific phobia types have been less pronounced than those from clinical samples.

The findings reported in Table 11.4 should be interpreted cautiously for a number of reasons. First, these studies are inconsistent with respect to how they dealt with individuals who reported having had a fear for as long as they could remember. The Craske, Burton, Rapee, Rygh, and Barlow (1989) study excluded anyone who reported that their phobia had been present for as long as they could recall, which probably inflated their reported onset ages. In contrast, for the 35% of cases where the individual reported having the fear for as long as he or she could remember, the Antony et al. (1997a) study had each participant estimate the earliest age at which he or she recalled having the fear. Finally, the other studies did not report how this issue was dealt with.

In addition, only the Antony et al. (1997a) study distinguished between the onset of the *fear* versus the onset of the *phobia* (with all the associated features, including clinically significant distress and functional impairment). Therefore, it is unclear in most studies whether the age of onset reported is for the fear or the phobia. This issue is not trivial; we

(Antony et al., 1997a) found that on average, there was a period of 9 years between the time when the fear began and the time when the fear began to cause enough distress and impairment to meet criteria for specific phobia. Onset ages for both fears and phobias in this study are reported in Table 11.4

Sex Differences

Specific fears and phobias have consistently been found to affect females more often than males in epidemiological samples (e.g., Bourdon et al., 1988; Curtis et al., 1998), clinical samples (Goisman et al., 1998; Himle et al., 1989; Thyer, Parrish, et al., 1985), and student samples (Cornelius & Averill, 1983). As shown in Table 11.5, the differences in prevalence across sexes are particularly strong for fears of animals, lightning, enclosed places, and darkness (Fredrikson et al., 1996; see also Chapter 1, Table 1.5). The prevalence for phobias of heights, flying, injections, dentists, and injury did not differ significantly between the sexes.

The underlying reason for differences in phobia prevalence across the sexes has been a subject of much speculation. Hartung and Widiger (1998) have emphasized the effects of sampling biases and biases within the DSM-IV criteria themselves on some of the sex differences observed in the research literature. We have previously discussed additional reasons why women may be more likely than men to report having certain specific phobias (Antony & Barlow, 1997), including a tendency for men to underreport their fears, sex differences in treatment-seeking patterns, and sex differences in the learning of fear through modeling.

There is evidence that, relative to women, men underreport their fears. Pierce and Kirkpatrick (1992) asked female and male college students to complete a fear survey on two occasions—first in a classroom setting, and next in a laboratory setting immediately before watching videotapes depicting various potentially fear-provoking scenes. Before

TABLE 11.5. Point Prevalence of Particular Specific Phobias in Women and Men, Based on a Questionnaire Survey of 1,000 Individuals

Phobia type	Prevalence (%)			χ^2
	Men	Women	Total	
Snakes	2.4	8.3	5.5	11.6**
Spiders	1.2	5.6	3.5	10.0**
Lightning	0.3	3.7	2.1	10.0**
Closed spaces	2.4	5.4	4.0	4.0*
Darkness	0.0	4.3	2.3	14.6***
Heights	6.3	8.6	7.5	1.3
Flying	1.8	3.2	2.6	1.4
Injections	1.2	1.9	1.6	<1
Dentists	2.1	2.1	2.1	<1
Injuries	2.4	4.0	3.3	1.4

Note. Adapted from Fredrikson, Annas, Fischer, and Wik (1996), copyright 1996, with kind permission from Elsevier Science Ltd, The Boulevard, Langford Lane, Kidlington, OX5 1GB, UK.
*$p < .05$. **$p < .01$. ***$p < .001$.

completing the fear survey for the second time, participants were told that their physiological responses to the videotape (e.g., heart rate) would be monitored to assess their truthfulness on the fear survey. Knowing that their truthfulness was being independently assessed, males' ratings were significantly higher on the second administration of the fear survey, whereas females' ratings did not change. These findings were interpreted as evidence that males underreport their fears to conform with traditional male gender roles. This explanation is consistent with findings by Arrindell, Kolk, Pickersgill, and Hageman (1993) indicating that high levels of self-reported masculinity were predictive of low levels of self-reported fear of a number of objects and situations (including animal fears). However, it should be noted that Arrindell et al. (1993) also found that biological sex was predictive of fear levels even after masculinity was controlled for.

Another explanation for sex differences in specific phobias is the possibility that women are more likely than men to seek treatment for their difficulties. This would account for the fact that sex differences are often larger in treatment samples than in epidemiological samples.

Sex differences in prevalence may also reflect actual differences between men and women in the susceptibility to develop phobias. Davey (1994b) proposed that sex differences in the prevalence of certain animal phobias may be related to a sex difference in disgust sensitivity, which, as reviewed later, has been shown to be elevated in people with phobias of spiders and certain other animals. Arrindell, Mulkens, Kok, and Vollenbroek (1999) failed to support this hypothesis after they controlled for other variables.

Finally, sex differences in the prevalence of specific phobias may be related to the possibility that woman and men are taught to deal differently with typical phobic stimuli. Traditionally, boys are often encouraged to take more risks (e.g., playing with spiders, hiking in high places) than girls are. In addition, women may have more role models for the development of fear than men do. It seems much more common in movies, television, and literature to see women avoiding phobic stimuli than it is to see men being frightened by these objects. Therefore, it is possible that in Western cultures, women *learn* to fear certain situations more strongly than do men. Of course, it is difficult to know the extent to which culture and the mass media are to blame for sex differences. It is possible that the media simply reflect differences that exist for other reasons (e.g., different predisposing factors).

Age Differences

A number of studies have examined differences in the prevalence of specific phobias across different adult age groups. In all cases, these have been cross-sectional studies; therefore, observed differences may have been due to cohort effects as well as to possible developmental changes in phobic symptomatology across the lifespan. In a Canadian epidemiological sample, Bland et al. (1988) found that the prevalence of specific phobias increased across ages and then decreased later in life. The prevalence rates peaked between ages 25 and 54, during which specific phobias affected between 7.9% and 8.8% of the sample. The prevalence of phobias was lower in younger and older participants, affecting 6.5% of those in the 18-to-24 age range and between 5.0% and 5.2% of those over age 55.

Fredrikson et al. (1996) examined differences in the prevalence of particular specific phobias in a group of younger adults (mean age = 29 years) and a group of older adults (mean age = 53.3 years). Phobias of darkness, enclosed places, flying, darkness, injections, injuries, and dentists were about equally prevalent in the two groups. However, phobias of storms and heights were more prevalent among older adults. This study also examined age differences in the intensity of fear, based on ratings on a visual analogue scale. Generally, younger adults rated their fears higher than older adults did for spiders and injections, and lower than older adults did for lightning, heights, and flying. Groups did not differ with respect to fear ratings for snakes, enclosed places, darkness, dentists, and injury.

Finally, Kirkpatrick (1984) examined changes in fear levels across six different age groups, ranging from 15–17 years to over 54 years. Patterns of fear across age groups differed between men and women.[3] For women, fears of deep water, looking down from high buildings, and strange dogs were greater in older groups than in younger groups. Fears of roller coasters, snakes, swimming, and high places on land tended to increase until about age 45, and then to decrease in older groups. For men, fears of deep water, spiders, and heights were the most commonly reported specific fears. Although they did not show a consistent pattern across different age groups, fears of these situations tended to be lower late in life than early in life.

In summary, it appears that the prevalence of specific phobias may vary across age groups. Furthermore, differences across ages appear to depend on the type of phobia as well as the sex of the individual.

Cultural and Geographic Differences

Several studies have examined the relationship between ethnicity and the prevalence of specific phobias. However, findings regarding cultural differences in specific phobias should be interpreted cautiously, in light of evidence that cultures differ with respect to social stigma regarding psychiatric illness (Fabrega, 1991), help seeking for psychological problems (Raguram & Bhide, 1985), and the ways in which anxiety and other emotions are defined and described (Mesquita & Frijda, 1992; Russell, 1991). Factors such as these may influence the responses that individuals give to standard psychiatric interviews.

Specific Phobias in African Americans

Neal, Lilly, and Zakis (1993) found that the content of fears among African American and white children (ages 6 to 12) was similar. However, despite the apparent similarity between these groups in the content of fears, there is evidence that the prevalence of specific phobias differs between African American and white adults. Based on data from the ECA study, Brown, Eaton, and Sussman (1990) found that phobic disorders (including specific phobias, agoraphobia, and social phobia) were more prevalent among African American than among white participants, even after demographic and socioeconomic factors were controlled for (see also Chapter 1, Table 1.5). In the NCS, Curtis et al. (1998) reported that being African American was a risk factor for having a greater number of specific phobias.

Specific Phobias in Hispanic Americans

Karno et al. (1989) examined the prevalence of phobias in different Hispanic and non-Hispanic groups in a sub-sample of individuals from the ECA study. The prevalence of specific phobias was 7.8% among Mexican Americans born in Mexico, 12.7% among

---

[3]Only items reflecting typical specific phobia situations for which at least 10% of individuals in a single age group reported terror were included. Therefore, the situations included for males and females are slightly different.

Mexican Americans born in the United States, and 6.8% among non-Hispanic whites born in the United States. Mexican Americans born in the United States were significantly more likely to have a specific phobia than non-Hispanic whites born in the United States. In a related study (Vega et al., 1998), recent Mexican immigrants were much less likely to have a specific phobia than Mexican Americans who had lived in the United States for many years or who were born in the United States. Finally, Curtis et al. (1998) found that in the NCS, being Hispanic was associated with an increased number of specific phobias diagnosed.

Specific Phobias in Different Countries

Ingman, Ollendick, and Akande (1999) examined differences in the prevalence of specific fears in children (ages 8 through 17) from two different African countries. Nigerian children reported higher fear ratings (on the Fear Survey Schedule for Children; Ollendick, 1983) than children from Kenya did. Furthermore, children from both countries had higher ratings than children from the United States, Australia, and China. Finally, Christian children living in Nigeria and Kenya reported higher levels of fear on certain factors than did Muslim children.

Chambers, Yeragani, and Keshavan (1986) studied the prevalence of specific phobias in adults living in India and the United Kingdom. Phobias of animals, darkness, and bad weather were more than twice as prevalent in India as in the United Kingdom. The pattern was reversed for certain other phobic disorders, including agoraphobia and social phobia, which were considerably more prevalent in the United Kingdom.

Finally, Davey et al. (1998) studied cultural differences in the factor structure of animal fears in people of Western and Asian cultures from seven different countries. Factor analyses indicated that animals fell into three main groups: fear-irrelevant (e.g., rabbits, cows), fear-relevant—fierce (e.g., lions, sharks), and disgust-relevant (e.g., spiders, mice). The core group of animals constituting the disgust-relevant category was similar across cultures.

Specific Phobias and Religion

Koenig, Ford, George, Blazer, and Meador (1993) examined the relationship between religion-related variables and the prevalence of specific phobias in a subset of ECA study participants. Variables such as frequency of church attendance, frequency of Bible study and prayer, and a tendency to tune in to religious television and radio programs were not related to the prevalence of specific phobias in any age groups. However, young adults who reported that religion was very important to them were more likely to be diagnosed with a specific phobia than those for whom religion was less important (a similar difference was found for individuals with OCD). This finding was not observed in middle-aged or older adults. This observation should be interpreted cautiously, because of the large number of comparisons that were examined in this study and the relatively small number of significant differences observed.

Urban–Rural Differences

In a study of 3,648 persons living near Piedmont, North Carolina, the prevalence of specific phobias was similar in urban and rural regions (George, Hughes, & Blazer, 1986). The similar rates of specific phobia in urban and rural locations were confirmed in a study of Mexican Americans living in California (Vega et al., 1998).

Summary and Conclusions

In summary, specific phobias appear to be more prevalent in African American and Hispanic American groups than in white Americans. In addition, there appears to be differences across countries in the prevalence of particular specific phobias. Finally, there is little evidence that the strength of an individual's religious convictions or whether he or she lives in a rural or urban location influences the likelihood of having a specific phobia.

DESCRIPTIVE PSYCHOPATHOLOGY

Physiological Response to the Phobic Situation

For most specific phobias, the typical response to encountering a phobic stimulus is a panic attack or a similar, panic-like reaction. In an unpublished study (Antony, 1994), individuals with four different phobia types reported the percentage of previous exposures during which they experienced a rush of fear accompanied by symptoms of arousal. The percentages were as follows: BII, 81.7%; heights, 88.0%; driving, 48.5%; and animals, 91.3%. Except for individuals with driving phobia, participants from each phobia type reported experiencing a panic-like reaction during almost all previous encounters with the phobic stimulus.

The same groups of patients were exposed to their phobic stimuli during a behavioral approach test (BAT) (Antony et al., 1997a). The percentages of participants in each group who experienced a panic attack during the BAT (based on DSM criteria) were as follows: BII, 50%; heights, 47%; driving, 36%; and animals, 20%. Taken together, these studies and others suggest that panic attacks are common among people with specific phobias (for a review, see Craske, 1991).

Commonly Experienced Symptoms

According to a study by Thyer and Himle (1987), the 10 strongest symptoms experienced by individuals with specific phobias during exposure to a phobic stimulus (in order) were fast heartbeat, tight muscles, an urge to run, rapid breathing, feeling of doom, feeling fidgety, trembling, shortness of breath, cold hands or feet, and a pounding sensation in the chest. These symptoms were similar to those reported by individuals with unexpected panic attacks, although the rank order of particular symptoms differed. Many of the symptoms experienced by individuals with different specific phobias (e.g., phobias of enclosed places, dentists, blood, animals) are similar across phobia types. However, again the ranking of particular symptoms (based on their intensity) appears to vary somewhat across groups (Hugdahl & Öst, 1985).

Vasovagal Syncope and BII Phobias

Although most phobia types are associated with increased arousal upon exposure to the phobic stimulus, BII phobias are associated with a unique pattern of responding. This consists of a diphasic response, in which heart rate and blood pressure increase initially for a few seconds or minutes, followed by a sudden decrease in arousal, often accompanied by fainting (for a review, see Page, 1994). The term "vasovagal syncope" (Lewis, 1932) has been used to describe the process by which heart rate and blood pressure suddenly fall— presumably due to activity in the vagus nerve, a parasympathetic nerve that innervates the chest and upper abdomen.

Öst, Sterner, and Lindahl (1984) examined the nature of the diphasic response in 18 patients with blood phobia presenting for treatment. Heart rate and blood pressure were monitored while subjects watched a film depicting surgery. As previously reported in numerous case studies (e.g., Babcock & Powell, 1982; Curtis & Thyer, 1983; Thyer & Curtis, 1985), patients showed an initial increase in arousal (during the instruction period), followed by a sharp decrease reaching a low point 4 minutes into the film. Some patients did not experience the initial increase in arousal. Five patients fainted or almost fainted during the film.

Friedman, Thayer, Borkovec, Tyrrell, et al. (1993) examined patterns of cardiac activity in individuals with blood phobia and individuals who experienced nonclinical panic attacks. Cardiac activity was studied in the context of several laboratory tasks that were not specifically related to panic attacks or blood (e.g., at rest, under threat of shock). Consistent with expectations, blood phobia and nonclinical panic attacks were associated with different patterns of cardiac activity. Whereas those who experienced panic attacks had (1) higher heart rates and lower heart rate variability, (2) unexpected associations among measures of cardiac activity, and (3) dominant sympathetic control of heart rate and lower vagal tone, those with blood phobia showed the opposite pattern on these variables.

To assess whether fainting is indeed unique to BII phobias, Öst (1992) examined the percentages of individuals with blood phobias ($n = 81$), injection phobias ($n = 59$), animal phobias ($n = 50$), dental phobias ($n = 60$), and claustrophobia ($n = 40$) with a history of fainting in the presence of the phobic situation. All participants met DSM-III or DSM-III-R criteria for specific phobia. Although 70% of subjects with blood phobias and 56% of those with injection phobias reported a history of fainting, none of the subjects in the other groups reported such a history, confirming the unique physiological response of individuals with blood and injection phobias.

Despite the diphasic response observed in many individuals with blood phobias, a substantial minority of blood phobias are not associated with a history of fainting (e.g., 30% in the study by Öst, 1992). Furthermore, Kleinknecht and Lenz (1989) identified a group of subjects who fainted in response to blood cues but did not report any fear of seeing blood. Of 103 college students who reported a history of fainting upon exposure to blood, 38% were classified as having a blood phobia, 28% were classified as having a blood fear, and 34% were classified as having neither. These results imply that fainting in response to blood may sometimes occur independently of fear. It seems likely, based on analyses presented in earlier chapters of this book, that most individuals who faint become anxious over fainting and develop blood phobia in response to their fainting (rather than the other way around). The analogy to developing anxiety over the next panic attack and its somatic cues, and thus to developing full-blown panic disorder, is described in Chapter 8. This is in contrast to nonclinical panic, where anxiety does not develop.

If this is true, one possibility is that individuals with nonclinical fainting experience the characteristic drop in heart rate and blood pressure without the initial increase (assuming that the initial increase is a reflection of anticipatory anxiety or fear). This possibility has yet to be examined. However, if this is so, fainting may not be a phobic *response* in blood phobia, but rather an anxiety *trigger* contributing to blood phobia in a similar manner to the relation of panic and anxiety in the etiology of panic disorder (see Chapter 10). In support of this hypothesis, scores on the Anxiety Sensitivity Index (ASI; Peterson & Reiss, 1993)—which measures anxiety over certain physical sensations, including faintness—predicted whether a person who fainted in response to blood desired treatment for blood phobia (Kleinknecht & Lenz, 1989).

An additional finding suggesting the independence of fear of blood and fainting in response to blood comes from a study by Schwartz, Adler, and Kaloupek (1987), in which groups of undergraduates with blood anxiety and with social anxiety showed increases in heart rate while watching films with social-evaluative themes, and decreases in heart rate while watching films with blood–injury content. These responses were independent of the content of subjects' fears.

If fainting in response to blood cues is an evolutionarily determined response that is independent of anxiety and fear, one might expect exposure-based treatments for blood phobia to decrease anxiety, but not necessarily to decrease fainting. However, Öst, Lindahl, Sterner, and Jerremalm (1984) found that exposure-based treatments for blood phobia were effective in reducing both anxiety and fainting; this suggests that anxiety and fainting are not entirely independent among individuals with BII phobias, perhaps because physiological processes associated with anxiety exacerbate the vasovagal response.

Focus of Apprehension

Fear of Anxiety Sensations

For more than two decades, researchers with an interest in anxiety disorders have been studying the ways in which "fear of fear" and the related construct "anxiety sensitivity" contribute to the experiences of fear, anxiety, and related problems (Goldstein & Chambless, 1978; Reiss, 1987, 1991; Taylor, 1999). Previously, behavioral conceptualizations of fear and anxiety had focused on the external objects and situations that trigger an individual's fear. With a growing literature on anxiety sensitivity, it is now clear that another important feature of anxiety disorders is the extent to which people are anxious about experiencing the physical symptoms of anxiety (particularly the physical symptoms of arousal). Anxiety sensitivity plays an important role in the pathogenesis of panic disorder and seems to play a significant, although smaller, role in other anxiety disorders as well (Taylor, Koch, & McNally, 1992).

Taylor, Koch, and McNally (1992) compared scores on the ASI (Peterson & Reiss, 1993) across six groups of people with different anxiety disorders, as well as a group of nonanxious controls. Although individuals with panic disorder had the highest scores on the ASI, other anxiety disorders were also associated with elevated scores relative to those of controls. In fact, specific phobia was the only anxiety disorder that was *not* associated with heightened anxiety sensitivity compared to the nonanxious group. In contrast, we found that individuals with specific phobias scored higher than nonanxious controls on the ASI, but lower than people in any other anxiety disorder group except social phobia (Rapee, Brown, Antony, & Barlow, 1992). Taken together, these data suggest that individuals with specific phobias may have some fear of experiencing symptoms of arousal, but not to the same degree as individuals with other anxiety disorders.

A limitation of these studies is their failure to examine differences across specific phobia types. As reviewed earlier, Curtis et al. (1989) proposed that specific phobia types differ with respect to their relationship with agoraphobia. Specifically, Curtis and colleagues hypothesized that agoraphobia shares more features with situational specific phobias than with other specific phobia types. If this is true, situational phobias might be expected to be associated with heightened levels of anxiety sensitivity, relative to other specific phobia types.

A number of studies have examined this possibility. We (Antony et al., 1997a) compared scores on the ASI across four types of specific phobias: heights, driving, animal, and blood–injection. Scores on the ASI ranged from 14.33 (blood–injection) to 20.73 (driving). Although the means were in the expected direction, differences across specific phobia groups were nonsignificant. A related study (Lehman, Hofmann, & Barlow, 1998) failed to find any differences in ASI scores across the four DSM-IV specific phobia types.

Still, there are several studies suggesting that fear of physical sensations varies across specific phobia types. Also, there is evidence that anxiety sensitivity is related to phobic behavior, particularly among people with claustrophobic fears. Craske and Sipsas (1992) found support for the hypothesis that situational phobias are associated with greater anxiety sensitivity than animal phobias are. Mean ASI scores were 19.8 for individuals without phobias ($n = 18$), 22.9 for individuals with animal phobias ($n = 19$), and 32.9 for individuals with claustrophobia ($n = 9$). Scores were significantly higher in the claustrophobia group than in the nonphobic group, whereas the animal phobia group did not differ from either of the other two groups with respect to ASI scores. In addition, anxiety sensitivity was significantly correlated with various measures of claustrophobic fear. Given that ASI scores in the claustrophobia group were in the same range as those found in panic disorder in other studies (e.g., Antony et al., 1997a), it is likely that low power accounted for the failure to find differences between individuals with claustrophobia and those with animal phobias.

Confirming a relationship between anxiety sensitivity and claustrophobic fear, Valentiner and colleagues found that an interaction between anxiety sensitivity and expected anxiety was predictive of avoidance behavior in claustrophobic situations (Valentiner, Telch, Ilai, & Hehmsoth, 1993; Valentiner, Telch, Petruzzi, & Bolte, 1996). In addition, Davey, Menzies, and Gallardo (1997) examined correlations between fear of physical sensations, as measured by the Body Sensations Questionnaire (BSQ; Chambless, Caputo, Bright, & Gallagher, 1984), and fear of heights or spiders in a student sample. Although BSQ scores were significantly correlated with avoidance of heights, they were not significantly correlated with fear or avoidance of spiders.

Response to Panic Induction Challenges

Compared to people with other anxiety disorders, people with panic disorder tend to respond with greater fear to biological challenges that induce uncomfortable sensations (e.g., lactate infusion, yohimbine injections, cholecystokinin injections, CO_2 inhalation) (see Antony & Swinson, 2000, for a review). Perhaps the most commonly used panic induction methods are CO_2 inhalation and voluntary hyperventilation. Moreover, there is evidence that the intensity of fear experienced during these challenges can be predicted by an individual's fear of anxiety sensations (Eke & McNally, 1996; Rapee, Brown, et al., 1992; Schmidt & Telch, 1994).

Several studies have examined the effects of CO_2 inhalation and hyperventilation on people with specific phobias, as well as the extent to which the response to these challenges varies across the anxiety disorders. As expected, we (Rapee, Brown, et al., 1992) found that individuals with specific phobias responded to these challenges with less fear than individuals with panic disorder. However, on a number of measures, the response of people with specific phobias was greater than that of nonanxious controls.

Three studies have compared specific phobia types on responses to respiratory challenges. Verburg, Griez, and Meijer (1994) compared 15 individuals with animal phobias to 15 individuals with situational or natural environment phobias (e.g., heights, enclosed places, storms, water) on their responses to a single inhalation of 35% CO_2-enriched air. In this study, the fear reported by individuals with situational and environmental phobias was significantly higher than that reported by controls, whereas those with animal phobias did not differ from controls.

Craske and Sipsas (1992) exposed individuals with spider/snake fears and claustrophobia to three situations: exposure to a live spider or snake, exposure to a small dark closet, and a hyperventilation challenge. As expected, fear-relevant exposures (e.g., exposing participants with animal phobias to their feared animals, exposing participants with claustrophobia to a closet) led to more fear symptoms than fear-irrelevant exposures. In addition, individuals with claustrophobia were more fearful of the hyperventilation challenge than were those in the spider/snake phobia group. In fact, the individuals with claustrophobia were as fearful of the hyperventilation challenge as they were of being in the closet.

In contrast to these studies, we found few significant differences among specific phobia types (animals, heights, driving, BII) in responses to hyperventilation and CO_2 inhalation (Antony, Brown, & Barlow, 1997b). On the few analyses for which there were differences, individuals with driving or height phobias tended to respond more strongly than individuals with animal or BII phobias.

Summary and Conclusions

Summarizing across studies, there is mixed evidence regarding sensation-focused fear and specific phobias. Generally, anxiety sensitivity tends to be lower in specific phobias than in panic disorder. Some studies have found heightened fear of sensations in people with specific phobias, relative to nonanxious controls, and others have failed to replicated this finding. Studies examining responses to hyperventilation and CO_2 inhalation have also been mixed. Among studies that have shown differences across specific phobia types, differences tend to be in the expected direction, with situational phobias (as well as phobias of heights) being associated with greater anxiety sensitivity and greater fear during panic induction challenges.

Specific Phobias and Disgust Sensitivity

Over the past few years, there has been a growing interest in the relationship between fear and disgust, particularly in the context of certain specific phobias (for a review, see Woody & Teachman, 2000). Specifically, heightened disgust sensitivity has been implicated in the development and maintenance of BII phobias and certain animal phobias. There is also limited evidence that other anxiety-related symptoms (e.g., trait anxiety and separation anxiety in children) are correlated with self-reported disgust sensitivity (Muris, Merckelbach, Schmidt, & Tierney, 1999).

Tolin, Lohr, Sawchuk, and Lee (1997) compared the disgust and fear responses of individuals with spider phobias, BII phobias, or no phobias to photographs of spiders and injections. Participants also completed questionnaires measuring disgust sensitivity. Generally, disgust sensitivity was higher in the two phobia groups than in the nophobia group. In response to injection photos, the reaction of participants with BII phobias was *primarily* one of disgust. The reaction of participants with spider phobias to spider photos was mostly one of fear, although disgust was also a strong component of the response. Merckelbach, Muris, de Jong, and de Jongh (1999) failed to replicate this study, finding either no correlation or only modest correlations between BII fear and disgust sensitivity in three separate samples.

As reviewed earlier, Davey et al. (1998) found that animals can be grouped into three basic categories: fear-irrelevant (e.g., rabbits), fear-relevant—fierce (including predatory animals such as wolves and bears), and disgust-relevant (including animals such as snakes, mice, slugs, and cockroaches). Disgust sensitivity appears to be correlated only with fear of animals in the disgust-relevant group (Ware, Jain, Burgess, & Davey, 1994). In addition, the tendency for disgust to be associated with these animals occurs across different cultures (Davey et al., 1998). Heightened disgust sensitivity in parents has been found to predict fear of disgust-relevant animals in children (Davey, Forster, & Mayhew, 1993; de Jong, Andrea, & Muris, 1997).

Disgust and Avoidance of Contamination

Several investigators have hypothesized that the relationship between disgust and certain phobic objects stems from a desire to avoid contamination and disease. In support of this view, Ware et al. (1994) found that fear of disgust-relevant animals was positively correlated with obsessive–compulsive washing, but not with other symptoms of OCD. Sawchuk, Lohr, Tolin, Lee, and Kleinknecht (2000) compared levels of disgust across groups of students with spider fears, students with BII fears, and nonfearful controls. Generally, levels of self-reported disgust were higher in the two fearful groups than in the nonfearful group. Furthermore, in contrast to the study by Ware et al. (1994), there was an association between levels of disgust and a fear of contamination among individuals with BII fears, but not among those with spider fears.

Generalized versus Stimulus-Specific Disgust Sensitivity

Recently, investigators have begun to question whether the disgust sensitivity observed in people with animal and BII phobias is generalized or just specific to the phobic stimulus. Mulkens, de Jong, and Merckelbach (1996) found that individuals with spider phobias were more likely than individuals without such phobias to report heightened disgust sensitivity on questionnaire measures, and to respond with more disgust during a behavioral test. They were also less inclined to eat a cookie that had been walked on by a spider, compared to individuals without a spider phobia. However, individuals from both groups were equally likely to drink from a dirty tea cup, suggesting that the heightened disgust sensitivity observed in the context of spider phobias may not generalize to non-spider-related situations.

Consistent with these findings, Thorpe and Salkovskis (1998a) found little evidence of a relationship between generalized disgust sensitivity and a phobic fear response in people with spider fears, although individuals with spider phobias did report heightened disgust in response to seeing spiders. The authors argued that phobias do not stem from a generalized disgust sensitivity. Instead, they hypothesized that when stimuli normally associated with disgust become the focus of phobic anxiety, the disgust response in reaction that that particular stimulus may increase.

In contrast to these findings, Sawchuk, Lee, Tolin, and Lohr (1997) compared responses of individuals with and without BII fears to watching films depicting maggots or neutral landscape scenes. Individuals with BII fears rated the maggot films as more disgusting than did the control participants. The disgust ratings following the maggot film were also higher than ratings of other emotions (e.g., fear, surprise, anger, etc.). These results suggest that the disgust sensitivity reported by individuals with BII fear may in fact be generalized, extending to situations other than blood and related stimuli.

Disgust Sensitivity and Fainting in BII Phobias

Kleinknecht, Kleinknecht, and Thorndike (1997) used structural equation modeling to examine BII stimuli. Analyses based on the Disgust Emotion Scale (Walls & Kleinknecht,

1996) found that disgust sensitivity was *negatively* correlated with fainting. Analyses based on the Disgust Scale (Haidt, McCauley, & Rozin, 1994) found no relationship between disgust and fainting. Neither result supported the hypothesis that higher disgust sensitivity would be predictive of fainting, although the intensity of BII fear was positively associated with fainting. In contrast, Hepburn and Page (1999) found that listening to narratives designed to induce images of disgust increased symptoms of fainting, but not of fear, during exposure to BII stimuli. However, narratives designed to induce images of fear led to increases in symptoms of both faintness and fear.

Disgust Sensitivity and Response to Treatment

Merckelbach, de Jong, Arntz, and Schouten (1993) examined differences in outcome following exposure-based treatment for individuals with spider phobias who were high or low in disgust sensitivity. Treatment was equally effective in both groups. Furthermore, there is evidence that disgust decreases following treatment of childhood spider phobias, in parallel with decreases in fear (de Jong, Andrea, & Muris, 1997).

Summary and Conclusions

It is fairly well established that BII phobias and certain animal phobias are associated with heightened disgust sensitivity, and that the disgust response may be related to a fear of disease or contamination, particularly for BII phobias. Evidence regarding the relationship between disgust sensitivity and fainting in response to BII stimuli is mixed. Furthermore, there is some evidence that the heightened disgust observed in spider phobias is situation-specific, whereas the disgust associated with BII fears may be more generalized. Finally, disgust sensitivity does not appear to have an impact upon treatment. In fact, there is evidence that following behavioral treatment, disgust decreases in parallel with fear.

Information Processing and Specific Phobia

As is the case with all of the anxiety disorders, a growing emphasis over the past 10 years of research on specific phobias has been in the area of information processing. Specifically, researchers have studied biases in attention, memory, and other cognitive processes.

Attention

Almost all studies examining attentional biases in specific phobias have been based on individuals with spider phobias, and in most cases researchers have relied on a modified version of the Stroop (1935) procedure. The modified Stroop task (Mathews & MacLeod, 1985) involves showing participants threat-related words (e.g., "snake," "blood") and neutral words (e.g., "desk," "light"), printed in different colors (e.g., red, green). The participant is instructed to name the *color* of each word as the word is presented, and the time taken to name each color is measured. Differences in the time taken to name the colors of threat-related and neutral words are generally assumed to reflect differences in the amount of attention that the participant is devoting to the word itself.

Most published studies based on the Stroop paradigm have found evidence of heightened attention to threat-related words in people with spider phobias (Kindt & Brosschot, 1997; Lavy & van den Hout, 1993; Lavy, van den Hout, & Arntz, 1993a; Watts, McKenna, Sharock, & Trezise, 1986). However, some studies, mostly based on other cognitive paradigms, have failed to find the expected attentional bias. Using a task requiring individuals with spider phobias to react quickly to targets presented with either fear-relevant or fear-irrelevant pictures, Merckelbach, Kenemans, Dijkstra, and Schouten (1993) found no evidence of an attentional bias among these participants, compared to controls. Wenzel and Holt (1999) also failed to demonstrate any attentional bias toward phobia-related words using a dot probe task in students with either spider or BII phobias.

Recently, investigators have begun to study attentional biases for stimuli other than words (e.g., pictures, live spiders). Stroop interference has been found for spider-related pictures in adults (Kindt & Brosschot, 1997; Lavy & van den Hout, 1993), although there is evidence that attentional biases for pictures may be weaker than biases for words (Lavy & van den Hout, 1993). In contrast, a study of children with spider phobias failed to find any attentional bias for pictures, although the expected bias for threat-related words was found (Kindt & Brosschot, 1999).

Thorpe and Salkovskis (1998b) conducted one of the only studies to examine attentional processes in the presence of the actual phobic stimulus. As quickly as possible, participants with spider phobias had to detect a target light that was located near a live tarantula. The tarantula and light were placed either near the door (which represented escape and safety) or away from the door. Reaction times were significantly shorter when the spider was located near the door. The authors interpreted this finding as evidence that when a threatening stimulus is located away from a safety stimulus, attention is divided between the treat and safety.

Investigators have also studied whether the attentional bias is present even when stimuli are presented in a masked form, preventing conscious identification of the stimulus. Results have been mixed. Whereas van den Hout, Tenney, Huygens, and de Jong (1997) found an attentional bias for masked spider-related words, Thorpe and Salkovskis (1997a) failed to replicate this finding. Furthermore, a study examining skin conductance responses of children with spider phobias to masked stimuli found no differences in responses to fear-relevant and fear-irrelevant pictures presented preattentively (Mayer, Merckelbach, & Muris, 1999).

A number of studies have examined the effect of exposure-based treatments on attentional biases. Although there is evidence that the spider Stroop effect is stable over time in untreated individuals (Kindt & Brosschot, 1998), several studies have found that treatment reduces interference on the spider Stroop task (Lavy & van den Hout, 1993; Lavy et al., 1993a; van den Hout et al., 1997; Thorpe & Salkovskis, 1997b; Watts, McKenna, et al., 1986).

Finally, a few studies have examined the relationship between disgust and attentional biases. The Stroop test failed to demonstrate an attentional bias for medical and disgust-related words, even under conditions of disgust provocation (Sawchuk, Lohr, Lee, & Tolin, 1999). Thorpe and Salkovskis (1998a) also failed to demonstrate a relationship between disgust and attentional biases in participants with spider phobias.

In summary, the evidence regarding attentional biases is mixed. Although such a bias is frequently found in experimental studies, the effect is fragile and has not always been replicated. To the extent that this bias exists, little is known about its function. However, some investigators have suggested that the attentional bias observed in specific phobias facilitates escape from danger (Lavy, van den Hout, & Arntz, 1993b).

Memory

As with attention, most studies on memory and specific phobias have been based on individuals with phobias of spiders. Watts, Trezise, and Sharrock (1986) found that individuals with spider phobias had poorer recognition of previously seen dead spiders mounted on cards than controls without phobias, although the effect was only found for larger spiders. Furthermore, this deficit improved following behavioral treatment. Watts and colleagues interpreted the finding as support for the hypothesis that people with phobias have poor focused attention for phobic stimuli. A study by Tolin, Lohr, Lee, and Sawchuk (1999) supports this hypothesis. Individuals with spider phobias, BII phobias, or no phobias were instructed to carefully study spider-related, BII-related, and neutral photographs for a subsequent recognition task. Participants with phobias showed decreased viewing times for phobic stimuli, suggesting poorer focused attention for phobic stimuli.

A number of researchers have recently begun more fine-grained studies of the relationship between phobias and memory. For example, Sawchuk et al. (1999) found an implicit memory bias for medical and disgust-related words among individuals with BII phobias. Among individuals with phobias, implicit memory was greater for phobia-related words than for neutral words.

As a test of the "attentional narrowing theory" of emotional memory, Wessel and Merckelbach (1997, 1998) studied memory for characteristics that are central versus peripheral to the phobic stimulus. This model suggests that fearful individuals narrow their attention toward the object of their fear (i.e., central details) and decrease their attention to other information (i.e., peripheral details). According to the model, recall for details that are central to the feared objects (e.g., the color of a spider) should be recalled better than details that are peripheral (e.g., the color of a table in the room).

Consistent with the model, Wessel and Merckelbach (1998) found that compared to participants without phobias, individuals with spider phobias had enhanced memory for threat-related stimuli (e.g., photos of spiders) than for non-threat-related stimuli (e.g., photos of babies and pens). In a related study involving exposure to a live spider, individuals with spider phobias had poorer memory for peripheral objects in a room (e.g., a clock) than did participants without phobias (Wessel & Merckelbach, 1997). However, there were no group differences in memory for central details (e.g., characteristics of the spider). This study therefore provided only partial support for the attentional narrowing hypothesis of emotional memory.

In summary, studies regarding memory and phobias have yielded mixed results, although these studies have tended to look at different aspects of memory. For example, studies of recognition for threat-related stimuli (e.g., Watts, Tresize, & Sharrock, 1986) have found limited evidence of deficits in recognition for phobia-related stimuli. In contrast, studies examining implicit memory and memory for fear-related characteristics of the phobic situation have found increased memory among individuals with phobias.

Other Cognitive Processes

Researchers from around the world have consistently shown that individuals with specific phobias have distorted beliefs regarding the objects and situations they fear. Furthermore, unlike studies of memory and attention, which have focused primarily on spider phobias, studies of distorted thinking have included a broad range of phobias. For example, Menzies and Clarke (1995a) found that compared to controls without phobias, individuals with height phobias provided higher estimates of the likelihood of falling from a ladder and of the injuries that would result from such a fall. This study confirmed previous findings (Marshall, Bristol, & Barbaree, 1992) showing a tendency for height phobias to be associated with distorted thinking about safety in high places. Furthermore, distorted thinking has been found in people with spider phobias (Jones & Menzies,

2000; Jones et al., 1996), dental phobias (Kent, 1985; Lindsay, Wege, & Yates, 1984), and a range of other specific phobias (Thorpe & Salkovskis, 1995; Radomsky, Teachman, Baker, & Rachman, 1996).

In addition, individuals with specific phobias (e.g., claustrophobia) are frequently inaccurate when reporting their expected fear level prior to entering a feared situation (Telch, Ilai, Valentiner, & Craske, 1994). Moreover, people who fear spiders tend to engage in deductive reasoning that confirms their fearful beliefs rather than reasoning that disconfirms their beliefs, which may be a factor in maintaining their fear (de Jong, Mayer, & van den Hout, 1997; de Jong, Weertman, Horselenberg, & van den Hout, 1997).

Individuals with specific phobias may also be more likely to assume high correlations between their feared stimulus and negative consequences. Pauli, Wiedemann, and Montoya (1998) presented participants with and without flying phobias with fear-relevant slides (e.g., airplane crash sites) and fear-irrelevant slides (e.g., airplanes in flight, mushrooms), followed randomly either by an electrical shock or by no electrical shock. Later, when estimating the covariation between the shock and each type of slide, individuals with flying phobias estimated higher degrees of covariation between the shock and fear-relevant slides, compared to control participants and compared to fear-irrelevant slides. Tendencies for perceiving an illusory correlation between fear-relevant stimuli and a negative consequence (e.g., shock) has also been demonstrated in people with spider phobias (de Jong, Merckelbach, & Arntz, 1995) and BII phobias (Pury & Mineka, 1997).

In addition to distorted beliefs, there is evidence of distorted perceptions in people with specific phobias. Rachman and Cuk (1992) found that individuals with snake and spider phobias tended to overestimate the degree of activity by their feared animals, and that these distorted cognitions decreased following treatment. However, they did not show evidence of distorted cognitions regarding the animals' size. Riskind, Moore, and Bowley (1995) confirmed previous findings suggesting that spider phobias are associated with a tendency to imagine that spiders are moving more rapidly. In addition, they found that individuals with spider phobias often assumed that spiders selectively moved toward them rather than other people in the same physical space. Perceptual distortions regarding feared stimuli have also been found for a broader range of fears, including snakes, heights, and enclosed places (Radomsky et al., 1996).

Finally, there is evidence that individuals can respond to phobic stimuli even when they are exposed to the stimuli outside of their awareness. Öhman and Soares (1994) studied the skin conductance responses of controls without phobias and individuals with phobias of snakes or spiders to photos of spiders, snakes, flowers, or mushrooms that were presented in either a masked or an unmasked format. Individuals with phobias showed increased responses to phobic stimuli presented either masked or unmasked, compared to controls and compared to neutral stimuli.

Physiological Correlates

Although there is a great deal of research on the physiological underpinnings of fear and anxiety (see Chapter 6), there is relatively little research that particularly addresses this aspect of specific phobias. Nevertheless, there is some evidence suggesting that important physical changes occur during exposure to phobic stimuli. An early study found that upon exposure to spiders, individuals with spider phobias experienced increased heart rates and greater heart rate variability compared to controls without phobias (Prigatano & Johnson, 1974). Furthermore, heart rate and skin conductance have been shown to increase as an individual with a snake phobia approaches a snake (Teghtsoonian & Frost, 1982).

In a more comprehensive study of 10 women with animal phobias, Nesse et al. (1985) found that when participants were exposed to their feared animals, increases were observed in their pulse rate, blood pressure, plasma norepinephrine, epinephrine, insulin, cortisol, and growth hormone. Changes were not observed in plasma glucagons or pancreatic polypeptide. Although the subjective and behavioral fear responses of all participants were intense and consistent, the authors noted that the cardiovascular and endocrine correlates varied considerably with respect to their intensity, timing, and consistency.

In addition, several studies have used positron emission tomography to examine patterns of brain activity during the experience of phobic fear. Generally, results have been somewhat inconsistent across studies. Mountz et al. (1989) found no differences between participants with and without animal phobias in their patterns of cerebral blood flow during exposure to feared animals, particularly after controlling for the effects of hyperventilation. Fredrikson et al. (1993) found that changes in cortical and thalamic cerebral blood flow were associated with viewing phobic stimuli, but not other aversive stimuli or neutral stimuli. Wik, Fredrikson, and Fischer (1997) found changes in cerebral blood flow in pathways involving the amygdala, thalamus, and striatum when individuals with phobias observed phobia-relevant scenes. Finally, Rauch et al. (1995) observed increased cerebral blood flow in the anterior cingulate cortex, insular cortex, anterior temporal cortex, somatosensory cortex, posterior medial orbito-frontal cortex, and thalamus.

Investigators have also begun to study the role of physiological correlates in determining outcome following behavioral treatment for specific phobias. Merckelbach, Muris, Pool, and de Jong (1998) found a correlation between right parietal hyperactivation on an electroencephalographic (EEG) assessment and pretreatment scores on a spider phobia assessment. However, EEG asymmetry was not correlated with posttreatment outcome measures. In addition, there is evidence that neuroendocrine function may be involved in the effects of exposure treatment for phobias (see Carr, 1996, for a review). For example, Arntz (1993) found that administration of naltrexone (an endorphin blocker) negatively affected approach toward a spider, but did not affect fear. The author concluded that endorphin release may stimulate approach behavior in the face of a feared stimulus, although fear is not directly reduced.

ETIOLOGY OF SPECIFIC PHOBIA

As discussed in Chapter 7, the etiology of most phobic disorders seems to involve the association of either a true or false alarm with an object or situation that has a high probability of acquiring phobic properties. Some of these objects or situations may have real danger or pain associated with them, or otherwise are "prepared" in some way for this type of association or learning (Seligman, 1971). Although the evidence for "prepared" learning in the etiology of specific phobias is still somewhat controversial (McNally, 1987), it has received increasing support over the decades, (e.g., Mineka, 1985b; Öhman, 1993), as outlined in some detail in Chapter 7. Also described in Chapter 7 are the modifications to paradigms of emotional learning or conditioning that incorporate cognitive variables, such as concepts of probability learning, information processing, attention, surprise, and short-term memory (e.g., Mineka & Zinbarg, 1996). In any case, the evidence is now very strong that the process of emotional learning is a fundamentally distinct process to which the principles of conditioning are particularly applicable (Bouton, Mineka, & Barlow, 2001). Evidence presented in Chapter 7 illustrates the contrast between emotional learning and the more usual conscious cognitive acquisition of what has been described as prepositional declarative knowledge dependent on verbal input. Specifically, emotional conditioning in general, and fear conditioning specifically, do not seem to depend on conscious awareness (e.g., LeDoux, 1996; Öhman, 1997) although obviously (and as described below), conditioning and propositional systems of acquiring fear do sometimes overlap and interact (Davey, 1997; Lovibond, 1993). Several factors, then, influence the etiology of specific phobia.

Family and Genetic Factors

It is well established that specific phobias run in families. For example, a family study by Fyer et al. (1990) found that specific phobias occur in 31% of first-degree relatives of individuals without specific phobias. Furthermore, familial transmission tended to be stronger for females than for males. Interestingly, the presence of a specific phobia did not increase the chances of having a different anxiety disorder. These findings were replicated in a second study from the same group (Fyer, Mannuzza, Chapman, Martin, & Klein, 1995).

A number of investigators have used twin studies to tease out the effects of genetic and environmental factors in the familial transmission of specific phobias. In one of the earliest twin studies of this type, Torgersen (1979) studied the concordance rates of five fear types in monozygotic and dizygotic twin pairs: fears of separation, animals, mutilation, social situations, and nature. In this study, both genetics and environment played a role in the strength and content of fears, although the effects of genetics were weaker for fears of separation. Since this study was published, several other studies have found support for the hypothesis that genetics and environment both play a role in the development of specific phobias (e.g., Neale et al., 1994; Phillips, Fulker, & Rose, 1987). However, at least one study (Skre, Onstad, Torgersen, Lygren, & Kringlen, 1993) found little support for a genetic contribution to specific phobias and concluded that environmental factors are most important.

Several recent twin studies have examined the effects of particular types of genetic and environmental influences on the transmission of phobias. After correcting for unreliability, Kendler, Karkowski, and Prescott (1999) found heritability estimates of 47% for animal phobias, 59% for BII phobias, and 46% for situational phobias. Although individual-specific environmental influences (e.g., traumatic events occurring in the phobic situation) were also very important, family-specific environmental influences (e.g., shared environmental factors) were not especially important. This confirmed earlier findings from the same group (Kendler, Neale, Kessler, Heath, & Eaves, 1992b). This finding was also confirmed by Page and Martin (1998), who found that genetic factors, unique environmental factors, and nonshared environmental factors were important for the transmission of BII phobias. Thus, as reviewed in some detail in Chapter 6, specific phobia seems to be the one disorder for which some evidence exists supporting a specific genetic contribution, in contrast to a nonspecific contribution to emotionality that underlies anxiety and depression generally. Most likely, what are inherited are specific defensive reactions (e.g., low threshold for alarm reactions or vasovagal responses), which then interact with (nonshared) environmental influences to set the stage for development of phobia.

Experiential Pathways to the Development of Specific Phobia

Interacting with genetic contributions to the development of specific phobia (see Chapter 7) is the influence of early experience. Rachman (1976b, 1977) suggested three possible pathways to fear: direct conditioning (e.g., experiencing a car accident), vicarious acquisition or observational learning (e.g., seeing another person experience a car accident or repeatedly watching someone else behave fearfully while driving), and information/instruction (e.g., reading or hearing about the dangers of driving). The direct conditioning pathway refers to firsthand, classical conditioning experiences, whereas the other two pathways are best considered indirect means of learning. In addition, Rachman acknowledged the role of biological constraints (reviewed above) and other factors that might mediate the development of fear, such as trait anxiety and preparedness.

Numerous studies have examined the frequency with which phobia acquisition can be accounted for by these three methods. A large number of studies have provided support for the model, showing that direct and indirect forms of phobia acquisition occur frequently across a wide range of phobia types (e.g., Di Nardo et al., 1988; Ehlers, Hofmann, Herda, & Roth, 1994; McNally & Steketee, 1985; Menzies & Clarke, 1993a; Merckelbach, Arntz, & de Jong, 1991; Merckelbach, Arntz, Arrindell, & de Jong, 1992; Merckelbach & Muris, 1997; Muris, Merckelbach, & Collaris, 1997; Muris, Steerneman, Merckelbach, & Meesters, 1996; Öst, 1985, 1991; Öst & Hugdahl, 1985; Rimm, Janda, Lancaster, Nahl, & Dittmar, 1977; Townend, Dimigen, & Fung, 2000).

Three observations are worth noting. Across most (but not all) of these studies, direct conditioning experiences tend to be more frequently reported than are either vicarious acquisition or informational onsets. Furthermore, as noted in Chapter 7, a significant proportion of participants in most studies fail to endorse any of these methods of acquisition. Finally, the percentages of individuals endorsing particular modes of phobia onset vary considerably across studies.

There are a number of possible reasons for the variability across studies. First, investigators have tended to use different rules for diagnosing phobias. In some studies full DSM criteria were necessary for inclusion, whereas other studies have tended to include anyone with a specific fear. In addition, studies have been inconsistent with respect to how they determined whether a particular causal event, was relevant. For example, some studies allowed for multiple events, whereas others forced participants to choose the most important causal event. Furthermore, many studies have ignored the timing of the causal event, and most studies have failed to pay attention to the functional relationship between the event and the phobia. For example, a bee sting that is followed immediately by the onset of a fear of bees is sometimes afforded the same degree of importance as a bee sting that occurs 10 years before or even 10 years after the phobia begins. Finally, some of the variability across studies may be accounted for by a lack of reliability in the retrospective self-reports that investigators have relied upon. For example, Taylor, Deane, and Podd (1999) found that individuals with driving phobias were inconsistent with respect to their reported modes of phobia acquisition over the course of two assessments separated by about a year.

Three advances in recent studies have led to improvements in the quality of research on phobia acquisition. First, there has been a trend to use more carefully diagnosed patients who meet full criteria for specific phobia. In addition, more studies have included comparison groups without phobias, to assess whether the frequency of conditioning events among individuals with phobias differs from the frequency among people without phobias. Finally, some researchers have begun to study phobia acquisition in children, using longitudinal assessments and interviews with both children and parents. This methodology avoids the problems of retrospective recall biases, particularly for phobias that begin in childhood.

For example, prospective studies of childhood water phobias (Poulton, Menzies, Craske, Langley, & Silva, 1999) and height phobias (Poulton, Davies, Menzies, Langley, & Silva, 1998) did not find a relationship between a history of relevant trauma before age 9 and the presence of fear at age 18. In fact, Poulton et al. (1998) found that childhood injury in a high place before the age of 9 was more often associated with a lack of fear in high places at age 18.

There is still some disagreement regarding the role of conditioning, vicarious acquisition, and informational learning in the development of phobias. Although it is clear that these pathways are important for the development of some phobias, it also seems that these pathways do not account for all phobias. Furthermore, the question of why some people but not others develop phobias following these experiences remains to be answered. Previously, we proposed several possible answers to this question, most of which remain to be verified by research (Antony & Barlow, 1997). These include such variables as previous exposure to the feared situation (before the learning event); subsequent exposure to the situation (after the learning event); the context of the event (e.g., stress at the time of the event, availability of social support, the individual's perception of control over the event); and individual-difference variables such as trait anxiety or a genetic predisposition. These ideas have been elaborated in the Bouton et al. (2001) paper.

In any case, and as noted in the first edition of this book (Barlow, 1988) and in Chapter 7, a larger number of individuals with specific phobia may experience a false alarm of such intensity that emotional learning occurs. That is, false alarms become strongly associated with the object or situation that set the occasion for the first false alarm. Anxiety that subsequently occurs in the presence of the object or situation occurs primarily over the possibility of having another (unpredictable) false alarm in the presence of the cues signaling the possibility of this alarm. In addition to the biological constraints and various moderators of the experience, such as previous exposure to the feared situation (reviewed above), other issues may interact to diminish or exacerbate emotional learning connected with this experience. For example, as reviewed in Chapter 7, blocking the overpowering action tendency of escape—which is inherently a part of the alarm reaction—serves to intensify the emotion. Thus, in situations where one perceives the possibility of being "trapped" (while driving, flying, crossing bridges, etc.), the prevention of easy escape in the event of false alarm could block the overwhelmingly powerful action tendency of escape intensifying and prolonging the alarm. As also reviewed in Chapter 7 and suggested in the first edition of this book, the occurrence of a false alarm may well be one of the "missing links" in a traumatic conditioning etiology of some phobias.

Thus, in our model of the etiology of specific phobia (see Figure 11.1), a relatively nonspecific genetic predisposition to experience anxiety or alarm responses (fear or panic), along with a psychological vulnerability to experience anxiety, may interact with several specific life experiences. First, the experience of stress due to negative life events may lead directly to a false alarm that becomes closely associated with specific predisposed or prepared situations. If the vulnerabilities line up correctly, and particularly if the individual has been sensitized in some way to the phobic situation through early learning experiences (a specific vulnerability), then anxiety will develop to the possibility of having additional alarm responses in this particular situation. As represented in Figure 11.1, several other experiential factors could similarly lead to the development of phobia. These include a direct traumatic conditioning experience, which seems to lead to a minority of phobias. In this context, a true alarm may occur during the actual dangerous event and result in subsequent false alarms (learned anxiety or conditioned anxiety), which could become the focus of anxious apprehension leading to phobia. As outlined above, vicarious experience and misinformation occurring in the fertile ground of biological and psychological vulnerabilities could also lead to the occurrence of true and/or false alarms, which could then become associated (conditioned) with the object or situation, and thus become the focus of subsequent anxiety.

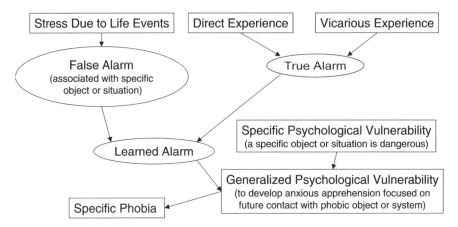

FIGURE 11.1. A model of the etiology of specific phobia.

On rare occasions, strongly learned (mis)information could be sufficient to trigger a phobia in the context of preexisting biological and psychological vulnerabilities. For example, Öst (1985) described the case of a woman with extremely severe snake phobia who had never encountered a snake in her life. Rather, she had been told repeatedly while growing up of the dangers of snakes in the high grass. She was encouraged to wear high rubber boots to guard against this imminent threat. Of course, one would expect that the intense anxiety and vigilance of someone repeatedly warned of the dangers of an object or situation will eventually lead to a full-blown alarm or panic when and if the person finally confronts the object or situation. Of course, a sense of unpredictability and uncontrollability of negative events, existing as a psychological vulnerability, may set the occasion for the above-described chain of events leading to the development of phobia. It is also important to note that the severity of the trauma, interacting with vulnerabilities and moderating variables reviewed above, may well determine whether the resulting disorder is specific phobia or posttraumatic stress disorder. As reviewed in Chapter 12, there are numerous examples of seemingly less severe traumatic events leading to posttraumatic stress disorder rather than specific phobia in some individuals, for whom, presumably, vulnerabilities and other psychological and contextual variables facilitate this development.

TREATMENT

Compared to other anxiety disorders, there is very little disagreement regarding the treatment of choice for specific phobias. Almost all experts agree that exposure to feared objects and situations is both necessary and sufficient for treating the vast majority of patients with this condition. In this section, we provide an overview of the literature on treatment of specific phobias. This review includes information on the efficacy of exposure-based treatments, of which there are several variations. In addition, we discuss the literature on alternative approaches to treatment that have been studied, including eye movement desensitization and reprocessing (EMDR), cognitive therapy, and pharmacotherapy.

Effects of Exposure-Based Treatment

Early exposure-based treatments for specific phobias were based on a procedure developed by Joseph Wolpe called "systematic desensitization" (Wolpe, 1958, 1973). Essentially, systematic desensitization involves teaching an individual to relax while exposing him or her to fear-producing images that gradually increase in intensity. Systematic desensitization has fallen out of favor in recent years for three main reasons. First, some studies have found that *in vivo* exposure is a more effective method of reducing fear than exposure in imagination is (Emmelkamp & Wessels, 1975; Mannion & Levine, 1984). Second, *in vivo* exposure is generally briefer than systematic desensitization, because time is not initially spent teaching the patient relaxation techniques and because steps on the exposure hierarchy are often taken more quickly than is the case in systematic desensitization.

Finally, although there is evidence that relaxation inhibits fear and arousal during exposure to feared objects and situations (McGlynn, Moore, Rose, & Lazarte, 1995; McGlynn, Moore, Lawyer, & Karg, 1999), there is little evidence that incorporating relaxation training into exposure-based treatments leads to improved outcomes. One study found that a subset of individuals with claustrophobia (those who tended to react physiologically rather than behaviorally) responded more to applied relaxation training (i.e., relaxation conducted in the context of exposure) than to standard *in vivo* exposure (Öst, Johansson, & Jerremalm, 1982). However, other studies have failed to find any benefit of adding relaxation training to exposure-based treatment for specific phobias (e.g., Öst, Lindahl, et al., 1984).

In vivo exposure to feared situations has been found to be effective for a wide range of specific phobias, including phobias of spiders (Hellström & Öst, 1995; Muris, Mayer, & Merckelbach, 1998; Öst, 1996b; Öst, Ferebee, & Furmark, 1997; Öst, Salkovskis, & Hellström, 1991), snakes (Gauthier & Marshall, 1977; Hepner & Cauthen, 1975), rats (Foa, Blau, Prout, & Latimer, 1977), thunder and lightning (Öst, 1978), water (Menzies & Clarke, 1993b), heights (Baker, Cohen, & Saunders, 1973; Bourque & Ladouceur, 1980), flying (Beckham, Vrana, May, Gustafson, & Smith, 1990; Howard, Murphy, & Clarke, 1983; Öst, Brandberg, & Alm, 1997), enclosed places (Öst et al., 1982; Craske, Mohlman, Yi, Glover, & Valeri, 1995), choking (Greenberg, Stern, & Weilburg, 1988), dental treatment (Gitin et al., 1996; Moore & Brødsgaard, 1994), blood (Öst, Fellenius, & Sterner, 1991), and balloons (Houlihan, Schwartz, Miltenberger, & Heuton, 1993).

There is considerable variability across studies with respect to the duration of treatment, the ages of participants, and the extent of therapist involvement—and yet the positive effects of exposure appear to be robust. In fact, for some phobias (e.g., phobias of animals, injections, dental treatment), a single session of *in vivo* exposure lasting 2–3 hours can lead to clinically significant improvement in all but a few patients (Gitin et al., 1996; Öst, 1989; Öst, Brandberg, & Alm, 1997; Öst, Salkovskis, & Hellström, 1991).

Group versus Individual Treatments

Very few studies have examined the use of group treatments for specific phobias. Öst (1996b) compared a single session of large-group treatment (seven to eight patients) to a single session of small-group treatment (three to four patients) for spider phobia. Both groups showed significant improvements after a single session lasting about 3 hours. In addition, gains were maintained or increased over the 1-year follow-up period. After 1 year, the percentages of individuals in the small and large groups with clinically significant improvement were 95% and 75%, respectively. Differences between the two group conditions were nonsignificant on most measures.

Degree of Therapist Involvement

Several studies have examined the question of whether exposure-based treatments can be effective without significant therapist contact. An early study found that systematic desensitization administered using a tape recording instead of a live therapist was quite effective for reducing fear of heights (Baker et al., 1973). However, a study of *in vivo* exposure for snake phobias (O'Brien & Kelley, 1980) found that individuals who received treatment that was either predominantly or exclusively therapist-assisted achieved a greater reduction in fear than individuals who attempted treatment with less therapist involvement.

More recent studies on individuals with spider phobias have yielded mixed findings. Öst, Salkovskis, and Hellström (1991) compared a single session of therapist-assisted exposure to treatment with a self-help manual for overcoming spider phobias. Using stringent criteria for identifying those with clinically significant improvement, the investigators concluded that 71% of those in the therapist-assisted group and only 6% in the self-help group were improved.

In a follow-up study, Hellström and Öst (1995) found that the way in which self-help treatment is administered affects outcome for individuals with spider phobias. In this study, five different treatments were compared: (1) a single session of therapist-assisted group exposure, (2) a spider-phobia-specific manual used in the home, (3) a spider-phobia-specific manual used in the clinic, (4) a nonspecific manual used in the home, and (5) a nonspecific manual used in the clinic. The percentages of individuals achieving clinically significant improvement were 80%, 10%, 63%, 9%, and 10%, respectively. These findings suggest that self-help treatments can be effective for a significant number of individuals when they are conducted in a clinic setting.

In the last decade, a number of self-help manuals have been published for individuals with a broad range of specific phobias (e.g., Antony, Craske, & Barlow, 1995a; Bourne, 1998a). Although these manuals are meant to be used in conjunction with the assistance of a therapist (Bourne, 1998b; Craske, Antony, & Barlow, 1997), it is possible that these treatments could be adapted for self-administration, particularly to be used in a clinic setting.

The Effect of Direct versus Indirect Exposure

Modeling of nonfearful behavior by a therapist is often considered an important part of therapist-assisted exposure for specific phobias (Antony & Swinson, 2000). However, observational learning in and of itself is probably not sufficient to effect clinically significant changes in most patients. In a study of group treatment for spider phobias, Öst, Ferebee, and Furmark (1997) compared direct exposure, direct observation (i.e., watching another individual being treated in person), and indirect observation (i.e., watching another person being treated on videotape). At posttreatment, the percentages of individuals with a clinically significant response to each of these treatments were 75%, 7%, and 33%, respectively. Improvements were maintained or slightly greater at 1-year follow-up. The findings in this study are consistent with previous findings that vicarious exposure alone is not effective for reducing childhood water phobias (Menzies & Clarke, 1993b).

Technology and the Treatment of Specific Phobias

In the past few years, clinicians have begun to take advantage of technological advances for the treatment of specific phobias. For example, it is now common practice to use videotapes to expose patients to feared stimuli. In addition, a number of investigators have begun to use virtual reality to expose patients to simulated situations involving heights (Rothbaum et al., 1995a, 1995b), flying (Kahan, Tanzer, Darvin, & Borer, 2000; Rothbaum, Hodges, & Smith, 1999; Rothbaum, Hodges, Watson, Kessler, & Opdyke, 1996; S. M. Smith, Rothbaum, & Hodges, 1999), spiders (Carlin, Hoffman, & Weghorst, 1997), and certain other fear-provoking situations (Rothbaum & Hodges, 1999).

To date, only two controlled studies have been published on virtual reality treatment for specific phobias. Rothbaum et al. (1995b) treated 12 college students with height fears in eight sessions of virtual reality exposure. Compared to 8 individuals in a wait-list control condition, those who were treated with virtual reality were significantly more improved. In a more recent study, Rothbaum, Hodges, Smith, Lee, and Price (2000) assigned 45 individuals with flying phobias to one of three conditions: (1) anxiety management training plus exposure to a virtual airplane; (2) anxiety management training plus exposure to a real airplane; or (3) wait-list control. Both treatment conditions were equally effective and were more effective than the wait-list condition. Although the authors concluded that virtual reality exposure and standard exposure are equally effective, a number of methodological limitations make such a conclusion premature. First, because both groups received anxiety management training (e.g., cognitive restructuring, breathing retraining, thought stopping), this study did not provide a "clean" comparison of virtual reality versus standard exposure. These other components of treatment may have blurred any differences that otherwise might have emerged. Second, the content of the exposure was different in the two exposure-based conditions. In the virtual reality condition, exposure involved simulations of takeoffs, landings, in-flight sounds, and various weather effects. In contrast, standard exposure involved being at the airport, sitting on a stationary airplane, and imagining exposure to flying. In other words, *in vivo* exposure to actual flights was not included.

Although these preliminary data concerning virtual reality are promising, more controlled studies with a broader range of phobias are needed. In addition, direct comparisons to the "gold standard" treatment (i.e., *in vivo* exposure) are also warranted. Even if virtual reality does not prove to be as effective as standard exposure-based treatments, it may still offer a treatment option for cases in which *in vivo* exposure is impractical or in which the patient refuses to enter the situation. Presumably, the quality and availability of virtual reality technology will improve in the coming years.

In addition to virtual reality, there are several other ways in which technology has been used to complement standard treatments for specific phobias. Computer-administered treatments have been studied for spider phobias (Nelissen, Muris, & Merckelbach, 1995; Smith, Kirkby, Montgomery, & Daniels, 1997) and dental phobia (Coldwell et al, 1998). In addition, radio contact (Levine & Wolpe, 1980) and mobile telephones (Flynn, Taylor, & Pollard, 1992) have been successfully used in the behavioral treatment of people with driving phobias.

Predictors of Response to Exposure-Based Treatment

In general, it has been difficult to identify variables that can help a clinician to predict whether a given individual will to respond to exposure therapy for a specific phobia. Because almost everyone with a specific phobia responds to treatment, there is a restricted range of outcomes in most treatment studies, making it difficult to identify particular predictors. For example, Hellström and Öst (1996) examined numerous variables—including age of onset, duration, method of onset, family history, anxiety, depression, heart rate, severity, and blood pressure—and found no stable predictors of outcome.

Still, a large number of other variables have been investigated as possible predictors of response to exposure-based treatments for specific phobias. Many of these have to do more with the ways in which treatment is conducted than with aspects of the patient. Some variables that have been studied include predictability and perceived control during the exposure practice; frequency of exposure practices; context of the exposure; whether the exposure occurs in response to the same stimulus or varied stimuli; the effects of distraction during exposure; and the effects of the individual's coping style. Each of these variables is discussed in turn.

Predictability and Perceived Control

Studies on perceived control during exposure in specific phobias have yielded inconsistent results. Craske, Bunt, Rapee, and Barlow (1991) found that giving patients with spider phobias control over the duration of an exposure trial had no effect on fear reduction. In a series of studies, McGlynn and colleagues investigated the effects of having the patient control his or her distance from a feared animal versus having the distance controlled by another individual. In the first of these studies, McGlynn, Rose, and Lazarte (1994) found that patient control over the distance from feared spiders or cockroaches was associated with higher levels of skin conductance and subjective fear. Rose, McGlynn, and Lazarte (1995) also found higher levels of skin conductance among those who could control their distance from a feared snake, particularly during early exposure trials. However, in a study of individuals with snake fears, McGlynn, Rose, and Jacobson (1995) failed to show any differences in either subjective fear ratings or skin conductance between participants who controlled their distance from the snake and those who did not control the distance themselves.

In contrast to research on perceived control, there is almost no research on the effects of predictable versus unpredictable exposure in people with specific phobias. An exception is an unpublished study by Lopatka (1989). In this study, individuals with snake fears were exposed to a live snake at either predictable or unpredictable intervals. Compared to predictable exposure, unpredictable exposure subsequently led to more avoidance of the snake. In addition, individuals who underwent unpredictable exposure were somewhat more likely than those who received predictable exposure to predict greater fear levels during later exposures to the snake.

Frequency of Exposure

Foa, Jameson, Turner, and Payne (1980) demonstrated that 10 daily exposure sessions are more effective for decreasing agoraphobic fear and avoidance than are 10 weekly sessions. In light of these findings, it has generally been accepted that massed exposure (with sessions scheduled close together) is a more effective method of fear reduction than is spaced exposure.

Recently, Michelle Craske and her colleagues have begun to examine the benefits of an expanding-spaced exposure schedule. In this paradigm, sessions begin close together and are gradually spread out as treatment progresses. In the first of two studies on the treatment of specific phobias, Rowe and Craske (1998a) found that massed exposure did indeed lead to significantly more fear reduction in a group of participants with spider phobias. However, they also found that an expanding-spaced schedule was less likely than a massed schedule to be associated with a return of fear following treatment. In contrast, a subsequent study based on individuals with height phobias (Lang & Craske, 2000) failed to replicate this finding.

Context of Exposure

A number of studies have examined the relationship between context and the effects of treatment. Mineka, Mystkowski, Hladek, and Rodriguez (1999) found that individuals with spider fears showed greater return of fear when tested in a different context from that in which treatment was administered. In a related study, Rodriguez, Craske, Mineka, and Hladek (1999) partially replicated these findings. The results of these studies are consistent with findings from animal studies (e.g., Bouton et al., 2001; Gunther, Denniston, & Miller, 1998) showing that treatment in multiple contexts can reduce the rate of relapse. Taken together, these studies suggest that people with specific phobias should be exposed to phobic stimuli in a variety of locations and situations.

Same-Stimulus and Varied-Stimulus Exposure

Rowe and Craske (1998b) studied the effects of using a variety of different spiders to treat individuals with spider phobias. Individuals exposed to only one spider experienced a greater reduction of fear over the course of treatment than did those exposed to four different spiders. However, when tested 3 weeks later, those who received the varied-stimulus treatment did not experience significant return of fear, whereas those who received the same stimulus treatment often showed a clear return of fear in response to seeing a spider.

Effects of Distraction during Exposure

Theoretical models of emotional processing (e.g., Foa & Kozak, 1986) suggest (1) that distraction can prevent fear from occurring, thereby leading to less intense fear during exposure to a feared stimulus as well as less thorough emotional and cognitive processing; and (2) that distraction interferes with the *long-term* reduction of fear following exposure-based treatments. Consistent with models of emotional processing, Craske, Street, Jayaraman, and Barlow (1991) found that fear ratings increased significantly more during a 6-minute focused exposure session than during a similar session during which participants were distracted.

However, studies investigating the effects of distraction on treatment outcome have yielded mixed results. Whereas some studies have found that distraction interferes with the effects of exposure (Weir & Marshall, 1980), other studies have found that specific phobia treatment works equally well regardless of whether the patient is distracted (Antony, McCabe, Leeuw, Sano, & Swinson, 2001). Furthermore, some studies have shown that the effects of distraction depend on other variables. For example, Rodriguez and Craske (1995) found that distraction interfered with fear reduction during high-intensity exposure but not low-intensity exposure.

The timing of the assessment may also influence whether distraction is shown to have an effect on outcome. Haw and Dickerson (1998) found that although distraction did not have any noticeable effects on emotional processing in the short term, individuals who underwent distraction during exposure showed more fear at follow-up than those who underwent focused exposure. In contrast, Penfold and Page (1999) found that distraction led to increased fear reduction within the exposure session, although after treatment ended, there were no differences between distracted-exposure and focused-exposure groups on a behavioral test.

Rodriguez and Craske (1993) reviewed the literature on distraction and exposure, and hypothesized several reasons for the inconsistent findings across studies. They suggested that these different findings may be due to differences in the nature of the attentional demand created by the distracting stimulus, as well as the affective quality of the distracting stimulus. Studies also differ with respect to the type of phobia investigated, the severity of the fear (e.g., analogue sample vs. patient sample), the timing of fear measurement (e.g., during exposure, following exposure, after a follow-up period), and the ways in which fear is measured (e.g., questionnaire measures vs. behavioral tests). Until researchers sort out the effects of these different variables, it will be difficult to understand the exact ways in which distraction affects treatment of specific phobias.

Individual-Difference Variables

Muris, Mayer, and Merckelbach (1998) found that trait anxiety was a significant predictor of outcome following a single-session treatment for a specific phobia of spiders. In contrast, imagery ability was not found to be a significant predictor of outcome (Merckelbach, de Jong, & Arntz, 1991).

Several studies have examined the effects on treatment outcome of a tendency to cope with threat by "monitoring" (i.e., a tendency to seek out and attend to threat-related information) versus "blunting" (i.e., a tendency to avoid exposure to threat-related information). In one study, Muris, Merckelbach, and de Jong (1995) found that participants who monitored had a smaller response to treatment of spider phobias than did those who blunted. In another study, Muris, de Jong, Merckelbach, and van Zuuren (1993a) found that "monitors" had a higher relapse rate than did "blunters" 1 week after being treated for spider phobias. Interestingly, these findings differed from those of Steketee, Bransfield, Miller, and Foa (1989), who found that "monitors" had a greater reduction of subjective anxiety within exposure sessions and a greater reduction of physiological arousal across sessions. To complicate the picture further, at least two studies have found no relationship between coping style and outcome following exposure therapy for specific phobias (Antony, McCabe, et al., in press; Muris, de Jong, Merckelbach, & van Zuuren, 1993b).

Eye Movement Desensitization and Reprocessing

Perhaps one of the most controversial developments in the behavioral treatment of anxiety disorders has been the recent introduction and promotion of EMDR (for recent reviews, see Cahill, Carrigan, & Frueh, 1999; de Jongh, Broeke, & Renssen, 1999; Lohr, Lilienfeld, Tolin, & Herbert, 1999; Lohr, Tolin, & Lilienfeld, 1998; Shapiro, 1999). EMDR involves having a patient imagine a feared scene while he or she is exposed to bilateral sensory stimulation. Usually, the procedure involves having the patient visually track the therapist's finger as it moves back and forth across the patient's visual field. However, the procedure can also involve listening to tones or other sounds as they are alternately played in each ear. EMDR was originally developed for the treatment of posttraumatic stress disorder, but several studies have also evaluated this treatment for people with specific phobias.

With at least one exception (Bates, McGlynn, Montgomery, & Mattke, 1996), early case studies suggested that EMDR might be useful for individuals with specific phobias of injections, blood, and medical situations (Kleinknecht, 1993; Lohr, Tolin, & Kleinknecht, 1995), claustrophobia (Lohr, Tolin, & Kleinknecht, 1996), and spider phobias (Muris & Merckelbach, 1995). However, in several of these reports (e.g., Lohr, Tolin, & Kleinknecht, 1995; Lohr et al., 1996; Muris & Merckelbach, 1995), the positive effects of EMDR appeared to be limited to subjective reports of fear, rather than indices of phobic avoidance and physiological measures.

Recently, larger group studies have confirmed the finding that EMDR appears to affect only subjective fear ratings (Muris, Merckelbach, Holdrinet, & Sijsenaar, 1998; Muris, Merckelbach, van Haaften, & Mayer, 1997). In addition, there is evidence that the active component of EMDR is imaginal exposure, and that the eye movements (or other forms of bilateral sensory simulation) are essentially irrelevant. Sanderson and Carpenter (1992) found no differences in the effectiveness of EMDR and imaginal exposure without eye movements. Moreover, studies that have compared EMDR to standard *in vivo* exposure for specific phobias have found that *in vivo* exposure leads to improvements on a broader range of measures (Muris, Merckelbach, Holdrinet, & Sijsenaar, 1998; Muris, Merckelbach, van Haaften, & Mayer, 1997).

In summary, the extent to which EMDR is effective is probably related to the effects of exposure. In light of the fact that *in vivo* exposure is more effective than EMDR and other forms of imaginal exposure, EMDR has little to offer for the treatment of specific phobias.

Applied Tension for BII Phobia

As discussed earlier, BII phobia is the only phobia type that is associated with fainting in response to the phobic situation. In two published case studies, Michael Kozak (Kozak & Miller, 1985; Kozak & Montgomery, 1981) first introduced muscle tension as a treatment for fainting induced by scenes of blood and injury. Since then, a number of controlled studies by Öst and colleagues have demonstrated that applied muscle tension is an effective treatment for BII phobias. Essentially, the treatment involves teaching the patient to tense the muscles of the body in order to raise his or her blood pressure. Once the skill is mastered, the patient is encouraged to use the technique while exposed to BII-related situations that tend to induce symptoms of faintness (Öst & Sterner, 1987). Originally, the treatment was designed to last five sessions (Öst & Sterner, 1987). However, Hellström, Fellenius, and Öst (1996) recently showed that a single session of applied tension along with a maintenance program of self-exposure is as effective as a five-session course of the same treatment.

Applied tension has been shown to be more effective than exposure alone for the treatment of blood phobia (Öst, Fellenius, & Sterner, 1991). In another study (Öst, Sterner, & Fellenius, 1989), few differences were found among applied tension, applied relaxation, and their combination for the treatment of blood phobia, although there was a nonsignificant tendency for the applied tension treatment to be more effective overall.

Cognitive Therapy

Although *in vivo* exposure is generally believed to be the treatment of choice for specific phobias, some investigators have examined the use of cognitive strategies either alone or in combination with exposure for treating phobias (for a review, see Craske & Rowe, 1997a). de Jongh et al. (1995) provided patients who had dental phobias with a single session of either cognitive restructuring or education about oral health and dental treatment.

Cognitive restructuring led to greater declines in fear than either the education condition or a wait-list control condition. One year later, both interventions were associated with additional significant declines in fear, although they were no longer significantly different.

In a related study, Jerremalm, Jansson, and Öst (1986) found that a cognitive intervention and applied relaxation (i.e., a combination of relaxation training with graduated *in vivo* exposure) were equally effective for treating dental phobia over nine group sessions. Although both treatments led to significant improvements overall, individual response patterns (i.e., whether participants were deemed to be "cognitive reactors" vs. "physiological reactors") did not predict improvements with one treatment or the other. Another study by Getka and Glass (1992) confirmed that cognitive strategies are useful for individuals with dental phobias.

Craske, Mohlman, et al. (1995) treated individuals with fears of enclosed places, spiders, or snakes with a combination of *in vivo* exposure and either relaxation training or cognitive restructuring of misappraisals regarding bodily sensations. Although both interventions were equally effective for treating spider and snake fears, individuals with claustrophobia benefited more from the addition of cognitive restructuring to change their beliefs regarding bodily sensations. However, 4 weeks following the end of treatment, this difference was no longer evident.

In a related study, Booth and Rachman (1992) compared *in vivo* exposure, interoceptive exposure (i.e., exposure to feared bodily sensations), and cognitive restructuring for the treatment of claustrophobia. On most measures, *in vivo* exposure was found to be the most effective treatment, and interoceptive exposure led to only small gains. Individuals who received cognitive therapy made significant gains relative to a control group, although these gains tended to be smaller than those made by individuals who received *in vivo* exposure. Regardless of the treatment condition, changes in anxious cognitions regarding claustrophobic situations tended to be associated with fear reduction during treatment (Shafran, Booth, & Rachman, 1993).

Panzarella and Garlipp (1999) provide a practical discussion of how cognitive strategies can be integrated into an exposure-based treatment program for BII phobias. In addition, step-by-step suggestions for combining cognitive strategies with exposure-based treatments for a range of specific phobias are provided by Antony and Swinson (2000).

Pharmacological Approaches

It is generally believed that medications offer little benefit in the treatment of specific phobias. In fact, models of emotional processing (e.g., Foa & Kozak, 1986) imply that medications should interfere with the effects of exposure-based treatments by preventing the individual's fear from increasing to a sufficient level.

An early study by Whitehead, Robinson, Blackwell, and Stutz (1978) found that adding diazepam had no effect on the time required to treat individuals with small-animal phobias. In a related study, Zoellner, Craske, Hussain, Lewis, and Echeveri (1996) found that adding alprazolam to exposure-based treatment for spider phobia had neither positive nor negative effects on outcome.

In contrast, Wilhelm and Roth (1997) found that taking alprazolam reduced self-reported anxiety in a group of individuals with flying phobias in the short term. However, having taken alprazolam rather than placebo during an initial flight led to greater fear during a second flight. In a similar study, Thom, Sartory, and Jöhren (2000) found that both cognitive-behavioral treatment and providing a benzodiazepine 30 minutes before dental treatment were effective for reducing fear experienced during dental surgery. However, benzodiazepine treatment was associated with greater relapse following dental treatment, whereas cognitive-behavioral therapy was associated with further improvements at follow-up. Taken together, these findings suggest that benzodiazepines are not effective long-term treatments for specific phobias and may even interfere with the therapeutic effects of exposure across sessions.

To date, no controlled studies have been published on the topic of antidepressants for specific phobias, although a single-case study by Abene and Hamilton (1998) found that fluoxetine led to a reduction in flying phobia for two individuals who were being treated for depression. Given that certain situational phobias (e.g., claustrophobia, driving phobia) share features of panic disorder with agoraphobia, it is possible that these specific phobia types might respond to treatment with antidepressants that have been shown to be useful for blocking panic attacks.

Relapse and Return of Fear

For the majority of patients, relapse following treatment of a specific phobia is thought to be rare (Öst, 1996a). However, one study that followed patients for an average of 12 years after treatment found that a considerable number of individuals experienced a clinically significant return of symptoms (Lipsitz, Mannuzza, Klein, Ross, & Fyer, 1999). In addition, it is well established that at least some return of fear in the presence of a particular stimulus often occurs (Craske, 1999; Rachman, 1989).

A number of variables have been shown to predict return of fear in people with specific phobias, although some findings have been inconsistent (Craske, 1999). Variables that have been shown to be associated with increased return of fear in at least some studies include distraction during exposure (Rose & McGlynn, 1997); a relatively quick reduction in fear during exposure (Rose & McGlynn, 1997); a relatively slow reduction in fear during exposure (Rachman & Lopatka, 1988; Rachman & Whittal, 1989), depression (Salkovskis & Mills, 1994); higher initial heart rate (Craske & Rachman, 1987); the spacing of exposure sessions (Rowe & Craske, 1998a); the extent to which the exposure stimuli are varied (Rowe & Craske, 1998b); and a tendency to show a covariation bias (i.e., a tendency to overassociate fear-relevant stimuli with aversive outcomes) immediately after treatment (de Jong, van den Hout, & Merckelbach, 1995). In addition, despite the hypothesis that incomplete fear reduction leads to greater return of fear, Rachman, Robinson, and Lopatka (1987) found the opposite to be true. Individuals with snake fear who experienced a 50% reduction in their fear following exposure were less likely to have their fear return than individuals who experienced a complete reduction in their fear.

CHAPTER 12

Posttraumatic Stress Disorder

TERENCE M. KEANE
DAVID H. BARLOW

One of the great questions in all of psychopathology concerns etiology. It is widely agreed that determining what causes emotional and behavioral disorders may ultimately lead to the development of preventive interventions that reduce the likelihood of a disorder's ever occurring. For this reason, the study of posttraumatic stress disorder (PTSD) is critically important in the study of psychopathology in general. With PTSD, it is possible to specify the onset of psychological and behavioral disturbance with good precision. As a result, it is a condition that may prove to be scientifically invaluable as we attempt to understand the relative contributions of constitutional factors, psychological parameters, and environmental contributants to the development of psychopathology.

Among the most important questions addressed in the past 20 years of research on PTSD is why some people develop this disabling psychological condition in the wake of exposure to traumatic life events when others, seemingly exposed to the same event, do not. To explain this, one needs to examine many different factors that make one person more vulnerable to developing PTSD following a particular traumatic stressor. Does rape "cause" PTSD? Does combat "cause" PTSD? The literature to date suggests that although these environmental events contribute to the development of PTSD, they generally interact with other factors to yield PTSD. To state it more accurately, we know the proximal or precipitating events (e.g., rape, combat) that activate this disorder in vulnerable individuals, but these events may not be sufficient to lead to the disorder in all exposed individuals. However, as the events become more severe in nature, the chances that they will lead to PTSD in people who experience them increase. As Sutker and Allain (1996) eloquently stated in their evaluation of the impact of torture experienced by U.S. former prisoners of war: "An accumulating literature suggests that as trauma events become universally brutal; more horrific, gruesome, and prolonged; and more threatening to life, the greater the likelihood that negative sequelae will develop. . . . Eventually all victims succumb to psychological distress." As the severity of a traumatic event increases, in other words, the role of personal or individual risk factors diminishes. For less severe (although still traumatic) events, constitutional, psychological, and environmental factors will all interact to determine who will and who will not develop PTSD. It is clear that PTSD or other negative psychological outcomes can arise in even the most emotionally stable and healthy individuals if the stressor is severe enough. The sudden death of a child constitutes one such stressor; prolonged torture represents another.

PTSD is characterized by high levels of anxiety, panic, and often depression. Yet the symptoms that appear to distinguish PTSD from other psychological disorders are the reliving experiences, such as a preoccupation with, nightmares about, and flashbacks recapitulating the precipitating event. These symptoms are typically present with an emotionally numb state, avoidance of cues that are reminders of the event, and a range of signs of elevated anxiety (such as insomnia, poor concentration, heightened startle reactions, hypervigilance for danger, and irritability).

When the disorder was initially conceptualized in the *Diagnostic and Statistical Manual of Mental Disorders*, third edition (DSM-III), traumatic events were considered extreme life stressors that were outside the range of normal human experience (American Psychiatric Association, 1980). However, several outstanding epidemiological studies since that time have yielded high prevalence rates of exposure to traumatic events in the general population, dismissing the idea that traumatic events were "outside the range of normal human experience." In contemporary society, traumatic events are frequent across age, race, gender, and socioeconomic status (Kessler, Sonnega, Bromet, Hughes, & Nelson, 1995).

HISTORY AND BACKGROUND

Historical depictions of PTSD can be traced to the story of Ulysses in Homer's *Iliad* and *Odyssey*, which are among the oldest literature in Western civilization (Shay, 1992). The devastating impact of fighting the Trojan War resulted in damaged character among many of those who survived. These changes were observed to be long-standing in nature and resulted in difficulties in returning to the warriors' homeland. Remarkably, the symptoms and behaviors described in Homer's works are similar to those observed among individuals with PTSD today.

Stephen Crane's description in *The Red Badge of Courage* of the psychological effects of combat experience in the American Civil War resulted in the term "soldier's heart." The effects of war were seen as a combination of the losses sustained in the war with the removal of soldiers from the interpersonal connections associated with their families, friends, and communities. Thus the adverse psychological consequences of combat, and of war more broadly, have been recognized for hundreds if not thousands of years.

Scientific study of war's effects reached new heights with World War II and its aftermath. Studies of combatants, former prisoners of war, survivors of the concentration camps and death camps, and resistance fighters indicated significant levels of psychological distress and mood disturbance among those who survived (e.g., Grinker & Spiegel, 1945). Although these conditions were not yet considered to be PTSD, they set the stage for the ultimate recognition of the long-term negative effects of exposure to traumatic stressors. This would, in time, lead to the construction of the PTSD diagnosis. Terms such as "shell shock," "combat fatigue," and "war neurosis" all seemed to capture the essence of war-related PTSD, though there was as yet no appreciation for how other traumatic life stressors produced the same psychological effects. It wasn't until Ann Burgess, working at Boston City Hospital, observed the impact of rape on women that the term "rape trauma syndrome" was coined (Burgess & Holmstrom, 1974). Concomitantly, American and Australian veterans of the Vietnam War were also searching for an understanding of their psychological distress following that politically difficult conflict. Advocates for these two disenfranchised populations (i.e., rape survivors and Vietnam veterans) teamed with scholars who had studied and treated World War II veterans and concentration camp survivors to create the synergy necessary to construct the diagnosis of PTSD.

Yet even before the great wars of the 20th century, anxiety as a response to severe stress was observed and labeled "traumatic neurosis" by Oppenheim (1892; cited by Kraepelin, 1896) or *Schreckneurose* (i.e., "fright neurosis") by Kraepelin (1896). Kraepelin considered this condition a separate clinical entity "composed of multiple nervous and psychic phenomenon arising as a result of severe emotional upheaval or sudden fright which build up great anxiety; it can therefore be observed after serious accidents and injuries, particularly fires, railway derailments, or collisions, etc." (Kraepelin, 1896; translation by Jablensky, 1985, p. 737). In view of the early and clear recognition of this emotional disorder, it is surprising that controversy regarding its validity emerged during the 1970s and 1980s (Figley, 1978; Goodwin & Guze, 1984). Although much of the initial controversy about PTSD's validity has ceased (Keane, Wolfe, & Taylor, 1987), the nature of the disorder still instigates considerable debate in the field (Yehuda & McFarlane, 1995).

Epidemiological studies now confirm that PTSD occurs following a wide range of extreme life events. War, rape, torture, crime, vehicular accidents, industrial accidents, sudden death of a loved one—all result in the development of PTSD in a certain proportion of those exposed. Many early examples of these reactions have been recorded over the centuries by those inclined to write them down. One of the better-known descriptions is the reaction of the famous 17th-century diarist, Samuel Pepys, after the Great Fire of London in 1666. This catastrophe resulted in substantial loss of life and property and in marked disorganization in the city, all of which was very well described by Pepys. Fully 6 months after the fire, he recorded: "It is strange to think how to this very day I cannot sleep a night without great terrors of fire; and this very night could not sleep to almost 2 in the morning through thoughts of fire" (quoted in Daly, 1983, p. 66). Insomnia, and recurring dreams of the event, are of course prominent features of PTSD as we know it today; however, Pepys also manifested mild depersonalization, as well as some characteristic guilt about saving himself and his property while others died (known as "survivors' guilt").

In addition to recurrent and intrusive recollections and dreams concerning the event, an individual may experience "flashback" episodes wherein he or she seems to experience a recurrence of at least a portion of the traumatic event. Individuals describe these experiences "as if it's happening all over again." These flashbacks can often contain input from all senses—sights, sounds, smells, tastes, and tactile sensations recapitulating the traumatic event—and they can be extraordinarily frightening.

Extreme distress and avoidance of cues or reminders of the event also accompany PTSD. This avoidance may involve an inability to remember aspects of the traumatic event itself. The debate over the nature of trauma memories has captured the attention of clinicians and cognitive psychologists the world over. The discussion hinges on the notion of "recovered memories," which are typically (but not exclusively) of child sexual abuse. Rancorous at times, this debate led the International Society for Traumatic Stress Studies to impanel a representative team of clinicians, researchers and scholars to study the matter. The senior editors of this effort (Roth & Friedman, 1998) concluded as follows, based on the available scientific evidence:

> We know that people forget childhood traumas and that this is not limited to people in treatment or to people whose trauma is sexual abuse. We also know that people can accurately recall memories of documented childhood trauma that they report having previously forgotten,

and that a wide range of triggers seem to be associated with these memories. Most memory recovery appears to be precipitated in situations that include cues that are similar to the original trauma and does not occur as a direct result of psychotherapy (i.e. memories implanted or imposed by a therapist). However, it is possible, and indeed many would argue likely, that therapists who fail to conform to accepted standards of practice may promote a "recovered memory" of an event that never occurred. (p. 23)

The issue of recovered memory has unfortunately been tied to the societal problems associated with childhood sexual abuse. Yet there is considerable clinical evidence across different types of traumatic events that individuals store memories for traumatic events in unusual ways. For example, news about an explosion aboard a U.S. aircraft carrier brought a World War II Navy veteran to seek counseling from the National Center for PTSD for a traumatic event he had experienced 45 years earlier, which he reportedly had not thought about since his return stateside. When the newscasts of the current explosion reminded him of the death and destruction that he experienced as a function of a Japanese kamikaze attack, he developed acute symptoms of PTSD. Did he forget this event? Did he distract himself effectively for nearly half a century? Did he take this opportunity to reveal the experience to others? This is the nature of the scientific debate and discussion regarding traumatic memory and what has been termed "recovered memory" of trauma. More scientific information is needed before firm conclusions can be drawn regarding the nature of recovered memories of traumatic events.

Additional symptoms of PTSD also include emotional numbing, described by patients as an inability to feel any positive emotions such as love, contentment, satisfaction, or happiness. As such, the emotional numbing is disruptive to intimate and interpersonal relationships. Conceptualizations of emotional numbing are rare, but Litz and his colleagues (Flack, Litz, Hsieh, Kaloupek, & Keane, 2000; Litz, 1992; Litz & Keane, 1989; Litz, Orsillo, Kaloupek, & Weathers, 2000) have approached this problem from an information-processing perspective. Employing experimental psychopathology paradigms and using epidemiological data, they have concluded that the intensity of the anxiety and arousal symptoms in patients with PTSD appears to drive the extent of the emotional numbing observed.

PTSD is further characterized by trouble sleeping, trouble concentrating, an enhanced startle reaction, and difficulty controlling anger. Hypervigilance for danger is yet another component of the condition. Finally, individuals with PTSD live for the present, rarely planning for the future. This sense of a foreshortened future has a significant impact on the development of life trajectories for the large number of children, adolescents, and young adults who are plagued with this disorder.

While the emotional aspects of PTSD are substantial, the societal, interpersonal, and psychosocial consequences are considerable. People who develop PTSD are more likely to utilize expensive medical services inappropriately, to earn less and divorce more often than the general population, and to become involved with the legal system; they also report greater dissatisfaction with their lives, have more trouble raising their children, and change jobs frequently (Koss, Koss, & Woodruff, 1991; Kulka et al., 1990). Thus exposure to traumatic events and the subsequent development of PTSD constitute a major problem for the public health of this nation and the world. When rates of exposure and PTSD are considered in conjunction with the costs associated with PTSD, efforts to prevent the occurrence of traumatic events and their psychological sequelae become a universal priority. The development of successful treatments for the survivors who develop PTSD also becomes an important public health goal. As with many disorders and conditions, we have accomplished more in terms of developing treatments than we have in prevention. This chapter outlines our achievements to date and the directions for further work.

INCIDENCE, PREVALENCE, AND COURSE

As noted above, when PTSD was initially conceptualized in the DSM-III, both it and the exposure to traumatic events were considered relatively rare conditions. Since the incorporation of PTSD into the diagnostic nomenclature, numerous epidemiological studies have been completed. In addition to examining the prevalence of PTSD, these studies have provided us with information on rates of exposure to traumatic life events, the rates of comorbidity of PTSD with other psychiatric conditions, and the distribution of PTSD among various subgroups of the population (e.g., adults, adolescents, children; males and females; minorities; and particular groups at risk, such as war veterans). They have also helped to establish factors that affect the onset and course of PTSD.

Most studies on the prevalence of traumatic events and PTSD have examined these rates in the United States. Few methodologically sound studies pursuing general population estimates of PTSD have been conducted in other parts of the world. Yet the vast majority of the wars, violence, and natural disasters occurring in the 20th and into the 21st centuries have actually occurred in the developing world. With increasing recognition of the health and economic costs associated with psychological morbidity across the world (Murray & Lopes, 1996), there is a growing acknowledgment of the need for regional and world estimates of psychiatric disorders, including PTSD.

PTSD in the General Population

The first study that attempted to examine the prevalence of PTSD in the general population was the Epidemiologic Catchment Area (ECA) study. Helzer, Robins, and McEvoy (1987) examined data from the St. Louis site only (of the five sites included in the study). As measured by the National Institute of Mental Health's Diagnostic Interview Schedule (DIS), the prevalence of PTSD was observed to be 1% of the general population. Rates of PTSD were higher in women than in men. Scholars criticized this study because of the limited sampling of the population, the manner in which traumatic events were elicited (i.e., asking the participants to categorize the events as traumatic), and the accuracy of the DIS PTSD module (Keane & Penk, 1988). Most leaders in the field felt that the findings were underestimates of PTSD.

Breslau, Davis, Andreski, and Peterson (1991) reported the results of a survey of 1,007 randomly selected members of a health maintenance organization (HMO) in the Detroit, Michigan area. The sample was one of young adults aged 21–30 years. Using an update of the DIS that attempted to address the limitations of the earlier version, they found a prevalence rate for the general population of 9.5%, with 11.3% in women and 5.6% in men. They also found that nearly 40% of the participants had experienced one or more of the traumatic events about which they inquired, a striking finding in itself.

As noted in Chapter 1, perhaps the most complete general population study was that conducted by Kessler and his colleagues (e.g., Kessler et al., 1995), the National Comorbidity Survey (NCS). The investigators interviewed 5,877 nationally representative individuals in the United States from the ages of 15 to 54 years, using an updated version of the DIS, while recording prevalence of different types of traumatic events and their impact. They found an overall prevalence rate of PTSD of 7.8%, with the rate for women (10.4%) more than twice that for men (5.0%). Estimates for trauma exposure indicated that about 60% of men were exposed to one or more traumatic events, while 51% of women were so exposed.

The NCS also provided information on the types of events most likely to lead to PTSD. Rape and combat were the life events most likely to produce PTSD. The sudden death of a loved one, a very common experience across the sample, was actually the single event that yielded the most cases of PTSD in NCS, even though combat and rape were more likely to result in PTSD from a probability perspective.

There were important demographic differences between those who did and did not develop PTSD. In addition to the large gender difference, Kessler et al. (1995) found a positive association between age and trauma exposure for males and females; as well, there was a slight negative correlation between age and PTSD. These findings indicate, expectedly, that as people age they are more likely to be exposed to traumatic events, but that when they are exposed at an older age there is a trend toward less likelihood of developing PTSD. Kessler et al. also found that marriage seemed to confer some level of protection, as those who were currently married, as opposed to previously married, separated, or widowed, had lower rates of PTSD even when trauma exposure was held constant.

Focusing upon sexual abuse of college-age women, Koss, Gidycz, and Wisniewski (1987) surveyed 3,187 college women about sexual assault and rape. They found that 15.4% of the sample reported that they had been raped, and that another 12.1% reported that someone had attempted to rape them. This study did not collect information about PTSD, but it did set the stage for the National Women's Study, which examined many types of traumatic events in women and corresponding psychological disorders. Kilpatrick, Edmunds, and Seymour (1992) studied 4,008 women, using telephone interviews and the DIS. Thirteen percent of the women of all ages reported a completed rape, 32% of these reported lifetime PTSD. Twelve percent of those raped still had rape-related PTSD at the time of the survey.

Being the target of, or otherwise affected by, a crime is another type of traumatic event that can lead to psychological distress. In a national study of exposure to crime among women in the United States, Resnick, Kilpatrick, Dansky, Saunders, and Best (1993) found that 36% of women reported being directly affected by crime at some point in their lives. Attempted rape or molestation was most frequently reported (14%); death of a friend or family member by homicide was next (13%); experiencing a completed rape was third highest (12.7%); and being physically assaulted was fourth highest (10%). They found an overall PTSD prevalence rate of 12% lifetime and nearly 5% current (within the past 6 months). Resnick et al. found, as have others, that exposure to interpersonal violence increased the likelihood that women developed PTSD. Overall, rates of lifetime (25.8%) and current (8.9%) PTSD were higher for those exposed to crime than for those not exposed (9.4% and 3.4%, respectively).

In a study of adults residing in four Southeastern urban communities, Norris (1992) examined rates of exposure to traumatic events and PTSD. She asked those interviewed in the survey whether they had been exposed to any of eight broad categories of traumatic events. Current rates of PTSD were reported to be 5%, with PTSD most likely to occur following sexual assault (14%), physical assault (13%), and motor vehicle accidents (12%). Clearly, the prevalence of exposure to traumatic events is far more common than anyone anticipated in 1980 when the diagnosis of PTSD was incorporated into the diagnostic nomenclature. Exposure to trauma is common. Even more surprising is that the rate of PTSD in the general population falls only behind the rates of alcoholism, major depression, and social phobia, making it the fourth most common psychiatric condition in the

United States. The high level of disability often associated with PTSD clearly makes it a major public health problem.

PTSD in Combatants

Clearly certain subgroups within our society are at increased risk for being exposed to traumatic life events and for subsequently developing PTSD. The soldiers we send to fight wars and to keep peace are among those most at risk. Orner (1992) reported that in Europe alone there have been over 60 incidents involving military action or terrorism since 1918. The total number of wars across the world in the last half of the 20th century was estimated in the early 1990s at about 150 (Zwi, 1991). Yet few countries have ever tried to assess the psychological toll of war.

The major exception to this was the Vietnam War. The National Vietnam Veterans Readjustment Study (NVVRS; Kulka et al., 1990) was the first time that any government attempted to systematically understand the psychological costs of participating in a war. Employing a two-stage methodology (Dohrenwend & Shrout, 1981), lay interviewers evaluated a representative sample of Vietnam theater veterans (VTVs; n = 1,632), a matched sample of Vietnam era veterans (VEVs; n = 716) and civilian comparison subjects (n = 668). In the second stage of the study, all individuals seen as positive cases in Stage 1 were again interviewed, this time by a clinician using a structured diagnostic instrument (the Structured Clinical Interview for DSM [SCID]; Spitzer, Williams, Gibbon, & First, 1985). A particularly impressive fact about the design of this study was its inclusion of samples of women, African Americans, and Hispanic Americans, which would permit an analysis of the impact of the war on these important subgroups of those who served in Vietnam.

The findings on exposure to traumatic events were rather striking. Sixty-four percent of the VTVs were exposed to one or more traumatic events in their lives in contrast to 48% among the VEVs and 45% among the civilians. Clearly, the exposure rates across all groups were high. To make the diagnosis of PTSD, the NVVRS investigators relied upon a triangulation approach that utilized information from the diagnostic interviews as well as several self-report questionnaires that were administered (e.g., the Mississippi Scale; Keane, Caddell, & Taylor, 1988). Findings indicated that more than 15% of male VTVs met criteria for current PTSD and 30% met criteria for lifetime PTSD. Among the female VTVS, 9% met criteria for current PTSD and 27% met criteria for lifetime PTSD. In all cases, these prevalence rates were 5–10 times higher than those found for the VEVs and the civilians. These findings indicated that there were approximately 479,000 cases of current PTSD and nearly 1 million cases of lifetime PTSD in America stemming from the Vietnam War alone.

The NVVRS also reported findings for African American and Hispanic groups that served in Vietnam, as noted above. Of the approximately 3.14 million Americans who served in Vietnam nearly 170,000 were Hispanic Americans and 350,000 were African Americans. There were different rates for current PTSD among the various ethnic and racial groups: For the European American/other group the prevalence of current PTSD was 13.7%, while for the African Americans it was 20.6% and the Hispanic Americans it was 27.9%. The differences were largely due to higher levels of combat exposure among the minorities. Gender differences were also apparent in the NVVRS: Female VTVs had lower rates of PTSD than did the males. However, much of this difference must be attributed to the different roles that women had in the military at that time (primarily nursing and clerical), the different types of stressors to which they were exposed, and the higher educational levels among the women.

The NVVRS was a rare study in that it had an instant effect on public policy toward war veterans in America. Based on the findings, Congress allocated increased resources to address the psychological and social effects of war on veterans. These programs continue today and serve veterans of all wars, conflicts, and peacekeeping missions. In recognition of the prevalence of sexual assault among women veterans, programs have expanded to address the needs of sexual assault survivors as well.

There has been considerable debate about the impact of the Persian Gulf War on the soldiers sent to free Kuwait. Sutker, Uddo, Brailey, and Allain (1993) examined a convenience sample of 215 troops sent to the Persian Gulf. They found a prevalence rate of 16–19% for PTSD. Wolfe, Brown, and Kelley (1993) conducted a longitudinal study of 2,344 Persian Gulf veterans and found prevalence rates of PTSD based upon the Mississippi Scale (Keane et al., 1988) of 4% for men and 9% for women. Perconte et al. (1993) found a prevalence rate of 16% among 439 reservists sent to the Persian Gulf, whereas a prevalence of less than 4% was found for reservists deployed elsewhere or who remained at home. Clearly, the exposure to combat and war-related traumatic events yielded discernible levels of PTSD among various Persian Gulf veteran cohorts. Still under discussion is the extent to which the military in the Persian Gulf was exposed to toxicants (e.g., depleted uranium, burning oil, pesticides), which might be responsible for the increased levels of disorder and disability observed following that war. It is likely that these factors all interacted with the stress of deployment, combat, and reentry to yield the diverse psychological and health problems in this most recent cohort of American veterans.

Since the end of the Cold War, the United States and other leading nations have intervened, often with the United Nations, in efforts to maintain peace in many areas of the world. Peacekeeping has its own set of associated stressors, and increasingly these are being recognized as leading to PTSD. For example, peacekeeping forces are often instructed not to fire unless others fire upon them; they are also asked to patrol areas that are often under tenuous control. It is reasonable, then, to ask whether peacekeeping duties can lead to PTSD. Litz, Orsillo, Friedman, Ehlich, and Batres (1997) examined a sample of 3,461 active-duty military troops who served in Somalia, a particularly gruesome peacekeeping assignment for U.S. soldiers. Studied shortly after their return to the United States, these soldiers manifested a prevalence rate of PTSD of 8%—a rate that didn't differ for men and women. Clearly, those who serve as peacekeepers across the world are at risk for developing PTSD, even though the actions are not seen as traditional combat.

PTSD in Disaster Contexts

There is a burgeoning literature supporting the idea that a wide range of natural disasters and accidents can lead to the development of PTSD. Green and her colleagues first studied the psychological impact of the collapse of the Buffalo Creek Dam in West Virginia in the late 1970s. Initially they found that 44% of the survivors reached criteria for PTSD. When the survivors were studied some 14 years later, 28% of the sample still met criteria for PTSD, indicating that the effects of this type of disaster are long-lasting (Green, Lindy, Grace, et al., 1990; Green, Grace, Lindy, et al., 1990).

Similarly, McFarlane (1989) studied the effects of bush fires in Australia. These fires often burn for days and weeks, leaving disaster in their wake and challenging even the best firefighting teams to predict or to control them. Death, injury, and destruction are commonplace. Examining 315 firefighters, McFarlane found prevalence rates of PTSD of 32%, 27%, and 30% respectively at 4, 11, and 29 months after the disaster. Again, therefore, high rates of PTSD followed a disaster—rates that were sustained for a substantial period of time following the exposure.

These are just a few of the many different types of disasters that have been studied successfully over the past 20 years. These elevated rates and figures are not unusual; rather they are more typical than not. Studies of Three Mile Island (Bromet et al., 1982), Chernobyl (Havenaar et al., 1997), and the Lockerbie air disaster (Brooks & McKinlay, 1992) all indicate pervasive traumatic reactions in survivors, regardless of age, gender, or socioeconomic status. The maturing epidemiological literature on the effects of trauma exposure and PTSD has yielded considerable evidence to suggest that these events themselves contribute substantially to the development of PTSD and related disability and dysfunction.

PTSD in Children

PTSD is also common in children and adolescents. Kilpatrick and Saunders (1999) conducted a nationally representative survey of adolescents that included diagnostic interviews. They found that in adolescents under the age of 18, the current prevalence rate of PTSD was 5% of the U.S. population. Again, prevalence was higher among females than among males. The events most likely to yield PTSD were abuse and violence, often at the hands of family members.

Although there is still no nationwide epidemiological study of psychiatric conditions in children, there are excellent studies of the exposure of children to violence. Bell and Jenkins (1993) studied 536 African American elementary students (grades 2, 4, 6, and 8) at three different schools in urban Chicago. Strikingly, 26% of the students had seen someone being shot, and 30% had observed someone being stabbed. Moreover, 75% of the students stated that they had been exposed to at least one violent crime. Similar reports of exposure to violence in children abound in the literature (e.g., Burton, Foy, Bwanausi, Johnson, & Moore, 1994; Singer, Anglin, Song, & Lunghofer, 1995).

There are many studies examining rates of stress and PTSD among specific subgroups of children and adolescents. For example, Saigh (1988) examined civilian adolescents during various periods of war stress in Lebanon. He found that as time intervals reflecting high levels of combat alternated with periods of peace, these children systematically reported elevations in anxiety and depression and low levels of assertiveness. These changes reflected functional impairments as well, with the children having increasing difficulties at home and at school as they experienced stress secondary to the war.

In their evaluations of the survivors of the Buffalo Creek Dam collapse, Green and her colleagues found that among the 179 children they studied, some 37% had "probable" PTSD. Following Hurricane Andrew, a natural disaster, La Greca, Silverman, Vernberg, and Prinstein (1996) found a 30% prevalence rate of PTSD at 3 months, 18% at 7 months, and 13% at the 10-month follow-up among school-age children. These studies of selected high-risk samples of the population indicate that when children and adolescents are exposed to the death and destruction accompanying technological and natural disasters, they experience high rates of PTSD.

The Armenian earthquake of 1988 was one of the most dramatic of the natural disasters studied to date, in part because of the high levels of destruction near the earthquake's epicenter. Goenjian et al. (1995) found a PTSD prevalence among the children closest to the epicenter (mean age = 13 years) of 95%; among those children at a moderate distance from the epicenter, there was a PTSD prevalence of 71%; and for those furthest from the destruction, there was a PTSD prevalence of 26%. The linear relationship between intensity of the experience and the development of PTSD demonstrates the powerful effect of the traumatic event per se in the development of this psychological condition.

Finally, Garrison, Weinrich, Hardin, Weinrich, and Wang (1993) found a prevalence rate of 5% current PTSD in over 1,200 students who had been exposed to a disastrous hurricane in South Carolina. In all of these studies on disasters, the selection of participants for inclusion in the sample was not representative of the general population in the areas studied. For this reason, conclusions must be drawn tentatively; yet these studies provide an excellent base from which additional studies might be conducted following major life stressors. Clearly, the evidence suggests that either technological or natural disasters can yield high rates of PTSD, and that (as in adults), the more directly children or adolescents are affected, the more likely they are to develop PTSD.

PTSD Following Childhood Sexual Abuse

Childhood sexual abuse is one crime that has gotten increasing attention in the scientific literature since the publication of the classic book *Father–Daughter Incest*, by psychiatrist Judith Herman (1981). Growing empirical data suggest that the true prevalence of childhood sexual assault and the resulting psychological impact of this abuse are both greater than initially thought (Finkelhor & Dziuba-Leatherman, 1994). Past studies were hampered in part by the reporting requirements of governmental agencies and in part by the reluctance of family members to come forward when evidence of abuse (especially intrafamilial abuse) is uncovered (Freyd, 1994). As well, there is still no nationwide study that has attempted to tackle the many technical, methodological, political, and ethical issues involved in investigating sexual abuse in children and its relationship to psychiatric disorder (e.g., PTSD). Still, a number of studies of convenience samples indicate the difficulties experienced by some children who are identified as having been sexually abused.

McLeer, Deblinger, Atkins, Foa, and Ralphe (1988) studied 32 patients at a university clinic for sexually abused children. Using a locally constructed interview, they found that 48% of the participants met DSM-III criteria for PTSD. Similarly, McLeer, Deblinger, Henry, and Orvaschel (1992) examined 92 children who had been sexually abused and reported that 44% of the children reached criteria for PTSD, with those abused by their parent or a trusted adult more likely to have PTSD than those abused by a stranger or older youth.

In New Zealand, Merry and Andrews (1994) studied 66 children 3 to 6 months following the index sexual abuse event. Some 64% of these children met criteria for a psychiatric condition, and 18% of the sample met criteria for PTSD. These findings support the concept that traumatic events can precipitate PTSD as well as other psychiatric conditions. Interestingly, in Canada, Wolfe, Sas, and Wekerle (1994) used a locally constructed PTSD scale to examine 90 children with court-documented childhood sexual abuse. In their sample, Wolfe et al. (1994) found that 49% met DSM criteria for PTSD—a considerably higher rate than in the Merry and Andrews (1994) study.

Methodological differences in the studies discussed above limit the extent of our conclusions about the prevalence rate of PTSD in the general population of children and adolescents. Particularly problematic is the absence of measures that are widely accepted for measuring PTSD in children and adolescents. Although there have been several excellent attempts to address this limitation (Fredrick, Pynoos, & Nader, 1992; Nader et al., 1998; Saigh, 1989), to date no single instrument has proved itself to be the assessment device of choice for children and adolescents. This has clearly limited the extent to which sound epidemiological studies of the prevalence of PTSD in children can be conducted.

A MODEL OF THE ETIOLOGY OF PTSD

As noted earlier, we do not yet know the "cause" of PTSD, but identification of the precipitating event or proximal cause is relatively simple. In this sense, the etiology of PTSD seems much more straightforward, based on the theoretical descriptions of anxiety and fear described in Chapters 7 and 8. Unlike specific phobia, where true alarms, false alarms, or (less often) simple transmission of information may develop into a phobic reaction, PTSD seems to emerge from one special chain of events. Intense basic emotions, such as true alarms (but also including rage or distress, resulting from the overwhelming effects of traumatic life events), lead to learned alarms. Learned alarms occur during exposure to situations that symbolize or resemble an aspect of the traumatic event. This is one of the defining features of PTSD in DSM-IV (American Psychiatric Association, 1994).

Among occasions that symbolize aspects of the traumatic event are anniversaries of the trauma. As in any phobic reaction, the development of learned alarms results in persistent avoidance of stimuli associated with the trauma, which is another defining feature of PTSD in DSM-IV. Other stimuli associated with the trauma include thoughts or feelings, as well as memories of the event.

Wirtz and Harrell (1987) provide support for the process of classical conditioning (learned alarms) within PTSD. They observed that survivors of physical assault were less distressed 6 months after the assault if they had experienced exposure to situations or stimuli that were part of (or resembled) the context of the original assault without experiencing another assault. Survivors who had not had the advantage of this exposure, on the other hand, maintained a high level of distress in the 6-month interim. This is what one would expect in classical conditioning. Others have noted the seeming importance of conditioning in the development of PTSD (Keane, Fairbank, Caddell, Zimering, & Bender, 1985; Orr et al., 2000), whether the trauma is combat-related, involves a physical assault such as sexual assault (e.g., Holmes & St. Lawrence, 1983; Kilpatrick, Veronen, & Best, 1985; Orr et al., 1998), or is the consequence of terrorism (Shalev et al., 2000).

This suggests an important similarity to panic disorder that has been alluded to above. In PTSD, the experience of affect itself is avoided to some extent; this is characterized clinically as a numbing of general responsiveness. This seems to be similar to the tendency of patients with panic disorder to avoid feelings such as those occasioned by movies, whether they be frightening, sad, or exciting. According to the conceptualizations presented above, fear is associated with interoceptive cues signaling the possible occurrence of another false alarm (learned alarm). The numbing of general responsiveness in PTSD would seem to represent avoidance of aversive emotional reactions or alarms (Jones & Barlow, 1990; Litz, 1992; Litz et al., 2000). Whether the sensitivity to or avoidance of interoceptive cues in panic and the numbing of general responsiveness in PTSD are identical psychopathological responses remains to be demonstrated.

In any case, the experience of alarm or other intense emotions is not sufficient in and of itself for the development of PTSD. Much as in other disorders, one must develop anxiety or the sense that these events, including one's own emotional reactions to them, are proceeding in an unpredictable, uncontrollable manner. When negative affect (including a sense of uncontrollability) develops, one enters the vicious cycle of anxious apprehension described in Chapter 3, and PTSD emerges.

This implies that a psychological and biological vulnerability to develop the disorder exists, as outlined in Chapter 8. There, it is also noted that anxiety is always moderated to some extent by variables such as the presence of adequate coping skills and social support. In PTSD (as indicated in the work of the Kings; see "Modeling the Prediction of PTSD," below), evidence already exists that these moderating variables play a role in determining whether the disorder develops or not. Therefore, these factors are represented explicitly in the model presented in this chapter, although it is assumed that these factors moderate the occurrence of other anxiety disorders to an equal extent. A model of the etiology of PTSD is presented in Figure 12.1. An elaboration of the evidence supporting various aspects of the model is presented below.

RISK FACTORS

Interest in risk factors has grown considerably in recent years. In their comprehensive and illuminating review of risk factors entitled "Coming to Terms with the Terms of Risk," Kraemer et al. (1997) define the various forms of risk factor analysis that accompany epidemiological studies. In particular, these authors emphasize that risk factors are true correlates of a particular disorder. Risk factors differ from simple correlates, in that they are found to precede the onset of the disorder itself. They are then considered to be candidates for "causal risk factors," or ones that contribute to the etiology of the disorder.

Interest in risk factor analysis is important, because the identification of risk factors may assist us in the development of preventative approaches for people who are at highest risk for developing the disorder. These interventions, in the case of PTSD, may precede the occurrence of a traumatic event or may help us to identify those people at greatest risk for developing PTSD when exposed to massive traumatic events such as country- or region-wide technological disasters (e.g., the Chernobyl nuclear disaster). The study of risk factors, then, takes many different forms, some of which are examined below for their relevance to helping us better understand the etiology of PTSD.

Family Studies

What factors might account for the development of PTSD in some individuals following exposure to a major life stressor, but not in others undergoing seemingly the same stressor?

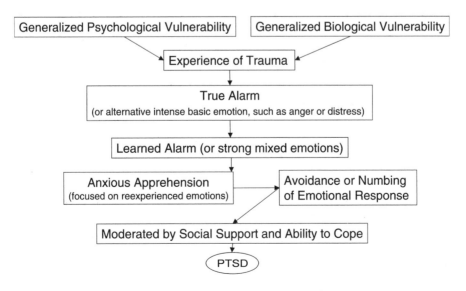

FIGURE 12.1. A model of the etiology of PTSD.

As reviewed above, a generalized biological vulnerability consisting of constitutional and hereditary variables is a major focus. Other contributing variables include the extent of exposure, the number of exposures to the same or similar traumatic events, the coping strategies of the individual, the availability of social support, and a generalized psychological vulnerability to developing anxiety/negative affect.

Examination of the evidence surrounding the constitutional/hereditary contributions to PTSD yields little systematic evidence to date that bears on this issue. Discriminating the predisposition for exposure to traumatic events from the predisposition to developing PTSD also represents a methodological and interpretive challenge. For example, people who are risk takers (e.g., skydivers) may actually be more likely to be exposed to traumatic events. Will they also be more or less likely to develop PTSD once exposed? Do the factors that predispose them to be risk takers function to prevent them from developing PTSD? These are questions of profound importance to accurately identifying those variables that contribute to the development of PTSD.

What has the literature told us about candidate risk factors for PTSD? Curran and Mallinson (1940) compared the family histories of 100 British soldiers returning from World War II with psychoneurosis to those of 50 surgical controls. Forty-five percent of the psychiatric casualties had a family member with a past psychiatric hospitalization, functional impairment, or a suicide attempt—a percentage considerably higher than that in the comparison group.

Cohen, White, and Johnson (1948) compared the family histories of 144 World War II service personnel with neurasthenia to those of 105 healthy comparisons, and 48 veterans and medical patients. The authors noted particularly high rates of neurasthenia in the mothers of the index group (58%), but also in the fathers (19%) and in the siblings (13%). The authors reported that no such histories were found in the comparison groups. Importantly, this study also interviewed a small subgroup of family members in the index group ($n = 15$) and confirmed the reports of the patients themselves. This was among the earliest efforts to incorporate family interviews into studies of family history of psychopathology.

Davidson, Swartz, Storck, Krishnan, and Hammett (1985) conducted the only family study to date of PTSD using contemporary methods of interviewing and diagnosis. Selecting patients from World War II with diagnoses of PTSD, they found familial rates of disorder in 66% of the participants. Of course, these patients were seeking help and may not truly represent PTSD in the general population; nonetheless, these data provide some preliminary support for the idea that there is a hereditary contribution to the development of PTSD. Similarly, in his examination of survivors of disastrous bush fires in Australia, McFarlane (1988) reported that 55% of those with PTSD had relatives with a psychiatric condition, whereas only 20% of those who did not develop PTSD reported such a family history.

In addition, two epidemiological studies indicated a possible family contribution to the development of PTSD. Davidson, Hughes, Blazer, and George (1991) examined the ECA data from the North Carolina site and observed that people with PTSD were three times more likely to report family psychiatric disorders than were comparison participants. In the Detroit HMO study, Breslau et al. (1991) observed elevations in reported family rates of several anxiety, mood, and psychotic disorders among those with PTSD. These epidemiological studies are all subject to problems with bias in retrospective recall. Although they do provide some important preliminary evidence, there is a need for future studies in this area to use contemporary methods of sampling, diagnosis, and family interviews, in order for more firm conclusions to be drawn on the role of constitutional/hereditary factors in the development of PTSD.

Twin studies have also provided some evidence supporting a constitutional basis for PTSD. True et al. (1993), using the Vietnam Veteran Twin Registry, found heritability factors for exposure to combat as well as to several of the PTSD symptoms. Yet this study used only questionnaire data in the analysis, and so strong conclusions must be deferred. Pitman and his colleagues (2000), using this same twin registry, attempted to elucidate the parameters that might underlie PTSD. Using a wide variety of laboratory tasks (e.g., psycho-physiological reactivity, evoked related potentials) and standardized diagnostic tools, they found little evidence for an inherited component for PTSD.

In summary, there is preliminary evidence suggesting that there may be a constitutional/hereditary component for PTSD. Yet most studies conducted to date have methodological and procedural limitations that compromise our capacity to draw strong inferences. Pitman et al. (2000) have presented only the preliminary analyses of their excellent twin study, and these did not seem to identify key constitutional variables. Additional studies will be required in order to identify those biological and physiological variables that interact with traumatic events to produce PTSD. At best, we can conclude that the presence of a family history of psychopathology increases the likelihood that one will develop PTSD once exposed to a traumatic event. Although the precise nature of this relationship remains to be further explored, it is likely that a generalized neurobiological tendency to react in an exaggerated manner to stress—described in Chapters 6 and 8 as associated with the development of all anxiety disorders and depression—also describes the generalized biological vulnerability to develop PTSD.

Demographic Risk Factors

Epidemiological studies of trauma exposure and PTSD provide one important way in which we can determine who develops PTSD following certain traumatic events. The NCS (Kessler et al., 1995), as noted earlier, included a representative sample of males and females between the ages of 15 and 54 from the 48 contiguous states. Information about PTSD was collected in face-to-face interviews on a subset of participants (5,877 of the 8,098 total). Consistent with prior research on women (Kilpatrick & Resnick, 1992), PTSD was found to vary as a function of the type of traumatic events experienced; rape, childhood physical abuse, and childhood neglect were the most likely events to lead to PTSD in this national sample. Each of these three types of events was also more likely to occur in women. Although men were more likely to report a traumatic event than women, women were more likely to report a traumatic event that was strongly linked to developing PTSD.

Breslau, Chilcoat, Kessler, Peterson, and Lucia (1999), in the Detroit HMO trauma study, examined the link between gender and PTSD in an effort to determine whether the higher prevalence of PTSD consistently observed among women is simply a function of the types of events to which they are differentially exposed. They found that the risk of developing PTSD among women was approximately twice that of men even when types of traumatic events were taken into account. Findings from the NCS supported these conclusions as well. The precise nature of the mechanism involved in the sex difference in PTSD has not yet been explained, but it is a consistent finding across most anxiety disorders, and is a question of such high importance that it will undoubtedly receive considerable attention in the future. Hypothetical explanations for a differential generalized psychological vulnerability based on gender are reviewed in Chapter 8.

In addition to gender, age has been examined as a risk factor for exposure to traumatic events and to developing PTSD. Among women, the NCS found no relationship between age and PTSD, and only a small relationship between age and exposure to traumatic events. In contrast, among men there was a strong positive correlation between age and PTSD, and this was due to increasing exposure to traumatic events over the lifespan.

The findings regarding race as a risk factor are somewhat complicated. To draw again upon the NCS data, African Americans and other minorities (Asian Americans and Native Americans) reported fewer exposures to traumatic events than did European Americans and Hispanic Americans. Yet these same groups (i.e., African Americans and other minorities) reported higher rates of PTSD following exposure. In the NVVRS, the study of the effects of the Vietnam War, prevalence of PTSD also varied by racial/ethnic subgroups. The prevalence rate among Hispanic Americans was about 28%; for African Americans, it was 21%; and for European Americans and others, it was 14%. These findings were largely, but not entirely, due to differences in rates of combat exposure. Other factors, especially among the Hispanic veterans, also contributed to the development of PTSD. These factors were never conclusively articulated and remain important to investigate. In sum, the role of race in the development of PTSD must take into account different levels of exposure to traumatic events. Yet even when this is done, there are still factors contributing to the differential rates of PTSD and trauma exposure that are observed in epidemiological studies. The differences found across race and gender are important for future research to address. They may provide important keys to solving the complex puzzle that PTSD presents.

There are other factors as well that relate to the development of PTSD. Several studies (the NCS, the NVVRS, and the Detroit HMO study) identify the prior existence of a psychiatric condition as a risk factor for the development of PTSD, once an individual is exposed to a traumatic event. In addition, the presence of an addictive disorder and/or of conduct disorder may well *lead* to exposure to traumatic events (Breslau et al., 1991; Kessler et al., 1995). This complex interaction is fundamental to our understanding of the effects of traumatic events and PTSD. Some psychological conditions, such as panic, depression, and social anxiety, can lead to the use of addictive agents (e.g., alcohol, heroin, cocaine); these can in turn create a lifestyle that results in exposure to assaultive violence, which then leads to the development of PTSD (Keane & Wolfe, 1990). Alternatively, a sexual assault can lead to the development of panic attacks, social anxiety, depression, or PTSD, which then leads to the use of addictive substances. Both patterns are commonly observed in epidemiological studies and provide important information for clinicians treating patients. The relationship between anxiety and substance use disorders is reviewed in some detail in Chapter 1. Careful assessment of the precipitating variables that contribute to a particular psychological condition can provide meaningful information about which condition to treat first in patients with multiple comorbid psychological disorders (e.g., Najavits, 2001).

Modeling the Prediction of PTSD

To understand more fully the factors associated with who does and who doesn't develop PTSD following a traumatic event, it would be necessary to assign individuals randomly to certain types of traumatic events and then follow them over time to record the effects on their lives. Such a strategy would allow us to disentangle some of the puzzles presented by epidemiological risk factor analyses (e.g., the finding that exposure to traumatic events does not appear to be random). Yet ethical standards do not permit research of this type. Structural equation modeling (SEM) is one statistical strategy that attempts to understand the direction of effects when many factors are involved in predicting an outcome.

SEM has been applied to the understanding of risk factors in PTSD primarily in war veterans. Psychologists Dan and Lynda King and their colleagues have applied SEM to a wide variety of theoretically driven variables in an effort to predict which men and women developed PTSD following the Vietnam War. Using the NVVRS data set, they created four war zone stressor variables: traditional combat, atrocities/abusive violence, perceived threat, and the malevolent environment of the war zone (King, King, Gudanowski & Vreven, 1995). Atrocities/abusive violence, perceived threat, and malevolent environment all had direct effects on PTSD outcome, with malevolent environment exerting the largest effect. Traditional combat had an indirect effect, influencing the development of PTSD primarily through the perceived threats that the individuals reported.

Next, King, King, Foy, and Gudanowski (1996) examined prewar factors, demographic variables, and war zone stressor variables and their relationship to PTSD. The prewar variables consisted of measures of family environment, childhood antisocial behavior, maturity at entry to Vietnam, and prior trauma exposure. For both men and women (the investigators derived separate equations for each), they found that war zone stressors remained important contributors to PTSD, but that additional variance was attributable to the prewar factors for men and women. The effect of prewar variables was greater for men than it was for women. For men, a prior history of trauma exposure and age at the time of trauma were important factors; for women, only the history of a prior traumatic event contributed to the development of PTSD. These findings accentuated the importance of family instability and of a previous trauma history contributing to a generalized psychological vulnerability (see Chapter 8) as determinants of who develops PTSD.

King, King, Fairbank, Keane, and Adams (1998) then used SEM to examine resilience and recovery factors with the NVVRS data set. They identified hardiness, structural social support, functional social support, and recent stressful life events as possible factors that would explain who developed chronic PTSD. When combined with the war zone stressor variables, they learned that the variables promoting resilience differed for men and women. For men, hardiness, structural support, functional support, and stressful life events all had direct effects on PTSD development. For women, only hardiness, functional support, and stressful life events did. The investigators concluded that there are complex patterns of direct and indirect effects of the wide range of variables they incorporated into their models, and that these patterns differed for men and women.

In the final report of their sequence of studies, King, King, Foy, Keane, and Fairbank (1999) aggregated the pretrauma risk factors, the four war zone stressors, and the posttrauma resilience and recovery variables to understand more comprehensively how these variables interact to lead to the development of PTSD. For female VTVs, these three categories of variables predicted 72% of the variability in PTSD as an outcome. Prewar trauma exposure, exposure to abusive violence and life threat during the war, and postwar additional life stressors and functional social support were the most significant factors in determining who among the women who served developed PTSD. Among the male VTVs, these researchers were able to account for 70% of the variance in PTSD as an outcome. The key variables among men were the same as for women, plus younger age at the time of service in the war, the malevolence of the war zone environment, and structural social support (i.e., number and types of supports). Thus, using only measures of environmental and psychological constructs, these researchers were able to identify important risk factors related to the development of PTSD. Future studies that would include constitutional, physiological, and measures of hereditary factors would improve the level of precision possible in prediction. Even still, the levels of precision obtained without the biological level of analysis are impressive indeed.

ASSESSMENT AND DIAGNOSIS

Since its inclusion in the DSM-III in 1980, there has been excellent progress in the psychological assessment of PTSD. Consisting of a wide array of symptoms, PTSD presents a significant challenge to those involved in the development of assessment instruments. Yet it is clear that this challenge has been successfully met with an assortment of high-quality diagnostic interviews and psychological tests (Keane, Weathers, & Foa, 2000; Weathers, Keane, & Davidson, 2001). The focus of this part of the chapter is on the recent progress attained in the assessment of trauma and PTSD in adults.

An Overview of Assessment

Increasingly, clinicians are recognizing that many patients in their clinical practice have experienced traumatic events. As a result, the psychological care of large numbers of patients in hospitals, clinics, and practices is complicated by the presence of PTSD. Accordingly, there has been growing interest among clinicians in the proper assessment and evaluation of patients with PTSD.

Clearly, PTSD is assessed for many different purposes, and the goals of a particular assessment can determine the approach selected by the professional. A common purpose for assessment is to screen large groups of individuals to determine the extent to which some proportion of individuals have been exposed to traumatic events and have symptoms associated with PTSD. A second purpose for assessment, and perhaps the most common, is the completion of a diagnostic workup that includes a differential diagnosis and treatment planning. Clinicians may also be involved in forensic evaluations, where diagnostic accuracy is of utmost importance. Researchers may be interested in the frequency of occurrence of PTSD and the risk factors and complications associated with it (as in epidemiological studies). Moreover, researchers may be interested in high levels of diagnostic accuracy when studying biological and psychological parameters of the disorder, as in case–control designed studies. Each clinical and research situation requires a different solution, depending upon the assessment goals of the professional.

All measures of a psychological disorder are imperfect (Gerardi, Keane, & Penk, 1989). Two measures of the error contained within a test are the concepts of "false positives" and "false negatives." A false positive occurs when a patient falls above the cutoff, but is not a true case. A false negative occurs when a patient falls below the given cutoff, yet is in fact a true case. Diagnostic utility is often described in terms of a test's "sensitivity" and "specificity." These are measures of a test's performance that take into account errors made in prediction. Sensitivity is the measure of a test's "true-positive" rate, or the probability that those with the disorder will score above a given cutoff score. Specificity is the "true-negative" rate of a test, or the probability that those without the disorder will score below the cutoff for the test. Sensitivity is low if the test yields too many false negatives, whereas specificity is low if the test yields too many false positives.

Selection of tests and diagnostic instruments should include an examination by the clinician of relevant data on their psychometric properties. Inspecting rates of false positives, false negatives, sensitivity, and specificity can also inform the clinician of how an instrument performs. Conclusions drawn in clinical assessment are most accurate if they take into account these limitations.

Efforts to diagnose and assess patients for the presence of PTSD can include a range of different methods. These include semistructured diagnostic interviews for PTSD and related comorbidity, psychological tests and questionnaires, psychophysiological measures, medical records, and the use of multiple informants regarding the patient's behavior and experiences. This approach has been referred to as a multimethod approach to the assessment of PTSD (Keane, Fairbank, Caddell, Zimering, & Bender, 1985).

Semistructured Diagnostic Interviews

In the practice of clinical research, it is standard to employ a semistructured diagnostic interview to insure that all PTSD symptomatology is reviewed in detail. Diagnostic interviews combine the virtues of defining precisely how a diagnosis was made with those of using interviews that have known psychometric properties (i.e., reliability and validity). The use of structured diagnostic interviews in the clinical setting is less common, with perhaps the single exception of clinical forensic practice, where it is strongly encouraged (Keane, 1995). Nonetheless, the use of diagnostic interviews in clinical settings may well improve diagnostic accuracy and improve treatment planning (Litz & Weathers, 1994). The use of broad-based diagnostic interviews that cover the range of high-frequency diagnoses will assist the clinician by providing an evaluation of not only the target disorder, but also the extent of clinical comorbidity that is present (Keane & Wolfe, 1990; Weiss, 1997). Some of the available diagnostic interviews and their psychometric properties are presented below.

Clinician-Administered PTSD Scale

Developed by the National Center for PTSD in Boston, the Clinician-Administered PTSD Scale (CAPS) was designed for use by trained, experienced clinicians (Blake et al., 1990). Consisting of 30 items, the CAPS assesses all 17 symptoms of PTSD, as well as a range of the frequently observed associated features. Also contained in the CAPS are ratings for social and occupational functioning and an assessment of the validity of the responses by the patient. Like several other interviews (see below), the CAPS provides both dichotomous and continuous scores. Unique features of the CAPS are that it contains separate ratings for frequency and intensity of each symptom, and that it possesses behaviorally anchored probe questions and scale values. Interviewers are trained to ask their own follow-up questions and to use their clinical judgment in arriving at the best ratings.

If administered completely (i.e., all questions regarding associated features, functional impairments, validity ratings), the CAPS takes approximately an hour to complete. If only the diagnostic symptoms are assessed, the time for administration is cut in half.

Psychometric data on the performance of the CAPS demonstrate unusual strength in identifying cases and noncases of PTSD. Across three clinicians and 60 separate male veteran subjects, Weathers et al. (1992) found test–retest correlations between .90 and .98. Internal consistency was equally impressive, with alpha at .94 across all three primary symptom clusters. Correlations with other established measures of PTSD yielded strong evidence for the construct validity of the CAPS. The correlation of the CAPS with the Mississippi Scale for Combat-Related PTSD was .91, with the Keane PTSD Scale of the Minnesota Multiphasic Personality Inventory—2 (MMPI-2) was .77, and with the SCID (see below) PTSD symptom score was .89. Correlations with a measure of antisocial personality disorder were low, as was predicted by the multitrait–multimethod study design.

When the CAPS was used as a continuous measure, it was found to have 84% sensitivity, 95% specificity, 89% efficiency, and a kappa of .78 against the SCID. When the CAPS was used as a diagnostic measure, a kappa of .72 was found as compared with the SCID diagnosis. Whether it is used as a diagnostic or a continuous measure, these findings establish the CAPS as a sound measure of PTSD with excellent psychometric properties. Replications of these findings with male and female survivors of motor vehicle accidents (Blanchard et al., 1995) and patients with serious mental illnesses of both genders (Mueser et al., 1999) indicated the generalizability of these results across populations, races, and genders. A recent publication has carefully explicated nine different scoring algorithms for the CAPS and their implications for diagnostic accuracy, reliability, and validity coefficients (Weathers, Ruscio, & Keane, 1999).

Structured Clinical Interview for DSM

The SCID (Spitzer, Williams, Gibbons, & First, 1994) is the most widely used interview to assess Axis I and Axis II psychiatric disorders. It consists of separate modules for the most common of the diagnostic categories. Although the administration of the full SCID can be time-consuming, it does provide information across a broad range of clinical conditions. In many clinical settings, the SCID is used to systematically assess only those conditions that are most frequently encountered. This is economical in terms of time and still provides an examination across key conditions. In working within the context of a trauma clinic, it is recommended that the anxiety disorder, mood disorder, and substance use disorder modules and the psychotic screen be employed. This provides a fairly comprehensive examination of those conditions that are frequently comorbid with PTSD, and it provides a systematic way in which to insure that a patient does not endorse signs of psychoses (conditions that would require a different initial set of clinical interventions).

The PTSD module of the SCID appears to be both clinically sensitive and reliable. Keane et al. (1998) examined the interrater reliability of the SCID by asking a second interviewer to listen to audiotapes of an initial interview. They found a kappa of .68 and agreement across lifetime, current, and "never" PTSD of 78%. Similarly, in a sample of patients who were reinterviewed within a week by a different clinician, they found a kappa of .66 and diagnostic agreement of 78%.

The SCID's primary limitation is that it permits only a dichotomous rating of a symptom (present or absent), placing clinicians in a forced-choice situation. Most clinicians agree that the psychological symptoms occur in a dimensional rather than a dichotomous fashion, and so the SCID seems limited by the use of the present–absent scoring algorithm. Several options have evolved in the field as a result of this limitation.

Anxiety Disorders Interview Schedule

The original Anxiety Disorders Interview Schedule (ADIS) was developed almost 20 years ago (Di Nardo, O'Brien, Barlow, Waddell, & Blanchard, 1983). It was revised for DSM-III-R (ADIS-R; Di Nardo & Barlow, 1988), and revised again for DSM-IV (ADIS-IV: Lifetime Version; Di Nardo, Brown, & Barlow, 1994; see Chapter 9). The ADIS is a structured diagnostic interview that focuses primarily on the anxiety and mood disorders. The ADIS uses a Likert-type scaling procedure for symptoms and is thus capable of being analyzed in multiple ways to determine the extent to which a symptom is present or absent. Psychometric properties of the ADIS PTSD module have been assessed in two separate studies, and there were mixed results. In the first study a small group of combat veterans was assessed by two independent interviewers. Blanchard, Gerardi, Kolb, and Barlow (1986) found excellent sensitivity (1.0) and specificity (.91) for the original ADIS. In a community-based study of the ADIS-R, the results were slightly less impressive, and the hit rates were less stable (Di Nardo, Moras, Barlow, Rapee, & Brown, 1993).

PTSD Interview

The PTSD Interview (Watson, Juba, Manifold, Kucala, & Anderson, 1991) yields both dichotomous and continuous scores. The authors report strong test–retest reliability (.95) and internal consistency (alpha = .92), as well as strong sensitivity (.89), specificity (.94), and kappa (.82) when this interview is compared with the DIS (Robins, Helzer, Croughan, & Ratcliff, 1981).

The PTSD Interview appears to have excellent psychometric properties, but differs in administrative format from most other diagnostic clinical interviews. With the PTSD Interview, the clinician provides the patient with a copy of the scale to read along with the interviewer. From this copy of the scale, the patient is asked to give to the clinician his or her rating on the Likert scale for each of the symptoms. This format has much in common with self-report questionnaires, but it deviates from the other diagnostic scales in that it does not allow clinicians to make ratings of their own and utilize their expertise and experience.

Structured Interview for PTSD

The Structured Interview for PTSD (SI-PTSD) was developed by Davidson, Smith, and Kudler (1989). Like the CAPS and the PTSD Interview, it yields both dichotomous (i.e., diagnostic) and continuous measures of PTSD symptoms. As a result, it appears to be a useful instrument for diagnosing PTSD and measuring symptom severity. Symptoms are rated by the clinician on 5-point Likert scales, and the focus for the clinician is on symptom severity. The SI-PTSD possesses initial probe questions and provides helpful follow-up questions to promote a more thorough understanding of the patient's symptom experiences. In a study of male combat veterans, the authors found sensitivity of .96 and specificity of .80, suggesting sound performance.

PTSD Symptom Scale—Interview

Developed by Foa, Riggs, Dancu, and Rothbaum (1993), the PTSD Symptom Scale—Interview (PSS-I) possesses many strong clinical features that warrant its consideration for clinical and research use. Consisting of the 17 criteria for the PTSD diagnosis, the PSS-I uses Likert-type rating scales for each of the criterion symptoms. It can be scored as a continuous and dichotomous measure of PTSD and takes approximately 20 minutes for completion. Administering this measure to 118 women with sexual assault histories, Foa, Riggs, et al. (1993) found excellent interrater reliability, diagnostic sensitivity of .88, and specificity of .96. Test–retest reliability over 1 month was also reported to be strong.

The advantages of the PSS-I are its relative brevity, its promising psychometric properties, and its use of Likert rating scales that provide both a dichotomous and a continuous scoring routine. Another strength of this interview is its development and validation with sexual assault survivors, a population of great interest and clinical importance.

Self-Report PTSD Questionnaires

Several self-report measures have been developed as time- and cost-efficient ways of obtaining information about PTSD symptomatology. These measures enjoy widespread acceptance and use due to ease of administration and scoring, and they are also useful adjuncts to the structured diagnostic instruments. They can also be invaluable when used as screens for PTSD. These measures are most frequently used as continuous measures of PTSD, but specific cutoff scores can be used in order to arrive at a diagnosis of PTSD.

PTSD Checklist

Developed by researchers at the National Center for PTSD in Boston, the PTSD Checklist (PCL) comes in two versions; one is for civilians, whereas the other is for military personnel. The scale contains the 17 items derived from the DSM diagnostic criteria, each scored on a 5-point Likert scale. Weathers, Litz, Herman, Huska, and Keane (1993) examined its psychometric properties and found excellent internal consistency (alpha = .97), excellent test–retest reliability over a 2- to 3-day period (.96), and strong correlations with other measures of PTSD. The association with the Mississippi Scale was .93, with the Keane PTSD Scale of the MMPI-2 was .77, and with the Impact of Event Scale (IES; see below) was .90. Blanchard, Jones-Alexander, Buckley, and Forneris (1996) used the PCL in their studies of motor vehicle accident survivors; they found that the correlation of the PCL with the CAPS was .93, and that its overall diagnostic efficiency was .90 when compared to the CAPS. The properties of the PCL with other populations have yet to be reported in the literature.

Impact of Event Scale

Initially developed by Horowitz, Wilner, and Alvarez (1979), the IES was revised by Weiss and Marmar (IES-R; 1997) to incorporate the symptoms of hyperarousal for PTSD (Criterion D). The original scale contained only reexperiencing symptoms and avoidance/numbing symptoms, and needed to be revised in order to parallel the diagnostic picture more closely. Although the authors have provided some preliminary data, more information is needed about the revision's reliability and validity. The original IES was the most frequently used measure of PTSD, and it possessed good psychometric properties. Similar studies with the IES-R will insure its continued use in clinics and research settings.

Mississippi Scale for Combat-Related PTSD

The Mississippi Scale (Keane et al., 1988) is a 35-item scale designed to measure combat-related PTSD. The items were selected from an initial pool of 200 items generated by experts to closely match the DSM-III criteria for the disorder. The Mississippi Scale has excellent psychometric properties, with an alpha of .94 and test–retest reliability of .97 over a 1-week interval. With a cutoff score of 107, the Mississippi Scale had strong sensitivity (.93) and specificity (.89).

These results were replicated in an independent laboratory by McFall, Smith, Mackay, and Tarver (1990), who found that the Mississippi Scale was highly correlated with the SCID PTSD module. These findings suggest that the Mississippi Scale, which is widely used in clinical and research settings serving veterans, is a valuable self-report tool.

Keane PTSD Scale of the MMPI-2

Originally derived from the MMPI Form R, the Keane PTSD Scale now consists of 46 items empirically drawn from the MMPI-2 (Keane, Malloy, & Fairbank, 1984; Lyons & Keane, 1992). The original report on the scale indicated that this Scale correctly classified some 82% of the 200 subjects in the study. Subsequent studies have confirmed these findings in combat veteran populations (Watson, Kucala, & Manifold 1986).

In terms of reliability, Graham (1990) found the Keane PTSD Scale to have strong internal consistency (.85–.87) and test–retest reliability (.86–.89). Although only a few studies have been conducted to date on this scale in nonveteran populations, the data presented appear to be promising (Koretzky & Peck, 1990). More research is needed in this area, especially in the area of forensic psychology, where the MMPI-2 is frequently employed because of its validity indices.

Penn Inventory for Posttraumatic Stress

The Penn Inventory is a 26-item questionnaire developed by Hammerberg (1992). Its psychometric properties have been examined in multiple trauma populations, and its specificity is comparable to that of the Mississippi Scale, while its sensitivity is only slightly lower. It has been used with accident survivors, veterans, and general psychiatric patients. It has been primarily employed with samples of male patients.

Posttraumatic Diagnostic Scale

Developed by Foa, Cashman, Jaycox, and Perry (1997), the Posttraumatic Diagnostic Scale (PTDS) is derived from the DSM criteria directly. The PTDS begins with a 12-question checklist to elucidate the traumatic events to which an individual might have been exposed. Next, the patient is asked to indicate which of the events experienced has bothered him or her the most in the past month. The patient then rates his or her reactions to the event at the time of its occurrence, in order to determine whether the event fits both Criterion A1 and Criterion A2. The patient next rates on a single 4-point scale the intensity *and* frequency of each of the 17 symptoms of PTSD he or she has experienced in the past 30 days. The final section of the scale asks for self-ratings of impairment across nine areas of life functioning.

The PTDS was validated on several populations, including combat veterans, accident survivors, sexual and nonsexual assault survivors, and persons experiencing other traumatic events. The psychometric analyses proved to be exceptional. For internal consistency, the coefficient alpha was .92 overall; test–retest reliability for the diagnosis of PTSD over a 2- to 3-week interval was also high (kappa = .74). For symptom severity, the test–retest correlation was .83. When the PTDS was compared to the SCID PTSD module, a kappa coefficient of .65 was obtained with 82% agreement; the sensitivity of the test was .89, whereas its specificity was .75. Clearly, this self-report scale functioned well in comparison to the clinician ratings obtained in the SCID. It is a useful self-report and screening device for measuring PTSD and its symptom components.

The use of these self-report questionnaires in a wide range of clinical and research contexts seems well supported by the extant data. It is clear that they can be successfully employed to measure PTSD symptoms when administering a structured diagnostic interview is not feasible or practical. Many of the measures can be used interchangeably, as the findings appear to be robust for the minor variations in methods and approaches involved. In selecting a particular instrument, the clinician is encouraged to examine the data for that instrument for the population on which it is to be employed. In so doing, the clinician is apt to maximize the accuracy and efficiency of the chosen test.

Psychophysiological Measures

Research on biologically based measures of PTSD has grown tremendously in the past 10 years. Findings suggest that PTSD alters a wide range of physiological functions (Yehuda,

1997) and may also affect structural components of the brain (particularly the hippocampus; Bremner et al., 1995; see Chapter 6). To date, these findings have not been subjected to rigorous psychometric testing (i.e. utility analyses) to determine the extent to which these deviations are predictive of PTSD and non-PTSD cases. The primary exceptions to this conclusion are findings in the area of psychophysiological reactivity, which from the start examined diagnostic accuracy (e.g. Blanchard, Kolb, Pallmeyer, & Gerardi, 1982; Malloy, Fairbank, & Keane, 1983; Pitman, Orr, Forgue, de Jong, & Claiborn, 1987).

The findings in this area clearly point to the capacity of psychophysiological indices to identify and classify cases of PTSD on the basis of reactivity to audio, audiovisual, and imagery-based cues. Measures have included heart rate, blood pressure, skin conductance, and electromyography. Studies covered the range of traumatic events and included motor vehicle accident survivors, combat veterans from available eras, female sexual assault survivors, and survivors of terrorism. In perhaps the largest study of its kind, Keane et al. (1998) examined the responses of over 1,000 combat veterans to audiovisual and imagery-based cues of combat experiences. The results supported the presence of elevated psychophysiological arousal and reactivity in the participants, more than two-thirds of whom were correctly classified as having or not having PTSD.

Clearly, psychophysiological assessment is expensive in terms of time, patient burden, and cost. Yet, in cases where much is at stake, it may be helpful to employ this assessment strategy clinically (cf. Prins, Kaloupek, & Keane, 1995). Widespread adoption of this method of assessment is not anticipated, however, due to the costs, the expertise required, and the success of more economical methods of assessment (such as the diagnostic interviews and the psychological tests that are available).

As more information is collected on measures of the hypothalamic–pituitary–adrenocortical axis, it is indeed possible that this system and measures of it could be useful adjuncts to the diagnosis of PTSD as well as other anxiety and mood disorders. In particular, indices of cortisol, norepinephrine, and their ratio appear ready for an intensive examination for their capacity to improve diagnostic hit rates for PTSD, above and beyond the use of diagnostic interviews and psychological tests (Yehuda, Giller, Levengood, Southwick, & Siever, 1995); however, questions of specificity relative to other anxiety disorders are likely to prove formidable.

Summary of Findings on Assessment

Diagnosing and assessing outcomes in PTSD constitute a topic of growing interest and concern in the mental health field (Wilson & Keane, 1997). Since the inclusion of PTSD in DSM-III, there has been considerable progress in understanding and evaluating the psychological consequences of exposure to traumatic events. Conceptual models of PTSD assessment have evolved (Keane et al., 1987; Sutker, Uddo-Crane, & Allain, 1991); psychological tests have been developed (Foa et al., 1997; Norris & Riad, 1997); diagnostic interviews have been validated (Davidson et al., 1989; Foa, Riggs, et al., 1993; Weathers et al., 1992); and subscales of existing tests have been created to assess PTSD (e.g., MMPI-2, Keane et al., 1984; Symptom Checklist 90—Revised, Saunders, Arata, & Kilpatrick, 1990). We can rightly conclude that the assessment tools available to evaluate PTSD are comparable to or better than those available for any disorder in the DSM. Multiple instruments have been developed to cover the range of needs of the clinician. The data on these instruments are nothing short of outstanding.

Clearly, the assessment of PTSD in clinic settings must focus on more than the presence–absence, and severity of PTSD. A comprehensive assessment strategy would certainly gather information about an individual's family history, life context, symptoms, beliefs, strengths, weaknesses, support system, and coping abilities (Newman, Kaloupek, & Keane, 1996). This would assist in the development of an effective treatment plan for the patient. The primary purpose of the present review has been to examine the quality of a range of different instruments used to diagnose and assess PTSD; of course, the comprehensive assessment of a patient also needs to include indices of social and occupational functioning. Finally, a satisfactory assessment ultimately relies upon the clinical, and interpersonal skills of the clinician, since many topics related to trauma are inherently difficult for a patient to disclose to others.

This part of the chapter is not intended to be comprehensive in its review of the psychometric properties of all instruments available. Its goal has been to provide a heuristic structure that clinicians might employ when selecting a particular instrument for their clinical purposes. By carefully examining the psychometric properties of an instrument, the clinician can make an informed decision about the appropriateness of a particular instrument for the task at hand. Instruments that provide a full utility analysis (i.e., sensitivity, specificity, hit rate, etc.) do much to assist clinicians in making their final judgments. Furthermore, instruments that are developed and evaluated on multiple trauma populations, across genders, and with different racial, cultural, and age groups are highly desirable; these are objectives for future study.

TREATMENT

Historical Precedents for Current Psychological Treatments

From a historical perspective, the work of Janet (1889) and Freud (1936) has most influenced the treatment of PTSD. The objectives of each approach have much in common with contemporary models of treatment, including the cognitive-behavioral treatments of today. Thus current models of treatment owe a substantive debt to these pioneers. As presented by Fenichel (1945), there are two components to the psychoanalytic treatment of "traumatic neurosis": (1) attempts to quiet the high levels of anxiety and reactivity to the event; and (2) attempts to reconstruct the details of the event with the accompanying emotional reactions, to promote mastery over memories of the event. The contemporary treatments of anxiety management training or AMT (i.e., stress management and stress inoculation treatments) and exposure therapies parallel the two aspects of treatment proposed by Fenichel in his classic text on psychoanalysis.

Janet's contributions, reanalyzed and discussed frequently since the inclusion of PTSD in DSM-III, focus on the phenomenology of symptoms often observed in traumatized patients. Janet was an early proponent of hypnosis and advocated its use in accessing the details of traumatic events. His recognition that a memory of a traumatic events is often fragmented and focused on particular aspects of the event at the expense of a more complete memory is one of his major contributions to our understanding of this subject. The inclusion of hypnosis as a viable treatment for traumatized people added a systematic and technical approach to achieving the psychoanalytic objective of reconstructing details of the event in order to achieve mastery over the event.

In the aftermath of World War II, the use of sodium amytal interviews to help patients recreate and recall details of traumatic war events became increasingly widespread. Again, the objective of these interviews was to identify critical elements of traumatic war events that were not reported by the patients, so that efforts to address the psychological sequelae of these events could begin. Typically, the events involved human devastation, atrocities, terror in the face of death and danger, and helplessness.

The issue of traumatic memories has become controversial in the contemporary study of PTSD. Some deny the idea that memories of traumatic events have distinctive characteristics in comparison to memories of other life events; some challenge the nature of the constructs often invoked to explain traumatic memories (e.g. dissociation or repression); others are vigorously holding to scientific standards, recognizing that work in this area has largely only attained the scientific status of clinical observation. Despite the debate, it is clear that thousands of clinicians over the lengthy history of psychotherapy have noted that during therapy traumatized patients do indeed come to understand the nature and details of past traumatic events, whether these events occurred in childhood (as in the case of incest) or in adulthood (as with war veterans). Additional research directly on the issue of traumatic memory would contribute immeasurably to our understanding of developmental psychopathology and to the treatment of PTSD. Roth and Friedman (1998) assembled a group of notable scholars to summarize the literature on memories of trauma on behalf of the International Society for Traumatic Stress Studies. Their report delineated the issues, examined the extant evidence on traumatic memories, and outlined the needs for future scientific study of traumatic memory. The full text of this report is available on the society's Web site (www.istss.org).

Current Psychological Treatments

Largely driven by the psychological and social problems of returning American Vietnam veterans, mental health practitioners established treatment programs to treat traumatic disorders for these large numbers of war veterans (e.g., Keane & Kaloupek, 1982). Concomitantly, clinical researchers began to understand more fully the psychological consequences of exposure to sexual assault and rape (Burgess & Holmstrom, 1974; Kilpatrick, Veronen, & Resick, 1979), and to develop treatments for these problems.

At the outset, conceptual models of PTSD borrowed from Mowrer's (1960) two-factor learning theory (Fairbank & Keane, 1982; Keane, Zimering, & Caddell, 1985; Kilpatrick, Resick, & Veronen, 1981), which posits that fear and other aversive emotions are learned through association via classical conditioning mechanisms. This is the first factor in the acquisition of aversive emotions. The second factor is that individuals will do whatever is necessary to escape from and to avoid cues that stimulate these aversive emotions.

Theoretical models have since increasingly accommodated cognitive factors (Brewin, Dalgleish, & Joseph, 1996; Ehlers & Clark, 2000; Foa, Steketee, & Rothbaum, 1989; Lang, 1977a; Litz & Keane, 1989; see Chapters 3, 7, and 8). Treatments deriving from the behavioral and the cognitive models are among the most widely recommended and evaluated today. Specifically, exposure therapies and AMT techniques have evolved as two of the most widely accepted treatment approaches for patients with PTSD. These cognitive-behavioral treatments are also the most likely to be empirically tested by their proponents.

Although group therapies, both structured and unstructured, and psychodynamically informed psychotherapy are also widely used to treat PTSD, few studies in the literature have documented the clinical efficacy of these approaches (Foa, Keane, & Friedman, 2000). The studies that do exist do not meet contemporary standards for strong evidence. For example, most studies do not involve the use of randomized controlled clinical trials, which are the standard means of evaluating treatments throughout health and mental health care. However, the parallels between the objectives of psychoanalytic approaches as delineated above and those of AMT and exposure therapies are unmistakable (i.e., directly reducing anxiety to cues of the event and mastering the memory).

A more recent approach to treating PTSD is eye movement desensitization and reprocessing (EMDR; Shapiro, 1989). This is essentially an atheoretical technique that was accidentally discovered to alter disturbing thoughts, feelings, and images (Shapiro, 1995). It has been applied to a broad range of psychological problems, but the bulk of the available research on its efficacy is with PTSD, and so it is discussed in this chapter.

Accordingly, this section on current psychological treatments for PTSD examines the data supporting the use of exposure therapies, AMT, and their combination with cognitive therapies, as well as EMDR. Other treatments for PTSD are in developing phases and, though important, do not yet have an empirical base (e.g., group therapies, interpersonal psychotherapy, psychodynamic therapy, acceptance and commitment therapy). Accordingly, these are not discussed at any length.

Exposure Therapies

There is a long, rich tradition for treating anxiety disorders with one or another of the exposure therapies, whether it be systematic desensitization, flooding, prolonged exposure, implosive therapy, or another form (e.g., Barlow, 1988; Levis, 1980; Rachman, 1980). Exposure therapy is applied to PTSD in two fundamental ways: by using *in vivo* exposure or imaginal exposure. *In vivo* exposure generally involves returning to the site of the traumatic event in order to reduce avoidance and promote mastery over the cues associated with the event. For example, if a person developed PTSD following a car accident, the therapist might consider returning to the scene of the accident with the patient during the course of a treatment regimen (Blanchard & Hickling, 1997).

Imaginal exposure is often used in treating PTSD when *in vivo* exposure isn't possible (e.g., returning to a distant location is impractical, returning to an earlier time in life isn't feasible). Cues are presented in imagery in an effort to describe details of an event or set of events from the perspective of the stimulus propositions, response propositions, and meaning propositions associated with the event (Lang, 1977a). Like *in vivo* exposure, imaginal exposure has as its goal the reduction of avoidance and the promotion of mastery. Concomitantly, in some cases it promotes recall of details of the traumatic event that were previously not reported. This is probably a result of the systematic use of the cues as reminders.

Keane and his colleagues were the first to apply exposure therapy to the treatment of PTSD. Initially, this application took the form of single-subject designed studies to document the effects of exposure to memories of the traumatic combat events experienced by veteran patients (Black & Keane, 1982; Fairbank & Keane, 1982; Keane & Kaloupek, 1982). Significant reductions in trauma symptoms, anxiety, and other related symptoms were noted as a function of these interventions. These case demonstrations were instructive because they employed a consistent conceptual model of PTSD in the implementation of a treatment; utilized systematic diagnostic measures for case identification; and measured outcome in replicable, standardized ways. Several of these cases also employed scientifically validated single-subject research methodologies (see Fairbank & Keane, 1982).

COMPARISONS AND COMBINATIONS WITH OTHER TREATMENTS. This preliminary work led to the development of a randomized clinical trial that compared two active treatments (imagery-based exposure therapy and AMT) to a wait-list condition in the treatment of combat-related PTSD in Vietnam veterans. The results of this study were clear-cut. Compared to the wait-list condition, those patients receiving imagery-based exposure therapy showed reductions on standard psychometric instruments and on clinician ratings of symptoms at the posttreatment assessment. Changes on these measures were maintained at a 6-month follow-up evaluation. Interestingly, the less intensive AMT resulted in so many treatment dropouts that data were not available for analyses (Keane, Fairbank, Caddell, & Zimering, 1989).

Brom, Kleber, and Defares (1989) also conducted a randomized clinical trial comparing three active treatments for 112 patients who had experienced a traumatic event and were seeking psychotherapy. The treatments were exposure therapy (i.e., systematic desensitization), hypnotherapy, and psychodynamic treatment. Patients were evaluated before treatment, immediately after treatment, and at a 3-month follow-up with standardized psychometric instruments. The patients receiving exposure therapy showed a reduction in symptoms at posttest that was maintained at the 3-month follow-up. While comparable levels of change were noted in the other two active treatment groups, all three groups demonstrated greater change than the wait-list condition.

Foa, Rothbaum, Riggs, and Murdoch (1991) examined exposure therapy, an AMT condition called "stress inoculation," supportive counseling, and a wait-list condition in the treatment of rape-induced PTSD. Measures included clinical ratings of symptoms and standardized psychometric inventories, all administered at pretreatment, posttreatment, and a 3.5-month follow-up. The stress inoculation treatment was superior to the counseling and wait-list conditions at posttest. However, at the follow-up, the patients receiving exposure therapy performed better on measures of PTSD than patients in the other conditions did.

Three additional studies with combat veterans with PTSD demonstrate the salutary effects of exposure therapy. First, Boudewyns and Hyer (1990) and Cooper and Clum (1989) demonstrated that the addition of exposure therapy to available treatments of PTSD improved outcome for patients. Next, Glynn et al. (1999) assessed the effects of adding a family-based skills training intervention to imaginal exposure therapy. Comparing exposure therapy with behavioral family therapy to exposure therapy alone and to a wait-list comparison group, they found that the exposure therapy resulted in significant declines in symptoms of anxiety, arousal, and reliving the traumatic event, but did not affect the avoidant or numbing symptoms of the disorder. These treatment gains were maintained at the 6-month follow-up. Importantly, the addition of 16 sessions of family behavioral treatment did not yield incremental treatment gains.

Other combinations of treatment also appear to have promise in the amelioration of PTSD symptomatology. For example, Frueh, Turner, Beidel, Mirabella, and Jones (1996) assembled a multicomponent treatment for combat-related PTSD. These investigators combined exposure therapy, AMT, and cognitive therapy into a package for treating war veterans. They found positive treatment effects in a preliminary clinical trial that awaits more rigorous scientific review. Other packages combining these three forms of therapy are discussed later.

More recently, studies have appeared in the literature examining the comparative effectiveness of various approaches to treatment, including exposure therapy. For example, Tarrier et al. (1999) examined exposure therapy and cognitive therapy in the treatment of outpatients with PTSD stemming from many different traumatic events. Seventy-two patients entered treatment, and 62 patients completed treatment. Both groups manifested significant improvement that was maintained at the 6-month follow-up period. Outcomes were favorable for both groups, although there was no difference between the two at conventional levels of significance. Unfortunately, there was no attention control or wait-list control against which these two active treatments could be compared.

Similarly, Foa, Dancu, et al. (1999) compared exposure therapy to AMT and then combined the two treatments. These three groups were compared to a wait-list control group. All three of these treatments effectively reduced symptoms of rape-related PTSD and resulted in functional improvement. There were no differences among the three treatment groups on outcome measures, but all three groups improved more than the wait-list comparison group did.

In a study that once again compared exposure therapy to cognitive therapy, Marks, Lovell, Noshirvani, Livanou, and Thrasher (1998) examined these two treatments alone and in combination in outpatients with PTSD secondary to a wide range of traumatic events. A relaxation therapy condition was employed as the primary comparison group. All three active treatment conditions showed significant improvement, and greater improvement than that observed in the relaxation group. The three active treatments did not differ from one another on the key outcome variables.

Several investigations have advanced the field of PTSD treatment, even though the methodology utilized in the outcome study limited the conclusions that could be drawn. Frank and Stewart (1983) reported the effects of systematic desensitization on women who had been raped and who developed significant psychological symptomatology. Compared to an untreated comparison group, those women treated with graduated exposure improved most on a range of anxiety and depression symptom measures.

Richards, Lovell, and Marks (1994) compared imaginal and *in vivo* exposure in a randomized study of survivors of diverse traumatic events. At the 12-month follow-up, patients reported consistent reductions in PTSD symptoms and improved social adjustment. These data further substantiate the effectiveness of exposure therapy for some patients, and also suggest that improvements in symptoms are also reflected in critical domains of life functioning. In summary, the extant data support the use of exposure therapy in the treatment of PTSD. In a previous review of this literature, Solomon, Gerrity, and Muff (1992) derived the same conclusion from data available at that time. Similar conclusions were drawn by Otto, Penava, Pollack, and Smoller (1996) in a more recent review of the literature.

As data continue to accrue on exposure therapy, there is a distinct need for studies to examine combinations of treatments, to employ measures that assess social and occupational functioning, and to address the impact of treatments on comorbid psychological conditions. Clearly, the available efficacy studies demonstrate the value of extending the use of exposure therapies to patients with PTSD. Because their rich tradition is deeply rooted in experimental psychology and has been tested in the treatment of many anxiety disorders, exposure therapy in its many formats should be given priority by clinicians encountering patients with PTSD. Future studies assessing the generalization of exposure therapy from laboratory trials (efficacy studies) to clinical settings (effectiveness studies) would be particularly welcome.

EXPOSURE THERAPY IN THE PREVENTION OF PTSD. In what may ultimately prove to be an important lesson for the treatment of individuals exposed to traumatic events, Foa, Hearst-Ikeda, and Perry (1995) examined the efficacy of a brief intervention to prevent the development of chronic PTSD. For women who had been recently raped, the authors developed a program based upon that which worked so well in earlier trials with chronic PTSD. Exposure therapy figured prominently in the package of treatments assembled. This package also included elements of education, breathing retraining, and cognitive restructuring. When patients receiving the package were compared to a matched control group, this study found that at 2 months after intervention only 10% of the treated group met criteria for PTSD, while 70% of the untreated comparison group did.

Similarly, Bryant, Harvey, Dang, Sackville, and Basten (1998) constructed a treatment package consisting of exposure therapy, cognitive restructuring, and AMT in the treatment of acute stress disorder, a disorder that follows exposure to traumatic events but precedes the development of PTSD (i.e., it occurs within a month of exposure). In a randomized controlled trial, they found that individuals provided with the five sessions of this package as compared to supportive counseling met criteria for PTSD less often (17%) than did those receiving supportive counseling (67%) at a 6-month follow-up evaluation.

Anxiety Management Training

Typically, AMT involves teaching patients an assortment of behavioral and cognitive strategies to enhance their capacity to manage the emotions associated with PTSD. Such skills may include relaxation training, breathing retraining, trauma education, guided self-dialogue, cognitive restructuring, and communication skills training. Some programs for PTSD have emphasized the incorporation of anger management training as a part of the skills taught to patients (Chemtob, Novaco, Hamada, & Gross, 1997; Keane et al., 1989), given the salience of this interpersonal problem among patients with PTSD.

The studies described above by Foa and colleagues (Foa, Rothbaum, et al., 1991; Foa, Dancu, et al, 1999) and Keane et al. (1989) compared exposure therapy to AMT. In the Keane et al. study, therapists were instructed to explicitly avoid discussing or processing the traumatic events of the patients, in an effort to minimize the amount of exposure provided in this treatment condition. Perhaps this severe restriction led to the high rates of dropout in the AMT condition. Although the treatment appeared to be face-valid in its emphasis on treating the precise symptoms of PTSD, it evidently didn't provide sufficient relief to the combat veterans enrolled in this trial. However, this treatment did result in significant reductions in symptoms for female rape victims in both of Foa and colleagues' studies. The long-term effects were just not as strong as those found for exposure therapy.

Some studies primarily employed one form of AMT, rather than a multifaceted treatment package. For example, Peniston (1986) completed a project examining the effects of biofeedback-assisted relaxation treatment for veterans with combat-related PTSD. This form of AMT did result in significant short-term positive effects for the experimental group, although the long-term effects of this intervention were not systematically investigated.

Similarly, Chemtob et al. (1997) presented data on the treatment of anger and rage in veterans with PTSD, using a randomized controlled clinical design. Although the sample size of this study was small, behavioral treatment employing an anger-focused version of AMT yielded impressive reductions on psychometric measures of anger and on laboratory measures (behavioral) of anger reactivity. Importantly, these changes were associated with reductions in the reexperiencing symptoms of PTSD.

Clearly, there is evidence to suggest that a skills training approach such as AMT can have a favorable impact on symptoms of PTSD. Although the data are neither as strong nor as consistent as those for exposure therapies, it seems reasonable to conclude that there is some empirical foundation for the use of AMT in treating PTSD. An application with possibly the strongest potential for treating PTSD is a combination of various forms of therapy that includes exposure therapy, cognitive therapy, and AMT.

Combinations of Exposure Therapy, Cognitive Therapy, and AMT

Resick and Schnicke (1992) have proffered a multidimensional behavioral treatment package for women who have rape-related PTSD. This package, entitled "cognitive processing therapy" (CPT), combines elements of exposure therapy, AMT, and cognitive restructuring. The cognitive therapy component of CPT involves addressing key cognitive distortions found among women who have been assaulted. In particular, these authors have designed interventions for addressing difficulties in safety, trust, power, self-esteem, and intimacy in the lives of survivors. In a preliminary evaluation of CPT, the authors compared outcomes at pretreatment, posttreatment, 3 months, and 6 months for a treatment group and a wait-list comparison group (no random assignment was used). On clinician ratings and psychometric inventories of PTSD, the patients receiving CPT improved markedly. At the posttreatment assessment, impressively, none of the treated patients met criteria for PTSD.

In a recently completed study, Resick, Nishith, and Astin (2000) reported on a comparison of CPT and exposure therapy in the treatment of rape-related PTSD. In general, the two treatments were equally effective and more effective than a wait-list control condition. CPT did also seem to reduce comorbid symptoms of depression, as well as those of PTSD.

Combination treatments that include an array of cognitive-behavioral strategies have the advantage of addressing multiple problems that people with PTSD may exhibit, as well as incorporating techniques that have considerable empirical support in the clinical literature. Keane, Fisher, Krinsley, and Niles (1994) described a treatment package including exposure therapy, AMT, and cognitive restructuring as central features of their approach to treating PTSD. This package employs a phase-oriented approach to treating severe and chronic PTSD that includes the following six phases: (1) behavioral stabilization; (2) trauma education; (3) AMT; (4) trauma focus work; (5) relapse prevention skills; and (6) aftercare procedures (see Table 12.1).

Although this approach has intuitive clinical appeal, it wasn't until psychologists Fecteau and Nicki (1999) examined such a package in a randomized clinical trial for PTSD secondary to motor vehicle accidents that the impact of a combination package such as that proposed by Keane et al. (1994) was assessed. Their intervention consisted of trauma education, relaxation training, exposure therapy, cognitive restructuring, and guided behavioral practice. Patients were randomly assigned to the intervention or to a wait-list comparison group and received some 8–10 sessions of individualized treatment. The results of the intervention were successful as measured by clinical ratings, self-report questionnaires, and a laboratory-based psychophysiological assessment procedure. Described by the authors as clinically as well as statistically significant, these treatment effects were maintained at the 6-month follow-up assessment.

Thus there appear to be at least three treatments with excellent empirical support for treating PTSD: exposure therapy, AMT, and cognitive therapy. These three approaches have excellent empirical support in well-controlled clinical trials (efficacy studies), manifest strong treatment effect sizes, and appear to work well across diverse populations of trauma survivors. Future studies to examine the effectiveness of these approaches in clinic settings (effectiveness studies) are warranted.

Eye Movement Desensitization and Reprocessing

EMDR is a technique designed by Shapiro (1989, 1995) that has received considerable attention from practitioners and academics alike. Worldwide training institutes are well attended by clinicians seeking to learn about EMDR and its use in PTSD. Although Shapiro (1995) alleges that this technique is helpful for treating a range of disorders, its use is often directly associated with PTSD.

TABLE 12.1. A Phase-Oriented Approach to the Cognitive-Behavioral Treatment of PTSD

Phase 1: Behavioral stabilization
- Alcohol and drug use addressed.
- Basic needs of food, shelter, and safety insured.
- Proximal crises precipitating treatment controlled.
- Acceptance of therapy and the therapeutic relationship.
- Pharmacological assistance considered to improve emotional control.

Phase 2: Trauma education
- Reactions, responses, and symptoms that follow trauma exposure explained.
- Patient's responses normalized.
- Common interpersonal, marital, and vocational effects explored.
- Physiological signs and symptoms reviewed.
- Anger as a counterconditioning agent to anxiety explained.

Phase 3: Anxiety management training (AMT)
- Breathing retraining taught.
- General relaxation training considered for patient.
- Identify those cognitive beliefs and distortions contributing to distress.
- Teach rational self-statements.
- Communication skills training surrounding the traumatic experience.
- Anger management skills considered.

Phase 4: Trauma focus work
- Systematic desensitization using AMT skills.
- Prolonged exposure to traumatic memories.
- Structured group therapy exposure sessions.
- Use of imagery and *in vivo* therapy and homework assignments to promote mastery and reduce avoidance.
- Systematic uncovering work.

Phase 5: Relapse prevention
- Management of trauma cues and anniversary reactions.
- Education about substance use when cues are triggered.
- Identifying and managing situations where control is compromised.
- Mobilization of social support systems.
- Teaching the use of appropriate communication skills to seek assistance when needed.
- Attention to the need for intimate relationships.

Phase 6: Aftercare services
- Use of community-based support, such as Alcoholics Anonymous and survivor groups.
- Community involvement and social activism to address the needs of other survivors.
- Teaching appropriate skills to access professional care when needed.

In the development of EMDR, Shapiro (1989) conducted a series of single-subject cases and open clinical trials, which suggested that this approach to treating the psychological effects of trauma exposure may promote recovery. From an operational perspective, the fundamentals of EMDR are (1) the evocation of trauma-relevant images and memories, (2) the psychological evaluation of the aversive qualities of these images/memories, (3) the identification (with or without therapist assistance) of an alternative cognitive appraisal of the image/memory, (4) examination of physiological reactions to the image/memory, (5) focusing on the idiographically determined positive appraisal of the image/memory, and (6) repeated sets of lateral eye movements while the patient is focusing on elements of the traumatic response or the alternative cognitive appraisal.

Examining the efficacy and effectiveness of EMDR is challenging. Its mechanism of action is not based on any contemporary theories of human behavior, learning, or cognitive science, although some discussion of Pavlovian neurophysiology is provided across publications (Shapiro, 1989, 1995). For this reason, it has been seriously criticized in the scientific literature (Herbert & Mueser, 1992; Keane, 1998; Lohr, Kleinknecht, Tolin, & Barrett, 1995; Lohr, Tolin, & Lilienfeld, 1998). Yet the absence of theory or a conceptual foundation is not sufficient to enable us to dismiss totally the preliminary findings on this technique. If there is efficacy, then serious scholars can assume responsibility for identifying the precise mechanism responsible for any effects observed. The question is therefore "Is there evidence for EMDR's efficacy?", and, more importantly, "Is EMDR more effective or efficient than tested techniques?"

Carlson, Chemtob, Rusnak, Hedlund, and Muraoka (1998) compared EMDR to biofeedback-assisted relaxation training and to routine clinical care. In this randomized clinical trial with combat veterans, the authors reported that at the 180-day follow-up, the group receiving EMDR showed greater clinical improvement than either of the two comparison groups on self-report, psychometric, and clinician-rated measures of PTSD.

Wilson, Becker, and Tinker (1995) reported on the treatment of traumatic memories in a heterogeneous sample of individuals recruited through newspaper advertisements and other means. Half of their subjects received EMDR, while the remaining half were placed on a waiting list. Of the 80 subjects in this study, fewer than half reached DSM criteria for PTSD. Following three 90-minute sessions of EMDR, the treated group demonstrated a greater reduction on psychometric measures and clinician ratings of symptoms than did the wait-list subjects.

Rothbaum (1997) utilized EMDR in a sample of female rape survivors with PTSD. She found strong treatment effects when the active treatment was compared to a wait-list comparison group. Similarly, Chemtob, Nakashima, Hamada, and Carlson (in press) found that EMDR was an effective treatment for PTSD in children who survived Hurricane Iniki on the island of Kauai in the state of Hawaii. This study also compared EMDR to a wait-list comparison group.

In an HMO setting, Marcus, Marquis, and Sakai (1997) found that EMDR was more effective than standard psychological care among individuals with PTSD due to diverse traumatic events. These findings are impressive because the study was conducted in a clinical setting, where control over the patient characteristics and therapist behavior (particularly for the experimental treatment) is difficult to attain.

Devilly, Spence, and Rapee (1998) compared EMDR to a similar type of treatment but without the eye movements in the treatment of combat-related PTSD in Australian Vietnam veterans. Each of these treatments was also compared to a supportive treatment comparison. The results of this study indicated that both active treatment groups improved equally; there was no apparent benefit to the inclusion in this treatment package of the eye movements per se. Pitman et al. (1996) also found no differences between EMDR with the eye movements and EMDR without the eye movements in the treatment of combat-related PTSD among American Vietnam veterans. These studies contribute to the growing skepticism about the value of the eye movement processes in achieving the outcomes observed to date in using EMDR with PTSD.

Other studies on EMDR's efficacy have been less encouraging. Projects by Boudewyns, Stwertka, Hyer, Albrecht, and Sperr (1993), Jensen (1994), and Vaughan et al. (1994) found only modest effects for EMDR. These studies all have significant methodological limitations, but they are comparable in quality and design to many of those projects providing the empirical support for this technique. One study by Renfrey and Spates (1994) found no differences between a group that received the eye movements and a similar group that didn't, contributing to the mounting evidence challenging their role in the treatment.

In summary, much work needs to be done before research will firmly support the use of EMDR in the treatment of PTSD. To date, there is not a single study supporting EMDR (as espoused by its developer) as a treatment superior to any of the existing treatments for PTSD, such as exposure therapy, AMT, or cognitive therapy. Such studies would provide needed evidence in the debate about the ultimate contribution of EMDR to the scientific and clinical literature (Chemtob, Tolin, van der Kolk, & Pitman, 2000; Lohr et al., 1998). Unlike the various forms of exposure therapy, which have a long tradition of ameliorating a range of anxiety-mediated clinical problems and which are embedded in the rich conceptual tradition of experimental psychology, EMDR falters seriously at the theoretical level. Needed are basic studies to examine the effects of eye movements (or other laterally alternating stimuli); small-scale, well-controlled efficacy studies that meet contemporary standards for treatment outcome research; and the formulation of a testable theory for the technique. Implicit in this latter recommendation are the development of a conceptual model of PTSD, and an explanation of how EMDR attempts to correct either the deficits or excesses involved in this disabling psychological condition.

To conclude the review of EMDR, it may be valuable to specify the possible strengths of this technique. First, EMDR does share some components of exposure therapy and cognitive therapy. These overlapping components should be identified and operationalized to promote our ability to study the approach more fully. Second, the technique builds assessment into the ongoing therapy process. Third, EMDR suggests that instructions to modify images and alter cognitive self-statements may be a reasonable treatment objective for patients with PTSD. Fourth, proponents of this technique have always noted the need for empirical documentation to support their approach.

If there is a fundamental weakness of EMDR, it stems from a distinct lack of integration with existing psychological models of psychopathology and psychotherapy. Although all existing models of PTSD clearly have their own limitations, it is incumbent upon the proponents of EMDR to hypothesize how their view of the problems associated with PTSD differs from others; how the theoretical mechanisms of their technique derive from behavioral theory and/or cognitive neuroscience; and how this technique functions to allay specific targeted symptoms or to create alternative cognitive structures of the traumatic event, and thus contributes to our understanding of this multidimensional disorder.

Psychopharmacological Treatments

Psychopharmacological treatments for PTSD are in the nascent stages of development. Although there have been numerous randomized placebo-controlled clinical trials across medication types, few studies have been replicated across research laboratories. Initial results of randomized clinical trials appeared to favor the use of the antidepressant amitriptyline (Davidson et al., 1990). More recently, two studies suggested that the selective serotonin reuptake inhibitor (SSRI) sertraline improved the symptom picture of patients with PTSD (Brady et al., 2000; Davidson, Landburg, et al., 1997). These patients (200 in each of the two trials) manifested significant improvement across clinician-rated and self-report outcome measures. Patients tolerated well the dosages (50–200 mg) utilized in the study; sleep problems (insomnia) were the primary complaints of the participants.

Similarly, van der Kolk et al. (1994) found fluoxetine to be effective in the treatment of PTSD in women. This randomized placebo-controlled clinical trial resulted in improvement in the numbing and arousal symptoms of PTSD, but little impact on the reliving or intrusive symptoms. Importantly, this trial also showed little effect on the PTSD symptoms of combat-related PTSD in males.

In these trials of the SSRIs the treatment effects were significantly smaller than those observed in the cognitive-behavioral treatment trials and in the psychotherapy trials more broadly. Clearly, there is a need for additional research on the neurobiology of PTSD, so that newer medications can be developed to target those neurobiological systems that experience dysregulation in PTSD. Virtually all neurobiological systems studied thus far are adversely affected by the presence of PTSD. Efforts to improve psychosocial functioning by indexing a single neurobiological system may be inadequate in the treatment of a disorder with this level of biological complexity.

Psychopharmacological treatment of PTSD is indeed in its earliest stages (Friedman, 2000). Yet there is some definite improvement in the symptom picture when the SSRIs are employed. It is also clear that relatively large treatment effects are found when patients are treated with cognitive-behavioral strategies. It seems logical, then, that trials combining SSRIs and cognitive-behavioral treatments should receive priority, to determine whether the interaction of these two approaches is superior to either one alone. With the use of contemporary methods of assessing outcome, it is likely that studies could detect both main effects and interaction effects that may improve psychological symptoms and psychosocial functioning in patients with PTSD.

In summary, the introduction of the SSRIs has spurred important new research on the treatment of PTSD. With the completion of several well-controlled, multisite clinical trials, and with the recent approval of sertraline for the treatment of PTSD by the Food and Drug Administration, the psychopharmacology of PTSD holds much promise for continuing and additional developments. Because PTSD is a disorder that affects as much as 8% of the general population, it is likely that pharmaceutical companies will continue to devote research and development efforts to finding more and more effective treatments for it. Clinical trials that examine the interactive effects of cognitive-behavioral treatments and psychopharmacological agents are clearly warranted in the next generation of treatment outcome studies.

Future Treatment Development

There is much to be learned about the treatment of PTSD. To be sure, there will be no simple answers for treating people who have experienced the most horrific events life offers. Undoubtedly, combinations of treatments as proposed by Keane et al. (1994) and Resick and Schnicke (1992) may prove to be the most powerful interventions.

As these treatment packages are developed, there is a need for additional work from perspectives other than cognitive-behavioral ones. Interpersonal psychotherapy (Klerman, Weissman, Rounsaville, & Chevron, 1984) and other short-term psychodynamically informed treatments need to be developed, evaluated, and then compared to existing behavioral and cognitive-behavioral treatments to determine which patients benefit most from these methods (Kudler, Blank, & Krupnick, 2000).

Similarly, there is a need to develop psychopharmacological interventions further so that they can be compared and contrasted with effective psychological methods, both individually and in combination. PTSD research in this area is only in the earliest stages of its development.

Finally, an assumption about the uniformity of traumatic events has been made in the literature in general (and throughout this chapter). Although it is reasonable to speculate that fundamental similarities exist among patients who have experienced diverse traumatic events and then develop PTSD, whether these patients will respond to clinical interventions in the same way is an empirical question that has yet to be addressed. Studies posing a question such as this would be a welcome addition to the clinical literature: Will people with PTSD resulting from combat, torture, genocide, and natural disasters all improve as well as those treated successfully following rape, motor vehicle accidents, and assaults? This is a crucial issue that requires additional scientific study in order to provide clinicians with the requisite evidence supporting the use of available techniques.

Worldwide, the problems associated with war, rape, violence, criminal assault, and disaster do not appear to be declining. As a result, sound public policy is needed to guide society's response to survivors of these experiences. PTSD in its most chronic form is a debilitating condition that affects individuals, their families, their communities, and their nations. Those who are the targets of violence may ultimately become perpetrators, thus contributing to the cycle of violence initially documented by Widom (1989). If this is so, then interventions need to be implemented to prevent the occurrence of violence (primary prevention) or to mitigate its effects once it occurs (secondary prevention). Reliance upon sound empirical work to devise and implement these prevention efforts may ultimately be the best solution to the problems associated with PTSD.

FUTURE STUDIES

The evidence on the prevalence of exposure to traumatic events and the prevalence of PTSD is excellent in the United States. Yet there are fundamental errors in assuming that these prevalence rates apply even to other Western, developed countries. Studies that examine the prevalence of PTSD and other disorders internationally are clearly needed. Implicit in this recommendation is the need to examine the extent to which current assessment instrumentation is culturally sensitive to the ways in which traumatic reactions are expressed internationally. Much work on this topic will be required before definitive conclusions regarding prevalence rates of PTSD internationally can be drawn.

Studies of the effectiveness of the psychological and pharmacological treatments across cultures and ethnic groups are also needed. What may be effective for Western populations may be inadequate or possibly even unacceptable treatment for people who reside in other areas of the world and who have different world views, beliefs, and perspectives. This issue will need to be more closely examined before we can draw definitive conclusions. With the world's refugee population exploding, many of whom undoubtedly have PTSD, there is a clear need to test available treatments to see whether they can alleviate suffering in these diverse populations as these strategies have done in the United States.

Another area of increasing research importance, and one worthy of considerable energy and effort, is the impact of PTSD on health outcomes. In an important preliminary study, Felitti et al. (1998) examined a large sample of outpatients enrolled in the Kaiser Permanente HMO ($n = 9,508$). They found that as individuals experienced increasing numbers of adverse childhood experiences, they were increasingly at risk for a range of mental and physical health problems. These problems included disease risk factors such as obesity, alcohol use, drug use, cigarette smoking, and risky sexual behavior. When individuals who had experienced four or more adverse childhood experiences were examined, important relationships between the events and disease conditions themselves emerged: These people were more likely to develop diabetes, emphysema, stroke, cancer, and cardiovascular disease. These were statistically found to be direct effects of the exposure, operating above and beyond the indirect effects of engaging in high-risk behaviors.

The relationship among traumatic events, PTSD, and health outcomes is important for a wide range of reasons. Stress has been implicated in many different illnesses for more than 100 years. Trauma exposure and PTSD provide an important arena for examining the interrelationship of stress and health. The level of stress and anxiety in PTSD is extreme, and the prevalence of the disorder in the population is high. It is distinctly likely that if we were to develop important leads in the interaction of stress and health, we might very well do so by examining those who have been exposed to traumatic life events. Currently the correlational evidence is strong that trauma exposure and PTSD result in increased service utilization, high-risk behavior, and even certain diseases (Schnurr, Friedman, Sengupta, Jankowski, & Holmes, 2000). The exact nature of the processes involved requires additional scientific inquiry. The possibility of unlocking the complex relationship among environmental events, stress, PTSD, and disease will challenge researchers at all levels of the analysis: cellular, organ, systemic, behavioral, and social. The prospect of addressing these issues successfully is among the most exciting enterprises facing clinical research today.

CHAPTER 13

Social Phobia (Social Anxiety Disorder)

STEFAN G. HOFMANN
DAVID H. BARLOW

Donny Osmond has been an overachiever since the day he started show business. After his childhood stint as lead singer of the Osmonds in the late 1960s, he became a teenage star with a string of early 1970s solo hits, and then had a late-1980s comeback hit. In a 1999 interview with *People* magazine, Osmond revealed:

> "I'd been a little nervous about every one of my performances all my life, but for as long as I can remember—whether I was onstage or in a business meeting—I knew that if I just got that applause at the end of the first song, a laugh when I made a joke, my nervousness would diminish, though never go away. Sometime around 1994, I began feeling a kind of anxiousness unlike anything I'd ever felt before. . . .
>
> "Once the fear of embarrassing myself grabbed me, I couldn't get loose. It was as if a bizarre and terrifying unreality had replaced everything that was familiar and safe. In the grip of my wildest fears, I was paralyzed, certain that if I made one wrong move, I would literally die. Even more terrifying, I'd have felt relieved to die. The harder I tried to remember the words, the more elusive they became. The best I could do was not black out, and I got through the show, barely, telling myself repeatedly, *Stay conscious, stay conscious.*
>
> "And these attacks of nerves weren't only about performing onstage. I remember being so wound up at the prospect of cohosting *Live with Regis and Kathie Lee* that I didn't sleep at all the night before and got nauseous before I went on. Another time, my anxiety was so overwhelming during my audition to play the voice of Hercules in the Disney animated feature, my performance was embarrassing. I started to wonder if I could continue a singing career at all." (quoted in "Broken Heartthrob," 1999, pp. 109–111)

Nowhere is the paradox of self-defeating behavior more evident than in cases of famous and well-paid performers—including entertainers such as Donny Osmond, Barbra Streisand, and Carly Simon, or professional athletes who may have to forfeit lucrative careers. However, severe social anxiety is not limited to people in the public eye. In fact, social phobia (social anxiety disorder) is the most common type of anxiety disorder and the third most common mental disorder in the population. Results from the National Comorbidity Survey indicate that the lifetime prevalence rate of social phobia is 13.3% (Kessler et al., 1994). The disorder often follows a chronic course (Amies, Gelder, & Shaw, 1983; Marks, 1970; Öst, 1987a), and results in substantial impairments in vocational and social functioning (Davidson, Hughes, George, & Blazer, 1993; Liebowitz, Gorman, Fyer, & Klein, 1985; Schneier, Johnson, Hornig, Liebowitz, & Weissman, 1992; Schneier et al., 1994; Stein, Walker, & Forde, 1996).

Despite the high prevalence and significant degree of interference with one's personal and professional life, this disorder has only recently become the focus of clinical research. In 1985, Liebowitz, Gorman, Fyer, and Klein published an article entitled "Social Phobia: Review of a Neglected Anxiety Disorder." Since then, the number of scientific publications on social phobia and social anxiety has been rapidly increasing from year to year.

At this writing, at least 11 books on the topic of social anxiety or social phobia have been written, most of them published in the middle or late 1990s (Beidel & Turner, 1998; Carmin, Pollard, & Flynn, 1992; Dayhoff, 2000; Heimberg, Liebowitz, Hope, & Schneier, 1995; Hofmann & DiBartolo, 2001; Hope, Heimberg, Juster, & Turk, 1999; Jefferson & Katzelnick, 1997; Leary & Kowalski, 1995; Marshall, 1994; Rapee & Sanderson, 1998; Schneier & Welkowitz, 1996; Stein, 1995). Moreover, medical journals are filled with advertisements for paroxetine, the first drug approved by the U.S. Food and Drug Administration (FDA) for social anxiety disorder. Characterizing this condition as a "neglected anxiety disorder" no longer seems appropriate. Increased public awareness, new findings on the prevalence of the disorder, and encouraging results from the treatment outcome literature may all have contributed to this explosion of research activity.

Many researchers, pharmaceutical companies, and professional organizations prefer the term "social anxiety disorder" over "social phobia," because the former more appropriately connotes a more pervasive and impairing disorder (Liebowitz, Heimberg, Fresco, Travers, & Stein, 2000). This trend is likely to continue. Nevertheless, we have chosen for this chapter the term "social phobia," to clearly distinguish individuals meeting the *Diagnostic and Statistical Manual of Mental Disorders* criteria for the disorder (DSM-III-R or DSM-IV) from socially anxious individuals with unknown diagnostic status. Our goal is to summarize and integrate the wealth of recent research findings on the psychopathology and treatment of social phobia and social anxiety, and to identify areas that require further research.

PSYCHOPATHOLOGY

Core Symptoms

Fears and anxieties in social situations have been noted and recorded throughout history, but the definition of social phobia as we know it today dates back only to 1966. At that time, Marks and Gelder (1966) described a condition in which an individual becomes very "anxious" in situations where he or she may be subject to scrutiny by others while performing a specific task. The most common situation of this type to which most people can relate is public speaking. But other types of situations also meet the definitional criteria, such as eating at a lunch counter or in any public restaurant; writing one's signature in front of a bank clerk; or, for males, urinating in a crowded men's room. What is common about each of these examples is that the individual is required to do something while knowing that others will be watching and, to some extent, evaluating the behavior. That this is truly a "social phobia" is clear, because these patients report no difficulty whatsoever eating, writing, or urinating in private. Only when others are watching does the behavior deteriorate.

Early theorists assumed that social anxiety is due to a deficit in social skills (Stravynski & Greenberg, 1989; Trower, Bryant, & Argyle, 1978). Although it is questionable whether socially anxious individuals are in fact deficient in any of their social skills (Clark & Arkowitz, 1975; Glasgow & Arkowitz, 1975; Halford & Foddy, 1982; Hofmann, Gerlach, Wender, & Roth, 1997; Rapee & Lim, 1992; Stopa & Clark, 1993), they do tend to appraise their own performance in social situations more negatively than nonanxious individuals do, even when actual differences in performance are accounted for (Alden & Wallace, 1995; Glasgow & Arkowitz, 1975; Rapee & Lim, 1992; Stopa & Clark, 1993). Furthermore, socially anxious people tend to interact with others in an "innocuously" social manner, which involves polite smiling, agreeableness, and increased head nodding (Leary, 1983a; Leary, Knight, & Johnson, 1987; Patterson & Ritts, 1997); they also make greater use of excuses and apologies (Edelman, 1987; Schlenker, 1987), and exhibit fewer behaviors of social cooperativeness and dominance (Walters & Hope, 1998), than do nonanxious controls. The last-mentioned study also found self-reported anxiety to be negatively correlated with commands, bragging, and interruptions during a social interaction (Walters & Hope, 1998) which is consistent with the notion that social anxiety is characterized by less social cooperation and dominance and greater submission and escape/avoidance (Trower & Gilbert, 1989). Other studies have shown that socially anxious individuals frequently doubt their ability to create desired impressions on others (Wallace & Alden, 1995), and they expect their performance to fall short of other people's expectations of them (Alden & Wallace, 1995; Wallace & Alden, 1991, 1997). Therefore, it has been suggested that social anxiety arises when people desire to make a particular impression on others, but doubt that they will be able to do so (Leary & Kowalski, 1995).

Epidemiological and community-based studies suggest that social phobia is more common in women than in men. For example, data from the National Comorbidity Survey indicate that the female-to-male ratio for social phobia is approximately 3:2 (Kessler et al., 1994). This study reported that the lifetime prevalence rate of social phobia was 15.5% for females and 11.1% for males. In most treatment settings, however, either the sexes are equally represented, or the majority of patients with social phobia are male (American Psychiatric Association [APA], 1994). Social phobia often begins in the midteens, but can also occur in early childhood. During childhood, social phobia is commonly associated with overanxious disorder (as defined by DSM-III-R), mutism, school refusal, separation anxiety, behavioral inhibition, and shyness (see Albano & Detweiler, 2001, and Francis & Radka, 1995, for reviews).

The disorder is common around the world. Interestingly, however, there are certain forms of social concerns that seem to be culturally specific. For example, a recent article in *The New York Times* (Sims, 2000) with the headline "Behold, the Fragrant Japanese Man!" provides an example of such cultural differences in social concerns. The article told the story of Mr. Karasawa, a 49-year-old auditor. "I am a very clean person, and in my mind, I know that I don't smell," Mr. Karasawa said. "But I'm wearing fragrance for the first time in my life, to eliminate any chance that I might offend someone." Mr. Karasawa is not alone. "Everywhere one looks in Japan, for instance, in magazines, newspapers and store windows and on billboards and television, there are advertisements for products that rid the body of odor."

Mr. Karasawa, as well as many other people in his country, may be suffering from *taijin kyofusho* (TKS)—an emotional disorder believed to be particularly prevalent in Japanese and Korean cultures and described in Chapter 1. Like individuals suffering from social phobia, patients with TKS are concerned about being observed, and consequently avoid a variety of social situations. The major difference from social phobia, however, is that a person with TKS is concerned about doing something or presenting an appearance that will offend or embarrass *others*. In contrast, social phobia is defined as the fear of embarrassing *oneself*. Examples of TKS may include individuals who fear that they would offend others by emitting offensive odors (as in Mr. Karasawa's case), blushing, staring inappropriately, and presenting an improper facial expression or physical deformity (Takahashi, 1989). Most patients with TKS only experience a single circumscribed fear, although the specific focus may change over time. More males than females (at the ratio of 3:2) present with this problem (Takahashi, 1989). TKS cases seem to vary on a continuum of severity from the highly prevalent but transient adolescent social concerns to delusional disorders (Kirmayer, 1991). TKS illustrates the importance of cultural influences on an individual's psychopathology (see Chapter 1). However, it remains uncertain whether such concerns are in fact culture-specific, or whether they occur (with different expressions) in all cultures (Kleinknecht, Dinnel, Kleinknecht, Hiruma, & Hirada, 1997). Clearly, more research is necessary on the cultural influences on social anxiety and social concerns.

Diagnostic Issues: Social Phobia, Social Phobia Subtypes, and Avoidant Personality Disorder

The concept of social phobia was elaborated over the years by Isaac Marks (e.g., Marks, 1969) and proved useful enough to be adopted in a full-scale fashion within the definitions of anxiety disorders in DSM-III (APA, 1980). In this earlier version of our diagnostic system, the disorder was classified as a "phobic disorder" together with agoraphobia and simple phobia (which has since been renamed specific phobia; see Chapter 11). Conceptually, social phobia was closely related to simple phobia. It was further assumed that an individual typically only has one social phobia. Interestingly, the fear of social interaction was not part of the definition, and the diagnosis of social phobia was ruled out if the person met criteria for avoidant personality disorder (APD). These diagnostic criteria underwent some changes in DSM-III-R (APA, 1987), which included a "generalized" subtype of social phobia if an individual fears "most social situations." Furthermore, a person could meet the diagnostic criteria for both APD and social phobia. These criteria have remained virtually unchanged in DSM-IV (APA, 1994).

The operational definition of "most social situations" varies considerably within the social phobia literature. For example, Turner, Beidel, and Townsley (1992) and Stemberger, Turner, Beidel, and Calhoun (1995) assigned individuals to the generalized subtype if they feared the most commonly occurring social situations, such as parties (social gatherings), initiating conversations, or maintaining conversations. A "specific" subtype (not specified in DSM-IV) was assigned if individuals feared only performance-oriented situations, such as giving speeches, speaking in meetings, eating or writing in public, and/or using public restrooms. Subjects from this group could fear multiple "specific" social situations, but should not fear more "general" social situations, such as parties or conversations.

Heimberg and colleagues discussed three possible subtypes of social phobia: generalized, "nongeneralized," and "circumscribed" (Heimberg, Holt, Schneier, Spitzer & Liebowitz, 1993). According to this definition, the individual with nongeneralized social phobia functions in at least one broad social domain without clinically significant anxiety. People with the circumscribed subtype of social phobia, on the other hand, experience anxiety in only one or two discrete situations. Due to the small number of individuals with circumscribed social phobia, previous studies either did not include the circumscribed subtype (Herbert,

Hope, & Bellack, 1992), or pooled them with the nongeneralized group (E. J. Brown, Heimberg, & Juster, 1995; Hofmann, Newman, Ehlers, & Roth, 1995; Hofmann & Roth, 1996; Holt, Heimberg, & Hope, 1992). Only a few studies included a subgroup corresponding to Heimberg, Holt, et al.'s (1993) "circumscribed" subtype (Heimberg, Hope, Dodge, & Becker, 1990; Levin et al., 1993; McNeil, Ries, Taylor, et al., 1995; Stein et al., 1996). In all of those studies, this subtype was restricted to individuals with anxiety about public speaking, the most commonly feared social situation. However, only the "generalized" subtype is specified in DSM-IV.

This brief review of the literature suggests that there are almost as many operational definitions of social phobia subtypes as there are research groups studying the disorder. Unfortunately, very little is known about the range of social situations to be used in subtyping individuals with social phobia. When examining the prevalence and overlap of social anxiety across different classes of situations, Holt, Heimberg, Hope, and Liebowitz (1992) identified four different domains: formal speaking/interaction, informal speaking/interaction, assertive interaction, and observation by others. Recent studies suggest that this schema can be useful for subtyping individuals with social phobia (Hofmann & Roth, 1996; Hofmann et al., 1999).

Validity of Diagnostic Subgroups

The literature consistently reports a high overlap between the generalized subtype of social phobia and APD (e.g., Heimberg, 1996; Schneier, Spitzer, Gibbon, Fyer, & Liebowitz, 1991). This is not overly surprising, given that six of the seven diagnostic criteria for APD include a social-interactional component. Thus many researchers have questioned the utility of maintaining two diagnostic categories on two separate DSM-IV axes. Studies have found that both diagnoses (the generalized subtype of social phobia and APD) are associated with a high level of social anxiety, poor overall psychosocial functioning, greater overall psychopathology, high trait anxiety, and depression (e.g., Boone et al., 1999; E. J. Brown et al., 1995; Herbert, Hope, & Bellack, 1992; Holt, Heimberg, & Hope, 1992; Tran & Chambless, 1995; Turner et al., 1992). It has therefore been suggested that these diagnoses may simply be different points on the social anxiety continuum of increasing severity: from specific (nongeneralized) social phobia, to generalized social phobia without APD, and then to generalized social phobia with APD (McNeil, 2001).

However, other studies suggest that not all differences in these diagnostic groupings can simply be explained by differences in the level of social anxiety. Some studies showed subgroup differences in age and mode of onset (E. J. Brown et al., 1995; Mannuzza et al., 1995; Stemberger et al., 1995), cognitive processing (Hofmann, Gerlach, Wender, & Roth, 1997; McNeil, Ries, Taylor, et al., 1995), and psychophysiological response during exposure (Boone et al., 1999; Heimberg, Hope, et al., 1990; Hofmann, Newman, Ehlers, & Roth, 1995; Levin et al., 1993). For example, Mannuzza et al. (1995) reported that patients with generalized social phobia had a significantly earlier age of onset of their social phobia (mean = 10.9 years) than patients with nongeneralized social phobia (mean = 16.9 years), with half of the former developing the disorder before age 10. Stemberger et al. (1995) further found that 56% of individuals with "specific" social phobia and 40% of those with generalized social phobia, but only 20% of nonanxious controls, reported the presence of traumatic conditioning experiences. Statistical analyses showed that the specific subtype percentage was significantly higher than that of the normal controls.

Other studies showed that individuals with generalized social phobia and those with the additional diagnosis of APD reported greater subjective anxiety, but exhibited less of a heart rate response to an impromptu speech task, than individuals with nongeneralized social phobia or those without APD as an additional diagnosis (Heimberg, Hope, et al., 1990; Hofmann, Newman, Ehlers, & Roth, 1995; Levin et al., 1993; Boone et al., 1999). One might therefore suggest that individuals with generalized social phobia (and those with the additional diagnosis of APD) experience more of an *anxiety* response, whereas people with nongeneralized social phobia (and also those without APD) experience more of a *fear* reaction (i.e., a response that is physiologically more robust and closely tied to specific stimulus situations) during social threat. It may also be possible that the subtype distinction is linked to embarrassment and shame, which may be more closely related to the generalized subtype of social phobia (and APD). Psychophysiological studies suggest that the feeling of embarrassment is associated with heart rate deceleration due to an increase in parasympathetic arousal (Buck & Parke, 1972; Buck, Parke, & Buck, 1970). Therefore, it has been suggested that in those with generalized (and "anxious") social phobias, this competing parasympathetic response may summate with fearful sympathetic activation to produce an emotional blend that leads to high subjective distress and low autonomic arousal (McNeil, Vrana, Melamed, Cuthbert, & Lang, 1993). Alternatively, as outlined in Chapter 3, these findings may reflect autonomic restriction associated with chronic anxious apprehension (e.g., Thayer, Freedman, & Borkovec, 1996).

Studies of comorbidity in patients with social phobia, most with the generalized subtype, evidence high levels of anxiety and depression. In the study reported in Chapter 9 (Brown, Campbell, Lehman, Grisham, & Mancill, 2001), 46% of 186 carefully diagnosed patients with social phobia met criteria for an additional Axis I disorder (see Table 9.5). More specifically, 45% met criteria for either an anxiety or mood disorder, 28% for an anxiety disorder alone, and 29% for a mood disorder alone (major depressive disorder or dysthymia). When one looks at individual disorders, the most frequent comorbid disorder by a substantial margin was one of the mood disorders, with 14% meeting criteria for major depressive disorder and 13% meeting criteria for dysthymia. If one looks at the comorbidity of mood disorders over a lifetime, fully 44% presenting with a principal diagnosis of social phobia had met criteria for a mood disorder at some point in their lives, with 44% meeting criteria for major depressive disorder and 17% for dysthymia. These data underscore the close relationship between social phobia and depression discovered in the structural equation modeling studies described in Chapter 3.

A MODEL OF THE ETIOLOGY OF SOCIAL PHOBIA

It has been suggested that social fears are the result of a biologically determined readiness to associate fear with angry, critical, or rejecting facial stimuli (Öhman, 1986; Öhman, Dimberg, & Öst, 1985b). In fact, angry faces and happy faces elicit different patterns of electromyographic activity in nonanxious individuals (Dimberg, 1982), and fear conditioning to angry faces shows much more resistance to extinction than do responses to happy or neutral expressions (Öhman & Dimberg, 1978; Dimberg, 1986). Interestingly, this conditioning effect is only obtained when the stimulus person directs his or her anger toward the subject; angry faces looking away are as ineffective as happy faces in conditioning paradigms (Dimberg & Öhman, 1983). This suggests that direct eye contact is crucial. In species such as our close relatives, the primates, direct eye contact seems to be very frightening. Furthermore, various species employ displays of eyes or eye-like spots to frighten potential predators. Among humans, the response to eye contact is obviously greatly altered by contextual and learning factors, but it seems to be there nevertheless. It has therefore been suggested that the fear of being watched among individuals with social phobia is an exaggeration of the normal human sensitivity to eyes (Marks, 1987).

Although this is an intriguing hypothesis, very little research has been conducted on this issue. A study by Merckelbach, van Hout, van den Hout, and Mersch (1989) compared nine individuals with social phobia and nine nonanxious controls in their eye blink rate and skin conductance response during exposure to slides of angry faces, happy faces, and neutral objects. The results showed that angry faces elicited greater skin conductance response and stronger inhibition of eye blink rate than the other stimuli in both groups. However, no difference was found between individuals with social phobia and nonanxious controls in their responses to these stimuli. This study was limited by the small sample size and the choice of the dependent variables. Future studies should include a fear conditioning phase prior to stimulus exposure, and should also include startle response and cardiovascular variables as additional dependent variables.

In contrast to psychophysiological data, there is some evidence that individuals with social phobia and nonanxious controls do differ in their memory for faces. In a study by Lundh and Öst (1996), a group of individuals with social phobia (most of them met criteria for the generalized subtype) and nonanxious controls were presented with a number of photos with faces and asked to judge whether the persons in the photos were critical or accepting. Following this encoding task, subjects were asked to perform an unrelated task for 5 minutes and were then unexpectedly presented with a facial recognition task. The results showed that individuals with social phobia recognized more of the critical than the accepting faces, whereas the controls tended to recognize more of the accepting than the critical faces. These findings demonstrate that individuals with social phobia show either a recognition bias or a response bias for critical faces. Interestingly, such an effect has not been found in studies that used words as stimulus material (e.g., Cloitre, Cancienne, Heimberg, Holt, & Liebowitz, 1995; Rapee, McCallum, Melville, Ravenscroft, & Rodney, 1994). Future studies should therefore explore whether words and faces (as well as voices) are processed differently. Signal detection analyses of subjects' responses could determine whether the results, if replicable, are due to a response bias or due to a true recognition bias.

In the first edition of this book (Barlow, 1988), it was postulated that individuals with specific phobia and individuals with PTSD experience true or false alarms, and develop anxiety over possible loss of control of their emotions on the basis of psychological and biological vulnerabilities. This anxiety is limited to anticipating the possibility of experiencing the fear or intense emotion once again in the form of flashbacks, panic attacks, and so on. Within the category of social phobia, an additional complication develops: Because of arousal-driven negative cognitive activity (or worry), the individual actually becomes distracted from the task at hand if some performance is necessary. This is consistent with results from the information-processing literature, which suggests that individuals with social phobia show an attentional and judgmental bias toward socially threatening information (see Heinrichs & Hofmann, 2001, for a review). Figure 13.1 summarizes the results from the information-processing literature on social phobia.

A number of studies further highlight the process of self-focused attention in socially anxious individuals confronted with fearful social situations (Beidel, Turner, & Dancu, 1985; Cacioppo, Glass, & Merluzzi, 1979; Glasgow & Arkowitz, 1975; Glass, Merluzzi, Biever, & Larsen, 1982; Hope, Gansler, & Heimberg, 1989; Mahone, Bruch, & Heimberg, 1993; Stopa & Clark, 1993). Studies have also shown that self-focused attention impairs performance in individuals with social phobia (Hope & Heimberg, 1988) and test-anxious individuals in a social-evaluative situation (Carver, Peterson, Follansbee, & Schier, 1983)

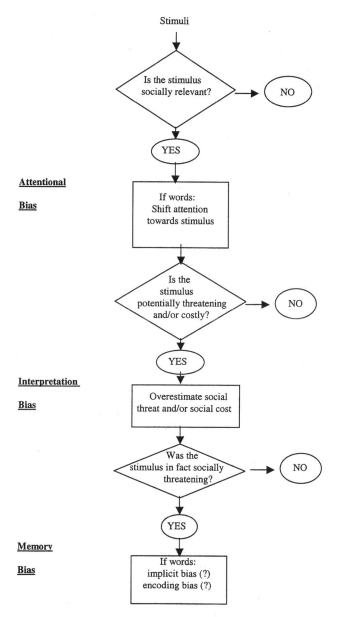

FIGURE 13.1. A summary of the information-processing literature on social phobia. Arrows represent the direction of information flow. The rectangular boxes refer to the output and types of information-processing biases. The diamonds reflect decision points. From Heinrichs and Hofmann (2001). Copyright by Elsevier Science. Reprinted by permission.

as outlined in Chapter 3, possibly because self-focus detracts attentional resources necessary from optimal task performance (Ingram, 1990).

The present model of the etiology of social phobia (Figure 13.2) follows very closely the models presented for other anxiety disorders in prior chapters. Specifically, for reasons of evolutionary significance, humans seem sensitive to anger, criticism, or other means of social disapproval. Therefore, most people are socially fearful at one time or another, par-

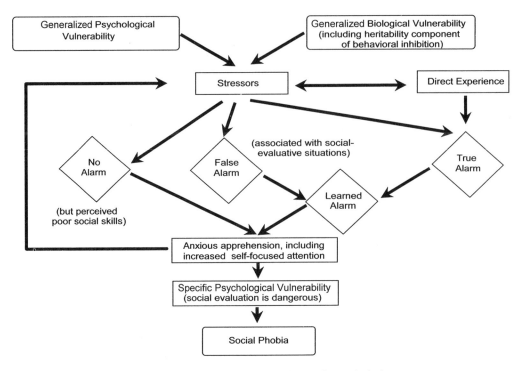

FIGURE 13.2. A model of the etiology of social phobia.

ticularly in adolescence, but few develop social phobia. To develop social phobia, one must be biologically and psychologically vulnerable to anxious apprehension. Evidence for a genetic contribution to social anxiety comes from family studies, twin studies, and high-risk studies (Fyer, Manuzza, Chapman, Liebowitz, & Klein, 1993; Horwath et al., 1995; Kendler, Neale, Kessler, Heath, & Eaves, 1992b; Mancini, van Ameringen, Szatmari, Fugere, & Boyle, 1996; Reich & Yates, 1988; Skre, Onstad, Torgersen, Lygren, & Kringlen, 1993). For example, the results of a direct family interview study showed that the risk of social phobia was approximately three times higher for relatives of probands with social phobia than for relatives of controls who were never mentally ill (Fyer et al., 1993). Furthermore, the twin study by Kendler et al. (1992b), which was based on over 1,000 female twin pairs, found substantial concordance rates for social phobia in identical (24%) and fraternal (15%) twin pairs. The study by Mancini et al. (1996) reported that 23% of the children (mean age = 11 years) of adults with social phobia met diagnostic criteria for social phobia.

The genetic disposition to develop social phobia may be nonspecific, as suggested in Chapter 6, but seems to be closely connected to certain temperament variables. Shyness, one of the most heritable temperament factors (Plomin & Daniels, 1985), seems to be closely related to social phobia (Turner, Beidel, & Townsley, 1990). However, the precise nature of this relationship remains uncertain. Another possible precursor of social phobia is behavioral inhibition, which refers to a child's fearfulness, timidity, and wariness when encountering novel people, objects, or events (Kagan, Reznick, & Snidman, 1988). The relationship of behavioral inhibition to neuroticism and other related temperaments has been reviewed in Chapter 2.

Numerous studies have found that behavioral inhibition in childhood is closely associated with social anxiety and social phobia in adolescence (Mick & Telch, 1998; Rosenbaum, Biederman, Pollock, & Hirshfeld, 1994; Rosenbaum, Biederman, Hirshfeld, Bolduc, & Chaloff, 1991; Schwartz, Snidman, & Kagan, 1999). For example, parents of children who were identified as inhibited at 21 months of age were significantly more likely to meet DSM-III diagnostic criteria for social phobia (17.5%) than were parents of uninhibited children (0%) or control parents whose children were neither inhibited or uninhibited (2.9%; Rosenbaum et al., 1991). These findings suggest that behaviorally inhibited children are more likely to have parents with social phobia. However, it has yet to be investigated whether parents with social phobia are also more likely to have behaviorally inhibited children, and whether behavioral inhibition in childhood leads to social phobia in adulthood. If this relationship between behavioral inhibition and social phobia holds true, future studies should identify factors that protect behaviorally inhibited children from developing social phobia in adulthood. Some of these protective factors restricting the development of anxiety generally have been described in Chapters 6 to 8. For example, it is possible that family factors and peer relationships constitute such protective factors. However, little empirical evidence exists on the specific relationship of those variables on social functioning during childhood and later adulthood (Masia & Morris, 1998; Rapee, 1997).

Our model assumes that relatively minor negative life events involving performance or social interactions can lead to anxiety, particularly if an alarm is associated with these social events. These factors then form the platform from which false and true alarms can develop. We assume that the pathway via true alarms is more common for individuals with a nongeneralized (specific, circumscribed) subtype of social phobia than for people with generalized social phobia. This assumption is consistent with the notion that individuals with nongeneralized social phobia exhibit more of a *fear* reaction (similar to individuals with specific phobias), whereas individuals with a generalized subtype experience more of an *anxiety* response, which may also involve feelings of embarrassment and shame. This distinction corresponds to Buss's (1980) classification of shy individuals into "fearful shys" and "self-conscious shys." According to this classification schema, one of the characteristic features of the former group is the fear of autonomic reactivity, whereas the second group is characterized by excessive "public self-awareness" (i.e., increased attention focused on public aspects of the self). This might explain why individuals with social phobia attribute their fear of public speaking more often to "panic attacks" than to fear of evaluation, traumatic events, or indirect conditioning events (Hofmann, Ehlers, & Roth, 1995). In contrast, our model assumes that the etiological pathway for the generalized subtype of social phobia is more likely to occur without alarm or via false alarms associated with social-evaluative situations. Supporting evidence for this claim comes from a study showing that, in contrast to individuals with generalized social phobia, those with a "specific" social phobia subtype are more likely to report the presence of traumatic conditioning experiences than controls are (Stemberger et al., 1995). The repeated experience of such false alarms may be the reason why individuals with social phobia often perceive a lack of internal control (Leung & Heimberg, 1996) and believe that events are controllable only by people other than themselves (Cloitre, Heimberg, Liebowitz, & Gitow, 1992). Once established, social phobia can persist for many years, if not indefinitely, in the absence of any treatment.

Contemporary theories of social anxiety and social phobia emphasize the role of cognitive processes and the focus of attention for the maintenance of the disorder (Clark & Wells, 1995; Leary & Kowalski, 1995; Rapee & Heimberg, 1997; Turner, Beidel, & Jacob, 1994). It has been suggested that effective psychological treatment changes the person's representation of the self in a more positive direction (Rapee & Heimberg, 1997). Supporting evidence comes from a study by Woody, Chambless, and Glass (1997), who reported a decrease in self-focused attention during the course of cognitive-behavioral group therapy (CGBT) in individuals with social phobia. However, external focus of attention remained unchanged. Furthermore, Hofmann (2000a) reported that individuals with social phobia who underwent exposure therapy reported a significant decline in negative self-focused thoughts, which was correlated with changes in self-reported social anxiety. Another study by Wells and Papageorgiou (1998b) showed that exposure therapy combined with instructions to focus on the external environment was more effective than standard exposure therapy. Wells et al. (1995) hypothesized that self-focused attention, or evaluating one's responding, in social phobia is part of an individual's misguided attempts to prevent an embarrassing and humiliating situation; however, this strategy interferes with the processing of information that could provide disconfirming evidence against negative beliefs. The model of anxious apprehension detailed in Chapter 3 considers self-focused attention to be a more fundamental component of the process of anxious apprehension in general, as represented in Figure 3.1. This is particularly problematic in social phobia, due to the "distracting" nature of the process.

ASSESSMENTS

Behavioral Assessment Tests

The performance hall quiets. The curtain opens to reveal a concert pianist ready to play. Video cameras start whirring. But this is no usual performance: The pianist has electrodes attached from head to toe to measure heart rate, respiration, and skin conductance. Furthermore, the person has been told, "Accomplished pianists and experts in behavioral assessment who have copies of your music will be evaluating your performance. At the sound of the buzzer, begin playing."

Although this scenario might have been daunting even to Vladimir Horowitz, it is in fact a standard procedure to assess musical performance anxiety among a group of accomplished pianists (Craske & Craig, 1984). Behavioral assessment tests (BATs) are frequently used. The BAT procedure has the advantage of allowing researchers to quantify anxiety simultaneously on various dimensions, including self-report, overt behavior, and psychophysiological responding. In their review of behavioral observation methods of social anxiety, Glass and Arnkoff (1989) identified five important issues: (1) nature of situation or interaction, (2) type of role-play assessment, (3) identity of partner or audience, (4) raters for observation and coding, and (5) choice of behavior being evaluated.

McNeil, Ries, and Turk (1995) have described three frequently employed types of standardized BATs: conversation with a same-gender stranger, conversation with an opposite-gender stranger, and an impromptu speech given to a small audience. Other situations sometimes include solving simple math problems on a chalkboard in front of an audience or discussing controversial topics with strangers (Hofmann, 2000a). Subjective anxiety ratings are typically obtained by using subjective units of discomfort (SUDs). Patients are then asked to give SUDs ratings before and after the BAT, and sometimes at regular intervals during the BAT. In addition, behavioral indicators (such as length of an impromptu speech) and physiological indicators (such as heart rate) are assessed before, during, and after the test.

Different BAT situations have been used. McNeil, Ries, and Turk (1995) have identified a number of dimensions BAT situations vary on, including the degree of role play (some exposure situations, such as public speaking, have greater "external validity" than others), the instructional control of interactions, the amount of preparation allowed, whether there are interruptions for anxiety ratings, the number and familiarity of interaction partners or audiences, whether these confederates are socially interactive or not, and whether avoidance or escape from the task is allowed and quantified.

Some researchers have used such situations individually tailored to a patient's greatest social anxiety (e.g., Heimberg, Hope, et al., 1990; Coles & Heimberg, 2000), because it has been argued that individually tailored BAT situations have the greatest external validity and clinical utility (Becker & Heimberg, 1988). However, such a procedure leads to significant methodological problems when one is comparing groups of individuals, because different social situations (e.g., saying no to a pressuring salesperson, asking a person out on a date, and speaking in front of a group of people) elicit slightly different emotional reactions (fear of rejection, embarrassment, fear of negative evaluation, etc.). Therefore, our recommendation is to include at least one standardized social test in a BAT. Of all social situations, public speaking is by far the most often feared in both the general population (Pollard & Henderson, 1988) and among individuals with social phobia (Mannuzza et al., 1995; Pollard & Henderson, 1988). Furthermore, an impromptu speech task shows good reliability (Beidel, Turner, Jacob, & Cooley, 1989), and has been included as a criterion for a multimethod index to assess social phobia improvement (Turner, Beidel, & Wolff, 1994) and social phobia end-state functioning (Turner, Beidel, Long, & Townsley, 1993).

Interviewer-Rated Scales

Psychopharmacological studies frequently use the Liebowitz Social Anxiety Scale (LSAS) to measure the severity of anxiety and avoidance in social situations (Liebowitz, 1987). This interviewer-rated scale consists of 24 items, which include a number of social-interactional situations (13 items) and performance situations (11 items). Each item is rated separately for fear and avoidance on a 4-point Likert scale. This scale has good psychometric properties (Heimberg et al., 1999), and numerous trials have demonstrated its clinical utility (e.g., Heimberg et al., 1998; Liebowitz et al., 1988, 1992; Pohl, Balon, Chapman, & McBride, 1998; Reich & Yates, 1988; Versiani et al., 1992).

Another interviewer-rated scale is the Brief Social Phobia Scale (Davidson, Potts, et al., 1991). This scale consists of seven items describing a number of common social situations that are rated on both fear and avoidance, and four items measuring physiological symptoms. Each item is rated on a 5-point Likert scale. The instrument has shown good psychometric properties (Davidson, Miner, et al., 1997).

Self-Report Scales

Several self-report measures of social anxiety and avoidance have been employed in previous research (for a review, see Herbert, Rheingold, & Brandsing, 2001). The most frequently used scales today include the Fear of Negative Evaluation Scale (FNE) and the Social Avoidance and Distress Scale (SADS) by Watson and Friend (1969); the Social Phobia Scale (SPS) and the Social Interaction Anxiety Scale (SIAS) by Mattick and Clarke (1998); and the Social Phobia and Anxiety Inventory (SPAI), with versions for adults (Turner, Beidel, Dancu, & Stanley, 1989) and for children between the ages of 8 and 17 (Beidel, Turner, & Morris, 1995).

The SADS and FNE, both in use since 1969, consist of 28 and 30 true–false items, respectively. Although these two instruments are among the most widely used social anxiety assessment measures, their appropriateness for patients with social phobia is questionable. For example, the two instruments seem to lack discriminant validity, because they correlate highly with general measures of emotional distress rather than with measures of social anxiety per se (Turner, McCanna, & Beidel, 1987; Turner & Beidel, 1988). The scales are also limited by the true–false format of their items (McNeil, Ries, & Turk, 1995), although the shorter 12-item version of the FNE (brief FNE) uses a 5-point Likert-type scale (Leary, 1983b). Finally, the scoring procedure of the SADS is most likely erroneous. Specifically, in Table 1 of Watson and Friend (1969), the scoring key of item 19 ("When my superiors want to talk with me, I talk willingly") of the 28-item scale is incorrectly labeled "true" (p. 450). It is unlikely that researchers who have used this scale in the past have detected this error, and it is unclear how much it affected the data pool of this instrument. Unfortunately, no erratum has ever been published.

The SPS and SIAS were designed to be used together in the assessment of social phobia. The SPS measures fears of being scrutinized or observed by others, whereas the SIAS assesses anxiety concerning interpersonal interactions. Specifically, research suggests that individuals who score high on the SPS primarily focus anxiety on somatic symptoms of arousal and possible harmful consequences associated with these symptoms, whereas individuals who score high on the SIAS are more anxious about social situations in general (Norton, Cox, Hewitt, & McLeod, 1997). The two scales consist of 20 items that are rated on a 0–4 point Likert scale. Several studies have reported that both scales are reliable and valid instruments (E. J. Brown et al., 1997; Heimberg, Mueller, Holt, Hope, & Liebowitz, 1992; Mattick & Clarke, 1998).

The SPAI consists of 109 items rated on a 7-point Likert-type scale to assess the cognitive, somatic, and behavioral aspects of social anxiety. This instrument consists of two subscales: the Social Phobia subscale and the Agoraphobia subscale. The latter subscale assesses anxiety associated with classic agoraphobic situations. A total score is derived by subtracting the Agoraphobia subscale score from the Social Phobia subscale score. This measure is capable of discriminating persons with social phobia from those with other anxiety disorders (Turner, Stanley, Beidel, & Bond, 1989) and from nonanxious controls (Beidel, Turner, Stanley, & Dancu, 1989). Test–retest and internal reliability have been high for this scale (Turner, Stanley, et al., 1989). Both convergent and discriminant validity of this instrument have also been demonstrated for both the adult version (Beidel, Borden, Turner, & Jacob, 1989; Turner, Beidel, et al., 1989) and the adolescent version (D. B. Clark et al., 1994).

Turner, Beidel, et al. (1989) recommended using the difference score as an indicator of social anxiety, because it results in better discrimination between patients with social phobia and patients with panic disorder. However, Herbert, Bellack, and Hope (1991) argued that the SPAI Social Phobia subscale is a better measure of social phobia, because it makes no theoretical assumptions about the relationship between social phobia and agoraphobia. Beidel and Turner (1992) in turn criticized the lack of empirical support for Herbert et al.'s (1991) recommendation and provided some theoretical reasons to support the use of the difference score. Herbert, Bellack, Hope, and Mueser (1992) suggested that the best SPAI subscale score depends on the intended use of the instrument (e.g., as a treatment outcome measure, as an assessment instrument for social phobia symptoms, or as a means of differentiating groups of individuals). However, this issue has not been completely resolved.

A recent study by Ries et al. (1998) compared the SPS, SIAS, and SPAI to each other and evaluated these instruments in patients with social phobia. These self-report measures were administered to 41 participants with social phobia. In addition, all patients underwent diagnostic assessments and two BATs. One of the tests consisted of a conversation task with a stranger of the opposite sex, and the other consisted of an impromptu speech task. After each task, positive and negative self-statements were measured with the original Social Interaction and Self-Statement Test (SISST; Glass et al., 1982) and a modification of it. Finally, 27 of the 41 participants received the same assessment again after 12 weekly sessions of CBGT. The results showed that, as expected, all three scales were significantly intercorrelated. However, Ries et al., also suggested that each of these instruments offers a unique contribution to the assessment of social phobia in terms of behavioral and cognitive self-report criteria, as well as distinction among subtypes. Specifically, the SIAS was consistently related to negative and positive self-reported thoughts in the speech and conversation test, whereas the SPS showed a significant negative relationship with time spent during the impromptu speech. The SIAS and the SPAI were most sensitive to treatment change and most useful for distinguishing social phobia subtypes.

Although reliable and valid, these measures are somewhat limited for research purposes, because they only provide an overall score as a general indicator of distress and avoidance in social situations. Despite the theoretical importance of cognitions in social phobia, a review of the literature suggests that fewer than three-quarters of the studies on social phobia utilized any type of cognitive assessment (Heimberg, 1994). This might be due to the fact that many of the available cognitive measures for social anxiety either are difficult to administer and score (such as the thought-listing procedure—see below), or are of questionable validity (such as the FNE, Watson & Friend, 1969; see Heimberg, 1994, for a critique of this scale). The only two instruments that were specifically designed to measure cognitions in individuals with social phobia are the SISST (Glass et al., 1982) and (more recently) the Self-Statement during Public Speaking Scale (SSPS; Hofmann & DiBartolo, 2000). The SISST is a frequently used structured self-statement test that is administered after an interaction task. The items were originally drawn from thought listings of a large student sample in response to frequently occurring problematic heterosexual social situations. The SSPS is a modified and abbreviated version of the SISST that can be administered without a BAT in order to measure positive and negative cognitions related to public speaking, the most commonly feared social situation. Preliminary data suggest that this 10-item instrument shows promising psychometric characteristics and is sensitive to treatment change.

Finally, the literature reports a number of other instruments that have occasionally been used in social phobia research. For example, the Personal Report of Confidence as a Speaker Scale, originally developed by Gilkinson (1942) and modified by Paul (1966), has been used to assess the fear of public speaking. An alternative scale to measure speech anxiety is the Personal Report of Communication Apprehension (Richmond & McCroskey, 1992). Other scales that are worth mentioning are the Interaction Anxiousness Scale and the Audience Anxiousness Scale by Leary (1983b); the Situation Questionnaire by Rehm and Marston (1968) to assess heterosexual social anxiety; the Stanford Shyness Survey (Zimbardo, 1977); the Social Reticence Scale (W. H. Jones, Briggs, & Smith, 1986); and the Self-Consciousness Scale (Fenigstein, Scheier, & Buss, 1975). Furthermore, some investigators have measured social phobia by using the Social Phobia subscale of the Fear Questionnaire (Marks & Mathews, 1979). A more detailed discussion of these scales can be found in McNeil, Ries, and Turk (1995). In summary, a number of self-report measures for social anxiety are available, each with different advantages and disadvantages.

Thought Listing

As discussed earlier, contemporary theories of anxiety in general, and theories of social anxiety and social phobia specifically, emphasize the role of cognitive processes and the focus of attention. Unfortunately, measuring self-focused attention is very complicated. Some studies have attempted to assess self-focused attention directly through questionnaires (Wells & Papageorgiou, 1998b; Woody et al., 1997). However, this assessment technique is problematic, because attention is necessarily altered in order to answer the question (Woody et al., 1997). Moreover, the existing instruments either assess the focus of attention (Woody et al., 1997) or the valence of thoughts (Glass et al., 1982) but not both, which makes it difficult to determine whether individuals with social phobia focus on positive or negative aspects of themselves or the situation. Some authors have therefore employed thought-listing techniques to study self-focused attention. When using these techniques, subjects are typically asked either to articulate or to write down their thoughts related to a simulated social situation (e.g., Bruch, Heimberg, & Hope, 1991; Cacioppo et al., 1979; Davison, Vogel, & Coffman, 1997; Heimberg, Bruch, Hope, & Dombeck, 1990; Hofmann, 2000a; Kendall & Hollon, 1981; Schwartz & Garamoni, 1989; Stopa & Clark, 1993). Although this assessment technique is useful for research purposes, its practical utility is limited due to the complicated administration and scoring procedure.

Self-Monitoring Forms

Self-monitoring forms, such as daily logs and diaries, are an integral part of any effective psychosocial treatment protocol for social phobia. Data from these forms provide valuable feedback for patients and therapists about treatment progress, and often lead to positive changes of behavior as a result of self-observation (e.g., Becker & Heimberg, 1988). A typical monitoring form gathers information on the date and time of a feared social event; the level of anxiety (on a Likert-type scale) at the beginning and end of the situation; and the maximum level of anxiety experienced during the event. In addition, these instruments may provide information on the time the patient stays in the social situation, whether or not the patient used any avoidance strategies, how the patient felt afterward, and whether or not the patient would enter the situation again. Additional measures may include feelings, thoughts, and perceived physiological arousal associated with a feared social situation. This information provides very valuable data related to treatment planning and treatment progress. Unfortunately, little research exists on the psychometric properties of such data.

PSYCHOLOGICAL TREATMENTS

A number of effective treatments are available to those who suffer from this debilitating disorder, such as cognitive therapy; cognitive-behavioral therapy (CBT), especially in group form (CBGT); exposure treatment; and social skills training (e.g., Heimberg, Dodge, et al., 1990; Heimberg et al., 1998; Heimberg, Salzman, Holt, & Blendell, 1993; Mattick & Peters, 1988; Turner, Beidel, Cooley, Woody, & Messer, 1994; Turner, Beidel, & Cooley-Quille, 1995). Of those interventions, Heimberg's CBGT for social phobia has been included in a list of empirically supported treatments by the Society of Clinical Psychology's (Division 12 of the American Psychological Association) Task Force on Promotion and Dissemination of Psychological Procedures (Chambless et al., 1996).

Moreover, the efficacy of CBGT has been demonstrated in a number of well-designed studies (Gelernter et al., 1991; Heimberg, Becker, Goldfinger, & Vermilyea, 1985; Heimberg, Dodge, et al., 1990; Heimberg, Salzman, et al., 1993; Heimberg et al., 1998). CBGT is typically administered by two therapists in 12 weekly 2.5-hour sessions (30 hours in total) to groups consisting of approximately six participants. In one of the earlier studies, Heimberg, Dodge, et al. (1990) compared CBGT to an alternative treatment called educational–supportive group psychotherapy, which was shown to equal CBGT in credibility. Results indicated that patients receiving CBGT were rated as less impaired by clinical interviewers than patients receiving the educational–supportive intervention, and reported less anxiety during a behavioral test at posttreatment assessment and 6-month follow-up. Patients in both treatments showed increases in positive cognition and decreases in negative cognition at posttreatment, but only patients receiving CBGT maintained this improvement at 6-month follow-up.

More recently, CBGT was compared to phenelzine (a monoamine oxidase inhibitor [MAOI] commonly used to treat social phobia), an educational–supportive group, and a pill placebo (Heimberg et al., 1998). The results of this study showed that more people responded to phenelzine and CBGT than to the pill placebo and the educational–supportive group therapy (this study is discussed in more detail later).

CBT (including CBGT) is based on the assumption that treatment progress occurs as a result of changes in cognitive schemata. More specifically, it is assumed that effective psychotherapy either directly modifies a patient's irrational beliefs, or deactivates them while making other schemata available. According to this model, individuals with social phobia believe that they are in danger of behaving in an inept and unacceptable fashion, and that such behavior will have disastrous consequences in terms of loss of status, loss of worth, and rejection (Clark & Wells, 1995; Rapee & Heimberg, 1997). This model predicts that once a situation is perceived as holding the potential for social evaluation, individuals with social phobia become preoccupied with negative thoughts about themselves and the way other people perceive them. The model also proposes that this negative impression typically occurs in the form of an image from an "observer" perspective, in which people with social phobia can see themselves as if from another person's vantage point. This model therefore predicts that treatment is most effective if it is aimed at changing dysfunctional cognitions directly and systematically via cognitive interventions.

Although some experimental studies seem to support the validity of certain aspects of this model (Stopa & Clark, 1993, 2000; Wells, Clark, & Ahmad, 1998; Wells & Papageorgiou, 1999), the treatment outcome literature does not provide strong corroborating evidence for it. For example, a number of review articles and meta-analyses showed that CBT is not more effective than exposure therapy alone, which does not specifically address negative cognitive appraisals and probability overestimation (Feske & Chambless, 1995; Gould, Buckminster, Pollack, Otto, & Yap, 1997; Taylor, 1996; Turner, Cooley-Quille, & Beidel, 1996). For example, the meta-analysis by Gould et al. (1997) showed that exposure interventions yielded the largest effect sizes, whether alone (effect size = 0.89) or in combination with cognitive restructuring (effect size = 0.80). Similar results were reported by Feske and Chambless (1995), who also found no evidence of differential dropout or relapse rates between the two treatment modalities. Another meta-analysis by Taylor (1996) compared the effect sizes of cognitive treatments, exposure treatments, CBT, social skills training, placebo treatments, and wait-list control groups. The results showed that the effect size of the wait-list control group was significantly smaller than the effect sizes of the different treatment conditions at posttreatment. Only combined cognitive restructuring–exposure treatments produced effect sizes that were significantly larger than those of placebo controls. However, the effect sizes of the different treatment conditions did not differ significantly from one another. Finally, the results of a dismantling study conducted by Hope, Heimberg, and Bruch (1995) also suggested that exposure alone is at least as effective as exposure plus cognitive intervention in the treatment of social phobia. This study randomly assigned 40 individuals with social phobia to either Heimberg's CBGT, an exposure condition without cognitive intervention, or a wait-list control group. As expected, individuals in both active treatments improved more than those in the wait-list control group. However, participants who received CBGT did not improve more than those who received exposure without cognitive intervention. In fact, individuals in the exposure-only condition improved even more than those who received CBGT on some measures.

These studies underline the importance of exposure intervention in the treatment of social phobia, and suggest that both CBT and exposure alone are effective treatments for social phobia. However, there is no clear advantage for CBT over exposure alone. Both treatment modalities seem to produce very similar pretreatment–posttreatment and pretreatment–follow-up effects for self-report measures of social phobia, cognitive symptoms, and depressed/anxious mood, with no evidence of differential dropout or relapse rates.

These data are consistent with our model of social phobia, which emphasizes the role of "false alarms" (Figure 13.2). Our model predicts that repeated and prolonged exposure to social threat in the absence of all manner of avoidance strategies (safety signals and behavior) will lead to an "unlearning" or extinction of the learned alarm response, improvement of perceived social skills, and decrease in anxious apprehension (including self-focused attention). These changes are more likely to occur if internal fear cues and all other significant contexts are systematically produced (e.g., Bouton, Mineka, & Barlow, 2001) and if the outcome of the social situation is unexpectedly positive, because it forces the person to reevaluate the actual threat of the social situation. Therefore, cognitive interventions may facilitate the fear reduction mechanism, but they cannot replace the effects of direct reality-testing exposure.

It should be pointed out that in practice, it is difficult to directly compare the efficacy of exposure treatment and cognitive therapy in isolation. Unexpected positive experiences during exposure to fearful social situations inevitably changes the patient's beliefs and attitudes about a situation, even without explicit cognitive restructuring techniques. Furthermore, it is methodologically difficult to control for the number of treatment sessions and the amount of exposure the patient receives, especially if both therapies are conducted within the same amount of time. By adding cognitive techniques to an exposure-based intervention, less time is available for exposure as compared to "pure" exposure therapy. This problem has typically not been adequately addressed in comparative treatment outcome studies. A notable exception is a study by Glass, Gottman, and Shmurak (1976), which compared different training programs for shy male undergraduate and graduate students. The study included "response acquisition training" (consisting of role plays and coaching), "cognitive self-statement modification training" (similar to cognitive therapy), and a combination of both training programs. In addition to a wait-list control group, two enhanced-treatment groups (enhanced response acquisition and enhanced cognitive self-statement modification) were used to control for the longer training time of the combined-treatment group. The results showed a significant treatment effect, but no length of treatment effect. Subjects who received cognitive self-statement modification showed better performance in role-play situations and made more phone calls than individuals from the other groups. These effects were maintained at a 6-month follow-up. Although these results are difficult to compare directly with contemporary treatment outcome studies on social phobia, due to the analogue nature of the participants (among other differences), the design used by Glass et al. could serve as a model for future dismantling studies.

It should also be noted that all published treatment outcome studies on social phobia have been based on cross-sectional assessments, which simply demonstrate good maintenance of gains *on average* following such interventions. However, little is known about the course of each individual's symptoms following treatment completion. Furthermore, the actual active treatment ingredient has yet to be determined. Exposure, cognitive intervention, and social skills training are frequently applied techniques, although different treatment protocols vary greatly in their emphasis on these components. This raises important questions about the mechanism of action of treatment (i.e., the mediators) and the predictors of treatment outcome (Hofmann, 2000b).

Another controversial area of social phobia treatment research concerns the issue of social phobia subtypes. Our model states that social threat leads principally to "anxiety" (an integrated affective and cognitively mediated anticipation of potential danger) in individuals with generalized social phobia and those with APD, and principally to "fear" or panic (a more basic and less cognitively mediated emotional response) in individuals with nongeneralized social phobia and those without APD, although anxiety may come to be focused on the next alarm response in a social context. Therefore, our model predicts that cognitive interventions may be more effective for the generalized subtype of social phobia and for individuals with APD than they are for individuals with nongeneralized social phobia and for those without APD, while exposure-based procedures are an essential part of treatment for any individual with social phobia.

Unfortunately, the current literature provides insufficient data to either corroborate or refute this hypothesis. Some studies suggest that the presence of a generalized subtype of social phobia and/or the additional Axis II diagnosis of APD (or a significant feature of it) will complicate psychosocial treatment and may dictate alternative approaches (e.g., Chambless, Tran, & Glass, 1997; Feske, Perry, Chambless, Renneberg, & Goldstein, 1996). In contrast, other studies have not found the generalized subtype of social phobia or APD to be predictive of poor psychosocial treatment outcome (E. J. Brown et al., 1995; Hofmann, Newman, Becker, Taylor, & Roth, 1995; Hope, Herbert, & White, 1995; Turner, Beidel, & Townsley, 1992). Turner, Beidel, Wolff, Spaulding, and Jacob (1996) reported that individuals with generalized and nongeneralized social phobia improved equivalently over treatment, but that the overall status of the generalized subtype was poorer than that of the nongeneralized subtype at posttreatment. A similar pattern was found when cases of social phobia with and without comorbid conditions were compared. Turner, Beidel, Wolff, Spaulding, and Jacob (1996) have suggested that the addition of social skills training to exposure intervention might improve the functional status of individuals with a generalized subtype of social phobia.

The inconsistent findings in the literature may be partly due to the small sample size in some of the studies, differences in the operational definition of the generalized subtype, and differences in the assessment procedures for APD. Systematic dismantling studies would provide valuable data. Furthermore, future studies investigating the moderating role of diagnostic subgroups of social phobia will need to consider the effects of treatment expectancy (Chambless et al., 1997; Safren, Heimberg, & Juster, 1997), homework compliance (Edelman & Chambless, 1995; Leung & Heimberg, 1996), and depression (Chambless et al., 1997), as well as those of therapeutic alliance, adherence and competence to the treatment protocol, sociodemographic variables, and diagnostic data.

For example, the study by Chambless et al. (1997) considered depression, treatment expectancy, personality disorder traits, clinical severity, and frequency of negative thoughts during social interactions as possible predictors for treatment outcome in 62 patients with social phobia. Treatment consisted of 12 weekly sessions following Heimberg's CBGT protocol (e.g., Heimberg, Dodge, et al., 1990). Participants were assessed at pretreatment, posttreatment, and 6-month follow-up. Outcome measures included self-report questionnaires and behavioral tests. The results showed that none of the predictors was related to outcome across all domains of measurement. However, higher levels of depression as measured with the Beck Depression Inventory (Beck & Steer, 1987), more APD traits, and lower treatment expectancy were each related to poorer treatment response on one or more outcome criteria. The most salient predictor for poor treatment outcome was depression. This raises important questions about the external validity of many of the existing psychotherapy outcome studies, because Heimberg and colleagues excluded patients with major depression from their research trials (Chambless et al., 1997, p. 235). Furthermore, the results of the Chambless et al. (1997) study showed that cognitive change (as measured with the SISST; Glass et al., 1982) was associated with change on self-report symptom measures, but lower rates of negative thinking at posttreatment did not predict better maintenance of treatment gains at follow-up. This again raises important questions about the validity of the existing cognitive model for social phobia.

PHARMACOLOGICAL TREATMENTS

With the recognition of social phobia as a prevalent and serious condition, the number of pharmacological studies has increased substantially in recent years. To date, the most common drug treatments for social phobia include MAOIs, which include both reversible (e.g., moclobemide) and irreversible (e.g., phenelzine) compounds; selective serotonin reuptake inhibitors (SSRIs); benzodiazepines; tricyclic and other antidepressants; and beta-blockers.

Monoamine Oxidase Inhibitors

The results of four double-blind placebo-controlled trials show evidence for the efficacy of phenelzine in social phobia (Gelernter et al., 1991; Heimberg et al., 1998; Liebowitz et al., 1992; Versiani et al., 1992). In the study by Liebowitz et al. (1992), 85 patients were treated with either phenelzine (at least 45 mg/day); atenolol, a beta-blocker (at least 50 mg/day); or placebo. Phenelzine was significantly more effective than atenolol and placebo. The results showed that 64% of patients receiving phenelzine, 30% of patients receiving atenolol, and 23% of those receiving placebo were classified as responders based on clinical global improvement ratings (Guy, 1976). Similar results were reported by Versiani et al. (1992), who compared the efficacy of phenelzine (on average 67.5 mg/day), moclobemide (on average 570.7 mg/day), and placebo for treating social phobia. After 8 weeks, both active drugs were more effective than placebo. In terms of scores on the LSAS, phenelzine was superior to moclobemide. At Week 16, 82% of the moclobemide-treated and 91% of the phenelzine-treated patients were markedly improved. Moclobemide, however, was better tolerated than phenelzine.

Two studies included cognitive-behavioral intervention in the study design (Gelernter et al., 1991; Heimberg et al., 1998; Liebowitz et al., 1999). Gelernter et al. (1991) randomly assigned 65 patients to one of four groups, each lasting for 12 weeks: phenelzine (on average 55 mg/day), alprazolam (on average 4.2 mg/day), placebo, or Heimberg's CBGT. The results showed no significant difference among the active treatments. However, all patients receiving pharmacotherapy also received exposure instructions.

More recently, Heimberg et al. (1998) recruited 133 patients for a study comparing phenelzine versus placebo, educational–supportive group therapy, or CBGT (Table 13.1). Dosage started at 15 mg/day and could be raised up to 90 mg/day. After 12 weeks, both phenelzine (65%) and CBGT (58%) had higher proportions of responders than the pill placebo (33%) or educational–supportive group therapy (27%), which served as a psychotherapy placebo condition. The criterion for treatment response was based on a 7-point rating of change on the Social Phobic Disorders Severity Change Form (Liebowitz et al., 1992) by an independent evaluator. Patients given a rating of 1 or 2 (markedly or moderately improved) were classified as responders. Responders to this acute trial entered a 6-month maintenance phase and a 6-month treatment-free phase (Liebowitz et al., 1999). Approximately two-thirds of the patients (20 of the 31 patients receiving phenelzine, and 21 of the 36 patients receiving CGBT) were classified as responders after 12 weeks of acute treatment and were therefore eligible to enter the maintenance phase of the study. Six patients in the phenelzine group and 7 patients in the CBGT group declined, leaving 14 responders after CBGT and 14 responders after phenelzine who were eligible to enter the maintenance phase. Patients receiving phenelzine were maintained on medication, which could be adjusted depending on the clinical state and side effects, but could not exceed a maximum dosage of 90 mg/day. Patients in the CBGT condition received monthly CBGT group sessions. No difference was found in relapse and dropout rates during maintenance between patients receiving CBGT (2 relapsers and 1 dropout) and patients receiving phenelzine (3 relapsers and 1 dropout). The remaining patients from the phenelzine group (10 of 14) and the CBGT group (11 of 14) were classified as responders at the postmaintenance assessment and therefore eligible to enter a 6-month treatment-free follow-up period. The analysis of the follow-up phase showed no difference between the groups in the dropout rates (1 patient in each group). However, the relapse rate was higher in the phenelzine group (3 of 14) than in the CBGT group (0 of 14). Due to the small sample size, this difference did not reach the conventional level of statistical significance ($p < .09$).

These data demonstrate the short-term efficacy of phenelzine and CBGT for the treatment of social phobia. However, there is some indication that patients receiving phenelzine are more likely to relapse than patients receiving CBGT after a treatment-free follow-up period. Furthermore, the use of irreversible MAOIs is limited by the risk of hypertensive crisis if dietary restrictions are not followed, and by their adverse effect profile. For ex-

TABLE 13.1. Comparison of Cognitive-Behavioral Group Treatment (CBGT), Phenelzine (PHEN), Pill Placebo (PLA), and Educational–Supportive Group Treatment (ES) in the Responder Rates of the Intent-to-Treat-Analyses after 12 Weeks of Acute Treatment, 6 Monthly Maintenance Sessions, and 6 Months of No-Treatment Follow-Up

Assessment	CBGT	PHEN	PLA	ES	Statistical comparisons
Posttreatment	58% (21/36)	65% (20/31)	33% (11/33)	27% (19/33)	CBGT, PHEN > PLA, ES**
Postmaintenance	79% (11/14)	79% (11/14)	Not assessed	Not assessed	CBGT = PHEN
6-month follow-up	91% (10/11)	50% (7/14)	Not assessed	Not assessed	CBGT ≥ PHEN*

Note. The table shows percentage (number) of individuals who were rated as moderately or markedly improved on the Social Phobic Disorders Severity Change Form (Liebowitz et al., 1992) among the total number of patients who entered the study. The data are from Heimberg et al. (1998) and Liebowitz et al. (1999).
*$p < .09$. **$p < .005$.

ample, Gelernter et al. (1991) reported that 95% of the patients who were taking phenelzine experienced at least one side effect, compared to 27% in the placebo group. Therefore, researchers have been testing the efficacy of reversible inhibitors of MAO-A, which do not require any dietary restrictions at the clinically recommended dosage. Furthermore, other side effects commonly observed in nonreversible MAOIs, such as fatigue and hypotension, seem to be less common and less severe. However, the clinical trials using reversible MAO-A inhibitors, such as moclobemide, have had mixed results (Katschnig, Stein, & Buller, 1997; Noyes et al., 1997; Versiani et al., 1992, 1996).

Selective Serotonin Reuptake Inhibitors

The promising results of studies using MAOIs for the treatment of social phobia have stimulated research on other antidepressants with better tolerability as potential treatments for social phobia. On May 11, 1999, the FDA approved paroxetine for the treatment of social phobia, making it the first (and so far only) medication approved for this disorder in the United States.

Stein et al. (1998) tested the efficacy of paroxetine in a 12-week, placebo-controlled, double-blind, and flexible-dose design that included 187 patients (Table 13.2). The initial daily dose of paroxetine was 20 mg, and this was increased weekly by 10 mg up to a maximum of 50 mg/day. The results showed that 55% of patients receiving paroxetine and 23.9% of those receiving placebo were classified as responders based on clinical global improvement ratings. On the average, the reduction from baseline on the LSAS total score was more than twice as large in the paroxetine group (39.1%) as in the placebo group (17.4%). In addition, various smaller studies have used other SSRIs with promising results, including fluvoxamine (van Vliet, den Boer, & Westenberg, 1994), sertraline (Katzelnick et al., 1995), and fluoxetine (Black, Uhde, & Tancer, 1992; Schneier, Chin, Hollander, & Liebowitz, 1992; Sternbach, 1990; van Ameringen, Mancini, & Streiner, 1993).

Benzodiazepines

To date, only two studies have tested the efficacy of benzodiazepines (e.g., clonazepam and alprazolam) to reduce social anxiety under double-blind conditions (Davidson, Potts, et al., 1993; Gelernter et al., 1991). The study by Davidson, Potts, et al. (1993) investigated the efficacy of clonazepam for the treatment of social phobia in a 10-week double-blind study including 75 patients at a mean dose of 2.4 mg/day. The results showed that 78% of the patients using clonazepam were classified as responders, compared to 20% of those receiving placebo. In addition, reports on a number of open trials support the efficacy of clonazepam (Munjack, Baltazar, Bohn, Cabe, & Appleton, 1990; Ontiveros &

TABLE 13.2. Comparison between Paroxetine (PAR) and Placebo (PLA) before and after 12 Weeks of Treatment

Assessment	PAR	PLA	Statistical comparisons
Responder rates	55% (50/91)	23.9% (22/92)	PAR > PLA
Decrease in LSAS from baseline	39.1%	17.4%	PAR > PLA

Note. The table shows the percentage of responders (much or very much improved on clinical global improvement ratings; Guy, 1976) and the decrease in the Liebowitz Social Anxiety Scale (LSAS; Liebowitz, 1987) scores from baseline. All p's < .05. The data are from Stein et al. (1998).

Fontaine, 1990; Reiter, Pollack, Rosenbaum, & Cohen, 1990). In contrast, the afore-mentioned study by Gelernter et al. (1991) reported that only 38% of patients receiving alprazolam at a mean dose of 4.2 mg/day were classified as responders, compared to 69% of those who received phenelzine. Two months after discontinuation of alprazolam, most patients experienced a recurrence of their social anxiety symptoms to baseline levels.

These studies illustrate the major disadvantage of using clonazepam or alprazolam for treating social anxiety, which can lead to physical dependence and a relatively high rate of relapse after (rapid) discontinuation. Clonazepam is usually easier to taper, possibly because of its longer half-life. Furthermore, benzodiazepines are contraindicated in patients who drink alcohol to reduce their social anxiety, due to the synergistic effects of these drugs with alcohol.

Tricyclic Antidepressants

Only limited data exist on the efficacy of tricyclic antidepressant medications for the treatment of social anxiety, such as imipramine (Benca, Matuzas, & Al-Sadir, 1986; Emmanuel, Johnson, & Villareal, 1998; Liebowitz, Gorman, Fyer, Campeas, et al., 1985; Zitrin, Klein, Woerner & Ross, 1983) and clomipramine (Beaumont, 1977; Pecknold, McClure, Appeltauer, Allan, & Wrzesinski, 1982; Versiani, Mundim, Nardi, & Liebowitz, 1988). These studies reported only small improvements in social anxiety due to the medication. For example, Emmanuel et al. (1998) treated 41 patients with imipramine or placebo over a period of 8 weeks, using a flexible-dose design. Only 2 of the 18 patients who received imipramine and 1 out of 23 patients receiving placebo improved. Similar results were reported after treating a series of 15 patients with imipramine at a mean dose of 17.4 mg/day (Simpson et al., 1998). Only 9 patients completed the study, while the other 6 withdrew due to intolerable side effects. The results showed that 20% of the patients were classified as responders, suggesting that imipramine is not an effective treatment for social phobia. These results are consistent with earlier case studies (Liebowitz, Gorman, Fyer, Campeas, et al., 1985; Zitrin, et al., 1983).

Similar conclusions can be drawn with regard to the use of clomipramine as a treatment for social phobia. For example, Versiani et al. (1988) treated six patients with social phobia in an open-label design with 175–250 mg/day of clomipramine. Although depressive and generalized anxiety symptoms showed some improvement, no positive change was observed in the social phobia symptoms. In fact, some patients developed even greater social anxiety due to a tremor that developed as a side effect of the medication. These studies suggest that the efficacy of imipramine and clomipramine in social phobia is very limited.

Other Antidepressants

Bupropion, a fairly novel antidepressant with dopamine agonist properties, has been reported to be effective for treating social phobia in a single case (Emmanuel, Lydiard, & Ballenger, 1991). Furthermore, buspirone, an anxiolytic drug with antidepressant properties, has been studied in one controlled trial (Clark & Agras, 1991) and two open-label trials (Munjack et al., 1990; Schneier et al., 1993). In the Clark and Agras (1991) study, 29 musicians with performance anxiety (all of whom met DSM-III-R criteria for social phobia) were either treated with (1) buspirone; (2) buspirone plus CBT; (3) a pill placebo; or (4) a pill placebo plus CBT. All treatments lasted for 6 weeks. At a moderate dose (30 mg/day), the drug was not any more effective than placebo and less effective than CBT. In contrast, Schneier et al. (1993) reported that patients who tolerated dosages of 45 mg/day or greater did experience modest benefit. The treatment phase of this study lasted for 12 weeks, and it was based on 22 patients.

Beta-Blockers

It is a commonly held belief that beta-blockers (such as propranolol or atenolol) are effective for treating social anxiety because they block the peripheral autonomic response to the anxiety-provoking stimulus. Therefore, these drugs have been widely used for treating performance anxiety since the 1970s (e.g., Gottschalk, Stone, & Gleser, 1974; Sittonen & Tanne, 1976). The results of a survey conducted on 2,212 professional musicians found that 27% of them reported using beta-blockers to treat their stage fright. The majority of them (70%) had obtained the medication without prescription (Fishbein, Middlestadt, & Ottati, 1988).

Despite the enthusiasm for these drugs to treat social anxiety, their efficacy has not been supported by double-blind studies (Liebowitz et al., 1992; Turner, Beidel, & Jacob, 1994). For example, Liebowitz et al. (1992) compared the effects of phenelzine, atenolol, and placebo for treating social phobia. As already reported earlier, the results showed no advantage for atenolol over placebo. Only 30% responded to atenolol, as compared to 64% of patients receiving phenelzine and 23% of patients taking a pill placebo. Similar results were also reported by Turner, Beidel, and Jacob (1994), who found no benefit for atenolol over pill placebo. The authors treated 72 individuals who had social phobia with either behavior therapy (flooding), atenolol (up to 100 mg/day), or a pill placebo for a period of 3 months. Flooding was superior to placebo on self-report measures, clinician ratings, behavioral assessment measures, and performance on composite indices, and also superior to atenolol on behavioral measures and composite indices. Subjects who improved during treatment maintained gains at the 6-month follow-up, regardless of whether they received flooding or atenolol. These data provide little empirical support for atenolol as a treatment of social phobia when used at a standing dose.

In contrast, Pohl, Balon, et al. (1998) reported some promising results after conducting a preliminary double-blind study using beta-blockers as needed or placebo for individuals with nongeneralized social phobia. The study compared 10 patients who received propranolol as needed with 8 patients who received placebo for a period of 6 weeks after a 2-week placebo lead-in period. The study used self-report measures and a patient diary as an outcome measure. Patient visits were scheduled at 2, 4, and 6 weeks. Participants who received propranolol reported less anxiety after both 4 and 6 weeks of treatment, and they rated their level of impairment as less severe after 6 weeks of treatment than patients on placebo. Furthermore, the propranolol group showed greater improvement on the LSAS than the placebo group. However, there were no differences in self-report measures of social anxiety. These results, albeit preliminary, suggest that beta-blockers, when administered as needed, may be clinically useful for treating individuals with a nongeneralized subtype of social phobia.

CHAPTER 14

Generalized Anxiety Disorder

LIZABETH ROEMER
SUSAN M. ORSILLO
DAVID H. BARLOW

In the first edition of this book (Barlow, 1988) it was noted that despite the apparent prevalence of chronic, general anxiety (according to estimates from primary care physicians), it had been difficult to successfully identify and classify individuals under the rubric of generalized anxiety disorder (GAD). At the time of that edition, GAD had just recently been classified as a separate, nonresidual category, based in part on the identification of worry (apprehensive expectation) as its central defining feature. This development, along with the diagnostic revisions that followed it, has dramatically increased our understanding of the nature of this disorder, its associated features, and its successful treatment. In large part, this improvement stems from extensive basic research on the phenomenon of worry, elucidating its nature, function, and maintaining factors.

Because worry and accompanying neurobiological features are common features across the anxiety disorders (see Chapter 3), GAD (centrally defined by worry) may in fact be the "basic" anxiety disorder. That is, our understanding of the etiological and maintaining factors of GAD may have implications for the understanding of all anxiety disorders. In fact, given the apparent close association between GAD and major depression (discussed below), the study of this disorder may indeed be relevant to the understanding and treatment of all emotional disorders.

We begin this chapter with a brief review of the history of the diagnosis of GAD, because the refinements in the diagnostic criteria for GAD have played an important role in enhancing our understanding and successful treatment of this disorder. We then review the epidemiology and demographic characteristics of GAD. A large portion of the chapter is devoted to reviewing research and theory regarding important characteristics and maintaining factors of GAD and worry; it is here that conceptualizations likely to be relevant to many (if not all) emotional disorders are introduced. The etiological model of GAD (similarly relevant across the anxiety disorders; see Chapter 8) is reviewed next. After a summary of major assessment tools commonly used with individuals diagnosed with GAD, we conclude with discussions of pharmacological and psychosocial interventions for GAD. We address the existing literature in these areas, as well as issues that are the focus of current theoretical and empirical inquiry.

DIAGNOSTIC CONSIDERATIONS

History of the diagnostic criteria

The diagnostic criteria for GAD have undergone extensive revision over the past 20 years. GAD was first introduced into the DSM system in the third edition of the *Diagnostic and Statistical Manual of Mental Disorders* (DSM-III; American Psychiatric Association, 1980). As noted in Chapter 9, for this revision the broad category of anxiety neurosis (which encompassed all individuals who experienced excessive anxiety over a prolonged period of time without marked phobic avoidance) was divided into the categories of panic disorder (described in Chapter 10) and GAD. In DSM-III, GAD was a residual category, meaning that patients could not be diagnosed as having GAD unless they did not meet the criteria for any other anxiety disorder. However, interrater reliability of this GAD diagnosis was only fair (kappa = .47; Di Nardo, O'Brien, Barlow, Waddell, & Blanchard, 1983). Furthermore, the 1-month duration criterion was thought to lead to overdiagnosis, because adjustment reactions to negative life events might result in transient GAD-like symptoms.

The residual status of GAD in DSM-III was also a potential source of diagnostic confusion; studies investigated whether in fact GAD would be more accurately conceptualized as an independent disorder. Although in one study symptoms of GAD were reported by individuals diagnosed with all other anxiety disorders (except simple phobia; Barlow, Blanchard, Vermilyea, Vermilyea, & Di Nardo, 1986), a second study found that only a small proportion of patients with anxiety disorders actually received an additional diagnosis of GAD when the diagnostic exclusionary rules that were part of the DSM-III hierarchy were dropped (Barlow, Di Nardo, Vermilyea, Vermilyea, & Blanchard, 1986). This discrepancy probably came about because diagnostic interviewers in the latter study considered the focus of reported apprehensive expectation (worry) in making a diagnosis. That is, individuals who reported worrying about future panic attacks (in the case of panic disorder) or social situations (in the case of social phobia) did not receive an additional diagnosis of GAD, while individuals who worried about multiple situations in addition to the focus of their principal diagnosis did. These findings suggested that GAD symptomatology was independent of other disorders, even though disorder-specific worry was also often a component of other diagnostic categories. This conclusion was consistent with clinical experience: Some patients with other anxiety disorders continued to exhibit general anxiety symptoms that interfered with their lives following successful treatment of their principal disorder, while others did not.

Based on these considerations, DSM-III-R (American Psychiatric Association, 1987) contained a revised definition of GAD in which the duration criterion was increased to 6 months and GAD was moved from the status of a residual category to its own category, centrally defined by unrealistic or excessive anxiety and worry (apprehensive expectation) about two or more life circumstances. The criteria specified that if another Axis I disorder was present, a diagnosis of GAD was only appropriate if the focus of anxiety and worry was unrelated to that disorder. The identification of apprehensive expectation or worry as the cardinal feature of this disorder had implications for our understanding of this disorder, as well as for the development of efficacious treatments. The resulting conceptual and empirical advances in our understanding of worry have been reviewed in Chapter 3 and are considered again in detail below. However, despite these conceptual advances, the reliability of GAD as a principal diagnosis remained only fair (kappa = .57; Di Nardo, Moras, Barlow, Rapee, & Brown, 1993).

Refinement of Diagnostic Criteria for DSM-IV

Between the publication of DSM-III-R and DSM-IV (American Psychiatric Association, 1994), extensive study of each element of the diagnostic criteria for GAD was conducted, resulting in refined, empirically based criteria in the current version of the DSM. These revisions have also guided research and theory in the area of GAD and worry.

Once worry had been identified as a central characteristic of GAD in DSM-III-R, researchers began investigating the content of worry that characterized individuals with GAD (e.g., Borkovec, Shadick, & Hopkins, 1991; Craske, Rapee, Jackel, & Barlow, 1989; Roemer, Molina, & Borkovec, 1997; Sanderson & Barlow, 1990). As noted in Chapter 3, these studies revealed few content differences between analogue and clinical GAD samples and their nonanxious counterparts; however, individuals with chronic worry reported more frequent worries across content areas, as well as more frequent unclassifiable or miscellaneous worries. In fact, studies found that individuals with GAD very commonly reported worrying about minor matters, and that the report of excessive worry about minor things effectively discriminated among individuals with GAD, individuals with other anxiety disorders, and nonanxious individuals (see Brown, Barlow, & Liebowitz, 1994, for a review; see also Abel & Borkovec, 1995; Sanderson & Barlow, 1990). Based on these findings, the DSM-IV criteria no longer specify worry about two or more spheres; instead, GAD worry is characterized as pervasive.

Studies have shown that, in addition to being pervasive, the worry associated with GAD is commonly perceived by individuals to be uncontrollable (Craske, Rapee, et al., 1989; Borkovec et al., 1991). Reports of worry as uncontrollable significantly discriminated individuals diagnosed with GAD from nonanxious controls, whereas reports that worry was unrealistic (one of the criteria in DSM-III-R) were less discriminating (Abel & Borkovec, 1995). Accordingly, the DSM-IV criteria have added that worry must be perceived as difficult to stop once it starts, and the unrealistic nature of worry is no longer part of the diagnostic criteria.

Finally, the most extensive revision in the DSM-IV diagnosis of GAD has been made to the 18 associated features (somatic symptoms) specified in DSM-III-R. An extensive multisite study exploring both the reliability and frequency of endorsement of these 18 symptoms revealed that the autonomic hyperactivity symptoms were the least reliable and least frequently endorsed symptoms among individuals with GAD (Marten et al., 1993). These findings were consistent with recent laboratory findings suggesting that GAD is *not* associated with autonomic hyperarousal (e.g., Hoehn-Saric, McLeod, & Zimmerli, 1989). In fact, studies suggest that worry *reduces* physiological arousal in response to a threatening stimulus (e.g., Borkovec & Hu, 1990). Based on Marten et al.'s findings, the most reliable and common symptoms of GAD (specifically, six symptoms representing seven of the DSM-III-R symptoms, because restlessness and feeling keyed up or on edge were combined) were identified. DSM-IV diagnosis requires endorsement of three of these six symptoms more days than not over a period of 6 months. Other studies using clinical (Abel & Borkovec, 1995; Brawman-Mintzer et al., 1994; T. A. Brown, Marten, & Barlow, 1995; Starcevic, Fallon, & Uhlenhuth, 1994) and analogue (Freeston, Dugas, Letarte, et al., 1996) samples support the association between these six symptoms and GAD. For instance, T. A. Brown, Marten, and Barlow (1995) found that the DSM-IV associated symptoms criterion significantly discriminated between patients with GAD and those with other anxiety disorders in a large sample of outpatients with anxiety disorders.

Nonetheless, some questions still remain regarding the associated somatic symptoms of GAD. As noted in Chapter 9, the associated symptoms of GAD almost entirely overlap with symptoms of depression. In fact, in the T. A. Brown, Marten, and Barlow (1995) study, the DSM-IV associated features criterion did not significantly discriminate patients with GAD from those with depressive disorders. Brown and his colleagues suggested raising the requirement to four of six symptoms, noting that in their sample this improved specificity without compromising sensitivity. Joormann and Stöber (1999) explored the relationship between the DSM-IV associated symptom criteria and measures of excessive worry and depression in a nonclinical sample. They found that the six symptoms showed differential relationships with worry and depression; muscle tension was particularly associated with worry, while difficulty concentrating was primarily related to depression. The specific relevance of muscle tension to GAD is supported by laboratory findings of elevated baseline levels of muscle tension in individuals with GAD compared to nonanxious controls (Hazlett, McLeod, & Hoehn-Saric, 1994; Hoehn-Saric et al., 1989).[1]

Although further refinement of the associated symptoms may still be needed (particularly in order to improve discrimination between GAD and mood disorders; T. A. Brown, Marten, & Barlow, 1995), the revisions made in DSM-IV have improved diagnostic reliability for GAD, as discussed in Chapter 9 (Brown, Di Nardo, Lehman, & Campbell, 2001). Interestingly, the most common source of disagreement in GAD diagnoses in this study was due to one interviewer's assigning a diagnosis of a mood disorder rather than GAD, confirming that research on reliable discrimination of GAD from the mood disorders is needed.

Although reliability and specificity of the diagnostic criteria for GAD seem to have improved from DSM-III-R to DSM-IV, it is important to note that the majority of individuals diagnosed with GAD according to DSM-III-R would similarly be diagnosed with GAD according to DSM-IV. In fact, one study found that all 40 clients diagnosed with GAD by two independent raters according to DSM-III-R criteria also met criteria for GAD as defined in DSM-IV (Abel & Borkovec, 1995). This suggests that descriptive psychopathology and intervention studies using individuals who meet DSM-III-R criteria (particularly when independent raters were used for diagnosis) will probably still apply to current definitions of GAD. Studies utilizing DSM-III criteria, however, are likely to include both individuals who would meet DSM-IV criteria and those with an insufficient duration of symptoms to meet current diagnostic criteria.

Although this chapter focuses on GAD in adulthood, it is worth noting that another change in the DSM-IV criteria was the omission of a diagnosis of childhood overanxious disorder; these symptoms are now subsumed under the GAD diagnosis. An initial study found support for the convergent and divergent validity of the diagnostic criteria (Tracey, Chorpita, Douban, & Barlow, 1997). However, children appeared to have difficulty determining whether their worry was uncontrollable, suggesting that parental report of this criterion may be particularly important. Also, muscle tension was infrequently endorsed by either children or their parents, suggesting that this symptom, which seems particularly important in GAD among adults, may not be as central to the disorder during childhood. The authors note that although analyses of their sample did not seem to suggest the need for refinement of the criteria for specific age ranges, their sample did not include children under the age of 7. Thus research needs to address whether the diagnostic criteria apply to children under the age of 7.

---

[1]Interestingly, Hazlett et al. (1994) found that individuals with GAD demonstrated a restricted variability in frontalis electromyographic variability during a stressor task, similar to the restriction in autonomic reactivity demonstrated by this group.

EPIDEMIOLOGY AND DEMOGRAPHIC FEATURES

Epidemiology

Historically, the lifetime prevalence rates for GAD have varied widely owing to the use of varying methodologies and significant changes in the criteria over time. Only three sites of the Epidemiologic Catchment Area study assessed for GAD, each using slightly different questions to determine the presence of symptoms. As reviewed briefly in Chapter 1, the estimated 1-year prevalence rate of GAD according to DSM-III criteria, without any diagnostic exclusions across these sites, was 3.8% (Blazer, Hughes, George, Swartz, & Boyer, 1991). As also noted in Chapter 1, the National Comorbidity Study (NCS) estimated prevalence rates of GAD in the United States, using DSM-III-R criteria and drawing from a representative sample of over 8,000 adults. The prevalence rates for current and lifetime GAD were 1.6% and 5.1%, respectively (Wittchen, Zhao, Kessler, & Eaton, 1994). These rates were based on diagnoses made without regard to diagnostic hierarchy rules; however, the NCS prevalence estimates did not change appreciably when the diagnostic hierarchy rules were imposed to exclude respondents whose GAD occurred exclusively during the course of a mood or psychotic disorder. Thus GAD, though less prevalent than social and simple (now specific) phobia, currently appears to be slightly more common in the general population than panic disorder (Kessler et al., 1994).

Epidemiological studies estimating the occurrence of GAD have also been conducted outside the United States. Prevalence estimates of 2.8% for current GAD and 5.4% for lifetime GAD based on DSM-III-R criteria were found in a population study conducted in Florence, Italy (Faravelli, Degl'Innocenti, & Giardinelli, 1989). A prevalence rate of 3.7% based on DSM-IV criteria was found in a two-stage epidemiological study of a rural area of South Africa (Bhagwanjee, Parekh, Paruk, Petersen, & Subedar, 1998).

GAD is significantly more common in primary care settings, with current and lifetime prevalence rates ranging from 3.5% and 14.5% among primarily low-income, African American females (Brantley, Mehan, Ames, & Jones, 1999) to 22% and 40% among high utilizers of medical care (Katon et al., 1990). Similar rates have been found in other countries, such as Africa (e.g., Hollifield, Katon, & Morojele, 1994). These findings are not surprising, given that approximately half of the respondents in the NCS study who reported seeking help for GAD did so in primary care settings (Wittchen et al., 1994).

Sociodemographic Features

Rates of GAD appear to be about twice as high among women as among men in both community (Wittchen et al., 1994) and clinical (Woodman, Noyes, Black, Schlosser, & Yagla, 1999; Yonkers, Warshaw, Massion, & Keller, 1996) samples. However, this finding may be culturally specific. The epidemiological study conducted in South Africa described above found higher prevalence rates of GAD among men (Bhagwanjee et al., 1998).

In the NCS, several other sociodemographic factors emerged as significantly associated with an increased risk for GAD. For example, previously married respondents had a significantly higher lifetime prevalence of GAD than either married or never-married respondents. Homemakers and other respondents not working outside the home (e.g., individuals who were permanently disabled or had retired early) had significantly higher prevalence of GAD than did other respondents. There was also a differential risk for GAD based on geographic location, with higher lifetime prevalence for GAD in the Northeast. In contrast, race and income levels were not uniquely associated with risk. Moreover, no relationship between risk for GAD and education, religion, and urbanicity were demonstrated.

Considerable controversy exists as to the typical age of onset of GAD, with reports in some samples ranging from age 2 to 61 (e.g., Yonkers et al., 1996). Several studies have found GAD to have an earlier age of onset than other anxiety disorders (e.g., Anderson, Noyes, & Crowe, 1984; Massion, Warshaw, & Keller, 1993; Noyes et al., 1992; Woodman et al., 1999). The Epidemiologic Catchment Area study found GAD (using DSM-III criteria with no exclusions) to be most prevalent among the youngest age group (Blazer et al., 1991). Furthermore, overanxious disorder (which, before the publication of DSM-IV, was considered to be the childhood presentation of GAD) has been found to be fairly common, with prevalence estimates ranging from 2.9% to 7.3% (e.g., Anderson, Williams, McGee, & Silva, 1987; Bowen, Offord, & Boyle, 1990; Kashani & Orvaschel, 1988).

In contrast, other studies seem to indicate that GAD is more common among older adults. For instance, in the NCS, current GAD was found to be most common in the oldest age group (≥ 45 years) and least common in the youngest age group (15–24 years; Wittchen et al., 1994). It is important to note that the methodology of the studies, as well as the nature of the sample (clinical vs. community), may significantly affect the age of onset reported. For instance, clinical studies may base their reported ages of onset on the age at which a patient first reports having been troubled by persistent worry. In contrast, other studies, such as the NCS, require the presence of full diagnostic criteria to designate an age of onset. However, the latter, more conservative methodology does not provide historical information about the gradual onset of GAD and the presence of subclinical levels that are likely to precede the full-blown development of the disorder (Brown, 1999). This apparent discrepancy in the literature about age of GAD onset has led researchers to conclude that there may be two distinct subtypes of GAD, with earlier and later onset, that are associated with distinct causal features and course.

Within a clinical data set, Hoehn-Saric, Hazlett, and McLeod (1993) found that 64% of patients experienced an early onset of GAD. In this early-onset group, 15% of participants reported that their symptoms started before the age of 10, with the remainder of the group reporting their onset between the ages of 10 and 19. In the late-onset group, 43% of the patients reported first experiencing symptoms between the ages of 20 and 29, 31% between the ages of 30 and 39, and 22% at or after age 40.

Several studies have compared participants diagnosed with early- and late-onset GAD derived from community and clinical sample. No sociodemographic differences were apparent between those with earlier- and later-onset GAD in the NCS study (Wittchen et al., 1994). However, in a clinical sample, more African Americans were found in the late-onset group, early-onset patients were younger, and there was a trend toward more females in this group (Hoehn-Saric et al., 1993).

With regard to proposed etiology, GAD with an earlier age of onset has been associated with a self-reported childhood history of fears; inhibited or avoidance behavior; developmental, academic, and social-interactional difficulties; and a disturbed home environment (Hoehn-Saric et al., 1993). In contrast, patients with late-onset GAD were significantly more likely to identify a precipitating stressful event that corresponded with the onset of their disorder (Hoehn-Saric et al., 1993). In terms of current symptom picture, early-onset GAD was shown to be associated with current problems in marital functioning, interpersonal sensitivity, depression (Hoehn-Saric et al., 1993), and a poorer course of GAD illness (Woodman et al., 1999).

Although these findings are intriguing, their implications are limited by several methodological factors. For instance, as discussed by Brown (1999), studies comparing patients with early- and late-onset GAD do not typically take into account the potential impact of patients' current age and the duration of their illness on their results. Furthermore, because GAD is such a chronic disorder with a known insidious onset, the reliability of the retrospective report of age of onset has been challenged (Brown, 1999). In a study of older adults (and thus a more homogeneous sample with regard to age), few factors were found to differ significantly between those patients with early- and late-onset GAD (Beck, Stanley, & Zebb, 1996).

Given that GAD can develop later in life, and that it is known to have a fairly chronic course (discussed in more detail below), it is not surprising that it is one of the most significant anxiety disorders among older adults. In the review of eight community studies of older adults (see Chapter 1), Flint (1994) found prevalence rates of GAD to range from 0.7% to 7.1 %. Based on this review, he concluded that although rates of anxiety disorders overall seem to be lower among older adults, the presence of GAD accounts for a large proportion of the anxiety seen in this age group.

Furthermore, GAD in older adults is clearly an important target of treatment. The symptom pattern and severity of GAD in older adults are like those of younger adults diagnosed with GAD, and unlike those of older adults without GAD; this finding dispels the notion that worry in this age group is part of the normal aging process and not reflective of psychopathology (Beck et al., 1996). In an even more sobering evaluation of the importance of targeting GAD in this segment of the population, Lenze et al. (2000) revealed that 25% of older adults with depression also met criteria for GAD, and that the additional presence of symptoms of GAD was associated with a higher level of suicidality.

Course

GAD symptoms typically persist over long periods of time, with a majority of patients describing an unremitting course of illness (Noyes et al., 1992). In a prospective longitudinal study of patients with DSM-III-R GAD, the remission rate of the disorder was .15 at 1 year and .25 at 2 years (Yonkers et al., 1996). Compared to patients with panic disorder at a 5-year follow-up to treatment, those with GAD were found to be more likely still to meet full criteria for their disorder and less likely to be in partial or full remission, or to have had a period of remission in the previous 5 years (Woodman et al., 1999).

Associated Features

In addition to comorbid Axis I conditions (reviewed briefly below and extensively in Chapter 9), GAD is associated with a number of factors that underscore the significance and impact of the disorder. GAD has been associated with impairment in role functioning, in social life, and in life satisfaction (Massion et al., 1993), as well as with an increased number of distressing minor life stressors (Brantley et al., 1999). In the NCS, about half of those diagnosed with GAD reported that the disorder caused significant interference in their life and activities (Wittchen et al., 1994). Two-thirds of the sample had sought help for their GAD, with 44% having received medication. Rates of professional help seeking, receiving medication, and life interference were all higher among individuals diagnosed with GAD along with comorbid conditions than among those with "pure" GAD.

Furthermore, GAD has been shown to be associated with a variety of somatic complaints, including chest pain (Carter & Maddock, 1992; Logue et al., 1993; Wulsin, Arnold, & Hillard, 1991) and irritable bowel syndrome (e.g., Lydiard, Fossey, Marsh, & Ballenger, 1993). These associated features frequently drive patients to present in primary care settings and may lead to inappropriate and costly medical testing and treatment, in addition to missed GAD diagnoses (Roy-Byrne, 1996; Roy-Byrne & Katon, 2000).

As mentioned in Chapter 1, economic analysis has in part confirmed this fear. Data from the NCS revealed that patients with GAD have a significant impact on direct medical service utilization and cost, particularly through visits to their family doctors and specialists (Greenberg et al., 1999). GAD is also associated with indirect costs at the workplace through lost productivity at work (Greenberg et al., 1999). Souêtre et al. (1994) indicated that health care and workplace costs are significantly higher among those with GAD and comorbid disorders as compared to "pure" GAD. However, the method by which participants were designated as having comorbid disorders or not, and the exclusion criteria used in this study, severely limit the implications of the findings.

CHARACTERISTICS AND CORRELATES OF WORRY AND GAD

As noted earlier, the DSM-III-R definition of GAD identified chronic, excessive worry as the central defining feature of GAD. Subsequent research on the nature of GAD has therefore focused predominantly on clarifying the nature and function of worry. Because worry is a common feature across the anxiety disorders (although it is significantly more frequent among individuals with GAD; Brown, Antony, & Barlow, 1992), a better understanding of worry may facilitate understanding of other anxiety disorders as well. For this reason, the research on worry has been previously reviewed in Chapter 3. We revisit it here specifically within the context of increasing our understanding of potential factors in the etiology and maintenance of GAD. We note when studies have shown that a particular characteristic is specific to GAD; however, even those characteristics that may apply across emotional disorders are likely to be important to our understanding of the etiological and maintaining factors of worry in GAD.

Prior to its inclusion in the diagnostic criteria for GAD, worry had been discussed as an element of test anxiety (e.g., Deffenbacher, 1980) and as an important factor in understanding and treating insomnia (e.g., Borkovec, 1982). From the latter area of study emerged a focus on the construct of worry itself (e.g., Borkovec, 1985b; Borkovec, Robinson, Pruzinsky, & DePree, 1983). In the early stages of this research, worry was defined in part as "an attempt to engage in mental problem-solving on an issue whose outcome is uncertain but contains the possibility of one or more negative outcomes" (Borkovec et al., 1983, p. 10). It was noted that worry commonly consisted of a series of "What if . . ." statements, and as such seemed to represent the first stage of problem solving (i.e., generating the problem) without the subsequent steps of successfully solving or coping with the problem (Borkovec, 1985b).

The Nature of Worry

As noted in the discussion of diagnostic criteria for GAD, studies have shown that individuals with GAD worry more frequently, excessively, and uncontrollably than their nonanxious counterparts, but not necessarily about dramatically different topics. One study of worry content found that both individuals with GAD and nonanxious controls reported frequent worry about family/interpersonal concerns (Roemer et al., 1997). However, individuals who endorsed GAD criteria (both clinical and analogue samples) were unique in their reports of a substantial number of unclassifiable (miscellaneous) events, such as worries about daily hassles. Thus a specific content area does not seem to characterize the worry of individuals diagnosed with GAD; instead, these individuals report a range of idiosyncratic worries, in addition to more worries in all content areas.

Although broad content categorization studies have not revealed significant differences between individuals with GAD and nonanxious controls, one study did reveal what may be an important theme associated with worry (Davey & Levy, 1998). Nonclinical volunteers were asked to catastrophize their current worries (i.e., to successively list the worrisome aspects of each worry—"What worries you about this?"). Scores on a measure of excessive worry were significantly correlated with the frequency of statements related to personal inadequacy, suggesting that this may be a type of concern particularly characteristic of individuals who worry excessively.

Studies have only recently begun to investigate developmental differences in worry content. Among a large stratified sample of adults 25 years and older, participants over 65 years of age reported a higher proportion of worries about health than did younger adults (Person & Borkovec, 1995). Approximately half of worries reported by 65 years and older were health-related, compared to only 7.3% of the worries reported by 25- to 44-year-olds.

A few studies have also explored worry content in children. One study of a large sample of children aged 7 to 12 (unselected for anxiety status) revealed that health, school, and personal harm were the most commonly reported worry topics, with worries related to physical harm being the most intense (Silverman, La Greca, & Wasserstein, 1995). A recent follow-up study (Weems, Silverman, & La Greca, 2000) found that similar worries were reported in a sample of children aged 6 to 16 who presented to an anxiety disorder clinic. However, these children reported significantly more frequent worries about disasters, and less frequent worries about future events, their classmates, personal harm, and war, than children in the normative sample reviewed above did. The clinical sample reported more intense worries about a number of topics, including "little things" and "other worries." Finally, Vasey, Crnic, and Carter (1994) specifically investigated the developmental course of worry content in their study of a nonclinical sample that included three age groups: children aged 5 to 6, 8 to 9, and 12 to 13 years. These authors found that although all age groups reported worries, this phenomenon was more prevalent among children in the latter two age ranges. Content of worry was found to change significantly across age groups. Younger children reported more frequent concerns about physical well-being, while older children reported more frequent concerns about competence, psychological well-being, and social evaluation. These findings among both children and older adults underscore the importance of continued study of worry content across different age groups, particularly in clinically defined samples.

Even fewer studies to date have addressed cultural differences in worry content. A recent study compared worry in Japanese American and European American older adults, revealing no significant differences in worry content between the two groups (Watari & Brodbeck, 2000). Similar to previous research on older adults, for both groups, health worries were most frequent. Another investigation administered Spanish translations of self-report measures of excessive worry and GAD diagnostic criteria to university students and educated professionals living in a major city of Peru (Diaz, 2000). No significant differences in worry content emerged between individuals who endorsed GAD diagnostic criteria and those who did not. Similar to findings reported above, individuals endorsing GAD criteria identified family/home/interpersonal and miscellaneous (unspecified) worries as most frequent. However, an interesting cultural difference in diagnostic criteria did emerge. Although prevalence rates for GAD as defined by the DSM-III-R criteria were comparable to those reported in U.S. populations, the rates were significantly lower when DSM-IV criteria were used (in contrast to the comparability reported by Abel & Borkovec,

1995). Closer examination of the data revealed that Peruvians who met all other DSM-IV criteria for GAD rarely endorsed the uncontrollability criterion. Diaz (2000) hypothesized that the Spanish translation used for this item was more closely associated to appraisals of being "crazy" or personally out of control, which individuals meeting all other GAD criteria did not feel characterized them. A better translation that specified difficulty in stopping worry, rather than being generally out of control, might have resulted in more comparable prevalence rates. These findings suggest that care needs to be taken in translating constructs from one culture to another. Clearly, considerably more research is needed on the nature of worry cross-culturally.

Although studies comparing worry content of clients with GAD to their nonanxious counterparts have not revealed striking differences, studies comparing clients with GAD to those with panic disorder have yielded some interesting distinctions. Breitholtz, Westling, and Öst (1998) elicited anxiety-related cognitions from patients diagnosed with GAD and those diagnosed with panic disorder (diagnoses were made with the Anxiety Disorders Interview Schedule—Revised [ADIS-R]). A semistructured interview was used to identify recent, most important anxious thoughts. These thoughts were then categorized into one of seven categories, which were subsequently collapsed into three: physical catastrophe (illness, injury, and death), mental catastrophe (loss of control and inability to cope), and other (shame, and other). Patients diagnosed with GAD reported significantly more worries in the mental catastrophe and other categories, while patients diagnosed with panic disorder reported significantly more worries in the physical catastrophe category. A subsequent study (Breitholtz, Johansson, & Öst, 1999) used a daily monitoring methodology to acquire cognitions from the same two clinical groups. These thoughts were then categorized into 10 categories. Individuals with GAD reported significantly more thoughts in the following categories: interpersonal conflict, competence (i.e., concerns about incompetence), acceptance (i.e., concerns about rejection by others), concern about others, and worry over minor matters. On the other hand, individuals with panic disorder again reported significantly more thoughts related to physical catastrophe. These findings suggest that while individuals with panic disorder are primarily worried about potential physical threat, individuals with GAD are more worried about a variety of potential aversive events that encompass interpersonal/social threats, threats to self-esteem and a sense of self-efficacy, and threats over minor matters. Interestingly, the latter study did not find a significant difference between groups in worry over worry itself ("meta-worry"), a factor that has been proposed as important in understanding GAD (Wells, 1995; discussed more fully below). Studies have yet to compare worry content among individuals with GAD and those with other emotional disorders (e.g., social phobia and major depression).

As noted in the discussion of changes in the diagnostic criteria of GAD, worry among individuals with GAD is characterized by its excessive and uncontrollable nature. Individuals with GAD commonly report that they worry more than they wish they did, or more than others feel they should. They also report substantial difficulty stopping their worry once it has started. Similarly, in a nonclinical population, individuals with high levels of worry reported more difficulty stopping worry once it started than did those with low levels (Tallis, Davey, & Capuzzo, 1994). This characteristic may contribute to the maintenance of worry, as attempts to control internal experiences may in fact paradoxically increase the frequency of those experiences (e.g., Roemer & Borkovec, 1993; but see Purdon, 1999, for a review of inconsistencies in this literature). In fact, Tallis, Davey, and Capuzzo (1994) found that individuals with high worry levels reported they were more likely to experience a return of worry after successful termination of a worry episode than those with low levels did.

Research on worry in both nonclinical and GAD populations has revealed another characteristic that relates to the functions of worry described below. Worry appears to be a primarily verbal/linguistic (as opposed to imaginal) activity (Borkovec, 1994a). For instance, in one study (Borkovec & Inz, 1990), both individuals with GAD and nonanxious controls reported a predominance of thoughts (vs. images) during an instructed worry period, and participants with GAD also reported significantly more frequent thoughts during a relaxing period than did their nonanxious counterparts. Following successful treatment, individuals with GAD showed patterns of thought and imagery more similar to those of nonanxious controls. Other investigators have similarly found an association between worry and reports of thoughts versus images (e.g., Freeston, Dugas, & Ladouceur, 1996; Tallis, Davey, & Capuzzo, 1994). Most strikingly, in an experimental study, Rapee (1993) found that a task involving verbal working memory interfered with worry, while a task involving visual–spatial working memory did not. The verbal/linguistic nature of worry is further supported by electroencephalographic studies that reveal elevated left frontal cortical activity among self-reported "worriers" during episodes of worry (Carter, Johnson, & Borkovec, 1986)—activity that is commonly associated with verbal, analytic processing. These findings expand the definition of worry provided at the beginning of this section; that is, worry is a primarily conceptual activity that involves the generation of multiple potential future catastrophes. But the question remains: Why do people engage in this activity?

The Function of Worry

Much of the research on GAD and worry over the past 10 years has focused on the function of worry and the factors that maintain this process. Some confusion has arisen in this literature, based in part on differences in definitions of worry. Some researchers (e.g., Davey, 1994a; Wells, 1999) have distinguished between constructive and maladaptive worry and have described the former as closely associated with successful coping and problem solving. Others (e.g., Borkovec, 1994a; Mathews, 1990) have distinguished worry from effective problem solving, stating that to the extent that cognitive planning is successful, it is more accurately described as preparatory coping rather than worry (Mathews, 1990). Consistent with the former position, Craske (1999) suggests that worry may be an initial stage in the anticipation of threat, in which arousal is reduced (as noted in Chapter 3 and discussed more fully below) and conceptual planning takes place. She suggests that worry may reduce threat imminence and therefore may be positively reinforced by the sense of control and minimization of risk it provides.[2] This proposal coincides with explanations provided by individuals with GAD for their worry (described more fully below), but research to date has failed to document any actual (as opposed to perceived) facilitative effects of worry on threat reduction or problem solving (Borkovec, Hazlett-Stevens, & Diaz, 1999). In fact, most studies on the process of worry have found that experimentally induced worry (in normative samples) has correlates similar to those of chronic, clinically significant worry. This suggests that comparable processes underlie both, although frequency and intensity clearly differ between individuals with a clinically significant degree of worry and nonanxious controls.

Nonetheless, one series of studies, described in Chapter 3, does provide apparent correlational evidence of an adaptive aspect to worry (Davey, Hampton, Farrell, & Davidson, 1992; Davey, 1993b). These studies demonstrated that when trait anxiety (which was

---

[2]In fact, minimization of risk and reduction of an unpleasant sense of uncontrollability might be better described as negatively reinforcing contingencies.

correlated .53 to .57 with a measure of content-specific student worry) was controlled for, worry was positively correlated with self-reports of active coping strategies. However, the zero-order correlations between worry and various avoidant coping strategies, and the strong correlations between worry and trait anxiety, suggest that worry is more strongly associated with impaired than with successful coping even in a student sample. The consistent finding in the literature of strong associations between worry and anxiety, coupled with the finding that experimental induction of a worrisome state results in state anxiety (and depression; Andrews & Borkovec, 1988), suggests that worry is unlikely to occur in the absence of heightened anxiety. Thus, although anxiety can be statistically separated from worry—revealing an adaptive aspect of worry (in some instances)—it remains unclear whether anxiety-free, adaptive worry exists in nature. Therefore, it seems most clarifying at this point to distinguish between two constructs: (1) the normative, adaptive process of identifying potential threats and actively problem solving or preparing to cope with these threats (i.e., "conceptual planning," Craske, 1999; "preparatory coping," Mathews, 1990); and (2) the process of worry, which is anxiety-laden and characterized by the generation of multiple potential future negative events, in the absence of effective attempts to actively solve problems or cope with these outcomes (Borkovec et al., 1983). What Craske (1999) calls "worry" may be a kind of preparatory coping that is effective as long as it does not escalate, reciprocally with anxiety, into a chain of worrisome thoughts as defined by Borkovec et al. (1983). It may even be the case that preparatory coping and worry are intricately intertwined at times, with preparatory coping escalating into worrisome episodes and worrisome episodes alleviated by more productive efforts at preparatory coping. For instance, Davey (1994a) suggests that the two may be related, in that (pathological) worry is an example of thwarted or exacerbated problem solving. More research is needed on both adaptive, conceptual planning and worry, in order to determine the relationship and boundaries between the two.

Although worry is distinct from effective coping and problem solving, it may function to prepare people to *attempt* to cope with future threat, as proposed in the first edition of this book. This is consistent with the definition of worry as generating potential future negative outcomes. However, if worry does not proceed past this point (to preparatory coping), it will not achieve successful coping. Mathews (1990) suggests that worry functions to maintain hypervigilance to personally relevant threat cues, but that this hypervigilance is followed by cognitive avoidance that precludes elaboration of threatening material (the "seek to avoid" process described in Chapter 3). As such, worry elicits a state of readiness in an individual, which may be negatively reinforced by the reduction of an uncomfortable state of unpredictability (Craske, 1999). However, because worry involves predictions of numerous negative events—many of which have a low probability of actually occurring (see Borkovec et al., 1999, for a review)—this sense of predictability is illusory. A wealth of information processing research on individuals with high trait anxiety and those with GAD supports the assertion that worry is associated with heightened attention to threat. Although this literature has been reviewed in depth in Chapter 3, we briefly highlight a few studies below.

Information-Processing Biases Associated with Worry and GAD

As reviewed in detail in Chapter 3, anxiety has been consistently associated with evidence of preattentive bias toward threatening material, confirming Mathews's (1990) assertion that worry serves to maintain hypervigilance to potential threat. Studies using the modified Stroop task have shown that participants with GAD are slower to color-name threat-related words, particularly those associated with their reported worries (Mogg, Mathews, & Weinman, 1989). Interference effects remain when Stroop words are masked (Mogg, Bradley, Millar, & White, 1995), and attentional bias has also been demonstrated with the dot probe paradigm (MacLeod, Mathews, & Tata, 1986). Taken together, these findings suggest that individuals who worry chronically are particularly likely to detect potential threat, which is likely to heighten cues for their worry and therefore perpetuate the process. Studies have shown, however, that interference effects are successfully reduced following cognitive-behavioral therapy for GAD (Mathews, Mogg, Kentish, & Eysenck, 1995; Mogg et al., 1995).

Studies of attentional bias have traditionally used only verbal stimuli, commonly threatening and nonthreatening words. However, a recent study used the dot probe methodology to investigate attentional biases to emotional faces among individuals with GAD in comparison to nonanxious controls (Bradley, Mogg, White, Groom, & de Bono, 1999). Participants were shown pairs of faces concurrently; each pair consisted of a neutral and an emotional (either threatening or happy) face. On each trial, a dot replaced one of the faces, and participants responded to the dot as quickly as possible; their reaction time was the dependent variable of interest. Individuals diagnosed with GAD demonstrated faster reaction times to dots that replaced threatening versus neutral faces, suggesting an attentive bias to threatening faces. The finding of an attentional bias toward threatening faces suggests a mechanism through which social-evaluative fears of individuals with GAD may be perpetuated.

In addition to being associated with an attentional bias toward threat, GAD, worry, and anxiety also seem to be associated with a tendency to perceive negative outcomes as likely and ambiguous situations as threatening (i.e., interpretative biases, as reviewed in Chapter 3). An early study revealed that anxious participants rated negative events as significantly more likely to happen than did controls, and also rated these events as more likely to happen to themselves than to others (Butler & Mathews, 1983). In another study, individuals with chronic worry produced more hypothetical catastrophic scenarios and rated these scenarios significantly more likely than did controls (Vasey & Borkovec, 1992). Similarly, MacLeod, Williams, and Bekerian (1991) found that participants with chronic worry reported higher subjective probabilities of negative events; also, those with extreme worry in the sample were more readily able to generate reasons why the negative events would happen than reasons why they would not. Interestingly, when participants with worry in this study were asked to generate reasons why an event would *not* occur, they subsequently reported lowered subjective probabilities for that event, suggesting that the generation of counterreasons for catastrophes may be a potential intervention for worry.

Individuals diagnosed with GAD are also likely to interpret ambiguous stimuli as threatening. For instance, individuals who met DSM-III criteria for GAD were significantly more likely to produce the threat-related spelling of aurally presented homophones (e.g., "slay/sleigh") than were nonanxious controls, with individuals who were in remission from GAD falling nonsignificantly in between the other two groups (Mathews, Richards, & Eysenck, 1989).

In contrast to the robust findings of threat-related biases in attention to and interpretation of stimuli among individuals with clinical anxiety/GAD, research on memory bias has failed to reveal consistent threat-related biases. Studies have not revealed threat-related biases in explicit memory among individuals with GAD, either on free-recall measures (e.g., Becker, Roth, Andrich, & Margraf, 1999) or recognition measures (e.g., Mogg et al., 1989). In contrast, anxious participants did exhibit threat-related biases in implicit memory; they completed more three-letter word stems with previously presented threatening words than their nonanxious counterparts did (Mathews, Mogg, May, & Eysenck, 1989). This bias for implicit but not explicit memory among individuals diagnosed with GAD was also demonstrated by MacLeod and McLaughlin (1995).

Mathews (1990) suggests that the repeated findings of attentional bias toward threat, coupled with an absence of explicit memory biases for threatening material, are consistent with his proposed theory on the function of worry. He suggests that worry functions to heighten awareness of potential threat, but that threat detection is followed by cognitive avoidance, such that the threat is not elaborated and therefore is not easily recalled. A great deal of research and theorizing in the area of worry has focused on the role that avoidance may play in maintaining both the process of worry and the threatening associations that seem to underlie it.

Worry as Cognitive Avoidance and Its Role in the Maintenance of Anxiety

As noted in Chapter 3, Borkovec and colleagues (e.g., Borkovec, 1994a; Borkovec et al., 1991, 1999) have combined research from the past 10 years into an integrated theory of worry in which its avoidant function plays a central role. Borkovec (1994a) posits that worry is maintained primarily through negative reinforcement. This reinforcement comes from two sources: (1) the nonoccurrence of predicted negative outcomes (which are primarily events with low base rates), and (2) actual reductions in somatic arousal that are associated with worry. Evidence for the latter function is found in several laboratory studies. For example, in contrast to other anxious states, neither chronic nor state worry is associated with increased sympathetic activation; instead, they are associated with reduced autonomic variability (Hoehn-Saric & McLeod, 1988; Connor & Davidson, 1998). Although this reduced variability (associated with decreased vagal tone [parasympathetic activity]; Thayer, Friedman, & Borkovec, 1996) has detrimental long-term consequences, the short-term effect of diminished activation is likely to be negatively reinforcing, increasing the frequency of worrisome responding. This hypothesized function of worry is further supported by the finding that GAD is associated with chronic tension, vigilance, and scanning symptoms, rather than with the increased autonomic symptoms found in all the other anxiety disorders (Brown, Barlow, & Liebowitz, 1994; Marten et al., 1993).

Borkovec (1994a) proposes that the association between worry and reduced arousal is due to the predominantly verbal/linguistic nature of worry, citing research that thoughts of feared stimuli are less arousing than images of the same stimuli (Vrana, Cuthbert, & Lang, 1986). Other laboratory studies also support the association between worry and reduced autonomic arousal, and particularly the association between thoughts and reduced arousal. Participants with public speaking phobias who worried prior to imagining giving a speech did not show increased heart rate during imaginal exposure, in contrast to those who relaxed prior to exposure (Borkovec & Hu, 1990). In a replication of this study (Borkovec, Lyonfields, Wiser, & Deihl, 1993), degree of thought during the worry period was negatively correlated with heart rate response. In another study, participants who worried after exposure to a gruesome film reported less anxiety immediately following this postprocessing period than those who engaged in imaginal rehearsal (Wells & Papageorgiou, 1995). However, a recent study by Peasley-Miklus and Vrana (2000) found that worrisome thinking itself was associated with a marginal *increase* in heart rate acceleration, compared to relaxing thinking. Furthermore, although phobic imagery was associated with less heart rate acceleration from the worrisome versus relaxing thinking periods (replicating Borkovec & Hu 1990), there were no differences between conditions when changes from a prethinking period baseline were compared. These authors suggest that worry may provide a more graduated increase in activation, which may be preferable to a quicker increase associated with the change from relaxed thinking to fearful imagery.

Taken in isolation, the data presented above may suggest a beneficial facet of worry: It seems to reduce autonomic arousal (or at least sudden increases in arousal). However, Borkovec (1994a) notes that reduced autonomic activation indicates a failure to fully access the fear associative network (Lang, 1985; see Chapter 2), and is thus likely to interfere with successful emotional processing (Foa & Kozak, 1986) and maintain threatening meanings. In other words, this reduction in arousal indicates an absence of functional exposure to fearful cues, and also possibly a failure to elaborate fearful information (similar to Mathews's theory discussed above). Thus the immediately positive effects of worry are counteracted by long-term negative effects in the form of continued threatening associations and an absence of new learning.

Several lines of research support these propositions. The Wells and Papageorgiou (1995) study described above found that although worry was associated with reduced anxiety immediately following the study, it was associated with increased intrusions over a 3-day period following viewing of the film. Similarly, in the Borkovec and Hu (1990) study, participants who engaged in relaxing thinking showed a nonsignificant decline in heart rate response to fearful images, while those who engaged in worry showed no such trend. In a study comparing individuals with GAD and nonanxious controls in a cued threat paradigm, controls demonstrated habituation to novel neutral stimuli, while individuals with GAD did not (Thayer, Friedman, Borkovec, Johnsen, & Molina, 2000). Finally, the consistent finding that both chronic and experimentally induced worry are associated with autonomic rigidity and reduced vagal tone (e.g., Lyonfields, Borkovec, & Thayer, 1995; Thayer et al., 1996) supports Borkovec's theory. That is, this psychophysiological state is associated with reduced flexibility in attention and affective regulation, suggesting a sustained state of vigilance and chronic anxiety that may preclude incorporation of new, nonanxious associations (Thayer et al., 2000).[3]

Interestingly, self-report data also support a cognitively avoidant function for worry. Borkovec and Roemer (1995) demonstrated that only one self-reported function of worry was uniquely related to self-reported GAD status: Participants who endorsed GAD criteria were more likely to report worrying to distract themselves from more emotional topics. This finding was replicated by Freeston, Rhéaume, Letarte, Dugas, and Ladouceur (1994). In addition, a measure of cognitive avoidance was found to significantly discriminate individuals diagnosed with GAD (by clinical interview) from a nonanxious control group (Dugas, Gagnon, Ladouceur, & Freeston, 1998).

Finally, Borkovec et al. (1999) note that worry is inherently avoidant by virtue of its focus on future, potential events, rather than present-moment circumstances.[4] The rigid habit of detecting and interpreting potential future threat, coupled with autonomic rigidity, interferes with the individual's ability to respond flexibly to current environmental contingencies. This is likely to interfere with both adaptive functioning and the ability to learn new associations and new responses. Thus, although a heightened ability to detect poten-

---

[3]It is important to note that autonomic rigidity has been associated with panic disorder and obsessive–compulsive disorder (OCD) as well (see Chapter 6 and Craske, 1999, for a review) so this is not necessarily a specific characteristic of GAD, but may be associated with worry throughout the anxiety disorders.

[4]The non-present-moment nature of worry is supported by a study comparing narrative analysis of streams of thought during experimentally induced worry and neutral thinking (Molina, Borkovec, Peasley, & Person, 1998). Worrisome thought was characterized by significantly fewer present-focused statements and less attention to environmental cues than neutral thinking was.

tial future threat may facilitate preparatory coping or conceptual planning, a rigid habit of attention to future outcomes precludes successful responding to current circumstances. Because these negative outcomes are long-term, they are unlikely to alter the frequency of worry unless attention is brought to them.

Positive Beliefs about Worry

In fact, individuals who worry chronically tend to believe that their worry serves positive functions. Investigators who have explored the reasons why such individuals engage in worry consistently find that these individuals believe their worry will help them prepare for, problem-solve in regard to, or superstitiously avoid the negative events they fear (Borkovec & Roemer, 1995; Cartwright-Hatton & Wells, 1997; Davey, Tallis, & Capuzzo, 1996; Freeston et al., 1994). Positive beliefs about worry have been significantly associated with GAD and worry in both clinical (Dugas et al., 1998) and nonclinical samples (e.g., Davey, Tallis, & Capuzzo, 1996). However, evidence suggests that worry does not reduce the likelihood of negative outcomes or increase the likelihood of effective coping (Borkovec et al., 1999); nor does it result in effective, concrete problem solving (Stöber, 1998). Nevertheless, because individuals with GAD typically predict events that are extremely unlikely, their belief in the superstitious efficacy of their worry is frequently reinforced by the nonoccurrence of feared outcomes, thereby strengthening this belief and increasing the frequency of their worry (Borkovec et al., 1999; Wells, 1995). As Borkovec et al. (1999) note, these beliefs in the functionality of worry may interfere with attention to the actual contingencies taking place, again precluding the possibility of new, flexible learning from experience.

Worry, GAD, Problem Solving, and Task Performance

Although individuals who worry chronically believe that the process facilitates problem solving, evidence suggests that it is more likely to detract from successful problem solving. As noted above, Davey et al. (1992) found that worry was positively correlated with low levels of problem-solving confidence and a low sense of personal control (both of which were subsumed under the construct of "poor problem orientation"), although this relationship disappeared when trait anxiety was controlled for. Dugas, Freeston, and Ladouceur (1997), also using a nonclinical sample, found that poor problem orientation significantly predicted levels of worry, even after mood state was controlled for. Similarly, Ladouceur, Blais, Freeston, and Dugas (1998) found that individuals with GAD reported lower levels of problem-solving confidence and personal control than a group of moderate worriers. Interestingly, one study found that experimental manipulation of problem-solving confidence resulted in the generation of more catastrophic steps, suggesting that low problem-solving confidence may in fact increase worry, rather than vice versa (Davey, Jubb, & Cameron, 1996). A final study suggests the relationship with poor problem orientation may be specific to GAD: Individuals with principal and additional diagnoses of GAD reported higher levels of poor problem orientation than did individuals with mixed anxiety disorders (predominantly OCD) (Ladouceur et al., 1999). Neither of these two studies found a relationship between worry or GAD and problem-solving skills. Taken together, these findings suggest that individuals who worry excessively and/or meet criteria for GAD are likely to have little confidence in their ability to solve problems or in their control over outcomes, although they exhibit no clear self-reported deficits in their ability to problem solve.

Although worry is not associated with problem-solving skill deficits, it does interfere with successful completion of certain types of tasks. In particular, worry seems to inhibit performance on ambiguous tasks. For instance, in an experimental investigation of stimulus categorization, participants who reported chronic worry exhibited slowed decision making in response to ambiguous stimuli, and nonanxious controls showed comparable deficits after they were instructed to worry for 15 minutes (Metzger, Miller, Cohen, Sofka, & Borkovec, 1990). Similarly, when instructed to count the number of e's in a word, individuals with high worry levels demonstrated significantly longer latencies than controls on trials where the word did not contain any e's (Tallis, Eysenck, & Mathews, 1991). Clinical observation also suggests that worry and GAD are associated with procrastination, although no formal studies of this relationship have been conducted to date (Borkovec et al., 1999).

Stöber (1998) provides an interesting explanation of how worry may interfere with successful problem solving. Drawing on research that finds "concrete" problem elaboration (identifying risks and consequences of problems) to be more likely to generate solutions than "abstract" problem elaboration, he reviews evidence that worry (in nonclinical populations) is associated with more abstract problem elaboration. This assertion is consistent with the predominance of thought activity in worry, given that images are more concrete than words. Stöber proposes that the absence of concreteness associated with worry is what impairs successful problem solving. This is a compelling theory, with clear implications for intervention, and thus is worthy of further study.

Finally, as noted above, Davey (1994a) proposes that pathological worry may best be understood as a type of thwarted problem solving. He posits that what would otherwise be adaptive problem solving may be detrimental in response to uncontrollable situations, or among individuals with poor problem-solving confidence, a negative cognitive style, and a tendency to perceive events as threatening. This theory is consistent with the evidence reviewed above, as well as the finding that worry is perceived as less adaptive to the extent that the target of worry is subjectively and objectively defined as uncontrollable (Davey, 1994c).

Worry, Predictability, Controllability and Uncertainty

As discussed in Chapters 3 and 8, a large body of research has shown that a sense of unpredictability and uncontrollability is an integral component of anxiety. Worry involves the prediction of potential future negative outcomes and is associated with the belief that this prediction allows for control over these outcomes (either through preparation for, effective problem solving of, or the ability to avoid the outcome; Borkovec & Roemer, 1995). As Craske (1999) suggests, this increased predictability and sense of control may reinforce the tendency to worry. However, as noted above, studies have shown that people with chronic worry tend to overestimate subjective risk. In fact, a diary study that tracked outcomes related to predicted worries revealed that both anxious and nonanxious individuals worried about unlikely outcomes. Both groups experienced outcomes better than those they predicted approximately 70% of the time (Diaz & Borkovec, cited in Borkovec et al., 1999), which provides even more evidence that worrying is not associated with accurate prediction of future events. Thus, as suggested in Chapter 3, worry may be an ineffective *attempt* at control, rather than a means by which controllability is achieved.

However, the illusion of predictability and control may be particularly reinforcing for individuals diagnosed with GAD. Ladouceur and colleagues have conducted a series of studies exploring the consistent association between intolerance of uncertainty and worry in both nonclinical and clinical populations (see Dugas, Buhr, & Ladouceur, in press, for a review). These researchers have found that self-reported intolerance of uncertainty predicts worry in nonclinical samples, above and beyond measures of anxiety and depression (Dugas et al., 1997). Also, intolerance of uncertainty significantly discriminated between a group of individuals diagnosed with GAD and a group of nonanxious controls (Dugas et al., 1998). Furthermore, intolerance of uncertainty was significantly higher among individuals with both principal and additional diagnoses of GAD than in a group with mixed anxiety disorders (predominantly OCD) (Ladouceur et al., 1999), suggesting that intolerance of uncertainty may be specific to GAD. Lastly, a treatment package designed specifically to target intolerance of uncertainty was efficacious in reducing GAD symptoms, compared to a wait-list control (Ladouceur et al., 2000). Moreover, time series analyses from this study and single-case studies indicate that intolerance of uncertainty most commonly changes before level of worry in this treatment package (Dugas et al., in press).

These findings suggest that individuals with GAD may be particularly uncomfortable with the uncertainty that results from an inability to predict the future. Although worry is not an accurate prediction of future events, it may provide an illusion of certainty that is particularly appealing for individuals who are intolerant of uncertainty. As such, the reduction in feeling uncertain that accompanies worry may be a particularly powerful reinforcer for these individuals.

Other Correlates of Worry and GAD That May Contribute to Its Maintenance

Negative Beliefs about Worry, Meta-Worry, and Efforts to Control Worry

The studies and theories reviewed above suggest that worry functions to heighten awareness of potential threat, and to reduce somatic activation and feelings of uncertainty in the short term. However, worry provides inaccurate predictions and interferes with successful processing, elaboration, and responsiveness to current environmental contingencies, thus maintaining threatening meanings over the long term. Although worry is perceived as effective in problem solving and preparation for threat, it seems to be particularly likely to interfere with successful responding in ambiguous situations. These findings provide compelling explanations for the frequent occurrence of worry and the perpetuation of worrisome cycles of responding among chronically anxious individuals.

However, other factors may also serve to exacerbate the cycle of worry. In particular, authors have noted that negative beliefs about worry—for instance, considering worry itself dangerous or undesirable—may further exacerbate the worry cycle (e.g., Davey, Tallis, & Capuzzo, 1996; Wells, 1999). These authors have identified several types of negative beliefs, including the belief that worry is associated with going crazy, the sense that worry is uncontrollable, and the tendency to worry about worry ("meta-worry"; Wells, 1999). Preliminary studies have indicated that negative beliefs are correlated with worry in nonclinical samples (Davey, Tallis, & Capuzzo, 1996; Wells & Carter, 1999). Also, self-reported beliefs that worry is uncontrollable and dangerous significantly discriminated between individuals (from a nonclinical sample) who endorsed GAD criteria and those who endorsed only somatic anxiety criteria, or no anxious symptoms at all (Davis & Valentiner, 2000). However, negative beliefs did not differ between a small sample of individuals with GAD and those with OCD (Cartwright-Hatton & Wells, 1997), nor was meta-worry significantly more frequent among a sample with GAD than among a sample with panic disorder (Breitholtz et al., 1999). Thus negative appraisals of worry may not be specific to GAD.

Although more research is needed on the role of negative appraisals of worry in the maintenance of worrisome responding in clinical samples, the potentially exacerbating role of attempts to control or suppress worry (likely to result from these negative appraisals) is consistent with theorizing and research in other areas of psychology. For instance, theories of OCD (see Chapter 15) suggest that among the factors exacerbating obsessions are the negative appraisal of these intrusive thoughts and the repeated efforts to suppress these thoughts. Experimental research in the area of thought suppression has suggested that in certain circumstances, attempts to avoid unwanted thoughts can paradoxically increase occurrence of these thoughts (Wegner, 1994). This phenomenon may be comparable to (typically unsuccessful) attempts made by individuals with chronic worry to avoid their worrisome thoughts (Roemer & Borkovec, 1993; Wells, 1995). Thus negative appraisals of worry may motivate attempts to stop worrying, but these attempts at cognitive control may paradoxically increase the frequency of worries. However, to date, laboratory studies of the effects of suppressing worrisome thoughts have not supported this prediction (see Purdon, 1999, for a review). Because worry itself appears to be a form of suppression, it is difficult to disentangle exactly what the targets of suppression are among individuals with GAD. Furthermore, negative consequences other than immediate increases in worry that may follow suppression attempts, such as increased negative appraisals of worry, feelings of uncontrollability, or negative affect, have yet to be studied (Purdon, 1999).

Hayes and colleagues (Hayes, Wilson, Gifford, Follette, & Strosahl, 1996; Hayes, Strosahl, & Wilson, 1999) have recently suggested that experiential avoidance, or repeated efforts to avoid uncomfortable internal experiences (such as thoughts and feelings), may be responsible for a host of psychological difficulties. These authors note that attempts to control internal experience are likely to be unsuccessful and to distract from a focus on environmental contingencies that are more likely to be under instrumental control. Both worry itself (in that it reduces somatic activation) and attempts to control worry may be forms of experiential avoidance that are self-perpetuating, and that distract from what would be more effective behavioral forms of responding to the environment. More research is needed to explore the role of experiential avoidance and thought suppression in GAD and other disorders; these areas may have important implications for prevention and intervention strategies (e.g., Roemer & Orsillo, in press).

Behavioral Avoidance in GAD

Unlike the other anxiety disorders, GAD appears to be most obviously associated with internal, cognitive, experiential forms of avoidance, as opposed to overt behavioral avoidance. However, an early study found that 64% of a sample of individuals diagnosed with GAD reported avoidance of specific situations (Butler, Gelder, Hibbert, Cullington, & Klimes, 1987). Not surprisingly, the most frequently avoided situations were social, but some clients also reported avoiding agoraphobic situations, being alone, and exercising, as well as miscellaneous specific situations. In addition, given the diffuse nature of GAD worry, it is likely that other, more subtle forms of avoidance are present among individuals with GAD. One study found that over half a sample of patients with GAD were habitually engaging in some form of preventative behavior associated with their worries, such as calling a loved one repeatedly to be sure he or she was safe (Craske, Rapee, et al., 1989). Similar to ritualistic behaviors in OCD, these actions may prevent corrective experiences regarding the small likelihood of predicted negative outcomes. Finally, some evidence exists that worry may slow behavioral responding in certain contexts, as noted in the discussion of slowed reaction times in ambiguous tasks and tendency to procrastinate among individuals with GAD.

Although GAD is often associated with a great deal of nervous activity (e.g., the preventative behaviors noted above), it may also be associated with behavioral inaction in valued directions, as desired goals are avoided for fear of failure or other negative outcome (Roemer & Orsillo, in press). As Borkovec et al. (1999) note, the chronic apprehension of potential future threat results in repeated fight-or-flight responses without any fighting or fleeing behaviors available. As such, the cognitive and physiological rigidity described above may be matched to a similar behavioral inactivity, in that fears are not faced directly and goals are not actively pursued. Just as constant attention to future fears versus present experience may interfere with new, flexible learning, the failure to approach either desired goals or feared situations may similarly inhibit new, nonanxious learning. These conjectures have yet to be fully empirically investigated, so their utility in understanding and treating GAD remains to be seen.

Interpersonal Correlates of GAD

Borkovec and colleagues (e.g., Borkovec, Alcaine, & Behar, in press; Newman, 2000) have recently expanded their conceptualization of GAD to the interpersonal realm. These authors note the high frequency of interpersonal worries among individuals with GAD (reviewed above) and the high rate of comorbid social phobia (reviewed below), suggesting that social-evaluative, interpersonal factors are prevalent among patients with GAD. In addition, preliminary investigations of interpersonal problems among clients with GAD reveal higher levels of rigidity and distress in their interpersonal relationships compared to those of nonanxious controls, as well as a particularly high frequency of overly nurturant, intrusive relationships among clients (Pincus & Borkovec, 1994, cited in Borkovec et al., in press). In addition, retrospective reports of childhood attachment among clients with GAD and a student sample who endorsed GAD criteria revealed more role-reversed/enmeshed relationships among these participants than among their nonanxious counterparts (Cassidy, 1995). Of course, this pattern of attachment may have implications for the etiology of anxiety generally, as well as the development of GAD specifically (see Chapter 8). An interpersonal style characterized by inflexible overinvolvement with others may be particularly characteristic of individuals with GAD, or may be characteristic of anxious individuals more broadly. More research is needed on the role of interpersonal factors in both the etiology and maintenance of GAD and other anxiety disorders.

THE RELATIONSHIP OF GAD TO OTHER PSYCHOLOGICAL DISORDERS

The comorbidity and discriminant validity of GAD in relation to other psychological disorders has been extensively reviewed in Chapter 9. Here we only briefly highlight important considerations regarding the relationship between GAD and other disorders.

As noted earlier in this chapter and in Chapter 9, there is both symptomatic overlap between GAD and other emotional disorders, and a great deal of co-occurrence between GAD and these disorders. Although these relationships have caused some to question whether in fact GAD is an independent disorder, several lines of research support the assertion that it is. Despite initial concerns about overlap between panic and GAD, numerous apparent distinctions between GAD and panic have been revealed; these have been reviewed in Chapters 3 and 4. Similarly, despite apparent symptom overlap, OCD and GAD can be easily distinguished by clinical interviewers (Brown, Moras, Zinbarg, & Barlow, 1993). Furthermore, although evidence suggests a close association between GAD and mood disorders (in terms of symptom level, comorbidity rates, and shared genetic vulnerability, as reviewed in Chapters 6 and 9 and above), evidence also exists for a distinction between the two. As discussed in Chapter 9, Brown, Chorpita, and Barlow (1998) found that a structural model in which GAD and major depressive disorder were separate factors was superior to one in which they weren't. And as noted in Chapter 6, although evidence suggests a shared genetic vulnerability for the two disorders, distinct environmental factors appear to be present (e.g., Kendler, 1996). Finally, an analysis of GAD only, major depression only, and comorbid samples from two large epidemiological samples indicated an independent, additive effect of GAD and major depression symptoms on functional impairment, supporting the distinction between the two disorders (Kessler, DuPont, Berglund, & Wittchen, 1999).

Even if GAD is distinct from the other emotional disorders, it is clear that it commonly co-occurs with them. In the large study reported in Chapter 9 (Brown, Campbell, Lehman, Grisham, & Mancill, 2001), fully 68% of 120 carefully diagnosed patients with a principal diagnosis of GAD met criteria for an additional Axis I disorder (see Table 9.5). More specifically, 65% met criteria for either an anxiety or mood disorder, 52% for any anxiety disorder, and 36% for any mood disorder. When one looks at specific disorders, 36% met criteria for social phobia and 18% for panic disorder with or without agoraphobia. Among the mood disorders, fully 26% met criteria for major depressive disorder. If one looks at the comorbidity of mood disorders occurring at any time in the lives of patients with a current principal diagnosis of GAD, the percentage increases to 73% for any mood disorder. In addition, fully 64% met criteria for major depressive disorder at some time in their lives. These data support the very close relationship between major depressive disorder and GAD described in Chapter 3. As noted in Chapter 1, the NCS revealed similarly high rates of comorbidity in a community (as opposed to Brown et al.'s clinical) sample. The NCS also revealed high rates of comorbid alcohol-related disorders among individuals with GAD.

The frequently documented degree of overlap between GAD and other emotional disorders has contributed to speculation that it may be the "basic" emotional disorder, so that understanding and effectively treating GAD would contribute to an understanding of other emotional disorders. In addition, it has been proposed that GAD may in fact be a risk factor for the development of subsequent comorbid conditions (e.g., Roy-Byrne & Katon, 1997). Initial evidence for the early onset of GAD, along with the observation that many individuals with GAD report having experienced symptoms "all their lives" (e.g., Rapee, 1991), supported the proposal that GAD precedes its comorbid disorders. However, more recent studies suggest a broader range of age of onset for GAD (as noted above), and variability regarding whether it precedes or follows comorbid conditions (e.g., Brawman-Mintzer et al., 1993; Yonkers et al., 1996).

In addition to the emotional disorders, two other types of comorbid conditions common in GAD should be mentioned. As noted in the section on demographic features of GAD, several studies have revealed a relationship between GAD and somatic complaints. These findings suggest that GAD often presents with concurrent somatic symptoms that may result in treatment seeking in a medical versus a psychiatric setting. Also, as with all anxiety disorders, comorbidity of alcohol and other substance use problems is not uncommon and is very important to assess (as reviewed in Chapter 1). As noted above, the NCS revealed high levels of comorbidity between GAD and alcohol-related disorders.

The high rates of comorbid disorders among individuals with GAD have important implications for both assessment and treatment. Clearly, individuals who present with chronic worry need to be assessed for a range of disorders, in order to differentially diagnose the presenting problem and to establish a clinical picture of comorbid symptomatology so that all clinical targets are identified. Also, as noted above, comorbidity seems to be associated with greater functional impairment among individuals with GAD. Despite findings that treatments for GAD evidence beneficial effects on comorbid (emotional) disorders as well (e.g., Borkovec, Abel, & Newman, 1995), more research is needed on how best to treat various combinations of comorbid disorders.

A MODEL OF THE ETIOLOGY OF GAD

We have noted that GAD is the "basic" anxiety disorder. This is because our understanding of the etiological and maintaining factors of GAD have implications for understanding all of the anxiety disorders (as well as major depression, in view of the close association and seeming common genesis of GAD and depressive disorders). It is in GAD that the cognitive–affective structure of anxiety described in Chapter 3 reaches its full clinical manifestation. As noted there, at the core of anxiety is an abiding sense of unpredictability and uncontrollability concerning future events that are perceived as potentially threatening or dangerous. The process of worry seems to be associated with (failed) attempts to predict potential future negative outcomes, and with the belief that this prediction allows for increased control over these outcomes through either preparation for the event, effective problem solving, or the ability to avoid the outcome (see above; see also Borkovec & Roemer, 1995). In this sense, GAD is similar to those forms of social phobia in which panic does not play an etiological role. Rather, the difficulty in some performance anxieties such as public speaking or erectile dysfunction is intense excessive chronic anxiety with a strong sense of loss of control and inappropriate attentional focus, as detailed in Chapter 3. In the case of the performance anxieties, such as erectile dysfunction, the focus of anxiety is solely on sexual performance. The processes and evidence supporting this observation have been fully described in Chapter 3. In GAD the focus is more diffuse, since by definition anxiety is focused across multiple small disruptions in one's life (hassles), resulting in avoidance, withdrawal, and/or a shifting, excessive process of worry. This generalized focus of anxiety, as it becomes chronic, insures that the process of nonproductive worry becomes the principal (failed) coping mechanism, since alternative efforts to focus on more discrete areas of concern (such as specific performance anxieties) are not available. Rather, individuals with GAD lurch from one crisis to another in their lives, attempting to impose whatever control they may over this dangerous chaotic state by using all mental means at their disposal.

For an overall depiction of the etiology of GAD, the reader is referred to Chapter 8 (and Figure 8.7), where the familiar pattern of generalized neurobiological and psychological vulnerabilities activated by negative or stressful life events contributing to the development of GAD is described in some detail. The origins of these vulnerabilities in the genome and early experience have been described in Chapter 8, as have likely patterns of interaction. Early family and twin studies suggested that GAD may be associated with a unique heritable vulnerability, since some of these studies reported that GAD tends to run in families (e.g., Noyes, Clarkson, Crowe, Yates, & McChesney, 1987; Noyes et al., 1992). A major twin study also supported this conclusion (Kendler, Neale, Kessler, Heath, & Eaves, 1992a). But, as discussed in some detail in Chapter 6, subsequent studies with a broader focus (e.g., Kendler, Neale, Kessler, Heath, & Eaves, 1992c; Kendler et al., 1995) confirm that what seems to be heritable is a nonspecific tendency to develop emotional disorders generally.

Within GAD the focus of anxiety remains on (usually) negative life events, rather than on discrete external events (phobic objects) or internal events (panic attacks), and an exquisite sensitivity to relatively minor hassles is manifested. As noted above, reactions to these events are accompanied by arousal associated with negative affect and a sense that these events are proceeding in an unpredictable, uncontrollable fashion, reflecting a psychological diathesis arising out of early experience, as detailed in Chapter 8. This process in turn is associated with a maladaptive shift in focus of attention from the task at hand to self-evaluative modes, resulting in further increases in arousal. Increased vigilance, narrowing of attention to the focus of concern, and other distortions in information processing (as detailed above and outlined in Chapter 3; see Figure 3.1) are consequences of a fundamental perception of lack of control over potential threats. The process of worry then becomes a negatively reinforcing, but maladaptive, attempt to control this spiraling process. As noted in Chapter 8, the presence of a generalized psychological vulnerability or a generalized neurobiological vulnerability in isolation is unlikely to lead to GAD. Rather, one is likely to see a personality style characterized by some combination of arousability, pessimism, low self-confidence and esteem, and lack of initiative—or, perhaps, no obvious manifestations. On the other hand, a synergism of generalized biological (genetic) and generalized psychological (early experience) vulnerabilities is most likely to lead to the clinical syndromes of GAD and depressive disorders, as outlined in Figure 8.7. A more specific description of the etiology of GAD is presented in Figure 14.1.

ASSESSMENT

The following is a brief overview of considerations and tools for the assessment of GAD. More extensive discussions of relevant considerations in assessment and reviews of specific measures are available elsewhere (e.g., Antony, Orsillo, & Roemer, 2001; Campbell & Brown, in press).

From the review of the literature above, it is clear that comprehensive assessment of GAD will involve multiple domains. In addition to assessment of the central diagnostic features of GAD (i.e., excessive, uncontrollable, pervasive worry) and its associated symptoms (restlessness and feeling keyed up or on edge, muscle tension, etc.), attention should be paid to comorbid anxious, depressive, and physical symptomatology (both to establish a differential diagnosis and to determine all necessary targets of treatment even if GAD is the principal complaint), as well as features proposed to maintain chronic worry (e.g., positive and negative beliefs about worry, cognitive avoidance, intolerance of uncertainty). Because the need to assess comorbid psychological and physical symptoms is constant across the anxiety disorders, this section focuses on assessment of GAD-specific features. That is, the diagnostic criteria and factors thought to perpetuate the disorder's central defining feature are discussed.

Interview-Based Measures

The most widely used interview measure of GAD is the Anxiety Disorders Interview Schedule for DSM-IV: Lifetime Version (ADIS-IV-L; Di Nardo, Brown, & Barlow, 1994), described in detail in Chapter 9. This semistructured interview provides diagnoses of both

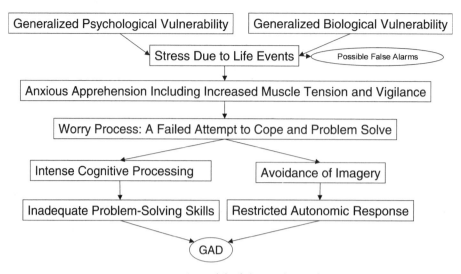

FIGURE 14.1. A model of the etiology of GAD.

current and lifetime GAD; diagnoses of other, often comorbid anxiety, mood, and substance use disorders; ratings of clinical severity of all disorders; and other information relevant to a diagnosis of GAD, such as frequency of preventative behaviors, worry about minor things, and percentage of the day typically spent worrying. Other commonly used diagnostic interviews (e.g., the Structured Clinical Interview for DSM-IV Axis I Disorders; First, Spitzer, Gibbon, & Williams, 1996) also contain GAD sections, but none as extensive as that of the ADIS-IV-L.

The Hamilton Anxiety Rating Scale (HARS; Hamilton, 1959, 1969) is another semi-structured interview commonly used to assess severity of anxious symptoms among individuals with GAD. This 14-item measure was specifically designed to assess the severity of symptomatology, not to determine the presence of an anxiety disorder. It contains two subscales, assessing Psychic (e.g., anxious apprehension, irritability) and Somatic symptoms. The latter subscale contains many autonomic symptoms, which are less likely to characterize GAD, possibly reducing overall severity scores on this measure for individuals with GAD. Although the HARS has shown good convergent validity (e.g., Maier, Buller, Philipp, & Heuser, 1988), questions regarding its discriminant validity have been raised. Studies have revealed high correlations between the HARS and measures of depression, and scores on the HARS failed to discriminate patients with GAD from those with major depressive disorder (Riskind, Beck, Brown & Steer, 1987). Even reformulated versions of the scale continue to have trouble discriminating anxiety and depression (Moras, Di Nardo, & Barlow, 1992). In addition, interrater reliability for HARS rating has been somewhat low (e.g., Maier et al., 1988; Moras et al., 1992). However, newly developed structured interview guides are associated with improved interrater reliability (Bruss, Gruenberg, Goldstein, & Barber, 1994; Shear, Vander Bilt, et al., 2001).

Self-Report Measures

The Penn State Worry Questionnaire (PSWQ; Meyer, Miller, Metzger, & Borkovec, 1990) is a widely used 16-item self-report questionnaire that assesses an individual's general tendency to worry excessively. It was specifically designed to assess intensity/excessiveness of worry without reference to specific content of the worries. Studies have revealed excellent psychometric properties in both nonclinical and clinical populations (see Molina & Borkovec, 1994, for a review), including strong discriminant validity even in samples with anxiety disorders (Brown et al., 1992). The scale has also been found to demonstrate good psychometric properties among older adults (Beck, Stanley, & Zebb, 1995). Finally, the PSWQ is sensitive to change following psychological treatment (e.g., Borkovec & Costello, 1993).

Other content-specific measures of worry have been developed. The Worry Domains Questionnaire (Tallis, Eysenck, & Mathews, 1992a) was specifically designed to assess nonpathological worry; it assesses the content domains of relationships, lack of confidence, aimless future, work, and finances. It may be a useful adjunct to the PSWQ in order to assess specific areas of worry (Tallis, Davey, & Bond, 1994). The Anxious Thoughts Inventory (Wells, 1994b) specifically assesses social and health worries; however, its psychometric properties have yet to be explored in a clinical sample. Finally, the Worry Scale for Older Adults (Wisocki, 1988), designed specifically to assess worry among older adults, assesses frequency of worry in the areas of social concerns, health, and finances, and any other significant topics of worry.

The aforementioned measures all focus on assessing worry, the central feature of GAD, rather than its full diagnostic criteria. Other scales have been designed specifically to assess the diagnostic criteria of GAD. The Generalized Anxiety Disorder Questionnaire (GADQ; Roemer, Borkovec, Posa, & Borkovec, 1995), based on DSM-III-R criteria, demonstrated adequate psychometric properties but a tendency to overdiagnose GAD among nonclinical samples (making it best used as a screening device). The revised version of this scale, the GADQ-IV (Newman, Zuellig, Kachin, & Constantino, 2000), assesses symptoms based on DSM-IV criteria with good reliability. This scale also provides a continuous score reflecting GAD symptom severity, in addition to a dichotomous score of whether an individual meets GAD criteria or not.

In addition to assessment of GAD-specific symptoms of worry and its associated features, assessment of general level of anxiety among patients with GAD is often helpful, particularly in monitoring change across treatment. In choosing an assessment measure, it is important to keep in mind that GAD is not characterized by the same level of autonomic arousal as other anxiety disorders. Therefore, measures like the Beck Anxiety Inventory (BAI; Beck, Epstein, Brown, & Steer, 1988), which consist of a number of arousal-type symptoms, may not be accurate in assessing the level of anxiety in GAD (Cox, Cohen, Direnfeld, & Swinson, 1996). Similarly, given the amount of overlap between GAD and symptoms of depression, anxiety measures that show poor discriminant validity in reference to measures of depression may also be problematic. Despite this, the Trait version of the State–Trait Anxiety Inventory (STAI; Spielberger, Gorsuch, Lushene, Vagg, & Jacobs, 1983), which has been found to predict depressive symptoms (Bieling, Antony, & Swinson, 1998), is a commonly used measure in treatment outcome studies for GAD.

The Depression Anxiety and Stress Scales (Lovibond & Lovibond, 1995) is a relatively new measure that may provide a more discriminating assessment of the anxiety associated with GAD. In addition to the Anxiety subscale, which assesses symptoms of anxious arousal similar to those included in the BAI, this measure contains a Tension/Stress subscale that assesses symptoms of difficulty relaxing, nervous arousal, being easily upset/agitated, and irritability. Scores on this subscale were significantly higher among patients with GAD than among patients diagnosed with panic disorder, social phobia, or specific phobia, suggesting that it may be a useful measure of anxiety among individuals with GAD (Brown, Chorpita, Korotitsch, & Barlow, 1997).

In addition to assessing GAD-specific symptoms (e.g., worry) and general levels of anxiety/stress, it may be useful to assess factors thought to be implicated in the maintenance of GAD. Several recently developed measures assess positive beliefs about worry: the Why Worry Questionnaire (Freeston et al., 1994), the Consequences of Worrying Scale (Davey, Tallis, & Capuzzo, 1996), and the Meta-Cognitions Questionnaire (Cartwright-Hatton & Wells, 1997). Attempts to control worry or other negative thoughts, along with general negative beliefs about worry and other negative thoughts (which may motivate attempts to control worry) are assessed in several relatively new measures: the Meta-Cognitions Questionnaire, the Thought Control Questionnaire (Wells & Davies, 1994), the White Bear Suppression Inventory (Wegner & Zanakos, 1994), the Anxious Thoughts Inventory, the Acceptance and Action Questionnaire (Hayes et al., 2001), and the Consequences of Worrying Scale. Some of these measures have only been explored in nonclinical samples at this point, and their clinical utility remains to be determined.

Finally, the Intolerance of Uncertainty Scale (IUS; Freeston et al., 1994) assesses the degree of difficulty coping with uncertainty in life, a factor proposed to relate to GAD. This scale shows good reliability and convergent validity in nonclinical samples (Freeston et al., 1994) and also significantly discriminates patients with GAD from a nonanxious control group (Dugas et al., 1998). Also, IUS scores were higher in samples of individuals with principal and additional diagnoses of GAD than in another sample with mixed anxiety disorders (mostly OCD) (Ladouceur et al., 1999). In addition, treatment sensitivity has been demonstrated following an intervention designed specifically to target intolerance of uncertainty (Ladouceur et al., 2000).

Self-Monitoring

Several self-monitoring forms have been developed specifically for use with patients with GAD. These forms are useful for initial assessment, for assessing changes throughout treatment, and as intervention tools themselves, in that they increase awareness of the cues and consequences associated with worry and anxiety. Thus clients can evaluate the contingencies that perpetuate their worry, develop alternative response options, and practice rapidly implementing these responses following anxiety-provoking cues. Craske, Barlow, and O'Leary (1992) describe a Worry Record that addresses these three aims. Each time the client experiences an increase in anxiety, he or she records the intensity and topic of worry, any associated symptoms, an event description, and a list of thoughts experienced. In addition, Borkovec et al. (1999) describe the use of a Worry Outcome Diary, in which clients record specific negative predictions weekly and then go back and assess whether the outcomes were as negative as they predicted and how well they coped with them. This allows clients to test their beliefs in the functionality of worry, in addition to providing a continual assessment of the content of their worries.

Assessment of Subtle Behavioral Avoidance

By definition, individuals diagnosed with GAD do not manifest overt phobic avoidance, so the types of behavioral assessment that have proved so useful in the phobic disorders are less relevant in work with this population. However, excessive worry and prediction of potential threat may lead individuals with GAD to refrain from engaging in various potentially threatening activities in order to reduce their anxiety. Thus it is important to carefully assess any more subtle forms of avoidance (e.g., to ask clients what activities they might engage in if they did not worry so much) and to address these situations in treatment. Techniques such as those used to assess valued directions in Hayes et al.'s (1999) Acceptance and Commitment Therapy might help determine areas in which an individual with GAD is restricting his or her behavior based on apprehension about possible future negative outcomes (e.g., becoming more intimate in relationships, pursuing a potential romantic partner or a promotion at work). These forms of avoidance clearly would not lend themselves to the same kind of assessment used in a behavioral avoidance test. To date, no formal means of assessing these areas have been developed; however, they remain important elements to keep in mind when working with individuals with GAD.

PHARMACOLOGICAL TREATMENTS

Pharamacological approaches to GAD or its diagnostic predecessor, anxiety neurosis, have been extensively studied over the course of the last 30 years. Three basic drug groups have been demonstrated to be efficacious in the treatment of GAD: benzodiazepines, azapirones, and antidepressants. Although other drugs such as antipsychotics and antihistamines have been considered, the data are too preliminary to establish their efficacy and safety.

Benzodiazepines

Starting in the 1970s, benzodiazepines became the most commonly used medications to treat anxiety neurosis or GAD. Literally hundreds of studies have documented the superiority of benzodiazepines over placebo in the short-term reduction of symptoms in 65–70% of patients diagnosed with GAD. However, fewer than two-thirds of patients treated with benzodiazepines actually experience a full remission of symptoms during treatment, and the reoccurrence of anxiety after treatment is fairly common (Schweizer & Rickels, 1996).

Benzodiazepines are thought to work by increasing gamma-aminobutyric acid inhibitory impulses in the central nervous system, which are mediated via benzodiazepine receptors (Möller, 1999). Their action is rapid, with most studies demonstrating an effect within the first week of treatment. Specific types of benzodiazepines differ primarily in terms of their rate of metabolism and the strength of their agonist properties. Although diazepam, a slowly metabolizing drug with a long half-life, was previously the most widely prescribed benzodiazepine (Shader & Greenblatt, 1993), concern over the potential side effects of longer-lasting benzodiazepines undoubtedly contributed to the increased popularity of alprazolam and other shorter-acting benzodiazepines in the late 1980s.

Benzodiazepines seem to be most effective in treating the somatic rather than the psychic (e.g., worry, irritability) symptoms of GAD (Pourmotabbed, McLeod, Hoehn-Saric, Hipsley, & Greenblatt, 1996; Rickels et al., 1982; Rickels, Downing, Schweizer, & Hassman, 1993). Given the recent diagnostic changes in GAD criteria emphasizing worry over the somatic symptoms in the conceptualization of the disorder, the utility of benzodiazepines for GAD may continue to decrease (Connor & Davidson, 1998). Furthermore, benzodiazepines may be less effective in patients with depressive symptoms (Rickels et al., 1993); this may be an important issue, given the high rate of comorbid depression associated with GAD.

The safety of benzodiazepine treatment has been debated vigorously throughout the literature. Typical side effects of the benzodiazepines include sedation (Shader & Greenblatt, 1993), impairment of psychomotor function (Pourmotabbed et al., 1996), and anterograde amnesia (Lucki, Rickels, & Geller, 1986). There is some evidence that chronic benzodiazepine use does not produce consistent problems with sedation and psychomotor functioning (Lucki et al., 1986); however, the cognitive effects of benzodiazepines are likely to vary, depending on the specific drug, the sensitivity of the tests, and the general health of the patient (Hart, Colenda, & Hamer, 1991). Nonetheless, evidence of anterograde amnesia exists both in patients treated for the first time with benzodiazepines and in those with a history of chronic use (Lucki et al., 1986). Although the clinical significance of this amnesia has not been fully established (Rickels & Schweizer, 1998), it certainly raises concern about the long-term, widespread use of such medications.

There is also significant controversy over the potential addictiveness of benzodiazepines (Möller, 1999). Although there does not appear to be evidence for the widespread abuse of benzodiazepines (e.g., Garvey & Tollefson, 1986), patients with a history of addiction, those with chronic physical illnesses, patients with dysthymic disorders and personality disorders, and patients with chronic sleep disorders may be at increased risk (Salzman, 1991, cited in Möller, 1999). Tolerance to the anxiolytic properties of benzodiazepines has not been demonstrated in studies with patients treated for 6 to 8 months (e.g., Rickels, Case, Downing, & Winokur, 1983; Rickels, Schweizer, Csanalosi, Case, & Chung, 1988). However, in clinical practice the course of GAD is typically chronic, and treatment can span years; thus prospective studies that assess the efficacy and safety of long-term maintenance treatment are sorely needed.

Another issue of concern with this class of drugs is the return of symptoms after medication is discontinued. The reemergence of original symptoms after treatment is thought to reflect a relapse, demonstrating the inability of benzodiazepines to "cure" GAD. The emergence of new or more intense symptoms is thought to imply physical dependence and withdrawal. In practice, these two events are difficult to differentiate due to overlapping symptoms. Also, they can occur simultaneously or sequentially in the same patient (Shader & Greenblatt, 1993).

Among patients receiving long-term treatment (>6 months) with benzodiazepines, 70–80% seem to experience a withdrawal syndrome (e.g., Rickels, Case, Schweizer, Swenson, & Fridman, 1986; Rickels et al., 1988). The severity of this withdrawal syndrome has been associated with a number of drug and patient factors. Higher dosages, shorter half-lives, longer duration of daily therapy, more rapid taper, higher pretaper anxiety or depression, higher levels of personality psychopathology, and concomitant alcohol and other substance use problems have all been associated with more severe withdrawal (Schweizer & Rickels, 1996).

The absence of research on the long-term efficacy and safety of benzodiazepine therapy has led some researchers to suggest alternative courses of therapy. For instance, Rickels and Schweizer (1998) have proposed intermittent short-term (2-week) therapy as an alternative for some patients. They developed this proposal based on the fact that 50–70% of patients in studies they reviewed (e.g., Rickels, 1985; Rickels et al., 1983, 1988) were able to remain in remission for periods of a few weeks up to 3 months after treatment. Although this is an interesting proposal, research is needed to examine the safety and efficacy of this approach.

The benzodiazepines that are currently marketed are fairly full agonists of the benzodiazepine receptor (Schweizer & Rickels, 1996). Partial benzodiazepine agonists have also recently been developed and tested, in the hope that they can produce anxiolytic effects without the negative side effects associated with full-agonist benzodiazepines. Abecarnil, a beta-carboline, has been shown to be effective in double-blind placebo-controlled studies using both DSM-III-R and DSM-IV criteria for GAD (Ballenger et al., 1991; Lydiard, Ballenger, & Rickels, 1997), and it has fewer withdrawal symptoms than benzodiazepines (Lydiard, Ballenger, & Rickels, 1997; Rickels, DeMartinis, & Aufdembrinke, 2000). However, other studies have failed to demonstrate the continued superiority of abecarnil over placebo (e.g., Aufdembrinke, 1998; Pollack, Worthington, Manfro, Otto, & Zucker, 1997; Rickels, DeMartinis, & Aufdembrinke, 2000). The authors of these studies attribute their inability to detect differences between the abecarnil and placebo groups to surprisingly high response rates found within their placebo groups. This phenomenon has been discussed in detail by Schweizer and Rickels (1997).

Azapirones

Azapirones are the second class of drugs that have demonstrated effective control over symptoms of GAD. In 1996, buspirone, one of the most commonly used azapirones, became the only nonbenzodiazepine approved by the U. S. Food and Drug Administration (FDA) for the treatment of GAD (Apter & Allen, 1999). Although other azapirones have been evaluated, no other drug in this class has consistently emerged as efficacious. Buspirone differs both structurally and pharmacologically from benzodiazepines, and is thought to work by binding to serotonin 5-HT$_{1A}$ receptors in the brain (Pecknold, 1994). Unlike benzodiazepines, buspirone does not appear to cause sedation (Cohn, Bowden, Fisher, & Rodos, 1986; Dement et al., 1991; Manfredi et al., 1991; Seidel, Cohen, Bliwise, & Dement, 1985) or deficits in psychomotor (e.g., Boulenger et al., 1989; Mattila, Aranko, & Seppala, 1982; Moskowitz & Smiley, 1982) or cognitive (e.g., Unrug-Neervoot, van Luijtelaar, & Coenen, 1992) performance, even among older individuals (Hart et al., 1991). Although there is some evidence that buspirone can accelerate performance decrements in prolonged and monotonous tasks, the pervasiveness and clinical significance of this potential side effect need more study (O'Hanlon, 1991). Finally, findings from both animal (Balster, 1990) and human (Cole, Orzack, Beake, Bird, & Bar-Tal, 1982; Griffith, Jasinski, Casten, & McKinney, 1986; Lader & Olajide, 1987; Sellers, Schneiderman, Romach, Kaplan, & Somer, 1992; Troisi, Critchfield, & Griffiths, 1993) studies suggest that buspirone has little abuse or dependence potential. The most common side effects of buspirone include dizziness, headaches, nervousness, paresthesia, diarrhea, and sweating (Enkelmann, 1991; Goa & Ward, 1986; Newton, Marunycz, Alderdice, & Napoliello, 1986).

Buspirone typically takes longer than benzodiazepines to produce symptom-reducing effects (e.g., Ansseau, Papart, Gérard, von Frenckell, & Franck, 1990; Boyer & Feighner, 1993; Cutler et al., 1993; Enkelmann, 1991; Feighner, Merideth, & Hendrickson, 1982; Rickels et al., 1988), although some studies have not found that difference (Pecknold et al., 1989; Strand et al., 1990). This slower onset of action may cause a higher dropout rate (Rickels et al., 1988).

In contrast to benzodiazepines, buspirone seems to have a stronger impact on psychic symptoms than on somatic symptoms (Rickels et al., 1982). Furthermore, buspirone seems to be relatively efficacious in reducing the depressive symptoms that commonly co-occur with GAD (Gammans et al., 1992; Sramek et al., 1996). However, the clinical significance of the antidepressant effect of buspirone remains unknown (Casacalenda & Boulenger, 1998).

Buspirone has been used to manage withdrawal or rebound anxiety in patients discontinuing benzodiazepine treatment, with mixed results (Ashton, Rawlins, & Tyrer, 1990; Delle Chiaie et al., 1995; Schweizer, Rickels, & Lucki, 1986; Udelman & Udelman, 1990). Patients previously and recently treated with benzodiazepines have been shown to be more likely to drop out of buspirone treatment prematurely, to report more adverse side effects, and to demonstrate less improvement than those without prior benzodiazepine treatment or those with remote (more than 1 month before) benzodiazepine treatment (DeMartinis, Rynn, Rickels, & Mandos, 2000).

Antidepressants

Given the presumed relationship between GAD and major depressive disorder, it is no surprise that antidepressants have been considered as a potential treatment. Controlled studies of patients diagnosed with GAD have demonstrated the efficacy of imipramine (Hoehn-Saric, McLeod, & Zimmerli, 1988; Rickels et al., 1993), a tricyclic antidepressant, and paroxetine (Rocca, Fonzo, Scotta, Zanalda, & Ravizza, 1997), a selective serotonin reuptake inhibitor, in treating patients with GAD and no comorbid major depression. Similar to buspirone, compared to benzodiazepines, antidepressants seem to take longer to show improvement and are more efficacious in reducing psychic as compared to somatic symptoms.

Venlafaxine, a combined serotonin and noradrenaline reuptake inhibitor, has also recently received FDA approval for the treatment of GAD (Schatzberg, 2000). Venlafaxine is a powerful antidepressant that is more easily tolerated than older tricyclic antidepressants (Sheehan, 1999). The safety and efficacy of this drug has been demonstrated among patients without comorbid depression in short (Davidson, DuPont, Hedges, & Haskins, 1999; Rickels, Pollack, Sheehan, & Haskins, 2000) and longer (6-month) controlled trials (Gelenberg et al., 2000). Although these results are promising, more research is needed.

Summary

At least three classes of medications offer potential efficacy in the short-term treatment of GAD. Several factors (including the prominence of somatic vs. psychic symptoms, patient acceptance, and side effects) potentially determine which drug may be best for a particular patient; however, more research is needed to determine better predictors of response (Schweizer & Rickels, 1996). Furthermore, there is a significant need for studies that assess the safety and effectiveness of medications for GAD as they are typically prescribed in practice. In a recent review of the literature, Mahe and Balogh (2000) found only eight drug studies conducted with patients diagnosed with GAD that reported more than a 2-month duration of treatment. These studies were also plagued with methodological limitations; the placebo groups in particular presented a number of problems. As discussed above, many studies have found a high rate of response among patients in the placebo group, which severely limits the conclusions that can be drawn from this body of research. Moreover, the placebo dropout rate is typically quite high, making group comparisons difficult or impossible (Mahe & Balogh, 2000).

PSYCHOSOCIAL TREATMENT

In the first edition of this book, psychosocial interventions were just being developed for GAD, and few (if any) controlled trials had been conducted. Since that time, several cognitive-behavioral treatment (CBT) packages have been developed, and evidence for their efficacy compared to both wait-list and nonspecific treatment conditions has accrued. In addition, the long-term maintenance of these treatment gains has been documented, suggesting that they may provide a particularly effective alternative to existing pharmacological interventions that fail to result in long-lasting symptom reduction. Although these accomplishments are impressive, studies that have investigated the rates of high end-state functioning (symptom levels within the range of a nonanxious population) following interventions for GAD reveal lower estimates than extant psychosocial treatments for other anxiety disorders (e.g., panic disorder and OCD). This suggests the need for continued treatment development in this area. Fortunately, several investigators have begun to develop new protocols that incorporate recent research on mechanisms and maintaining factors of chronic worry. We begin below with a review of findings from randomized controlled intervention trials, then briefly summarize some studies using alternative interventions or targeting alternative populations, and conclude with a discussion of recent proposals for newer treatments for GAD.

Findings from Randomized Controlled Studies

Although early research on interventions targeting general anxiety and tension (e.g., relaxation training), conducted prior to the definition of GAD as a diagnostic entity, has informed the components of existing treatments for GAD, we focus here only on studies utilizing the DSM criteria for GAD (beginning with DSM-III). Borkovec and Ruscio (2001) recently reviewed 13 randomized controlled GAD psychosocial treatment outcome studies, all of which included a CBT condition. The majority of studies investigated individual therapy, although two used a group format for intervention. Overall attrition was low (particularly in CBT conditions), and all studies included a 6- or 12-month follow-up assessment. Seven of the studies reviewed utilized DSM-III criteria for GAD, while the remaining six used DSM-III-R criteria. As we write this chapter, only one randomized controlled study using DSM-IV criteria has been published (Ladouceur et al., 2000, described below).

Borkovec and Ruscio's (2001) review indicated that CBT approaches yield significant changes (with large effect sizes) that are maintained or improved at a 6- to 12-month follow-up. The average effect size for anxiety (including worry) measures for CBT interventions was 2.48 at posttreatment and 2.44 at follow-up, while effect sizes for depression measures were 1.13 at posttreatment and 1.22 at follow-up. These findings suggest substantial therapeutic gains in both anxious and depressive symptomatology following CBT. Not surprisingly, given the chronic nature of this disorder, wait-list conditions showed minimal change from pre- to postassessment, resulting in large effect sizes when CBT was compared to a wait-list condition. More importantly, comparison of treatment effects of CBT versus nonspecific or alternative interventions (which consisted of one nonmanualized psychodynamic intervention and two trials using low doses of diazepam) revealed small to large effect sizes, with an average effect size of 0.71 for anxiety measures and 0.66 for depression measures at posttreatment. These diminished to small effects at follow-up (0.30 and 0.21, respectively). However, the authors note that the decrease in differential efficacy at follow-up is probably attributable due to clients in the nonspecific treatment conditions seeking alternative (possibly CBT) interventions. Finally, Borkovec and Ruscio note that some studies have found that a full package of CBT is more effective than its component parts (e.g., Butler, Fennell, Robson, & Gelder, 1991). However, others have found the dismantled and full packages comparable (e.g., Barlow, Rapee, & Brown, 1992).

Common Components of CBT Packages

Thus empirical evidence to date suggests that several multicomponent CBT interventions for GAD result in significant, relatively long-lasting improvement in both anxious and depressive symptomatology. These treatments vary in terms of the specific cognitive behavioral elements they contain, and very few dismantling studies have been conducted to isolate the necessary features of each treatment package.[5] However, certain common elements can be identified and are reviewed below.

PSYCHOEDUCATION. Similar to all CBT interventions, versions of CBT for GAD contain a substantial psychoeducational component. Clients are taught about the functional nature of anxiety and fear, but are told that anxiety can escalate in a cycle of physiological, cognitive, and behavioral habitual responses that maintain rather than diminish fear. Different elements of this model are emphasized, depending on the different emphases of the intervention (e.g., cognitive elements are highlighted in treatments that include cognitive restructuring components). Psychoeducation also includes a rationale for the given treatment, in order to increase expectancy and client commitment.

MONITORING/EARLY CUE DETECTION. Monitoring, too, is a common element across all CBT interventions. In the context of GAD treatments, the importance of recognizing cues associated with anxious responding early, in order to implement alternative coping strategies and reduce the cycle of anxious escalation, is emphasized in this component. Monitoring can focus on situational, physiological, cognitive, and behavioral cues associated with anxious responding, again varying depending on the focus of the specific intervention. Some specific techniques for monitoring in GAD have been reviewed in the "Assessment" section above.

APPLIED RELAXATION. Although applied relaxation is not a uniform element of GAD treatments, it is very commonly included in CBT packages for this disorder. Clients are taught multiple methods of relaxation (e.g., pleasant imagery, diaphragmatic breathing, cue-controlled relaxation, progressive muscle relaxation; Bernstein, Borkovec, & Hazlett-Stevens, 2000), which they practice daily. Clients are then taught to apply these relaxation strategies to anxiety-provoking situations, either imaginally or *in vivo* (Öst, 1987b). Multiple methods are emphasized in order to encourage flexible responding (e.g., Borkovec & Roemer, 1994).

IMAGINAL AND IN VIVO EXPOSURE/COPING SKILLS REHEARSAL. Due to the absence of a clear phobic target in GAD, the traditional exposure-based methods so integral to the successful treatment of other anxiety disorders (see Chapters 10–13 and Chapter 15) have not frequently been used in the treatment of GAD. However, exposure to feared stimuli either *in vivo* or imaginally has often been an element of the treatments that have been developed. This element has varied from more traditional graduated exposure to feared situations (e.g., Butler et al., 1991) to coping skills rehearsal components in which exposure is paired with rehearsal of acquired coping skills (e.g., cognitive restructuring and relaxation) until anxiety subsides. The latter form of exposure has been implemented both imaginally (e.g., self-control desensitization, Borkovec & Costello, 1993, based on Goldfried, 1971) and *in vivo* (Barlow et al., 1992). Some packages have also included a focus on increasing engagement in pleasurable activities (e.g., Butler, Cullington, Hibbert, Klimes, & Gelder, 1987), which may be considered exposure if individuals with GAD are thought to avoid engagement in pleasurable activities due to fear of disappointment or failure (e.g.,

---

[5]Notable exceptions are Butler et al.'s (1991) finding of superior efficacy for a cognitive behavioral intervention over a solely behavioral (relaxation plus *in vivo* exposure) intervention, and Borkovec and Costello's (1993) finding that a complex package including applied relaxation, cognitive restructuring, and self-control desensitization was superior to applied relaxation alone over the long term.

Roemer & Orsillo, in press). More recently, Borkovec et al. (in press) have emphasized the importance of increased attention to present-moment experience, particularly those experiences associated with one's values or with joy; this too might be considered a form of coping skills rehearsal.

COGNITIVE RESTRUCTURING. Finally, many treatments have incorporated cognitive restructuring elements as described by Beck and Emery with Greenberg (1985), targeting distorted cognitions and information-processing biases associated with GAD. These components typically involve identification of anxious thoughts and an encouragement to question the accuracy of interpretations and predictions. For GAD, an emphasis is often placed on increasing awareness of multiple perspectives, which complements the emphasis on multiple methods of relaxing (e.g., Borkovec & Costello, 1993). Both of these elements are thought to counter the rigidity of cognitive and emotional responding that characterizes GAD. In addition, strategies to counter catastrophizing or overestimating the probability of threat from minor events (e.g., exploring feared consequences through continual prompts of "And then what would be the worst thing? And how likely is that?") are often employed in order to explore the likelihood of clients' catastrophic predictions (e.g., Zinbarg, Craske, & Barlow, 1993). Cognitive components may also include planned behavioral experiments in which predictions are tested in order to determine their accuracy (e.g., Zinbarg et al., 1993, Butler et al., 1991). This element most likely combines cognitive restructuring and exposure, given that experiments necessarily involve approaching rather than avoiding feared cues.

Efficacy of Treatment Components

A recent randomized controlled study not included in Borkovec and Ruscio's (2001) review suggests that individual components of this comprehensive package may be comparable in terms of efficacy. Borkovec, Newman, Pincus, and Lytle (in press) compared cognitive therapy alone to self-control desensitization (including applied relaxation) alone to a combined package of these elements (with portions of sessions in each component condition devoted to supportive listening therapy, in order to equate therapist contact across conditions). Analyses at posttreatment and across follow-up periods (up to 24 months) revealed comparable improvement in anxiety symptoms and depression symptoms across conditions. At 6-month follow-up, the combined treatment was associated with significantly more clients categorized as meeting criteria for high end-state functioning, but this difference disappeared at 12- and 24-month follow-ups. These findings suggest that cognitive therapy and self-control desensitization are each efficacious in the treatment of GAD, and raise questions regarding whether this efficacy involves similar or different mechanisms of change. It should be pointed out that this trial involved considerably more therapy time than prior GAD outcome trials, and it may be that component elements can yield as much improvement as a combined package when extensive therapy in each component is provided. In fact, comparisons of within-group effect sizes from each of these elements to the average effect sizes for CBT packages reported in Borkovec and Ruscio's (2001) meta-analysis indicate that the elements equaled or exceeded the outcome of prior CBT conditions (T. D. Borkovec, personal communication, November 2000).

Very few studies have directly compared CBT and pharmacological approaches to treating GAD. Two studies have compared diazepam and CBT alone and in combination (with pill placebo controls); both found conditions that included CBT to be more efficacious than those without it (Power, Jerrom, Simpson, Mitchell, & Swanson, 1989; Power,

Simpson, Swanson, & Wallace, 1990). However, the diazepam condition involved a low fixed-dosage regimen, which probably minimized efficacy (Borkovec & Ruscio, 2001). A meta-analysis comparing effect sizes of pharmacological and CBT interventions for GAD found comparable effects for measures of anxiety, but significantly greater effects for CBT on measures of depression (Gould, Otto, Pollack, & Yap, 1997). However, the pharmacological studies reviewed consisted primarily of benzodiazepine trials, so these findings cannot be generalized to those classes of drugs that have been shown to be more efficacious in the treatment of depressive symptoms. On the other hand, CBT interventions demonstrated maintenance of gains at follow-up, while there was no evidence for sustained treatment effects following termination of pharmacotherapy. In summary, some evidence suggests that CBT interventions may be more beneficial (particularly over the long term), but overall little is known about comparative efficacy, particularly with newer classes of drugs. Even less is known about the impact of using pharmacological and psychosocial interventions in combination, which is a common clinical occurrence.

Clinical Significance and Predictors of Outcome

Despite the impressive gains made in the development of efficacious treatments for GAD over the past 10 years, to date it remains the least successfully treated of the anxiety disorders (Brown, Barlow, & Liebowitz, 1994). Although cognitive behavioral intervention is consistently associated with reliable, statistically significant change that is maintained at follow-up, it is typically associated with high end-state functioning in only 40–60% of a treated sample. Because definitions of high end-state functioning vary across samples, it is difficult to compare these proportions across studies. Nonetheless, it is helpful to review the highest reported percentages to date, in order to gain a sense of how effective our current interventions are at leaving clients with symptoms within the range of a nonanxious population after a follow-up period. Butler et al. (1991) defined good outcome as scores within the normal range on two anxiety measures and below clinical cutoff on a third. They found that 42% of their sample treated with CBT met these criteria at 6-month follow-up. Borkovec and Costello (1993) considered scores falling within the normative range on at least six of eight outcome measures as indicative of high end-state functioning; according to these criteria, 57.9% of clients receiving their cognitive-behavioral package reported high end-state functioning at 12-month follow-up. Ladouceur et al. (2000) defined high end-state functioning as scores within normative range on at least five of six outcome measures; 57.7% of their treated sample met these criteria at 12-month follow-up. Thus, even when cognitive behavioral interventions are at their most efficacious, more than 40% of treated samples fail to meet high end-state functioning at follow-up. One possible explanation for the limited effects may be that more treatment within each module is needed. Yet the study by Borkovec, Newman, et al. (in press) lengthened the treatment in an attempt to improve efficacy, but still resulted in high end-state functioning in less than half the participants. These findings suggest that it may be necessary to supplement existing cognitive-behavioral treatments with new elements in order to improve their efficacy.

Very few studies have analyzed factors predictive of outcome in clinical trials of psychosocial treatments for GAD. Several studies have found that expectancy ratings at the beginning of treatment predict outcome (e.g., Borkovec & Mathews, 1988; Borkovec & Costello, 1993), although others have failed to find a significant relationship between expectancy and outcome (e.g., Borkovec, Newman, et al., in press; Ladouceur et al., 2000). Credibility ratings prior to treatment have also been inconsistently related to outcome, with some studies finding a significant relationship (e.g., Borkovec, Newman, et al., in press) while others did not (Borkovec & Costello, 1993; Borkovec & Mathews, 1988). Early studies that included relaxation in treatment found that anxiety experienced during relaxation negatively predicted outcome and amount of relaxation positively predicted outcome (Borkovec, et al., 1987; Borkovec & Mathews, 1988). Finally, Borkovec, Newman, et al. (in press) explored the relationship between reports of interpersonal problems prior to and following therapy and measures of end-state functioning. They found that several dimensions of interpersonal problems reported prior to therapy, and especially after therapy, were significantly negatively correlated withend-state functioning at posttreatment and at 6- and 12-month follow-ups. These findings suggest that interpersonal problems (not targeted by the employed behavioral and cognitive therapies) may be particularly associated with poor outcome following treatment for GAD.

Studies Targeting Child or Geriatric Populations or Utilizing Alternative Interventions

Recently investigators have begun to conduct randomized controlled trials of CBT interventions for GAD among older adults. The first of these studies (Stanley, Beck, & Glassco, 1996) was included in Borkovec and Ruscio's (2001) review described above. Stanley and colleagues compared a comprehensive cognitive behavioral treatment (consisting of progressive relaxation, cognitive restructuring, and exposure components) and supportive psychotherapy, both administered in a group format. The study had a fairly high rate of attrition (33%). All participants demonstrated a significant decrease in measures of worry, anxiety, and depression and in proportion of comorbid diagnoses; however, no condition effects emerged on any of these measures. Thus this study provides some evidence for the efficacy of psychosocial intervention for older adults with GAD, but does not indicate that CBT is particularly efficacious in this population. In their review of cognitive behavioral therapy for GAD in older adults, Stanley and Novy (2000) report two other ongoing controlled investigations of CBT in this population. In one study, CBT is being compared to a minimal-contact control condition, and preliminary data indicate improvement in symptoms and quality of life among those in the CBT condition (Stanley, Beck, Novy, Averill, & Swann, 1997, as cited in Stanley & Novy, 2000). The second study involves a comparison of medical management alone to medical management plus CBT among individuals taking benzodiazepines regularly (Gorenstein, Papp, & Kleber, 1997, as cited in Stanley & Novy, 2000). Again, preliminary findings suggest efficacy of the CBT condition in the reduction of symptoms, and concurrently in the reduction of medication use.

Because the diagnosis of GAD was only recently extended to include children and adolescents, no controlled trials of GAD treatment for individuals under 18 exist. However, several randomized controlled studies of interventions for samples of children and adolescents with mixed anxiety disorders include participants diagnosed with overanxious disorder, which is likely to correspond highly with DSM-IV definitions of GAD in children. These studies suggest that psychosocial treatments may be beneficial for this age range as well. For instance, Kendall et al. (1997) conducted a controlled investigation that included 94 children aged 9 to 13 with anxiety disorders, 55 of whom were diagnosed with overanxious disorder. Their CBT intervention was significantly more efficacious than a wait-list control condition, with gains maintained at follow-up. Barrett, Dadds, and Rapee (1996) compared CBT and CBT plus a family management component to a wait-list control in a sample of 79 children aged 7 to 14, 30 of whom were diagnosed with overanxious disorder. Both interventions were efficacious, and these effects were maintained at follow-up. In addition, the family component was associated with significantly greater improvement on some outcome measures.

A few uncontrolled studies of psychosocial interventions for GAD are also worth noting. Crits-Christoph, Connelly, Azarian, Crits-Christoph, and Shappell (1996) conducted an open trial of supportive–expressive psychodynamic psychotherapy for GAD. Prior to their investigation, Durham et al. (1994) had conducted the only study that utilized a psychodynamic intervention for this disorder; however, the absence of a therapy manual for this condition limited the conclusions that could be drawn. Crits-Christoph et al. (1996), on the other hand, have developed a manualized treatment that specifically targets GAD, based in part on the research on interpersonal factors in GAD reviewed above. Their study included 26 patients who met DSM-IV criteria for GAD. Patients showed statistically significant change on measures of worry, anxiety, depression, and interpersonal problems. Effect sizes for the worry and anxiety measures ranged from 0.95 to 1.99; for the depression measures, effect sizes ranged from 1.09 to 1.15. This study suggests that supportive–expressive therapy may be effective in treating GAD and therefore warrants further study. Borkovec and colleagues have recently developed a treatment that integrates interpersonal and cognitive behavioral interventions; it is described in more detail below.

Another open trial was conducted on a sample that included individuals diagnosed with GAD according to DSM-III-R criteria. Kabat-Zinn and colleagues (1992) found that an 8-week group intervention based on mindfulness meditation led to a significant reduction in anxiety and depression among individuals meeting criteria for GAD and panic disorder. These reductions were maintained at 3-year follow-up (Miller, Fletcher, & Kabat-Zinn, 1995). These findings—coupled with a review of controlled studies of stress management interventions, which concludes that meditation techniques reduce anxiety, particularly its cognitive component (Lehrer & Woolfolk, 1993)—suggest that mindfulness meditation may be an efficacious component of psychosocial interventions for GAD.

Finally, a recent pilot study explored the effectiveness of computer-assisted therapy for GAD (Newman, Consoli, & Taylor, 1999). The authors propose that using a palmtop computer program to supplement treatment will increase the efficiency and cost-effectiveness of CBT for GAD. Three clients who met criteria for DSM-IV GAD were treated in a group format. The treatment was adapted from Borkovec and Costello (1993), but was reduced from 14 individual to 6 group sessions, thus substantially decreasing therapist contact time per person. The software developed for this protocol consisted of several modules: "diary only," "recognizing triggers" (consisting of identification of anxiety cues), and "therapy" (consisting of relaxation and cognitive therapy modules). The palmtop provided both continued assessments of anxiety levels and prompts for implementation of various aspects of the intervention, therefore extending active intervention beyond therapy sessions. This pilot study found that symptoms decreased after the intervention and that gains were maintained at 6-month follow-up. None of the clients met criteria for GAD at the 6-month follow-up. If controlled trials support this initial indication of efficacy, Newman and colleagues estimate a savings of between $630 and $1,057.50 per individual over standard individual CBT interventions. Clearly, this mode of intervention is worthy of further investigation.

Recent Developments/New Directions

As noted above, despite the gains made in developing efficacious psychosocial interventions for GAD, more work is needed in this area. Brown, Barlow, and Liebowitz (1994), in their review of current research in GAD, suggest that new treatments be developed that more specifically address the central features of GAD. Several research groups have undertaken this challenge, applying recent research and theory in the function of worry and associated features of GAD (as well as research and theory throughout the clinical field) to further refine cognitive behavioral/integrative psychosocial treatments of this chronic disorder. Many of these approaches share common features, but each investigative group also highlights specific elements and intervention strategies. A brief overview of the current status of their work is provided below; however, it should be kept in mind that these research programs are constantly evolving and refining their interventions.

Worry Exposure

In order to address the need for specific treatments based on conceptualizations of worry, Craske and colleagues (Craske et al., 1992; Craske, 1999; Zinbarg et al., 1993) have developed a cognitive-behavioral protocol that highlights imaginal exposure to feared catastrophic outcomes. These authors suggest that the impaired emotional processing associated with worry can be countered through prolonged exposure to feared catastrophic scenes, allowing successful processing to occur. This (approximately 30-minute) exposure is followed by a management phase in which cognitive and other coping strategies are employed in response to the imagined scene. The comprehensive treatment proposed by these authors also includes psychoeducation, self-monitoring, cognitive restructuring (which includes targeting of meta-worry; Craske, 1999), problem-solving training, and an emphasis on the prevention of worry-related behaviors (such as repeated checking or never leaving work until everything is done). This treatment package has yet to be empirically evaluated.

Integrating Interpersonal / Experiential Therapy

Borkovec has adapted his cognitive-behavioral treatment package in many ways to reflect empirical findings over the past 10 years (Borkovec, Alcaine, & Behar, in press): (1) cognitive and emotional flexibility have been highlighted; (2) an increased focus on present-moment experience has been added as a coping skill that is rehearsed; (3) worry's avoidant function has been addressed through the use of stimulus control approaches (Borkovec et al., 1983); and (4) beliefs about the functionality of worry have been challenged through systematic monitoring of worrisome predictions and behavioral experiments.

   However, Borkovec, Castonguay, and Newman (T. D. Borkovec, personal communication, June 2000) have recently further expanded this cognitive-behavioral treatment package by adding an interpersonal/experiential component. This development is based on two lines of research: (1) studies suggesting that worry interferes with emotional processing and present-moment focus, and (2) studies highlighting the interpersonal nature of worry and its association with interpersonal problems. Borkovec, Alcaine, and Behar (in press) propose that attention to interpersonal concerns will more effectively access the core fears that underlie the diffuse worry of clients with GAD. Thus increasing the depth of emotional experience and attending to interpersonal (including therapeutic relationship) factors (in conjunction with the cognitive-behavioral techniques reviewed above) is expected to more completely access the core elements that perpetuate GAD (Borkovec, Alcaine, & Behar, in press; Newman, 2000). These researchers have developed an interpersonal/experiential component of GAD treatment, based on Safran and Segal's (1990) integrative therapy. This treatment focuses on present phenomenological experience, identifying interpersonal needs, fears, beliefs, patterns of behavior, and emotional responses, and increasing flexible responding within these areas through a variety of interpersonal/experiential techniques (T. D. Borkovec, personal communication, June 2000). The treatment remains based in cognitive-behavioral/learning theory, but expands the focus of this model to include interpersonal schemata and behaviors and the importance of emotional experience (based on Safran & Segal, 1990). A controlled, additive design investigation is currently underway comparing CBT with the interpersonal/experiential component to CBT with a supportive listening component, to determine whether these additions improve outcome. Results from a small pilot open trial of the new combined treatment suggest outcomes on measures of anxiety and depression that are comparable or superior to the outcomes of prior CBT trials conducted by this group (T. D. Borkovec, personal communication, June 2000).

Targeting Intolerance of Uncertainty

Ladouceur and his colleagues have followed up their program of research exploring the role of intolerance of uncertainty in GAD with the development of a cognitive-behavioral protocol that specifically targets this phenomenon (Ladouceur et al., 2000). Central to their treatment rationale is the premise that worry and anxiety are driven in part by uncertainty and that uncertainty is inevitable. Therefore, treatment focuses on ways to recognize, accept, and implement coping strategies when clients are faced with uncertain situations. This intervention consists of cognitive and behavioral techniques targeting this goal, which include challenging erroneous (positive) beliefs about worry, problem orientation training, cognitive (worry) exposure, and relapse prevention. Clients are taught to distinguish between worries that are amenable to problem solving and those that aren't; problem orientation training is implemented for the former, and imaginal worry exposure for the latter. A recent controlled trial of this intervention (compared to a wait-list control) revealed statistically and clinically significant effects that were maintained at 12-month follow-up. As noted above, 57.7% of the sample met high end-state functioning criteria at 12-month follow-up.

Targeting Meta-Worry and Beliefs about Worry

Wells (1997, 1999) has developed metacognitive therapy, a cognitive intervention for GAD designed specifically to target the features he highlights in his model of this disorder: positive and negative beliefs about worry. He suggests that existing treatments have failed to focus on the beliefs that maintain this maladaptive process. He proposes the following sequence in addressing beliefs about worry (although he stresses that flexibility is important): modification of negative beliefs and appraisals regarding uncontrollability of worry, then modification of meta-worry and beliefs about the danger of worry, then identification and challenging of positive beliefs, and finally the introduction of alternative strategies for appraising threat (Wells, 1999). He outlines specific techniques for accomplishing each of these goals (Wells, 1997, 1999). Empirical evaluation of this approach has yet to be conducted.

Integrating Acceptance/Mindfulness Approaches

Finally, we have recently embarked on the development of a new integrative therapy for GAD that incorporates acceptance and mindfulness approaches into a traditional cognitive-behavioral protocol (e.g., Roemer & Orsillo, in press; Orsillo, Roemer, & Barlow, 2001). This work is based on an integration of the model of worry and GAD reviewed here (see also Borkovec, 1994a) and Hayes et al.'s (1999) model of experiential avoidance, coupled with others' work on the role of acceptance in psychotherapy (cf. Hayes, Jacobson, Follette,

& Dougher, 1994; Linehan, 1993a). Our intervention is based on findings regarding the experientially avoidant function of worry, as well as theorizing that worry is an unsuccessful effort at control (of both internal and external events; see Chapter 3). We propose that in addition to the techniques reviewed above, successful treatment of GAD should emphasize acceptance of unwanted internal experiences, coupled with action aimed at pursuing valued directions. In the current version of this intervention, typical elements of CBT are expanded to incorporate this perspective. Thus psychoeducation includes attention to the function of emotions and to the inherent paradox, as well as potential harm, in efforts to control internal experience (Hayes et al., 1999). Self-monitoring techniques emphasize a mindfulness approach by encouraging present-moment awareness in contrast to future-focused worry. Similarly, relaxation techniques are expanded to include various mindfulness exercises that specifically target increased present-moment awareness and acceptance of experience (e.g., Linehan, 1993b). Finally, our "mindful action" component combines more traditional elements of behavioral exposure and skills rehearsal with those techniques from Hayes et al.'s (1999) Acceptance and Commitment Therapy that facilitate identification of valued directions and encourage action in ways that are consistent with these values. Thus, rather than encouraging approach behaviors in order to reduce anxiety, we emphasize acting in valued ways regardless of one's internal experience. This distinction may be important, because efforts to reduce worry and anxiety are likely to perpetuate the cycle of anxious responding (e.g., Wells, 1995).

We have completed a small pilot study of an early (brief) version of this treatment protocol and found that two (of four) clients displayed substantial symptomatic reductions at posttreatment and another displayed moderate reductions, while the fourth missed several sessions and demonstrated little symptomatic improvement. Most striking was the observation that all four clients made substantial life changes throughout the course of therapy. We are currently in the process of revising the treatment and plan a controlled trial comparing it to a wait-list control to determine its efficacy. Then efforts will be made to dismantle the protocol, to determine whether mindfulness and acceptance elements enhance cognitive behavioral interventions for GAD.

Much remains to be learned regarding psychosocial treatments for GAD. In addition to the need to develop more consistently efficacious interventions (that result in higher proportions of clients within normal ranges on symptom measures), we need to determine active ingredients in our complex protocols and begin to explore mechanisms of change in order to enhance our understanding of basic processes in human emotional functioning. Furthermore, we need to examine the ability of our interventions to affect broader areas of functioning such as quality of life and interpersonal functioning. We have come a long way in our understanding of and ability to successfully treat GAD through programs of theory-driven basic research and controlled intervention trials. Continuing these approaches—and expanding to component control, additive, and parametric designs (Borkovec, 1994b), in addition to attention to implementation, effectiveness, and generalizability considerations—will insure our continued progress in this area.

CHAPTER 15

Obsessive–Compulsive Disorder

GAIL STEKETEE
DAVID H. BARLOW

Among anxiety disorders, obsessive–compulsive disorder (OCD) is often the one that generates very severe consequences. Patients who are hospitalized because of anxiety are most likely to be diagnosed with OCD. In fact, in recent years, several inpatient psychiatric units have been established around the country exclusively to treat OCD. These facilities provide specialized therapy to those who have not responded to standard pharmacological and behavioral treatments known to work for most people with this disorder. Chances are that these inpatients with severe OCD have comorbid debilitating conditions, such as major depression, other anxiety disorders, eating disorders, and personality disorders. These co-occurring conditions sometimes complicate the OCD symptoms, making it difficult for patients to respond to or even undertake standard therapies. For those with this condition, gaining control and predictability over the seemingly ubiquitous dangers in life leads them to resort to magic and rituals in vain attempts to reestablish safety or prevent a dreaded event. In OCD, danger appears in the form of a thought, image, or impulse that provokes intense discomfort. This thought or image is upsetting and is avoided, much as a person with a snake phobia avoids snakes. Usually obsessions occur many times a day, often continuously in severe cases.

The intensity, severity, and sometimes bizarre qualities of OCD are hard to appreciate without case illustrations. A 32-year-old married woman who had given birth 3 months before to her second child sought outpatient treatment when her checking of faucets, light switches, and buttons on her children's clothing increased sharply.[1] In addition, she complained of several magical rituals regarding numbers, and noted that certain items of clothing and other activities had become connected in her mind to the devil. These symptoms had begun in her mid-20s before her marriage, but had worsened recently with the stress of

---

[1]This case description is adapted from Steketee, G. (1998). Judy: A compelling case of obsessive–compulsive disorder. In R. P. Halgin & S. K. Whitbourne (Eds.), *A casebook in abnormal psychology* (pp. 58–71). Oxford: Oxford University Press. Copyright 1998 by Oxford University Press. Adapted by permission.

raising two children of her own, as well as two stepchildren, and in the face of financial instability. Neither she, a free-lance videographer, nor her husband, an art teacher, earned much money. Her obsessive fears focused mainly on the possibility that bad luck would happen to her loved ones, especially her children, unless she intervened. She associated bad luck with many types of situations. These obsessive triggers included the numbers 3 and 13; thoughts or words related to the devil, Satan, or black magic; violating Jewish religious rules regarding cooking and activity on the Sabbath, despite the fact that she and her husband were not orthodox practitioners; superstitious violations such as stepping on cracks; passing cemeteries or funeral homes; and saying something negative about someone. Like a number of individuals with OCD, she also felt that she was not entitled to "have a good time," and believed that feeling happy would be followed by bad outcomes.

To manage her fears, this patient performed a variety of repeating, undoing, and checking rituals. For example, if a bad thought about the devil occurred while dressing, she took off her clothes and started over until she dressed without the bad thought. She said "Amen" when passing graves or funerals, and stopped all activity whenever the clock indicated 13 minutes before or after the hour. She also checked when leaving home to make sure that no fire could occur and that the cat was safe. This required her to check each room several times for the cat, things that might fall on the cat, and potential causes of fire such as the stove or heaters. This patient agreed entirely that her symptoms were unreasonable and was highly motivated to reduce her behavior, since it interfered significantly with her ability to manage her household responsibilities and take care of her children, especially feeding, dressing, and playing with them. She reported feeling mildly depressed, and her self-esteem was quite low, but she did not meet criteria for any other psychological disorder.

The second case to be described here was more complex and more severe, and illustrates the wide range of behavior encountered in OCD. The patient was a 19-year-old single white male, a college freshman majoring in philosophy, who had withdrawn from school because of incapacitating ritualistic behaviors. The patient had an 8-year history of severe compulsive rituals. These included excessive hand washing and showering; ceremonial rituals for dressing and studying; compulsive placement of any objects handled; grotesque hissing, coughing, and head tossing while eating; and shuffling and wiping his feet while walking. These rituals interfered with every aspect of his daily functioning. The patient's condition had steadily deteriorated within the past 2 years; he was now isolating himself from family and friends, refusing meals, and neglecting his personal appearance. His hair was very long, as he had not allowed it to be cut in 5 years. He had never shaved or trimmed his beard. When he walked, he shuffled, taking small steps on his toes while continually looking back, checking and rechecking. On occasion he would run quickly in place. He had withdrawn his left arm completely from his shirt sleeve, as if he were crippled and his shirt was a sling.

Seven weeks prior to admission, his rituals had become so time-consuming and debilitating that he refused to engage in any personal hygiene, for fear that the associated rituals would interfere with the time needed to study. Almost continual showering became no showering. He stopped washing his hair, brushing his teeth, or changing his clothes. He left his room infrequently and, to avoid rituals associated with the toilet, had begun defecating on paper towels, urinating in paper cups, and storing the waste in a corner of the closet in his room. His eating habits had degenerated from eating with the family, to eating in an adjoining room, to eating in his own room. In the 2 months prior to admission, he had lost 20 pounds and would only eat late at night when others were asleep. He felt that eating was "barbaric"; this well described his grotesque eating rituals, consisting of hissing noises, coughs and hacks, and severe head tossing. His food intake had been narrowed to ice cream or a mixture of peanut butter, sugar, cocoa, milk, and mayonnaise. He considered several foods (e.g., cola, beef, and butter) contaminating, and would not eat these foods. He also had a long list of checking rituals associated with the placement of objects. Excessive time was spent checking and rechecking to see that wastebaskets and curtains were in place. These rituals had progressed to tilting of wastebaskets and twisting of curtains, which were checked periodically throughout the day.

DEFINITION AND DIFFERENTIAL DIAGNOSIS

Both of the cases described above fit very clearly within the definition of OCD in the *Diagnostic and Statistical Manual of Mental Disorders*, fourth edition (DSM-IV), where the disorder is characterized by "obsessions or compulsions [that] cause marked distress, are time consuming (take more than 1 hour a day), or significantly interfere with the person's normal routine, occupational (or academic) functioning, or usual social activities or relationships" (American Psychiatric Association, 1994, p. 423). Obsessions are defined as "recurrent and persistent thoughts, impulses, or images that are experienced, at some time during the disturbance, as intrusive and inappropriate and that cause marked anxiety or distress" (p. 422). Compulsions are defined as "repetitive behaviors (e.g., hand washing, ordering, checking) or mental acts (e.g., praying, counting, repeating words silently) that the person feels driven to perform in response to an obsession, or according to rules that must be applied rigidly" (p. 423). The behaviors or mental acts are designed to prevent or reduce discomfort and the likelihood of a dreaded event's occurring, but the compulsions are either unrealistic or clearly excessive. Interestingly, the definition of OCD given in DSM-IV remains quite similar to those from earlier versions of the DSM, as well as to psychiatric descriptions as early as Westphal's in 1878 (Insel, 1984).

The DSM-IV definition specifies that obsessions are not simply excessive worries about real-life problems, as in generalized anxiety disorder (GAD). The definition of GAD, as described in Chapter 14, highlights apprehensive expectation. Specifically, arousal-driven "worry," accompanied by somatic symptoms of anxiety, is the defining feature of GAD. To make this disorder more easily discriminated, apprehension must be focused on a number of events or activities (e.g., work performance). Rachman (1973) has described what he calls "morbid preoccupations," which are intrusive, repetitive ideas that differ from obsessions in that they are ego-syntonic, rational but exaggerated, realistic and current in content, and seldom resisted. This is a good description of worry within GAD. Although the definitions of these two anxiety disorders are clear and seemingly distinguishable, on occasion it proves difficult in practice to differentiate these cognitive phenomena. For example, Steketee, Grayson, and Foa (1987) observed that patients with OCD did not score significantly higher than those with GAD on the Checking subscale of the Maudsley Obsessional–Compulsive Inventory (MOCI). In fact, Ladouceur et al. (2000) have noted that patients with GAD also report using overt and covert strategies to reduce their anxiety, much as compulsions are used in OCD. This seems to support the phenomenological similarity of these two disorders.

Nevertheless, in principle, the distinction is clear. The troublesome thoughts and ideas of patients with GAD may be intrusive and repetitive, but they are current in content (if exaggerated beyond all reason), and therefore are not resisted. There is no quality of a phobic reaction to these thoughts. In OCD, on the other hand, the thoughts are often bizarre and alien to the individual. The thoughts themselves may produce a phobic or panic reaction and are most often avoided or resisted at all cost. In the prototypical example, then,

OCD is another phobic reaction; the phobic object is cognition. This differs from panic disorder, where the phobic reaction is to a somatic event. Even when the ideas become overvalued and are not necessarily resisted, the content seems distinguishable from the usual life circumstances that are the focus of GAD. The distinction is important, because there are significantly different treatment implications within both pharmacological and cognitive-behavioral approaches.

Most individuals with OCD recognize that their behavior is excessive or unreasonable, although this may not be true of young children who are unable to compare their behavior with that of others. Adults with OCD who have lost perspective on the rationality of their fears are considered to have "poor insight," a subtype that was added in DSM-IV. Problems with insight have also been labeled "overvalued ideas" (e.g., Foa, 1979; McKenna, 1984) when the person consistently overestimates the likelihood that the obsession is true. For example, a woman who really believes she will contaminate her children with cancer if she touches them because medical science cannot rule it out would be considered to have poor insight. A large-scale field trial has demonstrated that patients with OCD vary widely in their degree of insight (Foa & Kozak, 1995). In fact, as Rachman and de Silva (1978) have demonstrated, few individuals with OCD consider their obsessions to be totally senseless, especially when anxiety is high (Kozak & Foa, 1994).

According to DSM-IV, to distinguish obsessions from thought insertion or delusions characteristic of psychotic disorders, the person must recognize that the obsessions are the product of his or her own mind and not imposed from outside sources. Because of the frequent misidentification of OCD as schizophrenia in the past, Rachman and Hodgson (1980) have listed the distinctive features of OCD as compared to closely related conditions. Specifically, obsessions and compulsions are distinguished from intrusive or repetitive cognitions that may be associated with schizophrenia, organic disorders, or "morbid preoccupations." These distinctive features are listed in Table 15.1. In practice, bizarreness alone in obsessions or compulsions would not lead a clinician to suspect a psychotic process unless other psychotic symptoms were evident. For example, one young man's obsessions centered on whether he had, without realizing or intending it, climbed up a telephone pole, extracted material containing poisonous chemicals, and then put this material in someone's drink. Clearly his concerns were unusual, but careful assessment indicated no delusions associated with these fears. He recognized them to be groundless, despite his intense anxiety to be certain he had not engaged in such behavior. Nonetheless, OCD does co-occur with schizophrenia, albeit infrequently (Jenike, 1990; Tallis, 1995); and in some cases obsessions appear to be overtly delusional (Eisen & Rasmussen, 1993; Insel & Akiskal, 1986). In these cases, patients seem to lose altogether the sense that their obsessions are irrational and cease to resist them, leading some researchers to consider a diagnosis of reactive psychosis or perhaps even "obsessive" psychosis (see Kozak & Foa, 1994, for discussion).

Unfortunately, OCD symptoms that are overvalued or border on the delusional have been associated with more severe symptoms and a worse prognosis (Foa, 1979; Solyom, DiNicola, Sookman, & Luchins, 1985). However, some studies have not supported poor insight in OCD as a predictor of poor outcome (Başoğlu, Lax, Kasvikis, & Marks, 1988; Lelliott, Noshirvani, Başoğlu, Marks, & Monteiro, 1988). Furthermore, for patients who have OCD with psychotic features, Eisen and Rasmussen (1993) concluded that their poorer prognosis is due to the presence of schizophrenia-spectrum disorders rather than to lack of insight into obsessions. This corresponds with findings that patients with schizotypal personality traits, including ideas of reference and suspiciousness, may fare poorly in behavioral and pharmacological treatment (Jenike, Baer, Minichiello, Schwartz, & Carey, 1986; Minichiello, Baer, & Jenike, 1987). In light of concerns about prognosis for those with

TABLE 15.1. Distinctive Features of Obsessional–Compulsive Disorders and Their Relation to Schizophrenia, Organic Impairments, Morbid Preoccupations, and "Obsessional Personality"

Obsessions
    are unwanted
    have aggressive/sexual themes
    provoke internal resistance
    cause distress
    are recognized to be of internal origin
    are recognized to be senseless (insight)
    are ego-alien
    are associated with lack of confidence in memory or reality of memory
    are associated with depression

Compulsions are distinguished by repetitive, stereotyped behavior that
    is preceded or accompanied by a sense of compulsion that is recognized to be of internal origin
    provokes internal resistance
    is recognized to be senseless (insight)
    may cause embarrassment or distress
    is difficult to control over the long term

Schizophrenic conditions differ in that the intrusive ideas, images, or impulses are
    attributed to external forces
    not necessarily ego-alien
    not regarded as senseless (lack of insight)
    unlikely to provoke internal resistance

Organic impairments may involve repetitive ideas or acts that
    lack intellectual content
    lack intentionality
    have a mechanical and/or primitive quality

Morbid preoccupations (see Rachman, 1973) involve intrusive, repetitive ideas that are
    ego-syntonic
    rational (but exaggerated)
    realistic, and current in content
    seldom resisted

"Obsessional personality" traits
    show greater stability than obsessional disorders
    are ego-syntonic
    seldom cause distress
    are seldom accompanied by a sense of compulsion
    seldom provoke resistance

Note. From Rachman and Hodgson (1980). Copyright 1980 by Prentice-Hall, Inc. Reprinted by permission.

unrealistic convictions about their obsessive fears, researchers have proposed that cognitive approaches that include developing a rational perspective (see below) may be needed to address poor insight (cf. Salkovskis & Warwick, 1986). Further research will be needed to test this notion.

    Early reviews of the evidence for an association of OCD with biological conditions, such as physical trauma, epilepsy, other brain abnormalities, encephalitis, and Parkinson's disease, concluded that neurological factors are present in only a minority of cases (Rachman & Hodgson, 1980; Kettl & Marks, 1986). Successful behavioral treatment appeared to be independent of such factors. Since this time, Swedo, Rapaport, Cheslow, and Leonard (1989) have linked conditions such as Sydenham's chorea to the onset of OCD symptoms.

In these cases, bacterial and viral agents have been associated with the onset or exacerbation of OCD in some children, suggesting the possibility of an autoimmune dysfunction (Swedo & Kiessling, 1994). In addition to these findings, in the past 10 years extensive data from more sophisticated neuroimaging techniques suggest that OCD is associated with dysfunction in particular neural pathways. The most consistent findings across a variety of studies indicate that people with OCD show hyperactivity in the orbito-frontal region of the brain; basal ganglia involvement has been less commonly found. Of considerable interest are the findings from several studies that successful treatment (either behavioral interventions or medication) has resulted in normalization of activity in this region of the brain, with changes in OCD symptoms correlated with changes in brain functions (e.g., Baxter et al., 1992; J. M. Schwartz, Stoessel, Baxter, Martin, & Phelps, 1996).

CHARACTERISTICS

As with several other anxiety disorders, the age of onset for OCD is usually late adolescence to the early 20s, and it rarely begins after age 50 (Rachman & Hodgson, 1980; Rasmussen & Tsuang, 1986). However, OCD can erupt full-blown in childhood and has appeared even before age 5 (e.g., Jenike et al., 1986). OCD is more likely to begin earlier in boys, usually in midadolescence (Bellodi, Sciuto, Diaferia, Ronchi, & Smeraldi, 1992; Rapoport, 1989; Rasmussen & Eisen, 1990). In most research studies, the mean onset age for males ranged from 14 to 19.5 years, whereas the figures for females were 21 to 22 years. Thus, in studies of childhood OCD, boys outnumber girls by a factor of 2:1. However, this ratio becomes more equal for studies of adults, where women report having OCD slightly more frequently than men (Rasmussen & Eisen, 1990; Weissman et al., 1994).

In an effort to understand why OCD develops, some investigators have identified precipitants related to stressful (e.g., Kolada, Bland, & Newman, 1994; Rachman, 1997) and sometimes traumatic (de Silva & Marks, 1999; Rhéaume, Freeston, Leger, & Ladouceur, 1998) life experiences. Important developmental changes such as pregnancy and childbirth (Wisner, Peindl, Gigliotti, & Hanusa, 1999) may play a role, although these events may also coincide with biological changes that could also figure in OCD onset. In some cases, the content of the obsessions appears to be associated with the stressor, as in the case of new mothers who become fearful of harming their children (Wisner et al., 1999). However, it is noteworthy that in up to 40% of cases, no clear-cut precipitant can be identified.

Many investigators have sought to determine the course of OCD. In recent years, research on this topic has been made difficult by the ready availability of several effective treatments for OCD. Thus natural course is confounded with treatment outcome in most studies, so that it is difficult to know what might happen if OCD were left untreated. Studies before 1980 are probably more informative on this point than very recent ones, with the notable exception of a Scandinavian study described below. Furthermore, most studies are retrospective and thus methodologically less sound. In reviewing this research, Eisen and Steketee (1998) concluded that recent studies with prospective designs show findings similar to older ones: The majority of patients either continue to meet full criteria for OCD or retain significant symptoms of the disorder over long periods of time. Studies of children with OCD also support these findings. A recent study of a large cohort in Sweden has provided very important information about course and its predictors (Skoog & Skoog, 1999). When 144 people were followed approximately 40 years after their initial diagnosis with OCD, 83% had improved and 48% were considered recovered. This latter number included 20% who recovered completely and 28% who had only subclinical symptoms that did not meet diagnostic criteria. More than one-third had achieved their recovery within the first 10 years, leaving a larger number whose symptoms had persisted for decades.

In the Swedish study, early onset, low social functioning at the time of diagnosis, and persistent symptoms in the first few years predicted worse outcomes (Skoog & Skoog, 1999). Eisen and Steketee's (1998) review found surprisingly few predictors of course. Even age of onset is not a consistent predictor, although it appears that this may interact with gender so that men with early onset fare more poorly than women, whose onset tends to be several years later. Early onset in boys may especially predispose them to developmental difficulties in social and other life skills, making their course more severe, although research is needed to clarify this point. It is noteworthy that neither depressed nor anxious mood predicted course, but studies of comorbid diagnoses (especially major depression, anxiety disorders, and personality disorders) have not been conducted. Thus it is unclear whether some co-occurring conditions adversely affect the course of OCD itself.

It is clear from the case histories and definitions provided above that obsessions and compulsions represent situations in which strong anxiety and/or other negative emotions (e.g., guilt or disgust) have overtaken rational thinking and behavior. It is important to realize, however, that the intrusive thoughts, images, and impulses and compulsive activities that are the hallmarks of OCD are also present to a lesser degree in nearly 90% of the general population (Ladouceur et al., 2000; Rachman & de Silva, 1978; Salkovskis & Harrison, 1984). That is, ordinary people commonly experience intrusive ideas or engage in neutralizing actions as part of their everyday experience. However, most do not go on to develop OCD. What causes such ordinary experiences to develop into a severe and debilitating anxiety disorder? This chapter examines the important question of etiology after first describing the symptoms and features associated with OCD and comprehensive methods for assessing these. The models for explaining the development of OCD are far from complete at this stage of our research knowledge, but they do point to specific treatment strategies that have been demonstrated to be effective. Behavioral and biological models for understanding and treating OCD are reviewed in some detail, with attention to newer cognitive theories and interventions. These latter methods appear to be very promising and were not available at the time the first edition of this book (Barlow, 1988) was published.

PSYCHOPATHOLOGY

More than diagnosing any other anxiety disorder, diagnosing OCD can confound inexperienced clinicians because of the wide range of mental and behavioral symptoms characterizing this condition. Because of the unusual diversity of symptom patterns, investigators have tried to classify obsessions and compulsions into symptom subtypes. In early studies, researchers studied symptom type by accumulating a large number of cases and examining the content of the obsessions and compulsions. More recently, some studies have used factor-analytic methods to develop subscales of symptoms based on self-report questionnaires (e.g., Hodgson & Rachman, 1977; van Oppen, Hoekstra, & Emmelkamp, 1995), and others have applied multivariate clustering methods to determine which symptoms from an interview symptom checklist tend to cluster together (Baer, 1994; Calamari, Wiegartz, & Janeck, 1999; Leckman et al., 1997; Mataix-Cols, Rauch, Manzo, Jenike, & Baer, 1999; Summerfeldt, Richter, Antony, & Swinson, 1999). The findings from these studies, which examined hundreds of cases of OCD, are fairly consistent. They generally indicate that the following OCD subtypes are common: harming/religious/sexual obsessions and checking rituals; contamination obsessions and washing/cleaning rituals; and symmetry/ordering/certainty concerns and counting/repeating/checking compulsions. In these studies, hoarding of possessions typically appears as a separate symptom, not linked to other forms of OCD. Many patients displayed multiple obsessions and compulsions that often overlapped. This was especially true for checking and contamination-related symptoms, perhaps because many patients with OCD use both checking and washing rituals to reduce contamination fears. Clearly, it is difficult to classify patients with OCD solely according to their type of symptom. That is, terms like "checkers" or "washers" are misnomers, since most patients suffer from multiple symptoms.

Several descriptive studies have tried to categorize obsessions by their form rather than their content. For example, Akhtar, Wig, Verma, Pershad, and Verma (1975) pointed out that the content of an obsession may be about a child's safety, but the obsession may take any of several forms, including obsessive doubts ("Has something happened to him?"), fears ("Something might happen to him because of my negligence"), thinking ("If he plays outside, he might catch cold that might turn into pneumonia, and if that goes undiagnosed, then . . ."), and images ("Over and over I see him drowning!") (p. 345). An impulse along the same lines might be "What if I pick up this knife and stab him?" de Silva (1986) particularly emphasized the importance of images, and noted that these can occur as obsessions that provoke discomfort and also as compulsions that relieve this distress. For example, Rachman (1976a) described a young woman with the recurrent image of four people lying dead in an open grave. The compulsive or neutralizing image involved imagining the same four people standing or walking, quite healthy.

Unfortunately, efforts to identify the frequency of these various forms of OCD symptoms have produced quite inconsistent findings (Reed, 1985; Akhtar et al., 1975). This suggests disagreement in defining the forms, as well as possible confusion in distinguishing obsessions from mental compulsions. In the latter case, the complex interweavings of obsessions and subtle forms of neutralizing or rituals may be overlooked, especially when these have evolved into a seemingly endless pattern of rumination characterized by preoccupation, anxiety, guilt, and neutralizing. For example, a woman who reads about the death of a young family in a fire may form negative images, develop doubts, and otherwise ruminate about whether she might somehow be responsible and how she could have prevented it. Similarly, a student may ruminate about the adequacy of his studying and concentration, and also wonder endlessly whether he has behaved appropriately in social situations. In both such cases, innumerable corrective or self-reassuring thoughts (compulsions) are commonly interspersed with the fearful ruminations. Intense anxiety may not be associated with any particular part of the process; rather, the whole process itself is continually distressing, as fears alternate with calming efforts.

In general, it is not clear that identifying the form obsessions take will help determine what treatment to provide or whether the patient will benefit from treatment. Although this is an area that has not been well researched, at the present time both pharmacological and psychological interventions would be similar whether obsessions are doubts, impulses, thoughts, or images, and whether rituals are overt or covert. However, differentiating obsessions from mental compulsions is important for behavioral interventions, since different procedures are used to treat the anxiety-provoking intrusions and obsessions and anxiety-reducing compulsions and neutralizing strategies (see the later discussion of behavior therapy). It is also possible that the type of symptom (e.g., contamination, symmetry/ordering) may influence treatment, but so far evidence for this is quite limited. Possible exceptions are hoarding (Mataix-Cols et al., 1999; Black et al., 1999) and symmetry/ordering concerns, which appear to be more similar to tics and may have a stronger neurological basis (Rasmussen & Eisen, 1992a, 1992b). These symptoms occur more often in men and may respond less well to standard pharmacological or behavioral interventions found to be effective for other symptoms of OCD (see Ball, Baer, & Otto, 1996). However, this possibility remains speculative, and further research is needed.

In early research on OCD, investigators classified ritualistic behavior mainly according to the type of behavior, such as washing, cleaning, checking, repeating, ordering, and primary obsessional slowness. Several studies report somewhat different percentages of these types of rituals, although, as for obsessions, many patients present with more than one type. For example, Hodgson and Rachman (1977) used a factor-analytic technique to determine that 52% of their patients displayed some form of checking rituals, while 48% evidenced cleaning rituals. Rachman (1976a) pointed to an obvious difference between these two types of symptoms, in that washing rituals are aimed at restoring safety and control after contact with contaminants, whereas checking serves to prevent some future harm or catastrophe. However, systematic examination has not revealed any additional substantive differences between patients with these two types of symptoms (Steketee, Grayson, & Foa, 1985). Stern and Cobb (1978) noted that about half of their patients had "avoiding" rituals similar to the avoidance behavior manifested in phobic disorders, perhaps mainly in relation to contamination fears. They also found a large percentage with checking (38%) and repeating (40%) rituals, usually demonstrated by doing things by numbers, regardless of the type of activity being carried out. In Jenike et al.'s (1986) sample of 100 patients, a larger percentage (nearly 80%) had checking rituals, with washing/cleaning rituals also present in more than half (58%) and relatively few having counting rituals (21%). This large preponderance of checking rituals is not evident in other studies (Foa et al., 1983; Rachman & Hodgson, 1980).

In contrast to previous versions of diagnostic criteria for OCD, the DSM-IV criteria emphasize the potential presence of mental acts to mitigate obsessions, thereby recognizing the importance of covert rituals in this disorder. In fact, up to one-quarter of all patients presenting with OCD seem to have no motoric compulsions, but almost always present with some form of neutralizing thoughts that serve as compulsions (Mavissakalian, Turner, & Michelson, 1985). Freeston and Ladouceur (1997) have observed that patients with OCD exhibit many forms of neutralizing behaviors designed to reduce discomfort from obsessions. These include replacing one thought with another, reassuring oneself and/or seeking reassurance from others, saying "Stop!" to remove a thought, various forms of magical undoing, and thinking something through. These researchers are careful to note that often it is difficult to distinguish "coping strategies" from neutralizing acts, and therefore difficult for a therapist engaging in behavioral treatment to know when to permit a patient to continue to employ the method and when to restrict it.

A far less frequent but seemingly distinct form of ritualistic behavior, referred to as "primary obsessional slowness," was first identified and labeled by Rachman (1974). Essentially, this refers to a condition in which the individual behaves in slow motion. For example, Bilsbury and Morley (1979) described a patient who took 4 hours to get up in the morning. This patient did not repeat activities, but subdivided each activity involved in getting ready in the morning into a number of stages. He then narrated his progress through these stages. In this way, it took him 1 hour to get out of bed, 35 minutes to wash his face, and so on. What is unique about this behavioral pattern is that the excessive mental rehearsal involved in meticulously carrying out each small portion of behavior is intrusive, unpleasant, or resisted. The patient was simply making sure that he did everything properly by paying excessive attention to detail. It is not clear whether this problem should be considered a variant of OCD, and Rasmussen and Eisen (1992a) have suggested that it may have distinctive neurological substrates.

CULTURAL ASPECTS

It is interesting to note that clinicians, greatly puzzled by the bizarre content of many of these rituals, have often attributed them to excessive concern with cultural preoccupations. For example, it has been noted that the high percentage of cleaning rituals in Egypt or India may be due to the dictates of the Muslim religion in Egypt or the emphasis on cleanliness in India. In fact, patients from a variety of different cultures display remarkably similar forms of the disorder (e.g., washing, checking). Even the frequencies of specific forms of the disorder are similar across cultures. Insel's (1984) review of studies from England, Hong Kong, India, Egypt, Japan, and Norway showed OCD symptoms typical of U.S. and European studies, including fears of contamination accompanied by cleaning rituals; pathological doubt accompanied by checking; obsessional thoughts accompanied by neutralizing thoughts but no behavioral rituals; and, more rarely, primary obsessional slowness. According to a cross-national study by Weissman et al. (1994), the prevalence of OCD appears to be quite stable across different cultures represented in Canada, Finland, Taiwan, Africa, Puerto Rico, Korea, and New Zealand. Nonetheless, culture and possibly religion do appear to have some influence on the presentation of OCD. For example, some obsessive fears are quite culturally specific, such as fear of leprosy in Africa. Even in the United States and Europe, historical shifts occur in the focus of obsessive fears of disease, which mirror current media information within the culture. For example, 20 years ago, contamination fears were commonly focused on sexually transmitted diseases like syphilis and gonorrhea, whereas fears of AIDS have replaced these in recent years (see also Weissman et al., 1994).

Interestingly, most studies in the United States have not found differences in the prevalence of OCD based on race (Hispanic, African American, European American), although epidemiological research has indicated that OCD is slightly less common among African Americans than European Americans in the general population (Karno, Golding, Sorenson, & Burnham, 1988). This may be due to greater tolerance in some cultures for behavior that deviates from the norm (Castillo, 1997). In the United States, most patients in clinical settings are of European descent, suggesting that those from minority groups are underrepresented among treatment seeking samples. Friedman, Hatch, Paradix, Popkin, and Shalita (1995) have observed that African Americans with washing rituals may seek assistance more often from medical settings (e.g., dermatology clinics); they may also have more severe symptoms (Chambless & Williams, 1995). Thus culture does not seem to be important in the development of OCD, but it does appear to influence how the disorder is expressed and whether it is viewed as deviant behavior that requires treatment.

PREVALENCE AND CONTINUITY WITH NORMAL BEHAVIOR

> Whenever I walk in a London street,
> I'm ever so careful to watch my feet;
>   And I keep in the squares,
>   And the masses of bears,
> Who wait at the corners all ready to eat
> The sillies who tread on the lines of the street,
>   Go back to their lairs,
>   And I say to them, "Bears,
>   Just look how I'm walking in all of the squares!"
> And the little bears growl to each other, "He's mine,
> As soon as he's silly and steps on a line."

And some of the bigger bears try to pretend
That they came round the corner to look for a friend;
And they try to pretend that nobody cares
Whether you walk on the lines or squares.
But only the sillies believe their talk;
It's ever so portant how you walk.
And it's ever so jolly to call out, "Bears,
Just watch me walking in all the squares!"
                                          —A. A. Milne[2]

Do the fanciful and superstitious games of children so eloquently depicted by A. A. Milne have anything to do with the grotesque and debilitating life lived by the 19-year-old young man described earlier? How common are the clinical manifestations of obsessive–compulsive behavior? As recently as 1980, OCD was thought to be a rare condition. However, with the completion of the Epidemiologic Catchment Area study (see Chapter 1), this estimate increased substantially. The cross-national study by Weissman et al. (1994) identified figures of 1.1% to 1.8% for annual prevalence and 1.9% to 2.5% for lifetime prevalence—approximately 1 in 45 persons. Other epidemiological and community studies completed in the United States and abroad generally confirm these figures, making OCD up to twice as frequent as panic disorder without agoraphobia. Thus, like panic symptoms, worries, and social anxiety, obsessions and compulsions also occur on a continuum that includes mild forms of these symptoms. One indication of this is derived from a study of college students using a standard measure of OCD symptoms, the Yale–Brown Obsessive Compulsive Scale (Y-BOCS). Average scores on the Y-BOCS for college students ranged from 5 to 9 out of a possible 40, compared to a clinical cutoff score for OCD of 16 and above (Steketee, Frost, & Bogart, 1996). That these students frequently scored well above 0 (no symptoms) suggests that many had some degree of obsessive and compulsive symptoms.

Rachman and de Silva (1978) were the first to study subclinical obsessive–compulsive behavior. These investigators administered a questionnaire to 124 participants to determine the presence of intrusive, unacceptable thoughts and impulses, as well as their frequency, and whether they could be easily dismissed. The term "intrusion" was used in place of "obsession," since the latter connotes a clinical disorder, whereas the former refers to any thought, image, or impulse that intrudes into consciousness. Fully 80% of the sample reported intrusions, with a somewhat higher percentage in women than in men. When the intrusive thoughts of this nonclinical sample were compared to those experienced by a clinical sample with OCD, they contained almost identical content. Typical intrusions concerned impulses to attack and harm someone, thoughts about sexual assault or unacceptable sexual acts, or ruminations over the family being harmed by asbestos in the household. These "normal" thoughts and impulses are certainly familiar to any clinician working with OCD. Furthermore, "normal" and "abnormal" obsessions were similar in form and bore the same relationship to mood. That is, they occurred more frequently during periods of anxiety or depression. Finally, both clinical and nonclinical groups reported attempting to resist the thoughts, because they provoked discomfort and were considered ego-alien. Apart from these similarities, the clinical and nonclinical groups differed in several

---

[2]Milne, A. A. "Lines and squares." From A. A. Milne, *When we were very young* (pp. 14–15). New York: E. P. Dutton. Copyright 1924 by E. P. Dutton, renewed 1952 by E. P. Dutton. Reprinted by permission of the publisher, E. P. Dutton, a division of NAL Penguin Inc.

important respects. Clinical obsessions lasted longer and were more intense and frequent, thereby provoking more discomfort. They were also viewed as less acceptable and therefore were more strongly resisted, and perhaps because of this, more difficult to dismiss. Table 15.2 provides many examples of intrusions experienced by ordinary people who do not have OCD.

Subsequent studies have supported Rachman and de Silva's (1978) findings. In fact, Salkovskis and Harrison (1984) found a slightly higher percentage of nonclinical subjects who reported intrusive obsessional thoughts. Furthermore, Freeston, Ladouceur, Thibodeau, and Gagnon (1991) have determined that most people commonly report performing a variety of neutralizing strategies to relieve discomfort from intrusions. These are very similar to the ritualistic behaviors of people diagnosed with OCD. They include thinking logically about the intrusion, replacing one thought with another, seeking reassurance, saying "Stop!", and distraction. Thus these studies provide strong evidence that there are quantitative but not qualitative differences between those with clinical OCD and people who do not have the disorder. That is, obsessions are similar in form and content for both clinical and nonclinical groups, but obsessions in OCD are characterized by greater frequency, intensity, and discomfort. Both groups try to neutralize the behavior to reduce discomfort, but these efforts to resist intrusions are stronger and less successful among those with OCD.

Studies of nonclinical samples with compulsive checking behavior by Sher and Frost have also been informative (Frost, Sher, & Geen, 1986; Sher, Frost, & Otto, 1983; Sher, Mann, & Frost, 1984). These investigators found that 10–15% of college students scored in the clinical range on the Checking subscale of the MOCI. Interestingly, those students had a poorer memory for prior actions than those without compulsive checking did, and also had difficulty distinguishing between real and imagined events. The greater depression and anxiety in the checking sample suggests that such cognitive deficits may be mediated by negative mood and poorer concentration (Frost et al., 1986). Significantly, the investigators suggested that the checking behavior of nonclinical subjects was a reaction to general distress and may have been an attempt to reestablish control over the environment, consistent with the concerns over controlling thoughts and actions in OCD (Clark & Purdon, 1993). Interestingly, recent studies of clinical patients with OCD suggest that they suffer less from actual memory impairment than from decreased confidence in their memory (e.g., MacDonald, Antony, MacLeod, & Richter, 1997; McNally & Kohlbeck, 1993). This might also result from anxiety and lead to checking behavior, and perhaps other obsessive and compulsive symptoms.

COMORBIDITY

OCD and Personality Disorders

Perhaps because of the similarity in the diagnostic labels, many have assumed that OCD is related to obsessive–compulsive personality disorder (OCPD). However, the evidence for this is weak. Comprehensive reviews have consistently indicated that most patients with OCD do not meet criteria for comorbid OCPD (e.g., Baer & Jenike, 1992; Black, 1974; Pfohl & Blum, 1991), though they may have some features of this disorder. In fact, patients with OCD are just as likely to have another personality disorder (mainly in the "anxious" cluster) as OCPD. Interestingly, even early clinical observations have not strongly supported this hypothetical connection. One of the acknowledged experts on OCD in his

TABLE 15.2. Obsessions and Intrusive Thoughts Reported by Nonclinical Samples

Harming

Impulse to jump out of a high window
Idea of jumping in front of a car
Thought of running into oncoming traffic
Thought of poking something into my eyes
Idea of hurting someone I love
Impulse to push someone in front of a train
Wishing a person would die
Idea of taking a meat cleaver and threatening someone in the family
While holding a baby, having a sudden urge to kick it
Thought of dropping a baby
Impulse to harm or be violent toward children, especially smaller ones
Impulse to violently attack and kill someone
Thought of running up to the church altar and hitting people
Worrying that something goes wrong because of my own error
Image of hitting a car or pedestrian with my car
The thought that if I forget to say goodbye to someone, they might die
Idea that something terrible will happen because I'm not careful
Picturing a loved one dead
Picturing my mother dying of cancer
Imagining what it would be like if my brother died
Thought of my family being tortured in front of me
Idea of my sister being murdered by her boyfriend
Thought of throwing a baby down the stairs
Thought that I'd be less likely to have a plane crash if a relative had one
Thinking a loved one will die because I've thought about what I'd do if they did
Thought that thinking about a horrible thing happening to a child will cause it
Image of objects flying into my eye
Image of being in a car accident, trapped under water
Thoughts of smashing a table full of crafts made of glass

Contamination or disease

Fear of harm to husband and child through exposure to asbestos
Fear of harm to self through exposure to asbestos
Thought of catching a disease from public pools or other public places
Thoughts I may have caught a disease from touching toilet seat
Idea of contracting a disease from contact with person
Wanting to wash my hands
Idea that dirt is always on my hand

Inappropriate or unacceptable behavior

Urge to insult a friend for no apparent reason
Impulse to say something hurtful
Idea of swearing or yelling at my boss
Thought that I might have ruined a relationship with a friend
Thought of doing something embarrassing in public, like forgetting to wear a top
Impulse to say something nasty and damning to someone
Impulse to do something shameful or terrible
Idea of blaming a coworker for my own mistakes
A thought or image that is contrary to my moral and religious beliefs
Thought of intense anger toward someone, related to a past experience
Hoping someone doesn't succeed
Picturing myself singing inappropriately at a friend's funeral
Idea that I'll go out of control or do something out of character
Thought of blurting out something in church

(cont.)

TABLE 15.2. (*cont.*)

Thoughts of acts of violence in sex
Thought of "unnatural" sexual acts
Desire for sex with inappropriate partners
Image of a penis
Idea of having sex with ugly people on the bus
Idea of sex with a family member

Doubts about safety, memory, etc.

Thought that I haven't locked the house up properly
Idea of my apartment getting broken into while I'm not home
Idea of leaving my curling iron on the carpet and forgetting to pull out the plug
Idea of electrical appliances catching fire while I'm not home
Thought that I've left the heater and stove on
Image that my house has burned down and I've lost everything I own
Thoughts that I didn't correctly put out an open fire at my vacation home before leaving
Idea that I've left the car unlocked when I know I've locked it
Thought that I haven't put my car brake on properly and my car will crash into traffic while I'm away
Idea that a lost car key causes my car to be stolen
Idea that someone will break in and hurt me or my family
Thought that I have forgotten something I need when I actually checked
Thought that I haven't got any money when it's time to pay for something
Thinking I have left something important behind
Idea that objects are not arranged perfectly

Failure

Thought of being fired because I'm not perfect
Idea of being unsuccessful and not having a good future
Thought of becoming homeless or a derelict

Note. Examples were obtained from Rachman and de Silva (1978) and from unpublished research by Dana Thordarson, PhD, and Michael Kyrios, PhD (personal communications, 2000).

lifetime, Sir Aubrey Lewis (1936), concluded that obsessive or compulsive personality traits (e.g., excessive orderliness, conscientiousness, uncertainty, and cleanliness) were not found among patients with OCD at a greater frequency than among other psychiatric patients. He also observed that these traits are common among healthy people and, conversely, are not present in a substantial proportion of the premorbid personalities of patients with severe OCD. Furthermore, consistent with current reports, he pointed out that these traits are readily differentiated from symptoms of OCD, since they lack any immediate sense of subjective compulsion. That is, little affect or emotion is associated with these traits, which are experienced as ego-syntonic.

Although there appears to be no special link between OCD and OCPD, many patients with OCD also have at least one diagnosable personality disorder (Baer & Jenike, 1992; Black, Noyes, Pfohl, Goldstein, & Blum, 1993; Cassano, del Bruono, & Catapano, 1993; Mavissakalian, Hamann, & Jones, 1990; McKay, Neziroglu, Todaro, & Yaryura-Tobias, 1996; Steketee, Chambless, & Tran, 2001). In fact, the frequency of personality disorder diagnoses in research studies ranges quite widely (from 33% to 92%), probably because of the unreliability of personality diagnoses and the use of several different self-report and interview measures to assess them. Overall, it is not surprising that the most common Axis II disorders for OCD (indeed, for any anxiety disorder) appear to fall in the Cluster C ("anxious") group, including avoidant and especially dependent personality disorders, as well as OCPD. Interestingly, antisocial personality disorder, which is characterized by a general disregard for ordinary rules of social behavior, rarely appears among those with clinical OCD (Mavissakalian et al., 1990). This finding is consistent with recent observations that patients with OCD typically exhibit excessive responsibility (see the discussion of cognitive features of OCD below; Salkovskis, 1985)—a trait that is quite incompatible with antisocial behavior.

OCD and Other Axis I Disorders

Most studies of comorbidity indicate that more than half of patients with OCD have at least one other Axis I disorder (e.g., Rasmussen & Eisen, 1990; Lucey, Butcher, Clare, & Dinan, 1994), mainly mood and anxiety disorders. Comorbidity with specific phobias, social phobia, GAD, and panic disorder ranges from 25% to 60%, according to a large-scale epidemiological study (Weissman et al., 1994). Similar frequencies have been reported in clinical studies (Austin, Lydiard, Fossey, & Zealberg, 1990; Crino & Andrews, 1996; Eisen et al., 1999; Rasmussen & Eisen, 1991). In the large study reported in Chapter 9 (Brown, Campbell, Lehman, Grisham, & Mancill, in press), 57% of 77 carefully diagnosed patients with OCD met criteria for an additional Axis I disorder (see Table 9.5). More specifically, 53% met criteria for either an anxiety or mood disorder, 39% for an anxiety disorder alone, and 32% for a mood disorder alone (major depressive disorder or dysthymia). When one looks at individual disorders, 26% met criteria for social phobia and 22% for major depressive disorder. Concurrent posttraumatic stress disorder (PTSD) has also been reported, and it appears that the risk of OCD goes up considerably for people who are diagnosed with PTSD, compared to those without this disorder (Helzer, Robins, & McEvoy, 1987). In some cases, trauma appears to have precipitated the OCD symptoms (de Silva & Marks, 1999) and is likely to require special attention during treatment. When GAD co-occurs with OCD, patients appear to experience more pathological responsibility and indecisiveness (Abramowitz & Foa, 1998), and may be more likely to drop out of behavioral treatment (Chambless & Steketee, 1999).

Although eating disorders and hypochondriasis accompany OCD somewhat infrequently (10% or fewer of cases; Formea & Burns, 1995; Hsu, Kaye, & Weltzin, 1993; Savron et al., 1996), these disorders share features with OCD and can complicate the symptom picture. The fears and worries of those with anorexia nervosa or bulimia nervosa are focused on body weight, apparently influenced strongly by cultural norms of thinness for women who are far more prone to these disorders than men (Rothenberg, 1986). At times, however, fears of weight gain may lead to compulsive behaviors centering around eating, cooking, and exercise that are similar to OCD rituals. Likewise, in hypochondriasis, anxiety-provoking ideas are focused exclusively on the possibility of having an illness (e.g., AIDS) and are accompanied by excessive consultation with physicians and other reassurance-seeking behaviors that are akin to rituals. Hypochondriasis can be especially difficult to distinguish from OCD when individuals are fearful of having AIDS and engage in extensive avoidance behavior and rituals, including reassurance seeking from medical sources, to ward off this condition. When patients with OCD also exhibit excessive health concerns, they appear to have less insight into their obsessive fears than those without such concerns (Abramowitz, Brigidi, & Foa, 1999), potentially interfering with motivation and compliance in treatment.

Two other disorders have garnered clinical attention as potentially related to OCD. These are body dysmorphic disorder (BDD) and Tourette's disorder with accompanying tics. BDD is characterized by excessive preoccupation with presumed defects in appearance, such as thinning hair or an "ugly" nose. These appear to be nearly delusional (or at least overvalued) in nature, in that the individual rarely expresses insight into the excessive nature of his or her concern. Ritualistic behaviors (e.g., mirror checking and reassurance seeking) and avoidance of social situations are commonly observed in BDD, and resemble OCD compulsions and avoidance. Lifetime comorbidity of BDD with OCD appears to occur in 12% of cases (Simeon, Hollander, Stein, Cohen, & Aronowitz, 1995). Whether BDD should be considered a variant of OCD or is better classed with hypochondriasis as a somatoform disorder is a question that requires further study. Tourette's disorder appears to be genetically linked to OCD, in that the former rarely occurs in the absence of OCD symptoms (Leckman & Chittenden, 1990; Pauls, 1992). However, the reverse is not true. Only a small proportion (4–7%) of clinical patients who suffer from OCD also exhibit Tourette's (Eisen et al., 1999; Rasmussen & Eisen, 1991). Thus, for clinical purposes, Tourette's disorder is a relatively rare accompaniment to OCD, but its genetic connection is nonetheless important in identifying etiologies of OCD. Furthermore, because its presence implies important underlying neurological substrates, treatment of OCD that is comorbid with Tourette's disorder often requires specialized pharmacological interventions.

OCD and Depression

Nowhere is the relationship of anxiety and depression stronger than for OCD, and so we devote special attention here to the comorbidity of OCD with the depressive disorders. Up to 80% of patients with OCD may be currently depressed according to measures that assess severity of depressed mood. In addition, a diagnosable major depressive episode is also present in approximately one-quarter to one-third of cases (Barlow, Di Nardo, Vermilyea, Vermilyea, & Blanchard, 1986; Crino & Andrews, 1996; Weissman et al., 1994), with 22% meeting criteria in the data set discussed in Chapter 9 (see Table 9.5). Dysthymia accompanies OCD somewhat less frequently, with 10% meeting criteria in Table 9.5. Some recent evidence also suggests that bipolar disorder may accompany OCD almost as frequently as other forms of depression (Kruger, Cooke, Hasey, Jorna, & Persad, 1995), but more evidence is needed to confirm this finding. According to a recent report on a large cohort of patients, the likelihood of developing a mood disorder after the onset of OCD is second only to the likelihood of developing another type of anxiety disorder (Yaryura-Tobias et al., 2000). This relationship between OCD and depression is particularly evident if one examines lifetime diagnoses—that is, whether patients presenting with OCD have ever met criteria for another diagnosis during their lifetimes (see Table 9.6). There we see that fully 61% of patients experienced a major depressive disorder at some point in their lives, far exceeding the next most prevalent lifetime diagnosis (social phobia, at 27%).

Because of this high frequency of depression, some investigators have questioned whether OCD is simply a variant of a mood disorder (e.g., Insel, Zahn, & Murphy, 1985), and should be classified with mood rather than anxiety disorders. In addition to their high rates of comorbidity, the biological underpinnings of depression and OCD appear to be similar—for example, in nonsuppression on the dexamethasone suppression test and in sleep electroencephalographic findings (see Turner, Beidel, & Nathan, 1985). Furthermore, similarities of psychopharmacology treatments for OCD and depressed mood suggest a connection, although the specificity of selective serotonin reuptake inhibitors (SSRIs) over other types of antidepressants for OCD implies some clear differences between these disorders. Patients with OCD also seem to display a broader range of negative affect in addition to anxiety (e.g., low self-esteem, indecision, guilt, etc.). But these findings are difficult to interpret, for the same reasons outlined in previous chapters in regard to the relationship between anxiety and depression, and results across studies of biological and genetic characteristics are not always consistent. For example, Monteiro, Marks, Noshirvani, and Checkley (1986) found normal results on the dexamethasone suppression test in patients with OCD who were not depressed. Furthermore, most studies that chronicle the onset of OCD and of depression have indicated that depression typically develops after OCD (e.g., Rasmussen & Eisen, 1992b; Welner, Reich, Robins, Fishman, & Van Doren, 1976), although there are clearly some exceptions to this rule. In addition, successful treatment of OCD, whether pharmacological or psychological, very often results in reduction of depression as well (van Balkom et al., 1994; Foa, Steketee, Grayson, Turner, & Latimer, 1984). These findings suggest that depression is usually a secondary disorder, perhaps brought on by the debilitation produced by serious or incapacitating OCD symptoms.

A MODEL OF THE ETIOLOGY OF OCD

Any model of OCD must consider one firmly established, if paradoxical, fact: As we have noted earlier, despite the bizarreness and the debilitating nature of OCD in its severe forms, intrusive thoughts and even neutralizing compulsions are very common in the normal population. That stressful experiences prompt intrusive thoughts is hardly surprising. Horowitz (e.g., 1975) provided evidence that those who watched a stressful film experienced many more intrusive thoughts and images than those who did not see the film. Also, Parkinson and Rachman (1981a, 1981c) reported that mothers whose children were about to be admitted for surgery reported many more intrusive thoughts than mothers in a control group. These thoughts and images were not necessarily related to the upcoming surgery, suggesting that stressors are nonspecific producers of intrusions.

Not surprisingly, intrusive thoughts are much more common in the context of depressed and anxious mood (Farid, 1986; Rachman & Hodgson, 1980), both of which are common features of OCD. This could be due to increased accessibility of negatively valenced cognitions while experiencing negative mood states (Teasdale, 1983). Freeston, Rhéaume, and Ladouceur (1996) have postulated that negative mood increases the frequency and duration of intrusive thoughts, making it more difficult to dismiss or control them. Some evidence to support this has been presented in studies of thought suppression (Purdon, 1999), where it appears that efforts to suppress thoughts of an obsessional nature are associated with more anxiety and depressed mood. Thus stressful events may provide a pathway to intrusive thoughts via negative emotions (see Jones & Menzies, 1998b), though more research is needed to demonstrate this connection. There is also some evidence that compulsions may result from stress. For example, the animal behavior literature suggests that performance of certain stereotyped and ritualistic behaviors may be an innate response to stress (Mineka, 1985a). Such behaviors in humans are often considered efforts to control an unpredictable and therefore stressful environment.

What is needed, then, is a way to account for differences in severity of intrusive thoughts and related rituals between patients appearing at clinics and ordinary people who may be experiencing stress. Once again, both biological and psychological vulnerabilities are likely to be important. Specifically, individuals who go on to develop OCD are susceptible to reacting with a strong, biologically based emotional response to stress. Based on a general psychological vulnerability, negative life events and the effects of stress are quickly elaborated into anxiety and a sense that events are out of control. For example, stressors that appear to have both a biological and a psychological base for generating OCD symptoms in some women are pregnancy and childbirth (Diaz, Grush, Sichel, & Cohen, 1998). Intrusive thoughts, especially in relation to children, can emerge in the context of this stress. Chapter 8 has reviewed evidence that different anxiety disorders derive from a differential disposition to focus anxious apprehension on certain situations or events—in other words, a specific psychological vulnerability. For example, persons who develop social phobia are exposed as children to parents who display significantly more concerns with social evaluation than parents of those who develop agoraphobia do (Bruch, Heimberg, Berger, & Collins, 1987). Patients with OCD may undergo an etiological process similar to that of patients with phobias, who experience repeated, exaggerated misinformation in the context of biological and psychological anxiety proneness. In the case of OCD, enormous importance is placed on intrusive thoughts that are believed to be dangerous and/or indicators of "bad" or "abnormal" character (Obsessive Compulsive Cognitions Working Group [OCCWG], 1997, 2001).

Such negative self-evaluations appear to be commonly derived from excessive responsibility and the resulting guilt, usually developed during childhood. Salkovskis, Shafran, Rachman, and Freeston (1999) have proposed that an early broad sense of responsibility encouraged during childhood and rigid codes of conduct or duty required in school or religious education may predispose people to develop OCD symptoms. Such childhood experiences may encourage thought–action fusion, in which thoughts are equated with actions ("Thinking is as bad as doing"), and magical thinking, in which thoughts are believed to cause outcomes (e.g., imagining an accident increases its likelihood) (Rachman, 1993; Shafran, Thordarson, & Rachman, 1996), both common in OCD. For example, the woman described at the beginning of this chapter believed that merely thinking about abortion was the moral equivalent of having one. She then spent years attempting to prevent similar thoughts about actions that might harm others. In the second example, the college student finally admitted strong homosexual impulses, which were unacceptable to him and to his father (who was a minister). Many Catholic, Jewish, and fundamentalist Christian patients with OCD present with similar intolerant or rigid attitudes derived from their early family and religious training that they have applied inflexibly, even perfectionistically. That rigid beliefs may constitute a vulnerability factor for OCD is supported by the finding that the strength (but not type) of religious belief was associated with severity of OCD pathology (Steketee, Quay, & White, 1991).

Of course, the source of this sensitivity need not be religious experience, and the vast majority of individuals who hold fundamentalist religious beliefs do not develop OCD. Thus, as in any emotional disorder, the combination of biological and psychological vulnerabilities (including a disposition to focus anxiety in at least some cases) must line up correctly for the etiological process to ensue. Salkovskis (1985, 1989) concluded that intrusions only produce distress when they have some idiosyncratic meaning or salience to the individual experiencing them. It seems likely that extremely high standards imposed during childhood and/or excessively critical reactions from authority figures may also contribute to perfectionistic attitudes, feelings of guilt, and extreme beliefs in responsibility. These historical experiences are likely to have special influence when the person experiences an actual increase in duties and responsibility, as in stressful life changes (e.g., leaving home, marriage, birth of children, or increase in job responsibilities). Thus patients with OCD, perhaps especially those with checking rituals, appear to have learned that certain intrusive thoughts—which almost everyone eventually experiences under stress—are unacceptable because they signal potential danger for which they feel personally responsible.

Cognitive theorists have also postulated that people who develop OCD do so in part because they overestimate the likelihood and severity of danger in personally salient situations and are unable to tolerate uncertainty and ambiguity that could possibly signal threat (Foa & Kozak, 1986; Jones & Menzies, 1997; OCCWG, 1997, 2001; Rasmussen & Eisen, 1989). Kozak, Foa, and McCarthy (1987) have pointed to a problem with epistemological reasoning, in which people with OCD assume danger unless they can assure themselves of safety, whereas most people expect safety unless danger has been demonstrated. Doubting the veracity of one's experience is a hallmark of OCD, described in some of the earliest theories about this disorder (see Reed, 1985). Several laboratory studies have supported the excessive difficulty of those with OCD in making even simple decisions (e.g., Persons & Foa, 1984; Reed, 1985). These studies suggest that they require excessive information before making decisions and often doubt their actions, a concept that has also been linked to perfectionistic attitudes (see Frost & Steketee, 1997). It is possible that the doubting of actions and intolerance for ambiguity seen in OCD derives from difficulty with cognitive tasks, such as the ability to categorize, organize, and shift mental set (e.g., Savage et al., 1999).

Becoming anxious over internal cognitive stimuli, as opposed to somatic events (as in panic disorder) or external objects or situations (as in specific or social phobia), has other implications. Individuals with specific or social phobia have some control through avoidance over events signaling panic and anxiety. Many patients with panic disorder develop a series of safety signals that provide them with some sense of control over their next panic attack. But patients with OCD are most often continually buffeted with aversive, unacceptable mental intrusions that are not under their control. This has two consequences. First, they strongly resist these experiences and develop mental or behavioral strategies to neutralize them (compulsions). Second, the increasing anxiety sets the stage for false alarms, which inevitably become associated with the focus of their anxiety—specific thoughts. Indeed, some patients with OCD also experience panic reactions to these thoughts (see Chapter 4). They become vigilant to prevent or suppress such thoughts, in an attempt to gain some control over their internal environment. Unfortunately, such efforts may backfire. Wegner (1989) and others have provided some evidence that when ordinary people try to not think about unwanted thoughts, they paradoxically increase the salience of such ideas, making them even harder to dismiss (see Purdon, 1999). As Clark and Purdon (1993) have noted, when efforts to control or dismiss unacceptable thoughts fail, people resort to neutralizing rituals. It is also possible that depression plays an important role in this process, as we have indicated earlier. Research findings indicate that negative (obsessive) thoughts are more easily suppressed by other negative ones, and that depressive thoughts may fill the bill, further increasing the negative mood state for people with OCD (Salkovskis & Campbell, 1994; Wegner, 1989).

Since thoughts are inherently uncontrollable, it is no surprise that the utter helplessness engendered by this process results in a high frequency of reactive depression. As Sir Aubrey Lewis observed in 1966, "obsessional patients are in most cases depressed; their illness is a depressing one" (p. 1200). Thus, as we have noted earlier, the onset of OCD is typically followed by the development of a depressive condition (which may or may not reach the proportions of a major depressive disorder). Less frequently, the depressive disorder precedes the development of OCD (Coryell, 1981; Welner et al., 1976) and appears to be associated with a more episodic course characteristic of major depressive episodes (see Eisen & Steketee, 1998). It is possible that the experience of prior depression, along with accompanying stress, may have prompted intrusive thoughts in the first place. In any case, it seems likely that depression and OCD feed on and maintain each other, leading to a vicious downward spiral. As Rachman and Hodgson (1980) point out, for some patients the development of severe depression may be associated with a decrease in their obsessive–compulsive symptoms, perhaps due to the inhibiting qualities of a very severe, retarded depression.

Finally, questions on the etiology of specific forms of compulsion remain. In the face of overwhelmingly aversive, uncontrollable events, the origins of cognitive compulsions such as prayer or requests for reassurance seem clear. When the content of the obsession concerns contamination, cleaning rituals are easily explained. But the origins of checking rituals are less clear when they are not tied closely to the source of danger (e.g., checking the gas stove). Steketee et al. (1985) examined differences in the parental backgrounds of persons with washing and checking rituals, and came to the interesting conclusion that the mothers of "checkers" were significantly more meticulous and demanding than the mothers of "washers." Since both groups by definition had OCD, these data suggest a specifically learned disposition not only for the obsession, but also for the compulsive behavior chosen to neutralize or control it. That is, those with checking compulsions may have a learned tendency to react to stress or negative events by becoming meticulous, perhaps even perfectionistic. Indeed, perfectionism is a relatively common trait associated with OCD symptoms (Ferrari, 1995; Frost & Steketee, 1997; Frost, Steketee, Cohn, & Greiss, 1994; Rhéaume, Freeston, Dugas, Letarte, & Ladouceur, 1995). Interestingly, Hoover and Insel (1984) have also reported that the parents of patients with OCD emphasized cleanliness and perfection, again potentially linking family attitudes and behavior to the development of OCD. Obviously, these data are only preliminary and subject to retrospective distortion. It also seems likely that perfectionism is not exclusive to the etiology of OCD, but also plays a role in the development of other disorders (see Frost & Steketee, 1997).

In summary, the present model of OCD combines features of previous models of phobic disorders and GAD. Specifically, intense stress-related negative affect and neurobiological reactions are triggered by negative life events (biological vulnerability). The resulting intrusive thoughts, which are commonly experienced in the normal population (and other anxiety disorders) during periods of stress, are judged unacceptable; attempts are made to avoid or suppress these thoughts. Recurrence of these thoughts causes intensification of anxiety, with accompanying negative affect and a sense that these thoughts are proceeding in an unpredictable and uncontrollable fashion (generalized psychological vulnerability). The vicious negative feedback loop of anxiety then develops, with attention narrowed onto the content of the unacceptable thoughts themselves. The specific content of the obsessions is determined by learned dispositions that certain thoughts or images are unacceptable (specific psychological vulnerability). These thoughts become much like discrete phobic stimuli in their capacity to elicit alarm and even panic attacks. The severity of this process, relative to other anxiety disorders, makes it more likely to be accompanied by hopelessness and depression. Either depression occurs in reaction to the severity of OCD, or a prior depression is maintained because of this severity. A diagram of this process is presented in Figure 15.1.

ASSESSMENT

The several types of assessment tools for OCD fall into the categories of interview, self-report, and behavioral instruments. Physiological measures are seldom used in clinical practice with this disorder and are not reviewed here. Feske and Chambless (2000) provide an excellent detailed review of the measurement instruments described below.

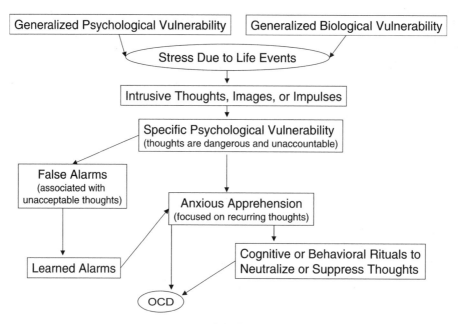

FIGURE 15.1. A model of the etiology of OCD.

Interview Measures

Among the several options for establishing a diagnosis of OCD according to DSM-IV, the Anxiety Disorders Interview Schedule for DSM-IV: Lifetime Version (ADIS-IV-L; Di Nardo, Brown, & Barlow, 1994) is the most useful for clinical purposes. This diagnostic schedule inquires about specific DSM-IV criteria for determining the presence of OCD and distinguishing it from other similar conditions as we have discussed above. In addition, it permits the clinician to obtain some detail about the type and severity of presenting obsessions and compulsions, including frequency, persistence, distress and resistance associated with these symptoms. The ADIS-IV-L also includes sections to determine environmental stressors (family, work, finances, health) and to identify those patients who lack insight into their obsessive fears, consistent with DSM-IV criteria for the insight modifier for OCD. These latter factors may be especially important in planning treatment.

An instrument mentioned earlier, the Y-BOCS (Goodman, Price, Rasmussen, Mazure, Delgado, et al., 1989; Goodman, Price, Rasmussen, Mazure, Fleischman, et al., 1989), has become the standard method for assessing the severity of OCD symptoms in both pharmacological and cognitive-behavioral treatment trials. It is also one of the most useful measures of OCD symptoms from a clinical standpoint. The interviewer begins by first defining obsessions and compulsions for the patient, so that these terms are clearly understood. Using the Y-BOCS Checklist, the assessor then questions the patient about 36 different types of obsessions and 23 types of compulsions. This list covers the following types of symptoms: harming, contamination/washing, sexual, hoarding/saving, religious, symmetry/exactness, somatic, and miscellaneous. After the patient has indicated whether any of these occur currently or have occurred in the past, the interviewer then rates the severity of the three main obsessions and also the three main compulsions on time spent, interference, distress, resistance, and perceived control over each. A summed score is obtained separately for Obsessions and for Rituals, and a total score includes both. A total score of 16 or above is considered to indicate clinical severity, and average scores for patients participating in treatment trials are usually in the mid-20s.

The reliability and validity of the interview Y-BOCS is well established, although some drawbacks have been noted. For example, internal consistency is not enhanced by the resistance items (Woody, Steketee, & Chambless, 1995), and patients who report mainly obsessions may score low on this measure (Kim, Dysken, & Katz, 1989). Potential revisions to the Y-BOCS are now being studied. A self-report version of the Y-BOCS and the Y-BOCS Checklist is also available, and appears useful for clinical and nonclinical samples (Steketee et al., 1996). S. Wilhelm (personal communication, 2000) has also begun testing of scales to score the severity of categories of OCD symptoms based on the Y-BOCS Checklist. This measure will help determine whether some symptoms change more than others during treatment. This may be especially important for determining whether some interventions (e.g., cognitive, behavioral, pharmacological) are more helpful for some types of symptoms than others.

Questionnaires and Rating Scales

Another instrument mentioned earlier, the MOCI (Hodgson & Rachman, 1977), has been used frequently in research trials. This brief 30-item questionnaire provides a total score and four subscales that assess Checking, Washing, Doubting/Conscientiousness, and Slowness/Repetition. In general, it possesses good test–retest reliability and internal consistency and adequate validity (Emmelkamp, Kraaijkamp, & van den Hout, 1999; Sanavio & Vidotto, 1985), but the Slowness and Doubting subscales performed more poorly. Feske and Chambless (2000) have recommended that the MOCI be used in conjunction with other instruments. Another commonly used questionnaire measure of severity of obsessions and compulsions is the Padua Inventory (Sanavio, 1988). The original form is somewhat lengthy at 60 items, but two revisions have been proposed, each considerably shorter. Based on a factor analysis and other psychometric testing, van Oppen, Hoekstra, and Emmelkamp (1995) recommended a 41-item scale that included several subscales assessing Contamination, Checking, Impaired Mental Control, and Urges and Worries. Also based on factor analyses of nonclinical samples, Burns, Keortge, Formea, and Sternberger (1996) reconfigured the scale into 39 items. Both methods appear to be useful strategies for assessing treatment outcome, especially for patients with ruminations and impulses that are not adequately assessed in other self-report measures such as the MOCI (Feske & Chambless, 2000).

A number of other questionnaires have been used in previous research studies, but are considered inferior to the Y-BOCS, Padua Inventory, and MOCI. The newly developed Obsessive–Compulsive Inventory (Foa, Kozak, Salkovskis, Coles, & Amir, 1998) contains 42 items arranged in seven subscales. It has shown satisfactory reliability and validity in a large sample of patients and nonpsychiatric controls, but has not yet been widely adopted. It is interesting to note that several of the instruments to assess OCD, including the widely used MOCI and Y-BOCS, have had difficulty discriminating OCD and depression—perhaps because OCD is so often accompanied by depressed mood.

Two questionnaires have recently been developed by an international consortium of researchers to identify and rate cognitive aspects of intrusive thoughts and obsessions (OCCWG, 1997, 2001). The 87-item Obsessional Beliefs Questionnaire includes dysfunctional assumptions or beliefs covering six domains: overimportance and control of thoughts, overestimation of threat, tolerance for uncertainty, responsibility, and perfectionism. In addition, the 31-item Interpretation of Intrusions Inventory asks patients to rate their immediate appraisal or interpretation when they have an intrusive/obsessive thought. This questionnaire focuses on three content areas: overimportance and control of thoughts, and responsibility. Studies of clinical and nonclinical subjects suggests good evidence of reliability and validity, but substantial overlap among some subscales that will require further investigation. These instruments were designed particularly to evaluate the effects of cognitive therapy for OCD.

Target Ratings and Self-Monitoring

Many of the studies of behavioral treatment for OCD have used Likert-type scales on which patients, therapists, and independent assessors rate the severity of specific OCD symptoms. These scales have generally shown good agreement among raters, but may be less stable than desirable. However, they are highly sensitive to treatment effects, probably because the symptoms rated are those selected for intervention. Use of these scales is recommended only in conjunction with other standardized instruments (see Feske & Chambless, 2000). Another method that allows ratings of idiosyncratic symptoms is self-monitoring of the frequency and duration of obsessions and compulsions, as well as the distress provoked by the obsessions. Ratings of distress called "subjective units of discomfort" (SUDs) usually range from 0 (no discomfort) to 100 (maximum/extreme distress). For anxiety disorders including OCD, where specific anxiety symptoms themselves constitute the targets for therapy, self-monitoring measures assume increased importance. One example of this type of form is presented in Figure 15.2. A frequency count of obsessions and/or rituals is especially useful for monitoring progress and compliance during behavioral treatment. However, when symptoms are lengthy rather than frequent, recording the duration of an obsession or ritual may be more relevant. When obsessive thoughts or rituals (e.g., checking or repeating) are too numerous to count, daily estimates of the total duration may be made, or the patient can time-sample their presence during preselected hours. Since compulsions are usually prevented during behavioral treatment, and therefore counting them is less useful, monitoring of urges to perform rituals becomes an important measure. This helps the therapist be sure that urges have diminished considerably and are unlikely to trigger rituals after treatment has ended.

Behavioral Measures

Direct behavioral observation and mechanical counting of rituals have been employed only in rare instances (e.g., Mills, Agras, Barlow, & Mills, 1973; Turner, Hersen, Bellack, & Wells, 1979), because they are difficult to design in a valid manner for many patients with OCD. Likewise, behavioral avoidance tests (BATs), which work well for assessing change in phobic behavior, have been used infrequently to assess changes in OCD symptoms after treatment. This is partly due to the wide variety of symptoms these patients display and the difficulty of constructing a stepwise task. Steketee, Chambless, Tran, Worden, and Gillis (1995) devised multiple-step/multiple-task behavioral tests for 50 patients with widely varying symptoms of OCD. This method used up to three tasks to reflect the main obsessive fears and rituals the patients reported. Each task had up to seven steps for which a rater determined whether patients did the task, how much anxiety they reported, and whether they engaged in any ritual. Examples of tasks included listening to media information pertinent to obsessions about harming others, thinking bad numbers, encounter-

Please record the actual *number of minutes* or *number of times* you perform rituals specified on this form. Please note the situation that led to your need to do the ritual, as well as the amount of discomfort on a scale from 0 to 100, where 0 means completely calm and 100 means extremely upset or disturbed. Please note the following suggestions from your therapist for keeping records of rituals: _____

_____

_____

Example:

Ritual A: _____*Washing*_____   Ritual B: _____*Checking for harm*_____

Time of day	Situation that led to ritual	Discomfort	Minutes ritualizing Ritual A	Ritual B
9:30 a.m.	Took out the garbage	70	4 min.	
11:30 a.m.	Bathroom—urination	80	5 min.	
1:00 p.m.	Drove car to town center	85		10 min.
4:00 p.m.	Used iron	60		2 min.
6:30 p.m.	Cleaning up after dinner: checking stove, oven, faucet	55		15 min.

Please record your rituals below:

Time of day	Situation that led to ritual	Discomfort	Minutes ritualizing Ritual A	Ritual B

FIGURE 15.2. Daily Self-Monitoring Form.

ing objects associated with death, doing laundry, touching money, and using public restroom facilities. These examples make it clear that BATs can be constructed for most types of OCD problems, including washing/cleaning, checking for harm, and "bad" thoughts, though more ingenuity may be required for patients whose obsessions are based mainly on internal rather than external cues. The investigators concluded that BATs were feasible and valid methods for assessing the effects of behavioral treatment for OCD.

TREATMENT

Three main types of treatment have been demonstrated to be effective for OCD. These are behavior therapy that includes exposure to feared situations and blocking rituals, cognitive therapy (CT—either rational–emotive therapy or Beckian CT), and medications that affect the serotonin system. Below we describe these methods and their effects on OCD symptoms, including considerations regarding combining treatment methods. Because cognitive therapies are relatively more recently developed for OCD, fewer studies of them have been conducted, so findings must be considered more tentative than for either behavioral or pharmacological therapies.

Behavioral Treatment

Although classifying symptoms according to content or type appears to have little heuristic value, determining the function of obsessions and compulsions has influenced the conceptualization of OCD and especially the application of behavioral treatment methods, developed over 30 years ago. That is, prolonged exposure procedures (described below) are applied to discomfort-provoking obsessions. Response prevention is intended to block rituals, and is therefore systematically applied to anxiety-reducing phenomena that include behavioral and mental compulsions, as well as other forms of neutralizing or undoing the obsessions. For functionally autonomous rituals, procedures involving shaping, pacing, and prompting have proven useful (Mavissakalian & Barlow, 1981). Although no one is quite sure why exposure is effective, it seems likely that extended periods of exposure permit emotional discomfort (usually anxiety) to dissipate, so that feared situations provoke less reaction. This in turn may alter the person's attitudes toward the situation and the expected outcomes. In any case, the major procedural issue in treatment is arranging for sufficient exposure to occur without interruption from neutralizing strategies.

Early studies using treatments successful with phobic behavior, such as systematic desensitization, yielded generally disappointing results with OCD (e.g., Beech & Vaughn, 1978; Cooper, Gelder, & Marks, 1965). A commonality among these studies was that they often ignored compulsive behavior associated with obsessions. A variety of early case studies took the opposite tack by attempting to block compulsive behavior (Marks, Crowe, Drewe, Young, & Dewhurst, 1969; Walton, 1960). Although some patients responded well, this strategy was also disappointing, and relapses occurred. In 1966, Victor Meyer reported results from a more comprehensive program in which rituals were prevented while the patients were exposed to circumstances that normally provoked distress and compulsive behavior. Clinical results from these early trials were very encouraging (e.g., Meyer, 1966; Meyer & Levy, 1973). This approach, which came to be known by the descriptive if unimaginative name of "exposure and response prevention" (ERP), generated a great deal of interest. Subsequent controlled studies have demonstrated quite clearly the effectiveness of this treatment for OCD, as summarized below.

Over the years, this treatment was further developed and investigated, first at the Maudsley Hospital in London by Rachman, Marks, and their colleagues (e.g., Marks, Bird, & Lindley, 1978; Rachman & Hodgson, 1980), and later by Foa and her colleagues in Philadelphia (e.g., Foa, Steketee, & Ozarow, 1985). Foa et al. (1983) summarized results for a large group of 50 patients with OCD who were treated with ERP. The majority (58%) were rated as "much improved," indicating that they showed gains of 70% or more on an independent assessor's rating scale of the patients' main OCD symptoms. Another 38% were classified as "improved" (gains of 30–70%), leaving very few patients who were considered failures. Long-term follow-ups ranging from 3 months to 3 years indicated the rate of failure increased to 24%, although most patients retained their improved status. Foa et al. (1983) commented that those classified as only "improved" were most likely to relapse.

Since the first report of this treatment, at least 30 open trials and controlled studies have investigated the effects of 10–20 sessions of ERP for OCD in more than 600 patients. Several meta-analyses have supported the efficacy of this treatment. van Balkom et al. (1994) reported that behavior therapy produced a very large average effect size of 1.46 and was significantly more effective than placebo. A meta-analysis by Abramowitz (1997) also showed that ERP was highly effective in reducing OCD symptoms and that more direct exposure was very strongly correlated with more benefits. Furthermore, a recent summary of five studies that assessed outcome with the now standard Y-BOCS showed that scores dropped from averages of 20–25 to a range of 10–17 (Steketee & Frost, 1998). Given that most patients who qualify for a diagnosis of OCD score above 16 on the Y-BOCS, this means that many of the patients treated with ERP no longer met criteria for the disorder. Most patients showed little if any relapse. Overall, these are impressive results for a disorder previously considered difficult to treat.

Several studies have examined variations on ERP treatments to determine the best method for delivering the therapy. It is clear that both exposure and response prevention are necessary. Because exposure activates the emotional response (usually anxiety) associated with obsessive fears and allows this response to habituate, it has its strongest effect on obsessions (Foa et al., 1984; Mills et al., 1973). In contrast, response prevention enables a patient to gain control over compulsions (e.g., Foa et al., 1984; Turner, Hersen, Bellack, Andrasik, & Capparell, 1980). Thus, from a clinical standpoint, the therapist can use the intensity of the discomfort reported at initial exposure and the degree of reduction in discomfort as indicators of progress during therapy. The patient's ability to restrict rituals while exposure is ongoing is another good reflection of the likely outcome of therapy (Abramowitz, 1996).

Treatment can be delivered with quite limited therapist involvement, and self-directed ERP may actually protect patients from relapse (e.g., Emmelkamp & Kraanen, 1977; Emmelkamp, van den Heuvell, Ruphan, & Sanderman, 1989). However, Abramowitz's (1996) meta analysis suggests that therapist-directed exposure is more effective. That ERP developed and tested in research settings can be delivered very effectively in routine clinical practice is a very important finding. Studying 36 clinic patients with OCD, Kirk (1983) implemented an unsystematic behavioral treatment that relied heavily on task assignments at home. Including 4 patients who dropped out of therapy, 75% were moderately improved or better, and very favorable results were evident for those with only mental rituals. For 81% of the patients, no further treatment was required up to 5 years after treatment. These results are presented in Table 15.3. In a more recent study, results for 110 clinical patients who received intensive ERP on an outpatient fee-for-service basis were compared to findings from controlled clinical research studies (Franklin, Abramowitz, Kozak, Levitt, & Foa, 2000). Benefits were comparable for both groups. These results are most encouraging to clinicians wanting to incorporate ERP into their outpatient practice.

TABLE 15.3. Outcome of Obsessive–Compulsive Problems after Treatment (Global Ratings)

	Outcome (global rating)				
	Worse	No change	Slightly improved	Moderately improved	Goal achieved
Compulsions					
Cleaning	—	1	1	1	1
Checking	—	—	1	2	5
Cleaning and checking	—	—	2	2	2
Slowness	—	—	1	—	1
All compulsions	—	1	5	5	9
Obsessions	—	—	1	1	12
Total (*n* = 36)	—	1 (8%)	6 (17%)	6 (17%)	21 (58%)

Note. Adapted from Kirk (1983). Copyright 1983 by Pergamon Journals, Ltd. Adapted by permission.

The optimum number of exposure sessions appears to be about 20, and these may occur as often as daily or as infrequently as once a week. Treatment can include direct exposure and also imagined exposure, which may be especially helpful to patients who worry greatly about catastrophic consequences related to their obsessions (e.g., damage due to fire, long-term illness or death, going to hell). The inclusion of specific strategies for preventing relapse in the face of natural stressors appears to help patients maintain long-term gains (Hiss, Foa, & Kozak, 1994). It is also clear that exposure can be effectively delivered in a group format, as several studies have shown (e.g., Fals-Stewart, Marks, & Schafer, 1993; van Noppen, Steketee, McCorkle, & Pato, 1997). Training family members to assist in treatment may also be advantageous, especially when family members are not anxious themselves and are able to provide support and supervision (Mehta, 1990; Thornicroft, Colson, & Marks, 1991; Van Noppen et al., 1997). Among the variations in treatment delivery is a novel self-treatment program using computerized assessment and treatment assistance, called "BT Steps." A recent study by Bachofen et al. (1999) indicated that of 21 patients who completed self-assessment, 10 went on to do at least two ERP sessions according to instructions over a 2-month period. These participants improved as much as is typical of patients treated with serotonin reuptake inhibitor (SRI) medications. As one might expect for an entirely self-directed therapy, those who showed clear motivation by completing the assessment phase in a timely fashion fared best in using this method.

Thus ERP has alleviated the suffering of many with this debilitating disorder. However, it is important to realize that this therapy may require considerable departures from the usual office-based outpatient treatment of anxiety disorders. Particularly in severe cases, the treatment is often rigorous and demanding for both therapist and patient. By actively blocking or preventing rituals that have come to be equated with everything that is safe and comfortable, the therapist is insisting that the patient confront his or her worst fears. But, unlike *in vivo* exposure treatments for those with phobic conditions, the experience is not over in an hour or two. Since patients are unable to use rituals to escape their overwhelming fears of disaster or thoughts of impending catastrophe, exposure is really in effect 24 hours a day for weeks at a time. This process has been described in detail elsewhere (Steketee, 1993), and is illustrated in the treatment of the two cases presented at the beginning of this chapter. In severe cases, round-the-clock supervision may be necessary to assist patients in refraining from the overwhelming temptation to ritualize their worst fears away. Inpatient therapy may be needed to assist such patients in ERP treatment, and the hospital staff may also include behavioral contingencies (rewards and withdrawal of privileges) in addition to ERP procedures. The process of treatment is illustrated below for the two patients described earlier, the first treated on an outpatient basis and the second in a hospital setting.

Case Study: Checking and Magical Rituals to Prevent Harm from the Devil

The 32-year-old Jewish woman who was fearful of situations associated with the devil was treated as an outpatient over the course of two periods of approximately 4 months each. A hiatus occurred after the first 4 months when finances ran low, but treatment resumed a few months later. Thereafter, sessions were spaced to every 2–3 weeks for discussion of continued improvement in OCD symptoms and issues of career, marriage, and children (during this time, she had her third child). The first several treatment sessions focused on identifying all of her obsessions and the associated rituals. To do this, the patient kept a log such as the one given in Figure 15.2 for a 1-week period.

A hierarchy was constructed according to the patient's expected anxiety level if she were prevented from doing a ritual. Although many different types of situations provoked obsessive fear, all of them hinged on harm that would befall her family, for which she would be responsible. Thus one hierarchy was constructed to include a wide variety of situations. From easier to harder, these were as follows: fastening snaps on children's clothes; dressing herself; turning on lights and faucets; thinking angry thoughts about her stepchildren; stepping on cracks; going up and down stairs with bad thoughts about others; leaving the house without checking; saying, writing, or doing activities associated with the numbers 3 and 13; cooking cheese with chicken; shopping on Saturday; driving by funeral homes and cemeteries without rituals; going into an occult shop; reading about devils; and writing and saying words she associated with the devil.

She worked on one or two of these situations per week and agreed to stop all of her rituals for each step. At her own request, she wrote out a brief contract outlining her obligations and signed it each week, to enhance her resolve to engage in the exposure and blocking of rituals. She made generally steady progress, with occasional slips that were usually related to stressful events occurring in her life (e.g., children ill, deadlines for work). However, although she considerably curtailed her rituals, she was unable to stop them completely, no matter how hard she tried and what plan was devised. She had much difficulty making herself persist in activities when the clock showed 13 minutes before or after the hour, and this took several weeks to master. She then worked on cooking and eating foods associated with the devil (devil's food cake, deviled eggs) and on writing and reading words associated with the devil. The patient also visited cemeteries and an occult shop with the therapist, where she purchased small items she associated with the devil. These she placed on her refrigerator and in her drawers at home. This exposure led to considerable anxiety about her children dying if she were not "good," and also to a review of her feelings of (misplaced) responsibility about her depressed father's suicide death by prescription drug overdose.

She gradually mastered her discomfort and made good progress, eventually reducing her rituals by more than 80% according to her own estimate. Her score on the MOCI decreased from 14 before treatment to 6—a clear improvement that satisfied her and enabled her to function well, although she never eliminated her symptoms completely. A follow-up appointment several years later confirmed that she experienced some obsessive thoughts, but ritualized infrequently. She described herself as quite satisfied with her improvement, which she estimated to be about 85%, compared to her OCD problem on first seeking treatment.

Case Study: Severe Multiple Washing and Checking Rituals

The 19-year-old young man described earlier was admitted to an inpatient unit where he received 24-hour-a-day supervision. One day's experience in the cafeteria convinced the staff that the other patients would not tolerate his grotesque eating patterns. Thus he spent all of his time on the unit, where rituals associated with eating, cleaning, and checking were monitored. Three sets of rituals were treated sequentially (Caldwell, McCrady, & Barlow, 1979). Since cleaning and washing rituals were the most severe, these were treated first. Prior to hospitalization, the patient had been spending up to 16 hours a day showering and engaging in other washing behavior. Several weeks before admission, he had begun avoiding the bathroom altogether and defecating and urinating in a corner of his closet, as noted at the beginning of the chapter. During baseline procedures in the hospital, the patient spent approximately 3 hours washing his hands. What followed was an elaborate 2-month-long ERP program in which contingency management procedures were introduced.

Throughout treatment, the patient was exposed once each hour for 16 hours a day to a series of contaminating substances (e.g., ashes, dirt, urine, and butter) that ordinarily produced hand washing. The patient was instructed to rub each substance over his arms and hands and let it remain for at least 30 seconds before excess was wiped (but not washed) off. As indicated in Figure 15.3, several additional steps were instituted during these 2 months. Since he spent long periods of time ritualizing while eating and showering, he was told (initially) that increased eating time would be contingent on decreased bathroom time. Specifically, he was given 30 minutes to shower, wash his hair, brush his teeth, and so on. He was further instructed (during Week 3) that response prevention would end when he could meet the 30-minute time limit, as well as refrain from defecating in his clothes for 7 days in a row (a practice he had taken up in the hospital to avoid bathroom rituals associated with bowel movements, since a convenient closet was no longer available). The third criterion involved sleeping in pajamas or other designated sleeping clothes, since he had begun wearing the same clothes 24 hours a day to avoid other rituals. During this phase, the patient experienced the contingency of reduced eating time (as well as the loss of piano-playing privileges) only once. As treatment progressed, staff involvement was systematically faded out, and he took increasing responsibility for his own behavior.

After completion of ERP for washing rituals, eating rituals were treated. Initially the patient ate only certain foods, as described earlier. While eating, he would engage in a variety of counting rituals with his utensils, attempt to expire all air from his lungs (which resulted in a variety of coughing and hissing sounds), and toss his head as if he were tossing his

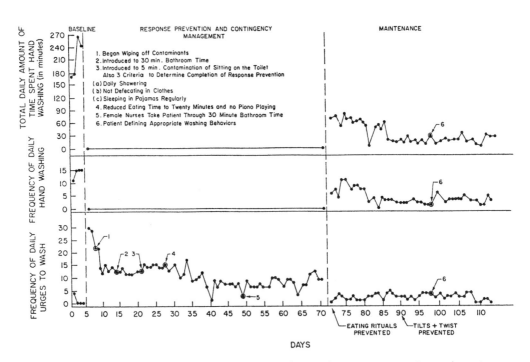

FIGURE 15.3. Hand-washing results during various phases of response prevention and contingency management treatment for a 19-year-old male with severe OCD. From Caldwell, McCrady, and Barlow (1979). Reprinted by permission of the authors.

long hair out of his face before taking a bite. A baseline phase was followed by a short phase in which his hair was tied in a ponytail. Monitoring of coughs, hisses, and head tosses demonstrated that his hair was not a factor in these rituals. During response prevention, the therapist stood directly behind him and gently held his head in place whenever head tossing was about to occur. He was also instructed not to cough or hiss at this time. Contingency management was also introduced, as indicated in Figure 15.3. As treatment progressed, staff members were faded out and the patient was gradually able to eat in the cafeteria, sitting with increasingly larger groups of people. Checking rituals associated with the wastebasket, curtains, and so forth, which were least severe in terms of interfering with functioning, were successfully treated during the last week of the program.

After a hospitalization that lasted approximately 4 months, the patient returned home. Although he returned to school and maintained his gains on rituals treated in the hospital for some time, he reestablished a variety of additional checking rituals that had been reported by his family but had not been present in the hospital. In addition, after several months in college, some ritualistic washing returned, although at a lower frequency and intensity than before hospitalization. He also began staring at his food during meals for long periods, although other eating rituals did not return.

Since this patient had one of the more severe cases of OCD we have encountered, Herculean efforts were required to attack the plethora of obsessions and compulsions. Despite 4 months of 24-hour-a-day supervision and active treatment, the patient was only 50–60% improved, relapsing to 20–30% improved after 6 months. In view of this patient's enormous suffering, any therapeutic gain was worth the effort. However, for some patients with extensive incapacitation from OCD who do not respond adequately to behavioral or medication treatment, it may be necessary to refer them for psychosurgery (Ananth, 1985).

Predictors of Outcome from Behavioral Treatment

Several investigators have now studied factors associated with the failure of ERP treatments for OCD. Surprisingly few predictors of outcome have emerged in this literature (Steketee & Shapiro, 1995). The difficulties in treating patients with overvalued ideation have been mentioned above and described in a seminal paper by Foa (1979). However, as Kozak and Foa (1994) reported in a later review of insight and OCD, poor insight has not actually predicted poor outcome in most studies, although very strong conviction that feared consequences would occur may be problematic (Foa, Abramowitz, Franklin, & Kozak, 1999). A major problem with this literature is that good measures of insight have only recently been developed. Thus more research using updated measures is needed to be certain of this finding. Another widely noted problem is the potential negative effect of initial depression on treatment outcome. Foa and her colleagues have provided some evidence suggesting that depressed patients habituate more slowly and less effectively to obsessive cues (Foa et al., 1983). However, a prospective study that tested medication and ERP effects in patients with OCD who were high and low on depression found no effect of depression on outcome (Foa, Kozak, Steketee, & McCarthy, 1992). Overall, studies that have examined mood state as a predictor of behavior therapy outcome have produced quite mixed findings, making it difficult to draw any conclusions (Steketee & Shapiro, 1995). However, the more severe version of depression reflected in a comorbid diagnosis of major depressive disorder does appear to adversely affect outcome (Eisen et al., 1999; Steketee et al., 2001). When severe depression accompanies OCD, it may be advisable to include interventions to address the depression.

Personality disorders have also been investigated as predictors of outcome in several studies. Some reports have identified conditions such as borderline (Hermesh, Shahar, & Munitz, 1987) and schizotypal (Minichiello et al., 1987) personality disorders as seriously interfering with successful treatment. The young man described above, who made only partial gains, may fit the description of a person with schizotypal personality disorder. Unfortunately, research efforts to replicate findings for personality disorders have been hampered by the relatively infrequent occurrence of any given personality disorder in clinical OCD samples of modest size (see Steketee et al., 2001). Thus results are again mixed and difficult to interpret. Only a large-scale multisite trial is likely to be able to provide definitive answers to questions about personality disorders that predict outcome.

Cases such as that of the young man described above and many of those summarized by Foa et al. (1985) are often failures from front-line clinicians, who then refer these difficult patients to specialized treatment centers. Thus it is possible that implementing approximations of these procedures in a standard everyday outpatient practice, with presumably less difficult patients, may produce superior results. Nevertheless, overall results from behavioral procedures, according to the studies reviewed above, are somewhat less favorable than for phobic disorders or panic disorder. As the principles established in Chapters 3 and 8 indicate, the most important task will be discovering how best to instill a sense of control and to shift attention away from negative affect associated with runaway cognitive processes. One such strategy may be cognitive therapy.

Cognitive Therapy

In recent years, the substantial interest in cognitive psychopathology of OCD has generated strong interest and research efforts to determine whether CT may be effective for this disorder. Standard ERP treatment undoubtedly alters some of the appraisals and beliefs we have described earlier for patients with OCD. For example, it seems very likely that ERP reduces patients' overestimation of the likelihood and severity of danger or harm from feared obsessive situations, especially in the case of contamination fears. Since most exposure therapies direct the patients to allow their fearful thoughts to occur freely, it may also attenuate some concerns about the importance or meaning of intrusive thoughts. Whether ERP also changes other types of beliefs, such as excessive responsibility, is not clear; to date, researchers have studied these effects only in a limited way. A recent study by Rhéaume and Ladouceur (2000) has provided initial evidence that change in beliefs preceded change in OCD symptoms in both ERP and CT, although the reverse sequence was also equally evident. Thus one important mechanism for change in both treatment methods may be cognitive change, but such change also appears to follow reductions in symptoms.

The first studies of CT were conducted by Emmelkamp and his colleagues (Emmelkamp & Beens, 1991; Emmelkamp, Visser, & Hoekstra, 1988), who tested the effect of rational–emotive therapy. They generally found that rational–emotive therapy was no more effective than ERP; but interestingly, however, it did produce significant reductions in OCD symptoms, though many clients continued to need further treatment during the follow-up period. When rational–emotive therapy was added to behavioral treatment, it did not confer any additional benefit. These studies were designed before recent elaborations of cognitive theories of OCD and before measures of cognition in OCD were developed. Thus the treatment method might not be considered very specific to the symptoms or psychopathology of OCD.

More recently, several controlled trials in different research settings have examined the effects of CT based on Beck's model. This method uses Socratic dialogue to identify and challenge beliefs that support OCD behavior, as well as a wide variety of additional cognitive challenge strategies designed to correct problematic beliefs of people with OCD. For example, patients who accept excessive responsibility for causing events beyond their control might be asked to indicate first what percentage of the responsibility they believe is their own fault. Then they are helped to identify all of the other people who realistically might bear any responsibility, and assign each the relevant portion of the "responsibility pie." When asked to reassign their own responsibility from what remains of the "pie," they are often surprised to find how little is left. Comparisons of old and new estimates help shape more realistic attitudes about their own responsibility.

In the Netherlands, van Oppen, de Haan, et al. (1995) developed a Beckian CT for OCD using the methods described above, and compared it with standard ERP for 57 patients with OCD. Patients in the CT group received exposure only in a very limited fashion, in the form of behavioral experiments conducted outside sessions to test their predictions about feared obsessive situations. Twelve sessions of CT appeared to produce more benefit than an equivalent amount of ERP, but the differences were not statistically significant. Fifty percent of patients in the CT group were considered recovered, compared to 28% in the ERP group. However, because the ERP treatment in this study was not as effective as in other research trials, it is possible that the effects of CT were overestimated. In France, Cottraux et al. (2001) found very good immediate and 1-year effects from a slightly longer (20-session) version of CT. Both CT and ERP produced equivalent and substantial benefits on obsessive and compulsive symptoms after 4 months and after 1 year, but CT produced more improvement in depressed mood. Both treatments also significantly reduced OCD beliefs, and changes in beliefs correlated with change in OCD symptoms for both therapies. Their design did not clarify whether change in beliefs was an important mechanism for producing change in OCD symptoms or merely a by-product of reduction in obsessive fears.

In Vancouver, McLean, Whittal, Thordarson, and Taylor (2001) compared a group version of CT to ERP. Treatment included 12 sessions conducted in a group format for 2.5 hours per session. Both treatments produced more benefit than a wait-list control condition, but ERP was marginally more effective than CT after treatment and at the 3-month follow-up. The degree of change after ERP was very similar to van Oppen, de Haan, et al.'s (1995) findings using the same measures of OCD symptoms, but results were considerably worse for CT. Furthermore, only one of several measures of beliefs associated with OCD changed with treatment, and there were no differences between ERP and CT on change in beliefs. These generally poor results for CT led the investigators to question whether CT, which must be individualized for each patient, should be delivered in a group format. Nonetheless, CT delivered in individual therapy appears to be a good alternative to ERP, especially for patients who are unwilling to engage in the latter more anxiety-provoking therapy. Combining CT with ERP has proven very effective in treating patients with OCD who had mental but not behavioral rituals ("pure obsessionals"). In a study by Freeston et al. (1997), the combination was substantially better than a wait-list control, and it produced an 84% success rate that was maintained 1 year later—an excellent outcome for this difficult-to-treat patient group.

Jones and Menzies (1998a) have provided some evidence that specialized CT without formal ERP for patients with contamination fears and washing rituals is also effective. Their treatment deviated somewhat from the CT used above in including techniques on attention focusing, corrective information from experts and from filmed interviews with workers who routinely exposed themselves to feared contaminants, and microbiological experiments to test for germs. These more novel methods designed to alter threat estimation were used in addition to the cognitive restructuring and probability estimation strategies used by other researchers of CT for OCD. The 21 patients given this therapy improved more than a wait-list control condition, but the degree of benefit was not as strong as patients treated in other ERP trials. It remains unclear whether CT is preferable to ERP for specific types of OCD symptoms, and prominent clinical researchers with experience in this area typically urge the use of a combination of these methods, rather than either one alone.

Pharmacological Treatment

Many different types of medications have been examined for efficacy in OCD, including anxiolytics, antidepressants, and even antipsychotic drugs. Generally these drugs have been studied in uncontrolled case studies or series of cases, and for the most part few medications that showed initial promise have withstood the more stringent tests of placebo-controlled trials. Exceptions to this are SRIs like clomipramine, and the even more specialized SSRIs, which include fluoxetine, fluvoxamine, sertraline, paroxetine, and citalopram. These medications have demonstrated good effects on OCD symptoms and in some cases have shown promise when combined with behavioral treatments. CT has not yet been tested in combination with medications to determine potentiating effects, probably because CT is a much newer psychosocial therapy for OCD. Below we examine the effects of SRIs and SSRIs compared to placebo and to other drugs. We also discuss the potential benefits and drawbacks of combining ERP with medications.

Effects of Serotonergic Medications for OCD

Pharmacological approaches to OCD initially focused on the SRI clomipramine. Early case reports and uncontrolled studies suggested its efficacy for OCD (see Ananth, 1985), and placebo-controlled trials and head-to-head comparisons with drugs made it clear that clomipramine was more effective than other types of tricyclics, such as nortriptyline and amitriptyline (e.g., Ananth, Pecknold, Van Den Steen, & Engelsmann, 1981; Mavissakalian, Turner, Michelson, & Jacob, 1985). There was some confusion about whether clomipramine actually improved OCD symptoms independently of its effect on depression. For example, Marks, Stern, Mawson, Cobb, and McDonald (1980) attributed most of clomipramine's effects to improvements in depression, since nondepressed patients with OCD improved very little. However, most studies indicted that clomipramine's benefits for OCD symptoms did not depend on improvement in depression (Insel et al., 1983; Mavissakalian, Turner, Michelson, & Jacob, 1985; Thorén, Åsberg, Cronholm, Jörnestedt, & Träskman, 1980).

   Although clomipramine has been the most extensively studied drug for OCD, according to meta-analyses and head-to-head comparisons, it does not appear to produce significantly stronger effects compared to other serotonergic medications (Abramowitz, 1997; Pigott & Seay, 1999; van Balkom et al., 1994). SSRIs have now largely replaced clomipramine as first-line drug treatments for OCD, because they are generally better tolerated by patients and show comparable antiobsessional effects. At the present time, fluvoxamine has probably been the most studied of the SSRI alternatives to clomipramine. Mundo, Maina, and Uslenghi's (2000) report of a multicenter trial comparing fluvoxamine with clomipramine indicated excellent results for both medications over a 10-week period— better than have been reported in many studies of medications. Patients' OCD symptoms were reduced by half on the Y-BOCS, and average scores were well below the clinical cutoff of 16. With its fewer side effects, fluvoxamine was also better tolerated by patients. In general, however, reviews of the comparative effectiveness of various SSRIs have indicated that there is relatively little difference among these medications. As with most drug treatments for emotional disorders, mechanisms of action are not yet clear. As Ananth (1985) pointed out, most studies indicate that SRI medication does not eradicate OCD or even the urge to perform the rituals. Rather, "the emotional force attached to the urge goes away" (p. 191). Further study of how these medications produce their effects will be useful in understanding the pathophysiology of OCD.

Effects of Medications and Behavioral Treatments

SSRI treatments have improved but not eliminated OCD symptoms, leaving open the question of whether their effects could be improved by the addition of behavior therapy. The first two studies of this type, both conducted in London, examined clomipramine and behavior therapy. Forty patients with OCD were randomly assigned to four groups, each receiving a variety of sequential treatments all of which included some behavior therapy (Marks et al., 1980; Rachman et al., 1979). Two groups received clomipramine, while the remaining two received placebo. The experimental design precluded a clean comparison of the separate and combined effect of medication and behavioral treatment, but the data did indicate that clomipramine had its primary effect on depressed mood, with weaker effects on obsessions and rituals. Behavioral treatments, on the other hand, manifested strong effects on compulsive behavior, but weaker effects on overall mood. The treatments did not seem to potentiate each other. After 2 years, the sample as a whole was significantly improved on all measures (Mawson, Marks, & Ramm, 1982), but any effects of clomipramine when compared to placebo had disappeared entirely. In fact, these effects had begun to diminish shortly after treatment, when the drug was discontinued. In fact, relapse appears to be a common outcome when SRI medications are withdrawn (O'Sullivan, Noshirvani, Marks, Monteiro, & Lelliot, 1991; Pato, Zohar-Kadouch, Zohar, & Murphy, 1988).

A second study by Marks et al. (1988) indicated that when combined with behavior therapy, clomipramine had a relatively limited additive effect that disappeared fairly quickly with additional behavior therapy. Again, exposure produced somewhat more benefit than clomipramine for OCD symptoms, and patients' depression did not influence benefits from either treatment.

Although the final outcome of a multicenter trial testing the separate and combined effects of clomipramine and intensive behavior therapy has not been published, preliminary findings are interesting. Foa, Liebowitz, and their colleagues found that combined treatment performed similarly to behavior therapy alone (responder rates were 71% and 85%, respectively) and better than clomipramine alone (50% responders) (Kozak, Liebowitz, & Foa, 2000). Having had behavior therapy appeared to protect patients from relapse when medications were withdrawn. The lower responder rates for combined therapy led the authors to raise concerns that adding SRIs to behavior therapy does little to enhance outcome, but adding behavior therapy to medications is helpful. Unfortunately, because this study excluded a large number of patients for various reasons, it is not clear how generalizable the finding will be to clinical samples.

Other studies have examined fluvoxamine in combination with behavioral treatment. Cottraux et al. (1989) contrasted this SSRI with behavior therapy versus the combination. All three groups improved approximately equally, with a slight advantage for the combined treatment at 6-month follow-up that disappeared by 11 months. More recently, van Balkom et al. (1998) reported that 16 weeks of fluvoxamine combined with either behavior therapy or CT produced positive benefits for OCD symptoms and also for depression. However, adding the drug to psychological treatments did not increase the degree of benefit beyond the psychological treatment alone—a finding similar to that reported by Kozak et al. (2000). Finally, Simpson, Gorfinkle, and Liebowitz (1999) used a small sample to determine whether the addition of an open trial of 17 sessions of ERP would reduce OCD symptoms further for those whose scores on the Y-BOCS indicated remaining clinically serious symptoms. All six patients who agreed to ERP treatment benefited, four rating themselves much improved and two very much improved, and all showing substantial reductions on the YBOCS.

Overall, findings from the limited trials of combined therapies do not indicate that combinations of medications and behavior therapy are better than behavioral treatment alone. They do appear to be better than medication alone, especially for preventing relapse. Even in the absence of empirical evidence arguing that behavioral treatments should be combined with medications, there may be some reasons to do so for individual patients. For example, for patients who are unwilling to engage in a treatment that is anxiety-provoking, medications that reduce discomfort from obsessions may enhance motivation for ERP. For patients who are already medicated, the very high likelihood of relapse on withdrawal suggests that behavior therapy may be useful in preventing relapse. This may be because patients learn specialized skills for tolerating obsessive anxiety and resisting rituals, which serve them well when stressors would otherwise overwhelm their capacity to cope.

References

Abel, G. G., Blanchard, E. B., & Barlow, D. H. (1981). The effects of stimulus modality, instructional set, and stimulus content on the objective measurement of sexual arousal in several paraphilias. *Behaviour Research and Therapy, 19,* 25–34.

Abel, J. L., & Borkovec, T. D. (1995). Generalizability of DSM-III-R generalized anxiety disorder to proposed DSM-IV criteria and cross-validation of proposed changes. *Journal of Anxiety Disorders, 9,* 303–315.

Abelson, J. L., & Nesse, R. M. (1994). Pentagastrin infusions in patients with panic disorder: I. Symptoms and cardiovascular responses. *Biological Psychiatry, 36,* 75–83.

Abelson, J. L., Nesse, R. M., & Vinik, A. J. (1994). Pentagastrin infusions in patients with panic disorder: II. Neuroendocrinology. *Biological Psychiatry, 36,* 84–96.

Abene, M. V., & Hamilton, J. D. (1998). Resolution of fear of flying with fluoxetine treatment. *Journal of Anxiety Disorders, 12,* 599–603.

Abercrombie, H. C., Larson, C. L., Ward, R. T., Schaefer, S. M., Holden, J. E., Perlman, S. B., Turski, P. A., Krahn, D. D., & Davidson, R. J. (1996). Metabolic rate in the amygdala predicts negative affect and depression severity in depressed patients: An FDG-PET study. *Neuroimage, 3*(2), S217.

Abrahamson, D. J., Barlow, D. H., & Abrahamson, L. S. (1989). Differential effects of performance demand and distraction on sexually functional and dysfunctional males. *Journal of Abnormal Psychology, 98*(3), 241–247.

Abrahamson, D. J., Barlow, D. H., Beck, J. G., Sakheim, D. K., & Kelly, J. P. (1985). The effects of attentional focus and partner responsiveness on sexual responding: Replication and extension. *Archives of Sexual Behavior, 14,* 361–371.

Abrahamson, D. J., Barlow, D. H., Sakheim, D. K., Beck, J. G., & Athanasiou, R. (1985). Effects of distraction on sexual responding in functional and dysfunctional men. *Behavior Therapy, 16,* 503–515.

Abramowitz, J. S. (1996). Variants of exposure and response prevention in the treatment of obsessive–compulsive disorder: A meta-analysis. *Behavior Therapy, 27,* 583–600.

Abramowitz, J. S. (1997). Effectiveness of psychological and pharmacological treatments for obsessive–compulsive disorder: A quantitative review. *Journal of Consulting and Clinical Psychology, 65,* 44–52.

Abramowitz, J. S., Brigidi, B. S., & Foa, E. B. (1999). Health concerns in patients with obsessive–compulsive disorder. *Journal of Anxiety Disorders, 13,* 529–539.

Abramowitz, J. S., & Foa, E. B. (1998). Worries and obsessions in individuals with obsessive–compulsive disorder with and without comorbid generalized anxiety disorder. *Behaviour Research and Therapy, 36,* 695–700.

Abramson, L. Y., Metalsky, G. I., & Alloy, L. B. (1989). Hopelessness and depression: A theory based subtype of depression. *Psychological Review, 96,* 358–392.

Abramson, L. Y., Seligman, M. E. P., & Teasdale, J. D. (1978). Learned helplessness in humans: Critique and reformulation. *Journal of Abnormal Psychology, 87,* 49–74.

Ader, R., & Grota, L. J. (1969). Effects of early experience on adrenocortical reactivity. *Physiology and Behavior, 4*, 303–305.

Adler, C. M., Craske, M. G., & Barlow, D. H. (1987). Relaxation-induced panic (RIP): When resting isn't peaceful. *Integrative Psychiatry, 5*, 94–112.

Agras, W. S. (1990). *The role of negative cognitions in panic disorder with or without agoraphobia* (Report to the DSM-IV Anxiety Disorders Work Group). Stanford, CA: Stanford University.

Agras, W. S., Chapin, H. N., & Oliveau, D. C. (1972). The natural history of phobia. *Archives of General Psychiatry, 26*, 315–317.

Agras, W. S., & Jacob, R. G. (1981). Phobia: Nature and measurement. In M. R. Mavissakalian & D. H. Barlow (Eds.), *Phobia: Psychological and pharmacological treatment.* New York: Guilford Press.

Agras, W. S., Leitenberg, H., & Barlow, D. H. (1968). Social reinforcement in the modification of agoraphobia. *Archives of General Psychiatry, 19*, 423–427.

Agras, W. S., Sylvester, D., & Oliveau, D. (1969). The epidemiology of common fears and phobia. *Comprehensive Psychiatry, 10*, 151–156.

Akhtar, S., Wig, N. N., Verma, V. K., Pershad, D., & Verma, S. K. (1975). A phenomenological analysis of symptoms in obsessive–compulsive neurosis. *British Journal of Psychiatry, 127*, 342–348.

Albano, A. M., Chorpita, B. F., & Barlow, D. H. (1996). Childhood anxiety disorders. In E. J. Mash & R. A. Barkley (Eds.), *Child psychopathology.* New York: Guilford Press.

Albano, A. M., & Detweiler, M. F. (in press). The developmental and clinical impact of social anxiety and social phobia in children and adolescents. In S. G. Hofmann & P. M. DiBartolo (Eds.), *From social anxiety to social phobia: Multiple perspectives.* Needham Heights, MA: Allyn & Bacon.

Alden, L. E., & Wallace, S. T. (1995). Social phobia and social appraisal in successful and unsuccessful social interactions. *Behaviour Research and Therapy, 33*, 497–505.

Allgulander, C. (1994). Suicide and mortality patterns in anxiety neurosis and depressive neurosis. *Archives of General Psychiatry, 51*, 708–712.

Allgulander, C., & Lavori, P. W. (1991). Excess mortality among 3302 patients with 'pure' anxiety neurosis. *Archives of General Psychiatry, 48*, 599–602.

Alloy, L. B., & Abramson, L. Y. (1979). Judgment of contingency in depressed and nondepressed students: Sadder but wiser? *Journal of Experimental Psychology: General, 108*(4), 441–485.

Alloy, L. B., & Clements, C. M. (1992). Illusion of control: Invulnerability to negative affect and depressive symptoms after laboratory and natural stressors. *Journal of Abnormal Psychology, 101*(2), 234–245.

Alloy, L. B., Kelly, K. A., Mineka, S., & Clements, C. M. (1990). Comorbidity of anxiety and depressive disorders: A helplessness–hopelessness perspective. In J. D. Maser & C. R. Cloninger (Eds.), *Comorbidity of mood and anxiety disorders.* Washington, DC: American Psychiatric Press.

American Psychiatric Association. (1980). *Diagnostic and statistical manual of mental disorders* (3rd ed.). Washington, DC: Author.

American Psychiatric Association. (1987). *Diagnostic and statistical manual of mental disorders* (3rd ed., rev.). Washington, DC: Author.

American Psychiatric Association. (1994). *Diagnostic and statistical manual of mental disorders* (4th ed.). Washington, DC: Author.

American Psychiatric Association. (1998). Practice guideline for the treatment of patients with panic disorder. American Journal of Psychiatry, *155*(Suppl. 5).

American Psychiatric Association. (2000). *Diagnostic and statistical manual of mental disorders* (4th ed., text revision). Washington, DC: Author.

Amering, M., Bankier, B., Berger, P., Griengle, H., Windhaber, J., & Katschnig, H. (1999). Panic disorder and cigarette smoking behavior. *Comprehensive Psychiatry, 40*, 35–38.

Amering, M., Katschnig, H., Berger, P., Windhaber, J., Baischer, W., & Dantendorfer, K. (1997). Embarrassment about the first panic attack predicts agoraphobia in panic disorder patients. *Behaviour Research and Therapy, 35*, 517–521.

Amies, P. L., Gelder, M. G., & Shaw, P. M. (1983). Social phobia: A comparative clinical study. *British Journal of Psychiatry, 142,* 174–179.

Ananth, J. (1985). Pharmaco-therapy of obsessive–compulsive disorder. In M. R. Mavissakalian, S. M. Turner, & L. Michelson (Eds.), *Obsessive–compulsive disorder: Psychological and pharmacological treatment.* New York: Plenum Press.

Ananth, J., Pecknold, J., Van Den Steen, N., & Engelsman, F. C. (1981). Double-blind comparative study of clomipramine and amitriptyline in obsessive neurosis. *Progress in Neuro-Psychopharmacology, 5,* 257–262.

Anastasiades, P., Clark, D. M., Salkovskis, P. M., Middleton, H., Hackmann, A., Gelder, M. G., & Johnson, D. W. (1990). Psychophysiological responses in panic and stress. *Journal of Psychophysiology, 4,* 331–338.

Anderson, D. J., Noyes, R., & Crowe, R. R. (1984). A comparison of panic disorder and generalized anxiety disorder. *American Journal of Psychiatry, 141,* 572–575.

Anderson, J. C., Williams, S. M., McGee, R., & Silva, P. A. (1987). DSM-III disorders in preadolescent children: Prevalence in a large sample from the general population. *Archives of General Psychiatry, 44,* 69–76.

Anderson, K. J. (1990). Arousal and the inverted-U hypothesis: A critique of Neiss's "reconceptualizing arousal. " *Psychological Bulletin, 107,* 96–100.

Andrews, G. (1990). Classification of neurotic disorders. *Journal of the Royal Society of Medicine, 83,* 606–607.

Andrews, G. (1996). Comorbidity in neurotic disorders: The similarities are more important than the differences. In R. M. Rapee (Ed.), *Current controversies in the anxiety disorders.* New York: Guilford Press.

Andrews, G., Stewart, G., Allen, R., & Henderson, A. S. (1990). The genetics of six neurotic disorders: A twin study. *Journal of Affective Disorders, 19,* 23–29.

Andrews, G., Stewart, G., Morris-Yates, A., Holt, P., & Henderson, A. S. (1990). Evidence for a general neurotic syndrome. *British Journal of Psychiatry, 157,* 6–12.

Andrews, V. H., & Borkovec, T. D. (1988). The differential effects of inductions of worry, somatic anxiety, and depression on emotional experience. *Journal of Behavior Therapy and Experimental Psychiatry, 19,* 21–26.

Anisman, H. (1984). Vulnerability to depression: Contribution of stress. In R. Post & J. Ballenger (Eds.), *Neurobiology of mood disorders.* Baltimore: Williams & Wilkins.

Ansseau, M., Papart, P., Gérard, M.-A., von Frenckell, R., & Franck, G. (1990). Controlled comparison of buspirone and oxazepam in generalized anxiety. *Neuropsychobiology, 24,* 74–78.

Antony, M. M. (1994). *Heterogeneity among specific phobia types in DSM-IV.* Unpublished doctoral dissertation, State University of New York at Albany.

Antony, M. M. (2000). [Frequency of specific phobia referrals in an anxiety disorders clinic]. Unpublished raw data, Anxiety Treatment and Research Centre, Hamilton, Ontario, Canada.

Antony, M. M., & Barlow, D. H. (1997). Social and specific phobias. In A. Tasman, J. Kay, & J. A. Lieberman (Eds.), *Psychiatry.* Philadelphia: Saunders.

Antony, M. M., Brown, T. A., & Barlow, D. H. (1997a). Heterogeneity among specific phobia types in DSM-IV. *Behaviour Research and Therapy, 35,* 1089–1100.

Antony, M. M., Brown, T. A., & Barlow, D. H. (1997b). Response to hyperventilation and 5.5% CO_2 inhalation of subjects with types of specific phobia, panic disorder, or no mental disorder. *American Journal of Psychiatry, 154,* 1089–1095.

Antony, M. M., Brown, T. A., Craske, M. G., Barlow, D. H., Mitchell, W. B., & Meadows, E. A. (1995). Accuracy of heartbeat perception in panic disorder, social phobia, and nonanxious subjects. *Journal of Anxiety Disorders, 9,* 355–371.

Antony, M. M., Craske, M. G., & Barlow, D. H. (1995a). *Mastery of your specific phobia: Client manual.* San Antonio, TX: Psychological Corporation/Graywind Publications Incorporated.

Antony, M. M., Craske, M. G., & Barlow, D. H. (1995b). *Mastery of your specific phobia: Client workbook.* San Antonio, TX: Psychological Corporation/Graywind Publications Incorporated.

Antony, M. M., McCabe, R. E., Leeuw, I., Sano, N., & Swinson, R. P. (2001). Effect of exposure and coping style on in vivo exposure for specific phobia of spiders. *Behaviour Research and Therapy, 39,* 1137–1150.

Antony, M. M., Meadows, E. A., Brown, T. A., & Barlow, D. H. (1994). Cardiac awareness before and after cognitive-behavioral treatment for panic disorder. *Journal of Anxiety Disorders, 8,* 341–350.

Antony, M. M., Moras, K., Meadows, E. A., Di Nardo, P. A., Utech, J. E., & Barlow, D. H. (1994). The diagnostic significance of the functional impairment and subjective distress criterion: An illustration with the DSM-III-R anxiety disorders. *Journal of Psychopathology and Behavioral Assessment, 16,* 253–263.

Antony, M. M., Orsillo, S. M., & Roemer, L. (Eds.). (2001). *Practitioner's guide to empirically-based measures of anxiety.* New York: Kluwer Academic/Plenum.

Antony, M. M., Roth, D., Swinson, R. P., Huta, V., & Devins, G. M. (1998). Illness intrusiveness in individuals with panic disorder, obsessive compulsive disorder, or social phobia. *Journal of Nervous and Mental Disease, 186,* 311–315.

Antony, M. M., & Swinson, R. P. (1996). Anxiety disorders and their treatment: A critical review of the evidence-based literature. Ottawa: Health Canada.

Antony, M. M., & Swinson, R. P. (2000). *Phobic disorders and panic in adults: A guide to assessment and treatment.* Washington, DC: American Psychological Association.

Apter, J. T., & Allen, L. A. (1999). Buspirone: Future directions. *Journal of Clinical Psychopharmacology, 19,* 86–93.

Arena, J. G., Blanchard, E. B., Andrasik, F., Cotch, B. A., & Myers, P. E. (1983). Reliability of psychophysiological assessment. *Behaviour Research and Therapy, 21,* 447–460.

Argyle, N., Deltito, J., Allerup, P., Maier, W., Albus, M., Nutzinger, D., Rasmussen, S., Ayuso, J. L., & Bech, P. (1991). The Panic-Associated Symptoms Scale: Measuring the severity of panic disorder. *Acta Psychiatrica Scandinavica, 83,* 20–26.

Arnow, B. A., Taylor, C. B., Agras, W. S., & Telch, M. J. (1985). Enhancing agoraphobia treatment outcome by changing couple communication patterns. *Behavior Therapy, 16,* 452–467.

Arntz, A. (1993). Endorphins stimulate approach behaviour, but do not reduce subjective fear: A pilot study. *Behaviour Research and Therapy, 31,* 403–405.

Aronson, T. A., & Craig, T. J. (1986). Cocaine precipitation of panic disorder. *American Journal of Psychiatry, 143,* 643–645.

Arrindell, W. A. (1980). Dimensional structure and psychopathology correlates of the Fear Survey Schedule (FSS-III) in a phobic population: A factorial definition of agoraphobia. *Behaviour Research and Therapy, 18,* 229–242.

Arrindell, W. A., Kolk, A. M., Pickersgill, M. J., & Hageman, W. J. J. M. (1993). Biological sex, sex role orientation, masculine sex role stress, dessimulation and self-reported fears. *Advances in Behaviour Research and Therapy, 15,* 103–146.

Arrindell, W. A., Mulkens, S., Kok, J., & Vollenbroek, J. (1999). Disgust sensitivity and the sex difference in fears to common indigenous animals. *Behaviour Research and Therapy, 37,* 273–280.

Ashton, C. H., Rawlins, M. D., & Tyrer, S. P. (1990). A double-blind placebo-controlled study of buspirone in diazepam withdrawal in chronic benzodiazepine users. *British Journal of Psychiatry, 157,* 232–238.

Asmundson, G. J. G. (1999). Anxiety sensitivity and chronic pain: Empirical findings, clinical implications, and future directions. In S. Taylor (Ed.), *Anxiety sensitivity: Theory, research, and treatment of the fear of anxiety.* Mahwah, NJ: Erlbaum.

Asmundson, G. J. G., Sandler, L. S., Wilson, K. G., & Walker, J. R. (1992). Selective attention toward physical threat in patients with panic disorder. *Journal of Anxiety Disorders, 6*(4), 295–303.

Asmundson, G. J. G., & Stein, M. B. (1994a). Resting cardiovascular measures in patients with panic disorder and social phobia and health control subjects: Relationship to habitual exercise frequency. *Anxiety, 1,* 26–30.

Asmundson, G. J. G., & Stein, M. B. (1994b). Triggering the false suffocation alarm in panic disorder patients by using a voluntary breath-holding procedure. *American Journal of Psychiatry, 151,* 264–266.

Asmundson, G. J. G., & Stein, M. B. (1994c). A preliminary analysis of pulmonary function in panic disorder: Implications for the dyspnea–fear theory. *Journal of Anxiety Disorders, 8*(1), 63–39.

Asmundson, G. J. G., & Stein, M. B. (1994–1995). Dot-probe evaluation of cognitive processing biases in patients with panic disorder: A failure to replicate and extend. *Anxiety, 1,* 123–128.

Aufdembrinke, B. (1998). Abecarnil, a new beta-carboline, in the treatment of anxiety disorders. *British Journal of Psychiatry,* (Suppl. 34), 55–63.

Austin, L. S., Lydiard, R. B., Fossey, M. D., & Zealberg, J. J. (1990). Panic and phobic disorders in patients with obsessive compulsive disorder. *Journal of Clinical Psychiatry, 51,* 456–458.

Babcock, H. H., & Powell, D. H. (1982). Vasovagal fainting: Deconditioning an autonomic syndrome. *Psychosomatics, 23,* 969–970.

Bach, A. K., Brown, T. A., & Barlow, D. H. (1999). The effects of false negative feedback on efficacy expectancies and sexual arousal in sexually functional males. *Behavior Therapy, 30,* 79–95.

Bachofen, M., Nakagawa, A., Marks, I. M., Park, J.-M., Greist, J. H., Baer, L., Wenzel, K. W., Parkin, J. R., & Dottl, S. L. (1999). Home self-assessment and self-treatment of obsessive–compulsive disorder using a manual and a computer-conducted telephone interview: Replication of a U.K.–U.S. study. *Journal of Clinical Psychiatry, 60,* 545–549.

Baddeley, A. D. (1986). *Working memory.* Oxford: Clarendon Press.

Baer, L. (1994). Factor analysis of symptom subtypes of obsessive compulsive disorder and their relation to personality and tic disorders. *Journal of Clinical Psychiatry, 55,* 18–23.

Baer, L., & Jenike, M. (1992). Personality disorders: Obsessive compulsive disorder. *Psychiatric Clinics of North America, 15,* 803–812.

Baker, B. L., Cohen, D. C., & Saunders, J. T. (1973). Self-directed desensitization for acrophobia. *Behaviour Research and Therapy, 11,* 79–89.

Baker, S. L., Patterson, M. D., & Barlow, D. H. (in press). Panic disorder and agoraphobia. In M. M. Antony & D. H. Barlow (Eds.), *Handbook of assessment and treatment planning: Empirically supported strategies for psychological disorders.* New York: Guilford Press.

Bakish, D., Hooper, C. L., Filteau, M.-J., Charbonneau, Y., Fraser, G., West, D. L., Thibaudeau, C., & Raine, D. (1996). A double-blind placebo-controlled trial comparing fluvoxamine and imipramine in the treatment of panic disorder with or without agoraphobia. *Psychopharmacology Bulletin, 32,* 135–141.

Bakish, D., Saxena, B. M., Bowden, R., & D'Souza, J. (1993). Reversible monoamine oxidase-A inhibitors in panic disorder. *Clinical Neuropsychopharacology, 16*(Suppl. 2), S77–S82.

Ball, S. G., Baer, L., & Otto, N. W. (1996). Symptom subtypes of obsessive–compulsive disorder in behavioral treatment studies: A quantitative review. *Behaviour Research and Therapy, 34,* 47–51.

Ballenger, J. C. (1994). Overview of pharmacotherapy of panic disorder. In B. E. Wolfe & J. D. Maser (Eds.), *Treatment of panic disorder: A consensus development conference.* Washington, DC: American Psychiatric Press.

Ballenger, J. C. (1997). Panic disorder in the medical setting. *Journal of Clinical Psychiatry, 58*(Suppl. 2), 13–17.

Ballenger, J. C., Burrows, G. D., DuPont, R. L., Lesser, I. M., Noyes, R., Pecknold, J. C., Rifkin, A., & Swinson, R. P. (1988). Aprazolam in panic disorder and agoraphobia: Results from a multicenter trial. I: Efficacy in short-term treatment. *Archives of General Psychiatry, 45,* 413–422.

Ballenger, J. C., McDonald, S., Noyes, R., Rickels, K., Sussman, N., Woods, S., Patin, J., & Singer, J. (1991). The first double-blind, placebo-controlled trial of a partial benzodiazepine agonist abecarnil (ZK 112-119) in generalized anxiety disorder. *Psychopharmacology Bulletin, 27,* 171–179.

Ballenger, J. C., Peterson, G. A., Laraia, M., Hucek, A., Lake, C. R., Jimerson, D., Cox, D. J., Trockman, C., Shipe, J. R., & Wilkinson, C. (1984). A study of plasma catecholamines in agoraphobia and the relationship of serum, tricyclic levels to treatment response. In J. C. Ballenger (Ed.), *Biology of agoraphobia.* Washington, DC: American Psychiatric Press.

Ballenger, J. C., Wheadon, D. E., Steiner, M., Bushnell, W., & Gergel, I. (1998). Double-blind fixed-dose, placebo controlled study of paroxetine in the treatment of panic disorder. *American Journal of Psychiatry, 155,* 36–42.

Balster, R. L. (1990). Abuse potential of buspirone and related drugs. *Journal of Clinical Psychopharmacology, 10*(Suppl. 3), 31–37.

Bandelow, B. (1995). Assessing the efficacy of treatments for panic disorder and agoraphobia: I. The Panic and Agoraphobia Scale. *International Clinical Psychopharmacology, 10,* 73–81.

Bandelow, B. (1999). *Panic and Agoraphobia Scale (PAS) manual.* Seattle, WA: Hogrefe & Huber.

Bandura, A. (1969). *Principles of behavior modification.* New York: Holt, Rinehart & Winston.

Bandura, A. (1977). *Social learning theory.* Englewood Cliffs, NJ: Prentice-Hall.

Bandura, A. (1986). *Social foundations of thought and action.* Englewood Cliffs. NJ: Prentice-Hall.

Bandura, A. (1988). Self-efficacy conception of anxiety. *Anxiety Research, 1,* 77–98.

Bandura, A., Adams, N. E., Hardy, A. B., & Howells, G. N. (1980). Tests of the generality of self-efficacy theory. *Cognitive Therapy and Research, 4,* 39–66.

Bandura, A., Taylor, C. B., Williams, S. L., Mefford, I. N., & Barchas, J. D. (1985). Catecholamine secretion as a function of perceived coping self-efficacy. *Journal of Consulting and Clinical Psychology, 53,* 406–414.

Barfield, R., & Sachs, B. (1968). Sexual behavior: Stimulation by painful electric shock to skin in male rats. *Science, 161,* 392–395.

Barloon, T. J., & Noyes, R., Jr. (1997). Charles Darwin and panic disorder. *Journal of the American Medical Association, 277*(2), 138–141.

Barlow, D. H. (1978). Aversive procedures. In W. S. Agras (Ed.), *Behavior modification: Principles and clinical applications* (2nd ed.). Boston: Little, Brown.

Barlow, D. H. (Ed.). (1981). *Behavioral assessment of adult disorders.* New York: Guilford Press.

Barlow, D H. (1986). Causes of sexual dysfunction: The role of anxiety and cognitive interference. *Journal of Consulting and Clinical Psychology, 54,* 140–148.

Barlow, D. H. (1988). *Anxiety and its disorders: The nature and treatment of anxiety and panic.* New York: Guilford Press.

Barlow, D. H. (1991a). Disorders of emotion. *Psychological Inquiry, 2*(1), 58–71.

Barlow, D. H. (1991b). The nature of anxiety: Anxiety, depression, and emotional disorders. In R. M. Rapee & D. H. Barlow (Eds.), *Chronic anxiety: Generalized anxiety disorder and mixed anxiety–depression.* New York: Guilford Press.

Barlow, D. H. (2000). Unraveling the mysteries of anxiety and its disorders from the perspective of emotion theory. *American Psychologist, 55*(11), 1247–1263.

Barlow, D. H. (Ed.). (2001). *Clinical handbook of psychological disorders: A step-by-step treatment manual* (3rd ed.). New York: Guilford Press.

Barlow, D. H., Blanchard, E. B., Vermilyea, J. A., Vermilyea, B. B., & Di Nardo, P. A. (1986). Generalized anxiety and generalized anxiety disorder: Description and reconceptualization. *American Journal of Psychiatry, 143,* 40–44.

Barlow, D. H., Brown, T. A., & Craske, M. C. (1994). Definitions of panic attacks and panic disorder in the DSM-IV: Implications for research. *Journal of Abnormal Psychology, 103*(3), 553–564.

Barlow, D. H., Chorpita, B. F., & Turovsky, J. (1996). Fear, panic, anxiety, and disorders of emotion. In D. A. Hope (Ed.), *Nebraska Symposium on Motivation: Vol. 43. Perspectives on anxiety, panic, and fear.* Lincoln: University of Nebraska Press.

Barlow, D. H., Cohen, A. S., Waddell, M., Vermilyea, J. A., Klosko, J. S., Blanchard, E. B., & Di Nardo, P. A. (1984). Panic and generalized anxiety disorders: Nature and treatment. *Behavior Therapy, 15,* 431–449.

Barlow, D. H., & Craske, M. G. (1988b). The phenomenology of panic. In S. Rachman & J. D. Maser (Eds.), *Panic: Psychological perspectives*. Hillsdale, NJ: Erlbaum.

Barlow, D. H., & Craske, M. G. (2000). *Mastery of your anxiety and panic (MAP-3): Client work-book for anxiety and panic* (3rd ed.). San Antonio, TX: Graywind/Psychological Corporation.

Barlow, D. H., Craske, M. G., Cerny, J. A., & Klosko, J. S. (1989). Behavioral treatment of panic disorder. *Behavior Therapy, 20*, 261–282.

Barlow, D. H., Di Nardo, P. A., Vermilyea, B. B., Vermilyea, J. A., & Blanchard, E. B. (1986). Comorbidity and depression among the anxiety disorders: Issues in diagnosis and classification. *Journal of Nervous and Mental Disease, 174*, 63–72.

Barlow, D. H., & Durand, V. M. (1999). *Abnormal psychology: An integrative approach* (2nd ed.). Pacific Grove, CA: Brooks/Cole.

Barlow, D. H., Gorman, J. M., Shear, M. K., & Woods, S. W. (2000). Cognitive-behavioral therapy, imipramine, or their combination for panic disorder: A randomized controlled trial. *Journal of the American Medical Association, 283*, 2529–2536.

Barlow, D. H., Hayes, S. C., & Nelson, R. O. (1984). *The scientist–practitioner: Research and accountability in clinical and educational settings*. New York: Pergamon Press.

Barlow, D. H., & Hersen, M. (1984). *Single case experimental designs: Strategies for studying behavior change* (2nd ed.). New York: Pergamon Press.

Barlow, D. H., & Lehman, C. (1996). Advances in the psychosocial treatment of anxiety disorders: Implications for national health care. *Archives of General Psychiatry, 53*, 727–735.

Barlow, D. H., Levitt, J. T., & Bufka, L. F. (1999). The dissemination of empirically supported treatments: A view to the future. *Behaviour Research and Therapy, 37*, S147–S162.

Barlow, D. H., & Mavissakalian, M. R. (1981). Directions in the assessment and treatment of phobia: The next decade. In M. R. Mavissakalian & K. H. Barlow (Eds.), *Phobia: Psychological and pharmacological treatment*. New York: Guilford Press.

Barlow, D. H., O'Brien, G. T., & Last, C. G. (1984). Couples treatment of agoraphobia. *Behavior Therapy, 15*, 41–58.

Barlow, D. H., O'Brien, G. T., Last, C. G., & Holden, A. E. (1983). Couples treatment of agoraphobia: Initial outcome. In K. D. Craig & R. I. McMahon (Eds.), *Advances in clinical behavior therapy*. New York: Brunner/Mazel.

Barlow, D. H., Rapee, R. M., & Brown, T. A. (1992). Behavioral treatment of generalized anxiety disorder. *Behavior Therapy, 23*, 551–570.

Barlow, D. H., Sakheim, D. K., & Beck, J. G. (1983). Anxiety increases sexual arousal. *Journal of Abnormal Psychology, 92*, 49–54.

Barlow, D. H., Vermilyea, J. A., Blanchard, E. B., Vermilyea, B. B., Di Nardo, P. A., & Cerny, J. A. (1985). The phenomenon of panic. *Journal of Abnormal Psychology, 94*, 320–328.

Barlow, D. H., & Waddell, M. T. (1985). Agoraphobia. In D. H. Barlow (Ed.), *Clinical handbook of psychological disorders: A step-by-step treatment manual*. New York: Guilford Press.

Barlow, D. H., & Wolfe, B. E. (1981). Behavioral approaches to anxiety disorders: A report on the NIMH–SUNY Albany research conference. *Journal of Consulting and Clinical Psychology, 49*, 448–454.

Barnard, P. J., & Teasdale, J. D. (1991). Interacting cognitive subsystems: A systematic approach to cognitive–affective interaction and change. *Cognition and Emotion, 5*(1), 1–39.

Barnett, M. A., King, L. M., & Howard, J. A. (1979). Inducing affect about self or other: Effects on generosity of children. *Developmental Psychology, 15*(2), 164–167.

Barrett, P. M., Dadds, M. R., & Rapee, R. M. (1996). Family treatment of childhood anxiety: A controlled trial. *Journal of Consulting and Clinical Psychology, 64*, 333–342.

Barrett, P. M., Rapee, R. M., Dadds, M. M., & Ryan, S. M. (1996). Family enhancement of cognitive style in anxious and aggressive children. *Journal of Abnormal Child Psychology, 24*, 187–203.

Barsky, A. J., Cleary, P. D., Sarnie, M. K., & Ruskin, J. N. (1994). Panic disorder, palpitations, and the awareness of cardiac activity. *Journal of Nervous and Mental Disease, 182*(2), 63–71.

Barsky, A. J., Delamater, B. A., & Orav, J. E. (1999). Panic disorder patients and their medical care. *Psychosomatics, 40*, 50–56.

Bartol, C. R. (1975). Extraversion and neuroticism and nicotine, caffeine, and drug intake. *Psychological Reports, 36*, 1007–1010.

Başoğlu, M., Lax, T., Kasvikis, Y., & Marks, I. M. (1988). Predictors of improvement in obsessive–compulsive disorder. *Journal of Anxiety Disorders, 2*, 299–317.

Başoğlu, M., Marks, I. M., & Sengun, S. (1992). A prospective study of panic and anxiety in agoraphobia with panic disorder. *British Journal of Psychiatry, 160*, 57–64.

Bates, L. W., McGlynn, F. D., Montgomery, R. W., & Mattke, T. (1996). Effects of eye-movement desensitization versus no treatment on repeated measures of fear of spiders. *Journal of Anxiety Disorders, 6*, 555–569.

Baxter, L., Schwartz, J., Bergman, K., Szuba, M., Guze, B., Mazziota, J., Alazraki, A., Selin, C., Huan-Kwang, F., Munford, P., & Phelps, M. (1992). Caudate glucose metabolic rate changes with both drug and behavior therapy for obsessive–compulsive disorder. *Archives of General Psychiatry, 49*, 681–689.

Beauclair, L., Fontaine, R., Annable, L., Holobow, N., & Chouinard, G. (1994). Clonazepam in the treatment of panic disorder: A double-blind, placebo-controlled trial investigating the correlation between clonazepam concentrations in plasma and clinical response. *Journal of Clinical Psychopharmacology, 14*, 111–118.

Beaumont, G. (1977). A large open multicenter trial of clomipramine in the management of phobic disorders. *Journal of International Medical Research, 5*, 116–129.

Bechara, A., Tranel, D., Damasio, H., Adolphs, R., Rockland, C., & Dumasir, A. R. (1995). Double dissociation of conditioning and declarative knowledge relative to the amygdala and hippocampus in humans. *Science, 269*, 1115–1118.

Beck, A. T. (1972). *Depression: Causes and treatment*. Philadelphia: University of Pennsylvania Press.

Beck, A. T. (1993). Cognitive therapy: Past, present and future. *Journal of Consulting and Clinical Psychology, 61*(2), 194–198.

Beck, A. T., & Clark, D. A. (1997). An information processing model of anxiety: Automatic and strategic processes. *Behaviour Research and Therapy, 35*, 40–58.

Beck, A. T., & Emery, G., with Greenberg, R. L. (1985). *Anxiety disorders and phobias: A cognitive perspective*. New York: Basic Books.

Beck, A. T., Epstein, N., Brown, G., & Steer, R. A. (1988). An inventory for measuring clinical anxiety: Psychometric properties. *Journal of Consulting and Clinical Psychology, 56*, 893–897.

Beck, A. T., Sokol, L., Clark, D. A., Berchick, R., & Wright, F. (1992). A crossover study of focused cognitive therapy for panic disorder. *American Journal of Psychiatry, 149*, 778–783.

Beck, A. T., & Steer, G. (1987). *Manual for the revised Beck Depression Inventory*. San Antonio, TX: Psychological Corporation.

Beck, A. T., Steer, R. A., Sanderson, W. C., & Skeie, T. M. (1991). Panic disorder and suicidal ideation and behavior: Discrepant findings in psychiatric outpatients. *American Journal of Psychiatry, 148*, 1195–1199.

Beck, J. G., & Barlow, D. H. (1984). Current conceptualizations of sexual dysfunction: A review and an alternative perspective. *Clinical Psychology Review, 4*, 363–378.

Beck, J. G., & Barlow, D. H. (1986a). The effects of anxiety and attentional focus on sexual responding: I. Physiological patterns in erectile dysfunction. *Behaviour Research and Therapy, 24*, 9–17.

Beck, J. G., & Barlow, D. H. (1986b). The effects of anxiety and attentional focus on sexual responding: II. Cognitive and affective patterns in erectile dysfunction. *Behaviour Research and Therapy, 24*, 9–26.

Beck, J. G., Barlow, D. H., & Sakheim, D. K. (1983). The effects of attentional focus and partner arousal on sexual responding in functional and dysfunctional men. *Behaviour Research and Therapy, 21*, 1–8.

Beck, J. G., Barlow, D. H., Sakheim, D. K., & Abrahamson, D. J. (1984). A cognitive processing account of anxiety and sexual arousal: The role of selective attention, thought content, and affective states. Paper presented at the 92nd Annual Convention of the American Psychological Association, Toronto.

Beck, J. G., Barlow, D. H., Sakheim, D. K., & Abrahamson, D. J. (1987). Shock threat and sexual arousal: The role of selective attention, thought content, and affective states. *Psychophysiology, 24,* 165–172.

Beck, J. G., & Berisford, M. A. (1992). The effects of caffeine on panic patients: Response components of anxiety. *Behavior Therapy, 23*(3), 405–422.

Beck, J. G., Berisford, M. A., Taegtmeyer, H., & Bennett, A. (1990). Panic symptoms in chest pain without coronary artery disease: A compaarison with panic disorder. *Behavior Therapy, 21,* 241–252.

Beck, J. G., & Shipherd, J. C. (1997). Repeated exposure to interoceptive cues: Does habituation of fear occur in panic disorder patients? A preliminary report. *Behaviour Research and Therapy, 35,* 551–557.

Beck, J. G., Shipherd, J. C., & Zebb, B. J. (1997). How does interoceptive exposure for panic disorder work?: An uncontrolled case study. *Journal of Anxiety Disorders, 11,* 541–556.

Beck, J. G., & Stanley, M. A. (1997). Anxiety disorders in the elderly: The emerging role of behavior therapy. *Behavior Therapy, 28,* 83–100.

Beck, J. G., Stanley, M. A., & Zebb, B. J. (1995). Psychometric properties of the Penn State Worry Questionnaire in older adults. *Journal of Clinical Geropsychology, 1,* 33–42.

Beck, J. G., Stanley, M. A., & Zebb, B. J. (1996). Characteristics of generalized anxiety disorder in older adults: A descriptive study. *Behaviour Research and Therapy, 34,* 225–234.

Beck, J. G., Taegtmeyer, H., Berisford, M. A., & Bennett, A. (1989). Chest pain without coronary artery disease: An exploratory comparison with panic disorder. *Journal of Psychopathology and Behavioral Assessment, 11*(3), 209–220.

Becker, E. S., Roth, W., Andrich, M., & Margraf, J. (1999). Explicit memory in anxiety disorders. *Journal of Abnormal Psychology, 108,* 153–163.

Becker, R. E., & Heimberg, R. G. (1988). Assessment of social skills. In A. S. Bellack & M. Hersen (Eds.), *Behavioral assessment: A practical handbook* (3rd ed.). New York: Pergamon Press.

Beckham, J. C., Vrana, S. R., May, J. G., Gustafson, D. J., & Smith, G. R. (1990). Emotional processing and fear measurement synchrony as indicators of treatment outcome in fear of flying. *Journal of Behavior Therapy and Experimental Psychiatry, 21,* 153–162.

Beech, H. R., & Vaughn, M. (1978). *Behavioral treatment of obsessional states.* New York: Wiley.

Beidel, D. C., Borden, J. W., Turner, S. M., & Jacob, R. G. (1989). The Social Phobia and Anxiety Inventory: Concurrent validity with a clinic sample. *Behaviour Research and Therapy, 27,* 573–576.

Beidel, D. C., & Turner, S. M. (1992). Scoring the Social Phobia and Anxiety Inventory: Comments on Herbert et al. (1991). *Journal of Psychopathology and Behavioral Assessment, 14,* 377–379.

Beidel, D. C., & Turner, S. M. (1998). *Shy children, phobic adults. Nature and treatment of social phobia.* Washington, DC: American Psychological Association.

Beidel, D. C., Turner, S. M., & Dancu, C. V. (1985). Physiological, cognitive, and behavioral aspects of social anxiety. *Behaviour Research and Therapy, 23,* 109–117.

Beidel, D. C., Turner, S. M., & Morris, T. L. (1995). A new inventory to assess childhood social anxiety and phobia: The Social Phobia and Anxiety Inventory for Children. *Psychological Assessment, 7,* 73–79.

Beidel, D. C., Turner, S. M., Jacob, R. G., & Cooley, M. R. (1989). Assessment of social phobia: Reliability of an impromptu speech task. *Journal of Anxiety Disorders, 3,* 149–158.

Beidel, D. C., Turner, S. M., Stanley, M. A., & Dancu, C. V. (1989). The Social Phobia and Anxiety Inventory: Concurrent and external validity. *Behavior Therapy, 20,* 417–427.

Beitman, B. D., DeRosear, L., Basha, I., Flaker, G., & Corcoran, C. (1987). Panic disorder in cardiology patients with atypical or non-anginal chest pain: A pilot study. *Journal of Anxiety Disorders, 1,* 277–282.

Beitman, B. D., Lamberti, J. W., Mukerji, V., DeRosear, L., Basha, I., & Schmid, L. (1987). Panic disorder in chest pain patients with angiographically normal coronary arteries: A pilot study. *Psychosomatics, 28,* 480–484.

Bell, C. C., & Jenkins, E. J. (1993). Community violence and children on Chicago's south side. *Psychiatry: Interpersonal and Biological Processes, 56*, 46–54.

Bellodi, L., Perna, G., Caldirola, D., Arancio, C., Bertani, A., & DiBella, D. (1998). CO_2 induced panic attacks: A twin study. *American Journal of Psychiatry, 155*, 1184–1188.

Bellodi, L., Sciuto, G., Diaferia, G., Ronchi, P., & Smeraldi, E. (1992). Psychiatric disorders in the families of patients with obsessive–compulsive disorder. *Psychiatry Research, 42*, 111–120.

Benca, R., Matuzas, W., & Al-Sadir, J. (1986). Social phobia, MVP, and response to imipramine. *Journal of Clinical Psychopharmacoloy, 6*, 50–51.

Benedikt, V. (1870). Ober platzschwindel. *Allgemeine Wiener Medizinische Zeitung, 15*, 488.

Benshoof, B. G. (1987). *A comparison of anxiety and depressive symptomatology in the anxiety and affective disorders.* Unpublished doctoral dissertation, State University of New York at Albany.

Berg, C. Z., Shapiro, N., Chambless, D. L., & Ahrens, A. H. (1998). Are emotions frightening?: II. An analogue study of fear of emotion, interpersonal conflict, and panic onset. *Behaviour Research and Therapy, 36*, 3–15.

Bergman, R. L., & Craske, M. G. (1994, November). *Covert verbalization and imagery in worry activity.* Poster session presented at the 28th Annual Convention of the Association for Advancement of Behavior Therapy, San Diego, CA.

Berkson, J. (1946). Limitations of the application of fourfold table analysis to hospital data. *Biometrics Bulletin, 2*, 47–53.

Bernstein, D. A., Borkovec, T. D., & Hazlett-Stevens, H. (2000). *New directions in progressive relaxation training: A guidebook for helping professionals.* Westport, CT: Praeger.

Berscheid, E., & Walster, E. (1974). A little bit about love. In T. Huston (Ed.), *Foundations of interpersonal attraction.* New York: Academic Press.

Bhagwanjee, A., Parekh, A., Paruk, Z., Petersen, I., & Subedar, H. (1998). Prevalence of minor psychiatric disorders in an adult African rural community in South Africa. *Psychological Medicine, 28*, 1137–1147.

Biaggio, M. K. (1987). Therapeutic management of anger. *Clinical Psychology Review, 7*, 663–675.

Bibb, J. L., & Chambless, D. L. (1986). Alcohol use and abuse among diagnosed agoraphobics. *Behaviour Research and Therapy, 24*, 49–58.

Biber, B., & Alkin, T. (1999). Panic disorder subtypes: Differential responses to CO_2 challenge. *American Journal of Psychiatry, 156*, 739–744.

Biederman, J., Rosenbaum, J., Bolduc-Murphy, E. A., Faraone, S. V., Chaloff, J., Hirshfeld, D. R., & Kagan, J. (1993). A three-year follow-up of children with and without behavioral inhibition. *Journal of the American Academy of Child and Adolescent Psychiatry, 32*, 814–821.

Biederman, J., Rosenbaum, J., Hirshfeld, D. R., Faraone, S. V., Bolduc, E. A., Gersten, M., Meminger, S. R., Kagan, F., Snidman, N., & Reznick, S. (1990). Psychiatric correlates of behavioral inhibition in young children of parents with and without psychiatric disorders. *Archives of General Psychiatry, 47*, 21–26.

Bieling, P. J., Antony, M. M., & Swinson, R. P. (1998). The State–Trait Anxiety Inventory, Trait Version: Structure and content re-examined. *Behaviour Research and Therapy, 36*, 777–788.

Bignami, G. (1965). Selection for high and low rates of conditioning in the rat. *Animal Behavior, 13*, 221–227.

Bilsbury, C., & Morley, S. (1979). Obsessional slowness: A meticulous replication. *Behaviour Research and Therapy, 17*, 405–408.

Biocca, L. J. (1985). The relationship among locus of control, perceived parenting, and sex-role attributes in adolescence. *Dissertation Abstracts International, 47*, 2193B.

Birchall, H. M. (1996). Just how common are common fears? *Anxiety, 2*, 303–304.

Bjork, R. A., & Bjork, E. L. (1992). A new theory of disuse and an old theory of stimulus fluctuation. In A. Healy, S. Kosslyn, & R. Shiffrin (Eds.), *From learning processes to cognitive processes: Essays in honor of William Estes* (Vol. 2). Hillsdale, NJ: Erlbaum.

Black, A. (1974). The natural history of obsessional patterns. In H. R. Beech (Ed.), *Obsessional states.* London: Methuen.

Black, B., Uhde, T. W., & Tancer, M. E. (1992). Fluoxetine for the treatment of social phobia [Letter to the editor]. *Journal of Clinical Psychopharmacology, 12*, 293–295.

Black, D. W., Monahan, P., Gable, J., Blum, N., Clancy, G., & Baker, P. (1998). Hoarding and treatment response in 38 nondepressed subjects with obsessive–compulsive disorder. *Journal of Clinical Psychiatry, 59*, 420–425.

Black, D. W., Monahan, P., Wesner, R., Gabel, J., & Bowers, W. (1996). The effect of fluvoxamine, cognitive therapy, and placebo on abnormal personality traits in 44 patients with panic disorder. *Journal of Personality Disorders, 10*, 185–194.

Black, D. W., Noyes, R., Pfohl, B., Goldstein, R., & Blum, N. (1993). Personality disorder in obsessive–compulsive volunteers, well comparison subjects, and their first-degree relatives. *American Journal of Psychiatry, 150*, 1226–1232.

Black, D. W., Wesner, R., Bowers, W., & Gabel, J. (1993). A comparison of fluvoxamine, cognitive therapy, and placebo in the treatment of panic disorder. *Archives of General Psychiatry, 50*, 44–50.

Black, D. W., Wesner, R. B., Gabel, J., Bowers, W., & Monahan, P. (1994). Predictors of short-term treatment response in 66 patients with panic disorder. *Journal of Affective Disorders, 30*, 233–241.

Black, J. L., & Keane, T. M. (1982). Implosive therapy in the treatment of combat related fears in a World War II veteran. *Journal of Behavior Therapy and Experimental Psychiatry, 13*, 163–165.

Blake, D. D., Weathers, F. W., Nagy, L. M., Kaloupek, D. G., Charney, D. S., & Keane, T. M. (1990). *The Clinician-Administered PTSD Scale—IV*. Boston: National Center for PTSD—Behavioral Science Division.

Blanchard, E. B., & Epstein, L. H. (1977). *A biofeedback primer*. Reading, MA: Addison-Wesley.

Blanchard, E. B., Gerardi, R. J., Kolb, L. C., & Barlow, D. H. (1986). The utility of the Anxiety Disorders Interview Schedule (ADIS) in the diagnosis of the post-traumatic stress disorder (PTSD) in Vietnam veterans. *Behaviour Research and Therapy, 24*, 577–580.

Blanchard, E. B., & Hickling, E. J. (1997). *After the crash: Assessment and treatment of motor vehicle accident survivors*. Washington, DC: American Psychological Association.

Blanchard, E. B., Hickling, E. J., Taylor, A. E., Forneris, C., Loos, W., & Jaccard, J. (1995). Psychiatric morbidity associated with motor vehicle accidents. *Journal of Nervous and Mental Disease, 183*, 495–504.

Blanchard, E. B., Jones-Alexander, J., Buckley, T. C., & Forneris, C. A. (1996). Psychometric properties of the PTSD Checklist (PCL). *Behaviour Research and Therapy, 34*, 669–673.

Blanchard, E. B., Kolb, L. C., Pallmeyer, T. P., & Gerardi, R. J. (1982). A psychophysiological study of post traumatic stress disorder in Vietnam veterans. *Psychiatric Quarterly, 54*, 220–229.

Blanchard, J. J., & Brown, S. B. (1998). Structured diagnostic interview schedules. In C. R. Reynolds (Ed.), *Comprehensive clinical psychology: Vol. 3. Assessment*. New York: Elsevier.

Bland, R. C., Orn, H., & Newman, S. C. (1988). Lifetime prevalence of psychiatric disorders in Edmonton. *Acta Psychiatrica Scandinavica, 77*(Suppl. 338), 24–32.

Blashfield, R. K. (1990). Comorbidity and classification. In J. D. Maser & C. R. Cloninger (Eds.), *Comorbidity of mood and anxiety disorders*. Washington, DC: American Psychiatric Press.

Blazer, D. G., George, L., & Hughes, D. (1991). The epidemiology of anxiety disorders: An age comparison. In C. Salzman & B. Liebowitz (Eds.), *Anxiety disorders in the elderly*. New York: Springer.

Blazer, D. G., Hughes, D., George, L. K., Swartz, M., & Boyer, R. (1991). Generalized anxiety disorder. In L. N. Robins & D. A. Regier (Eds.), *Psychiatric disorders in America: The Epidemiolgic Catchment Area study*. New York: Free Press.

Boadle-Biber, M. C., Singh, V. B., Corley, K. C., Phan, T., & Dilts, C. V. (1993). Evidence that corticotropin-release factor within the extended amygdala mediates the activation of tryptophan hydroxylase produced by sound stress in the rat. *Brain Research, 628*, 105–114.

Bolles, R. C., & Fanselow, M. S. (1980). A perceptual–defensive–recuperative model of fear and pain. *Behavioral and Brain Sciences, 3*, 291–323.

Bond, A., & Lader, M. H. (1979). Benzodiazepines and aggression. In M. Sandier (Ed.), *Psychopharmacology of aggression*. New York: Raven Press.

Bonn, J. A., Harrison, J., & Rees, W. (1971). Lactate-induced anxiety: Therapeutic application. *British Journal of Psychiatry, 119,* 468–470.

Bonn, J. A., Readhead, C. P. A., & Timmons, B. H. (1984). Enhanced adaptive behavioral response in agoraphobic patients pretreated with breathing retraining. *Lancet, ii,* 665–669.

Boomsma, D. I., Martin, N. G., & Neale, M. C. (Eds.). (1989). Genetic analysis of twin and family data: Structural equation modeling using LISREL [Special issue]. *Behavioral Genetics, 19.*

Boone, M. L., McNeil, D. W., Masia, C. L., Turk, C. L., Carter, L. E., Ries, B. J., & Lewin, M. R. (1999). Multimodal comparisons of social phobia subtypes and avoidant personality disorder. *Journal of Anxiety Disorders, 13,* 271–292.

Booth, R., & Rachman, S. (1992). The reduction of claustrophobia: I. *Behaviour Research and Therapy, 30,* 207–221.

Borden, J. W., Lowenbraun, P. B., Wolff, P. L., & Jones, A. (1993). Self-focused attention in panic disorder. *Cognitive Therapy and Research, 17*(5), 413–425.

Boren, J. L., Gallup, G. G., Suarez, S. D., Wallnau, L. B., & Gagliardi, G. J. (1979). Pargyline and tryptophan enhancement of tonic immobility: Paradoxical attenuation with combined administration. *Pharmacology, Biochemistry and Behavior, 11,* 17–22.

Borkovec, T. D. (1978). Self-efficacy: Cause or reflection of behavioural change? *Advances in Behaviour Research and Therapy, 1,* 177–193.

Borkovec, T. D. (1979). Pseudo (experimental) insomnia and idiopathic (objective) insomnia: Theoretical and therapeutic issues. *Advances in Behaviour Research and Therapy, 2,* 27–55.

Borkovec, T. D. (1982). Insomnia. *Journal of Consulting and Clinical Psychology, 50,* 880–895.

Borkovec, T. D. (1985a). The role of cognitive and somatic cues in anxiety and anxiety disorders: Worry and relaxation-induced anxiety. In A. H. Tuma & J. S. Maser (Eds.), *Anxiety and the anxiety disorders*. Hillsdale, NJ: Erlbaum.

Borkovec, T. D. (1985b). Worry: A potentially valuable concept. *Behaviour Research and Therapy, 23,* 481–482.

Borkovec, T. D. (1994a). The nature, functions, and origins of worry. In G. C. L. Davey & F. Tallis (Eds.), *Worrying: Perspectives on theory, assessment, and treatment*. New York: Wiley.

Borkovec, T. D. (1994b). Between-group therapy outcome research: Design and methodology. In L. S. Onken & J. D. Blaine (Eds.), *Behavioral treatments for drug abuse and dependence* (NIDA Research Monograph No. 137). Rockville, MD: National Institute on Drug Abuse.

Borkovec, T. D., Abel, J. L., & Newman, H. (1995). Effects of psychotherapy on comorbid conditions in generalized anxiety disorder. *Journal of Consulting and Clinical Psychology, 63,* 479–483.

Borkovec, T. D., Alcaine, O., & Behar, E. (in press). Avoidance theory of worry and generalized anxiety disorder. In R. G. Heimberg, C. L. Turk, & D. S. Mennin (Eds.), *Generalized anxiety disorder: Advances in research and practice*. New York: Guilford Press.

Borkovec, T. D., & Costello, E. (1993). Efficacy of applied relaxation and cognitive-behavioral therapy in the treatment of generalized anxiety disorder. *Journal of Consulting and Clinical Psychology, 61,* 611–619.

Borkovec, T. D., Hazlett-Stevens, H., & Diaz, M. L. (1999). The role of positive beliefs about worry in generalized anxiety disorder and its treatment. *Clinical Psychology and Psychotherapy, 6,* 126–138.

Borkovec, T. D., & Hu, S. (1990). The effect of worry on cardiovascular response to phobic imagery. *Behaviour Research and Therapy, 28,* 69–73.

Borkovec, T. D., & Inz, J. (1990). The nature of worry in generalized anxiety disorder: A predominance of thought activity. *Behaviour Research and Therapy, 28*(2), 153–158.

Borkovec, T. D., Lyonfields, J. D., Wiser, S. L., & Deihl, L. (1993). The role of worrisome thinking in the suppression of cardiovascular response to phobic imagery. *Behaviour Research and Therapy, 31,* 321–324.

Borkovec, T. D., & Mathews, A. M. (1988). Treatment of non-phobic anxiety disorders: A comparison of nondirective, cognitive, and coping desensitization therapy. *Journal of Consulting and Clinical Psychology, 56,* 877–884.

Borkovec, T. D., Mathews, A. M., Chambers, A., Ebrahimi, S., Lytle, R., & Nelson, R. (1987). The effects of relaxation training with cognitive or nondirective therapy and the role of relaxation-induced anxiety in the treatment of generalized anxiety. *Journal of Consulting and Clinical Psychology, 55,* 883–888.

Borkovec, T. D., Newman, M. G., Pincus, A., & Lytle, R. (in press). A component analysis of cognitive behavioral therapy for generalized anxiety disorder and the role of interpersonal problems. *Journal of Consulting and Clinical Psychology.*

Borkovec, T. D., Robinson, E., Pruzinsky, T., & DePree, J. A. (1983). Preliminary exploration of worry: Some characteristics and processes. *Behaviour Research and Therapy, 21,* 9–16.

Borkovec, T. D., & Roemer, L. (1994). Generalized anxiety disorder. In R. T. Ammerman & M. Hersen (Eds.), *Handbook of prescriptive treatments for adults.* New York: Plenum Press.

Borkovec, T. D., & Roemer, L. (1995). Perceived functions of worry among generalized anxiety disorder subjects: Distraction from more emotionally distressing topics? *Journal of Behavior Therapy and Experimental Psychiatry, 26,* 25–30.

Borkovec, T. D., & Ruscio, A. M. (2001). Psychotherapy for generalized anxiety disorder. *Journal of Clinical Psychiatry, 62,* 37–45.

Borkovec, T. D., Shadick, R. N., & Hopkins, M. (1991). The nature of normal and pathological worry. In R. M. Rapee & D. H. Barlow (Eds.), *Chronic anxiety: Generalized anxiety disorder and mixed anxiety–depression.* New York: Guilford Press.

Boudewyns, P. A., & Hyer, L. (1990). Physiological response to combat memories and preliminary treatment outcome in Vietnam veteran PTSD patients treated with direct therapeutic exposure. *Behavior Therapy, 21,* 63–87.

Boudewyns, P. A., Stwertka, S. A., Hyer, L. A., Albrecht, J. W., & Sperr, E. V. (1993). Eye movement desensitization for PTSD of combat: A treatment outcome pilot study. *The Behavior Therapist, 16,* 29–33.

Bouknight, D. P., & O'Rourke, R. A. (2000). Current management of mitral valve prolapse. *American Family Physician, 61,* 3353–3354.

Boulenger, J. P., Squillace, K., Simon, P., Herrou, M., Leymarie, P., & Zarifan, E. (1989). Buspirone and diazepam: Comparison of subjective, psychomotor, and biological effects. *Neuropsychobiology, 22,* 83–89.

Boulenger, J. P., Uhde, T. W., Wolff, E. A., & Post, R. M. (1984). Increased sensitivity to caffeine in patients with panic disorders. *Archives of General Psychiatry, 41,* 1067–1071.

Bourdon, K. H., Boyd, J. H., Rae, D. S., Burns, B. J., Thompson, J. W., & Locke, B. Z. (1988). Gender differences in phobias: Results of the ECA community study. *Journal of Anxiety Disorders, 2,* 227–241.

Bourne, E. J. (1998a). *Overcoming specific phobia: A hierarchy and exposure-based protocol for the treatment of all specific phobias (client manual).* Oakland, CA: New Harbinger.

Bourne, E. J. (1998b). *Overcoming specific phobia: A hierarchy and exposure-based protocol for the treatment of all specific phobias (therapist protocol).* Oakland, CA: New Harbinger.

Bourque, P., & Ladouceur, R. (1980). An investigation of various performance-based treatments with acrophobics. *Behaviour Research and Therapy, 18,* 161–170.

Bouton, M. E. (1991). Context and retrieval in extinction and in other examples of interference in simple associative learning. In L. Dachowski & C. F. Flaherty (Eds.), *Current topics in animal learning: Brain, emotion, and cognition.* Hillsdale, NJ: Erlbaum.

Bouton, M. E. (1993). Context, time, and memory retrieval in the interference paradigms of Pavlovian learning. *Psychological Bulletin, 114,* 80–99.

Bouton, M. E., Mineka, S., & Barlow, D. H. (2001). A modern learning-theory perspective on the etiology of panic disorder. *Psychological Review, 108*(1), 4–32.

Bowen, R. C., Cipywnyk, D., D'Arcy, C., & Keegan, D. (1984). Alcoholism, anxiety disorders and agoraphobia. *Alcoholism: Clinical and Experimental Research, 8,* 48–50.

Bowen, R. C., D'Arcy, C., & Orchard, R. C. (1991). The prevalence of anxiety disorders among patients with mitral valve prolapse syndrome and chest pain. *Psychosomatics, 32*, 400–406.

Bowen, R. C., Offord, D. R., & Boyle, M. H. (1990). The prevalence of overanxious disorder and separation anxiety disorder: Results from the Ontario Child Health Study. *Journal of the American Academy of Child and Adolescent Psychiatry, 29*, 753–758.

Bower, G. H. (1981). Mood and memory. *American Psychologist, 36*, 129–148.

Bowlby, J. (1969). *Attachment and loss: Vol. 1. Attachment.* New York: Basic Books.

Bowlby, J. (1973). *Attachment and loss: Vol. 2. Separation: Anxiety and anger.* New York: Basic Books.

Bowlby, J. (1980). *Attachment and loss: Vol. 3. Loss: Sadness and depression.* New York: Basic Books.

Bowlby, J. (1982). *Attachment and loss: Vol. 1. Attachment* (2nd ed.). New York: Basic Books.

Boyd, J. H. (1986). Use of mental health services for the treatment of panic disorder. *American Journal of Psychiatry, 143*(12), 1569–1574.

Boyd, J. H., Burke, J. D., Gruenberg, E., Holzer, C. E., Rae, D. S., George, L. K., Karno, M., Stolzman, R., McEvoy, L., & Nestadt, G. (1984). Exclusion criteria of DSM-III: A study of co-occurrence of hierarchy-free syndromes. *Archives of General Psychiatry, 41*, 983–989.

Boyer, W. (1994). Serotonin uptake inhibitors are superior to imipramine in alleviating panic attacks: A meta-analysis. In G. Darcourt, J. Mendlewicz, & N. Brunello (Eds.), *Current therapeutic approaches to panic and other anxiety disorders* (Vol. 8). Basel: Karger.

Boyer, W. F., & Feighner, J. P. (1993). A placebo-controlled double-blind multicenter trial of two doses of ipsapirone versus diazepam in generalized anxiety disorder. *International Clinical Psychopharmacology, 8*, 173–176.

Bradley, B. P., Mogg, K., Millar, N., & White, J. (1995). Selective processing of negative information: Effects of clinical anxiety, concurrent depression, and awareness. *Journal of Abnormal Psychology, 104*(3), 532–536.

Bradley, B. P., Mogg, K., White, J., Groom, C., & de Bono, J. (1999). Attentional bias for emotional faces in generalized anxiety disorder. *British Journal of Clinical Psychology, 38*, 267–278.

Bradley, M. M., Cuthbert, B. N., & Lang, P. J. (1996). Lateralized startle probes in the study of emotion. *Psychophysiology, 33*, 156–161.

Bradwejn, J., & Koszycki, D. (1994). Imipramine antagonism of the panicogenic effects of cholecystokinin in panic disorder patients. *American Journal of Psychiatry, 151*, 261–263.

Bradwejn, J., Koszycki, D., Couetoux du Tertre, A., van Megen, H., den Boer, J., Westenberg, H., & Annable, L. (1994). The panicogenic effects of cholecystokinin-tetrapeptide are antagonized by L-365,260, a central cholecystokinin receptor antagonist, in patients with panic disorder. *Archives of General Psychology, 51*, 486–493.

Bradwejn, J., Koszycki, D., & Shriqui, C. (1991). Enhanced sensitivity to cholecystokinin tetrapeptide in panic disorder: Clinical and behavioral findings. *Archives of General Psychology, 48*, 603–610.

Bradwejn, J., LeGrand, J. M., Koszycki, D., Bates, J. H. T., & Bourin, M. (1998). Effects of cholecystokinin tetrapeptide on respiratory function in healthy volunteers. *American Journal of Psychiatry, 155*, 280–282.

Brady, K. T., Pearlstein, T., Asnis, G. M., Baker, D., Rothbaum, B., & Sikes, C. R. (2000). Efficacy and safety of sertraline treatment of posttraumatic stress disorder: A randomized controlled trial. *Journal of the American Medical Association, 28*, 563–564.

Brannon, L., & Feist, J. (1997). *Health psychology: An introduction to behavior and health* (3rd ed.). Pacific Grove, CA: Brooks/Cole.

Brantley, P. J., Mehan, D. J., Ames, S. C., & Jones, G. N. (1999). Minor stressors and generalized anxiety disorder among low-income patients attending primary care clinics. *Journal of Nervous and Mental Disease, 187*, 435–440.

Brawman-Mintzer, O., Lydiard, R. B., Crawford, M. M., Emmanuel, N., Payeur, R., Johnson, M., Knapp, R. G., & Ballenger, J. C. (1994). Somatic symptoms in generalized anxiety disorder with and without comorbid psychiatric symptoms. *American Journal of Psychiatry*, *151*, 930–932.

Brawman-Mintzer, O., Lydiard, R. B., Emmanuel, N., Payeur, R., Johnson, M., Roberts, J., Jarrell, M. P., & Ballenger, J. C. (1993). Psychiatric comorbidity in patients with generalized anxiety disorder. *American Journal of Psychiatry*, *150*, 1216–1218.

Breggin, P. R. (1964). The psychophysiology of anxiety with a review of the literature concerning adrenaline. *Journal of Nervous and Mental Disease*, *139*, 558–568.

Brehm, J., Gatz, M., Goethals, G., McCrimmon, W., & Ward, L. (1978). Physiological arousal and interpersonal attraction. *JSAS: Catalog of Selected Documents in Psychology*, *8*, 63.

Breier, A., Charney, D. S., & Heninger, G. R. (1984). Major depression in patients with agoraphobia and panic disorder. *Archives of General Psychiatry*, *41*, 1129–1135.

Breier, A., Charney, D. S., & Heninger, G. R. (1986). Agoraphobia with panic attacks. *Archives of General Psychiatry*, *43*, 1029–1036.

Breitholtz, E., Johansson, B., & Öst, L.-G. (1999). Cognitions in generalized anxiety disorder and panic disorder patients: A prospective approach. *Behaviour Research and Therapy*, *37*, 533–544.

Breitholtz, E., Westling, B. E., & Öst, L.-G. (1998). Cognitions in generalized anxiety disorder and panic disorder patients. *Journal of Anxiety Disorders*, *12*, 567–577.

Bremner, J. D. (1999). Does stress damage the brain? *Biological Psychiatry*, *45*, 797–805.

Bremner, J. D., Licinio, J., Darnell, A., Krystal, J. H., Owens, M. J., Southnick, S. M., Nemeroff, C. B., & Charney, D. S. (1997). Elevated CSF corticotropin-releasing factor concentrations in posttraumatic stress disorder. *American Journal of Psychiatry*, *154*, 624–629.

Bremner, J. D., Randall, P. R., Capelli, S., Scott, T., McCarthy, G., & Charney, D. S. (1995). Deficits in short-term memory in adult survivors of childhood abuse. *Psychiatry Research*, *59*, 97–107.

Bremner, J. D., Randall, P. R., Scott, T. M., Bronen, R. A., Seibyl, J. P., Southwick, S. M., Delaney, R. C., McCarthy, G., Charney, D. S., & Innis, R. B. (1995). MRI-based measurement of hippocampal volume in patients with combat-related posttraumatic stress disorder. *American Journal of Psychiatry*, *152*, 973–981.

Bremner, J. D., Randall, P. R., Vermetten, E., Staib, L., Bronen, R. A., Mazure, C., Capelli, S., McCarthy, G., Innis, R. B., & Charney, D. S. (1997). MRI-based measurement of hippocampal volumle in posttraumatic stress disorder related to childhood physical and sexual abuse: A preliminary report. *Biological Psychiatry*, *41*, 23–32.

Bremner, J. D., Vermetten, E., Southwick, S. M., Krystal, J. H., & Charney, D. S. (1998). Trauma, memory, and dissociation: An integrative formulation. In J. D. Bremner & C. Marmar (Eds.), *Trauma, memory, and dissociation*. Washington, DC: American Psychiatric Press.

Breslau, N. (1985). Depressive symptoms, major depression and generalized anxiety: A comparison of self-reports on DES-D and results from diagnostic interviews. *Psychiatry Research*, *15*, 219–229.

Breslau, N., Chilcoat, H. D., Kessler, R. C., Peterson, E. L., & Lucia, V. C. (1999). Vulnerability to assaultive violence: Further specification of the sex difference in post-traumatic stress disorder. *Psychological Medicine*, *29*, 813–821.

Breslau, N., Davis, G. C., Andreski, P., & Peterson, E. L. (1991). Traumatic events and posttraumatic stress disorder in an urban population of young adults. *Archives of General Psychiatry*, *48*, 216–222.

Brewin, C. R., Dalgleish, T. & Joseph, S. (1996). A dual representation theory of posttraumatic stress disorder. *Psychological Review*, *103*, 670–686.

Briddell, D. W., Rimm, D. C., Caddy, G. R., Krawitz, G., Shalis, D., & Wunderlin, R. J. (1978). The effects of alcohol and cognitive set on sexual arousal to deviant stimuli. *Journal of Abnormal Psychology*, *87*, 418–430.

Broadhurst, P. L. (1975). The Maudsley reactive and nonreactive strains of rats: A survey. *Behavior Genetics*, *5*, 299–320.

Brockner, J., & Swap, W. C. (1983). Resolving the relationships between placebos, misattribution, and insomnia: An individual-differences perspective. *Journal of Personality and Social Psychology*, *45*, 32–42.

"Broken Heartthrob. " (1999, May 17). *People*, pp. 107–112.

Brom, D., Kleber, R. J., & Defares, P. B. (1989). Brief psychotherapy for posttraumatic stress disorders. *Journal of Consulting and Clinical Psychology*, 57, 607–612.

Bromet, E. J., Parkinson, P., Schulberg, K. et al. (1982). Mental health of residents near the Three Mile Island reactor: A comparative study of selected groups. *Journal of Preventive Psychiatry*, 1, 225–276.

Broocks, A., Bandelow, B., Pekrun, G., George, A., Meyer, T., Bartmann, U., Hillmer-Vogel, U., & Ruether, E. (1998). Comparison of aerobic exercise, clomipramine, and placebo in the treatment of panic disorder. *American Journal of Psychiatry*, 155, 603–609.

Brooks, N., & McKinlay, W. W. (1992). Mental health consequences of the Lockerbie disaster. *Journal of Traumatic Stress*, 5, 527–543.

Brooks, R. B., Baltazar, P. L., & Munjack, D. J. (1989). Co-occurrence of personality disorders with panic disorder, social phobia, and generalized anxiety disorder: A review of the literature. *Journal of Anxiety Disorders*, 3, 259–285.

Brown, D. R., Eaton, W. W., & Sussman, L. (1990). Racial differences in prevalence of phobic disorders. *Journal of Nervous and Mental Disease*, 178, 434–441.

Brown, E. J., Heimberg, R. G., & Juster, H. R. (1995). Social phobia subtype and avoidant personality disorder: Effect on severity of social phobia, impairment, and outcome of cognitive behavioral treatment. *Behavior Therapy*, 26, 467–489.

Brown, E. J., Turovsky, J., Heimberg, R. G., Juster, H. R., Brown, T. A., & Barlow, D. H. (1997). Validation of the Social Interaction Anxiety Scale and the Social Phobia Scale across the anxiety disorders. *Psychological Assessment*, 9, 21–27.

Brown, F. W. (1942). Heredity in the psychoneurosis (summary). *Proceedings of the Royal Society of Medicine*, 35, 785–790.

Brown, G. W. (1993). The role of life events in the etiology of depressive and anxiety disorders. In A. C. Stanford, P. Salmon, & J. A. Gray (Eds.), *Stress: From synapse to syndrome*. London: Academic Press.

Brown, G. W., & Harris, T. O. (1989). Depression. In G. W. Brown & T. O. Harris (Eds.), *Life events and illness*. New York: Guilford Press.

Brown, T. A. (1996). Validity of the DSM-III-R and DSM-IV classification systems for anxiety disorders. In R. M. Rapee (Ed.), *Current controversies in the anxiety disorders*. New York: Guilford Press.

Brown, T. A. (1997). The nature of generalized anxiety disorder and pathological worry: Current evidence and conceptual models. *Canadian Journal of Psychiatry*, 42(8), 817–825.

Brown, T. A. (1999). Generalized anxiety disorder and obsessive–compulsive disorder. In T. Millon, P. H., Blaney, & R. D. Davis (Eds.), *Oxford textbook of psychopathology*. New York: Oxford University Press.

Brown, T. A. (in press). The classification of anxiety disorders: Current status and future directions. In D. J. Stein & E. Hollander (Eds.), *Textbook of anxiety disorders*. Washington, DC: American Psychiatric Press.

Brown, T. A., Antony, M. M., & Barlow, D. H. (1992). Psychometric properties of the Penn State Worry Questionnaire in a clinical anxiety disorders sample. *Behaviour Research and Therapy*, 30, 33–38.

Brown, T. A., Antony, M. M., & Barlow, D. H. (1995). Diagnostic comorbidity in panic disorder: Effect on treatment outcome and course of comorbid diagnoses following treatment. *Journal of Consulting and Clinical Psychology*, 63, 408–418.

Brown, T. A., & Barlow, D. H. (1992). Comorbidity among anxiety disorders: Implications for treatment and DSM-IV. *Journal of Consulting and Clinical Psychology*, 60, 835–844.

Brown, T. A., & Barlow, D. H. (1995). Long-term outcome in cognitive-behavioral treatment of panic disorder: Clinical predictors and alternative strategies for assessment. *Journal of Consulting and Clinical Psychology*, 63, 754–765.

Brown, T. A., Barlow, D. H., & Liebowitz, M. R. (1994). The empirical basis of generalized anxiety disorder. *American Journal of Psychiatry*, 151(9), 1272–1280.

Brown, T. A., & Cash, T. F. (1989). The phenomenon of panic in nonclinical populations: Further evidence and methodological considerations. *Journal of Anxiety Disorders, 3,* 139–148.

Brown, T. A., & Cash, T. F. (1990). The phenomenon of nonclinical panic: Parameters of panic, fear, and avoidance. *Journal of Anxiety Disorders, 4,* 15–29.

Brown, T. A., Campbell, L. A., Lehman, C. L., Grisham, J. R., & Mancill, R. B. (2001). Current and lifetime comorbidity of the DSM-IV anxiety and mood disorders in a large clinical sample. *Journal of Abnormal Psychology, 110,* 49–58.

Brown, T. A., Chorpita, B. F., & Barlow, D. H. (1998). Structural relationships among dimensions of the DSM-IV anxiety and mood disorders and dimensions of negative affect, positive affect, and autonomic arousal. *Journal of Abnormal Psychology, 107,* 179–192.

Brown, T. A., Chorpita, B. F., Korotitsch, W., & Barlow, D. H. (1997). Psychometric properties of the Depression Anxiety Stress Scales (DASS) in clinical samples. *Behaviour Research and Therapy, 35,* 79–89.

Brown, T. A., & Deagle, E. A. (1992). Structured interview assessment of nonclinical panic. *Behavior Therapy, 23,* 75–85.

Brown, T. A., Di Nardo, P. A., & Barlow, D. H. (1994). *Anxiety Disorders Interview Schedule for DSM-IV (ADIS-IV).* San Antonio, TX: Psychological Corporation/Graywind Publications Incorporated.

Brown, T. A., Di Nardo, P. A., Lehman, C. L., & Campbell, L. A. (2001). Reliability of DSM-IV anxiety and mood disorders: Implications for classification of emotional disorders. *Journal of Abnormal Psychology, 110,* 49–58.

Brown, T. A., Dowdall, D. J., Côté, G., & Barlow, D. H. (1994). Worry and obsessions: The distinction between generalized disorder and obsessive–compulsive disorder. In G. C. L. Davey & F. Tallis (Eds.), *Worrying: Perspectives on theory, assessment, and treatment.* New York: Wiley.

Brown, T. A., Marten, P. A., & Barlow, D. H. (1995). Discriminant validity of the symptoms constituting the DSM-III-R and DSM-IV associated symptom criterion of generalized anxiety disorder. *Journal of Anxiety Disorders, 9,* 317–328.

Brown, T. A., Marten, P. A., & Barlow, D. H. (1996). Empirical evaluation of the panic symptom ratings in DSM-III-R panic disorder. In T. A. Widiger, A. J. Frances, H. A, Pincus, R. Ross, M. B. First, W. Davis, & M. Kline (Eds.), *DSM-IV sourcebook* (Vol. 4). Washington, DC: American Psychiatric Association.

Brown, T. A., Moras, K., Zinbarg, R. E., & Barlow, D. H. (1993). Diagnostic and symptom distinguishability of generalized anxiety disorder and obsessive–compulsive disorder. *Behavior Therapy, 24,* 227–240.

Brown, T. A., O'Leary, T. A., & Barlow, D. H. (2001). Generalized anxiety disorder. In D. H. Barlow (Ed.), *Clinical handbook of psychological disorders: A step-by-step treatment manual* (3rd ed.). New York: Guilford Press.

Bruce, M., Scott, N., Shine, P., & Lader, M. (1992). Anxiogenic effects of caffeine in patients with anxiety disorders. *Archives of General Psychiatry, 49*(11), 867–869.

Bruce, T. J., & Barlow, D. H. (1990). The nature and role of performance anxiety in sexual dysfunction. In H. Leitenberg (Ed.), *Handbook of social anxiety.* New York: Plenum Press.

Bruce, T. J., Spiegel, D. A., & Hegel, M. T. (1999). Cognitive-behavioral therapy helps prevent relapse and recurrence of panic disorder following alprazolam discontinuation: A long-term follow-up of the Peoria and Dartmouth studies. *Journal of Consulting and Clinical Psychology, 67,* 151–156.

Bruce, T. J., Spiegel, D. A., Gregg, S. F., & Nuzzarello, A. (1995). Predictors of alprazolam discontinuation with and without cognitive behavioral therapy for panic disorder. *American Journal of Psychiatry, 152,* 1156–1160.

Bruch, M. A., & Heimberg, R. G. (1994). Differences in perceptions of parental and personal characteristics between generalized and nongeneralized social phobics. *Journal of Anxiety Disorders. 8,* 155–168.

Bruch, M. A., Heimberg, R. G., Berger, P., & Collins, T. M. (1987). *Parental and personal origins of social evaluative threat: Differences between social phobics and agoraphobics.* Unpublished manuscript.

Bruch, M. A., Heimberg, R. G., & Hope, D. A. (1991). States of mind model and cognitive change in treated social phobics. *Cognitive Therapy and Research, 15*, 429–441.

Bruder, G. E., Fong, R., Tenke, C. E., Leite, P., Towey, J. P., Stewart, J. E., McGrath, P. J., & Quitkin, F. M. (1997). Regional brain asymmetries in major depression with or without an anxiety disorder: A quantitative electroencephalographic study. *Biological Psychiatry, 41*, 939–948.

Bruss, G. S., Gruenberg, A. M., Goldstein, R. D., & Barber, J. P. (1994). Hamilton Anxiety Rating Scale interview guide: Joint interview and test–retest methods for inter-rater reliability. *Psychiatry Research, 53*, 191–202.

Bryant, B. K., & Trockel, J. F. (1976). Personal history of control of psychological stress related to locus of control orientation among college women. *Journal of Consulting and Clinical Psychology, 44*, 266–271.

Bryant, R. A., Harvey, A. G., Dang, S. T., Sackville, T., & Basten, C. (1998). Treatment of acute stress disorder: A comparison of cognitive-behavioral therapy and supportive counseling. *Journal of Consulting and Clinical Psychology, 66*, 862–866.

Buchwald, A. M., & Rudick-Davis, D. (1993). The symptoms of major depression. *Journal of Abnormal Psychology, 102*(2), 197–205.

Buck, R., & Parke, R. D. (1972). Behavioral and physiological response to the presence of a friendly or neutral person in two types of stressful situations. *Journal of Personality and Social Psychology, 24*, 143–153.

Buck, R., Parke, R. D., & Buck, M. (1970). Differences in the cardiac response to the environment in two types of stressful situations. *Psychonomic Science, 18*, 95–96.

Bufka, L. F., & Hofmann, S. G. (1999). Modifying CBT to treat panic disorder in patients with schizophrenia. *Cognitive and Behavioral Practice, 6*, 10–15.

Buglass, P., Clarke, J., Henderson, A. S., Dreitman, D. N., & Presley, A. S. (1977). A study of agoraphobic housewives. *Psychological Medicine, 7*, 73–86.

Buigues, J., & Vallejo, J. (1987). Therapeutic response to phenelzine in patients with panic disorder and agoraphobia with panic attacks. *Journal of Clinical Psychiatry, 48*, 55–59.

Burgess, A. W., & Holmstrom, L. (1974). Rape trauma syndrome. *American Journal of Psychiatry, 131*, 981–986.

Burgess, A. W., & Holmstrom, L. L. (1976). Coping behavior of the rape victim. *American Journal of Psychiatry, 133*, 413–417.

Burgess, I. S., Jones, L. W., Robertson, S. A., Radcliffe, W. N., Emerson, E., Lawler, P., & Crowe, T. J. (1981). The degree of control exerted by phobic and non-phobic verbal stimuli over the recognition behaviour of phobic and non-phobic subjects. *Behaviour Research and Therapy, 19*, 233–234.

Burish, T. G., & Carey, M. P. (1986). Conditioned aversive responses in cancer chemotherapy patients: Theoretical and developmental analysis. *Journal of Consulting and Clinical Psychology, 54*, 593–600.

Burke, K. C., Burke, J. D., Jr., Regier, D. A., & Rae, D. S. (1990). Age at onset of selected mental disorders in five community populations. *Archives of General Psychiatry, 47*, 511–518.

Burns, L. E., Thorpe, C. L., & Cavallaro, L. A. (1986). Agoraphobia 8 years after behavioral treatment: A follow-up study with interview, self-report, and behavioral data. *Behavioral Therapy, 17*, 580–591.

Burns, L. G., Keortge, S. G., Formea, G. M., & Sternberger, L. G. (1996). Revision of the Padua Inventory of obsessive compulsive disorder symptoms: Distinctions between worry, obsessions, and compulsions. *Behaviour Research and Therapy, 34*, 163–173.

Burton, D., Foy, D. W., Bwanausi, C., Johnson, J., & Moore, L. (1994). The relationship between traumatic exposure, family dysfunction, and post-traumatic stress symptoms in male juvenile offenders. *Journal of Traumatic Stress, 7*, 83–93.

Buss, A. H. (1980). *Self-consciousness and social anxiety*. San Francisco: Freeman.

Butler, G., Cullington, A., Hibbert, G., Klimes, I., & Gelder, M. (1987). Anxiety management for persistent generalized anxiety. *British Journal of Psychiatry, 151*, 535–542.

Butler, G., Fennell, M., Robson, P., & Gelder, M. (1991). Comparison of behavior therapy and cognitive behavior therapy in the treatment of generalized anxiety disorder. *Journal of Consulting and Clinical Psychology, 59*, 167–175.

Butler, G., Gelder, M., Hibbert, G., Cullington, A., & Klimes, I. (1987). Anxiety management: Developing effective strategies. *Behaviour Research and Therapy, 25*, 517–522.

Butler, G., & Mathews, A. (1983). Cognitive processes in anxiety. *Advances in Behaviour Research and Therapy, 5*, 51–62.

Butler, P. D., Weiss, J. M., Stout, J. C., & Nemeroff, C. B. (1990). Corticotropin-releasing factor produces fear-enhancing and behavioral activating effects following infusion into the locus coeruleus. *Journal of Neuroscience, 10*(1), 176–183.

Byrne, D. (1977). Social psychology and the study of sexual behavior. *Journal of Personality and Social Psychology, 3*, 3–30.

Byrne, D. (1983a). The antecedents, correlates and consequences of erotophobia–erotophilia. In C. M. Davis (Ed.), *Challenges in sexual science.* Philadelphia: Society for the Scientific Study of Sex.

Byrne, D. (1983b). Sex without contraception. In D. Byrne & W. A. Fisher (Eds.), *Adolescents, sex, and contraception.* Hillsdale, NJ: Erlbaum.

Bystritsky, A., Ackerman, D. L., & Pasnau, R. O. (1991). Low dose desipramine treatment of cocaine-related panic attacks. *Journal of Nervous and Mental Disease, 179*, 755–758.

Bystritsky, A., Craske, M., Maidenberg, E., Vapnik, T., & Shapiro, D. (1995). Ambulatory monitoring of panic patients during regular activity: A preliminary report. *Biological Psychiatry, 38*, 684–689.

Bystritsky, A., Rosen, R. M., Murphy, K. J., Bohn, P., Keys, S. A., & Vapnik, T. (1994–1995). Double-blind pilot trial of desipramine versus fluoxetine in panic patients. *Anxiety, 1*, 287–290.

Cacioppo, J. T., Glass, C. R., & Merluzzi, T. V. (1979). Self-statement and self-evaluations: A cognitive-response analysis of heterosexual anxiety. *Cognitive Therapy and Research, 3*, 249–262.

Cahill, S. P., Carrigan, M. H., & Frueh, B. C. (1999). Does EMDR work? And if so, why?: A critical review of controlled outcome and dismantling research. *Journal of Anxiety Disorders, 13*, 5–33.

Calamari, J. E., Wiegartz, P. S., & Janeck, A. S. (1999). Obsessive–compulsive disorder subgroups: A symptom-based clustering approach. *Behaviour Research and Therapy, 37*, 113–127.

Caldwell, A. T., McCrady, B. S., & Barlow, D. H. (1979). *The effects of response prevention and contingency management in the treatment of obsessive–compulsive behavior.* Unpublished manuscript.

Callaway, E., & Stone, G. (1960). Re-evaluating the focus of attention. In L. Uhr & J. G. Miller (Eds.), *Drugs and behavior.* New York: Wiley.

Cameron, O. G., & Hudson, C. (1986). Influence of exercise on anxiety level in patients with anxiety disorders. *Psychosomatics, 27*, 720–723.

Campbell, L. A., & Brown, T. A. (in press). Assessment of generalized anxiety disorder. In M. M. Antony & D. H. Barlow (Eds.), *Handbook of assessment and treatment planning for psychological disorders.* New York: Guilford Press.

Campbell, S. B. (1986). Developmental issues in childhood anxiety. In R. Gittelman (Ed.), *Anxiety disorders of childhood.* New York: Guilford Press.

Campbell, S. B., Sanderson, R., & Laverty, S. G. (1964). Characteristics of a conditioned response in human subjects during extinction trials following a single traumatic conditioning trial. *Journal of Abnormal and Social Psychology, 66*, 627–639.

Cannon, W. B. (1927). *Bodily changes in pain, hunger, fear and rage.* New York: Appleton-Century-Crofts.

Cannon, W. B. (1929). *Bodily changes in pain, hunger, fear and rage* (2nd ed.). New York: Appleton-Century-Crofts.

Cannon, W. B. (1942). Voodoo death. *American Anthropologist, 44*, 169–181.

Carey, G. (1982). Genetic influences on anxiety neurosis and agoraphobia. In R. J. Mathew (Ed.), *The biology of anxiety.* New York: Brunner/Mazel.

Carey, G., & Gottesman, I. I. (1981). Twin and family studies of anxiety, phobic, and obsessive disorders. In D. F. Klein & J. G. Rabkin (Eds.), *Anxiety: New research and changing concepts.* New York: Ravlen Press.

Carlin, A. S., Hoffman, H. G., & Weghorst, S. (1997). Virtual reality and tactile augmentation in the treatment of spider phobia: A case report. *Behaviour Research and Therapy, 35,* 153–158.

Carlson, J. G., Chemtob, C. M., Rusnak, K., Hedlund, N. L., & Muraoka, M. Y. (1998). Eye movement desensitization and reprocessing (EMDR) treatment for combat-related posttraumatic stress disorder. *Journal of Traumatic Stress, 11,* 3–24.

Carmin, C. N., Pollard, C. A., & Flynn, T. (1992). *Dying of embarrassment: Help for social anxiety and phobia.* Oakland, CA: New Harbinger.

Carr, J. E. (1996). Neuroendocrine and behavioral interaction in exposure treatment of phobic avoidance. *Clinical Psychology Review, 16,* 1–15.

Carr, R. E. (1998). Panic disorder and asthma: Causes, effects and research implications. *Journal of Psychosomatic Research, 44,* 43–52.

Carr, R. E. (1999). Panic disorder and asthma. *Journal of Asthma, 36,* 143–152.

Carr, R. E., Lehrer, P. M., Jackson, A., & Hochron, S. M. (1996). Effect of physiological stress on airway impedence in individuals with asthma and panic disorder. *Journal of Abnormal Psychology, 105,* 137–141.

Carr, R. E., Lehrer, P. M., Rausch, L., & Hochron, S. M. (1994). Anxiety sensitivity and panic attacks in an asthmatic population. *Behaviour Research and Therapy, 32,* 411–418.

Carter, C. S., & Maddock, R. J. (1992). Chest pain in generalized anxiety disorder. *International Journal of Psychiatry in Medicine, 22,* 291–298.

Carter, C. S., Fawcett, J., Hertzman, M., Papp, L. A., Jones, W., Patterson, W. M., Swinson, R. P., Weise, C. C., Maddock, R. J., Denahan, A. Q., & Leibowitz, M. (1995). Adinazolam-SR in panic disorder with agoraphobia: Relationship of daily dose to efficacy. *Journal of Clinical Psychopharmacology, 56,* 202–210.

Carter, M. M., & Barlow, D. H. (1995). Learned alarms: The origins of panic. In W. O'Donohue & L. Krasner (Eds.), *Theories of behavior therapy: Exploring behavior change.* Washington, DC: American Psychological Association Press.

Carter, M. M., Hollon, S. D., Carson, R., & Shelton, R. C. (1995). Effects of a safe person on induced distress following a biological challenge in panic disorder with agoraphobia. *Journal of Abnormal Psychology, 104,* 156–163.

Carter, M. M., Turovsky, J., & Harlow, D. H. (1994). Interpersonal relationships in panic disorder with agoraphobia: A review of empirical evidence. *Clinical Psychology: Science and Practice, 1,* 25–34.

Carter, W. R., Johnson, M. C., & Borkovec, T. D. (1986). Worry: An electrocortical analysis. *Advances in Behaviour Research and Therapy, 8,* 193–204.

Carton, J. S., & Nowicki, S. (1994). Antecedents of individual differences in locus of control of reinforcement: A critical review. *Genetic, Social, and General Psychology Monographs, 120,* 31–38.

Cartwright-Hatton, S., & Wells, A. (1997). Beliefs about worry and intrusions: The Meta-Cognitions Questionnaire and its correlates. *Journal of Anxiety Disorders, 11,* 279–296.

Carver, C. S., Blaney, P. H., & Scheier, M. F. (1979). Focus of attention, chronic expectancy, and responses to a feared stimulus. *Journal of Personality and Social Psychology, 37,* 1186–1195.

Carver, C. S., Peterson, L. M., Follansbee, D. J., & Scheier, M. F. (1983). Effects of self-directed attention on performance and persistence among persons high and low in test anxiety. *Cognitive Therapy and Research, 7,* 333–354.

Carver, C. S., & Scheier, M. F. (1981). *Attention and self-regulation: A control theory approach to human behavior.* New York: Springer-Verlag.

Carver, C. S., & Scheier, M. F. (1991). A control-process perspective on anxiety. In R. Schwarzer & R. A. Wicklund (Eds.), *Anxiety and self-focused attention.* New York: Harwood.

Casacalenda, N., & Boulenger, J. P. (1998). Pharmacologic treatments effective in generalized anxiety disorder and major depressive disorder: Clinical and theoretical implications. *Canadian Journal of Psychiatry, 43*, 722–730.

Cassano, D., del Bruono, G., & Catapano, F. (1993). The relationship between obsessive compulsive personality and obsessive compulsive disorder: Data obtained by the Personality Disorder Examination. *European Psychiatry, 8*, 219–221.

Cassano, G. B., Michelini, S., Shear, M. K., Coli, E., Maser, J. D., & Frank, E. (1997). The panic–agoraphobia spectrum: A descriptive approach to the assessment and treatment of subtle symptoms. *American Journal of Psychiatry, 154*(Suppl. 6), 27–38.

Cassano, G. B., Petracca, A., Perugi, G., Nisista, C., Musetti, L., Mengali, F., & McNair, D. M. (1988). Clomipramine for panic disorder: I. The first 10 weeks of a long-term comparison with imipramine. *Journal of Affective Disorders, 14*, 123–127.

Cassens, G., Roffman, M., Kuruc, A., Orsulak, P., & Schildkraut, J. (1980). Norepinephrine metabolism induced by environmental stimuli previously paired with inescapable shock. *Science, 209*, 1138–1140.

Cassidy, J. (1995). Attachment and generalized anxiety disorder. In D. Cicchetti & S. Toth (Eds.), *Rochester Symposium on Developmental Psychopathology: Vol. 6. Emotion, cognition and representation* (pp. 343–370). Rochester, NY: University of Rochester Press.

Castillo, R. (1997). *Culture and mental illness: A client centered approach.* Pacific Grove, CA: Brooks/Cole.

Cella, D. F., Pratt, A., & Holland, J. C. (1986). Persistent anticipatory nausea, vomiting, and anxiety cured Hodgkin's disease patients after completion of chemotherapy. *American Journal of Psychiatry, 143*, 641–643.

Cerny, J. A., Barlow, D. H., Craske, M. G., & Himadi, W. G. (1987). Couples treatment of agoraphobia: A two-year follow-up. *Behavior Therapy, 18*, 401–415.

Chambers, J., Yeragani, V. K., & Keshavan, M. S. (1986). Phobias in India and the United Kingdom: A transcultural study. *Acta Psychiatrica Scandinavica, 74*, 388–391.

Chambless, D. L. (1990). Spacing of exposure sessions in treatment of agoraphobia and simple phobia. *Behavior Therapy, 21*, 217–229.

Chambless, D. L., Caputo, G. C., Bright, P., & Gallagher, R. (1984). Assessment of fear of fear in agoraphobics: The Body Sensations Questionnaire and the Agoraphobic Cognitions Questionnaire. *Journal of Consulting and Clinical Psychology, 52*, 1090–1097.

Chambless, D. L., Caputo, G., Gracely, S., Jasin, E., & Williams, C. (1985). The Mobility Inventory for agoraphobia. *Behaviour Research and Therapy, 23*, 35–44.

Chambless, D. L., Cherney, J., Caputo, G. C, & Rheinstein, B. J. G. (1987). Anxiety disorders and alcoholism: A study with inpatient alcoholics. *Journal of Anxiety Disorders, 1*, 29–40.

Chambless, D. L., Goldstein, A. A., Gallagher, R., & Bright, P. (1986). Integrating behavior therapy and psychotherapy in the treatment of agoraphobia. *Psychotherapy: Theory, Research, and Practice, 3*, 150–159.

Chambless, D. L., & Mason, J. (1986). Sex, sex-role stereotyping, and agoraphobia. *Behaviour Research and Therapy, 24*, 231–235.

Chambless, D. L., Renneberg, B., Goldstein, A., & Gracely, E. J. (1992). MCMI-diagnosed personality disorders among agoraphobic outpatients: Prevalence and relationship to severity and treatment outcome. *Journal of Anxiety Disorders, 6*, 193–211.

Chambless, D. L., Sanderson, W. C., Shoham, V., Johnson, S. B., Pope, K. S., Crits-Christoph, P., Baker, M., Johnson, B., Woody, S., Sue, S., Beutler, L., Williams, D. A., & McCurry, S. (1996). An update on empirically validated treatments. *The Clinical Psychologist, 49*, 5–18.

Chambless, D. L., & Steketee, G. (1999). Expressed emotion and behavior therapy outcome: A prospective study with obsessive–compulsive and agoraphobic outpatients. *Journal of Consulting and Clinical Psychology, 67*, 658–665.

Chambless, D. L., Tran, G. Q., & Glass, C. R. (1997). Predictors of response to cognitive-behavioral group therapy for social phobia. *Journal of Anxiety Disorders, 11*, 221–240.

Chambless, D. L., & Williams, K. E. (1995). A preliminary study of African Americans with agoraphobia: Symptom severity and outcome of treatment with in vivo exposure. *Behavior Therapy, 26*, 501–515.

Chan, C. K. Y., & Lovibond, P. F. (1996). Expectancy bias in trait anxiety. *Journal of Abnormal Psychology, 105*, 637–647.

Chandler, T. A., Wolf, F. M., Cook, B., & Dugovics, D. A. (1980). Parental correlates of locus of control in fifth graders: An attempt at experimentation in the home. *Merrill–Palmer Quarterly 26*, 183–195.

Chang, S. C. (1997). Social anxiety (phobia) and east Asian culture. *Depression and Anxiety, 5*, 115–120.

Chaplin, E. W., & Levine, B. A. (1981). The effects of total exposure duration and interrupted versus continued exposure in flooding therapy. *Behavior Therapy, 12*, 360–368.

Chappell, P. B., Smith, M. A., Kilts, C. D., Bissette, G., Ritchie, J., Anderson, C., & Nemeroff, C. B. (1986). Alterations in CRF-like immunoreactivity in discrete rat brain regions after acute and chronic stress. *Journal of Neuroscience, 6*, 2908–2914.

Charney, D. S., & Heninger, G. R. (1985). Noradrenergic function and the mechanism of action of antianxiety treatment. *Archives of General Psychiatry, 42*, 458–467.

Charney, D. S., & Heninger, G. R. (1986a). Abnormal regulation of noradrenergic function in panic disorders. *Archives of General Psychiatry, 43*, 1042–1054.

Charney, D. S., & Heninger, G. R. (1986b). Serotonin function in panic disorders: The effect of intravenous tryptophan in healthy subjects and patients with panic disorder before and during alprazolam treatment. *Archives of General Psychiatry, 43*, 1059–1065.

Charney, D. S., Heninger, G. R., & Breier, A. (1984). Noradrenergic function in pain attacks. *Archives of General Psychiatry, 41*, 751–763.

Charney, D. S., Heninger, G. R., & Jatlow, P. I. (1985). Increased anxiogenic effects of caffeine in panic disorders. *Archives of General Psychiatry, 42*, 223–243.

Charney, D. S., & Woods, S. W. (1989). Benzodiazepine treatment of panic disorder: A comparison of alprazolam and lorazepam. *Journal of Clinical Psychiatry, 50*, 418–423.

Charney, D. S., Woods, S. W., Goodman, W. K., & Heninger, G. R. (1987). Serotonin function in anxiety: II. Effects of the serotonin agonist MCPp in panic disorder patients and healthy subjects. *Psychopharmacology, 92*, 14–24.

Chemtob, C. M., Nakashima, J., Hamada, R. S., & Carlson, J. (in press). Brief treatment for elementary school children with disaster related posttraumatic stress disorder: A field study. *Journal of Clinical Psychology.*

Chemtob, C. M., Novaco, R. W., Hamada, R. S., & Gross, D. M. (1997). Cognitive behavioral treatment of severe anger in posttraumatic stress disorder. *Journal of Consulting and Clinical Psychology, 65*, 184–189.

Chemtob, C. M., Tolin, D. F., van der Kolk, B. A., & Pitman, R. K. (2000). Eye movement desensitization and reprocessing. In E. B. Foa, T. M. Keane, & M. J. Friedman (Eds.), *Effective treatments for PTSD: Practice guidelines from the International Society for Traumatic Stress Studies.* New York: Guilford Press.

Chen, E., Lewin, M. R., & Craske, M. G. (1996). Effects of state anxiety on selective processing of threatening information. *Cognition and Emotion, 10*(3), 225–240.

Chen, Y.-W., & Dilsaver, S. C. (1995). Comorbidity of panic disorder in bipolar illness: Evidence from the Epidemiologic Catchment Area survey. *American Journal of Psychiatry, 152*, 280–282.

Chorpita, B. F., Albano, A. M., & Barlow, D. H. (1998). The structure of negative emotions in a clinical sample of children and adolescents. *Journal of Abnormal Psychology, 107*, 74–85.

Chorpita, B. F., & Barlow, D. H. (1998). The development of anxiety: The role of control in the early environment. *Psychological Bulletin, 124*(1), 3–21.

Chorpita, B. F., Brown, T. A., & Barlow, D. H. (1998a). Diagnostic reliability of the DSM-III-R anxiety disorders: Mediating effects of patient and diagnostician characteristics. *Behavior Modification, 22*, 307–320.

Chorpita, B. F., Brown, T. A., & Barlow, D. H. (1998b). Perceived control as a mediator of family environment in etiological models of childhood anxiety. *Behavior Therapy, 29,* 457–476.

Chosak, A. (2000). *A multiple baseline across subjects evaluation of a panic control treatment for claustrophobia.* Unpublished doctoral dissertation, State University of New York at Albany.

Chrousos, G. P. (1995). The hypothalamic–pituitary–adrenal axis and immune-mediated inflammation. *New England Journal of Medicine, 332,* 1351–1362.

Chrousos, G. P. (1998). Stressors, stress, and neuroendocrine integration of the adaptive response. *Annals of the New York Academy of Sciences, 851,* 311–335.

Chrousos, G. P., & Gold, P. W. (1992). The concept of stress and stress system disorders: Overview of physical and behavioral homeostasis. *Journal of the American Medical Association, 267,* 1244–1252.

Clark, D. A., & Purdon, C. (1993). New perspectives for a cognitive theory of obsessions. *Australian Psychology, 28,* 161–167.

Clark, D. A., Steer, R. A., & Beck, A. T. (1994). Common and specific dimensions of self-reported anxiety and depression: Implications for the cognitive and tripartite models. *Journal of Abnormal Psychology, 103,* 645–654.

Clark, D. B., & Agras, W. S. (1991). The assessment and treatment of performance anxiety in musicians. *American Journal of Psychiatry, 148,* 598–605.

Clark, D. B., Turner, S. M., Beidel, D. C., Donovan, J. E., Kirisci, L., & Jacob, R. G. (1994). Reliability and validity of the Social Phobia and Anxiety Inventory for adolescents. *Psychological Assessment, 6,* 135–140.

Clark, D. M. (1986). A cognitive approach to panic. *Behaviour Research and Therapy, 24,* 461–470.

Clark, D. M. (1988). A cognitive model of panic attacks. In S. Rachman & J. D. Maser (Eds.), *Panic: Psychological perspectives.* Hillsdale, NJ: Erlbaum.

Clark, D. M. (1990). *Can cognitions be used to discriminate between panic disorder and other anxiety disorders?* (Report to the DSM-IV Anxiety Disorders Work Group). Oxford: Warneford Hospital, University of Oxford.

Clark, D. M., Salkovskis, P. M., & Anastasiades, P. (1990). *Cognitive mediation of lactate induced panic.* Paper presented at the 24th Annual Convention of the Association for Advancement of Behavior Therapy, San Francisco.

Clark, D. M., Salkovskis, P. M., & Chalkley, A. J. (1985). Respiratory control as a treatment for panic attacks. *Journal of Behavior Therapy and Experimental Psychiatry, 16,* 23–30.

Clark, D. M., Salkovskis, P. M., Hackmann, A., Middleton, H., Anastasiades, P., & Gelder, M. (1994). A comparison of cognitive therapy, applied relaxation, and imipramine in the treatment of panic disorder. *British Journal of Psychiatry, 164,* 759–769.

Clark, D. M., Salkovskis, P. M., Hackmann, A., Wells, A., Ludgate, J., & Gelder, M. (1999). Brief cognitive therapy for panic disorder: A randomized controlled trial. *Journal of Consulting and Clinical Psychology, 67,* 583–589.

Clark, D. M., Salkovskis, P. M., Öst, L.-G., Breitholtz, E., Koehler, K. A., Westling, B. E., Jeavons, A., & Gelder, M. (1997). Misinterpretation of body sensations in panic disorder. *Journal of Consulting and Clinical Psychology, 65,* 203–213.

Clark, D. M., & Wells, A. (1995). A cognitive model of social phobia. In R. G. Heimberg, M. R. Liebowitz, D. A. Hope, & F. R. Schneier (Eds.), *Social phobia: Diagnosis, assessment and treatment.* New York: Guilford Press.

Clark, J. V., & Arkowitz, H. (1975). Social anxiety and self-evaluation of interpersonal performance. *Psychological Report, 36,* 211–221.

Clark, L. A., & Watson, D. (1991). Tripartite model of anxiety and depression: Psychometric evidence and taxonomic implications. *Journal of Abnormal Psychology, 100,* 316–336.

Clark, L. A., Watson, D., & Mineka, S. (1994). Temperament, personality, and the mood and anxiety disorders. *Journal of Abnormal Psychology, 103,* 103–116.

Clark, L. A., Watson, D., & Reynolds, S. (1995). Diagnosis and classification of psychopathology: Challenges to the current system and future directions. *Annual Review of Psychology, 46,* 121–153.

Clayton, P. J. (1993). Suicide in panic disorder and depression. *Current Therapeutic Research, 54,* 825–831.

Cloitre, M., Cancienne, J., Heimberg, R. G., Holt, C. S., & Liebowitz, M. R. (1995). Memory bias does not generalize across anxiety disorders. *Behaviour Research and Therapy, 33,* 305–307.

Cloitre, M., Heimberg, R. H., Liebowitz, M. R., & Gitow, A. (1992). Perceptions of control in panic disorder and social phobia. *Cognitive Therapy and Research, 16,* 569–577.

Cloitre, M., Shear, M. K., Cancienne, J., & Zeitlein, S. B. (1994). Implicit and explicit memory for catastrophic associations to bodily sensation words in panic. *Cognitive Therapy and Research, 18,* 225–240.

Cloninger, C. R. (1986). A unified biosocial theory of personality and its role in the development of anxiety states. *Psychiatric Developments, 5,* 167–226.

Clum, G. A., Broyles, S., Borden, J., & Watkins, P. L. (1990). Validity and reliability of the panic attack symptoms and cognitions questionnaires. *Journal of Psychopathology and Behavioral Assessment, 12,* 233–245.

Cohen, A. S., Barlow, D. H., & Blanchard, E. B. (1985). The psychophysiology of relaxation-associated panic attacks. *Journal of Abnormal Psychology, 94,* 96–101.

Cohen, M. E., Badal, D. W., Kilpatrick, A., Reed, E. W., & White, P. D. (1951). The high familial prevalence of neurocirculatory asthenia (anxiety neurosis, effort syndrome). *American Journal of Human Genetics, 3,* 126–158.

Cohen, M. E., & White, P. D. (1947). Studies of breathing, pulmonary ventilation and subjective awareness of shortness of breath (dyspnea) in neurocirculatory asthenia, effort syndrome, anxiety neurosis. *Journal of Clinical Investigation, 26,* 520.

Cohen, M. E., & White, P. D. (1950). Life situations, emotions and neurocirculatory asthenia (anxiety neurosis, neurasthenia, effort syndrome). In H. G. Wolff (Ed.), *Life stress and bodily disease* (Nervous and Mental Disease, Research Publication No. 29). Baltimore: Williams & Wilkins.

Cohen, M. E., White, P. D., & Johnson, R. E. (1948). Neurocirculatory asthenia, anxiety neurosis or the effort syndrome. *Archives of Internal Medicine, 81,* 260–281.

Cohen, S. D., Monteiro, W., & Marks, I. M. (1984). Two-year follow-up of agoraphobics after exposure and imipramine. *British Journal of Psychiatry, 144,* 276–281.

Cohn, J. B., Bowden, C. L., Fisher, J. G., & Rodos, J. J. (1986). Double-blind comparison of buspirone and clorazepate in anxious outpatients. *American Journal of Medicine, 80*(Suppl. 3B), 10–16.

Coldwell, S. E., Getz, T., Milgrom, P., Prall, C. W., Spadafora, A., & Ramsey, D. S. (1998). CARL: A LabVIEW 3 computer program for conducting exposure therapy for the treatment of dental injection fear. *Behaviour Research and Therapy, 36,* 429–441.

Cole, D. A., Peeke, L. G., Martin, J. M., Truglio, R., & Seroczynski, A. D. (1998). A longitudinal look at the relation between depression and anxiety in children and adolescents. *Journal of Consulting and Clinical Psychology, 66*(3), 451–460.

Cole, D. A., & Turner, J. E. (1993). Models of cognitive mediation and moderation in child depression. *Journal of Abnormal Psychology, 102,* 271–281.

Cole, J. O., Orzack, M. H., Beake, B. Bird, M., & Bar-Tal, Y. (1982). Assessment of the abuse liability of buspirone in recreational sedative users. *Journal of Clinical Psychiatry, 43,* 69–75.

Coles, M. E., & Heimberg, R. G. (2000). Patterns of anxious arousal during exposure to feared situations in individuals with social phobia. *Behaviour Research and Therapy, 38,* 405–424.

Connor, K. M., & Davidson, J. R. T. (1998). Generalized anxiety disorder: Neurobiological and pharmacotherapeutic perspectives. *Biological Psychiatry, 44,* 1286–1294.

Cook, E. W., III, Hodes, R. L., & Lang, P. J. (1986). Preparedness and phobia: Effects of stimulus content on human visceral conditioning. *Journal of Abnormal Psychology, 95,* 195–207.

Cook, M., & Mineka, S. (1989). Observational conditioning of fear to fear-relevant versus fear-irrelevant stimuli in rhesus monkeys. *Journal of Abnormal Psychology, 98,* 448–459.

Cook, M., Mineka, S., Wolkenstein, B., & Laitch, K. (1985). Observational conditioning of snake fears in unrelated rhesus monkeys. *Journal of Abnormal Psychology, 94,* 591–610.

Cooper, J. E., Gelder, M. G., & Marks, I. M. (1965). Results of behavior therapy in 77 psychiatric patients. *British Medical Journal, i,* 1222–1225.

Cooper, N. A., & Clum, G. A. (1989). Imaginal flooding as a supplementary treatment for PTSD in combat veterans: A controlled study. *Behavior Therapy, 20,* 381–391.

Coplan, J. D., Andrew, M. W., Rosenblum, L. A., Owens, M. J., Friedman, S., Gorman, J. M., & Nemeroff, C. B. (1996). Persistent elevations of cerebrospinal fluid concentrations of corticotropin-releasing factor in adult nonhuman primates exposed to early life stressors: Implications for the pathophysiology of mood and anxiety disorders. *Proceedings of the National Academy of Science USA, 93,* 1619–1623.

Coplan, J. D., Goetz, R., Klein, D. F., Papp, L. A., Fyer, A. J., Liebowitz, M. R., Davies, S. O., & Gorman, J. M. (1998). Plasma cortisol concentrations preceding lactate-induced panic: Psychological, biochemical, and physiological correlates. *Archives of General Psychiatry, 55,* 130–136.

Coplan, J. D., Gorman, J. M., & Klein, D. F. (1992). Serotonin-related functions in panic–anxiety: A critical overview. *Neuropsychopharmacology, 6,* 189–200.

Coplan, J. D., & Klein, D. F. (1996). Pharmacological probes in panic disorder. In H. G. M. Westenberg, J. A. den Boer, & D. L. Murphy (Eds.), *Advances in the neurobiology of anxiety disorders.* New York: Wiley.

Coplan, J. D., Rosenbaum, L. A., & Gorman, J. M. (1995). Primate models of anxiety: Longitudinal perspectives. *Psychiatric Clinics of North America, 18,* 727–743.

Coplan, J. D., Sharman, T., Rosenblum, L. A., Friedman, S., Bassoff, T. B., Barbour, R. L., & Gorman, J. M. (1992). Effects of sodium lactate infusion on cisternal lactate and carbon dioxide levels in non-human primates. *American Journal of Psychiatry, 149,* 1369–1373.

Coplan, J. D., Trost, R. C., Owens, M. J., Cooper, T. B., Gorman, J. M., Nemeroff, C. B., & Rosenblum, L. A. (1998). Cerebrospinal fluid concentrations of somatostatin and biogenic amines in grown primates reared by mothers exposed to manipulated foraging conditions. *Archives of General Psychiatry, 55,* 473–477.

Cornelius, R. R., & Averill, J. R. (1983). Sex differences in fear of spiders. *Journal of Personality and Social Psychology, 45,* 377–383.

Coryell, W. (1981). Obsessive–compulsive disorder and primary unipolar depression. *Journal of Nervous and Mental Disease, 169,* 220–224.

Coryell, W. (1997). Hypersensitivity to carbon dioxide as a disease-specific trait marker. *Biological Psychiatry, 41,* 259–263.

Coryell, W., Noyes, R., & Clancy, J. (1982). Excess mortality in panic disorder: A comparison with primary unipolar depression. *Archives of General Psychiatry, 39,* 701–703.

Coryell, W., Noyes, R., & House, J. D. (1986). Mortality among outpatients with anxiety disorders. *American Journal of Psychiatry, 143,* 508–510.

Costa, P. T., & McCrae, R. R. (1988). Personality in adulthood: A six-year longitudinal study of self-reports and spouse ratings on the NEO Personality Inventory. *Journal of Personality and Social Psychology, 54,* 853–863.

Costello, C. G. (1992). Research on symptoms versus research on syndromes: Arguments in favour of allocating more research time to the study of symptoms. *British Journal of Psychiatry, 60,* 304–308.

Côté, G., Gauthier, J. G., Laberge, B., Cormier, H. J., & Plamondon, J. (1994). Reduced therapist contact in the cognitive behavioral treatment of panic disorder. *Behavior Therapy, 25,* 123–145.

Cottraux, J., Mollard, E., Bouvard, M., Marks, I., Sluys, M., Nury, A. M., Douge, R., & Cialdella, P. (1989). A controlled study of fluvoxamine and exposure in obsessive compulsive disorder. *International Clinical Psychopharmacology, 5,* 1–14.

Cottraux, J., Note, I. D., Cungi, C., Legeron, P., Heim, F., Cheinweiss, L., Bernard, G., & Bouvard, M. (1995). A controlled study of cognitive behaviour therapy with buspirone or placebo in panic disorder with agoraphobia. *British Journal of Psychiatry, 167,* 635–641.

Cottraux, J., Note, I., Yao, S. N., Lafont, S., Note, B., Mollard, E., Bouvard, M., Sauteraud, A., Bourgeois, M., & Dartigues, J.-F. (2001). A controlled trial of cognitive therapy versus intensive behavior therapy in obsessive compulsive disorder. *Psychotherapy and Psychosomatics, 70.*

Cowley, D. S., & Arana, G. W. (1990). The diagnostic utility of lactate sensitivity in panic disorder. *Archives of General Psychiatry, 47,* 277–284.

Cox, B. J., Borger, S. C., & Enns, M. W. (1999). Anxiety sensitivity and emotional disorders: Psychometric studies and their theoretical implications. In S. Taylor (Ed.), *Anxiety sensitivity: Theory, research, and treatment of the fear of anxiety.* Mahwah, NJ: Erlbaum.

Cox, B. J., Cohen, E., Direnfeld, D. M., & Swinson, R. P. (1996). Does the Beck Anxiety Inventory measure anything beyond panic attack symptoms? *Behaviour Research and Therapy, 34,* 949–954.

Cox, B. J., Direnfeld, D. M., Swinson, R. P., & Norton, R. G. (1994). Suicidal ideation and suicide attempts in panic disorder and social phobia. *American Journal of Psychiatry, 151,* 882–887.

Cox, B. J., Endler, N. S., & Swinson, R. P. (1995). An examination of levels of agoraphobic severity in panic disorder. *Behaviour Research and Therapy, 33,* 57–62.

Cox, B. J., Norton, G. R., Dorward, J., & Fergusson, P. A. (1989). The relationship between panic attacks and chemical dependencies. *Addictive Behaviors, 14*(1), 53–60.

Cox, B. J., Norton, R., Swinson, R. P., & Endler, N. S. (1990). Substance abuse and panic-related anxiety: A critical review. *Behaviour Research and Therapy, 28,* 385–393.

Cox, B. J., Parker, J. D., & Swinson, R. P. (1996). Confirmatory factor analysis of the Fear Questionnaire with social phobia patients. *British Journal of Psychiatry, 168,* 497–499.

Cox, B. J., Swinson, R. P., Parker, J. D., Kuch, K., & Reichman, J. T. (1993). Confirmatory factor analysis of the Fear Questionnaire in panic disorder with agoraphobia patients. *Psychological Assessment, 5,* 235–237.

Crandall, V. C., Katkovsky, W., & Crandall, V. J. (1965). Children's belief in their own control of reinforcements in intellectual–academic achievement situations. *Child Development, 36,* 91–109.

Cranston-Cuebas, M. A., & Barlow, D. H. (1990). Cognitive and affective contributions to sexual functioning. In J. Bancroft (Ed.), *Annual review of sex research.* Philadelphia: Society for the Scientific Study of Sex.

Cranston-Cuebas, M. A., & Barlow, D. H. (1995). *Attentional focus and the misattribution of male sexual arousal.* Unpublished manuscript.

Cranston-Cuebas, M. A., Barlow, D. H., Mitchell, W. B., & Athanasiou, R. (1993). Differential effects of a misattribution manipulation on sexually functional and dysfunctional males. *Journal of Abnormal Psychology, 102,* 525–533.

Craske, M. G. (1991). Phobic fear and panic attacks: The same emotional states triggered by different cues? *Clinical Psychology Review, 11,* 599–620.

Craske, M. G. (1993). [Ambulatory monitoring of panic disorder patients with nocturnal panic, and self-report comparison of panic disorder patients with and without nocturnal panic]. Unpublished raw data.

Craske, M. G. (1999). Anxiety disorders: Psychological approaches to theory and treatment. Boulder, CO: Westview Press.

Craske, M. G., Antony, M. M., & Barlow, D. H. (1997). *Mastery of your specific phobia: Therapist guide.* San Antonio, TX: Psychological Corporation/Graywind Publications Incorporated.

Craske, M. G., & Barlow, D. H. (1988). A review of the relationship between panic and avoidance. *Clinical Psychology Review, 8,* 667–685.

Craske, M. G., & Barlow, D. H. (1989). Nocturnal panic. *Journal of Nervous and Mental Disease, 177*(3), 160–167.

Craske, M. G., & Barlow, D. H. (1990). Nocturnal panic: Response to hyperventilation and CO_2 challenges. *Journal of Abnormal Psychology, 99,* 302–307.

Craske, M. G., & Barlow, D. H. (2000). *Mastery of your anxiety and Panic (MAP-3): Agoraphobia supplement.* San Antonio, TX: Psychological Corporation/Graywind Publications Incorporated.

Craske, M. G., & Barlow, D. H. (2001). Panic disorder and agoraphobia. In D. H. Barlow (Ed.), *Clinical handbook of psychological disorders: A step-by-step treatment manual* (3rd ed.). New York: Guilford Press.

Craske, M. G., Barlow, D. H., Clark, D. M., Curtis, G. C., Hill, E. M., Himle, J. A., Lee, Y.-J., Lewis,

J. A., McNally, R. J., Öst, L.-G., Salkovskis, P. M., & Warwick, H. M. C. (1996). Specific (simple) phobia. In T. A. Widiger, A. J. Frances, H. A. Pincus, R. Ross, M. B. First, & W. W. Davis (Eds.), *DSM-IV sourcebook* (Vol. 2). Washington, DC: American Psychiatric Association.

Craske, M. G., Barlow, D. H., & Meadows, E. (2000). *Mastery of your anxiety and panic: Therapist guide for anxiety, panic, and agoraphobia (MAP-3)*. San Antonio, TX: Graywind/Psychological Corporation.

Craske, M. G., Barlow, D. H., & O'Leary, T. (1992). *Mastery of your anxiety and worry*. San Antonio, TX: Psychological Corporation/Graywind.

Craske, M. G., Brown, T. A., Meadows, E. A., & Barlow, D. H. (1995). Uncued and cued emotions and associated distress in a college sample. *Journal of Anxiety Disorders, 9*(2), 125–137.

Craske, M. G., Bunt, R., Rapee, R. M., & Barlow, D. H. (1991). Perceived control and controllability during in vivo exposure: Spider phobics. *Journal of Anxiety Disorders, 5*, 285–292.

Craske, M. G., Burton, T. M., Rapee, R. M., Rygh, J., & Barlow, D. H. (1989). *Simple phobics presenting for treatment: What are their fears?* Unpublished manuscript.

Craske, M. G., & Craig, K. D. (1984). Musical performance anxiety: The three-system model and self-efficacy theory. *Behaviour Research and Therapy, 22*, 267–280.

Craske, M. G., & Freed, S. (1995). Expectations about arousal and nocturnal panic. *Journal of Abnormal Psychology, 104*, 567–575.

Craske, M. G., & Kreuger, M. (1990). The prevalence of nocturnal panic in a college population. *Journal of Anxiety Disorders, 4*, 125–139.

Craske, M. G., Maidenberg, E., & Bystritsky, A. (1995). Brief cognitive-behavioral versus non directive therapy for panic disorder. *Journal of Behavior Therapy and Experimental Psychiatry, 26*, 113–120.

Craske, M. G., Miller, P. P., Rotunda, R., & Barlow, D. H. (1990). A descriptive report of features of initial unexpected panic attacks in minimal and extensive avoiders. *Behaviour Research and Therapy, 28*, 395–400.

Craske, M. G., Mohlman, J., Yi, J., Glover, D., & Valeri, S. (1995). Treatment of claustrophobia and snake/spider phobias: Fear of arousal and fear of context. *Behaviour Research and Therapy, 33*, 197–203.

Craske, M. G., Poulton, R., Tsao, J. C. I., & Plotkin, D. (2001). Paths to panic-agoraphobia: An exploratory analysis from age 3 to 21 in an unselected birth cohort. *American Journal of Child and Adolescent Psychiatry, 40*, 556–563.

Craske, M. G., & Rachman, S. J. (1987). Return of fear: Perceived skill and heart rate responsivity. *British Journal of Clinical Psychology, 26*, 187–199.

Craske, M. G., Rachman, S. J., & Tallman, K. (1986). Mobility, cognitions and panic. *Journal of Psychopathology and Behavioral Assessment, 8*, 199–210.

Craske, M. G., Rapee, R. M., & Barlow, D. H. (1988). The significance of panic-expectancy for individual patterns of avoidance. *Behavior Therapy, 19*, 577–592.

Craske, M. G., Rapee, R. M., Jackel, L., & Barlow, D. H. (1989). Qualitative dimensions of worry in DSM-III-R generalized anxiety disorder subjects and nonanxious controls. *Behaviour Research and Therapy, 27*, 397–402.

Craske, M. G., & Rowe, M. K. (1997a). A comparison of behavioral and cognitive treatments for phobias. In G. C. L. Davey (Ed.), *Phobias: A handbook of theory, research, and treatment*. Chichester, England: Wiley.

Craske, M. G., & Rowe, M. K. (1997b). Nocturnal panic. *Clinical Psychology: Science and Practice, 4*, 153–174.

Craske, M. G., Sanderson, W. C., & Barlow, D. H. (1987). The relationships among panic, fear, and avoidance. *Journal of Anxiety Disorders, 1*, 153–160.

Craske, M. G., & Sipsas, A. (1992). Animal phobias versus claustrophobias: Exteroceptive versus interoceptive cues. *Behaviour Research and Therapy, 30*, 569–581.

Craske, M. G., Street, L. L., & Barlow, D. H. (1989). Instructions to focus upon or distract from internal cues during exposure treatment of agoraphobic avoidance. *Behaviour Research and Therapy, 27*, 663–672.

Craske, M. G., Street, L. L., Jayaraman, J., & Barlow, D. H. (1991). Attention versus distraction during in vivo exposure: Snake and spider phobias. *Journal of Anxiety Disorders, 5*, 199–211.

Craske, M. G., Zarate, R., Burton, T., & Barlow, D. H. (1993). Specific fears and panic attacks: A survey of clinical and nonclinical samples. *Journal of Anxiety Disorders, 7*, 1–19.

Crino, R., & Andrews, G. (1996). Obsessive compulsive disorder and Axis I comorbidity. *Journal of Anxiety Disorders, 10*, 37–46.

Crits-Cristoph, P., Connelly, M. B., Azarian, K., Crits-Christoph, K., & Shappell, S. (1996). An open trial of brief supportive expressive psychotherapy in the treatment of generalized anxiety disorder. *Psychotherapy, 33*, 418–430.

Cross-National Collaborative Panic Study, Second Phase Investigators. (1992). Drug treatment of panic disorder. *British Journal of Psychiatry, 160*, 191–202.

Crowe, R. R., Noyes, R., Pauls, D. L., & Slymen, D. J. (1983). A family study of panic disorder. *Archives of General Psychiatry, 40*, 1065–1069.

Crowe, R. R., Noyes, R., Samuelson, S., Wesner, R. B., & Wilson, A. F. (1990). Close linkage between panic disorder and α-haptoglobin excluded in 10 families. *Archives of General Psychiatry, 47*, 377–380.

Crowe, R. R., Noyes, R., Wilson, A. F., Elston, R. C., & Ward, L. J. (1987). A linkage study of panic disorder. *Archives of General Psychiatry, 44*, 933–937.

Crowe, R. R., Pauls, D. L., Slymen, D. J., & Noyes, R. (1980). A family study of anxiety neurosis: Morbidity risk in families of patients. *Archives of General Psychiatry, 37*, 77–79.

Crowe, R. R., Wang, Z., Noyes, R., Albrecht, B. E., Darlison, M. G., Baily, M. E., Johnson, K. J., & Zoega, T. (1997). Candidate gene study of eight GABA$_A$ receptor subunits in panic disorder. *American Journal of Psychiatry, 154*, 1096–1100.

Curran, D., & Mallinson, W. P. (1940). War-time psychiatry and economy in manpower. *Lancet, ii*, 738–743.

Curtis, G. C., Buxton, M., Lippman, D., Nesse, R., & Wright, I. (1976). "Flooding in vivo" during the circadian phase of minimal cortisol secretion: Anxiety and therapeutic success without adrenal cortical activation. *Biological Psychiatry, 11*, 101–107.

Curtis, G. C., Hill, E. M., & Lewis, J. A. (1990). *Heterogeneity of DSM-III-R simple phobia and the simple phobia/agoraphobia boundary: Evidence from the ECA study* (Report to the DSM-IV Anxiety Disorders Work Group). Ann Arbor: University of Michigan.

Curtis, G. C., Himle, J. A., Lewis, J. A., & Lee, Y. (1989). *Specific situational phobias: Variant of agoraphobia?* (Report to the DSM-IV Anxiety Disorders Work Group). Ann Arbor: University of Michigan.

Curtis, G. C., Magee, W. J., Eaton, W. W., Wittchen, H.-U., & Kessler, R. C. (1998). Specific fears and phobias: Epidemiology and classification. *British Journal of Psychiatry, 173*, 212–217.

Curtis, G. C., & Thyer, B. (1983). Fainting on exposure to phobic stimuli. *American Journal of Psychiatry, 140*, 771–774.

Cutler, N. R., Sramek, J. J., Hesselink, J. M. K., Krol, A., Roeschen, J., Rickels, K., & Schweizer, E. (1993). A double-blind, placebo-controlled study comparing the efficacy and safety of ipsapirone versus lorazepam in patients with generalized anxiety disorder: A prospective multicenter trial. *Journal of Clinical Psychopharmacology, 13*, 429–437.

Cutler, S. E., & Nolen-Hoeksema, S. (1991). Accounting for sex differences in depression through female victimizations: Childhood sexual abuse. *Sex Roles, 24*, 425–438.

DaCosta, J. M. (1871). On irritable heart: A clinical study of a form of functional cardiac disorder and its consequences. *American Journal of Medical Science, 61*, 17–52.

Dager, S. R., Comess, K. A., Saal, A. K., & Dunner, D. L. (1986). Mitral valve prolapse in a psychiatric setting: Diagnostic assessment, research and clinical implications. *Integrative Psychiatry, 4*, 211–223.

Daiuto, A. D., Baucom, D. H., Epstein, N., & Dutton, S. S. (1998). The application of behavioral couples therapy to the assessment and treatment of agoraphobia: Implications of empirical research. *Clinical Psychology Review, 18*, 663–687.

Daly, R. J. (1983). Samuel Pepys and post-traumatic stress disorder. *British Journal of Psychiatry,* *143,* 64–68.

Danyko, S. J., McKay, D. R., & Neziroglu, F. A. (1995). Facto structure of the Yale–Brown Obsessive Compulsive Scale: A two dimensional measure. *Behaviour Research and Therapy, 33,* 133–144.

Darwin, C. R. (1872). *The expression of the emotions in man and animals.* London: John Murray.

Dattilio, F. M. (1994). Paradoxical intention as a proposed alternative in the treatment of panic disorder. *Journal of Cognitive Psychotherapy, 8*(1), 33–40.

Davey, G. C. L. (1992). Classical conditioning and the acquisition of human fears and phobias: A review and synthesis of the literature. *Advances in Behaviour Research and Therapy, 14,* 29–66.

Davey, G. C. L. (1993a). Factors influencing self-rated fear to a novel animal. *Cognition and Emotion, 7,* 461–471.

Davey, G. C. L. (1993b). A comparison of three worry questionnaires. *Behaviour Research and Therapy, 31,* 51–56.

Davey, G. C. L. (1994a). Pathological worrying as exacerbated problem solving. In G. C. L. Davey & F. Tallis (Eds.), *Worrying: Perspectives on theory, assessment, and treatment.* New York: Wiley.

Davey, G. C. L. (1994b). Self-reported fears to common indigenous animals in an adult UK population: The role of disgust sensitivity. *British Journal of Psychology, 85,* 541–554.

Davey, G. C. L. (1994c). Trait factors and ratings of controllability as predictors of worrying about significant life stressors. *Personality and Individual Differences, 16,* 379–384.

Davey, G. C. L. (1994d). Worrying, social problem-solving abilities, and problem-solving confidence. *Behaviour Research and Therapy, 32,* 327–330.

Davey, G. C. L. (1997). A conditioning model of phobias. In G. C. L. Davey (Ed.), *Phobias: A handbook of theory, research, and treatment.* Chichester, England: Wiley.

Davey, G. C. L., Forster, L., & Mayhew, G. (1993). Familial resemblances in disgust sensitivity and animal phobias. *Behaviour Research and Therapy, 31,* 41–50.

Davey, G. C. L., Hampton, J., Farrell, J., & Davidson, S. (1992). Some characteristics of worrying: Evidence for worrying and anxiety as separate constructs. *Personality and Individual Differences, 13,* 133–147.

Davey, G. C. L., Jubb, M., & Cameron, C. (1996). Catastrophic worrying as a function of changes in problem-solving confidence. *Cognitive Therapy and Research, 20,* 333–344.

Davey, G. C. L., & Levy, S. (1998). Catastrophic worrying: Personal inadequacy and a perseverative iterative style as features of the catastrophizing process. *Journal of Abnormal Psychology, 107,* 576–586.

Davey, G. C. L., McDonald, A. S., Hirisave, U., Prabhu, G. G., Iwawaki, S., Jim, C. I., Merckelbach, H., de Jong, P. J., Leung, P. W. L., & Reimann, B. C. (1998). A cross-cultural study of animal fears. *Behaviour Research and Therapy, 36,* 735–750.

Davey, G. C. L., Menzies, R., & Gallardo, B. (1997). Height phobia and biases in the interpretation of bodily sensations: Some links between acrophobia and agoraphobia. *Behaviour Research and Therapy, 35*(11), 997–1001.

Davey, G. C. L., & Tallis, F. (Eds.). (1994). *Worrying: Perspectives on theory, assessment, and treatment.* New York: Wiley.

Davey, G. C. L., Tallis, F., & Capuzzo, N. (1996). Beliefs about the consequences of worrying. *Cognitive Therapy and Research, 20,* 499–520.

Davidson, J. R. T., DuPont, R. L., Hedges, D., & Haskins, J. T. (1999). Efficacy, safety, and tolerability of venlafaxine extended release and buspirone in outpatients with generalized anxiety disorder. *Journal of Clinical Psychiatry, 60,* 528–535.

Davidson, J. R. T., Hughes, D., Blazer, D. G., & George, L. K. (1991). Post-traumatic stress disorder in the community: An epidemiological study. *Psychological Medicine, 21,* 713–721.

Davidson, J. R. T., Hughes, D. L., George, L. K., & Blazer, D. G. (1993). The epidemiology of social phobia: Findings from the Duke Epidemiological Catchment Area study. *Psychological Medicine, 23,* 709–718.

Davidson, J. R. T., Kudler, H., Smith, R., Mahoney, S. L., Hammett, E. B., Saunders, W. B., &

Cavenar, J. O. (1990). Treatment of posttraumatic stress disorder with amitriptyline and placebo. *Archive of General Psychiatry, 47*, 259–266.

Davidson, J. R. T., Landburg, P. D., Pearlstein, T., Weisler, R., Sikes, C., & Farfel, G. M. (1997). Double-blind comparison of sertraline and placebo in patients with posttraumatic stress disorder (PTSD). *Abstracts of the American College of Neuropsychopharmacology, 36th Annual Meeting*, San Juan, Puerto Rico.

Davidson, J. R. T., Miner, C. M., DeVeaugh-Geiss, J., Tupler, L. A., Colket, J. T., & Potts, N. L. S. (1997). The Brief Social Phobia Scale: A psychometric evaluation. *Psychological Medicine, 27*, 161–166.

Davidson, J. R. T., & Moroz, G. (1998). Pivotal studies of clonazepam in panic disorder. *Psychopharmacology Bulletin, 34*, 169–174.

Davidson, J. R. T., Potts, N. L. S., Richichi, E. A., Ford, S. M., Krishnan, R. R., Smith, R., & Wilson, W. H. (1991). The Brief Social Phobia Scale. *Journal of Clinical Psychiatry, 52*, 48–51.

Davidson, J. R. T., Potts, N. L. S., Richichi, E. A., Krishnan, R. R., Ford, S. M., Smith, R., & Wilson, W. H. (1993). Treatment of social phobia with clonazepam and placebo. *Journal of Clinical Psychopharmacology, 13*, 423–428.

Davidson, J. R. T., Smith, R. D., & Kudler, H. S. (1989). Validity and reliability of the DSM III criteria for posttraumatic stress disorder: Experience with a structured interview. *Journal of Nervous and Mental Disease, 177*, 336–341.

Davidson, J. R. T., Swartz, M., Storck, M., Krishnan, R. R., & Hammett, E. (1985). A diagnostic and family study of posttraumatic stress disorder. *American Journal of Psychiatry, 142*, 90–93.

Davidson, R. J. (1992). Emotion and affective style: Hemispheric substrates. *Psychological Science, 1*, 39–43.

Davidson, R. J. (1993a). Cerebral asymmetry and emotion: Methodological conundrums. *Cognition and Emotion, 7*, 115–138.

Davidson, R. J. (1993b). The neuropsychology of emotion and affective style. In M. Lewis & J. Haviland (Eds.), *Handbook of emotions*. New York: Guilford Press.

Davidson, R. J., & Tomarken, A. J. (1989). Laterality and emotion: An electrophysiological approach. In F. Boller & J. Grafman (Eds.), *Handbook of neuropsychology*. Amsterdam: Elsevier.

Davis, M. (1997). The neurophysiological basis of acoustic startle modulation: Research on fear motivation and sensory gating. In P. J. Lang, R. F. Simons, & M. T. Balaban (Eds.), *Attention and orienting: Sensory and motivational processes*. Mahwah, NJ: Erlbaum.

Davis, M. (1998). Are different parts of the extended amygdala involved in fear versus anxiety? *Biological Psychiatry, 44*, 1239–1247.

Davis, R. N., & Valentiner, D. P. (2000). Does meta-cognitive theory enhance our understanding of pathological worry and anxiety? *Personality and Individual Differences, 29*, 513–526.

Davis, W. L., & Phares, E. J. (1969). Parental antecedents of internal–external control of reinforcement. *Psychological Reports, 24*, 427–436.

Davison, G. C., Vogel, R. S., & Coffman, S. G. (1997). Think-aloud approaches to cognitive assessment and articulated thoughts in simulated situations paradigm. *Journal of Consulting and Clinical Psychology, 6*, 950–958.

Dayhoff, S. A. (2000). *Diagonally-parked in a parallel universe: Working through social anxiety*. Placitas, NM: Effectiveness-Plus.

de Beurs, E., van Balkom, A. J., Lange, A., Koele, P., & van Dyke, R. (1995). Treatment of panic disorder with agoraphobia: Comparison of fluvoxamine, placebo, and psychological panic management combined with exposure and of exposure in vivo alone. *American Journal of Psychiatry, 152*, 683–691.

de Beurs, E., van Dyke, R., Lange, A., & van Balkom, A. J. (1999). Long-term outcome of pharmacological and psychological treatment for panic disorder with agoraphobia: A two-year naturalistic follow-up. *Acta Psychiatrica Scandinavica, 99*, 59–67.

Deffenbacher, J. L. (1980). Worry and emotionality in test anxiety. In I. G. Sarason (Ed.), *Test anxiety: Theory, research and application*. Hillside, NJ: Erlbaum.

Deffenbacher, J. L. (1992, February). *Cognitive-behavioral approaches to anger reduction*. Paper presented at the Banff International Conference on the Behavioral Sciences, Banff, Alberta, Canada.

de Jong, G. M., & Bouman, T. K. (1995). Panic disorder: A baseline period. Predictability of agoraphobic avoidance behavior. *Journal of Anxiety Disorders, 9,* 185–199.

de Jong, P. J., Andrea, H., & Muris, P. (1997). Spider phobia in children: Disgust and fear before and after treatment. *Behaviour Research and Therapy, 35,* 559–562.

de Jong, P. J., Mayer, B., & van den Hout, M. (1997). Conditional reasoning and phobic fear: Evidence for a fear-confirming reasoning pattern. *Behaviour Research and Therapy, 35,* 507–516.

de Jong, P. J., Merckelbach, H., & Arntz, A. (1995). Covariation bias in phobic women: The relationship between a priori expectancy, on-line expectancy, autonomic responding, and a posteriori contingency judgment. *Journal of Abnormal Psychology, 104,* 55–62.

de Jong, P. J., van den Hout, M., & Merckelbach, H. (1995). Covariation bias and return of fear. *Behaviour Research and Therapy, 33,* 211–213.

de Jong, P. J., Weertman, A., Horselenberg, R., & van den Hout, M. (1997). Deductive reasoning and pathological anxiety: Evidence for a relatively strong "belief bias" in phobic subjects. *Cognitive Therapy and Research, 21,* 647–662.

de Jongh, A., Broeke, E. T., & Renssen, M. R. (1999). Treatment of specific phobias with eye movement desensitization and preprocessing (EMDR): Protocol, empirical status and conceptual issues. *Journal of Anxiety Disorders, 13,* 69–85.

de Jongh, A., Muris, P., Horst, G. T., van Zuuren, F., Schoenmakers, N., & Makkes, P. (1995). One-session cognitive treatment of dental phobia: Preparing dental phobics for treatment by restructuring negative cognitions. *Behaviour Research and Therapy, 33,* 947–954.

Delle Chiaie, R. D., Pancheri, P., Casacchia, M., Stratta, P., Kotzalidis, G. D., & Zibellini, M. (1995). Assessment of the efficacy of buspirone in patients affected by generalized anxiety disorder, shifting to buspirone from prior treatment with lorazepam: A placebo-controlled, double-blind study. *Journal of Clinical Psychopharmacology, 15,* 12–19.

DeMartinis, N. A., Schweizer, E., & Rickels, K. (1996). An open-label trial of nefazodone in high comorbidity panic disorder. *Journal of Clinical Psychiatry, 57,* 245–248.

DeMartinis, N. A., Rynn, M., Rickels, K., & Mandos, L. (2000). Prior benzodiazepine use and buspirone response in the treatment to generalized anxiety disorder. *Journal of Clinical Psychiatry, 61,* 91–94.

Dement, W. C., Seidel, W. F., Cohen, S. A., Bailey, R., Rountree, M., & Yost, D. (1991). Effects of alprazolam, buspirone and diazepam on daytime sedation and performance. *Clinical Drug Investigation, 3,* 148–156.

Denenberg, V. H. (1964). Critical periods, stimulus input, and emotional reactivity: A theory of infantile stimulation. *Psychological Review, 71,* 335–351.

Derogatis, L. R., Lipman, R. S., & Covi, L. (1973). SCL-90: An outpatient psychiatric rating scale. Preliminary report. *Psychopharmacological Bulletin, 9,* 13–25.

Derryberry, D., & Rothbart, M. K. (1984). Emotion, attention, and temperament. In C. E. Izard, J. Kagan, & R. B. Zajonc (Eds.), *Emotion, cognition, and behavior.* New York: Cambridge University Press.

de Ruiter, C., Rijken, H., Garssen, B., & Kraaimaat, F. (1989). Breathing retraining, exposure, and a combination of both in the treatment of panic disorder with agoraphobia. *Behaviour Research and Therapy, 27,* 663–672.

de Silva, P. (1986). Obsessional–compulsive imagery. *Behaviour Research and Therapy, 24,* 333–350.

de Silva, P., & Marks, I. M. (1999). The role of traumatic experiences in the genesis of obsessive–compulsive disorder. *Behaviour Research and Therapy, 37,* 941–951.

de Silva, P., & Rachman, S. J. (1984). Does escape behaviour strengthen agoraphobic avoidance?: A preliminary study. *Behaviour Research and Therapy, 22,* 87–91.

Devilly, G. J., Spence, S. H., & Rapee, R. M. (1998). Statistical and reliable change with eye movement desensitization and reprocessing: Treating trauma within a veteran population. *Behavior Therapy, 29,* 435–455.

Diaferia, G., Sciuto, G., Perna, G., Barnardeschi, L., Battaglia, M., Rusmini, S., & Bellodi, L. (1993). DSM-III-R personality disorders in panic disorder. *Journal of Anxiety Disorders*, 7, 153–161.

Diaz, M. L. (2000). *Exploring generalized anxiety disorder and worry in Peru*. Unpublished doctoral dissertation, Pennsylvania State University.

Diaz, S. F., Grush, L. R., Sichel, D. A., & Cohen, L. S. (1998). Obsessive–compulsive disorder in pregnancy and the puerperium. In L. J. Dickstein, M. B. Riba, & J. M. Oldham (Eds.), *Review of psychiatry* (Vol. 16). Washington, DC: American Psychiatric Press.

Dienstbier, R. A. (1989). Arousal and physiological toughness: Implications for mental and physical health. *Psychological Review*, 96(1), 84–100.

Diethelm, K. (1991). *Mutter–Kind-Interaktion: Entwicklung von ersten Kontrolluberzeugungen* [Mother–child interaction: Development of early control beliefs]. Bern, Switzerland: Huber.

DiLalla, L. F., Kagan, J., & Reznick, S. J. (1994). Genetic etiology of behavioral inhibition among 2-year-old children. *Infant Behavior and Development*, 17, 405–412.

Dimberg, U. (1982). Facial reactions to facial expressions. *Psychophysiology*, 19, 643–647.

Dimberg, U., & Öhman, A. (1983). The effects of directional facial cues on electrodermal conditioning to facial stimuli. *Psychophysiology*, 20, 160–167.

Dimsdale, J. E., & Moss, J. (1980). Plasma catecholamines and stress and exercise. *Journal of the American Medical Association*, 243, 340–342.

Di Nardo, P. A., & Barlow, D. H. (1988). *Anxiety Disorders Interview Schedule—Revised (ADIS-R)*. Albany: Phobia and Anxiety Disorders Clinic, State University of New York.

Di Nardo, P. A., Brown, T. A., & Barlow, D. H. (1994). *Anxiety Disorders Interview Schedule for DSM-IV: Lifetime Version (ADIS-IV-L)*. San Antonio, TX: Psychological Corporation/ Graywind Publications Incorporated.

Di Nardo, P. A., Guzy, L. T., Jenkins, J. A., Bak, R. M., Tomasi, S. F., & Copland, M. (1988). Etiology and maintenance of dog fears. *Behaviour Research and Therapy*, 26, 241–244.

Di Nardo, P. A., Moras, K., Barlow, D. H, Rapee, R. M., & Brown, T. A. (1993). Reliability of DSM-III-R disorder categories using the Anxiety Disorders Interview Schedule—Revised (ADIS-R). *Archives of General Psychiatry*, 50, 251–256.

Di Nardo, P. A., O'Brien, G. T., Barlow, D. H., Waddell, M. T., & Blanchard, E. B. (1983). Reliability of the DSM-III anxiety disorder categories using a new structured interview. *Archives of General Psychiatry*, 40, 1070–1074.

Dobson, K. S. (1985). The relationship between anxiety and depression. *Clinical Psychology Review*, 5, 307–324.

Doctor, R. M. (1982). Major results of a large-scale pretreatment survey of agoraphobics. In R. L. DuPont (Ed.), *Phobia: A comprehensive summary of modern treatments*. New York: Brunner/ Mazel.

Dohrenwend, B. P., & Shrout, P. E. (1981). Toward the development of a two-stage procedure for case identification and classification in psychiatric epidemiology. *Research in Community and Mental Health*, 2, 295–323.

Dolski, I. V., Malmstadt, J. R., Schaefer, S. M., Larson, C. L., Abercrombie, H. C., Ward, R. T., Truski, P. A., Perlman, S. B., Holden, J. T., & Davidson, R. J. (1996). EEG-defined left versus right frontally activated groups differ in metabolic asymmetry in the amygdala. *Psychophysiology*, 33, S35–544.

Domjan, M., Huber-McDonald, M., & Holloway, K. S. (1992). Conditioning copulatory behavior to an artificial object: Efficacy of stimulus fading. *Animal Learning and Behavior*, 20, 350–362.

Donnell, C. D., & McNally, R. J. (1990). Anxiety sensitivity and panic attacks in a nonclinical population. *Behaviour Research and Therapy*, 28, 83–85.

Dreessen, L., Arntz, A., Luttels, C., & Sallaerts, S. (1994). Personality disorders do not influence the results of cognitive-behavior therapies for anxiety disorders. *Comprehensive Psychiatry*, 35, 265–274.

Drury, A. N. (1919). The percentage of carbon dioxide in the alveolar air and the tolerance to accumulating carbon dioxide in cases of so-called "irritable heart" of soldiers. *Heart (London)*, 7, 165–173.

Dugas, M. J., Buhr, K., & Ladouceur, R. (in press). The role of intolerance of uncertainty in the etiology and maintenance of generalized anxiety disorder. In R. G. Heimberg, C. L. Turk, & D. S. Mennin (Eds.), *Generalized anxiety disorder: Advances in research and practice*. New York: Guilford Press.

Dugas, M. J., Freeston, M. H., & Ladouceur, R. (1997). Intolerance of uncertainty and problem orientation in worry. *Cognitive Therapy and Research, 21*, 593–606.

Dugas, M. J., Gagnon, F., Ladouceur, R., & Freeston, M. H. (1998). Generalized anxiety disorder: A preliminary test of a conceptual model. *Behaviour Research and Therapy, 36*, 215–226.

Dumas, J. E., LaFreniere, P. J., & Serketich, W. J. (1995). "Balance of power": A transactional analysis of control in mother–child dyads involving socially competent, aggressive, and anxious children. *Journal of Abnormal Psychology, 104*, 104–113.

Dunner, D. L., Ishiki, D., Avery, D. H., Wilson, L. G., & Hyde, T. S. (1986). Effect of alprazolam and diazepam on anxiety and panic attacks in panic disorder: A controlled study. *Journal of Clinical Psychiatry, 47*, 458–460.

DuPont, R. L., Rice, D. P., Miller, L. S., Shiraki, S. S., Rowland, C. R., & Harwood, H. J. (1996). Economic costs of anxiety disorders. *Anxiety, 2*, 167–172.

Durham, R. C., Murphy, T., Allen, T., Richard, K., Treliving, L. R., & Fenton, G. W. (1994). Cognitive therapy, analytic psychotherapy and anxiety management training for generalized anxiety disorder. *British Journal of Psychiatry, 165*, 315–323.

Dutton, D. G., & Aron, A. P. (1974). Some evidence for heightened sexual attraction under conditions of high anxiety. *Journal of Personality and Social Psychology, 30*, 510–517.

Duval, S., & Wicklund, R. A. (1972). *A theory of objective self-awareness*. New York: Academic Press.

Dworkin, B. R. (1993). *Learning and physiological regulation*. Chicago: University of Chicago Press.

Easterbrook, J. A. (1959). The effect of emotion on cue utilization and the organization of behavior. *Psychological Review, 66*, 183–201.

Easton, J. D., & Sherman, D. G. (1976). Somatic anxiety attacks and propranolol. *Archives of Neurology, 33*, 689–691.

Eaton, W. W., Dryman, A., & Weissman, M. M. (1991). Panic and phobia. In L. N. Robins & D. A. Regier (Eds.), *Psychiatric disorders in America: The Epidemiological Catchment Area study*. New York: Free Press.

Eaton, W. W., Kessler, R. C., Wittchen, H.-U., & Magee, W. J. (1994). Panic and panic disorder in the United States. *American Journal of Psychiatry, 151*, 413–420.

Eaves, L., & Eysenck, H. J. (1976). Genetic and environmental components of inconsistency and unrepeatability in twins' responses to a neuroticism questionnaire. *Behavior Genetics, 6*, 145–160.

Edelman, R. E., & Chambless, D. L. (1995). Adherence during sessions and homework in cognitive-behavioral group treatment of social phobia. *Behaviour Research and Therapy, 33*, 573–577.

Edelman, R. J. (1987). *The psychology of embarrassment*. Chichester, England: Wiley.

Ehlers, A. (1993). Somatic symptoms and panic attacks: A retrospective study of learning experiences. *Behaviour Research and Therapy, 31*, 269–278.

Ehlers, A., & Breuer, P. (1992). Increased cardiac awareness in panic disorder. *Journal of Abnormal Psychology, 101*, 371–382.

Ehlers, A., & Breuer, P. (1996). How good are patients with panic disorder at perceiving their heartbeats? *Biological Psychology, 42*, 165–182.

Ehlers, A., & Clark, D. M. (2000). A cognitive model of posttraumatic stress disorder. *Behavior Research and Therapy, 38*, 319–345.

Ehlers, A., Feigenbaum, W., Florin, I., & Margraf, J. (1995, July). *Efficacy of exposure in vivo in panic disorder with agoraphobia in a clinical setting*. Paper presented at the World Congress of Behavioural and Cognitive Therapies, Copenhagen, Denmark.

Ehlers, A., Hofmann, S. G., Herda, C. A., & Roth, W. T. (1994). Clinical characteristics of driving phobia. *Journal of Anxiety Disorders, 8*, 323–339.

Ehlers, A., Margraf, J., & Roth, W. T. (1987). Interaction of expectancy and physiological stressors in a laboratory model of panic. In D. Hellhammer & I. Florin (Eds.), *Psychological and biological approaches to the understanding of human disease: Vol. 2. Neuronal control of bodily function-basic and clinical aspects.* Göttingen, Germany: Hogrefe.

Ehlers, A., Margraf, J., Davies, S., & Roth, W. T. (1988). Selective processing of threat cues in subjects with panic attacks. *Cognition and Emotion, 2,* 201–219.

Ehlers, A., Margraf, J., Roth, W. T., Taylor, C. B., Maddock, R. J., Sheikh, J., Kobell, M. L., McClenahan, K. L., Gossard, D., Blowers, G. H., Agras, W. S., & Kopell, B. S. (1986). Lactate infusions and panic attacks: Do patients and controls respond differently? *Psychiatry Research, 17,* 295–308.

Eisen, J. L., Goodman, W. K., Keller, M. B., Warshaw, M. G., DeMarco, L. M., Luce, D. D., & Rasmussen, S. A. (1999). Patterns of remission and relapse in obsessive–compulsive disorder: A 2-year prospective study. *Journal of Clinical Psychiatry, 60,* 346–351.

Eisen, J. L., & Rasmussen, S. A. (1993). Obsessive compulsive disorder with psychotic features. *Journal of Clinical Psychiatry, 54,* 373–379.

Eisen, J. L., & Steketee, G. (1998). Course of illness in obsessive–compulsive disorder. In L. J. Dickstein, M. B. Riba, & J. M. Oldham (Eds.), *Review of psychiatry* (Vol. 16). Washington, D. C. : American Psychiatric Press.

Eke, M., & McNally, R. J. (1996). Anxiety sensitivity, suffocation fear, trait anxiety, and breath-holding duration as predictors of response to carbon dioxide challenge. *Behaviour Research and Therapy, 34,* 603–607.

Ekman, P. (1992). Are there basic emotions? *Psychological Review, 99,* 550–553.

Ekman, P. (1994). Strong evidence for universals in facial expressions: A reply to Russell's mistaken critique. *Psychological Bulletin, 115,* 268–287.

Ekman, P., & Davidson, R. J. (Eds.). (1994). *The nature of emotion: Fundamental questions.* New York: Oxford University Press.

Ekman, P., Levenson, R., & Friesen, W. (1983). Autonomic nervous system activity distinguishes among emotions. *Science, 221,* 1208–1210.

Elam, M., Yoa, T., Thoren, P., & Svensson, T. H. (1981). Hypercapnia and hypoxia: Chemoreceptor-roediated control of locus ceruleus neurons and splanchnic, sympathetic nerves. *Brain Research, 222,* 373–381.

Elder, G. H. (1974). The children of the Great Depression: Social change in life experience. Chicago: University of Chicago Press.

Emde, R. N. (1980). Levels of meaning for infant emotions: A biosocial view. In W. A. Collins (Ed.), *Minnesota Symposia on Child Psychology: Vol. 13. Development of cognition, affect and social relations.* Hillsdale, NJ: Erlbaum.

Emde, R. N., Gaensbauer, T. J., & Harmon, R. J. (1976). *Emotional expressions in infancy.* New York: International Universities Press.

Emde, R. N., Kligman, D. H., Reich, J. H., & Wade, T. D. (1978). Emotional expression in infancy: Initial studies of social signaling and an emergent model. In M. Lewis & L. Rosenblum (Eds.), *The Development of affect.* New York: Plenum Press.

Emmanuel, N. P., Johnson, M., & Villareal, G. (1998). *Imipramine in the treatment of social phobia: A double-blind study.* Poster presented at the 36th Meeting of the American College of Neuropsychopharmacology, Waikoloa, HI.

Emmanuel, N. P., Lydiard, R. B., & Ballenger, J. C. (1991). Treatment of social phobia with bupropion. *Journal of Clinical Psychopharmacology, 11,* 276–277.

Emmelkamp, P. M. G. (1982). *Phobic and obsessive–compulsive disorders: Theory, research, and practice.* New York: Plenum Press.

Emmelkamp, P. M. G., & Beens, H. (1991). Cognitive therapy with obsessive–compulsive disorder: A comparative evaluation. *Behaviour Research and Therapy, 29,* 293–300.

Emmelkamp, P. M. G., Kraaijkamp, H. J. M., & van den Hout, M. A. (1999). Assessment of obsessive–compulsive disorder. *Behavior Modification, 23,* 269–279.

Emmelkamp, P. M. G., & Kraanen, J. (1977). Obsessional ruminations: A comparison between thought stopping and prolonged exposure in imagination. *Behaviour Research and Therapy, 15*, 491–495.

Emmelkamp, P. M. G., & Kuipers, A. C. M. (1979). Agoraphobia: A follow-up study four years after treatment. *British Journal of Psychiatry, 128*, 86–89.

Emmelkamp, P. M. G., & Ultee, K. A. (1974). A comparison of "successive approximation" and "self-observation" in the treatment of agoraphobia. *Behavior Therapy, 5*, 606–613.

Emmelkamp, P. M. G., van den Heuvell, C. V. L., Ruphan, M., & Sanderman, R. (1989). Home based treatment of obsessive–compulsive patients: Intersession interval and therapist involvement. *Behaviour Research and Therapy, 27*, 89–93.

Emmelkamp, P. M. G., Van Dyck, R., Bitter, M., Heins, R., Onstein, E. J., & Eisen, B. (1992). Spouse-aided therapy with agoraphobia. *British Journal of Psychotherapy, 160*, 51–56.

Emmelkamp, P. M. G., Visser, S., & Hoekstra, R. J. (1988). Cognitive therapy vs. exposure in vivo in the treatment of obsessive–compulsives. *Cognitive Therapy and Research, 12*, 103–114.

Emmelkamp, P. M. G., & Wessels, H. (1975). Flooding in imagination vs. flooding in vivo: A comparison with agoraphobics. *Behaviour Research and Therapy, 13*, 7–15.

Enkelmann, R. (1991). Alprazolam versus buspirone in the treatment of outpatients with generalized anxiety disorder. *Psychopharmacology, 105*, 428–432.

Evans, L., Schneider, P., Ross-Lee, L., Wiltshire, B., Eadie, M., Kenaidy, J., & Hoey, H. (1986). Plasma serotonin levels in agoraphobia. *American Journal of Psychiatry, 142*, 267.

Eysenck, H. J. (Ed.). (1960). *Behaviour therapy and the neuroses.* Oxford: Pergamon Press.

Eysenck, H. J. (1961). *The handbook of abnormal psychology.* New York: Basic Books.

Eysenck, H. J. (Ed.). (1967). *The biological basis of personality.* Springfield, IL: Charles C Thomas.

Eysenck, H. J. (1970). *The structure of human personality.* London: Methuen.

Eysenck, H. J. (1979). The conditioning model of neurosis. *Behavioral and Brain Sciences, 2*, 155–199.

Eysenck, H. J. (1981). *A model for personality.* New York: Springer-Verlag.

Eysenck, M. W. (1992). *Anxiety: The cognitive perspective.* Hillsdale, NJ: Erlbaum.

Eysenck, M. W., Mogg, K., May, J., Richards, A., & Mathews, A. (1991). Bias in interpretation of ambiguous sentences related to threat in anxiety. *Journal of Abnormal Psychology, 100*, 144–150.

Fabrega, H. (1991). Psychiatric stigma in non-Western societies. *Comprehensive Psychiatry, 32*, 534–551.

Fairbank, J. A., & Keane, T. M. (1982). Flooding for combat-related stress disorders: Assessment of anxiety reduction across traumatic memories. *Behavior Therapy, 13*, 499–510.

Fals-Stewart, W., Marks, A. P., & Schafer, J. (1993). A comparison of behavioral group therapy and individual behavior therapy in treating obsessive–compulsive disorder. *Journal of Nervous and Mental Disease, 181*, 189–193.

Faravelli, C. (1985). Life events preceding the onset of panic disorder. *Journal of Affective Disorders, 9*, 103–105.

Faravelli, C., Guerinni Degl'Innocenti, B., & Giardinelli, L. (1989). Epidemiology of anxiety disorders in Florence. *Acta Psychiatrica Scandinavica, 79*, 308–312.

Faravelli, C., & Pallanti, S. (1989). Recent life events and panic disorder. *American Journal of Psychiatry, 146*(5), 622–626.

Faravelli, C., Pallanti, S., Biondi, F., Paterniti, S., & Scarpato, M. A. (1992). Onset of panic disorder. *American Journal of Psychiatry, 149*, 827–828.

Farid, B. T. (1986). Obsessional symptomatology and adverse mood states. *British Journal of Psychiatry, 149*, 108–112.

Fava, G. A., Grandi, S., & Canestrari, R. (1988). Prodromal symptoms in panic disorder with agoraphobia. *American Journal of Psychiatry, 145*, 1564–1567.

Fava, G. A., Zielezny, M., Savron, G., & Grandi, S. (1995). Long-term effects of behavioural treatment for panic disorder and agoraphobia. *British Journal of Psychiatry, 166*, 87–92.

Fava, M., & Rosenbaum, J. F. (1998). Anger attacks in depression. *Depression and Anxiety, 8*, 59–63.

Fava, M., Anderson, K., & Rosenbaum, J. F. (1990). "Anger attacks": Possible variants of panic and major depressive disorders. *American Journal of Psychiatry, 147*, 867–870.

Fecteau, G., & Nicki, R. (1999). Cognitive behavioral treatment of post traumatic stress disorder after motor vehicle accident. *Behavioral and Cognitive Psychotherapy, 27*, 201–214.

Feigenbaum, W. (1988). Long-term efficacy of ungraded versus graded massed exposure in agoraphobics. In I. Hand & H.-U. Wittchen (Eds.), *Panic and phobias: Treatments and variables affecting course and outcome*. Berlin: Springer-Verlag.

Feighner, J. P., Merideth, C. H., & Hendrickson, G. A. (1982). A double-blind comparison of buspirone and diazepam in outpatients with generalized anxiety disorder. *Journal of Clinical Psychiatry, 43*, 103–107.

Feldman, J. M., Giardino, N. D., & Lehrer, P. M. (2000). Asthma and panic disorder. In D. I. Mostofsky & D. H. Barlow (Eds.), *The management of stress and anxiety in medical disorders*. Boston: Allyn & Bacon.

Felitti, V. J., Anda, R. F., Nordenberg, D., Williamson, D. F., Spitz, A. M., Edwards, V., Koss, M. P., & Marks, J. S. (1998). Relationship of childhood abuse and household dysfunction to many of the leading causes of death in adults: The Adverse Childhood Experiences (ACE) Study. *American Journal of Preventive Medicine, 14*, 245–258.

Fenichel, O. (1945). *The psychoanalytic theory of neurosis*. New York: Norton.

Fenigstein, A., & Carver, C. S. (1978). Self-focusing effects of heartbeat feedback. *Journal of Personality and Social Psychology, 36*, 1241–1250.

Fenigstein, A., Scheier, M. F., & Buss, A. H. (1975). Public and private self-consciouness: Assessment and theory. *Journal of Consulting and Clinical Psychology, 43*, 522–527.

Ferrari, J. R. (1995). Perfectionism cognitions with nonclinical and clinical samples. *Journal of Social and Behavioral Personality, 10*, 143–156.

Feske, U., & Chambless, D. L. (1995). Cognitive behavioral versus exposure only treatment for social phobia: A meta-analysis. *Behavior Therapy, 26*, 695–720.

Feske, U., & Chambless, D. L. (2000). A review of assessment measures for obsessive–compulsive disorder. In W. K. Goodman, M. Rudorfer, & J. D. Maser (Eds.) *Obsessive compulsive disorder: Contemporary issues in treatment*. Mahwah, NJ: Erlbaum.

Feske, U., & de Beurs, E. (1997). The Panic Appraisal Inventory: Psychometric properties. *Behaviour Research and Therapy, 35*, 875–882.

Feske, U., Perry, K. J., Chambless, D. L., Renneberg, B., & Goldstein, A. J. (1996). Avoidant personality disorder as predictor for severity and treatment outcome among generalized social phobics. *Journal of Personality Disorder, 10*, 174–184.

Fewtrell, W. D. (1984). Relaxation and depersonalization. *British Journal of Psychiatry, 145*, 217.

Fifer, S. K., Mathias, S. D., Patrick, D. L., Majonson, P. D., Lubeck, D. P., & Buesching, D. P. (1994). Untreated anxiety among adult primary care patients in a health maintenance organization. *Archives of General Psychiatry, 51*, 740–750.

Figley, C. R. (1978). Symptoms of delayed combat stress among a college sample of Vietnam veterans. *Military Medicine, 143*, 107–110.

Fink, M., Taylor, M. A., & Volavka, J. (1970). Anxiety produced by lactate. *New England Journal of Medicine, 281*, 1429–1440.

Finkelhor, D., & Dzuiba-Leatherman, J. (1994). Victimization of children. *American Psychologist, 49*, 173–183.

Finlay-Jones, R., & Brown, G. W. (1981). Types of stressful life event and the onset of anxiety and depressive disorders. *Psychological Medicine, 11*, 801–815.

First, M. B., Spitzer, R. L., Gibbon, M., & Williams, J. B. W. (1996). *Structured Clinical Interview for DSM-IV Axis I Disorders—Patient Edition (SCID-I/P, Version 2.0)*. New York: Biometrics Research Department, New York State Psychiatric Institute.

First, M. B., Spitzer, R. L., Gibbon, M., & Williams, J. B. W. (1997). *Structured Clinical Interview for DSM-IV Axis I Disorders (SCID-I): Clinician version.* Washington, DC: American Psychiatric Press.

Fishbein, M., Middlestadt, S. E., & Ottati, V. (1988). Medical problems among International Conference of Symphony and Opera Musicians (ICSOM): Overview of a national survey. *Medical Problems of Performing Arts, 3,* 1.

Fisher, M. F. K. (1978). The wind chill factor or, a problem of mind and matter. In S. Cahill (Ed.), *Women and fiction 2: Short stories by and about women.* New York: New American Library.

Flack, W. F., Litz, B. T., Hsieh, F. Y., Kaloupek, D. G., & Keane, T. M. (2000). Predictors of emotional numbing revisited: A replication and extension. *Journal of Traumatic Stress, 13,* 611–618.

Fleet, R. P., Dupuis, G., Marchand, A., Burelle, D., Arsenault, A., & Beitman, B. D. (1996). Panic disorder in emergency department chest pain patients: Prevalence, comorbidity, suicidal ideation, and physician recognition. *American Journal of Medicine, 101,* 371–378.

Fleiss, J. L., Nee, J. C. M., & Landis, J. R. (1979). Large sample variance of kappa in the case of different sets of raters. *Psychological Bulletin, 86,* 974–977.

Flint, A. J. (1994). Epidemiology and comorbidity of anxiety disorders in the elderly. *American Journal of Psychiatry, 151(5),* 640–649.

Flint, A., Koszycki, D., Vaccarino, F., Cadieux, A., Boulenger, P., & Bradwejn, J. (1998). The effect of aging on cholecystokinin-induced panic. *American Journal of Psychiatry, 155,* 283–285.

Flint, J., Corley, R., DeFries, J. C., Fulker, D. W., Gray, J. A., Miller, S., & Collins, A. C. (1995). A simple genetic basis for a complex psychological trait in laboratory mice. *Science, 269,* 1432–1435.

Flynn, T. M., Taylor, P., & Pollard, C. A. (1992). Use of mobile phones in the behavioral treatment of driving phobias. *Journal of Behavior Therapy and Experimental Psychiatry, 23,* 299–302.

Foa, E. B. (1979). Failure in treating obsessive–compulsives. *Behaviour Research and Therapy, 17,* 169–176.

Foa, E. B., Abramowitz, J. S., Franklin, M. E., & Kozak, M. J. (1999). Feared consequences, fixity of belief, and treatment outcome in patients with obsessive–compulsive disorder. *Behavior Therapy, 30,* 717–724.

Foa, E. B., Blau, J. S., Prout, M., & Latimer, P. (1977). Is horror a necessary component of flooding (implosion)? *Behaviour Research and Therapy, 15,* 397–402.

Foa, E. B., Cashman, L., Jaycox, L., & Perry, K. (1997). The validation of a self-report measure of posttraumatic stress disorder: The Posttraumatic Diagnostic Scale. *Psychological Assessment, 9,* 445–451.

Foa, E. B., Dancu, C. V., Hembree, E. A., Jaycox, L. H., Meadows, E. A., & Street, G. P. (1999). A comparison of exposure therapy, stress inoculation training, and their combination for reducing posttraumatic stress disorder in female assault victims. *Journal of Consulting and Clinical Psychology, 67,* 194–200.

Foa, E. B., Feske, U., Murdock, T. B., Kozak, M. J., & McCarthy, P. R. (1991). Processing of threat-related information in rape victims. *Journal of Abnormal Psychology, 100(2),* 156–162.

Foa, E. B., Grayson, J. B., Steketee, G., Doppelt, H. G., Turner, R. M., & Latimer, P. L. (1983). Success and failure in the behavioral treatment of obsessive–compulsives. *Journal of Consulting and Clinical Psychology, 15,* 287–297.

Foa, E. B., Hearst-Ikeda, D., & Perry, K. J. (1995). Evaluation of a brief cognitive-behavioral program for the prevention of chronic PTSD in recent assault victims. *Journal of Consulting and Clinical Psychology, 63,* 948–955.

Foa, E. B., Jameson, J. S., Turner, R. M., & Payne, L. L. (1980). Massed versus spaced exposure sessions in the treatment of agoraphobia. *Behaviour Research and Therapy, 18,* 333–338.

Foa, E. B., Keane, T. M., & Friedman, M. J. (Eds.). (2000). *Effective treatments for PTSD: Practice guidelines from the International Society for Traumatic Stress Studies.* New York: Guilford Press.

Foa, E. B., & Kozak, M. J. (1986). Emotional processing of fear: Exposure to corrective information. *Psychological Bulletin, 99,* 20–35.

Foa, E. B., & Kozak, M. J. (1995). DSM-IV field trial: Obsessive–compulsive disorder. *American Journal of Psychiatry, 152,* 90–96.

Foa, E. B., Kozak, M. J., Salkovskis, P. M., Coles, M. E., & Amir, N. (1998). The validation of a new obsessive–compulsive disorder scale: The Obsessive–Compulsive Inventory. *Psychological Assessment, 10,* 206–214.

Foa, E. B., Kozak, M. J., Steketee, G., & McCarthy, P. R. (1992). Treatment of depressive and obsessive compulsive symptoms in OCD by imipramine and behavior therapy. *British Journal of Clinical Psychology, 31,* 279–292.

Foa, E. B., & McNally, R. J. (1986). Sensitivity to feared stimuli in obsessive–compulsives: A dichotic listening analysis. *Cognitive Therapy and Research, 10,* 477–485.

Foa, E. B., Riggs, D., Dancu, C., & Rothbaum, B. O., (1993). Reliability and validity of a brief instrument for assessing posttraumatic stress disorder. *Journal of Traumatic Stress, 6,* 459–474.

Foa, E. B., Rothbaum, B. O., Riggs, D. S., & Murdock, T. B. (1991). Treatment of posttraumatic stress disorder in rape victims: A comparison between cognitive-behavioral procedures and counseling. *Journal of Consulting and Clinical Psychology, 59,* 715–723.

Foa, E. B., Steketee, G. S., Grayson, J. B., Turner, R. M., & Latimer, P. R. (1984). Deliberate exposure and blocking of obsessive–compulsive rituals: Immediate and long term effects. *Behaviour Therapy, 15,* 450–472.

Foa, E. B., Steketee, G. S., & Ozarow, B. J. (1985). Behavior therapy with obsessive–compulsives: From theory to treatment. In M. R. Mavissakalian, S. M. Turner, & L. Michelson (Eds.), *Obsessive–compulsive disorders: Psychological and pharmacological treatment.* New York: Plenum Press.

Foa, E. B., Steketee, G., & Rothbaum, B. O. (1989). Behavioral/cognitive conceptualizations of post-traumatic stress disorder. *Behavior Therapy, 20,* 155–176.

Fonagy, P., Leigh, T., Steele, M., Steele, H., Kennedy, R., Mattoon, G., Target, M., & Gerber, A. (1996). The relation of attachment status, psychiatric classification, and response to psychotherapy. *Journal of Consulting and Clinical Psychology, 64,* 22–31.

Formea, G., & Burns, L. (1995). Relation between the syndromes of bulimia nervosa and obsessive compulsive disorder. *Journal of Psychopathology and Behavioral Assessment, 17,* 167–176.

Forsman, L. (1981). Habitual catecholamine excretion and its relation to habitual distress. *Biological Psychiatry, 11,* 83–97.

Forsyth, J. P., & Eifert, G. H. (1996). Systematic alarms in fear conditioning: I. A reappraisal of what is being conditioned. *Behavior Therapy, 27*(3), 441–462.

Forsyth, J. P., & Eifert, G. H. (1998). Response intensity in content-specific fear conditioning comparing 20% versus 13% CO_2-enriched air as unconditioned stimuli. *Journal of Abnormal Psychology, 107,* 291–304.

Forsyth, J. P., Eifert, G. H., & Thompson, R. N. (1996). Systematic alarms in fear conditioning: II. An experimental methodology using 20% carbon dioxide inhalation as an unconditioned stimulus. *Behavior Therapy, 27,* 391–415.

Forsyth, J. P., Lejuez, C. W., & Finlay, C. (2000). Anxiogenic effects of repeated administrations of 20% CO_2-enriched air: Stability within sessions and habituation across time. *Journal of Behavior Therapy and Experimental Psychiatry, 31,* 103–121.

Fox, N. A. (1991). If it's not left, it's right. *American Psychologist, 46,* 863–872.

Frances, A., Widiger, T., & Fyer, M. R. (1990). The influence of classification methods on comorbidity. In J. D. Maser & C. R. Cloninger (Eds.), *Comorbidity of mood and anxiety disorders.* Washington, DC: American Psychiatric Press.

Francis, D., Diorio, J., Liu, D., & Meany, M. J. (1999). Nongenomic transmission across generations of maternal behavior and stress responses in the rat. *Science, 286,* 1155–1158.

Francis, G., & Radka, D. F. (1995). Social anxiety in children and adolescents. In M. Stein (Ed.), *Social phobia: Clinical and research perspectives.* Washigton, DC: American Psychiatric Press.

Frank, E., & Stewart, B. D. (1983). Treating depression in victims of rape. *Clinical Psychologist, 36*, 95–98.

Franklin, M. E., Abramowitz, J. S., Kozak, M. J., Levitt, J. T., & Foa, E. B. (2000). Effectiveness of exposure and ritual prevention for obsessive compulsive disorder: Randomized versus non-randomized samples. *Journal of Consulting and Clinical Psychology, 68*, 594–602.

Fredrick, C., Pynoos, R., & Nader, K. (1992). *Childhood PTSD Reaction Index (CPTS-RI)*. (Available from R. Pynoos, 760 Westwood Plaza, Los Angeles, CA 90024; or K. Nader, P.O. Box 2251, Laguna Hills, CA 92654.

Fredrikson, M., Annas, P., & Wik, G. (1997). Parental history, aversive exposure and the development of snake and spider phobia in women. *Behaviour Research and Therapy, 35*, 23–28.

Fredrikson, M., Annas, P., Fischer, H., & Wik, G. (1996). Gender and age differences in the prevalence of specific fears and phobias. *Behaviour Research and Therapy, 26*, 241–244.

Fredrikson, M., Wik, G., Greitz, T., Eriksson, L., Stone-Elander, S., Ericson, K., & Sedvall, G. (1993). Regional cerebral blood flow during experimental phobic fear. *Psychophysiology, 30*, 126–130.

Freedman, M. D., Leary, T. F., Ossorio, A. G., & Coffey, H. S. (1951). The interpersonal dimension of personality. *Journal of Personality, 20*, 143–161.

Freedman, R. R., Ianni, P., Ettedgui, E., & Puthezhath, N. (1985). Ambulatory monitoring of panic disorder. *Archives of General Psychiatry, 42*, 244–250.

Freeston, M. H., Dugas, M. J., & Ladouceur, R. (1996). Thoughts, images, worry, and anxiety. *Cognitive Therapy and Research, 20*(3), 265–273.

Freeston, M. H., Dugas, M. J., Letarte, H., Rhéaume, J., Blais, F., & Ladouceur, R. (1996). Physical symptoms associated with worry in a nonclinical population. *Journal of Anxiety Disorders, 10*, 365–377.

Freeston, M. H., & Ladouceur, R. (1997). What do patients do with their obsessional thoughts? *Behaviour Research and Therapy, 5*, 335–348.

Freeston, M. H., Ladouceur, R., Gagnon, F., Thibodeau, N., Rhéaume, J., Letarte, H., & Bujold, A. (1997). Cognitive-behavioral treatment of obsessive thoughts: A controlled study. *Journal of Consulting and Clinical Psychology, 65*, 405–413.

Freeston, M. H., Ladouceur, R., Thibodeau, H., & Gagnon, F. (1991). Cognitive intrusions in a nonclinical population: I. *Behaviour Research and Therapy, 29*, 585–597.

Freeston, M. H., Rhéaume, J., & Ladouceur, R. (1996). Correcting faulty appraisals of obsessional thoughts. *Behaviour Research and Therapy, 34*, 433–446.

Freeston, M. H., Rhéaume, J., Letarte, H., Dugas, M. J., & Ladouceur, R. (1994). Why do people worry? *Personality and Individual Differences, 17*, 791–802.

Freud, S. (1936). *The basic writings of Sigmund Freud.* New York: Random House.

Freud, S. (1940). The justification for detaching from neurasthenia a particular syndrome: The anxiety-neurosis (J. Rickman, Trans.). In *Collected papers* (Vol. 1). New York: Basic Books. (Original work published 1895)

Freud, S. (1959). Inhibitions, symptoms and anxiety. In J. Strachey (Ed. and Trans.), *The standard edition of the complete psychological works of Sigmund Freud* (Vol. 20). London: Hogarth Press. (Original work published 1926)

Freud, S. (1962). Obsessions and phobias: Their psychical mechanism and their aetiology. In J. Strachey (Ed. and Trans.), *The standard edition of the complete psychological works of Sigmund Freud* (Vol. 3). London: Hogarth Press. (Original work published 1895)

Freud, S. (1963). Introductory lectures on psycho-analysis: Lecture 25. Anxiety. In J. Strachey (Ed. and Trans.), *The standard edition of the complete psychological works of Sigmund Freud* (Vol. 16). London: Hogarth Press. (Original work published 1917)

Freyd, J. (1994). Betrayal trauma: Traumatic amnesia as an adaptive response to childhood abuse. *Ethics and Behavior, 4*, 307–329.

Fried, R. (1994). Respiration in clinical psychophysiology: How to assess clinical parameters in breathing and their change with treatment. In J. G. Carlson, R. A. Seifert, & N. Birbaumer (Eds.), *Clinical applied psychophysiology.* New York: Plenum Press.

Fried, R., & Grimaldi, J. (1993). *The psychology and physiology of breathing in behavioral medicine, clinical psychology, and psychiatry*. New York: Plenum Press.

Friedman, B. H., Thayer, J. F., Borkovec, T. D., & Lyonfields, J. (1993). *Psychophysiological assessment of generalized anxiety disorder*. Paper presented at the annual meeting of the Midwestern Psychological Association, Chicago.

Friedman, B. H., Thayer, J. F., Borkovec, T. D., Tyrrell, R. A., Johnson, B.-H., & Columbo, R. (1993). Autonomic characteristics of non-clinical panic and blood phobia. *Biological Psychiatry, 34*, 298–310.

Friedman, M. J. (2000). *Posttraumatic Stress Disorder: The Latest Assessment and Treatment Strategies*. Kansas City, MO: Clinical Compacts.

Friedman, S. (Ed.). (1997). *Cultural issues in the treatment of anxiety*. New York: Guilford Press.

Friedman, S., Hatch, M., Paradis, C. M., Popkin, M., & Shalita, A. R. (1995). Obsessive compulsive disorders in two black ethnic groups: Incidence in an urban dermatology clinic. *Journal of Anxiety Disorders, 7*, 343–348.

Friedman, S., Jones, J. C., Chernen, L., & Barlow, D. H. (1992). Suicidal ideation and suicide attempts among patients with panic disorder: A survey of two outpatient clinics. *American Journal of Psychiatry, 149*(5), 680–685.

Friedman, S., Paradis, C. M., & Hatch, M. (1994). Characteristics of African-American and white patients with panic disorder and agoraphobia. *Hospital and Community Psychiatry, 45*(8), 798–803.

Friedman, S., Sunderland, G. S., & Rosenblum, L. A. (1988). A nonhuman primate model of panic disorder. *Psychiatry Research, 23*(1), 65–75.

Frohlich, E. D., Tarazi, R. C., & Duston, H. P. (1969). Hyperdynamic beta-adrenergic circulatory state. *Archives of Internal Medicine, 123*, 1–7.

Frost, R. O., Sher, K. J., & Geen, T. (1986). Psychotherapy and personality characteristics of non-clinical compulsive checkers. *Behaviour Research and Therapy, 24*, 133–143.

Frost, R. O., & Steketee, G. (1997). Perfectionism in obsessive compulsive disorder patients. *Behaviour Research and Therapy, 35*, 291–296.

Frost, R. O., Steketee, G., Cohn, L., & Greiss, K. (1994). Personality traits in subclinical and non-obsessive compulsive volunteers and their parents. *Behaviour Research and Therapy, 32*, 47–56.

Frueh, B. C., Turner, S. M., Beidel, D. C., Mirabella, R. F., & Jones, W. J. (1996).Trauma management therapy: A preliminary evaluation of a multicomponent behavioral treatment for chronic combat related PTSD. *Behaviour Research and Therapy, 34*, 533–543.

Fuller, I. L., & Thompson, W. R. (1978). *Foundations of behavior genetics*. St. Louis: Mosby.

Fyer, A. J. (1995). *Schedule for Affective Disorders and Schizophrenia—Lifetime Anxiety version, updated for DSM-IV* [SADS-LA-IV]. New York: Anxiety Disorders Clinic, New York State Psychiatric Institute.

Fyer, A. J., Endicott, J., Mannuzza, S., & Klein, D. F. (1985). *Schedule for Affective Disorders and Schizophrenia: Lifetime Version* (modified for the study of anxiety disorders). New York: Anxiety Disorders Clinic, New York State Psychiatric Institute.

Fyer, A. J., Mannuzza, S., Chapman, T. F., Liebowitz, M. R., & Klein, D. F. (1993). A direct interview family study of social phobia. *Archives of General Psychiatry, 50*, 286–293.

Fyer, A. J., Mannuzza, S., Chapman, T. F., Martin, L. Y., & Klein, D. F. (1995). Specificity in familial aggregation of phobic disorders. *Archives of General Psychiatry, 52*, 564–573.

Fyer, A. J., Mannuzza, S., Gallops, M. S., Martin, L. Y., Aaronson, C., Gorman, J. G., Liebowitz, M. R., & Klein, D. F. (1990). Familial transmission of simple phobias and fears: A preliminary report. *Archives of General Psychiatry, 47*, 252–256.

Fyer, A. J., Mannuzza, S., Martin, L. Y., Gallops, M. S., Endicott, J., Schleyer, B., Gorman, J., Liebowitz, M. R., & Klein, D. F. (1989). Reliability of anxiety assessment: II. Symptom assessment. *Archives of General Psychiatry, 46*, 1102–1110.

Fyer, A. J., & Rassnick, H. (1990). *Frequency and symptom thresholds for panic disorder* (Report to the DSM-IV Anxiety Disorders Work Group). New York: New York State Psychiatric Institute.

Gaffney, F. A., Fenton, B. J., Lane, L. D., & Lake, R. (1988). Hemodynamic, ventilatory, and biochemical responses of panic patients and normal controls with sodium lactate infusion and spontaneous panic attacks. *Archives of General Psychiatry, 45,* 53–60.

Gallup, G. G., Jr. (1974). Animal hypnosis: Factual status of a fictional concept. *Psychological Bulletin, 81,* 836–853.

Gammans, R. E., Stringfellow, J. C., Hvizdos, A. J., Seidehamel, R. J., Cohn, J. B., Wilcox, C. S., Fabre, L. F., Pecknold, J. C., Smith, W. T., & Rickels, K. (1992). Use of buspirone in patients with generalized anxiety disorder and coexisting depressive symptoms. *Neuropsychobiology, 25,* 193–201.

Garcia, J., McGowan, B. K., & Green, K. F. (i972). Biological constraints on conditioning. In A. H. Black & W. F. Prokasy (Eds.), *Classical conditioning II: Current research and theory.* New York: Appleton-Century-Crofts.

Garfield, S. L., Gershon, S., Sletten, I., Sundland, D. W., & Ballows, S. (1967). Chemically induced anxiety. *International Journal of Neuropsychiatry, 3,* 426–433.

Garmezy, N. (1986). Developmental aspects of children's responses to the stress of separation and loss. In M. Rutter, C. E. Izard, & P. B. Reid (Eds.), *Depression in young people: Developmental and clinical perspectives.* New York: McGraw-Hill.

Garmezy, N., & Rutter, M. (1983). *Stress, coping, and development in children.* New York: McGraw-Hill.

Garrison, C. Z., Weinrich, M. W., Hardin, S. B., Weinrich, S., & Wang, L. (1993). Posttraumatic stress disorder in adolescents after a hurricane. *American Journal of Epidemiology, 138,* 522–530.

Garssen, B., Buikhuisen, M., & van Dyck, R. (1996). Hyperventilation and panic attacks. *American Journal of Psychiatry, 153,* 513–518.

Garssen, B., de Beurs, E., Buikhuisen, M., van Balkom, A., Lange, A., & van Dyck, R. (1996). On distinguishing types of panic. *Journal of Anxiety Disorders, 10,* 173–184.

Garssen, B., de Ruiter, C., & van Dyck, R. (1992). Breathing retraining: A rational placebo? *Clinical Psychology Review, 12,* 141–153.

Garssen, B., vanVeenendaal, W., & Bloemink, R. (1983). Agoraphobia and the hyperventilation syndrome. *Behaviour Research and Therapy, 21,* 643–649.

Garvey, M. J., & Tollefson, G. D. (1986). Prevalence of misuse of prescribed benzodiazepines in patients with primary anxiety disorder or major depression. *American Journal of Psychiatry, 143,* 1601–1603.

Gater, R., Tansella, M., Korten, A., Tiemens, B. G., Mavreas, V. G., & Olatawura, M. O. (1998). Sex differences in the prevalence and detection of depressive and anxiety disorders in general health care settings. *Archives of General Psychiatry, 55,* 405–413.

Gauthier, J., & Marshall, W. L. (1977). The determination of optimal exposure to phobic stimuli in flooding therapy. *Behaviour Research and Therapy, 15,* 403–410.

Geer, J. H., Davison, G. C., & Gatchel, R. I. (1970). Reduction of stress in humans through nonveridical perceived control of aversive stimulation. *Journal of Personality and Social Psychology, 16*(4), 731–738.

Geer, J. H., & Fuhr, R. (1976). Cognitive factors in sexual arousal: The role of distraction. *Journal of Consulting and Clinical Psychology, 44,* 238–243.

Gelder, M. G., & Marks, I. M. (1966). Severe agoraphobia: A controlled prospective trial of behavioral therapy. *British Journal of Psychiatry, 112,* 309–319.

Gelder, M. G., & Marks, I. M. (1968). Desensitization and phobias: A crossover study. *British Journal of Psychiatry, 114,* 323–328.

Gelder, M. G., Marks, I. M., & Wolff, H. H. (1967). Desensitization and psychotherapy in the treatment of phobic states: A controlled inquiry. *British Journal of Psychiatry, 113,* 53–73.

Gelenberg, A. J., Lydiard, R. B., Rudolph, R. L., Aguiar, L, Haskins, J. T., & Salinas, E. (2000). Efficacy of venlafaxine extended-release capsules in nondepressed outpatients with generalized anxiety disorder. *Journal of the American Medical Association, 283,* 3082–3088.

Gelernter, C. S., Uhde, T. W., Cimbolic, P., Arnkoff, D. B., Vittone, B. J., Tancer, M. E., & Bartko, J. J. (1991). Cognitive-behavioral and pharmacological treatment for social phobia: A controlled study. *Archives of General Psychiatry, 48,* 938–945.

Geller, I., & Seifter, J. (1960). The effects of meprobamate, barbituates, *d*-amphetamine and promazine on experimentally induced conflict in the rat. *Psychopharmacologia, 1,* 482–492.

George, L. K., Hughes, D. C., & Blazer, D. G. (1986). Urban/rural differences in the prevalence of anxiety disorders. *American Journal of Social Psychiatry, 6,* 249–258.

Geracioti, T. D., & Post, R. M. (1991). Onset of panic disorder associated with rare use of cocaine. *Biological Psychiatry, 29,* 403–406.

Gerardi, R., Keane, T. M., & Penk, W. E. (1989). Utility: Sensitivity and specificity in developing diagnostic tests of combat-related post-traumatic stress disorder (PTSD). *Journal of Clinical Psychology, 45,* 691–703.

Gershuny, B. S., & Sher, K. J. (1998). The relation between personality and anxiety: Findings from a 3-year prospective study. *Journal of Abnormal Psychology, 107*(2), 252–262.

Getka, E. J., & Glass, C. R. (1992). Behavioral and cognitive-behavioral approaches to the reduction of dental anxiety. *Behavior Therapy, 23,* 433–448.

Ghosh, A., & Marks, I. M. (1987). Self-treatment of agoraphobia by exposure. *Behavior Therapy, 18,* 3–16.

Gibbons, F. X. (1991). Self-evaluation and self-perception: The role of attention in the experience of anxiety. In R. Schwarzer & R. A. Wicklund (Eds.), *Anxiety and self-focused attention.* New York: Harwood.

Gilkinson, H. (1942). Social fears as reported by students in college speech classes. *Speech Monographs, 9,* 141–160.

Gilligan, S. G., & Bower, G. H. (1984). Cognitive consequences of emotional arousal. In C. E. Izard, J. Kagan, & R. B. Zajonc (Eds.), *Emotions, cognition, and behavior.* New York: Cambridge University Press.

Gillis, M. M., Haaga, D. A., & Ford, G. T. (1995). Normative values for the Beck Anxiety Inventory, Fear Questionnaire, Penn State Worry Questionnaire, and Social Phobia and Anxiety Inventory. *Psychological Assessment, 7,* 450–455.

Ginsburg, G. S., & Silverman, W. K. (2000). Gender role orientation and fearfulness in children with anxiety disorders. *Journal of Anxiety Disorders, 14,* 57–67.

Gitin, N. M., Herbert, J. D., & Schmidt, C. (1996, November). *One-session in vivo exposure for odontophobia.* Paper presented at the 30th Annual Convention of the Association for Advancement of Behavior Therapy, New York.

Gittelman, R., & Klein, D. F. (1985). Childhood separation anxiety and adult agoraphobia. In A. H. Tuma & J. D. Maser (Eds.), *Anxiety and the anxiety disorders.* Hillsdale, NJ: Erlbaum.

Gittelman-Klein, R. (1975). Psychiatric characteristics of the relatives of school phobic children. In D. Siv-Sankar (Ed.), *Mental health in children* (Vol. 1). New York: P. J. D.

Gittelman-Klein, R. (1995). Is panic disorder associated with childhood separation anxiety disorder? *Clinical Neuropharmacology, 18*(2), S7–S14.

Gittelman-Klein, R., & Klein, D. F. (1973). School phobia: Diagnostic considerations in the light of imipramine effects. *Journal of Nervous and Mental Disease, 156,* 199–215.

Glasgow, R. E., & Arkowitz, H. (1975). The behavioral assessment of male and female social competence in dyadic interactions. *Behavior Therapy, 6,* 488–498.

Glass, C. R., & Arnkoff, D. B. (1989). Behavioral assessment of social anxiety and social phobia. *Clinical Psychology Review, 9,* 75–90.

Glass, C. R., Gottman, J. M., & Shmurak, S. H. (1976). Response-acquisition and cognitive self-statement modification approaches to dating skills training. *Journal of Counseling Psychology, 23,* 520–526.

Glass, C. R., Merluzzi, T. V., Biever, J. L., & Larsen, K. H. (1982). Cognitive assessment of social anxiety: Development and validation of a self-statement questionnaire. *Cognitive Therapy and Research, 6,* 37–55.

Glynn, S. M., Eth, S., Randolph, E. T., Foy, D. W., Urbaitis, M., Boxer, L., Paz, G. G., Leong, G. B., Firman, G., Salk, J. D., Katzman, J. W., & Crothers, J. (1999). A test of behavioral family therapy to augment exposure for combat-related posttraumatic stress disorder. *Journal of Consulting and Clinical Psychology, 67,* 243–251.

Goa, K. L., & Ward, A. (1986). Buspirone: A preliminary review of its pharmacological properties and therapeutic efficacy as an anxiolytic. *Drugs, 32,* 114–129.

Goenjian, A. K., Pynoos, R. S., Steinberg, A. M., Najarian, L. M., Asarnow, J. R., Karayan, I., Ghurabi, M., & Fairbanks, L. A. (1995). Psychiatric comorbidity in children after the 1988 earthquake in Armenia. *Journal of the American Academy of Child and Adolescent Psychiatry, 34,* 1174–1184.

Goetz, R. R., Gorman, J., Dillon, D,., Papp, L., Hollander, E., Fyer, A., Liebowitz, M., & Klein, D. F. (1989). Do panic disorder patients indiscriminately endorse somatic complaints? *Psychiatry Research, 29*(2), 207–213.

Goetz, R. R., Klein, D. F., & Gorman, J. M. (1994). Consistencies between recalled panic and lactate-induced panic. *Anxiety, 1,* 31–36.

Goetz, R. R., Klein, D. F., & Gorman, J. M. (1996). Symptoms essential to the experience of sodium lactate-induced panic. *Neuropsychopharmacology, 14*(5), 355–366.

Goisman, R. M., Allsworth, J., Rogers, M. P., Warshaw, M. G., Goldenberg, I., Vasile, R. G., Rodriguez-Villa, F., Mallya, G., & Keller, M. B. (1998). Simple phobia as a comorbid anxiety disorder. *Depression and Anxiety, 7,* 105–112.

Goisman, R. M., Goldenberg, I., Vasile, R. G., & Keller, M. B. (1995). Comorbidity of anxiety disorders in a multicenter anxiety study. *Comprehensive Psychiatry, 36,* 303–311.

Goisman, R. M., Rogers, M. P., Steketee, G. S., Warshaw, M. G., Cuneo, P., & Keller, M. B. (1993). Utilization of behavioral methods in a multicenter anxiety disorders study. *Journal of Clinical Psychiatry, 54,* 213–218.

Goisman, R. M., Warshaw, M. G., & Keller, M. B. (1999). Psychosocial treatment prescriptions for generalized anxiety disorder, panic disorder, and social phobia, 1991–1996. *American Journal of Psychiatry, 156,* 1819–1821.

Goisman, R. M., Warshaw, M. G., Steketee, G. S., Fierman, E. J., Rogers, M. P., Goldenberg, I., Weinshenker, N. J., Vasile, R. G., & Keller, M. B. (1995). DSM-IV in the disappearance of agoraphobia without a history of panic disorder: New data on a controversial diagnosis. *American Journal of Psychiatry, 152,* 1438–1443.

Goldberg, R., Morris, P., Christian, F., Badger, J., Chabot, S., & Edlund, M. (1990). Panic disorder in cardiac outpatients. *Psychosomatics, 31,* 168–173.

Goldfried, M. R. (1971). Systematic desensitization as training in self-control. *Journal of Consulting and Clinical Psychology, 37,* 228–234.

Goldsmith, H. H. (1994). Parsing the emotional domain from a developmental perspective. In P. Ekman & R. J. Davidson (Eds.), *The nature of emotion: Fundamental questions.* New York: Oxford University Press.

Goldsmith, H. H., & Gottesman, I. I. (1981). Origins of variation in behavioral style: A longitudinal study of temperament in young twins. *Child Development, 52,* 91–103.

Goldstein, A. J., & Chambless, D. L. (1978). A reanalysis of agoraphobia. *Behavior Therapy, 9,* 47–59.

Goldstein, I. B. (1964). Physiological responses in anxious women patients: A study of autonomic activity and muscle tension. *Archives of General Psychiatry, 10,* 382–388.

Goldstein, S., Halbreich, U., Asnis, G. M., Endicott, J., & Alvir, J. (1987). The hypothalamic–pituitary–adrenal system in panic disorder. *American Journal of Psychiatry, 144,* 1320–1323.

Good, B. J., & Kleinman, A. M. (1985). Culture and anxiety: Cross-cultural evidence for the patterning of anxiety disorders. In A. H. Tuma & J. D. Maser (Eds.), *Anxiety and the anxiety disorders.* Hillsdale, NJ: Erlbaum.

Goodman, W. K., Price, L. H., Rasmussen, S. A., Mazure, C., Delgado, P., Heninger, G. R., & Charney, D. S. (1989). The Yale–Brown Obsessive Compulsive Scale: II. Validity. *Archives of General Psychiatry, 46,* 1012–1016.

Goodman, W. K., Price, L. H., Rasmussen, S. A., Mazure, C., Fleischman, R. L., Hill, C. L., Heninger, G. R., & Charney, D. A. (1989). The Yale–Brown Obsessive Compulsive Scale: I. Development, use, and reliability. *Archives of General Psychiatry, 46,* 1006–1011.

Goodwin, D. W., & Guze, S. B. (1984). *Psychiatric diagnosis.* New York: Oxford University Press.

Gordon, D. A., Nowicki, S., & Wichern, F. (1981). Observed maternal and child behaviors in a dependency-producing task as a function of children's locus of control orientation. *Merrill–Palmer Quarterly, 27,* 43–51.

Gorman, J. M., Askanazi, J., Liebowitz, M. R., Fyer, A. J., Stein, J., Kinney, J. M., & Klein, D. F. (1984). Response to hyperventilation in a group of patients with panic disorder. *American Journal of Psychiatry, 141,* 857–861.

Gorman, J. M., Battista, D., Goetz, R. R., Dillon, D. J., Liebowitz, M. R., Fyer, A. J., Snadberg, D., & Klein, D. F. (1989). A comparison of sodium bicarbonate and sodium lactate infusion in the induction of panic attacks. *Archives of General Psychiatry, 46,* 145–150.

Gorman, J. M., Fyer, A. J., Kinney, J., & Klein, D. F. (1988). Ventilatory physiology of patients with panic disorder. *Archives of General Psychiatry, 45,* 31–39.

Gorman, J. M., Goetz, R. R., Dillon, D., Liebowitz, M. R., Fyer, A. J., Davies, S., & Klein, D. F. (1990). Sodium D-lactate infusion of panic disorder patients. *Neuropsychopharmacology, 3,* 181–189.

Gorman, J. M., Kent, J., Martinez, J., Browne, S., Coplan, F., & Papp, L. A. (2001). Physiological changes during carbon dioxide inhalation in patients with panic disorder, major depression, and premenstrual dysphoric disorder. *Archives of General Psychiatry, 58,* 125–131.

Gorman, J. M., & Klein, D. F. (1985). In reply to effect of acute β–adrenergic blockade on lactate-induced panic. *Archives of General Psychiatry, 42,* 104–105.

Gorman, J. M., Levy, G. F., Liebowitz, M. R., McGrath, P., Appleby, I. L., Dillon, D. J., Davies, J. O., & Klein, D. F. (1983). Effect of acute β–adrenergic blockade on lactate-induced panic. *Archives of General Psychiatry, 40,* 1079–1082.

Gorman, J. M., & Papp, L. A. (1990). Respiratory physiology of panic. In J. C. Ballenger (Ed.), *Neurobiology of panic disorder.* New York: Wiley-Liss.

Gorman, J. M., Papp, L. A., Coplan, J. D., Martinez, J. M., Lennon, S., Goetz, R. R., Ross, D., & Klein, D. F. (1994). Anxiogenic effects of CO_2 and hyperventilation in patients with panic disorder. *American Journal of Psychiatry, 151,* 547–553.

Gorman, M. R., Liebowitz, J. M., Gorman, J. M., Fyer, A., Dillon, D., Levitt, M., & Klein, D. F. (1986). Possible mechanisms for lactate's induction of panic. *American Journal of Psychiatry, 143,* 495–502.

Gotlib, I. H., Ranginath, C., & Rosenfeld, J. P. (1998). Frontal EEG alpha asymmetry, depression, and cognitive functioning. *Cognition and Emotion, 12,* 449–478.

Gottesman, I. I. (1991). *Schizophrenia genesis: The origins of madness.* New York: Freeman.

Gottschalk, L. A., Stone, W. N., & Gleser, C. G. (1974). Peripheral versus central mechanisms accounting for antianxiety effects of propranolol. *British Journal of Psychiatry, 36,* 47–51.

Gould, E., Tanapat, P., McEwen, B. S., Flugge, G., & Fuchs, E. (1998). Proliferation of granule cell precursors in the dentate gyrus of adult monkeys is diminished by stress. *Proceedings of the National Academy of Sciences USA, 95,* 3168–3171.

Gould, R. A., Buckminster, S., Pollack, M. H., Otto, M. W., & Yap, L. (1997). Cognitive-behavioral and pharmacological treatment for social phobia: A meta-analysis. *Clinical Psychology: Science and Practice, 4,* 291–306.

Gould, R. A., Otto, M. W., & Pollack, M. H. (1995). A meta-analysis of treatment outcome for panic disorder. *Clinical Psychology Review, 15,* 819–844.

Gould, R. A., Otto, M. W., Pollack, M. H., & Yap, L. (1997). Cognitive behavioral and pharmacological treatment of generalized anxiety disorder: A preliminary meta-analysis. *Behavior Therapy, 28,* 1–21.

Graeff, F. G., Guimaraes, F. S., DeAndrade, T. G. C. S., & Deakin, J. F. W. (1996). Role of 5-HT in stress, anxiety, and depression. *Pharmacology, Biochemistry and Behavior, 54,* 129–141.

Graham, J. R. (1990). MMPI-2: *Assessing personality and psychopathology*. New York: Oxford University Press.

Granger, D. A., Weisz, J. R., & Kauneckis, D. (1994). Neuroendocrine reactivity, internalizing behavior problems, and control-related cognitions in clinic-referred children and adolescents. *Journal of Abnormal Psychology, 103*, 267–276.

Gray, J. A. (1971). *The psychology of fear and stress*. London: Weidenfeld & Nicholson.

Gray, J. A. (1982). *The neuropsychology of anxiety*. New York: Oxford University Press.

Gray, J. A. (1985). Issues in the neuropsychology of anxiety. In A. H. Tuma & J. D. Maser (Eds.), *Anxiety and the anxiety disorders*. Hillsdale, NJ: Erlbaum.

Gray, J. A. (1987). *The psychology of fear and stress* (2nd ed.). Cambridge, England: Cambridge University Press.

Gray, J. A. (1991). Fear, panic, and anxiety: What's in a name? *Psychological Inquiry, 2*(1), 72–96.

Gray, J. A., & McNaughton, N. (1996). The neuropsychology of anxiety: Reprise. In D. A. Hope (Ed.), *Nebraska Symposium on Motivation: Vol. 43. Perspectives on anxiety, panic, and fear*. Lincoln: University of Nebraska Press.

Grayson, I. B., Foa, E. B., & Steketee, G. (1982). Habituation during exposure treatment: Distraction versus attention-focusing. *Behaviour Research and Therapy, 20*, 323–328.

Green, B. L., Grace, M. C., Lindy, J. D., et al. (1990). Buffalo Creek survivors in the second decade: Comparison with unexposed and nonlitigant groups. *Journal of Applied Social Psychology, 20*, 1033–1050.

Green, B. L., Lindy, J. D., Grace, M. C., Glazer, G., Leonard, A., Korol, M., & Windget, C. (1990). Buffalo Creek survivors in the second decade: Stability of stress symptoms. *American Journal of Orthopsychiatry, 60*, 43–54.

Green, D. P., Goldman, S. L., & Salovey, P. (1993). Measurement error masks bipolarity in affect ratings. *Journal of Personality and Social Psychology, 64*, 1029–1041.

Green, D. P., & Salovey, P. (1999). In what sense are positive and negative affect independent?: A reply to Tellegen, Watson, and Clark. *Psychological Science, 10*, 304–306.

Green, D. P., Salovey, P., & Truax, K. M. (1999). Static, dynamic, and causative bipolarity of affect. *Journal of Personality and Social Psychology, 76*, 856–857.

Greenberg, D. B., Stern, T. A., & Weilburg, J. B. (1988). The fear of choking: Three successfully treated cases. *Psychosomatics, 29*, 126–129.

Greenberg, P. E., Sisitsky, T., Kessler, R. C., Finkelstein, S. N., Berndt, E. R., Davidson, J. R. T., Ballenger, J. C., & Fyer, A. J. (1999). The economic burden of anxiety disorders in the 1990s. *Journal of Clinical Psychiatry, 60*(7), 427–435.

Greenberg, R. L. (1988). Panic disorder and agoraphobia. In J. G. Williams & A. T. Beck (Eds.) *Cognitive therapy in clinical practice: An illustrative casebook*. London: Routledge.

Grey, S., Sartory, G., & Rachman, S. (1979). Synchronous and desynchronous changes during fear reduction. *Behaviour Research and Therapy, 10*, 124–133.

Griez, E., & van den Hout, M. A. (1986). CO_2 inhalation in the treatment of panic attacks. *Behaviour Research and Therapy, 24*, 145–150.

Griez, E., & Verburg, K. (1999). The current status of respiration in panic disorder. In D. J. Nutt, J. C. Ballenger, & J.-P. Lépine (Eds.), *Panic disorder: Clinical diagnosis, management and mechanisms*. London: Martin Dunitz.

Griffith, J., Jasinski, D., Casten, G., & McKinney, G. (1986). Investigation of the abuse liability of buspirone in alcohol dependent patients. *American Journal of Medicine, 80*(Suppl. 3B), 30–35.

Grilo, C. M., Money, R., Barlow, D. H., Goddard, A. W., Gorman, J. M., Hofmann, S. G., Papp, L. A., Shear, M. K., & Woods, S. W. (1998). Pretreatment patient factors predicting attrition from a multicenter randomized controlled treatment study for panic disorder. *Comprehensive Psychiatry, 39*, 323–332.

Grinker, R., & Spiegel, J. P. (1945). *Men under stress*. Philadelphia: Blakiston.

Gross, J. J. (1999). Emotion and emotion regulation. In L. A. Pervin & O. P. John (Eds.), *Handbook of personality: Theory and research* (2nd ed.). New York: Guilford Press.

Gross, J. J., & Munoz, R. F. (1995). Emotion regulation and mental health. *Clinical Psychology: Science and Practice, 2*(2), 151–164.

Grosz, H. J., & Farmer, B. B. (1969). Blood lactate in the development of anxiety symptoms: A critical examination of Pitts and McClure's hypothesis and experimental study. *Archives of General Psychiatry, 21,* 611–619.

Grosz, H. J., & Farmer, B. B. (1972). Pitts and McClure's lactate anxiety study revised. *British Journal of Psychiatry, 120,* 415–418.

Grunhaus, L., Gloger, S., Rein, A., & Lewis, B. S. (1982). Mitral valve prolapse and panic attacks. *Israel Journal of Medical Sciences, 18,* 221–223.

Guarnaccia, P. J., Canino, G., Rubio-Stipec, M., & Bravo, M. (1993). The prevalence of *ataques de nervios* in the Puerto Rico Disaster Study. *Journal of Nervous and Mental Disease, 181,* 157–165.

Guarnaccia, P. J., Rubio-Stipec, M., & Canino, G. J. (1989). *Ataques de nervios* in the Puerto Rican Diagnostic Interview Schedule: The impact of cultural categories on psychiatric epidemiology. *Culture, Medicine, and Psychiatry, 13,* 275–295.

Gunnar, M. R. (1994). Psychoendocrine studies of temperament and stress in early childhood: Expanding current models. In J. E. Bates & T. D. Wachs (Eds.), *Temperament: Individual differences at the interface of biology and behavior.* Washington, DC: American Psychological Association.

Gunnar, M. R., Larson, M., Hertsgaard, L., Harris, L. M., & Broderson, L. (1992). The stressfulness of separation among 9-month-old infants: Effects of social context variables and infant temperament. *Child Development, 63,* 290–303.

Gunther, L. M., Denniston, J. C., & Miller, R. R. (1998). Conducting exposure treatment in multiple contexts can prevent relapse. *Behaviour Research and Therapy, 36,* 75–91.

Gurvits, T. G., Shenton, M. R., Hokama, H., & Ohta, H. (1996). Magnetic resonance imaging study of hippocampal volume in chronic combat-related posttraumatic stress disorder. *Biological Psychiatry, 40,* 192–199.

Guy, W. (1976). *Early Clinical Drug Evaluation Unit (ECDEU) assessment manual for psychopharmacology* (rev. ed., DHEW Publication No. 76-338). Rockville, MD: National Institute of Mental Health.

Hafner, R. I. (1976). Fresh symptom emergence after intensive behavior therapy. *British Journal of Psychiatry, 129,* 378–383.

Haggard, E. (1943). Some conditions determining adjustment during and readjust following experimentally induced stress. In S. Tomkins (Ed.), *Contemporary psychopathology.* Cambridge, MA: Harvard University Press.

Hahn, S., Kroenke, K., Spitzer, R., Brody, D., Williams, J., Linzer, M., & de Gruy, F. V., III. (1996). The difficult patient: Prevalence, psychopathology, and functional impairment. *Journal of General Internal Medicine, 11,* 1–8.

Haidt, J., McCauley, C., & Rozin, P. (1994). Individual differences in sensitivity to disgust: Scale sampling seven domains of disgust elicitors. *Personality and Individual Differences, 16,* 701–713.

Halford, K., & Foddy, M. (1982). Cognitive and social skills correlates of social anxiety. *British Journal of Clinical Psychology, 21,* 17–28.

Hallam, R. S. (1985). *Anxiety: Psychological perspectives on panic and agoraphobia.* New York: Academic Press.

Hamada, T., Koshino, Y., Misawa, T., Isaki, K., & Gejyo, F. (1998). Mitral valve prolapse and autonomic function in panic disorder. *Acta Psychiatrica Scandinavica, 97,* 139–143.

Hamilton, M. (1959). The assessment of anxiety states by rating. *British Journal of Medical Psychology, 32,* 50–55.

Hamilton, M. (1960). A rating scale for depression. *Journal of Neurology, Neurosurgery, and Psychiatry, 23,* 56–62.

Hamilton, M. (1969). Diagnosis and rating of anxiety. *British Journal of Psychiatry,* Special Publication No. 3, 76–79.

Hamm, A. O., & Vaitl, D. (1996). Affective learning: Awareness and aversion. *Psychophysiology,* *33,* 698–710.

Hammen, C., Adrian, C., & Hiroto, D. (1988). A longitudinal test of the attributional vulnerability model in children at risk for depression. *British Journal of Clinical Psychology, 27,* 37–46.

Hammerberg, M., (1992). Penn Inventory for posttraumatic stress disorders: Psychometric properties. *Psychological Assessment: A Journal of Consulting and Clinical Psychology, 4,* 67–76.

Hand, I., Lamontagne, Y., & Marks, I. M. (1974). Group exposure (flooding) in vivo for agoraphobics. *British Journal of Psychiatry, 124,* 588–602.

Hannum, R. D., Rosellini, R. A., & Seligman, M. E. (1976). Learned helplessness in the rat: Retention and immunization. *Developmental Psychology, 12,* 449–454.

Harrison, B. I. (1985). *Anxiety provoked ideation in phobic and nonphobic panickers.* Unpublished bachelor of arts (honors) thesis, University of Winnipeg.

Hart, R. P., Colenda, C. C., & Hamer, R. M. (1991). Effects of buspirone and alprazolam on the cognitive performance of normal elderly subjects. *American Journal of Psychiatry, 148,* 73–77.

Hartung, C. M., & Widiger, T. A. (1998). Gender differences in the diagnosis of mental disorders: Conclusions and controversies in the DSM-IV. *Psychological Bulletin, 123,* 260–278.

Haslam, M. T. (1974). The relationship between the effect of lactate infusion on anxiety states and their amelioration by carbon dioxide inhalation. *British Journal of Psychiatry, 125,* 88–90.

Hauri, P., Friedman, M., Ravaris, R., & Fisher, J. (1985). Sleep in agoraphobia with panic attacks. In M. H. Chafe, D. J. McGinty, & R. Wilder-Iones (Eds.), *Sleep research.* Los Angeles: BIS/BRS.

Hauri, P., Friedman, R., & Ravaris, C. (1989). Sleep in patients with spontaneous panic attacks. *Sleep, 2,* 323–337.

Havenaar, J. M., Rumyantzeva, G. M., van den Brink, W. P., Nico, W., van den Bout, J., van Engeland, H., & Koeter, M. W. J. (1997). Long-term mental health effects of the Chernobyl disaster: An epidemiologic survey in two former Soviet regions. *American Journal of Psychiatry, 154,* 1605–1607.

Haw, J., & Dickerson, M. (1998). The effects of distraction on desensitization and reprocessing. *Behaviour Research and Therapy, 36,* 765–769.

Hayes, S. C., Bissett, R. T., Strosahl, K., Follette, W. C., Polusney, M. A., Pistorello, J., Toarmino, D., Batten, S. V., Dykstra, T. A., Stewart, S. H., Zvolensky, M. J., Eifert, G. H., Bond, F. W., & Bergan, J. (2001). *Psychometric properties of the Acceptance and Action Questionnaire (ACT).* Manuscript in preparation.

Hayes, S. C., Jacobson, N. S., Follette, V. M., & Dougher, M. J. (Eds.). (1994). *Acceptance and change: Content and context in psychotherapy.* Reno, NV: Context Press.

Hayes, S. C., Strosahl, K. D., & Wilson, K. G. (1999). *Acceptance and commitment therapy: An experiential approach to behavior change.* New York: Guilford Press.

Hayes, S. C., Wilson, K. G., Gifford, E. V., Follette, V. M., & Strosahl, K. (1996). Experiential avoidance and behavioral disorders: A functional dimensional approach to diagnosis and treatment. *Journal of Consulting and Clinical Psychology, 64,* 1152–1168.

Hayward, C., Killen, J. D., Hammer, L. D., Litt, I. F., Wilson, D. M., Simmonds, B., & Taylor, C. B. (1992). Pubertal stage and panic attack history in sixth- and seventh-grade girls. *American Journal of Psychiatry, 149,* 1239–1243.

Hayward, C., Killen, J. D., Kraemer, H. C., & Taylor, C. B. (2000). Predictors of panic attacks in adolescents. *Journal of the American Academy of Child and Adolescent Psychiatry, 39*(2), 1–8.

Hayward, C., Killen, J. D., Kraemer, H. C., Blair-Greiner, A., Strachowski, D., Cunning, D., & Taylor, C. B. (1997). Assessment and phenomenology of nonclinical panic attacks in adolescent girls. *Journal of Anxiety Disorders, 11,* 17–32.

Hayward, P., Wardle, J., & Higgitt, A. (1989). Benzodiazepine research: Current findings and practical consequences. *British Journal of Clinical Psychology, 28,* 307–327.

Hazlett, R. L., McLeod, D. R., & Hoehn-Saric, R. (1994). Muscle tension in generalized anxiety disorder: Elevated muscle tonus or agitated movement? *Psychophysiology, 31,* 189–195.

Hegel, M. T., & Ahles, T. A. (1992). Behavioral analysis and treatment of reflexive vomiting associated with visceral sensations: A case study of interoceptive conditioning? *Journal of Behavioural Therapy and Experimental Psychiatry, 23*(3), 237–242.

Hegel, M. T., & Ferguson, R. J. (1997). Psychophysiological assessment of respiratory function in panic disorder: Evidence for a hyperventilation subtype. *Psychosomatic Medicine, 59,* 224–230.

Heide, F. J., & Borkovec, T. D. (1983). Relaxation-induced anxiety: Paradoxical anxiety enhancement due to relaxation training. *Journal of Consulting and Clinical Psychology, 51,* 171–182.

Heide, F. J., & Borkovec, T. D. (1984). Relaxation-induced anxiety: Mechanisms and theoretical implications. *Behaviour Research and Therapy, 22,* 1–12.

Heim, C., & Nemeroff, C. B. (1999). The impact of early adverse experiences on brain systems involved in the pathophysiology of anxiety and affective disorders. *Biological Psychiatry, 46*(11), 1509–1522.

Heimberg, R. G. (1994). Cognitive assessment strategies and the measurement of outcome of treatment for social phobia. *Behaviour Research and Therapy, 32,* 269–280.

Heimberg, R. G. (1996). Social phobia, avoidant personality disorder and the multiaxial conceptualization of interpersonal anxiety. In P. M. Salkovskis (Ed.), *Trends in cognitive and behavioral therapies.* New York: Wiley.

Heimberg, R. G., Becker, R. E., Goldfinger, K., & Vermilyea, J. A. (1985). Treatment of social phobia by exposure, cognitive restructuring, and homework assignments. *Journal of Nervous and Mental Disease, 173,* 236–245.

Heimberg, R. G., Bruch, M. A., Hope, D. A., & Dombeck, M. (1990). Evaluating the states of mind model: Comparison to an alternative model and effects of method of cognitive assessment. *Cognitive Therapy and Research, 14,* 543–557.

Heimberg, R. G., Dodge, C. S., Hope, D. A., Kennedy, C. R., Zollo, L. J., & Becker, R. E. (1990). Cognitive behavioral treatment for social phobia: Comparison with a credible placebo control. *Cognitive Therapy and Research, 14,* 1–23.

Heimberg, R. G., Holt, C. S., Schneier, F. R., Spitzer, R. L., & Liebowitz, M. R. (1993). The issue of subtypes in the diagnosis of social phobia. *Journal of Anxiety Disorders, 7,* 249–269.

Heimberg, R. G., Hope, D. A., Dodge, C. S., & Becker, R. E. (1990). DSM-III-R subtypes of social phobia: Comparison of generalized social phobics and public speaking phobics. *Journal of Nervous and Mental Disease, 178,* 172–179.

Heimberg, R. G., Horner, K. J., Juster, H. R., Safren, S. A., Brown, E. J., Schneier, F. R., & Liebowitz, M. R. (1999). Psychometric properties of the Liebowitz Social Anxiety Scale. *Psychological Medicine, 29,* 199–212.

Heimberg, R. G., Liebowitz, M. R., Hope, D. A., & Schneier, F. R. (Eds.). (1995). *Social phobia: Diagnosis, assessment, and treatment.* New York: Guilford Press.

Heimberg, R. G., Liebowitz, M. R., Hope, D. A., Schneier, F. R., Holt, C. S., Welkowitz, L. A., Juster, H. R., Campeas, R., Bruch, M. A., Cloitre, M., Falloon, B., & Klein, D. F. (1998). Cognitive behavioral group therapy vs. phenelzine therapy for social phobia. *Archives of General Psychiatry, 55,* 1133–1141.

Heimberg, R. G., Mueller, G., Holt, C. S., Hope, D. A., & Liebowitz, M. R. (1992). Assessment of anxiety in social interaction and being observed by others: The Social Interaction Anxiety Scale and the Social Phobia Scale. *Behavior Therapy, 23,* 53–73.

Heimberg, R. G., Salzman, D. G., Holt, C. S., & Blendell, K. A. (1993). Cognitive behavioral group treatment for social phobia: Effectiveness at five-year follow-up. *Cognitive Therapy and Research, 17,* 325–339.

Heinrichs, N., & Hofmann, S. G. (2000). Information processing in social phobia: A critical review and preliminary model. *Clinical Psychology Review.*

Heinrichs, N., Spiegel, D. A., & Hofmann, S. G. (in press). Panic disorder with agoraphobia. In F. Bond & W. Dryden (Eds.), *Handbook of brief cognitive behavior therapy.* Chichester, England: Wiley.

Heit, S., Owens, M. J., Plotsky, P., & Nemeroff, C. B. (1997). Corticotropin-releasing factor, stress, and depression. *The Neuroscientist, 3,* 186–194.

Heller, W., & Nitschke, J. (1997). Regional brain activity in emotion: A framework for understanding cognition in depression. *Cognition and Emotion, 11*, 637–661.

Heller, W., Nitschke, J. B., Etienne, M. A., & Miller, G. A. (1997). Patterns of regional brain activity differentiate types of anxiety. *Journal of Abnormal Psychology, 106*(3), 376–385.

Hellström, K., Fellenius, J., & Öst, L.-G. (1996). One versus five sessions of applied tension in the treatment of blood phobia. *Behaviour Research and Therapy, 34*, 101–112.

Hellström, K., & Öst, L.-G. (1995). One-session therapist directed exposure vs. two forms of manual directed self-exposure in the treatment of spider phobia. *Behaviour Research and Therapy, 33*, 959–965.

Hellström, K., & Öst, L.-G. (1996). Prediction of outcome in the treatment of specific phobia: A cross validation study. *Behaviour Research and Therapy, 34*, 403–411.

Helzer, J. E., Robins, L. N. & McEvoy, L. (1987). Post-traumatic stress disorder in the general population: Findings of the Epidemiologic Catchment Area survey. *New England Journal of Medicine, 317*, 1630–1634.

Hepburn, T., & Page, A. C. (1999). Effects of images about fear and disgust upon responses to blood–injury phobic stimuli. *Behavior Therapy, 30*, 63–77.

Hepner, A., & Cauthen, N. R. (1975). Effect of subject control and graduated exposure on snake phobias. *Journal of Consulting and Clinical Psychology, 43*, 297–304.

Herbert, J. D., Bellack, A. S., & Hope, D. A. (1991). Concurrent validity of the Social Phobia and Anxiety Inventory. *Journal of Psychopathology and Behavioral Assessment, 13*, 357–368.

Herbert, J. D., Bellack, A. S., Hope, D. A., & Mueser, K. T. (1992). Scoring the Social Phobia and Anxiety Inventory: Reply to Beidel and Turner. *Journal of Psychopathology and Behavioral Assessment, 14*, 381–383.

Herbert, J. D., Hope, D. A., & Bellack, A. S. (1992). Validity of the distinction between generalized social phobia and avoidant personality disorder. *Journal of Abnormal Psychology, 101*, 332–339.

Herbert, J. D., & Mueser, K. T. (1992). Eye movement desensitization: A critique of the evidence. *Journal of Behavior Therapy and Experimental Psychiatry, 23*, 169–174.

Herbert, J. D., Rheingold, A. A., & Brandsma, L. L. (2001). Assessment of social anxiety and social phobia. In S. G. Hofmann & P. M. DiBartolo (Eds.), *From social anxiety to social phobia: Multiple perspectives*. Needham Heights, MA: Allyn & Bacon.

Herman, J. L. (1981). *Father–daughter incest*. Cambridge, MA: Harvard University Press.

Hermesh, H., Shahar, A., & Munitz, H. (1987). Obsessive–compulsive disorder and borderline personality disorder. *American Journal of Psychiatry, 144*, 120–121.

Hershberg, S. G., Carlson, G. A., Cantwell, D. P., & Strober, M. (1982). Anxiety and depressive disorders in psychiatrically disturbed children. *Journal of Clinical Psychiatry, 43*(9), 358–361.

Hibbert, G. A. (1984). Hyperventilation as a cause of panic attacks. *British Medical Journal, 288*, 263–264.

Hibbert, G. A. (1986). The diagnosis of hyperventilation using ambulatory carbon dioxide monitoring. In J. H. Lacey & D. A. Sturgeon (Eds.), *Proceedings of the 15th European Conference on Psychosomatic Research*. London: Libbey.

Hibbert, G., & Pilsbury, D. (1989). Hyperventilation: Is it a cause of panic attacks? *British Journal of Psychiatry, 155*, 805–809.

Higgins, E. (1994). A review of unrecognized mental illness in primary care: Prevalence, natural history, and efforts to change the course. *Archives of Family Medicine, 3*, 908–917.

Himle, J. A., McPhee, K., Cameron, O. G., & Curtis, G. C. (1989). Simple phobia: Evidence for heterogeneity. *Psychiatry Research, 28*, 25–30.

Hinton, D., Ba, P., Peou, S., & Um, K. (2000). *A common Khmer syndrome: Orthostatically induced panic attacks*. Manuscript.

Hinton, D., Ba, P., Peou, S., & Um, K. (2000). Panic disorder among Cambodian refugees attending a psychiatric clinic. *General Hospital Psychiatry, 22*, 437–444.

Hinton, D., Um, K., & Ba, P. (in press-a). *Kyol Goeu* ("Wind Overload") Part I: *Kyol Goeu* and orthostatic panic among Khmer refugees attending a psychiatric clinic; or cultural syndromes catastrophic cognitions, and the generation of panic. *Transcultural Psychiatry.*

Hinton, D., Um, K., & Ba, P. (in press-b). *Kyol Goeu* ("Wind Overload") Part II: The prevalence, characteristics, and mechanisms of *Kyol Goeu* ("Wind Overload") and near-*Kyol Goeu* episodes of Khmer patients attending a psychiatric clinic. *Transcultural Psychiatry.*

Hirschfeld, R. M. A. (1996). Placebo response in the treatment of panic disorder. *Bulletin of the Menninger Clinic, 60*(2), A76–A86.

Hirshfeld, D. R., Rosenbaum, J. F., Biederman, J., Bolduc, E. A., Faraone, S. V., Snidman, N., Reznick, J. S., & Kagan, J. (1992). Stable behavioral inhibition and its association with anxiety disorder. *Journal of the American Academy of Child and Adolescent Psychiatry, 31,* 103–111.

Hiss, H., Foa, E. B., & Kozak, M. J. (1994). Relapse prevention program for treatment of obsessive–compulsive disorder. *Journal of Consulting and Clinical Psychology, 62,* 801–808.

Hodgson, R. J., & Rachman, S. (1977). Obsessional–compulsive complaints. *Behaviour Research and Therapy, 15,* 389–395.

Hoehn-Saric, R. (1981). Characteristics of chronic anxiety patients. In D. F. Klein & J. G. Rabkin (Eds.), *Anxiety: New research and changing concepts.* New York: Raven Press.

Hoehn-Saric, R., Hazlett, R. L., & McLeod, D. R. (1993). Generalized anxiety disorder with early and late onset of anxiety symptoms. *Comprehensive Psychiatry, 34,* 291–298.

Hoehn-Saric, R., & McLeod, D. R. (1988). The peripheral sympathetic nervous system: Its role in normal and pathologic anxiety. *Psychiatric Clinics of North America, 11,* 375–386.

Hoehn-Saric, R., & McLeod, D. R. (1991). Clinical management of generalized anxiety disorder. In W. Coryell & G. Winokur (Eds.), *The clinical management of anxiety disorders.* New York: Oxford University Press.

Hoehn-Saric, R., McLeod, D. R., & Hipsley, P. (1995). Is hyperarousal essential to obsessive–compulsive disorder?: Diminished physiologic flexibility, but not hyperarousal, characterizes patients with obsessive–compulsive disorder. *Archives of General Psychiatry, 52,* 688–693.

Hoehn-Saric, R., McLeod, D. R., & Zimmerli, W. D. (1988). Differential effects of alprazolam and imipramine in generalized anxiety disorder: Somatic versus psychic symptoms. *Journal of Clinical Psychiatry, 49,* 293–301.

Hoehn-Saric, R., McLeod, D. R., & Zimmerli, W. D. (1989). Somatic manifestations in women with generalized anxiety disorder: Psychophysiological responses to psychological stress. *Archives of General Psychiatry, 46,* 1113–1119.

Hoehn-Saric, R., McLeod, D. R., & Zimmerli, W. D. (1991). Psychophysiological response patterns in panic disorder. *Munksgaard Scientific Journals, 83*(1), 4–11.

Hoffart, A. (1997). Interpersonal problems among patients suffering from panic disorder with agoraphobia before and after treatment. *British Journal of Medical Psychology, 70,* 149–157.

Hoffart, A., & Hedley, L. M. (1997). Personality traits among panic disorder with agoraphobia patients before and after symptom-focused treatment. *Journal of Anxiety Disorders, 11,* 77–87.

Hoffart, A., Friis, S., & Martinsen, E. W. (1992). Assessment of fear of fear among agoraphobic patients: The Agoraphobic Cognitions Scales. *Journal of Psychopathology and Behavioral Assessment, 14,* 175–187.

Hoffman, J. A., & Teyber, E. C. (1979). Some relationships between sibling age, space, and personality. *Merrill–Palmer Quarterly, 25,* 77–80.

Hofmann, S. G. (2000a). Self-focused attention before and after exposure treatment of social phobia. *Behaviour Research and Therapy, 38,* 717–725.

Hofmann, S. G. (2000b). Treatment of social phobia: Potential mediators and moderators. *Clinical Psychology: Science and Practice, 7*(1), 3–16.

Hofmann, S. G., Albano, A. M., Heimberg, R. G., Tracey, S., Chorpita, B. F., & Barlow, D. H. (1999). Subtypes of social phobia in adolescents. *Depression and Anxiety, 9,* 15–18.

Hofmann, S. G., & Barlow, D. H. (1996). Ambulatory psychophysiological monitoring: A potentially useful tool when treating panic relapse. *Cognitive and Behavioral Practice, 3,* 53–61.

Hofmann, S. G., & Barlow, D. H. (1999). The costs of anxiety disorders: Implications for psychosocial interventions. In N. E. Miller & K. M. Magruder (Eds.), *Cost-effectiveness of psychotherapy: A guide for practitioners, researchers, and policymakers*. New York: Oxford University Press.

Hofmann, S. G., & Bufka, L. F. (2000). Cognitive-behavioral treatment of panic in patients with schizophrenia: Preliminary findings. *Journal of Cognitive Psychotherapy: An International Quarterly, 14*, 27–37.

Hofmann, S. G., & DiBartolo, P. M. (2000). An instrument to assess self-statements during public speaking: Scale development and psychometric properties. *Behavior Therapy, 31*, 499–515.

Hofmann, S. G., & DiBartolo, P. M. (2001). *From social anxiety to social phobia. Multiple perspectives*. Needham Heights, MA: Allyn & Bacon.

Hofmann, S. G., Ehlers, A., & Roth, W. T. (1995). Conditioning theory: A model for the etiology of public speaking anxiety? *Behaviour Research and Therapy, 33*, 567–571.

Hofmann, S. G., Gerlach, A., Wender, A., & Roth, W. T. (1997). Speech disturbances and gaze behavior during public speaking in subtypes of social phobia. *Journal of Anxiety Disorders, 11*, 573–585.

Hofmann, S. G., Lehman, C. L., & Barlow, D. H. (1997). How specific are specific phobias? *Journal of Behavior Therapy and Experimental Psychiatry, 28*, 233–240.

Hofmann, S. G., Newman, M. G., Becker, E., Taylor, C. B., & Roth, W. T. (1995). Social phobia with and without avoidant personality disorder: Preliminary behavior therapy outcome findings. *Journal of Anxiety Disorders, 9*, 427–438.

Hofmann, S. G., Newman, M. G., Ehlers, A., & Roth, W. T. (1995). Psychophysiological differences between subtypes of social phobia. *Journal of Abnormal Psychology, 104*, 224–231.

Hofmann, S. G., & Roth, W. T. (1996). Issues related to social anxiety among controls in social phobia research. *Behavior Therapy, 27*, 79–91.

Hofmann, S. G., Shear, M. K., Barlow, D. H., Gorman, J. M., Hershberger, D., Patterson, M., & Woods, S. W. (1998). Effects of panic disorder treatments on personality disorder characteristics. *Depression and Anxiety, 8*, 14–20.

Holden, A. E., & Barlow, D. H. (1986). Heart rate and heart rate variability recorded in vivo in agoraphobics and nonphobics. *Behavior Therapy, 17*, 26–42.

Holden, A. E., & O'Brien, G. T., Barlow, D. H., Stetson, D., & Infantino, A. (1983). Self-help manual for agoraphobia: A preliminary report of effectiveness. *Behavior Therapy, 14*, 545–556.

Hollifield, M., Katon, W., & Morojele, N. (1994). Anxiety and depression in an outpatient clinic in Lesotho, Africa. *International Journal of Psychiatry in Medicine, 24*, 179–188.

Hollifield, M., Katon, W., Spain, D., & Pule, L. (1990). Anxiety and depression in a village in Lesotho, Africa: A comparison with the United States. *British Journal of Psychiatry, 156*, 343–350.

Hollis, K. L. (1997). Contemporary research on Pavlovian conditioning: A "new" functional analysis. *American Psychologist, 52*, 956–965.

Holmberg, G., & Gershon, S. (1961). Autonomic and psychiatric effects of yohimbine hydrochloride. *Psychopharmacologia, 2*, 93–106.

Holmes, M. R., & St. Lawrence, J. S. (1983). Treatment of rape-induced trauma: Proposed behavioral conceptualization and review of the literature. *Clinical Psychology Review, 3*, 417–433.

Holmgren, A., & Strom, G. (1959). Blood lactate concentration in relation to absolute and relative work load in normal men, and in mitral stenosis, atrial septal defect and vasoregulatory asthenia. *Acta Medica Scandinavica, 163*, 185–193.

Holt, C. S., Heimberg, R. G., & Hope, D. A. (1992). Avoidant personality disorder and the generalized subtype of social phobia. *Journal of Abnormal Psychology, 101*, 318–325.

Holt, C. S., Heimberg, R. G., Hope, D. A., & Liebowitz, M. R. (1992). Situational domains of social phobia. *Journal of Anxiety Disorders, 6*, 63–77.

Holt, P. E., & Andrews, G. (1989a). Hyperventilation and anxiety in panic disorder, social phobia, GAD, and normal controls. *Behaviour Research and Therapy, 27*, 453–460.

Holt, P. E., & Andrews, G. (1989b). Provocation of panic: Three elements of the panic reaction in four anxiety disorders. *Behaviour Research and Therapy, 27*, 253–261.

Hoon, P., Wincze, J., & Hoon, E. (1977). A test of reciprocal inhibition: Are anxiety and sexual arousal in women mutually inhibitory? *Journal of Abnormal Psychology, 86*, 65–74.

Hoover, C. F., & Insel, T. R. (1984). Families of origin in obsessive–compulsive disorder. *Journal of Nervous and mental Disease, 172*, 207–215.

Hope, D. A., Gansler, D. A., & Heimberg, R. G. (1989). Attentional focus and causal attributions in social phobia: Implications from social psychology. *Clinical Psychology Review, 9*, 49–60.

Hope, D. A., & Heimberg, R. G. (1988). Public and private self-consciousness and social phobia. *Journal of Personality Assessment, 52*, 626–639.

Hope, D. A., Heimberg, R. G., & Bruch, M. A. (1995). Dismantling cognitive-behavioral group therapy for social phobia. *Behaviour Research and Therapy, 33*, 637–650.

Hope, D. A., Heimberg, R. G., & Klein, J. F. (1990). Social anxiety and the recall of interpersonal information. *Journal of Cognitive Psychotherapy, 4*, 185–195.

Hope, D. A., Heimberg, R. G., Juster, H. R., & Turk, C. L. (1999). *Managing social anxiety: A cognitive-behavioral therapy approach.* San Antonio, TX: Psychological Corporation/ Graywind Publications Incorporated.

Hope, D. A., Herbert, J. D., & White, C. (1995). Diagnostic subtype, avoidant personality disorder, and efficacy of cognitive-behavioral group therapy for social phobia. *Cognitive Therapy and Research, 19*, 399–417.

Hope, D. A., Rapee, R. M., Heimberg, R. G., & Dombeck, M. J. (1990). Representations of the self in social phobia: Vulnerability to social threat. *Cognitive Therapy and Research, 14*, 177–189.

Hopper, J. L., Judd, F. K., Derrick, P. L., & Burrows, G. D. (1986). A family study of panic disorder. *Genetic Epidemiology, 4*, 33–41.

Hornig, C. D., & McNally, R. J. (1995). Panic disorder and suicide attempt: A reanalysis of data from the Epidemiologic Catchment Area study. *British Journal of Psychiatry, 167*, 76–79.

Horowitz, M. J. (1975). Intrusive and repetitive thoughts after experimental stress. *Archives of General Psychiatry, 32*, 1457–1463.

Horowitz, M. J., Siegel, B., Holen, A., Bonanno, G. A., Milbrath, C., & Stinson, C. H. (1997). Diagnostic criteria for complicated grief disorder. *American Journal of Psychiatry, 154*, 904–910.

Horowitz, M. J., Wilner, N., & Alvarez, W. (1979). Impact of Event Scale: A measure of subjective stress. *Psychosomatic Medicine, 41*, 209–218.

Horwath, E., Johnson, J., & Hornig, C. D. (1993). Epidemiology of panic disorder in African-Americans. *American Journal of Psychiatry, 150*, 465–469.

Horwath, E., Lish, J. D., Johnson, J., Hornig, C. D., & Weissman, M. M. (1993). Agoraphobia without panic: Clinical reappraisal of an epidemiological finding. *American Journal of Psychiatry, 150*, 1496–1501.

Horwath, E., & Weissman, M. M. (1997). Epidemiology of anxiety disorders across cultural groups. In S. Friedman (Ed.), *Cultural issues in the treatment of anxiety.* New York: Guilford Press.

Horwath, E., Wolk, S. I., Goldrein, R. B., Wickramaratne, P., Sobin, C., Adams, P., Lish, J. D., & Weissman, M. M. (1995). Is the comorbidity between social phobia and panic disorder due to familial cotransmission or other factors? *Archives of General Psychiatry, 52*, 574–582.

Houlihan, D., Schwartz, C., Miltenberger, R., & Heuton, D. (1993). The rapid treatment of a young man's balloon (noise) phobia using in vivo flooding. *Journal of Behavior Therapy and Experimental Psychiatry, 24*, 233–240.

Howard, W. A., Murphy, S. M., & Clarke, J. C. (1983). The nature and treatment of fear of flying: A controlled investigation. *Behavior Therapy, 14*, 557–567.

Hsu, L. K., Kaye, W., & Weltzin, T. (1993). Are the eating disorders related to obsessive–compulsive disorder? *International Journal of Eating Disorders, 14*, 305–318.

Hudson, C. J. (1981). Agoraphobia in Alaskan Eskimos. *New York State Journal of Medicine, 81*, 224–225.

Hudson, J. I., & Pope, H. G. (1990). Affective spectrum disorder: Does antidepressant response identify a family of disorders with a common pathophysiology? *American Journal of Psychiatry, 147*, 552–564.

Huey, S. R., & West, S. G. (1983). Hyperventilation: Its relation to symptom experience and to anxiety. *Journal of Abnormal Psychology, 92,* 422–432.

Hugdahl, K., & Öst, L.-G. (1985). Subjectively rated physiological and cognitive symptoms in six different clinical phobias. *Personality and Individual Differences, 6,* 175–188.

Hull, J. G., & Young, R. D. (1983). Self-consciousness, self-esteem, and success–failure as determinants of alcohol consumption in male social drinkers. *Journal of Personality and Social Psychology, 44,* 1097–1109.

Hume, W. I. (1973). Physiological measures in twins. In G. Claridge, S. Canter, & W. I. Hume (Eds.), *Personality differences and biological variations: A study of twins.* Oxford: Pergamon Press.

Ingman, K. A., Ollendick, T. H., & Akande, A. (1999). Cross-cultural aspects of fears in African children and adolescents. *Behaviour Research and Therapy, 37,* 337–345.

Ingram, R. E. (1990). Self-focused attention in clinical disorders: Review and a conceptual model. *Psychological Bulletin, 107,* 156–176.

Ingram, R. E., Miranda, J., & Segal, Z. V. (1998). *Cognitive vulnerability to depression.* New York: Guilford Press.

Inkeles, A. (1983). *Exploring individual modernity.* New York: Columbia University Press.

Insel, T. R. (Ed.). (1984). *New findings in obsessive–compulsive disorder.* Washington, DC: American Psychiatric Press.

Insel, T. R. (1986). The neurobiology of anxiety: A tale of two systems. In B. F. Shaw, Z. V. I. Segal, T. M. Vallis, & F. E. Cashman (Eds.), *Anxiety disorders: Psychological and biological perspectives.* New York: Plenum Press.

Insel, T. R., & Akiskal, H. S. (1986). Obsessive–compulsive disorder with psychotic features: A phenomenology analysis. *American Journal of Psychiatry, 143,* 1527–1533.

Insel, T. R., Murphy, D. L., Cohen, R. M., Alterman, I., Kilts, C., & Linnoila, M. (1983). Obsessive–compulsive disorder: A double blind trial of clomipramine and clorgyline. *Archives of General Psychiatry, 40,* 605–612.

Insel, T. R., Scanlan, J., Champoux, M., & Suomi, S. J. (1988). Rearing paradigm in a nonhuman primate affects response to B-CCE challenge. *Psychopharmacology, 96,* 81–86.

Insel, T. R., Zahn, T., & Murphy, D. L. (1985). Obsessive–compulsive disorder: An anxiety disorder? In A. H. Tuma & J. D. Maser (Eds.), *Anxiety and the anxiety disorders.* Hillsdale, NJ: Erlbaum.

Ironson, G., Taylor, C. B., Boltwood, M., Bartzokis, T., Dennis, C., Chesney, M., Spitzer, S., & Segall, G. M. (1992). Effects of anger on left ventricular ejection fraction in coronary artery disease. *American Journal of Cardiology, 70,* 281–285.

Izard, C. E. (Ed.). (1971). *The face of emotion.* New York: Appleton-Century-Crofts.

Izard, C. E. (1977). *Human emotions.* New York: Plenum Press.

Izard, C. E. (1991). *The psychology of emotions.* New York: Plenum Press.

Izard, C. E. (1992). Basic emotions, relations among emotions, and emotion–cognition relations. *Psychological Review, 99,* 561–565.

Izard, C. E. (1993). Four systems for emotion activation: Cognitive and noncognitive processes. *Psychological Review, 100,* 68–90.

Izard, C. E. (1994). Innate and universal facial expressions: Evidence from developmental and cross-cultural research. *Psychological Bulletin, 115,* 288–299.

Izard, C. E., & Blumberg, M. A. (1985). Emotion theory and the role of emotions in anxiety in children and adults. In A. H. Tuma & J. D. Maser (Eds.), *Anxiety and the anxiety disorders.* Hillsdale, NJ: Erlbaum.

Izard, C. E., Kagan, J., & Zajonc, R. B. (Eds.). (1984). *Emotions, cognition, and behavior.* New York: Cambridge University Press.

Izard, C. E., & Youngstrom, E. A. (1996). The activation and regulation of fear and anxiety. In D. A. Hope (Ed.), *Nebraska Symposium on Motivation: Vol. 43. Perspectives on anxiety, panic, and fear.* Lincoln: University of Nebraska Press.

Jablensky, A. (1985). Approaches to the definition and classification of anxiety and related disorders in European psychiatry. In A. H. Tuma & J. D. Maser (Eds.), *Anxiety and the anxiety disorders*. Hillsdale, NJ: Erlbaum.

Jacobs, S. (1993). *Pathologic grief: Maladaptation to loss*. Washington, DC: American Psychiatric Press.

Jacobs, S., Hansen, F., Berkman, L., Kasi, S., & Ostfield, A. (1989). Depressions of bereavement. *Comprehensive Psychiatry*, *30*(3), 218–224.

Jacobsen, P. B., Bovbjerg, D. H., Schwartz, M. D., Andrykowski, M. A., Futterman, A. D., Gilewski, T., Norton, L., & Redd, W. H. (1993). Formation on food aversions in cancer patients receiving repeated infusion of chemotherapy. *Behaviour Research and Therapy*, *31*(8), 739–748.

Jacobsen, P. B., Bovbjerg, D. H., Schwartz, M. D., Hudis, C. A., Gilewski, T. A., & Norton, L. (1995). Conditioned emotional distress in women receiving chemotherapy for breast cancer. *Journal of Consulting and Clinical Psychology*, *63*, 108–114.

Jacobson, R., & Edinger, J. D. (1982). Side effects of relaxation treatment. *American Journal of Psychiatry*, *139*, 952–953.

James, W. (1890). *The principles of psychology*. New York: Holt.

Janet, P. (1889). *L'automatisme psychologique*. Paris: Alcan.

Jansson, L., Jerremalm, L., & Öst, L.-G. (1986). Follow-up of agoraphobic patients treated with exposure in vivo or applied relaxation. *British Journal of Psychiatry*, *149*, 486–490.

Jansson, L., & Öst, L.-G. (1982). Behavioral treatments for agoraphobia: An evaluative review. *Clinical Psychology Review*, *2*, 311–336.

Jardine, R., Martin, N. G., & Henderson, A. S. (1984). Genetic covariation between neuroticism and the symptoms of anxiety and depression. *Genetic Epidemiology*, *1*, 89–107.

Jefferson, J. W., & Katzelnick, D. J. (1997). *Social phobia: A guide*. (Middleton, WI: Dean Foundation for Health Research and Education.

Jenike, M. A. (1990). Predictors of treatment failure. In M. A. Jenike, L. Baer, & W. E. Minichiello (Eds.), *Obsessive–compulsive disorders: Theory and management*. Chicago: Year Book Medical.

Jenike, M. A., Baer, L., Ballantine, H. T., Martuza, R. L., Tynes, S., Giriunas, I., Buttolph, L., & Cassem, N. H. (1991). Cingulotomy for refractory obsessive–compulsive disorder: A long-term follow-up of 33 patients. *Archives of General Psychiatry*, *48*, 548–555.

Jenike, M. A., Baer, L., Minchiello, W. E., Schwartz, E. E., & Carey, R. J. (1986). Concomitant obsessive–compulsive disorder and schizotypal personality disorders. *American Journal of Psychiatry*, *143*, 306–311.

Jensen, J. A. (1994). An investigation of eye movement desensitization and reprocessing (EMD/R) as a treatment for posttraumatic stress disorder (PTSD) symptoms of Vietnam combat veterans. *Behavior Therapy*, *25*, 311–325.

Jerremalm, A., Jansson, L., & Öst, L.-G. (1986). Individual response patterns and the effects of different behavioral methods in the treatment of dental phobia. *Behaviour Research and Therapy*, *24*, 587–596.

Johnson, J., Weissman, M. M., & Klerman, G. L. (1990). Panic disorder, comorbidity, and suicide attempts. *Archives of General Psychiatry*, *47*, 805–808.

Johnstone, E. C., Bourne, R. C., Crow, T. J., Frith, C. D., Gamble, S., Lofthouse, R., Owen, F., Owens, D. G. C., Robinson, J., & Stevens, M. (1981). The relationship between clinical response, psychophysiological variables and plasma levels of amitriptyline and diazepam in neurotic outpatients. *Psychopharmacology*, *72*, 233–240.

Joiner, T. E., Jr. (1996). A confirmatory factor analytic nivestigation of the tripartite model of depression and anxiety in college students. *Cognitive Therapy and Research*, *20*, 521–539.

Joiner, T. E., Jr., Catanzaro, S. J., & Laurent, J. (1996). Tripartite structure of positive and negative affect, depression, and anxiety in child and adolescent psychiatric inpatients. *Journal of Abnormal Psychology*, *105*, 401–409.

Joiner, T. E., Jr., Steer, R. A., Beck, A. T., Schmidt, N. B., Rudd, M. D., & Catanzaro, S. J. (1999). Physiological hyperarousal: Construct validity of a central aspect of the tripartite model of depression and anxiety. *Journal of Abnormal Psychology*, *108*, 290–298.

Jones, J. C., & Barlow, D. H. (1990). The etiology of posttraumatic stress disorder. *Clinical Psychology Review, 10,* 299–328.

Jones, J. C., Bruce, T. J., & Barlow, D. H. (1986, November). *The effects of four levels of "anxiety" on sexual arousal in sexually functional and dysfunctional men.* Poster presented at the 20th Annual Convention of the Association for Advancement of Behavior Therapy, Chicago.

Jones, M., & Mellersh, V. (1946). Comparison of exercise response in anxiety states and normal controls. *Psychosomatic Medicine, 8,* 180–187.

Jones, M. K., & Menzies, R. G. (1997). The cognitive mediation of obsessive–compulsive handwashing. *Behaviour Research and Therapy, 35,* 843–850.

Jones, M. K., & Menzies, R. G. (1998a). Danger ideation reduction therapy (DIRT) for obsessive–compulsive washers: A controlled trial. *Behaviour Research and Therapy, 36,* 959–970.

Jones, M. K., & Menzies, R. G. (1998b). The relevance of associative learning pathways in the development of obsessive–compulsive washing. *Behaviour Research and Therapy, 36,* 273–283.

Jones, M. K., & Menzies, R. G. (2000). Danger expenctancies, self-efficacy and insight in spider phobia. *Behaviour Research and Therapy, 38,* 585–600.

Jones, M. K., Whitmont, S., & Menzies, R. G. (1996). Danger expectancies and insight in spider phobia. *Anxiety, 2,* 179–185.

Jones, W. H., Briggs, S. R., & Smith, T. G. (1986). Shyness: Conceptualization and measurement. *Journal of Personality and Social Psychology, 51,* 629–639.

Joormann, J., & Stöber, J. (1999). Somatic symptoms of generalized anxiety disorder for the DSM-IV: Associations with pathological worry and depression symptoms in a nonclinical sample. *Journal of Anxiety Disorders, 13,* 491–503.

Joyce, P. R., Bushnell, J. A., Oakley-Brown, M. A., Wells, J. E., & Hornblow, A. R. (1989). The epidemiology of panic symptomotology and agoraphobic avoidance. *Comprehensive Psychiatry, 30,* 303–312.

Kabat-Zinn, J., Massion, A. O., Kristeller, J., Peterson, L. G., Fletcher, K. E., Pbert, L., Lenderking, W. R., & Santorelli, S. F. (1992). Effectiveness of a meditation-based stress reduction program in the treatment of anxiety disorders. *American Journal of Psychiatry, 149,* 936–943.

Kagan, J. (1989). Temperamental contributions to social behavior. *American Psychologist, 44,* 668–674.

Kagan, J. (1994). *Galen's prophecy.* New York: Basic Books.

Kagan, J. (1997). Temperament and the reactions to unfamiliarity. *Child Development, 68,* 139–143.

Kagan, J., Gibbons, J. L., Johnson, M. O., Reznick, J. S., & Snidman, N. (1990). A temperamental disposition to the state of uncertainty. In J. E. Rolf & A. S. Masten (Eds.), *Risk and protective factors in the development of psychopathology.* New York: Cambridge University Press.

Kagan, J., Reznick, J. S., & Snidman, N. (1986). Biological bases of childhood shyness. *Science, 240,* 167–171.

Kagan, J., Reznick, J. S., & Snidman, N. (1987). The physiology and psychology of behavioral inhibition. *Child Development, 58,* 1459–1473.

Kagan, J., Reznick, J. S., & Snidman, N. (1988). Biological bases of childhood shyness. *Science, 240,* 167–171.

Kagan, J., & Snidman, N. (1991). Temperamental factors in human development. *American Psychologist, 46,* 856–862.

Kagan, J., & Snidman, N. (1999). Early childhood predictors of adult anxiety disorders. *Biological Psychiatry, 46,* 1536–1541.

Kagan, J., Snidman, N., & Arcus, D. M. (1992). Initial reactions to unfamiliarity. *Current Directions in Psychological Science, 1*(6), 171–174.

Kagan, J., Snidman, N., & Arcus, D. M. (1998). Childhood derivatives of high and low reactivity in infancy. *Child Development, 69,* 1483–1493.

Kahan, M., Tanzer, J., Darvin, D., & Borer, F. (2000, March). *Fear of flying: Cognitive behavioral therapy using virtual reality exposure.* Paper presented at the meeting of the Anxiety Disorders Association of America, Washington, DC.

Kahn, R. J., McNair, D. M., Lipman, R. S., Covi, L., Rickels, K., Downing, R., Fisher, S., & Frankenthaler, L. M. (1986). Imipramine and chlordiazepoxide in depressive and anxiety disorders. *Archives of General Psychiatry, 43,* 79–85.

Kahn, R. S., Wetzler, S., van Praag, H. M., Asnis, G. M., & Strauman, T. (1988). Behavioral indications for serotonin receptor hypersensitivity in panic disorder. *Psychiatry Research, 25,* 101–104.

Kahneman, D. (1973). *Attention and effort.* Englewood Cliffs, NJ: Prentice-Hall.

Kalin, N. H., Shelton, S. E., & Davidson, R. J. (2000). Cerebrospinal fluid corticotropin-releasing hormone levels are elevated in monkeys with patterns of brain activity associated with fearful temperament. *Biological Psychiatry, 47,* 579–585.

Kalin, N. H., Shelton, S. E., Rickman, M., & Davidson, R. J. (1998). Individual differences in freezing and cortisol in infant and mother rhesus monkeys. *Behavioral Neuroscience, 112,* 251–254.

Kamieniecki, G. W., Wade, T., & Tsourtos, G. (1997). Interpretive bias for benign sensations in panic disorder with agoraphobia. *Journal of Anxiety Disorders, 11*(2), 141–156.

Kandel, E. R. (1983). From metapsychology to molecular biology: Explorations into the nature of anxiety. *American Journal of Psychiatry, 140,* 1277–1293.

Kandel, E. R., Jessell, T. M., & Schacter, S. (1991). Early experience and the fine tuning of synaptic connections. In E. R. Kandel, J. H. Schwartz, & T. M. Jessell (Eds.), *Principles of neural science* (3rd ed.). New York: Elsevier.

Kantor, J. S., Zitrin, C. M., & Zeldis, S. M. (1980). Mitral valve prolapse syndrome in agoraphobia patients. *American Journal of Psychiatry, 137,* 467–469.

Kaplan, H. S. (1974). *The new sex therapy.* New York: Brunner/Mazel.

Karajgi, B., Rifkin, A., Doddi, S., & Kolli, R. (1990). The prevalence of anxiety disorders in patients with chronic obstructive pulmonary disease. *American Journal of Psychiatry, 147,* 200–201.

Karno, M., Golding, J. M., Burnam, M. A., Hough, R. L., Escobar, J. I., Wells, K. M., & Boyer, R. (1989). Anxiety disorders among Mexican Americans and non-Hispanic whites in Los Angeles. *Journal of Nervous and Mental Disease, 177,* 202–209.

Karno, M., Golding, J. M., Sorenson, S. B., & Burnham, A. B. (1988). The epidemiology of obsessive–compulsive disorder in five U. S. communities. *Archives of General Psychiatry, 45,* 1094–1099.

Kashani, J. H., & Orvaschel, H. (1988). Anxiety disorders in mid-adolescence: A community sample. *American Journal of Psychiatry, 145,* 960–964.

Katerndahl, D. A., & Realini, J. P. (1993). Lifetime prevalence of panic states. *American Journal of Psychiatry, 150,* 246–249.

Katerndahl, D. A., & Realini, J. P. (1995). Where do panic attack sufferers seek care? *Journal of Family Practice, 40,* 237–243.

Katerndahl, D. A., & Realini, J. P. (1997). Comorbid psychiatric disorders in subjects with panic attacks. *Journal of Nervous and Mental Disease, 185,* 669–674.

Katon, W. (1996). Panic disorder: Relationship to high medical utilization, unexplained physical symptoms, and medical costs. *Journal of Clinical Psychiatry, 57,* 11–22.

Katon, W., Hall, M., Russo, J., Cormier, L., Hollifield, M., Vitaliano, P., & Beitman, B. (1988). Chest pain: Relationship of psychiatric illness to coronary arteriographic results. *American Journal of Medicine, 84,* 1–9.

Katon, W., Vitaliano, P., Russo, J., Cormier, L., Anderson, K., & Jones, M. (1986). Panic disorder: Epidemiology in primary care. *Journal of Family Practitioners, 23,* 233–239.

Katon, W., Vitaliano, P., Russo, J., Jones, M., & Anderson, K. (1987). Panic disorder: Spectrum of severity and somatization. *Journal of Nervous and Mental Disease, 175,* 12–19.

Katon, W., Von Korff, M., Lin, E., Lipscomb, R., Russo, J., Wagner, E., & Polk, E. (1990). Distressed high utilizers of medical care: DSM-III-R diagnoses and treatment needs. *General Hospital Psychiatry, 12,* 355–362.

Katschnig, H. (1999). Anxiety neurosis, panic disorder or what? In D. J. Nutt, J. C. Ballenger, & J.-P. Lépine (Eds.), *Panic disorder: Clinical diagnosis, management and mechanisms.* London: Martin Dunitz.

Katschnig, H., & Amering, M. (1994). The long-term course of panic disorder. In B. E. Wolfe & J. D. Maser (Eds.), *Treatment of panic disorder: A consensus development conference*. Washington, DC: American Psychiatric Press.

Katschnig, H., Amering, M., Stolk, J. M., Klerman, G. L., Garvey, M., Roth, M., & Solyom, C. (1995). Long-term follow-up after a drug trial for panic disorder. *British Journal of Psychiatry, 167*, 487–494.

Katschnig, H., Stein, M. B., & Buller, R. (1997). Moclobemide in social phobia: A double-blind, placebo-controlled clinical study. *European Archives of Psychiatry and Clinical Neuroscience, 247*, 71–80.

Katzelnick, D. J., Kobak, K. A., Greist, J. H., Jefferson, J. W., Mantle, J. M., & Serlin, R. C. (1995). Sertraline for social phobia: A double-blind, placebo-controlled crossover study. *American Journal of Psychiatry, 152*, 1368–1371.

Kawachi, I., Colditz, G. A., Ascherio, A., Rimm, E. B., Giovannucci, E., Stampfer, M. J., & Willett, W. C. (1994). Prospective study of phobic anxiety and risk of coronary heart disease in men. *Circulation, 9*, 1992–1997.

Kawachi, I., Sparrow, D., Vokonas, P. S., & Weiss, S. T. (1994). Symptoms of anxiety and risk of coronary heart disease: The Normative Aging Study. *Circulation, 90*, 2225–2229.

Kawachi, I., Sparrow, D., Vokonas, P. S., & Weiss, S. T. (1995). Decreased heart rate variability in men with phobic anxiety (data from the Normative Aging Study). *American Journal of Cardiology, 75*, 882–885.

Keane, T. M. (1995). Guidelines for the forensic psychological assessment of posttraumatic stress disorder claimants. In R. I. Simon (Ed.), *Posttraumatic stress disorder in litigation: Guidelines for forensic assessment*. Washington, DC: American Psychiatric Press.

Keane, T. M. (1998). Psychological and behavioral treatments of post-traumatic stress disorder. In P. E. Nathan & J. M. Gorman (Eds.), *A guide to treatments that work*. New York: Oxford University Press.

Keane, T. M., Caddell, J. M., & Taylor, K. L. (1988). Mississippi Scale for Combat-Related Posttraumatic Stress Disorder: Three studies in reliability and validity. *Journal of Consulting and Clinical Psychology, 56*, 85–90.

Keane, T. M., Fairbank, J. A., Caddell, J. M., & Zimering, R. T. (1989). Implosive (flooding) therapy reduces symptoms of PTSD in Vietnam combat veterans. *Behavior Therapy, 20*, 245–260.

Keane, T. M., Fairbank, J. A., Caddell, J. M., Zimering, R. T., & Bender, M. E. (1985). A behavioral approach to assessing and treating posttraumatic stress disorder in Vietnam veterans. In C. R. Figley (Ed.), *Trauma and its wake*. New York: Brunner/Mazel.

Keane, T. M., Fisher, L. M., Krinsley, K. E., & Niles, B. L. (1994). Posttraumatic stress disorder. In M. Hersen & R. T. Ammerman. (Eds.), *Handbook of prescriptive treatments for adults*. New York: Plenum Press.

Keane, T. M., & Kaloupek, D. G. (1982). Imaginal flooding in the treatment of posttraumatic stress disorder. *Journal of Consulting and Clinical Psychology, 50*, 138–140.

Keane, T. M., Kolb, L. C., Kaloupek, D. G., Orr, S. P., Blanchard, E. B., Thomas, R. G., Hsieh, F. Y., & Lavori, P. W. (1998). Utility of psychophysiology measurement in the diagnosis of posttraumatic stress disorder: Results from a Department of Veterans Affairs cooperative study. *Journal of Consulting and Clinical Psychology, 66*, 914–923.

Keane, T. M., Malloy, P. F., & Fairbank, J. A. (1984). Empirical development of an MMPI subscale for the assessment of combat-related posttraumatic stress disorder. *Journal of Consulting and Clinical Psychology, 52*, 888–891.

Keane, T. M., & Penk, W. E. (1988). Some concerns about the prevalence of PTSD in the general population [Letter to the editor]. *New England Journal of Medicine, 318*, 1690–1691.

Keane, T. M., Weathers, F. W., & Foa, E. B. (2000). Diagnosis and assessment. In E. B. Foa, T. M. Keane, & M. J. Friedman (Eds.), *Effective treatments for PTSD: Practice guidelines from the International Society for Traumatic Stress Studies*. New York: Guilford Press.

Keane, T. M., & Wolfe, J. (1990). Comorbidity in post-traumatic stress disorder: An analysis of community and clinical studies. *Journal of Applied Social Psychology, 20*, 1776–1788.

Keane, T. M., Wolfe, J., & Taylor, K. L. (1987). Post-traumatic stress disorder: Evidence for diagnostic validity and methods of psychological assessment. *Journal of Clinical Psychology, 43,* 32–43.

Keane, T. M., Zimering, R. T., & Caddell, J. M. (1985). A behavioral formulation of posttraumatic stress disorder in Vietnam veterans. *The Behavior Therapist, 8,* 9–12.

Kearney, C. A., Albano, A. M., Eisen, A. R., Allen, W. D., & Barlow, D. H. (1997). The phenomenology of panic disorder in youngsters: An empirical study of a clinical sample. *Journal of Anxiety Disorders, 11,* 49–62.

Kearney, C. A., Drabman, R. S., Joransen, J. A., Lange, S., et al. (1996). Mitral valve prolapse and symptoms of negative affectivity in adolescents. *Children's Health Care, 25,* 133–141.

Keller, M. B. (1994). *Harvard–Brown Anxiety Disorder Research Program.* Unpublished manuscript.

Keller, M. B., & Baker, L. (1992). The clinical course of panic disorder and depression. *Journal of Clinical Psychiatry, 53,* 5–8.

Keller, M. B., Lavori, P. W., Mueller, T. I., Endicott, J., Coryell, W., Hirschfeld, R. M. A., & Shea, T. (1992). Time to recovery, chronicity, and levels of psychopathology in major depression: A 5-year prospective follow-up of 431 subjects. *Archives of General Psychiatry, 49,* 809–816.

Keller, M. B., Yonkers, K. A., Warshaw, M. G., Pratt, L. A., Golan, J., Mathews, A. O., White, K., Swartz, A., Reich, J, & Lavori, P. (1994). Remission and relapse in subjects with panic disorder and agoraphobia: A prospective short interval naturalistic follow-up. *Journal of Nervous and Mental Disorders, 182,* 290–296.

Kelly, D. H. W. (1966). Measurement of anxiety by forearm blood flow. *British Journal of Psychiatry, 112,* 789–798.

Kelly, P., Mitchel-Heggs, N., & Sherman, D. (1971). Anxiety in the effects of sodium lactate assessed clinically and physiologically. *British Journal of Psychiatry, 119,* 468–470.

Kenardy, J., Evans, L., & Oei, T. P. S. (1988). The importance of cognitions in panic attacks. *Behavior Therapy, 19,* 471–483.

Kenardy, J., Fried, L., Kraemer, H. C., & Taylor, C. B. (1992). Psychological precursors of panic attacks. *British Journal of Psychiatry, 160,* 668–673.

Kenardy, J., & Taylor, C. B. (1999). Expected versus unexpected panic attacks: A naturalistic prospective study. *Journal of Anxiety Disorders, 13,* 435–445.

Kendall, P. C., & Butcher, J. N. (1982). *Handbook of research methods in clinical psychology.* New York: Wiley.

Kendall, P. C., Flannery-Schroeder, E., Panichelli-Mindel, S. M., Southam-Gerow, M., Henin, A., & Warman, M. (1997). Therapy for youths with anxiety disorders: A second randomized clinical trial. *Journal of Consulting and Clinical Psychology, 65,* 366–380.

Kendall, P. C., & Hollon, S. D. (1981). Assessing self-referent speech: Methods in the measurement of self-statements. In P. C. Kendall & S. D. Hollon (Eds.), *Assessment strategies for cognitive-behavioral interventions.* New York: Academic Press.

Kendall, P. C., & Watson, D. (Eds.). (1989). *Anxiety and depression: Distinctive and overlapping features.* San Diego, CA: Academic Press.

Kendell, R. E. (1975). *The role of diagnosis in psychiatry.* Oxford: Blackwell.

Kendler, K. S. (1995). Genetic epidemiology in psychiatry. *Archives of General Psychiatry, 52,* 895–899.

Kendler, K. S. (1996). Major depression and generalised anxiety disorder: Same genes, (partly) different environments—revisited. *British Journal of Psychiatry, 168*(Suppl. 30), 68–75.

Kendler, K. S., Heath, A. C., Martin, N. G., & Eaves, L. J. (1986). Symptoms of anxiety and depression in a volunteer twin population. *Archives of General Psychiatry, 43,* 213–221.

Kendler, K. S., Heath, A. C., Martin, N. G., & Eaves, L. J. (1987). Symptoms of anxiety and symptoms of depression: Same genes, different environments? *Archives of General Psychiatry, 44,* 451–457.

Kendler, K. S., Karkowski, L. M., & Prescott, C. A. (1999). Fear and phobias: Reliability and heritability. *Psychological Medicine, 29,* 539–553.

Kendler, K. S., Neale, M. C., Kessler, R. C., Heath, A. C., & Eaves, L. J. (1992a). Generalized anxiety disorder in women: A population-based twin study. *Archives of General Psychiatry, 49,* 267–272.

Kendler, K. S., Neale, M. C., Kessler, R. C., Heath, A. C., & Eaves, L. J. (1992b). The genetic epidemiology of phobias in women: The interrelationship of agoraphobia, social phobia, situational phobia, and simple phobia. *Archives of General Psychiatry, 49,* 273–281.

Kendler, K. S., Neale, M. C., Kessler, R. C., Heath, A. C., & Eaves, L. J. (1992c). Major depression and generalized anxiety disorder: Same genes, (partly) different environments? *Archives of General Psychiatry, 49,* 716–722.

Kendler, K. S., Walters, E. E., Neale, M. C., Kessler, R. C., Heath, A. C., & Eaves, L. J. (1995). The structure of genetic and environmental risk factors for six major psychiatric disorders in women: Phobia, generalized anxiety disorder, panic disorder, bulimia, major depression, and alcoholism. *Archives of General Psychiatry, 52,* 374–382.

Kennedy, B., & Schwab, J. (1997). Utilization of medical specialists by anxiety disorder patients. *Psychosomatics, 38,* 109–112.

Kennedy, R. (1976). Self-induced depersonalization syndrome. *American Journal of Psychiatry, 133,* 1326–1328.

Kent, G. (1985). Cognitive processes in dental anxiety. *British Journal of Clinical Psychology, 24,* 259–264.

Kessler, R. C. (1997). The effects of stressful life events on depression. *Annual Review of Psychology, 48,* 191–214. (Chapter Seven)

Kessler, R. C., Crum, R. M., Warner, L. A., Nelson, C. B., Schulenberg, J., & Anthony, J. C. (1997). Lifetime co-occurrence of DSM-III-R alcohol abuse and dependence with other psychiatric disorders in the National Comorbidity Survey. *Archives of General Psychiatry, 54,* 313–321.

Kessler, R. C., DuPont, R. L., Berglund, P., & Wittchen, H.-U. (1999). Impairment in pure and comorbid generalized anxiety disorder and major depression at 12 months in two national surveys. *American Journal of Psychiatry, 156,* 1915–1923.

Kessler, R. C., McGonagle, K. A., Zhao, S., Nelson, C. B., Hughes, M., Eshleman, S., Wittchen, H.-U., & Kendler, K. S. (1994). Lifetime and 12-month prevalence of DSM-III-R psychiatric disorders in the United States: Results from the National Comorbidity Survey. *Archives of General Psychiatry, 51,* 8–19.

Kessler, R. C., Nelson, C. B., McGonagle, K. A., Lui, J., Swartz, M., & Blazer, D. G. (1996). Comorbidity of DSM-III-R major depressive disorder in the general population: Results from the National Comorbidity Survey. *British Journal of Psychiatry, 168,* 17–30.

Kessler, R. C., Sonnega, A., Bromet, E., Hughes, M., & Nelson, C. B. (1995). Posttraumatic stress disorder in the National Comorbidity Survey. *Archives of General Psychiatry, 52,* 1048–1060.

Kessler, R. C., Stang, P. E., Wittchen, H.-U., Stein, M., & Walters, E. E. (1999). Lifetime comorbidities between social phobia and mood disorders in the U.S. National Comorbidity Survey. *Psychological Medicine, 29,* 555–567.

Kessler, R. C., Stang, P. E., Wittchen, H.-U., Ustan, T. B., Roy-Byrne, P. P., & Walters, E. E. (1998). Lifetime panic–depression comorbidity in the National Comorbidity Survey. *Archives of General Psychiatry, 55,* 801–808.

Kessler, R. C., Zhao, S., Katz, S. J., Kouzis, A. C., Frank, R. G., Edlund, M., & Leaf, P. (1999). Past-year use of outpatient services for psychiatric problems in the National Comorbidity Survey. *American Journal of Psychiatry, 156,* 115–123.

Kettl, P. A., & Marks, I. M. (1986). Neurological factors in obsessive–compulsive disorder: Two case reports and a review of the literature. *British Journal of Psychiatry, 149,* 315–319.

Khawaja, N. G., & Oei, T. P. S. (1992). Development of a Catastrophic Cognition Questionnaire. *Journal of Anxiety Disorders, 6,* 305–318.

Kierkegaard, S. (1944). *The concept of dread* (W. Lowrie, Trans.). Princeton, NJ: Princeton University Press. (Original work published 1844)

Kilpatrick, D. G., Edmunds, C. N., & Seymour, A. K. (1992). *Rape in America: A report to the nation.* Arlington, VA: National Victim Center.

Kilpatrick, D. G., Resick, P. A., & Veronen, L. J. (1981). Effects of a rape experience: A longitudinal study. *Journal of Social Issues, 37*, 105–122.

Kilpatrick, D. G., & Resnick, H. S. (1992). Posttraumatic stress disorder associated with exposure to criminal victimization in clinical and community populations, In J. R. T. Davidson & E. B. Foa (Eds.), *Posttraumatic stress disorder: DSM-IV and beyond*. Washington, DC: American Psychiatric Press.

Kilpatrick, D. G., & Saunders, B. E. (1999). *Prevalence and consequences of child victimization: Results from the National Survey of Adolescents*. Washington, DC: National Institute of Justice.

Kilpatrick, D. G., Veronen, L. J., & Best, C. L. (1985). Factors predicting psychological distress among rape victims. In C. R. Figley (Ed.), *Trauma and its wake*. New York: Brunner/Mazel.

Kilpatrick, D. G., Veronen, L. J., & Resick, P. A. (1979). Assessment of the aftermath of rape: Changing pattern of fear. *Journal of Behavioral Assessment, 1*, 133–147.

Kim, J. A., Siegel, S., & Patenall, V. R. A. (1999). Drug-onset cues as signals: Intraadministration associations and tolerance. *Journal of Experimental Psychology: Animal Behavior Processes, 25*, 491–504.

Kim, S. W., Dysken, M. W., & Katz, R. (1989). Rating scales for obsessive compulsive disorder. *Psychiatric Annals, 19*, 74–79.

Kindt, M., & Brosschot, J. F. (1997). Phobia-related cognitive bias for pictorial and linguistic stimuli. *Journal of Abnormal Psychology, 106*, 644–648.

Kindt, M., & Brosschot, J. F. (1998). Stability of cognitive bias for threat cues in phobia. *Journal of Psychopathology and Behavioral Assessment, 20*, 351–367.

Kindt, M., & Brosschot, J. F. (1999). Cognitive bias in spider-phobic children: Comparison of a pictorial and a linguistic spider Stroop. *Journal of Psychopathology and Behavioral Assessment, 21*, 207–220.

King, D. W., King, L. A., Foy, D. W., & Gudanowski, D. M. (1996). Prewar factors in combat-related posttraumatic stress disorder: Structural equation modeling with a national sample of female and male Vietnam veterans. *Journal of Consulting and Clinical Psychology, 64*, 520–531.

King, D. W., King, L. A., Foy, D. W., Keane, T. M., & Fairbank, J. A. (1999). Posttraumatic stress disorder in a national sample of female and male Vietnam veterans: Risk factors, war-zone stressors, and resilience–recovery variables. *Journal of Abnormal Psychology, 108*, 164–170.

King, D. W., King, L. A., Gudanowski, D. M., & Vreven, D. L. (1995). Alternative representations of war zone stressors: Relationships to posttraumatic stress disorder in male and female Vietnam veterans. *Journal of Abnormal Psychology, 104*, 184–196.

King, L. A., King, D. W., Fairbank, J. A., Keane, T. M., & Adams, G. A. (1998). Resilience–recovery factors in post-traumatic stress disorder among female and male Vietnam veterans: Hardiness, postwar social support, and additional stressful life events. *Journal of Personality and Social Psychology, 74*, 420–434.

King, R., Margraf, J., Ehlers, A., & Maddock, R. (1986). Panic disorder—overlap with symptoms of somatization disorder. In I. Hand & H.-U. Wittchen (Eds.), *Panic and phobias: Empirical evidence of theoretical models and longterm effects of behavioral treatments*. Berlin: Springer-Verlag.

Kirk, J. W. (1983). Behavioural treatment of obsessive–compulsive patients in routine clinical practice. *Behaviour Research and Therapy, 21*, 57–62.

Kirkpatrick, D. R. (1984). Age, gender and patterns of common intense fears among adults. *Behaviour Research and Therapy, 22*, 141–150.

Kirmayer, L. (1991). The place of culture in psychiatric nosology: *Taijin kyofusho* and DSM-III-R. *Journal of Nervous and Mental Disease, 179*, 19–28.

Klein, D. F. (1964). Delineation of two drug responsive anxiety syndromes. *Psychopharmacologia, 5*, 397–408.

Klein, D. F. (1981). Anxiety reconceptualized. In D. F. Klein & J. G. Rabkin (Eds.), *Anxiety: New research and changing concepts*. New York: Raven Press.

Klein, D. F. (1983). Reply to panic attacks in phobia treatment studies. *Archives of General Psychiatry, 40,* 1151–1152.

Klein, D. F. (1993). False suffocation alarms, spontaneous panics, and related conditions: An integrative hypothesis. *Archives of General Psychaitry, 50,* 306–317.

Klein, D. F., & Fink, M. (1962). Psychiatric reaction patterns to imipramine. *American Journal of Psychiatry, 119,* 432–438.

Klein, D. F., & Klein, H. M. (1989). The substantive effect of variations in panic measurement and agoraphobia definition. *Journal of Anxiety Disorders, 3,* 45–56.

Klein, E., Cnaani, E., Harel, T., Braun, S., & Ben-Haim, S. A. (1995). Altered heart rate variablility in panic disorder patients. *Society of Biological Psychiatry, 37,* 18–24.

Klein, E., Zohar, J., Geraci, M. F., Murphy, D. L., & Uhde, T. W. (1991). Anxiogenic effects of m-CPP in patients with panic disorder: Comparison to caffeine's anxiogenic effects. *Biological Psychiatry, 30,* 973–974.

Kleinknecht, R. A. (1993). Rapid treatment of blood and injection phobias with eye movement desensitization. *Journal of Behavior Therapy and Experimental Psychopathology, 24,* 211–217.

Kleinknecht, R. A., Dinnel, D. L., Kleinknecht, E. E., Hiruma, N., & Harada, N. (1997). Cultural factors in social anxiety: A comparison of social phobia symptoms and *taijin kyofusho*. *Journal of Anxiety Disorders, 11*(2), 157–177.

Kleinknecht, R. A., Kleinknecht, E. E., & Thorndike, R. M. (1997). The role of disgust and fear in blood and injection-related fainting symptoms: A structural equation model. *Behaviour Research and Therapy, 35,* 1075–1087.

Kleinknecht, R. A., & Lenz, J. (1989). Blood/injury fear, fainting, and avoidance of medically related situations: A family correspondence study. *Behaviour Research and Therapy, 27,* 537–547.

Klerman, G. L. (1992). Drug treatment of panic disorder: Reply to comment by Marks and associates. *British Journal of Psychiatry, 161,* 465–471.

Klerman, G. L., Weissman, M., Ouellette, R., Johnson, J., & Greenwald, S. (1991). Panic attacks in the community: Social morbidity and health care utilization. *Journal of the American Medical Association, 265,* 742–746.

Klerman, G. L., Weissman, M. M., Rounsaville, B. J., & Chevron, E. (1984). *Interpersonal psychotherapy of depression.* New York: Basic Books.

Klieger, D. M., & Franklin, M. E. (1993). Validity of the Fear Survey Schedule in phobia research: A laboratory test. *Journal of Psychopathology and Behavioral Assessment, 15,* 207–217.

Klonoff, E. A., Polefrone, J. M., Dambrocia, J. P., & Nochomovitz, M. L. (1986). *Treatment of panic attacks associated with chronic obstructive pulmonary disease (COPD).* Paper presented at the 20th Annual Convention of the Association for Advancement of Behavior Therapy, Chicago.

Klosko, J. S., Barlow, D. H., Tassinari, R., & Cerny, J. A. (1990). A comparison of alprazolam and behavior therapy in treatment of panic disorder. *Journal of Consulting and Clinical Psychology, 58,* 77–84.

Knott, V., Bakish, D., Lusk, S., & Barkely, J. (1997). Relaxation-induced EEG alterations in panic disorder patients. *Journal of Anxiety Disorders, 11,* 365–376.

Ko, G. N., Elsworth, J. D., Roth, R. H., Rifkin, B. G., Leigh, H., & Redmond, E. (1983). Panic induced elevation of plasma MHPG levels in phobic–anxious patients: Effects of clonidine and imipramine. *Archives of General Psychiatry, 40,* 424–430.

Koenig, H. G., Ford, S. M., George, L. K., Blazer, D. G., & Meador, K. G. (1993). Religion and anxiety disorder: An examination and comparison of associations in young, middle-aged, and elderly adults. *Journal of Anxiety Disorders, 7,* 321–342.

Kolada, J., Bland, R., & Newman, S. (1994). Obsessive compulsive disorder. *Acta Psychiatrica Scandinavica, 89,* 24–35.

Kopin, I. (1984). Avenues of investigation for the role of catecholamines in anxiety. *Psychopathology, 17,* 83–97.

Korchin, S. (1964). Anxiety and cognition. In C. Scheerer (Ed.), *Cognition: Theory, research, and practice.* New York: Harper & Row.

Koretzky, M. B., & Peck, A. H. (1990). Validation and cross-validation of the PTSD subscale of the MMPI with civilian trauma victims. *Journal of Clinical Psychology, 46,* 296–300.

Koss, M. P., Gidycz, C. A., & Wisniewski, N. (1987). The scope of rape: Incidence and prevalence of sexual aggression and victimization in a national sample of higher education students. *Journal of Consulting and Clinical Psychology, 55,* 162–170.

Koss, M. P., Koss, P. G., & Woodruff, W. J. (1991). Deleterious effects of criminal victimization on women's health and medical utilization. *Archives of Internal Medicine, 151,* 342–347.

Koszycki, D., Zacharko, R. M., LeMelledo, J. M., & Bradwejn, J. (1998). Behavioral, cardiovascular, and neuroendocrine profiles following CCK-4 challenge in healthy volunteers: A comparison of panickers to non-panickers. *Depression and Anxiety, 8,* 1–7.

Kovacs, M., Gatsonis, C., Paulauskas, S. L., & Richards, C. (1989). Depressive disorders in childhood: IV. A longitudinal study of comorbidity with and risk for anxiety disorders. *Archives of General Psychiatry, 46,* 776–782.

Kozak, M. J., & Foa, E. B. (1994). Obsessions, overvalued ideas, and delusions in obsessive–compulsive disorder. *Behaviour Research and Therapy, 32,* 343–353.

Kozak, M. J., Foa, E. B., & McCarthy, P. (1987). Assessment of obsessive–compulsive disorder. In C. Last & M. Hersen (Eds.). *Handbook of anxiety disorders.* NY: Pergamon Press.

Kozak, M. J., Liebowitz, M., & Foa, E. B. (2000). Cognitive behavior therapy and pharmacotherapy for OCD: The NIMH-sponsored collaborative study. In W. K. Goodman, M. V. Rudorfer, & J. D. Maser (Eds.), *Obsessive–compulsive disorder: Contemporary issues in treatment.* Mahwah, NJ: Erlbaum.

Kozak, M. J., & Miller, G. A. (1985). The psychophysiological process of therapy in a case of injury-scene-elicited fainting. *Journal of Behavior Therapy and Experimental Psychiatry, 16,* 139–145.

Kozak, M. J., & Montgomery, G. K. (1981). Multimodal behavioral treatment of recurrent injury-scene elicited fainting (vasodepressor syncope). *Behavioural Psychotherapy, 9,* 316–321.

Kraemer, H. C. (1992). *Evaluating medical tests: Objective and quantitative guidelines.* Newbury Park, CA: Sage.

Kraemer, H. C., Kazdin, A. E., Offord, D. R., Kessler, R. C., Jensen, P. S., & Kupfer, D. J. (1997). Coming to terms with the terms of risk. *Archives of General Psychiatry, 54,* 337–343.

Kraepelin, E. (1896). *Psychiatrie: Vol. 5 Auflage.* Leipzig: Barth.

Krampen, G. (1982). Schulische and familiare Entwicklungsbedingungen von Kontrolluberzeugungen [School and familial conditions for developing control beliefs]. *Schweizerische Zeitschrift für Psychologie und ihre Andwendugen, 41,* 16–35.

Kring, A. M., & Bachorowski, J. (1999). Emotions and psychopathology. *Cognition and Emotion, 13*(5), 575–599.

Kruger, S., Cooke, R., Hasey, G., Jorna, T., & Persad, E. (1995). Comorbidity of obsessive compulsive disorder with bipolar disorder. *Journal of Affective Disorders, 34,* 117–120.

Kudler, H. S., Blank, A. S., & Krupnick, J. L. (2000). Psychodynamic therapy. In E. B. Foa, T. M. Keane, & M. J. Friedman (Eds.), *Effective treatments for PTSD: Practice guidelines from the International Society for Traumatic Stress Studies.* New York: Guilford Press.

Kulka, R. A., Schlenger, W. E., Fairbank, J. A., Hough, R. L., Jordan, B. K., Marmar, C. R., & Weiss, D. S. (1990). *Trauma and the Vietnam war generation: Report of findings from the National Vietnam Veterans Readjustment Study.* New York: Brunner/Mazel.

Kushner, M. G., Abrams, K., & Borchardt, C. (2000). The relationship between anxiety disorders and alcohol use disorders: A review of major perspectives and findings. *Clinical Psychology Review, 20*(2), 149–171.

Kushner, M. G., & Beitman, B. D. (1990). Panic attacks without fear: An overview. *Behavior Research and Therapy, 28,* 469–479.

Kushner, M. G., Beitman, B. D., & Bartels, K. M. (1990). *Panic attacks without fear: A report to the DSM-IV Task Force* (Report to the DSM-IV Anxiety Disorders Work Group). Columbia: University of Missouri–Columbia.

Kushner, M. G., Sher, K. J., & Beitman, B. D. (1990). The relation between alcohol problems and the anxiety disorders. *American Journal of Psychiatry, 147,* 685–695.

Kushner, M. G., Sher, K. J., & Erickson, D. J. (1999). Prospective analysis of the relation between DSM-III anxiety disorders and alcohol use disorders. *American Journal of Psychiatry, 156(5),* 723–732.

Labbate, L. A., Pollack, M. H., Otto, M. W., Langenauer, S., & Rosenbaum, J. F. (1994). Sleep panic attacks: An association with childhood anxiety and adult psychopathology. *Biological Psychiatry, 36,* 57–60.

Laberge, B., Gauthier, J. G., Côté, G., Plamondon, J., & Cormier, H. J. (1993). Cognitive-behavioral therapy of panic disorder with secondary major depression: A preliminary investigation. *Journal of Consulting and Clinical Psychology, 61,* 1028–1037.

Ladd, C. O., Huot, R. L., Thrivikraman, K. V., Nemeroff, C. B., Meaney, M. J., & Plotsky, P. M. (2000). Long-term behavioral and neuroendocrine adaptations to adverse early experience. In E. A. Meyer & C. B. Saper (Eds.), *Progress in brain research: Vol. 122. The biological basis for mind–body interactions.* Amsterdam: Elsevier.

Lader, M., & Olajide, D. (1987). A comparison of buspirone and placebo in relieving benzodiazepine withdrawal symptoms. *Journal of Clinical Psychopharmacology, 7,* 11–15.

Lader, M. H. (1967). Palmar skin conductance measures in anxiety and phobic states. *Journal of Psychosomatic Research, 11,* 271–281.

Lader, M. H. (1975). *The psychophysiology of mental illness.* London: Routledge & Kegan Paul.

Lader, M. H. (1980a). Psychophysiological studies in anxiety. In G. D. Burrows & D. Davies (Eds.), *Handbook of studies on anxiety.* Amsterdam: Elsevier/North-Holland.

Lader, M. H. (1980b). The psychophysiology of anxiety. In H. van Praag, M. H. Lader, O. Rafaelsen, & E. Sachar (Eds.), *Handbook of biological psychiatry.* New York: Marcel Dekker.

Lader, M. H. (1985). Benzodiazephines, anxiety, and catecholamines: A commentary. In A. H. Tuma & J. D. Maser (Eds.), *Anxiety and the anxiety disorders.* Hillsdale, NJ: Erlbaum.

Lader, M. H., & Mathews, A. (1970). Physiological changes during spontaneous panic attacks. *Journal of Psychosomatic Research, 14,* 377–382.

Lader, M. H., & Wing, L. (1964). Habituation of the psycho-galvanic reflex in patients with anxiety states and in normal subjects. *Journal of Neurology, Neurosurgery and Psychiatry, 27,* 210–218.

Lader, M. H., & Wing, L. (1966). *Physiological measures, sedative drugs, and morbid anxiety.* London: Oxford University Press.

Ladouceur, R., Blais, F., Freeston, M. H., & Dugas, M. J. (1998). Problem solving and problem orientation in generalized anxiety disorder. *Journal of Anxiety Disorders, 12(2),* 139–152.

Ladouceur, R., Dugas, M. J., Freeston, M. H., Léger, E., Gagnon, F., & Thibodeau, N. (2000). Efficacy of a new cognitive-behavioral treatment for generalized anxiety disorder: Evaluation in a controlled clinical trial. *Journal of Consulting and Clinical Psychology, 68,* 957–964.

Ladouceur, R., Dugas, M. J., Freeston, M. H., Rhéaume, J., Blais, F., Boisvert, J. M., Gagnon, F., & Thibodeau, N. (1999). Specificity of generalized anxiety disorder symptoms and processes. *Behavior Therapy, 30,* 191–207.

Ladouceur, R., Freeston, M. H., Rhéaume, J., Dugas, M. J., Gagnon, F., Thibodeau, N., & Fournier, S. (2000). Strategies used with intrusive thoughts: A comparison of OCD patients with anxious and community controls. *Journal of Abnormal Psychology, 109,* 179–187.

La Greca, A. M., Silverman, W. K., Vernberg, E. M., & Prinstein, M. J. (1996). Symptoms of post-traumatic stress in children after Hurricane Andrew: A prospective study. *Journal of Consulting and Clinical Psychology, 64,* 712–723.

Landy, F. J., & Gaupp, L. A. (1971). A factor analysis of the FSS-III. *Behaviour Research and Therapy, 9,* 89–93.

Lang, A. J., & Craske, M. G. (2000). Manipulations of exposure-based therapy to reduce return of fear: A replication. *Behaviour Research and Therapy, 38,* 1–12.

Lang, A. J., Craske, M. G., & Bjork, R. A. (1999). Implications of a new theory of disuse for the treatment of emotional disorders. *Clinical Psychology: Science and Practice, 6,* 80–94.

Lang, P. J. (1968). Fear reduction and fear behavior: Problems in treating a construct. In J. M. Shlien (Ed.), *Research in psychotherapy* (Vol. 3). Washington, DC: American Psychological Association.

Lang, P. J. (1977a). Imagery in therapy: An information processing analysis of fear. *Behavior Therapy, 8,* 862–886.

Lang, P. J. (1977b). Physiological assessment of anxiety and fear. In J. D. Cone & R. A. Hawkins (Eds.), *Behavioral assessment: New directions in clinical psychology.* New York: Brunner/Mazel.

Lang, P. J. (1978). Anxiety: Toward a psychophysiological definition. In H. S. Akiskal & W. L. Webb (Eds.), *Psychiatric diagnosis: Exploration of biological predictors.* New York: Spectrum.

Lang, P. J. (1979). A bio-informational theory of emotional imagery. *Psychophysiology, 16,* 495–512.

Lang, P. J. (1984). Cognition in emotion: Concept and action. In C. Izard, J. Kagan, & R. Zajonc (Eds.), *Emotion, cognition, and behavior.* New York: Cambridge University Press.

Lang, P. J. (1985). The cognitive psychophysiology of emotion: Fear and anxiety. In A. H. Tuma & J. D. Maser (Eds.), *Anxiety and the anxiety disorders.* Hillsdale, NJ: Erlbaum.

Lang, P. J. (1994a). The motivational organization of emotion: Affect–reflex connections. In S. H. M. Van Goozen, N. E. Van de Poll, & J. A. Sergeant (Eds.), *Emotions: Essays on emotion theory.* Hillsdale, NJ: Erlbaum.

Lang, P. J. (1994b). The varieties of emotional experience: A meditation on James–Lange theory. *Psychological Review, 101*(2), 211–221.

Lang, P. J. (1995). The emotion probe: Studies of motivation and attention. *American Psychologist, 50,* 372–385.

Lang, P. J., Bradley, M. M., & Cuthbert, B. N. (1990). Emotion, attention, and the startle reflex. *Psychological Review, 97,* 377–395.

Lang, P. J., Bradley, M. M., & Cuthbert, B. N. (1997). Motivated attention: Affect, activation, and action. In P. J. Lang & R. F. Simons (Eds.), *Attention and orienting: Sensory and motivational processes.* Mahwah, NJ: Erlbaum.

Lang, P. J., Bradley, M. M., & Cuthbert, B. N. (1998). Emotion, motivation, and anxiety: Brain mechanisms and psychophysiology. *Biological Psychiatry, 44,* 1248–1263.

Lang, P. J., Bradley, M. M., Fitzsimmons, J. R., Cuthbert, B. N., Scott, J. D., Moulder, B., & Nangia, V. (1998). Emotional arousal and activation of the visual cortex: An fMRI analysis. *Psychophysiology, 35,* 199–210.

Lang, P. J., Cuthbert, B. N., & Bradley, M. M. (1998). Measuring emotion in therapy: Imagery, activation, and feeling. *Behavior Therapy, 29,* 655–674.

Lang, P. J., Davis, M., & Öhman, A. (2000). Fear and anxiety: Animal models and human cognitive psychophysiology. *Journal of Affective Disorders, 61*(3), 137–159.

Lansky, D., & Wilson, G. T. (1981). Alcohol, expectations, and sexual arousal in males: An information processing analysis. *Journal of Abnormal Psychology, 90,* 35–45.

Last, C. G., Barlow, D. H., & O'Brien, G. T. (1984). Precipitants of agoraphobia: Role of stressful life events. *Psychological Reports, 54,* 567–570.

Latimer, L. (1977). Carbon dioxide as a reciprocal inhibitor in the treatment of neurosis. *Journal of Behavior Therapy and Experimental Psychiatry, 8,* 83–85.

Lavy, E., & van den Hout, M. (1993). Selective attention evidenced by pictorial and linguistic Stroop tasks. *Behavior Therapy, 24,* 645–657.

Lavy, E., van den Hout, M., & Arntz, A. (1993a). Attentional bias and spider phobia: Conceptual and clinical issues. *Behaviour Research and Therapy, 31,* 17–24.

Lavy, E., van den Hout, M., & Arntz, A. (1993b). Attentional bias and facilitated escape: A pictorial test. *Advances in Behaviour Research and Therapy, 15,* 279–289.

Lazarus, R. S. (1968). Emotions and adaptation: Conceptual and empirical relations. In W. J. Arnold (Ed.), *Nebraska Symposium on Motivation* (Vol. 16). Lincoln: University of Nebraska Press.

Lazarus, R. S. (1984). On the primacy of cognition. *American Psychologist, 39,* 124–129.

Lazarus, R. S. (1991). Progress on a cognitive–motivational–relational theory of emotion. *American Psychologist, 46,* 819–834.

Lazarus, R. S. (1995). Vexing research problems inherent in cognitive-mediational theories of emotion—and some solutions. *Psychological Inquiry, 6*, 183–196.

Lazarus, R. S., Averill, J. R., & Opton, E. M., Jr. (1970). Towards a cognitive theory of emotion. In M. Arnold (Ed.), *Feelings and emotion*. New York: Academic Press.

Leary, M. R. (1983a). A brief version of the Fear of Negative Evaluation Scale. *Personality and Social Psychology Bulletin, 9*, 371–375.

Leary, M. R. (1983b). Social anxiousness: The construct and its measurement. *Journal of Personality Assessment, 47*, 66–75.

Leary, M. R., Knight, P. D., & Johnson, K. A. (1987). Social anxiety and dyadic conversation: A verbal response analysis. *Journal of Social and Clinical Psychology, 5*, 34–50.

Leary, M. R., & Kowalski, R. M. (1995). *Social anxiety*. New York: Guilford Press.

Leary, T. F. (1957). *Interpersonal diagnosis of personality: A functional theory and methodology for personality evaluation*. New York: Ronald Press.

Leckman, J. F., & Chittenden, E. (1990). Gilles de la Tourette's syndrome and some forms of obsessive compulsive disorder may share a common genetic diathesis. *Encephale, 16*, 321–323.

Leckman, J. F., Grice, D. E., Boardman, J., Zhang, H., Vitale, A., Bondi, C., Alsobrook, J., Peterson, B. S., Cohen, D. J., Rasmussen, S. A., Goodman, W. K., McDougle, C. J., & Pauls, D. L. (1997). Symptoms of obsessive–compulsive disorder. *American Journal of Psychiatry, 154*, 911–917.

Leckman, J. F., Weissman, M. M., Merikangas, K. R., Pauls, D. L., & Prusoff, B. A. (1983). Panic disorder and major depression. *Archives of General Psychiatry, 40*, 1055–1060.

Lecrubier, Y., Bakker, A., Dunbar, G., & Judge, R., for the Collaborative Panic Study Investigators. (1997). A comparison of paroxetine, clomipramine, and placebo in the treatment of panic disorder. *Acta Psychiatrica Scandinavica, 95*, 145–152.

LeDoux, J. E. (1987). Emotion. In F. Plum (Ed.), *Handbook of physiology: Section I. The nervous system*. Bethesda, MD: American Physiological Society.

LeDoux, J. E. (1995). In search of an emotional system in the brain: Leaping from fear to emotion to consciousness. In M. S. Gazzaniga (Ed.), *The cognitive neurosciences* (pp. 1049–1062). Cambridge, MA: MIT Press.

LeDoux, J. E. (1996). *The emotional brain: The mysterious underpinnings of emotional life*. New York: Simon & Schuster.

LeDoux, J. E. (1998). Fear and the brain: Where have we been, and where are we going? *Biological Psychiatry, 44*, 1229–1238.

Lee, M. A., & Cameron, O. G. (1986). Anxiety, Type A behavior, and cardiovascular disease. *International Journal of Psychiatry in Medicine, 16*(2), 123–129.

Lee, M. A., Cameron, O. G., & Greden, J. F. (1985). Anxiety and caffeine consumption in people with anxiety disorders. *Psychiatry Research, 15*, 211–217.

Lehman, C. L., Brown, T. A., & Barlow, D. H. (1998). Effects of cognitive behavioral treatment for panic disorder with agoraphobia on concurrent alcohol abuse. *Behavior Therapy, 29*, 423–433.

Lehman, C. L., Hofmann, S. G., & Barlow, D. H. (1998, November). *Do individuals with a situational subtype of specific phobia show greater anxiety sensitivity?* Paper presented at the 32nd Annual Convention of the Association for Advancement of Behavior Therapy, Washington, DC.

Lehman, C. L., Patterson, M. D., Brown, T. A., & Barlow, D. H. (1998, November). *Lifetime alcohol use disorders in patients with anxiety or mood disorders*. Paper presented at the 32nd Annual Convention of the Association for Advancement of Behavior Therapy, Washington, DC.

Lehrer, P. M., & Woolfolk, R. L. (1993). Specific effects of stress management techniques. In P. M. Lehrer & R. L. Woolfolk (Eds.), *Principles and practice of stress management* (2nd ed.). New York: Guilford Press.

Leitenberg, H., Agras, W. S., Edwards, J. A., Thompson, L. E., & Wincze, J. P. (1970). Practice as a psychotherapeutic variable: An experimental analysis within single cases. *Journal of Psychiatric Research, 7*, 215–225.

Lelliott, P. T., Noshirvani, H. F., Başoğlu, M., Marks, I. M., & Monteiro, W. O. (1988). Obsessive–compulsive beliefs and treatment outcome. *Psychological Medicine, 18*, 697–702.

Lenze, E. J., Mulsant, B. H., Shear, M. K., Schulberg, H. C., Dew, M. A., Begley, A. E., Pollock, B. G., & Reynolds, C. F. (2000). Comorbid anxiety disorders in depressed elderly patients. *American Journal of Psychiatry, 157*, 722–728.

Leon, A. C., Portera, L., & Weissman, M. M. (1995). The social costs of anxiety disorders. *British Journal of Psychiatry, 166*(Suppl. 27), 19–22.

Lépine, J. P., & Pélissolo, A. (1999). Epidemiology, comorbidity and genetics of panic disorder. In D. J. Nutt, J. C. Ballenger, & J. P. Lepine (Eds.) *Panic disorder: Clinical diagnosis, management and mechanisms.* London: Martin Dunitz.

Lesch, K. P., Bengel, D., Heils, A., Sabol, S. Z., Greenberg, B. D., Petri, S., Benjamin, J., Muller, C. R., Hamer, D. H., & Murphy, D. L. (1996). Association of anxiety-related traits with a polymorphism in the serotonin transporter gene regulatory region. *Science, 274*, 1527–1531.

Lesser, I. M., Rubin, R. T., Pecknold, J. C., Rifkin, A., Swinson, R. P., Lydiard, R. B., Burrows, G. D., Noyes, R., & DuPont, R. L. (1988). Secondary depression in panic disorder and agoraphobia: I. Frequency, severity, and response to treatment. *Archives of General Psychiatry, 45*, 437–443.

Leung, A. W., & Heimberg, R. H. (1996). Homework compliance, perceptions of control, and outcome of cognitive-behavioral treatment of social phobia. *Behaviour Research and Therapy, 34*, 423–432.

Leventhal, H. (1991). Emotion: Prospects for conceptual and empirical development. In R. G. Lister & H. J. Weingartner (Eds.), *Perspectives on cognitive neuroscience.* New York: Oxford University Press.

Leventhal, H., Brown, D., Shachan, S., & Engquist, G. (1979). Effect of preparatory information about sensations, threat of pain and attention on cold pressor distress. *Journal of Personality and Social Psychology, 37*, 688–714.

Levin, A. P., Liebowitz, M. R., Fyer, A. J., Gorman, J. M., & Klein, D. F. (1984). Lactate induction of panic: Hypothesized mechanisms and recent findings. In J. C. Ballenger (Ed.), *Biology of agoraphobia.* Washington, DC: American Psychiatric Press.

Levin, A. P., Saoud, J. B., Strauman, T., Gorman, J. M., Fyer, A., Crawford, R., & Liebowitz, M. R. (1993). Responses of "generalized" and "discrete" social phobics during public speaking. *Journal of Anxiety Disorders, 7*, 207–221.

Levine, B. A., & Wolpe, J. (1980). In vivo desensitization of a severe driving phobia through radio contact. *Journal of Behavior Therapy and Experimental Psychiatry, 11*, 281–282.

Levine, S. (1960). Stimulation in infancy. *Scientific American, 202*, 80–86.

Levis, D. J. (1980). The learned helplessness effect: An expectancy, discrimination deficit, or motivational-induced persistence? *Journal of Research in Personality, 14*, 158–169.

Lewinsohn, P. M., Gotlib, I. H., & Seeley, J. R. (1995). Adolescent psychopathology: IV. Specificity of psychosocial risk factors for depression and substance abuse in older adolescents. *Journal of the American Academy of Child and Adolescent Psychiatry, 34*(9), 1221–1229.

Lewinsohn, P. M., Gotlib, I. H., Lewinsohn, M., Seeley, J. R., & Allen, N. B. (1998). Gender differences in anxiety disorders and anxiety symptoms in adolescents. *Journal of Abnormal Psychology, 107*(1), 109–117.

Lewis, A. (1936). Problems of obsessional illness. *Proceedings of the Royal Society of Medicine, 29*, 325–336.

Lewis, A. (1966). Obsessional disorder. In R. Scott (Ed.), *Price's textbook of the practice of medicine* (10th ed.). London: Oxford University Press.

Lewis, A. (1980). Problems presented by the ambiguous word "anxiety" as used in psychopathology. In G. D. Burrows & B. Davies (Eds.), *Handbook of studies on anxiety.* Amsterdam: Elsevier/North-Holland.

Lewis, M. (1993). The emergence of human emotions. In M. Lewis & J. M. Haviland (Eds.), *Handbook of emotions.* New York: Guilford Press.

Lewis, T. (1917). *Medical research committee: Report upon soldiers returned as cases of "disordered action of the heart" (D. A. H.) or "valvular disease of the heart" (V. D. H.)*. London: His Majesty's Stationery Office.

Lewis, T. (1932). Vasovagal syncope and the carotid sinus mechanism. *British Medical Journal, i,* 873–876.

Ley, R. (1985). Blood, breath, and fears: A hyperventilation theory of panic attacks and agoraphobia. *Clinical Psychology Review, 5,* 271–285.

Ley, R. (1988). Panic attacks during sleep: A hyperventilation-probability model. *Journal of Behavior Therapy and Experimental Psychiatry, 19,* 181–192.

Ley, R. (1992). The many faces of Pan: Psychological and physiological differences among three types of panic attacks. *Behaviour Research and Therapy, 30,* 347–357.

Ley, R., & Walker, H. (1973). Effects of carbon dioxide–oxygen inhalation on heart rate, blood pressure, and subjective anxiety. *Journal of Behavior Therapy and Experimental Psychiatry, 4,* 223–228.

Liddell, A., Locker, D., & Burman, D. (1991). Self-reported fears (FSS-II) of subjects aged 50 years and over. *Behaviour Research and Therapy, 29,* 105–112.

Liddell, H. S. (1949). The role of vigilance in the development of animal neurosis. In P. Hoch & I. Zubin (Eds.), *Anxiety.* New York: Grune & Stratton.

Lidren, D. M., Watkins, P. L., Gould, R. A., Clum, G. A., Asterino, M., & Tullach, H. L. (1994). A comparison of bibliotherapy and group therapy in the treatment of panic disorder. *Journal of Consulting and Clinical Psychology, 62,* 865–869.

Liebowitz, M. R. (1987). Social phobia. *Modern Problems in Pharmacopsychiatry, 22,* 141–173.

Liebowitz, M. R., Fyer, A. J., Gorman, J. M., Dillon, D., Appleby, I. L., Levy, G., Anderson, S., Levitt, M., Palij, M., Davies, S. O., & Klein, D. F. (1984). Lactate provocation of panic. *Archives of General Psychiatry, 41,* 764–770.

Liebowitz, M. R., Gorman, J. M., Fyer, A. J., Campeas, R., Levin, A., Davies, S., & Klein, D. F. (1985). Psychopharmacological treatment of social phobia. *Psychopharmacological Bulletin, 21,* 610–614.

Liebowitz, M. R., Gorman, J. M., Fyer, A. J., Campeas, R., Levin, A., Davies, S., & Klein, D. F. (1988). Pharmacotherapy of social phobia: An interim report of a placebo-controlled comparison of phenelzine versus atenolol. *Journal of Clinical Psychiatry, 49,* 242–257.

Liebowitz, M. R., Gorman, J. M., Fyer, A. J., & Klein, D. F. (1985). Social phobia: Review of a neglected anxiety disorder. *Archives of General Psychiatry, 42,* 729–736.

Liebowitz, M. R., Gorman, J. M., Fyer, A. J., Levitt, M., Dillon, D., Levy, P., Appleby, I. L., Anderson, S., Palij, M., Davies, S. O., & Klein, D. F. (1984). Lactate provocation of panic attacks: II. Biochemical and physiological findings. *Archives of General Psychiatry, 42,* 709–719.

Liebowitz, M. R., Heimberg, R. G., Fresco, D. M., Travers, J., & Stein, M. B. (2000). Social phobia or social anxiety disorder: What's in the name? [Letter to the editor]. *Archives of General Psychiatry, 57,* 191–192.

Liebowitz, M. R., Heimberg, R. G., Schneier, F. R., Hope, D. A., Davies, S., Holt, C. S., Goetz, D., Juster, H. R., Lin, S., Bruch, M., Marshall, R. D., & Klein, D. F. (1999). Cognitive-behavioral group therapy versus phenelzine in social phobia: Long-term outcome. *Depression and Anxiety, 10,* 89–98.

Liebowitz, M. R., & Klein, D. F. (1979). Clinical psychiatric conferences: Assessment and treatment of phobic anxiety. *Journal of Clinical Psychology, 40,* 486–492.

Liebowitz, M. R., Salman, E., Jusino, C. M., Garfinkel, R., Street, L., Cardenas, D. L., Silvestre, J., Fyer, A. J., Carrasco, J. L., Davies, S., Guarnaccia, P., & Klein, D. F. (1994). *Ataque de nervios* and panic disorder. *American Journal of Psychiatry, 151*(6), 871–875.

Liebowitz, M. R., Schneier, F., Campeas, R., Hollander, E., Hatterer, J., Fyer, A., Gorman, J., Papp, L., Davies, S., Gully, R., & Klein, D. F. (1992). Phenelzine vs. atenolol in social phobia: A placebo-controlled comparison. *Archives of General Psychiatry, 49,* 290–300.

Líndal, E., & Stefánsson, J. G. (1993). The lifetime prevalence of anxiety disorders in Iceland as estimated by the US National Institute of Mental Health Diagnostic Interview Schedule. *Acta Psychiatrica Scandinavica, 88,* 29–34.

Lindemann, E., & Finesinger, I. E. (1938). The effect of adrenaline and mecholyl in states of anxiety in psychoneurotic patients. *American Journal of Psychiatry, 95,* 353–370.

Lindesay, J. (1991). Phobic disorders in the elderly. *British Journal of Psychiatry, 159,* 531–541.

Lindsay, S. J. E., Wege, P., & Yates, J. (1984). Expectations of sensations, discomfort, and fear in dental treatment. *Behaviour Research and Therapy, 22,* 99–108.

Lindsley, O. B. (1951). Emotion. In S. S. Stevens (Ed.), *Handbook of experimental psychology.* New York: Wiley.

Linehan, M. M. (1993a). *Cognitive-behavioral treatment of borderline personality disorder.* New York: Guilford Press.

Linehan, M. M. (1993b). *Skills training manual for treating borderline personality disorder.* New York: Guilford Press.

Linko, E. (1950). Lactate acid response to muscular exercise in neurocirculatory asthenia. *Annales Medicinae Internae Fenniae, 39,* 161–176.

Lint, D. W., Taylor, C. B., Fried-Behar, L., & Kenardy, J. (1995). Does ischemia occur with panic attacks? *American Journal of Psychiatry, 152,* 1678–1680.

Lipsitz, J. D., Mannuzza, S., Klein, D. F., Ross, D. C., & Fyer, A. J. (1999). Specific phobia 10–16 years after treatment. *Depression and Anxiety, 10,* 105–111.

Lipsitz, J. D., Martin, L. Y., Mannuzza, S., Chapman, T. F., Liebowitz, M. R., Klein, D. F., & Fryer, A. J. (1994). Childhood separation anxiety disorder in patients with adult anxiety disorders. *American Journal of Psychiatry, 151*(6), 927–929.

Litz, B. T. (1992). Emotional numbing in combat-related post-traumatic stress disorder: A clinical review and reformulation. *Clinical Psychology Review, 12,* 417–432.

Litz, B. T., & Keane, T. M. (1989). Information processing in anxiety disorders: Application to the understanding of post-traumatic stress disorder. *Clinical Psychology Review, 9,* 243–257.

Litz, B. T., Orsillo, S. M., Friedman, M., Ehlich, P., & Batres, A. (1997). Posttraumatic stress disorder associated with peacekeeping duty in Somalia for U. S. military personnel. *American Journal of Psychiatry, 154,* 178–184.

Litz, B. T., Orsillo, S. M., Kaloupek, D., & Weathers, F. (2000). Emotional processing in posttraumatic stress disorder. *Journal of Abnormal Psychology, 109,* 26–39.

Litz, B. T., & Weathers, F. W. (1994). The diagnoses and assessment of post-traumatic stress disorder in adults. In M. B. Williams & J. F. Sommer (Eds.). *The handbook of posttraumatic therapy.* Westport, CT: Greenwood Press.

Livesley, W. J., Schroeder, M. L., Jackson, D. N., & Jang, K. L. (1994). Categorical distinctions in the study of personality disorder: Implications for classification. *Journal of Abnormal Psychology, 103,* 6–17.

Logue, M. B., Thomas, A. M., Barbee, J. G., Hoehn-Saric, R., Maddock, R. J., Schwab, J., Smith, R. D., Sullivan, M., & Beitman, B. D. (1993). Generalized anxiety disorder patients seek evaluation for cardiological symptoms at the same frequency as patients with panic disorder. *Journal of Psychiatric Research, 27,* 55–59.

Lohr, J. M., Kleinknecht, R. A., Tolin, D. F., & Barrett, R. H. (1995). The empirical status of the clinical application of eye movement desensitization and reprocessing. *Journal of Behavior Therapy and Experimental Psychiatry, 26,* 285–302.

Lohr, J. M., Lilienfeld, S. O., Tolin, D. F., & Herbert, J. D. (1999). Eye movement desensitization and reprocessing: An analysis of specific versus non-specific treatment factors. *Journal of Anxiety Disorders, 13,* 185–207.

Lohr, J. M., Tolin, D. F., & Kleinknecht, R. A. (1995). Eye movement desensitization of medical phobias: Two case studies. *Journal of Behavior Therapy and Experimental Psychiatry, 26,* 141–151.

Lohr, J. M., Tolin, D. F., & Kleinknecht, R. A. (1996). An intensive design investigation of eye movement desensitization and reprocessing of claustrophobia. *Journal of Anxiety Disorders, 10,* 73–88.

Lohr, J. M., Tolin, D. F., & Lilienfeld, S. O. (1998). Efficacy of eye movement desensitization and reprocessing: Implications for behavior therapy. *Behavior Therapy, 29,* 123–156.

Lopatka, C. L. (1989). *The role of unexpected events in avoidance.* Unpublished master's thesis, State University of New York at Albany.

Louie, A. K., Lannon, R. A., & Ketter, T. A. (1989). Treatment of cocaine-induced panic disorder. *American Journal of Psychiatry, 146,* 40–44.

Louie, A. K., Lannon, R. A., Rutzick, E. A., Browne, D., Lewis, T. B., & Jones, R. (1996). Clinical features of cocaine-induced panic. *Society of Biological Psychiatry, 40,* 938–940.

Lovibond, P. F. (1993). Conditioning and cognitive-behaviour therapy. *Behaviour Change, 10,* 119–130.

Lovibond, S. H., & Lovibond, P. F. (1995). *Manual for the Depression Anxiety Stress Scales.* Sydney: Psychology Foundation of Australia.

Lucey, J., Bucher, G., Clare, A., & Dinan, T. (1994). The clinical characteristics of patients with obsessive compulsive disorder: A descriptive study of an Irish sample. *Irish Journal of Psychiatry, 11,* 11–14.

Lucki, I., Rickels, K., & Geller, A. M. (1986). Chronic use of benzodiazepines and psychomotor and cognitive test performance. *Psychopharmacology, 88,* 426–433.

Lum, L. C. (1975). Hyperventilation: The tip of the iceberg. *Journal of Psychosomatic Research, 19,* 375–383.

Lum, L. C. (1976). The syndrome of habitual chronic hyperventilation. In O. W. Hill (Ed.), *Modern trends in psychosomatic medicine* (Vol. 3). London: Butterworths.

Lundh, L.-G., & Öst, L.-G. (1996). Recognition bias for critical faces in social phobics. *Behaviour Research and Therapy, 34,* 787–794.

Luten, A., Ralph, J. A., & Mineka, S. (1997). Pessimistic attributional style: Is it specific to depression versus anxiety versus negative affect? *Behaviour Research and Therapy, 35*(8), 703–719.

Lydiard, R. B., Ballenger, J. C., & Rickels, K. (1997). A double-blind evaluation of the safety and efficacy of abecarnil, alprazolam, and placebo in outpatients with generalized anxiety disorder. *Journal of Clinical Psychiatry, 58*(Suppl. 11), 11–18.

Lydiard, R. B., Fossey, M. D., Marsh, W., & Ballenger, J. C. (1993). Prevalence of psychiatric disorders in patients with irritable bowel syndrome. *Psychosomatics, 34,* 229–234.

Lydiard, R. B., Lesser, I. M., Ballenger, J. C., Rubin, R. T., Laraia, M. T., & DuPont, R. (1992). A fixed-dose study of alprazolam 2 mg, alprazolam 6 mg, and placebo in panic disorder. *Journal of Clinical Psychopharmacology, 12,* 96–103.

Lydiard, R. B., Morton, W. A., Emmanuel, N. P., Zealberg, J. J., Laraia, M. T., Stuart, G. W., O'Neil, P. M., & Ballenger, J. C. (1993). Preliminary report: Placebo-controlled, double-blind study of the clinical and metabolic effects of desipramine in panic disorder. *Psychopharmacology Bulletin, 29,* 183–188.

Lydiard, R. B., Pollack, M. H., Judge, R., Michelson, D., & Tamura, R. (1997, September). *Fluoxetine in panic disorder: A placebo-controlled study.* Paper presented at the 10th Annual Convention of the European College of Neuropsychopharmacology, Vienna.

Lyonfields, J. D., Borkovec, T. D., & Thayer, J. F. (1995). Vagal tone in generalized anxiety disorder and the effects of aversive imagery and aversive thinking. *Behavior Therapy, 26,* 457–460.

Lyons, J. A., & Keane, T. M. (1992). Keane PTSD Scale: MMPI and MMPI-2 update. *Journal of Traumatic Stress, 5,* 111–117.

MacDonald, P. A., Antony, M., MacLeod, C. M., & Richter, M. A. (1997). Memory and confidence in memory judgments among individuals with obsessive compulsive disorder and nonclinical controls. *Behaviour Research and Therapy, 35,* 497–505.

Mackintosh, N. J. (1975). A theory of attention: Variations in the associability of stimuli with reinforcement. *Psychological Review, 82,* 276–298.

MacLean, P. D. (1963). Phylogenesis. In P. H. Knapp (Ed.), *Expression of the emotions in man.* New York: International Universities Press.

MacLeod, A. K., Williams, J. M. G., & Bekerian, D. A. (1991). Worry is reasonable: The role of explanations in pessimism about future personal events. *Journal of Abnormal Psychology, 100,* 478–486.

MacLeod, C. (1991). Clinical anxiety and the selective encoding of threatening information. *International Review of Psychiatry, 3,* 279–292.

MacLeod, C., Mathews, A., & Tata, P. (1986). Attentional bias in emotional disorders. *Journal of Abnormal Psychology, 95,* 15–20.

MacLeod, C., & McLaughlin, K. (1995). Implicit and explicit memory bias in anxiety: A Conceptual replication. *Behaviour Research and Therapy, 33*(1), 1–14.

Magee, W. J., Eaton, W. W., Wittchen, H.-U., McGonagle, K. A., & Kessler, R. C. (1996). Agoraphobia, simple phobia, and social phobia in the National Comorbidity Survey. *Archives of General Psychiatry, 53,* 159–168.

Mahe, V., & Balogh, A. (2000). Long-term pharmacological treatment of generalized anxiety disorder. *International Clinical Psychopharmacology, 15,* 99–105.

Mahgoub, O. M., & Abdel-Hafeiz, H. B. (1991). Pattern of obsessive–compulsive disorder in eastern Saudi Arabia. *British Journal of Psychiatry, 158,* 840–842.

Mahone, E. M., Bruch, M. A., & Heimberg, R. G. (1993). Focus of attention and social anxiety: The role of negative self-thoughts and perceived positive attributes of the other. *Cognitive Therapy and Research, 17,* 209–224.

Maidenberg, E., Chen, E., Craske, M., Bohn, P., & Bystritsky, A. (1996). Specificity of attentional bias in panic disorder and social phobia. *Journal of Anxiety Disorders, 10,* 529–541.

Maier, S. F., & Seligman, M. E. P. (1976). Learned helplessness: Theory and evidence. *Journal of Comparative and Physiological Psychology, 88,* 554–564.

Maier, W., Buller, R., Philipp, M., & Heuser, I. (1988). The Hamilton Anxiety Scale: Reliability, validity and sensitivity to change in anxiety and depressive disorders. *Journal of Affective Disorders, 14,* 61–68.

Maier, W., Lichtermann, D., Minges, J., Örlein, A., & Franke, P. (1993). A controlled family study in panic disorder. *Journal of Psychiatric Research, 27*(Suppl. 1), 79–87.

Malloy, P. F., Fairbank, J. A., & Keane, T. M. (1983). Validation of a multimethod assessment of posttraumatic stress disorders in Vietnam veterans. *Journal of Consulting and Clinical Psychology, 51,* 488–494.

Malmo, R. B., Shagass, C., David, I. F., Cleghorn, R. A., Graham, B. F., & Goodman, A. I. (1948). Standardized pain stimulation as controlled stress in physiological studies of psychoneurosis. *Science, 108,* 509–511.

Malmo, R. B., Shagass, C., & Heslam, R. M. (1951). Blood pressure response to repeated brief stress in psychoneurosis: A study of adaptation. *Canadian Journal of Psychology, 5,* 167–179.

Mancini, C., van Ameringen, M., Szatmari, P., Fugere, C., & Boyle, M. (1996). A high-risk pilot study of the children of adults with social phobia. *Journal of the American Academy of Child and Adolescent Psychiatry, 35,* 1511–1517.

Mandler, G. (1966). Anxiety. In D. L. Sills (Ed.), *International encyclopedia of the social sciences.* New York: Macmillan.

Mandler, G. (1975). *Mind and emotion.* New York: Wiley.

Mandler, G. (1984). *Mind and body: Psychology of emotion and stress.* New York: Norton.

Manfredi, R. L., Kales, A., Vgontzas, A. N., Bixler, E. O., Isaac, M. A., & Falcone, C. M. (1991). Buspirone: Sedative or stimulant effect? *American Journal of Psychiatry, 148,* 1213–1217.

Mannion, N. E., & Levine, B. A. (1984). Effects of stimulus representation and cue category level on exposure (flooding) therapy. *British Journal of Clinical Psychology, 23,* 1–7.

Mannuzza, S., Aronowitz, B., Chapman, T., Klein, D. F., & Fyer, A. J. (1992). Panic disorder and suicide attempts. *Journal of Anxiety Disorders, 6,* 261–274.

Mannuzza, S., Fyer, A. J., Martin, L. Y., Gallops, M. S., Endicott, J., Gorman, J. M., Liebowitz, M. R., & Klein, D. F., (1989). Reliability of anxiety assessment: I. Diagnostic agreement. *Archives of General Psychiatry, 46,* 1093–1101.

Mannuzza, S., Schneier, F. R., Chapman, T. F., Liebowitz, M. R., Klein, D. F., & Fyer, A. J. (1995). Generalized social phobia: Reliability and validity. *Archives of General Psychiatry, 52,* 230–237.

Maple, S., Bradshaw, C. M., & Szabadi, E. (1981). Pharmacological responsiveness of sweat glands in anxious patients and healthy volunteers. *British Journal of Psychiatry, 141,* 154–161.

Marchand, A., Goyer, L. R., Dupuis, G., & Mainguy, N. (1998). Personality disorders and the outcome of cognitive-behavioural treatment of panic disorder with agoraphobia. *Canadian Journal of Behavioural Science, 30,* 14–23.

Marcus, S. V., Marquis, P., & Sakai, C. (1997). Controlled study of treatment of PTSD using EMDR in an HMO setting. *Psychotherapy: Theory, Research, Practice, Training, 34,* 307–315.

Marcus, S. V, Olfson, M., Pincus, H., Shear, M., & Zarin, D. (1997). Self-reported anxiety, general medical conditions, and disability bed days. *American Journal of Psychiatry, 154,* 1766–1768.

Margraf, I., Taylor, C. B., Ehlers, A., Roth, W. T., & Agras, W. S. (1987). Panic attacks in the natural environment. *Journal of Nervous and Mental Disease, 175,* 558–565.

Margraf, J., & Schneider, S. (1991, November). *Outcome and active ingredients of cognitive-behavioral treatments for panic disorder.* Paper presented at the annual meeting of the Association for Advancement of Behavior Therapy, New York.

Markowitz, J. S., Weissman, M. M., Ouellette, R., Lish, J. D., & Klerman, G. L. (1989). Quality of life in panic disorder. *Archives of General Psychiatry, 46,* 984–992.

Marks, I. M. (1969). *Fears and phobias.* London: Heinemann.

Marks, I. M. (1970). The classification of phobic disorders. *British Journal of Psychiatry, 116,* 377–386.

Marks, I. M. (1971). Phobic disorders four years after treatment: A prospective follow-up. *British Journal of Psychiatry, 129,* 362–371.

Marks, I. M. (1978). *Living with fear.* New York: McGraw-Hill.

Marks, I. M. (1981). *Cure and care of neurosis: Theory and practice of behavioral psychotherapy.* New York: Wiley.

Marks, I. M. (1986). Genetics of fear and anxiety disorders. *British Journal of Psychiatry, 149,* 406–418.

Marks, I. M. (1987). *Fears, phobias, and rituals: Panic, anxiety, and their disorders.* New York: Oxford University Press.

Marks, I. M., Bird, J., & Lindley, P. (1978). Behavioural nurse therapists 1978—developments and implications. *Behavioural Psychotherapy, 6,* 25–36.

Marks, I. M., Birley, J. L. T., & Gelder, M. G. (1966). Modified leucotomy in severe agorophobia: A controlled serial inquiry. *British Journal of Psychiatry, 112,* 757–769.

Marks, I. M., Crowe, E., Drewe, E., Young, J., & Dewhurst, W. G. (1969). Obsessive–compulsive neurosis in identical twins. *British Journal of Psychiatry, 15,* 991–998.

Marks, I. M., & Gelder, M. G. (1966). Different ages of onset in varieties of phobia. *American Journal of Psychiatry, 123,* 218–221.

Marks, I. M., Grey, S., Cohen, S. D., Hill, R., Mawson, D., Ramm, E. M., & Stern, R. S. (1983). Imipramine and brief therapist-aided exposure in agoraphobics having self-exposure homework: A controlled trial. *Archives of General Psychiatry, 40,* 153–162.

Marks, I. M., & Lader, M. (1973). Anxiety states (anxiety neurosis): A review. *Journal of Nervous and Mental Disease, 156,* 3–18.

Marks, I. M., Lelliott, P., Basoglu, M., Noshirvani, H., Monteiro, W., Cohen, D., & Kasvikis, Y. (1988). Clomipramine, self exposure and therapist-aided exposure for obsessive compulsive rituals. *British Journal of Psychiatry, 152,* 522–534.

Marks, I. M., Lovell, K., Noshirvani, H., Livanou, M., & Thrasher, S. (1998). Treatment of post-traumatic stress disorder by exposure and/or cognitive restructuring: A controlled study. *Archives of General Psychiatry, 55,* 317–325.

Marks, I. M., & Mathews, A. M. (1979). Brief standard self-rating for phobic patients. *Behaviour Research and Therapy, 17,* 263–267.

Marks, I. M., Stern, R. S., Mawson, D., Cobb, J., & McDonald, R. (1980). Clomipramine and exposure for obsessive compulsive rituals. *British Journal of Psychiatry, 136,* 1–25.

Marks, I. M., Swinsan, R. P., Basaglu, M., Kuch, K., Nashirvani, H., O'Sullivan, G., Lelliott, P. T., Kirby, M., McNamee, G., Sengun, S., & Wickwire, K. (1993). Alprazolam and exposure alone and combined in panic disorder with agoraphobia: A controlled study in London and Toronto. *British Journal of Psychiatry, 162,* 776–787.

Marshall, G. (1976). *The affective consequences of "inadequately explained" physiological arousal.* Unpublished doctoral dissertation, Stanford University.

Marshall, G., & Zimbardo, P. G. (1979). Affective consequences of inadequately explained physiological arousal. *Journal of Personality and Social Psychology, 37,* 970–998.

Marshall, J. R. (1994). *Social phobia: From shyness to stage fright.* New York: Basic Books.

Marshall, W. L. (1985). The effects of variable exposure in flooding therapy. *Behavior Therapy, 16,* 117–135.

Marshall, W. L., Bristol, D., & Barbaree, H. E. (1992). Cognitions and courage in the avoidance behavior of acrophobics. *Behaviour Research and Therapy, 30,* 463–470.

Marsland, D. W., Wood, M., & Mayo, F. (1976). Content of family practice: A data bank for patient care, curriculum, and research in family practice—526,196 patient problems. *Journal of Family Practice, 3,* 25–68.

Marten, P. A., & Barlow, D. H. (1991, November). *Differences in dimensions of fantasy between sexually functional and dysfunctional males: Preliminary results and treatment implications.* Poster presented at the 25th Annual Convention of the Association for Advancement of Behavior Therapy, New York.

Marten, P. A., & Barlow, D. H. (1993). Implications of clinical research for psychotherapy integration in the treatment of anxiety disorders. *Journal of Psychotherapy Integration, 3,* 297–311.

Marten, P. A., Brown, T. A., Barlow, D. H., Borkovec, T. D., Shear, M. K., & Lydiard, R. B. (1993). Evaluation of the ratings comprising the associated symptom criterion of DSM-III-R generalized anxiety disorder. *Journal of Nervous and Mental Disease, 181,* 676–682.

Martin, I. (1983). Human classical conditioning. In A. Gale and J. Edward (Eds.), *Physiological correlates of human behavior: Vol. 2. Attention and performance.* London: Academic Press.

Martin, I., & Levey, A. B. (1985). Conditoning, evaluations, and cognitions: An axis of integration. *Behaviour Research and Therapy, 23,* 167–175.

Martin, N. G., Jardine, R., Andrews, G., & Heath, A. C. (1988). Anxiety disorders and neuroticism: Are there genetic factors specific to panic? *Acta Psychiatrica Scandinavica, 77,* 698–706.

Martinsen, E. W., Raglin, J. S., Hoffart, A., & Friis, S. (1998). Tolerance to intensive exercise and high levels of lactate in panic disorder. *Journal of Anxiety Disorders, 12,* 333–342.

Maser, J. D. (1985). List of phobias. In A. H. Tuma & J. D. Maser (Eds.), *Anxiety and the anxiety disorders.* Hillsdale, NJ: Erlbaum.

Maser, J. D., & Gallup, G. G. (1974). Tonic immobility in the chicken: Catalepsy potentiation by uncontrollable shock and alleviation by imipramine. *Psychosomatic Medicine, 36,* 199–205.

Masia, C. L., & Morris, T. L. (1998). Parental factors associated with social anxiety: Methodological limitations and suggestions for integrated behavioral research. *Clinical Psychology: Science and Practice, 5,* 211–228.

Maslach, C. (1979a). The emotional consequences of arousal without reason. In C. E. Izard (Ed.), *Emotions in personality and psychopathology.* New York: Plenum Press.

Maslach, C. (1979b). Negative emotional biasing of unexplained emotional arousal. *Journal of Personality and Social Psychology, 37,* 953–969.

Massion, A., Warshaw, M., & Keller, M. (1993). Quality of life and psychiatric morbidity in panic disorder versus generalized anxiety disorder. *American Journal of Psychiatry, 150,* 600–607.

Masten, A. S., Best, K. M., & Garmezy, N. (1991). Resilience and development: Contributions from the study of children who overcome adversity. *Development and Psychopathology, 2,* 425–444.

Masters, W. H., & Johnson, V. E. (1970). *Human sexual inadequacy.* Boston: Little, Brown.

Mataix-Cols, D., Rauch, S. L., Manzo, P. A., Jenike, M. A., & Baer, L. (1999). Use of factor-analyzed symptom dimensions to predict outcome with serotonin reuptake inhibitors and placebo in the treatment of obsessive–compulsive disorders. *American Journal of Psychiatry, 156,* 1409–1416.

Mathew, R. J., Ho, B. T., Francis, D. J., Taylor, D. L., & Weinman, M. L. (1982). Catecholamines and anxiety. *Acta Psychiatrica Scandinavica, 65,* 142–147.

Mathew, R. J., Ho, B. T., Kralik, P., Taylor, D. L., & Claghorn, J. L. (1981). Catecholamines and monoamine oxidase activity in anxiety. *Acta Psychiatrica Scandinavica, 63,* 245–252.

Mathews, A. M. (1978). Fear-reduction research and clinical phobias. *Psychological Bulletin, 85,* 390–404.

Mathews, A. M. (1990). Why worry?: The cognitive function of anxiety. *Behaviour Research and Therapy, 28,* 455–468.

Mathews, A. (1997). Information processing biases in emotional disorders. In D. M. Clark & C. G. Fairburn (Eds.), *Science and practice of cognitve-behavior therapy.* Oxford: Oxford University Press.

Mathews, A. M., Gelder, M. G., & Johnston, D. W. (1981). *Agoraphobia: Nature and treatment.* New York: Guilford Press.

Mathews, A. M., & MacLeod, C. (1985). Selective processing of threat cues in anxiety states. *Behaviour Research and Therapy, 23,* 563–569.

Mathews, A. M., & MacLeod, C. (1986). Discrimination of threat cues without awareness in anxiety states. *Journal of Abnormal Psychology, 95,* 131–138.

Mathews, A. M., & MacLeod, C. (1994). Cognitive approaches to emotion and emotional disorders. *Annual Review of Psychology, 45,* 25–50.

Mathews, A. M., Mogg, K., Kentish, J., & Eysenck, M. (1995). Effect of psychological treatment on cognitive bias in generalized anxiety disorder. *Behaviour Research and Therapy, 33,* 293–303.

Mathews, A. M., Mogg, K., May, J., & Eysenck, M. (1989). Implicit and explicit memory bias in anxiety. *Journal of Abnormal Psychology, 98,* 236–240.

Mathews, A. M., Richards, A., & Eysenck, M. (1989). Interpretation of homophones related to threat in anxiety states. *Journal of Abnormal Psychology, 98,* 31–34.

Mathews, A. M., Teasdale, J., Munby, M., Johnston, D., & Shaw, P. (1977). A home-based treatment program for agoraphobia. *Behavior Therapy, 8,* 915–924.

Mathias, S., Fifer, S., Mazonson, P., Lubeck, D., Buesching, D., & Patrick, D. (1994). Necessary but not sufficient: The effect of screening and feedback on outcomes of primary care patients with untreated anxiety. *Journal of General Internal Medicine, 9,* 606–615.

Mattia, J. I., Heimberg, R. G., & Hope, D. A. (1993). The revised Stroop color-naming task in social phobics. *Behaviour Research and Therapy, 31*(3), 305–313.

Mattick, R. P., & Clarke, J. C. (1998). Development and validation of measures of social phobia scrutiny fear and social interaction anxiety. *Behaviour Research and Therapy, 36,* 455–470.

Mattick, R. P., & Peters, L. (1988). Treatment of severe social phobia: Effects of guided exposure with and without cognitive restructuring. *Journal of Consulting and Clinical Psychology, 56,* 251–260.

Mattila, M. J., Aranko, K., & Seppala, T. (1982). Acute effects of buspirone and alcohol on psychomotor skills. *Journal of Clinical Psychiatry, 43*(Suppl. 12), 56–60.

Mavissakalian, M. R. (1993). Combined behavioral therapy and pharmacotherapy of agoraphobia. *Journal of Psychiatric Research, 27,* 179–191.

Mavissakalian, M. R. (1996a). Antidepressant medications for panic disorder. In M. R. Mavissakalian & R. F. Prien (Eds.), *Long-term treatments of anxiety disorders.* Washington, DC: American Psychiatric Press.

Mavissakalian, M. R. (1996b). Phenomenology of panic attacks: Responsiveness of individual symptoms to imipramine. *Journal of Clinical Psychopharmacology, 16,* 233–237.

Mavissakalian, M. R., & Barlow, D. H. (Eds.). (1981). *Phobia: Psychological and pharmacological treatment.* New York: Guilford Press.

Mavissakalian, M. R., & Hamann, M. S. (1986). DSM-III personality disorder in agoraphobia. *Comprehensive Psychiatry, 27,* 471–479.

Mavissakalian, M. R., & Hamann, M. S. (1987). DSM-III personality disorder in agoraphobia: II. Changes with treatment. *Comprehensive Psychiatry, 28,* 356–361.

Mavissakalian, M. R., Hamann, M., & Jones, B. (1990). Correlates of DSM-III personality disorder in obsessive compulsive disorder. *Comprehensive Psychiatry, 31,* 481–489.

Mavissakalian, M. R., & Michelson, L. (1983). Self-directed in vivo exposure practice in behavioral and pharmacological treatments of agoraphobia. *Behavior Therapy, 14,* 506–519.

Mavissakalian, M. R., & Michelson, L. (1986). Two-year follow-up of exposure and imipramine treatment of agoraphobia. *American Journal of Psychiatry, 143,* 1106–1112.

Mavissakalian, M. R., & Perel, J. M. (1989). Imipramine dose–response relationship in panic disorder with agoraphobia: Preliminary findings. *Archives of General Psychiatry, 46,* 127–131.

Mavissakalian, M. R., & Perel, J. M. (1992a). Protective effects of imipramine maintenance treatment in panic disorder with agoraphobia. *American Journal of Psychiatry, 149,* 1053–1057.

Mavissakalian, M. R., & Perel, J. M. (1992b). Clinical experiments in maintenance and discontinuation of imipramine therapy in panic disorder with agoraphobia. *Archives of General Psychiatry, 49,* 318–323.

Mavissakalian, M. R., & Perel, J. M. (1995). Imipramine treatment of panic disorder with agoraphobia: Dose ranging and plasma level-response relationships. *American Journal of Psychiatry, 152,* 673–682.

Mavissakalian, M. R., & Perel, J. M. (1999). Long-term maintenance and discontinuation of imipramine therapy in panic disorder with agoraphobia. *Archives of General Psychiatry, 56,* 821–827.

Mavissakalian, M. R., Turner, S. M., & Michelson, L. (1985). Future directions in the assessment and treatment of obsessive–compulsive disorder. In M. R. Mavissakalian, S. M. Turner, & L. Michelson (Eds.), *Psychological and pharmacological treatment of obsessive–compulsive disorder.* New York: Plenum Press.

Mavissakalian, M. R., Turner, S. M., Michelson, L., & Jacob, R. (1985). Tricyclic antidepressants in obsessive–compulsive disorder: Antiobsessional or antidepressant agents? *American Journal of Psychiatry, 142,* 572–576.

Mawson, D., Marks, I. M., & Ramm, L. (1982). Clomoipramine and exposure for chronic obsessive–compulsive rituals: III. Two year follow-up and further readings. *British Journal of Psychiatry, 140,* 11–18.

May, R. (1979). *The meaning of anxiety.* New York: Washington Square Press.

Mayer, B., Merckelbach, H., & Muris, P. (1999). Spider-phobic children do not react with masked skin conductance responses to masked phobic stimuli. *Journal of Psychopathology and Behavioral Assessment, 21,* 237–248.

Mazza, D. L., Martin, D., Spacavento, L., Jacobsen, J., & Gibbs, H. (1986). Prevalence of anxiety disorders in patients with mitral valve prolapse. *American Journal of Psychiatry, 143,* 349–352.

McCallum, W. C., & Walter, W. G. (1968). The effects of attention and distraction on the cintingent negative variation in normal and neurotic subjects. *Electroencephalography and Clinical Neurophysiology, 25,* 319–329.

McCauley, E., Mitchell, J. R., Burke, P., & Moss, S. (1988). Cognitive attributes of depression in children and adolescents. *Journal of Consulting and Clinical Psychology, 56,* 903–908.

McElroy, S. L., Keck, P. E., Pope, H. G., Hudson, J. L. Faedda, G. L., & Swann, A. C. (1992). Clinical and research implications of the diagnosis of dysphoric or mixed mania or hypomania. *American Journal of Psychiatry, 149*(12), 1633–1644.

McFall, M. E., Smith, D. E., Mackay, P. W., & Tarver, D. J. (1990). Reliability and validity of Mississippi Scale for Combat-Related Posttraumatic Stress Disorder. *Psychological Assessment, 2,* 114–121.

McFarlane, A. C. (1988). The etiology of post-traumatic stress disorders following a natural disaster. *British Journal of Psychiatry, 152,* 116–121.

McFarlane, A. C. (1989). The prevention and management of the psychiatric morbidity of natural disasters: An Australian experience. *Stress Medicine, 5,* 29–36.

McGlynn, F. D., Moore, P. M., Lawyer, S., & Karg, R. (1999). Relaxation training inhibits fear and arousal during in vivo exposure to phobia-cue stimuli. *Journal of Behavior Therapy and Experimental Psychiatry, 30,* 155–168.

McGlynn, F. D., Moore, P. M., Rose, M. P., & Lazarte, A. (1995). Effects of relaxation training on fear and arousal during in vivo exposure to a caged snake among DSM-III-R simple (snake) phobics. *Journal of Behavior Therapy and Experimental Psychiatry, 26,* 1–8.

McGlynn, F. D., Rose, M. P., & Jacobson, N. (1995). Effects of control and of attentional instructions on arousal and fear during exposure to phobia-cue stimuli. *Journal of Anxiety Disorders, 9,* 451–461.

McGlynn, F. D., Rose, M. P., & Lazarte, A. (1994). Control and of attention during exposure influence arousal and fear among insect phobias. *Behavior Modification, 18,* 371–388.

McGuffin, P., & Reich, T. (1984). Psychopathology and genetics. In H. E. Adams & P. B. Sutker (Eds.), *Comprehensive handbook of psychopathology.* New York: Plenum Press.

McKay, D., Neziroglu, F., Todaro, J., & Yaryura-Tobias, J. A. (1996). Changes in personality disorders following behavior therapy for obsessive–compulsive disorder. *Journal of Anxiety Disorders, 10,* 47–57.

McKenna, P. J. (1984). Disorders with overvalued ideas. *British Journal of Psychiatry, 145,* 579–585.

McLean, P. D., Whittal, M. L., Thordarson, D. S., & Taylor, S. (2001). Cognitive versus behavioral therapy in the group treatment of obsessive compulsive disorder. *Journal of Consulting and Clinical Psychology, 69,* 205–214.

McLeer, S. V., Deblinger, E., Atkins, M. S., Foa, E. B., & Ralphe, R. (1988). Post-traumatic stress disorder in sexually abused children. *Journal of the American Academy of Child and Adolescent Psychiatry, 27,* 650–654.

McLeer, S. V., Deblinger, E. B., Henry, D., & Orvaschel, H. (1992). Sexually abused children at high risk for post-traumatic stress disorder. *Journal of the American Academy of Child and Adolescent Psychiatry, 31,* 875–879.

McNair, D. M., Lorr, M., & Droppleman, L. F. (1971). *Manual: Profile of Mood States.* San Diego, CA: Educational and Industrial Testing Services.

McNally, R. J. (1987). Preparedness and phobias: A review. *Psychological Bulletin, 101,* 283–303.

McNally, R. J. (1994). *Panic disorder: A critical analysis.* New York: Guilford Press.

McNally, R. J. (1996). Cognitive bias in the anxiety disorders. In D. A. Hope (Ed.), *Nebraska Symposium on Motivation: Vol. 43. Perspectives on anxiety, panic, and fear.* Lincoln: Nebraska University Press.

McNally, R. J. (1999). Anxiety sensitivity and information-processing biases for threat. In S. Taylor (Ed.), *Anxiety sensitivity: Theory, research, and treatment of the fear of anxiety.* Mahwah, NJ: Erlbaum.

McNally, R. J., & Eke, M. (1996). Anxiety, sensitivity, suffocation fear, and breath-holding duration as predictors of response to carbon dioxide challenge. *Journal of Abnormal Psychology, 105,* 146–149.

McNally, R. J., & Foa, E. B. (1987). Cognition and agoraphobia: Bias in the interpretation of threat. *Cognitive Therapy and Research, 11,* 567–581.

McNally, R. J., Hornig, C. D., & Donnell, C. D. (1995). Clinical versus non-clinical panic: A test of suffocation false alarm theory. *Behaviour Research and Therapy, 33,* 127–131.

McNally, R. J., Hornig, C. D., Otto, M. W., & Pollack, M. H. (1997). Selective encoding of threat in panic disorder: Application of a dual priming paradigm. *Behaviour Research and Therapy, 35*(6), 543–549.

McNally, R. J., & Kohlbeck, P. A. (1993). Reality monitoring in obsessive–compulsive disorder. *Behaviour Research and Therapy, 31,* 249–253.

McNally, R. J., & Lorenz, M. (1987). Anxiety sensitivity in agoraphobics. *Journal of Behavior Therapy and Experimental Psychiatry, 18,* 3–11.

McNally, R. J., & Louro, C. E. (1992). Fear of flying in agoraphobia and simple phobia: Distinguishing features. *Journal of Anxiety Disorders, 6,* 319–324.

McNally, R. J., & Steketee, G. S. (1985). The etiology and maintenance of severe animal phobias. *Behaviour Research and Therapy, 23,* 431–435.

McNamara, H., & Fisch, R. (1964). Effect of high and low motivation on two aspects of attention. *Perceptual and Motor Skills, 19,* 571–578.

McNeil, D. W. (2001). Terminology and evolution of the constructs. In S. G. Hofmann & P. M. DiBartolo (Eds.), *From social anxiety to social phobia: Multiple perspectives.* Needham Heights, MA: Allyn & Bacon.

McNeil, D. W., Ries, B. J., Taylor, L. J., Boone, M. L., Carter, L. E., Turk, C. L., & Lewin, M. R. (1995). Comparison of social phobia subtypes using Stroop tests. *Journal of Anxiety Disorders, 9,* 47–57.

McNeil, D. W., Ries, B. J., & Turk, C. L. (1995). Behavioral assessment: Self- and other-report, physiology, and overt behavior. In R. G. Heimberg, M. R. Liebowitz, D. A. Hope, & F. R. Schneier (Eds.), *Social phobia: Diagnosis, assessment, and treatment.* New York: Guilford Press.

McNeil, D. W., Vrana, S. R., Melamed, B. G., Cuthbert, B. N., & Lang, P. J. (1993). Emotional imagery in simple and social phobia: Fear versus anxiety. *Journal of Abnormal Psychology, 102,* 212–225.

McPherson, F. M., Brougham, L., & McLaren, S. (1980). Maintenance of improvement in agoraphobic patients treated by behavioral methods: Four-year follow-up. *Behaviour Research and Therapy, 18,* 150–152.

Meehl, P. E. (1995). Bootstrap taxometrics: Solving the classification problem in psychopathology. *American Psychologist, 50,* 266–275.

Mehta, M. (1990). A comparative study of family-based and patient-based behavioral management in obsessive–compulsive disorder. *British Journal of Psychiatry, 157,* 133–135.

Meisler, A. W., & Carey, M. P. (1991). Depresed affect and male sexual arousal. *Archives of Sexual Behavior, 20,* 541–554.

Mendlewicz, J., Papadimitriou, G., & Wilmotte, J. (1993). Family study of panic disorder: Comparison with generalized anxiety disorder, major depression, and normal subjects. *Psychiatric Genetics, 3,* 73–78.

Menzies, R. G., & Clarke, J. C. (1993a). The etiology of fear of heights and its relationship to severity and individual response patterns. *Behaviour Research and Therapy, 31,* 355–365.

Menzies, R. G., & Clarke, J. C. (1993b). A comparison of in vivo and vicarious exposure in the treatment of childhood water phobia. *Behaviour Research and Therapy, 31,* 9–15.

Menzies, R. G., & Clarke, J. C. (1993c). The etiology of childhood water phobia. *Behaviour Research and Therapy, 31*(5), 499–501.

Menzies, R. G., & Clarke, J. C. (1995a). Danger expectancies and insight in acrophobia. *Behaviour Research and Therapy, 33,* 215–221.

Menzies, R. G., & Clarke, J. C. (1995b). The etiology of acrophobia and its relationship to severity and individual response patterns. *Behaviour Research and Therapy, 33,* 795–803.

Menzies, R. G., & Clarke, J. C. (1995c). The etiology of phobias: A nonassociative account. *Clinical Psychology Review, 15,* 23–48.

Menzies, R. G., Harris, L. M., & Jones, M. K. (1998). Evidence from three fearful samples for a poor insight type in specific phobia. *Depression and Anxiety, 8,* 29–32.

Merckelbach, H., Arntz, A., & de Jong, P. (1991). Conditioning experiences and spider phobics. *Behaviour Research and Therapy, 29,* 333–335.

Merckelbach, H., Arntz, A., Arrindell, W. A., & de Jong, P. J. (1992). Pathways to spider phobia. *Behaviour Research and Therapy, 30,* 543–546.

Merckelbach, H., de Jong, P., & Arntz, A. (1991). Imagery ability and exposure in vivo in spider phobia. *Behaviour Research and Therapy, 29,* 203–205.

Merckelbach, H., de Jong, P. J., Arntz, A., & Schouten, E. (1993). The role of evaluative learning and disgust sensitivity in the etiology and treatment of spider phobia. *Advances in Behaviour Research and Therapy, 15,* 243–255.

Merckelbach, H., Kenemans, J. L., Dijkstra, A., & Schouten, E. (1993). No attentional bias for pictoral stimuli in spider-fearful subjects. *Journal of Psychopathology and Behavioral Assessment, 15*, 197–206.

Merckelbach, H., & Muris, P. (1997). The etiology of childhood spider phobia. *Behaviour Research and Therapy, 35*, 1031–1034.

Merckelbach, H., Muris, P., de Jong, P. J., & de Jongh, A. (1999). Disgust sensitivity, blood–injection–injury fear, and dental anxiety. *Clinical Psychology and Psychotherapy, 6*, 279–285.

Merckelbach, H., Muris, P., Pool, K., & de Jong, P. J. (1998). Resting EEG asymmetry and spider phobia. *Anxiety, Stress, and Coping, 11*, 213–223.

Merckelbach, H., van Hout, W., van den Hout, M. A., & Mersch, P. P. (1989). Psychophysiological and subjective reactions of social phobics and normals to facial stimuli. *Behaviour Research and Therapy, 27*, 289–294.

Merry, S. N., & Andrews, L. K. (1994). Psychiatric status of sexually abused children 12 months after disclosure of abuse. *Journal of the American Academy of Child and Adolescent Psychiatry, 33*, 939–944.

Mesquita, B., & Frijda, N. H. (1992). Cultural variations in emotions: A review. *Psychological Bulletin, 112*, 179–204.

Meston, C. M., & Gorzalka, B. B. (1996). Differential effects of sympathetic activation on sexual arousal in sexually dysfunctional and functional women. *Journal of Abnormal Psychology, 105*(4), 582–591.

Metzger, R. L., Miller, M. L., Cohen, M., Sofka, M., & Borkovec, T. D. (1990). Worry changes decision-making: The effect of negative thoughts on cognitive processing. *Journal of Clinical Psychology, 46*, 78–88.

Meyer, T. J., Miller, M. L., Metzger, R. L., & Borkovec, T. D. (1990). Development and validation of the Penn State Worry Questionnaire. *Behaviour Research and Therapy, 28*, 487–495.

Meyer, V. (1966). Modification of expectations in cases with obsessional rituals. *Behaviour Research and Therapy, 4*, 273–280.

Meyer, V., & Gelder, M. G. (1963). Behaviour therapy and phobic disorders. *British Journal of Psychiatry, 109*, 19–28.

Meyer, V., & Levy, R. (1973). Modification of behavior in obsessive–compulsive disorders. In H. E. Adams & P. Unikel (Eds.), *Issues and trends in behavior therapy*. Springfield, IL: Charles C Thomas.

Michels, R., Frances, A., & Shear, M. K. (1985). Psychodynamic models of anxiety. In A. H. Tuma & J. D. Maser (Eds.), *Anxiety and the anxiety disorders*. Hillsdale, NJ: Erlbaum.

Michelson, D., Lydiard, R. B., Pollack, M. H., Tamura, R. N., Hoog, S. L., Tepner, R., Demitrack, M. A., & Tollefson, G. D. (1998). Outcome assessment and clinical improvement in panic disorder: Evidence from a randomized controlled trial of fluoxetine and placebo. The Fluoxetine Panic Disorder Study Group. *American Journal of Psychiatry, 155*, 1570–1577.

Michelson, L. K., & Mavissakalian, M. R. (1985). Psychophysiological outcome of behavioral and pharmacological treatments of agoraphobia. *Journal of Consulting and Clinical Psychology, 53*, 229–236.

Mick, M. A., & Telch, M. J. (1998). Social anxiety and history of behavioral inhibition in young adults. *Journal of Anxiety Disorders, 12*, 1–20.

Miller, J. J., Fletcher, K., & Kabat-Zinn, J. (1995). Three-year follow-up and clinical implications of a mindfulness meditation-based stress reduction intervention in the treatment of anxiety disorders. *General Hospital Psychiatry, 17*, 192–200.

Miller, L. C., Murphy, R., & Buss, A. H. (1981). Consciousness of body: Private and public. *Journal of Personality and Social Psychology, 41*(2), 397–406.

Miller, N. E. (1980). A perspective on the effects of stress and coping on disease and health. In S. Levine & H. Ursin (Eds.), *Coping and health*. New York: Plenum Press.

Miller, S. M. (1979). Controllability and human stress: Method, evidence, and theory. *Behaviour Research and Therapy, 17*, 287–304.

Miller, W. R. (1975). Psychological deficit in depression. *Psychological Bulletin, 82*, 238–260.

Mills, H. L., Agras, W. S., Barlow, D. H., & Mills, J. R. (1973). Compulsive rituals treated by response prevention. *Archives of General Psychiatry, 28,* 524–529.

Milne, A. A. (1952). Lines and squares. In A. A. Milne, *When we were very young.* New York: E. P. Dutton. (Original work published 1924)

Mineka, S. (1985a). Animal models of anxiety-based disorders: Their usefulness and limitations. In A. H. Tuma & J. D. Maser (Eds.), *Anxiety and the anxiety disorders.* Hillsdale, NJ: Erlbaum.

Mineka, S. (1985b). The frightful complexity of the origins of fear. In F. R. Bruch & J. B. Overmier (Eds.), *Affect, conditioning, and cognition: Essays on the determinants of behavior.* Hillsdale, NJ: Erlbaum.

Mineka, S. (1985b). The frightful complexity of the origins of fears. In F. R. Brach & J. B. Overmier (Eds.), *Affect, conditioning, and cognition: Essays on the determinants of behavior.* Hillsdale NJ: Erlbaum.

Mineka, S. (1987). A primate model of phobic fears. In H. Eysenck & I. Martin (Eds.), *Theoretical foundations of behavior therapy.* New York: Plenum Press.

Mineka, S., & Cook, M. (1993). Mechanisms involved in the observational conditioning of fear. *Journal of Experimental Psychology: General, 122,* 23–38.

Mineka, S., Cook, M., & Miller, S. (1984). Fear conditioned with escapable and inescapable shock: The effects of a feedback stimulus. *Journal of Experimental Psychology: Animal Behavior Processes, 10,* 307–323.

Mineka, S., Davidson, M., Cook, M., & Keir, R. (1984). Observational conditioning of snake fear in rhesus monkeys. *Journal of Abnormal Psychology, 93,* 355–372.

Mineka, S., Gunnar, M., & Champoux, M. (1986). Control and early socioemotional development: Infant rhesus monkeys reared in controllable versus uncontrollable environments. *Child Development, 57,* 1241–1256.

Mineka, S., & Kihlstrom, J. (1978). Unpredictable and uncontrollable aversive events. *Journal of Abnormal Psychology, 87,* 256–271.

Mineka, S., Mystkowski, J. L., Hladek, D., & Rodriguez, B. I. (1999). The effects of changing contexts on return of fear following exposure therapy for spider fear. *Journal of Consulting and Clinical Psychology, 67,* 599–604.

Mineka, S., Watson, D., & Clark, L. A. (1998). Comorbidity of anxiety and unipolar mood disorders. *Annual Review of Psychology, 49,* 377–412.

Mineka, S., & Zinbarg, R. (1996). Conditioning and ethological models of anxiety disorders: Stress in dynamic-context anxiety models. In D. A. Hope (Ed.), *Nebraska Symposium on Motivation: Vol. 43. Perspectives on anxiety, panic, and fear.* Lincoln: University of Nebraska Press.

Minichiello, W., Baer, L., & Jenike, M. A. (1987). Schizotypal personality disorder: A poor prognostic indicator for behavior therapy in the treatment of obsessive compulsive disorder. *Journal of Anxiety Disorders, 1,* 273–276.

Mitchell, W. B., DiBartolo, P. M., Brown, T. A., & Barlow, D. H. (1998). Effects of positive and negative mood on sexual arousal in sexually functional males. *Archives of Sexual Behavior, 27*(2), 197–207.

Mitchell, W. B., Marten, P. A., Williams, D. M., & Barlow, D. H. (1990, November). *Control of sexual arousal in sexual dysfunctional males.* Paper presented at the 24th Annual Convention of the Association for Advancement of Behavior Therapy, San Francisco.

Modigh, K., Westburg, P., & Ericksson, E. (1992). Superiority of clomipramine over imipramine in the treatment of panic disorder: A placebo-controlled trial. *Journal of Clinical Psychopharmacology, 12,* 251–261.

Mogg, K., Bradley, B. P., Millar, N., & White, J. (1995). A follow-up study of cognitive bias in generalized anxiety disorder. *Behaviour Research and Therapy, 33,* 927–935.

Mogg, K., Bradley, B. P., Williams, R., & Mathews, A. (1993). Subliminal processing of emotional information in anxiety and depression. *Journal of Abnormal Psychology, 102,* 304–311.

Mogg, K., Gardiner, J. M., Stavrou, A., & Golombok, S. (1992). Recollective experience and Recognition memory for threat in clinical anxiety states. *Bulletin of the Psychonomic Society, 30*(2), 109–112.

Mogg, K., Mathews, A., & Weinman, J. (1987). Memory bias in clinical anxiety. *Journal of Abnormal Psychology, 96*, 94–98.

Mogg, K., Mathews, A., & Weinman, J. (1989). Selective processing of threat cues in anxiety states: A replication. *Behaviour Research and Therapy, 27*, 317–323.

Mohler, H., & Okada, T. (1977). Benzodiazepine receptor: Demonstration in the central nervous system. *Science, 198*, 849.

Molina, S., & Borkovec, T. D. (1994). The Penn State Worry Questionnaire: Psychometric properties and associated characteristics. In G. C. L. Davey & F. Tallis (Eds.), *Worrying: Perspectives on theory, assessment, and treatment.* New York: Wiley.

Molina, S., Borkovec, T. D., Peasley, C., & Person, D. (1998). Content analysis of worrisome streams of consciousness in anxious and dysphoric participants. *Cognitive Therapy and Research, 22*, 109–123.

Möller, H.-J. (1999). Effectiveness and safety of benzodiazepines. *Journal of Clinical Psychopharmacology, 19*(Suppl. 2), 2–11.

Monteiro, W., Marks, I. M., Noshirvani, H., & Checkley, S. (1986). Normal dexamethasone suppression test in obsessive compulsive disorder. *British Journal of Psychiatry, 148*, 326–329.

Moore, R., & Brødsgaard, I. (1994). Group therapy compared with individual desensitization for dental anxiety. *Community Dentistry and Oral Epidemiology, 22*, 258–262.

Moore, R. Y. (1973). Retinohypothalamic projection in mammals: A comparative study. *Brain Research, 49*, 403–409.

Moran, C., & Andrews, G. (1985). The familial occurrence of agoraphobia. *British Journal of Psychiatry, 146*, 262–267.

Moras, K., Di Nardo, P. A., & Barlow, D. H. (1992). Distinguishing anxiety and depression: Reexamination of the reconstructed Hamilton Scales. *Psychological Assessment, 4*, 224–227.

Moras, K., Di Nardo, P. A., Brown, T. A., & Barlow, D. H. (1995). *Comorbidity, functional impairment, and depression among the DSM-III-R anxiety disorders.* Unpublished manuscript, State University of New York at Albany.

Moreau, D. M., & Weissman, M. M. (1992). Panic disorder in children and adolescents: A review. *American Journal of Psychiatry, 149*, 1306–1314.

Morokoff, P. J., & Heiman, J. R. (1980). Effects of erotic stimuli on sexually functional and dysfunctional women: Multiple measures before and after therapy. *Behaviour Research and Therapy, 18*, 127–137.

Moroz, G., & Rosenbaum, J. F. (1999). Efficacy, safety, and gradual discontinuation of clonazepam in panic disorder: A placebo-controlled, multicenter study using optimized dosages. *Journal of Clinical Psychiatry, 60*, 604–612.

Morris, J. S., Öhman, A., & Dolan, R. J. (1998). Conscious and unconscious emotional learning in the human amygdala. *Nature, 393*, 467–470.

Morrow, G. R., & Dobkin, P. L. (1988). Anticipatory nausea and vomiting in cancer patients undergoing chemotherapy treatment: Prevalence, etiology, and behavioral interventions. *Clinical Psychology Review, 8*, 517–556.

Moskowitz, H., & Smiley, A. (1982). Effects of chronically administered buspirone and diazepam on driving-related skills performance. *Journal of Clinical Psychiatry, 43*(Suppl. 12), 45–55.

Mostofsky, D. I., & Barlow, D. H. (Eds.). (2000). *The management of stress and anxiety in medical disorders.* Boston: Allyn & Bacon.

Mountz, J. M., Modell, J. G., Wilson, M. W., Curtis, G. C., Lee, M. A., Schmaltz, S., & Kuhl, D. E. (1989). Positron emission tomographic evaluation of cerebral blood flow during state anxiety in simple phobia. *Archives of General Psychiatry, 46*, 501–504.

Mowrer, O. H. (1947). On the dual nature of learning: A reinterpretation of "conditioning" and "problem solving. " *Harvard Educational Review, 17*, 102–148.

Mowrer, O. H. (1950). *Learning theory and the personality dynamics.* New York: Arnold Press.

Mowrer, O. H. (1960). *Learning theory and the symbolic processes.* New York: Wiley.

Mowrer, O. H., & Viek, P. (1948). An experimental analogue of fear from a sense of helplessness. *Journal of Abnormal Social Psychology, 83*, 193–200.

Mueser, K. T., Salyers, M., Rosenberg, S. D., Ford, J., Fox, L., & Auciello, P. (1999). *Reliability of trauma and PTSD assessments in persons with severe mental illness.* Manuscript submitted for publication.

Mulkens, S. A. N., de Jong, P. J., & Merckelbach, H. (1996). Disgust and spider phobia. *Journal of Abnormal Psychology, 105,* 464–468.

Mullan, M. J., Gurling, H. M. D., Oppenheim, B. S., & Murray, R. M. (1986). The relationship between alcoholism and neurosis: Evidence from a twin study. *British Journal of Psychiatry, 148,* 435–441.

Mullaney, J. A., & Trippett, C. J. (1979). Alcohol dependence and phobias: Clinical description and relevance. *British Journal of Psychiatry, 135,* 565–573.

Munby, J., & Johnston, D. W. (1980). Agoraphobia: The long-term follow-up of behavioral treatment. *British Journal of Psychiatry, 137,* 418–427.

Mundo, E., Maina, G., & Uslenghi, C. (2000). Multicentre, double-blind comparison of fluvoxamine and clomipramine in the treatment of obsessive-compulsive disorder. *International Clinical Psychopharmacology, 15,* 69–76.

Munjack, D. J. (1984). The onset of driving phobias. *Journal of Behavior Therapy and Experimental Psychiatry, 15,* 305–308.

Munjack, D. J., Baltazar, P. L., Bohn, P. B., Cabe, D. D., & Appleton, A. A. (1990). Clonazepam in the treatment of social phobia: A pilot study. *Journal of Clinical Psychiatry, 51*(Suppl. 5), 35–40.

Muris, P., de Jong, P. J., Merckelbach, H., & van Zuuren, F. (1993a). Is exposure therapy outcome affected by a monitoring coping style? *Advances in Behaviour Research and Therapy, 15,* 291–300.

Muris, P., de Jong, P. J., Merckelbach, H., & van Zuuren, F. (1993b). Monitoring coping style and exposure outcome in spider phobics. *Behavioural and Cognitive Psychotherapy, 21,* 329–333.

Muris, P., Mayer, B., & Merckelbach, H. (1998). Trait anxiety as a predictor of behaviour therapy outcome in spider phobia. *Behavioural and Cognitive Psychotherapy, 26,* 87–91.

Muris, P., & Merckelbach, H. (1995). Treating spider phobia with eye-movement desensitization and reprocessing: Two case reports. *Journal of Anxiety Disorders, 9,* 439–449.

Muris, P., Merckelbach, H., & Collaris, R. (1997). Common childhood fears and their origins. *Behaviour Research and Therapy, 35,* 929–937.

Muris, P., Merckelbach, H., & de Jong, P. J. (1995). Exposure therapy outcome in spider phobics: Effects of monitoring and blunting coping styles. *Behaviour Research and Therapy, 33,* 461–464.

Muris, P., Merckelbach, H., Holdrinet, I., & Sijsenaar, M. (1998). Treating phobic children: Effects of EMDR versus exposure. *Journal of Consulting and Clinical Psychology, 66,* 193–198.

Muris, P., Merckelbach, H., Schmidt, H., & Tierney, S. (1999). Disgust sensitivity, trait anxiety and anxiety disorders symptoms in normal children. *Behaviour Research and Therapy, 37,* 953–961.

Muris, P., Merckelbach, H., van Haaften, H., & Mayer, B. (1997). Eye movement desensitization and reprocessing versus exposure in vivo: A single-session crossover study of spider-phobic children. *British Journal of Psychiatry, 171,* 82–86.

Muris, P., Schmidt, H., & Merckelbach, H. (1999). The structure of specific phobia symptoms among children and adolescents. *Behaviour Research and Therapy, 37,* 863–868.

Muris, P., Steerneman, P., Merckelbach, H., & Meesters, C. (1996). The role of parental fearfulness and modeling in children's fear. *Behaviour Research and Therapy, 34,* 265–268.

Murray, C. J. L., & Lopes, A. D. (1996). *The global burden of disease.* Cambridge, MA: Harvard University Press.

Murray, E. J., & Foote, F. (1979). The origins of fear and snakes. *Behaviour Research and Therapy, 17,* 489–493.

Musson, R. F., & Alloy, L. B. (1988). Depression and self-directed attention. In L. B. Alloy (Ed.), *Cognitive processes in depression.* New York: Guilford Press.

Mutchler, K., Crowe, R. R., Noyes, R., & Wesner, R. W. (1990). Exclusion of the tyrosine hydroxy-lase gene in 14 panic disorder pedigrees. *American Journal of Psychiatry, 147,* 1367–1369.

Myers, J. K., Weissman, M. M., Tischler, G. L., Holzer, C. E., III, Leaf, P. J., Orvaschel, H., Anthony, J. C., Boyd, J. H., Burke, J. D., Jr., Kramer, M., & Stoltzman, R. (1984). Six-month prevalence of psychiatric disorders in three communities. *Archives of General Psychiatry, 41,* 959–967.

Nachmias, M., Gunnar, M., Mangelsdorf, S., Parritz, R. H., & Buss, K. (1996). Behavioral inhibition and stress reactivity: The moderating role of attachment security. *Child Development, 67,* 508–522.

Nader, K., Newman, E., Weathers, F. W., Kaloupek, D. G., Kriegler, J., Blake, D. D., & Pynoos, R. (1998). *Clinician-Administered PTSD Scale for Children and Adolescents for DSM-IV.* (Available from E. Newman, Department of Psychology, University of Tulsa, 600 S. College Avenue, Tulsa, OK 74104).

Nagy, L. M., Krystal, J. H., Woods, S. W., & Charney, D. S. (1989). Clinical and medication outcome after short-term alprazolam and behavioral group treatment in panic disorder: 2.5 year naturalistic follow-up study. *Archives of General Psychiatry, 46,* 993–999.

Nair, N. P., Bakish, D., Saxena, B., Amin, M., Schwartz, G., & West, T. E. (1996). Comparison of fluvoxamine, imipramine, and placebo in the treatment of outpatients with panic disorder. *Anxiety, 2,* 192–198.

Najavits, L. M. (2001). *Seeking safety: A treatment for PTSD and substance abuse.* New York: Guilford Press.

Neal, A. M., Lilly, R. S., & Zakis, S. (1993). What are African American children afraid of? *Journal of Anxiety Disorders, 7,* 129–139.

Neal, A. M., Nagle-Rich, L., & Smucker, W. D. (1994). The presence of panic disorder among African American hypertensives: A pilot study. *Journal of Black Psychology, 20,* 29–35.

Neal, A. M., & Turner, S. M. (1991). Anxiety disorders research with African Americans: Current status. *Psychological Bulletin, 109*(3), 400–410.

Neal-Barnett, A. M., & Smith, J., Sr. (1997). African Americans. In S. Friedman (Ed.), *Cultural issues in the treatment of anxiety.* New York: Guilford Press.

Neale, J. M., & Katahn, M. (1968). Anxiety, choice and stimulus uncertainty. *Journal of Personality, 36*(2), 235–245.

Neale, M. C., Walters, E. E., Eaves, L. J., Kessler, R. C., Heath, A. C., & Kendler, K. S. (1994). Genetics of blood–injury fears and phobias: A population-based study. *American Journal of Medical Genetics, 54,* 326–334.

Neff, D. F., & Blanchard, E. B. (1987). A multi-component treatment for irritable bowel syndrome. *Behavior Therapy, 18,* 70–83.

Nelissen, I., Muris, P., & Merckelbach, H. (1995). Computerized exposure and in vivo exposure treatments of spider fear in children: Two case reports. *Journal of Behavior Therapy and Experimental Psychiatry, 26,* 153–156.

Nelles, W. B., & Barlow, D. H. (1988). Do children panic? *Clinical Psychology Review, 8,* 359–372.

Nemeroff, C. B. (1996). The corticotropin-releasing factor (CRF) hypothesis of depression: New findings and new directions. *Molecular Psychiatry, 1,* 336–342.

Nesse, R. M., Cameron, O. G., Curtis, G. C., & Lee, M. (1986). How antipanic drugs might work. *American Journal of Psychiatry, 143,* 945.

Nesse, R. M., Cameron, O. G., Curtis, G. C., McCann, D. S., & Huber-Smith, M. J. (1984). Adrenergic function in patients with panic anxiety. *Archives of General Psychiatry, 41,* 771–776.

Nesse, R. M., Curtis, G. C., Thyer, B. A., McCann, D. S., Huber-Smith, M. J., & Knopf, R. F. (1985). Endocrine and cardiovascular responses during phobic anxiety. *Psychosomatic Medicine, 47,* 320–332.

Newman, C. F., Beck, J. G., & Beck, A. T. (1990, November). *Efficacy of cognitive therapy in reducing panic attacks and medication.* Presented at the 24th Annual Meeting of the Association for Advancement of Behavior Therapy, San Francisco, CA.

Newman, E., Kaloupek, D. G., & Keane, T. M. (1996). Assessment of posttraumatic stress disorder in clinical and research settings. In B. A. van der Kolk, A. C. McFarlane, & L. Weisaeth (Eds.), *Traumatic stress: The effects of overwhelming experiences on mind, body, and society.* New York: Guilford Press.

Newman, M. G. (2000). Recommendations for a cost-offset model of psychotherapy allocation using generalized anxiety disorder as an example. *Journal of Consulting and Clinical Psychology, 68,* 549–555.

Newman, M. G., Consoli, A. J., & Taylor, C. B. (1999). A palmtop computer program for the treatment of generalized anxiety disorder. *Behavior Modification, 23,* 597–619.

Newman, M. G., Zuellig, A. R., Kachin, K. E., & Constantino, M. J. (2000). *The reliability and validity of the GAD-Q-IV: A revised self-report measure.* Manuscript submitted for publication.

Newton, R. E., Marunycz, J. D., Alderdice, M. T., & Napoliello, M. J. (1986). Review of the side-effect profile of buspirone. *American Journal of Medicine, 80*(Suppl. 3B), 17–21.

Ngui, P. W. (1969). The *koro* epidemic in Singapore. *Australian and New Zealand Journal of Psychiatry, 3,* 263–266.

Nolen-Hoeksema, S. (1987). Sex differences in unipolar depression: Evidence and theory. *Psychological Bulletin, 101*(2), 259–282.

Nolen-Hoeksema, S. (1990). *Sex differences in depression.* Stanford, CA: Stanford University Press.

Nolen-Hoeksema, S., & Girgus, J. S. (1994). The emergence of gender differences in depression during adolescence. *Psychological Bulletin, 115,* 424–443.

Nolen-Hoeksema, S., Girgus, J. S., & Seligman, M. E. P. (1986). Learned helplessness in children: A longitudinal study of depression, achievement, and attributional style. *Journal of Personality and Social Psychology, 51,* 435–442.

Nolen-Hoeksema, S., Girgus, J. S., & Seligman, M. E. P. (1992). Predictors and consequences of childhood depressive symptoms: A 5-year longitudinal study. *Journal of Abnormal Psychology, 101,* 405–422.

Nolen-Hoeksema, S., Wolfson, A., Mumme, D., & Guskin, K. (1995). Helplessness in children of depressed and nondepressed mothers. *Developmental Psychology, 31,* 377–387.

Norris, F. H., (1992). Epidemiology of trauma: Frequency and impact of different potentially traumatic events on different demographic groups. *Journal of Consulting and Clinical Psychology, 60,* 409–418.

Norris, F. H. & Riad, J. K. (1997). Standardized self report measures of civilian trauma and posttraumatic stress disorder. In J. P. Wilson & T. M. Keane (Eds.), *Assessing psychological trauma and PTSD.* New York: Guilford Press.

Norton, G. R., Cox, B. J., Hewitt, P. L., & McLeod, L. (1997). Personality factors associated with generalized and non-generalized social anxiety. *Personality and Individual Differences, 22,* 655–660.

Norton, G. R., Cox, B. J., & Malan, J. (1992). Nonclinical panickers: A critical review. *Clinical Psychology Review, 12,* 121–139.

Norton, G. R., Dorward, J., & Cox, B. J. (1986). Factors associated with panic attacks in nonclinical subjects. *Behavior Therapy, 17,* 239–252.

Norton, G. R., Harrison, B., Hauch, J., & Rhodes, L. (1985). Characteristics of people with infrequent panic attacks. *Journal of Abnormal Psychology, 94,* 216–221.

Norton, G. R., Pidlubny, S. R., & Norton, P. J. (1999). Prediction of panic attacks and related variables. *Behavior Therapy, 30,* 319–330.

Norton, G. R., Rhodes, L., Hauch, J., & Kaprowy, E. A. (1985). Characteristics of subjects experiencing relaxation and relaxation-induced anxiety. *Journal of Behavior Therapy and Experimental Psychiatry, 16,* 211–216.

Norton, G. R., Rockman, G. E., Luy, B., & Marion, T. (1993). Suicide, chemical abuse and panic attacks: A preliminary report. *Behaviour Research and Therapy, 31,* 37–40.

Novaco, R. W. (1975). *Anger control: The development and evaluation of an experimental treatment.* Lexington, MA: Heath.

Novaco, R. W. (1994). Clinical problems of anger and its assessment and regulation through a stress coping skills approach. In W. O'Donohue & L. Krasner (Eds.), *Handbook of psychological skills training: Clinical techniques and applications*. Needham Heights, MA: Allyn & Bacon.

Nowicki, S., & Strickland, B. R. (1973). A locus of control scale for children. *Journal of Consulting and Clinical Psychology, 40*(1), 148–154.

Nowlis, V., & Nowlis, H. (1956). The description and analysis of mood. *Annals of the New York Academy of Sciences, 65*, 345–355.

Noyes, R. (1991). Suicide and panic disorder: A review. *Journal of Affective Disorders, 22*, 1–11.

Noyes, R., Burrows, G. D., Reich, J. H., Judd, F. K., Garvey, M. J., Norman, T. R., Cook, B. L., & Marriott, P. (1996). Diazepam versus alprazolam for the treatment of panic disorder. *Journal of Clinical Psychiatry, 57*, 349–355.

Noyes, R., Jr., & Clancy, J. (1976). Anxiety neurosis: A 5 year follow-up. *Journal of Nervous and Mental Disease, 162*, 200–205.

Noyes, R., Jr., Clancy, J., Hoenk, P. R., & Slymen, D. J. (1980). The prognosis of anxiety neurosis. *Archives of General Psychiatry, 37*, 173–178.

Noyes, R., Jr., Clarkson, C., Crowe, R. R., Yates, W. R., & McChesney, C. M. (1987). A family study of generalized anxiety disorders. *American Journal of Psychiatry, 144*, 1019–1024.

Noyes, R., Jr., Crowe, R. R., & Harris, E. L. (1986). Relationship between panic disorder and agoraphobia. *Archives of General Psychiatry, 43*, 227–232.

Noyes, R., Jr., Crowe, R. R., Harris, E. L., Hamra, B. J., McChesney, C. M., & Chaudhry, D. R. (1986). Relationship between panic disorder and agoraphobia: A family study. *Archives of General Psychiatry, 43*, 227–232.

Noyes, R., DuPont, R. L., Pecknold, J. C., Rifkin, A., Rubin, R. T., Swinson, R. P., Ballenger, J. C., & Burrows, G. D. (1988). Alprazolam in panic disorder and agoraphobia: Results from a multicenter trial. II: Patient acceptance, side effects, and safety. *Archives of General Psychiatry, 45*, 423–428.

Noyes, R., Moroz, G., Davidson, J. R., Liebowitz, M. R., Davidson, A., Siegel, J., Bell, J., Cain, J. W., Curlik, S. M., Kent, T. A., Lydiard, R. B., Mallinger, A. G., Pollack, M. H., Rapaport, M., Rasmussen, S. A., Hedges, D., Schweizer, E., & Uhlenhuth, E. H. (1997). Moclobemide in social phobia: A controlled dose-response trial. *Journal of Clinical Psychopharmacology, 17*, 247–254.

Noyes, R., Woodman, C., Garvey, M. J., Cook, B. L., Suelzer, M., Clancy, J., & Anderson, D. J. (1992). Generalized anxiety disorder versus panic disorder: Distinguishing characteristics and patterns of comorbidity. *Journal of Nervous and Mental Disease, 180*, 369–370.

Nugent, K., & Mineka, S. (1994). The effect of high and low trait anxiety on implicit and explicit memory tasks. *Cognition and Emotion, 8*(2), 147–163.

Nunn, G. D. (1988). Concurrent validity between the Nowicki–Strickland Locus of Control Scale and the State–Trait Anxiety Inventory for Children. *Educational and Psychological Measurement, 48*, 435–438.

Nutt, D. J. (1986). Increased central alpha adrenoceptor sensitivity in panic disorder. *Psychopharmacology, 90*, 268–269.

Nutt, D. J., Glue, P., Lawson, C., & Wilson, S. (1990). Flumazenil provocation of panic attacks. *Archives of General Psychiatry, 46*, 917–925.

Nutt, D. J., & Lawson, C. (1992). Panic attacks: A neurochemical overview of models and mechanisms. *British Journal of Psychiatry, 160*, 165–178.

O'Brien, G. T., & Barlow, D. H. (1984). Agoraphobia. In S. M. Turner (Ed.), *Behavioral treatment of anxiety disorders*. New York: Plenum Press.

O'Brien, T. P., & Kelley, J. E. (1980). A comparison of self-directed and therapist-directed practice for fear reduction. *Behaviour Research and Therapy, 18*, 573–579.

Obsessive Compulsive Cognitions Working Group (OCCWG). (1997). Cognitive assessment of obsessive–compulsive disorder. *Behaviour Research and Therapy, 35*, 667–681.

Obsessive Compulsive Cognitions Working Group (OCCWG). (2001). Development and initial validation of the Obsessive Beliefs Questionnaire and the Interpretation of Intrusions Inventory. *Behaviour Research and Therapy, 39*, 987–1006.

O'Connor, P. J., Smith, J. C., & Morgan, W. P. (2000). Physical activity does not provoke panic attacks in patients with panic disorder: A review of the evidence. *Anxiety, Stress, and Coping, 13,* 333–353.

Oehrberg, S., Christiansen, P. E., Behnke, K., Borup, A. L., Severin, B., Soegaard, J., Calberg, H., Judge, R., Ohrstrom, J. K., & Manniche, P. M. (1995). Paroxetine in the treatment of panic disorder: A randomised, double-blind, placebo-controlled study. *British Journal of Psychiatry, 167,* 374–379.

O'Hanlon, J. F. (1991). Review of buspirone's effects on human performance and related variables. *European Neuropsychopharmacology, 1,* 489–501.

O'Hanlon, J. F., & Beatty, J. (1976). Catecholamine correlates of radar monitoring performance. *Biological Psychiatry, 4,* 293–303.

Öhman, A. (1986). Face the beast and fear the face: Animal and social fears as prototypes for evolutionary analyses of emotion. *Psychophysiology, 23,* 123–145.

Öhman, A. (1993). Stimulus prepotency and fear: Data and theory. In N. Birbaumer & A. Öhman (Eds.), *The organization of emotion: Cognitive, clinical and psychophysiological perspectives.* Toronto: Hogrefe.

Öhman, A. (1996). Preferential pre-attentive processing of threat in anxiety: Preparedness and attentional biases. In R. M. Rapee (Ed.), *Current controversies in the anxiety disorders.* New York: Guilford Press.

Öhman, A. (1997). Unconscious pre-attentive mechanisms in the activation of phobic fear. In G. C. L. Davey (Ed.), *Phobias: A handbook of theory, research, and treatment.* Chichester, England: Wiley.

Öhman, A. (1999). Distinguishing unconscious from conscious emotional processes: Methodological considerations and theoretical implications. In T. Dalgleish & M. Power (Eds.), *Handbook of cognition and emotion.* Chichester, England: Wiley.

Öhman, A., & Dimberg, U. (1978). Facial expressions as conditioned stimuli for electrodermal responses: A case of "preparedness"? *Journal of Personality and Social Psychology, 36,* 1251–1258.

Öhman, A., Dimberg, U., & Öst, L.-G. (1985a). Animal and social phobias: A laboratory model. In P. O. Sjoden & S. Bates (Eds.), *Trends in behavior therapy.* New York: Academic Press.

Öhman, A., Dimberg, U., & Öst, L.-G. (1985b). Animal and social phobias: Biological constraints on learned fear responses. In S. Reiss & R. R. Bootzin (Eds.), *Theoretical issues in behavior therapy.* Orlando, FL: Academic Press.

Öhman, A., Erixon, G., & Lofburg, I. (1975). Phobias and preparedness: Phobic versus neutral pictures as conditional stimuli for human autonomic responses. *Journal of Abnormal Psychology, 84,* 41–45.

Öhman, A., Flykt, A., & Lundqvist, D. (in press) Unconscious emotion: Evolutionary perspectives, psycho physiological data and neuropsychological mechanisms. In R. Lane & L. Nadel (Eds.), *Cognitive neuroscience of emotion.* New York: Oxford University Press.

Öhman, A., & Mineka, S. (2001). Fears, phobias, and preparedness: Toward an evolved module of fear and fear learning. *Psychological Review, 108,* 483–522.

Öhman, A., & Soares, J. J. F. (1994). "Unconscious anxiety": Phobic responses to masked stimuli. *Journal of Abnormal Psychology, 103,* 231–240.

Öhman, A., & Soares, J. J. F. (1998). Emotional conditioning to masked stimuli: Expectancies for aversive outcomes following non-recognized fear-relevant stimuli. *Journal of Experimental Psychology: General, 127,* 69–82.

Ollendick, T. H. (1983). Reliability and validity of the revised fear Survey for Children (FSSC-R). *Behaviour Research and Therapy, 21,* 395–399.

Ollendick, T. H., Yule, W., & Ollier, K. (1991). Fears in British children and their relationship to manifest anxiety and depression. *Journal of Child Psychiatry, 32,* 321–331.

Ontiveros, A., & Fontaine, R. (1990). Social phobia and clonazepam. *Canadian Journal of Psychiatry, 35,* 439–441.

Oppenheim, B. S. (1918). Report on neurocirculatory asthenia and its management. *Military Surgeon, 42,* 711–744.

Orner, R. J. (1992). Post-traumatic stress disorders and European war veterans. *British Journal of Clinical Psychology, 31*, 387–403.

Orr, S. P., Lasko, N. B., Metzger, L. J., Berry, N. J., Ahern, C. J., & Pitman, R. K. (1998). Physiological assessment of women with PTSD resulting from childhood sexual abuse. *Journal of Consulting and Clinical Psychology, 66*, 906–913.

Orr, S. P., Metzger, L. J., Lasko, N. B., Macklin, M. L., Peri, T., & Pitman, R. K. (2000). De novo conditioning in trauma-exposed individuals with and without post-traumatic stress disorder. *Journal of Abnormal Psychology, 109*, 290–298.

Orsillo, S. M., Roemer, L., & Barlow, D. H. (2001). *Integrating mindfulness and acceptance into the cognitive-behavioral treatment of generalized anxiety disorder: A case study.* Manuscript submitted for publication.

Orvaschel, H., Lewinsohn, P. M., & Seeley, J. R. (1995). Continuity of psychopathology in community sample of adolescents. *Journal of the American Academy of Child and Adolescent Psychiatry, 34*(11), 1525–1535.

Orwin, A. (1973). The running treatment: A preliminary communication on a new use for an old therapy (physical activity) in the agoraphobic syndrome. *British Journal of Psychiatry, 122*, 175–179.

Öst, L.-G. (1978). Behavioral treatment of thunder and lightning phobias. *Behaviour Research and Therapy, 16*, 197–207.

Öst, L.-G. (1985). Mode of acquisition of phobias. *Acta Universitatis Uppsaliensis (Abstracts of Uppsala Dissertations from the Faculty of Medicine), 529*, 1–45.

Öst, L.-G. (1987a). Age of onset in different phobias. *Journal of Abnormal Psychology, 96*, 223–229.

Öst, L.-G. (1987b). Applied relaxation: Description of a coping technique and review of controlled studies. *Behaviour Research and Therapy, 25*, 397–409.

Öst, L.-G. (1989). One-session treatment for specific phobias. *Behaviour Research and Therapy, 27*, 1–7.

Öst, L.-G. (1991). Acquisition of blood and injection phobia and anxiety response patterns in clinical patients. *Behaviour Research and Therapy, 29*, 323–332.

Öst, L.-G. (1992). Blood and injection phobia: Background and cognitive, physiological, and behavioral variables. *Journal of Abnormal Psychology, 101*, 68–74.

Öst, L.-G. (1996a). Long term effects of behavior therapy for specific phobia. In M. R. Mavissakalian & R. F. Prien (Eds.), *Long term treatments of the anxiety disorders.* Washington, DC: American Psychiatric Press.

Öst, L.-G. (1996b). One-session group treatment for spider phobia. *Behaviour Research and Therapy, 34*, 707–715.

Öst, L.-G., Brandberg, M., & Alm, T. (1997). One versus five sessions of exposure in the treatment of flying phobia. *Behaviour Research and Therapy, 35*, 987–996.

Öst, L.-G., Fellenius, J., & Sterner, U. (1991). Applied tension, exposure *in vivo*, and tension-only in the treatment of blood phobia. *Behaviour Research and Therapy, 29*, 561–574.

Öst, L.-G., Ferebee, I., & Furmark, T. (1997). One-session group therapy of spider phobia: Direct versus indirect treatments. *Behaviour Research and Therapy, 35*, 721–732.

Öst, L.-G., & Hugdahl, K. (1981). Acquisition of phobias and anxiety response patterns in clinical patients. *Behaviour Research and Therapy, 19*, 439–447.

Öst, L.-G., & Hugdahl, K. (1983). Acquisition of agoraphobia, mode of onset and anxiety response patterns. *Behaviour Research and Therapy, 21*, 623–631.

Öst, L.-G., & Hugdahl, K. (1985). Acquisition of blood and dental phobia and anxiety response patterns in clinical patients. *Behaviour Research and Therapy, 23*, 27–34.

Öst, L.-G., Johansson, J., & Jerremalm, A. (1982). Individual response patterns and the effects of different behavioral methods in the treatment of claustrophobia. *Behaviour Research and Therapy, 20*, 445–460.

Öst, L.-G., Lindahl, I.-L., Sterner, U., & Jerremalm, A. (1984). Exposure in vivo vs. applied relaxation in the treatment of blood phobia. *Behaviour Research and Therapy, 22*, 205–216.

Öst, L.-G., Salkovskis, P. M., & Hellström, K. (1991). One-session therapist directed exposure vs. self-exposure in the treatment of spider phobia. *Behavior Therapy, 22,* 407–422.

Öst, L.-G., & Sterner, U. (1987). Applied tension: A specific behavioural method for treatment of blood phobia. *Behaviour Research and Therapy, 25,* 25–30.

Öst, L.-G., Sterner, U., & Fellenius, J. (1989). Applied tension, applied relaxation, and the combination in the treatment of blood phobia. *Behaviour Research and Therapy, 27,* 109–121.

Öst, L.-G., Sterner, U., & Lindahl, I.-L. (1984). Physiological responses in blood phobics. *Behaviour Research and Therapy, 22,* 109–117.

Öst, L.-G., Westling, B. E., & Hellstrom, K. (1993). Applied relaxation, exposure in vivo and cognitive methods in the treatment of panic disorder with agoraphobia. *Behaviour Research and Therapy, 31,* 279–287.

O'Sullivan, G., Noshirvani, H., Marks, I., Monteiro, W., & Lelliott, P. (1991). Six-year follow-up after exposure and clomipramine therapy for obsessive–compulsive disorder. *Journal of Clinical Psychiatry, 52,* 150–155.

O'Sullivan, G. H., Swinson, R., Kuch, K., Marks, I. M., Basoglu, M., & Noshirvani, H. (1996). Alprazolam withdrawal symptoms in agoraphobia with panic disorder: Observations from a controlled Anglo-Canadian study. *Journal of Psychopharmacology, 10,* 101–109.

Otto, M. W., Penava, S. J., Pollack, R. A., & Smoller, J. W. (1996). Cognitive-behavioral and pharmacologic perspectives on the treatment of posttraumatic stress disorder. In M. H. Pollack, M. W. Otto, & J. F. Rosenbaum (Eds.), *Challenges in clinical practice: Pharmacologic and psychosocial strategies.* New York: Guilford Press.

Otto, M. W., Pollack, M. H., Meltzer-Brody, S., & Rosenbaum, J. F. (1992). Cognitive-behavioral therapy for benzodiazepine discontinuation in panic disorder patients. *Psychopharmacology Bulletin, 28,* 123–130.

Otto, M. W., Pollack, M. H., & Sabatino, S. A. (1996). Maintenance of remission following cognitive behavior therapy for panic disorder: Possible deleterious effects of concurrent medication treatment. *Behavior Therapy, 27,* 473–482.

Otto, M. W., Pollack, M. H., Sachs, G. S., O'Neil, C. A., & Rosenbaum, J. F. (1992). Alcohol dependence in panic disorder patients. *Journal of Psychiatric Research, 26*(1), 29–38.

Otto, M. W., Pollack, M. H., Sachs, G. S., Teiter, S. R., Meltzer-Brody, S., & Rosenbaum, J. F. (1993). Discontinuation of benzodiazepine treatment: Efficacy of cognitive-behavioral therapy for patients with panic disorder. *American Journal of Psychiatry, 150,* 1485–1490.

Overmier, J. B., & Seligman, M. E. P. (1967). Effects of inescapable shock upon subsequent escape and avoidance behavior. *Journal of Comparative and Physiological Psychology, 63,* 23–33.

Owens, M. J., Mulchahey, J. J., Stout, S. C., & Plotsky, P. M. (1997). Molecular and neurobiological mechanisms in the treatment of psychiatric disorders. In A. Tasman, J. Kay, & J. A. Lieberman (Eds.) *Psychiatry* (Vol. 1). Philadelphia: Saunders.

Page, A. C. (1994). Blood–injury phobia. *Clinical Psychology Review, 14,* 443–461.

Page, A. C., & Martin, N. G. (1998). Testing a genetic structure of blood–injury–injection fears. *American Journal of Medical Genetics, 81,* 377–384.

Palace, E. M. (1995). A cognitive–physiological process model of sexual arousal and response. *Clinical Psychology: Science and Practice, 2*(4), 370–384.

Palace, E. M., & Gorzalka, B. B. (1990). The enhancing effects of anxiety on arousal in sexually dysfunctional and functional women. *Journal of Abnormal Psychology, 99*(4), 403–411.

Panayiotou, G., & Vrana, S. R. (1998). Effects of self-focused attention on the startle reflex, heart rate, and memory performance among socially anxious and nonanxious individuals. *Psychophysiology, 35*(3), 328–336.

Panksepp, J. (1982). Toward a general psychobiological theory of emotions. *Behavioral and Brain Sciences, 5,* 407–422.

Panzarella, C., & Garlipp, J. (1999). Integration of cognitive techniques into an individualized application of behavioral treatment of blood–injection–injury phobia. *Cognitive and Behavioral Practice, 6,* 200–211.

Papp, L. A., Klein, D. F., & Gorman, J. M. (1993). Carbon dioxide sensitivity, hyperventilation, and panic disorder. *American Journal of Psychiatry, 150,* 1149–1157.

Papp, L. A., Klein, D. F., Martinez, J., Schneier, F., Cole, R., Liebowitz, M. R., Hollander, E., Fyer, A. J., Jordan, F., Gorman, J. M. (1993). Diagnostic and substance specificity of carbon-dioxide-induced panic. *American Journal of Psychiatry, 150,* 250–257.

Papp, L. A., Schneier, F. R., Fyer, A. J., Liebowitz, M. R., Gorman, J. M., Coplan, J. D., Campeas, R., Fallon, B. A., & Klein, D. F. (1997). Clomipramine treatment of panic disorder: Pros and cons. *Journal of Clinical Psychiatry, 58,* 423–425.

Papp, L. A., Sinha, S. S., Martinez, J. M., Coplan, J. D., Amchin, J., & Gorman, J. M. (1998). Low-dose venlafaxine treatment in panic disorder. *Psychopharmacology Bulletin, 34,* 207–209.

Paradis, C. M., Friedman, S., & Hatch, M. (1997). Isolated sleep paralysis in African Americans with panic disorder. *Cultural Diversity and Mental Health, 3*(1), 69–76.

Paradis, C. M., Hatch, M., & Friedman, S. (1994). Anxiety disorders in African Americans: An update. *Journal of the National Medical Association, 86,* 609–612.

Parker, G. (1979). Reported parental characteristics of agoraphobics and social phobics. *British Journal of Psychiatry, 135,* 555–560.

Parker, G. (1983). *Parental overprotection: A risk factor in psychosocial development.* New York: Grune & Stratton.

Parker, G., Tupling, H., & Brown, L. B. (1979). A parental bonding instrument. *British Journal of Psychiatry, 52,* 1–11.

Parkinson, L., & Rachman, S. (1981a). Intrusive thoughts: The effects of an uncontrived stress. *Advances in Behaviour Research and Therapy, 3,* 111–118.

Parkinson, L., & Rachman, S. (1981b). Speed of recovery from an uncontrived stress. *Advances in Behaviour Research and Therapy, 3,* 119–123.

Parkinson, L., & Rachman, S. (1981c). The nature of intrusive thoughts. *Advances in Behaviour Research and Therapy, 3,* 101–110.

Pato, M., Zohar-Kadouch, R., Zohar, J., & Murphy, D. (1988). Return of symptoms after discontinuation of clomirparmine in patients with obsessive compulsive disorder. *American Journal of Psychiatry, 145,* 1521–1525.

Patterson, M. L., & Ritts, V. (1997). Social and communicative anxiety: A review and meta-analysis. In B. R. Burleson (Ed.), *Communication yearbook 20.* Thousand Oaks, CA: Sage.

Paul, G. (1966). *Insight vs. desensitization in psychotherapy.* Stanford, CA: Stanford University Press.

Paul, S. M., & Skolnick, P. (1978). Rapid changes in brain benzodiazepine receptors after experimental seizures. *Science, 202,* 892–894.

Paul, S. M., & Skolnick, P. (1981). Benzodiazepine receptors and psychopathological states: Towards a neurobiology of anxiety. In D. F. Klein & J. Rabkin (Eds.), *Anxiety: New research and changing concepts.* New York: Raven Press.

Pauli, P., Dengler, W., Wiedemann, G., Montoya, P., Flor, H., Birbaumer, N., & Buchkremer, G. (1997). Behavioral and neurophysiological evidence for altered processing of anxiety-related words in panic disorder. *Journal of Abnormal Psychology, 106,* 213–220.

Pauli, P., Marquardt, C., Hartl, L., Nutzinger, D. O., Holzl, R., & Strian, F. (1991). Anxiety induced by cardiac perceptions in patients with panic attacks: A field study. *Behaviour Research and Therapy, 29,* 137–145.

Pauli, P., Wiedemann, G., & Montoya, P. (1998). Covariation bias in flight phobics. *Journal of Anxiety Disorders, 12,* 555–565.

Pauls, D. (1992). The genetics of obsessive compulsive disorder and Gilles de la Tourette's syndrome. *Psychiatric Clinics of North America, 15,* 759–766.

Pearce, J. M., & Hall, G. (1980). A model for Pavlovian learning: Variations in the effectiveness of conditioned but not of unconditioned stimuli. *Psychological Review, 87,* 532–552.

Peasley-Miklus, C., & Vrana, S. R. (2000). Effect of worrisome and relaxing thinking on fearful emotional processing. *Behaviour Research and Therapy, 38,* 129–144.

Pecknold, J. C. (1994). Serotonin 5-HT$_{1a}$ agonists: A comparative review. *CNS Drugs, 2,* 234–251.

Pecknold, J. C., Matas, M., Howarth, B. G., Ross, C., Swinson, R., Vezeau, C., & Ungar, W. (1989). Evaluation of buspirone as an antianxiety agent: Buspirone and diazepam versus placebo. *Canadian Journal of Psychiatry*, *34*, 766–771.

Pecknold, J. C., McClure, D. J., Appeltauer, L., Allan, T., & Wrzesinski, L. (1982). Does tryptophan potentiate clomipramine in the treatment of agoraphobic and social phobic patients? *British Journal of Psychiatry*, *140*, 484–490.

Pecknold, J. C., Swinson, R. P., Kuch, K., & Lewis, C. P. (1988). Alprazolam in panic disorder and agoraphobia: Results from a multicenter trial. Discontinuation effects. *Archives of General Psychiatry*, *45*, 429–436.

Penfold, K., & Page, A. C. (1999). The effect of distraction on within-session anxiety reduction during brief in vivo exposure for mild blood–injection fears. *Behavior Therapy*, *30*, 607–621.

Peniston, E. G. (1986). EMG biofeedback-assisted desensitization treatment for Vietnam combat veterans with post-traumatic stress disorder. *Clinical Biofeedback and Health: An International Journal*, *9*, 35–41.

Perconte, S. T., Wilson, A. T., Pontius, E. B., Dietrick, A. L., Kirsch, C., & Sparacino, C. (1993). Psychological and war stress symptoms among deployed and non-deployed reservists following the Persian Gulf War. *Military Medicine*, *158*, 516–521.

Perna, G., Bertani, A., Arancio, C., Ronchi, & Bellodi, L. (1995). Laboratory response of patients with panic and obsessive–compulsive disorders to 35% CO_2 challenges. *American Journal of Psychiatry*, *152*, 85–89.

Perna, G., Bertani, A., Politi, E., Columbo, G., & Bellodi, L. (1997). Asthma and panic attacks. *Biological Psychiatry*, *42*, 625–630.

Perna, G., Caldirola, D., Arancio, C., & Bellodi, L. (1997). Panic attacks: A twin study. *Psychiatry Research*, *66*, 665–673.

Person, D., & Borkovec, T. D. (1995, August). *Anxiety disorders in the elderly*. Paper presented at the 103rd Annual Convention of the American Psychological Association, New York.

Persons, J., & Foa, E. (1984). Processing of fearful and neutral information by obsessive compulsives. *Behaviour Research and Therapy*, *22*, 259–265.

Pervin, L. A. (1963). The need to predict and control under conditions of threat. *Journal of Personality*, *31*, 570–585.

Peterson, R. A., & Heilbroner, R. L. (1987). The Anxiety Sensitivity Index: Construct validity and factor analytic structure. *Journal of Anxiety Disorders*, *3*, 25–32.

Peterson, R. A., & Reiss, S. (1993). *Anxiety Sensitivity Index Revised test manual*. Worthington, OH: IDS.

Pfohl, B., & Blum, N. (1991). Obsessive compulsive personality disorder: A review of available data and recommendations for DSM-IV. *Journal of Personality Disorders*, *5*, 363–375.

Phillips, K., Fulker, D. W., & Rose, R. J. (1987). Path analysis of seven fear factors in adult twin and sibling pairs and their parents. *Genetic Epidemiology*, *4*, 345–355.

Pierce, K. A., & Kirkpatrick, D. R. (1992). Do men lie on fear surveys? *Behaviour Research and Therapy*, *30*, 415–418.

Pigott, T. A., & Seay, S. M. (1999). A review of the efficacy of selective serotonin reuptake inhibitors in obsessive–compulsive disorder. *Journal of Clinical Psychiatry*, *60*, 101–106.

Pilsbury, D., & Hibbert, G. (1987). An ambulatory system for long-term continuous monitoring of transcutaneous pCO_2. *Bulletin of European Physiopathology and Respiration*, *23*, 9–13.

Pine, D. S., Coplan, J. D., Papp, L. A., Klein, R. G., Martinez, J. M., Kovalenko, P., Tancer, N., Moreau, D., Dummit, E. S., III, Shaffer, D., & Klein, D. F. (1998). Ventilatory physiology of children and adolescents with anxiety disorders. *Archives of General Psychiatry*, *55*, 123–129.

Pine, D. S., Weese-Myer, D. E., Silvestri, J. M, Davies, M., Whitaker, A., & Klein, D. F. (1994). Anxiety and congenital central hypoventilation syndrome. *American Journal of Psychiatry*, *151*, 864–870.

Pitman, R. K. (2000). *A twin study of biological markers for posttraumatic stress disorder*. Unpublished manuscript, available from Research Service at VA Medical Center, Manchester, NH.

Pitman, R. K., & Orr, S. P. (1986). Test of the conditioning model of neurosis. Differential aversive conditioning of angry and neutral facial expressions in anxiety disorder patients. *Journal of Abnormal Psychology, 95,* 208–213.

Pitman, R. K., Orr, S. P., Altman, B., Longpre, R. E., Poire, H., & Macklin, M. (1996). Emotional processing during eye movement desensitization and reprocessing therapy of Vietnam veterans with chronic posttraumatic stress disorder. *Comprehensive Psychiatry, 37,* 419–429.

Pitman, R. K., Orr, S. P., Forgue, D. F., de Jong, P. J., & Claiborn, J. (1987). Psychophysiologic assessment of posttraumatic stress disorder imagery in Vietnam combat veterans. *Archives of General Psychiatry, 44,* 970–975.

Pitts, F. N., & Alan, R. (1979). Beta-adrenergic receptor blocking drugs in psychiatry. In W. E. Fann, I. Karacan, A. D. Pokomy, & R. L. Williams (Eds.), *Phenomenology and treatment of anxiety.* New York: Spectrum.

Pitts, F. N., & & McClure, J. N. (1967). Lactate metabolism in anxiety neurosis. *New England Journal of Medicine, 277,* 1329–1336.

Plomin, R., & Daniels, D. (1985). Origins of individual differences in infant shyness. *Developmental Psychology, 21,* 118–121.

Plomin, R., DeFries, J. C., McClearn, G. E., & Rutter, M. (1997). *Behavioral genetics: A primer* (3rd ed.). New York: Freeman.

Plomin, R., & Stocker, C. (1989). Behavioral genetics and emotionality. In J. S. Reznick (Ed.), *Perspectives on behavioral inhibition.* Chicago: University of Chicago Press.

Plutchik, R. (1980). *Emotion: A psychoevolutionary synthesis.* New York: Harper & Row.

Plutchik, R., & Conte, H. R. (Eds.). (1997). *Circumplex models of personality and emotions.* Washington, DC: American Psychological Association.

Pohl, R. B., Balon, R., Chapman, P., & McBride, J. (1998). *A new patient diary to study performance anxiety.* Poster presented at the 151st Annual Convention of the American Psychiatric Association, Toronto.

Pohl, R. B., Wolkow, R. M., & Clary, C. M. (1998). Sertraline in the treatment of panic disorder: A double-blind multicenter trial. *American Journal of Psychiatry, 155,* 1189–1195.

Pohl, R. B., Yeragani, V., Balon, R., Ortiz, A., & Aleem, A. (1990). Isoproterenol-induced panic: A beta-adrenergic model of panic anxiety. In J. C. Ballenger (Ed.), *Frontiers of clinical neuroscience: Vol. 8. Neurobiology of panic disorder.* New York: Wiley-Liss.

Pollack, M. H., Kradin, R., Otto, M. W., Worthington, J., Gould, R., Sabatino, S. A., & Rosenbaum, J. F. (1996). Prevalence of panic in patients referred for pulmonary function testing at a major medical center. *American Journal of Psychiatry, 153,* 110–113.

Pollack, M. H., Otto, M. W., Kaspi, S. P., Hammerness, P. G., & Rosenbaum, J. F. (1994). Cognitive behavior therapy for treatment-refractory panic disorder. *Journal of Clinical Psychiatry, 55,* 200–205.

Pollack, M. H., Otto, M. W., Rosenbaum, J. F., Sachs, G., O'Neil, C., Asher, R., & Meltzer-Brody, S. (1990). Longitudinal course of panic disorder: Findings from the Massachusetts General Hospital naturalistic study. *Journal of Clinical Psychiatry, 51,* 12–16.

Pollack, M. H., Otto, M. W., Worthington, J. J., Manfro, G. G., & Wolkow, R. (1998). Sertraline in the treatment of panic disorder. *Archives of General Psychiatry, 55,* 1010–1016.

Pollack, M. H., Worthington, J. J., Manfro, G. G., Otto, M. W., & Zucker, B. G. (1997). Abecarnil for the treatment of generalized anxiety disorder: A placebo-controlled comparison of two dosage ranges of abecarnil and buspirone. *Journal of Clinical Psychiatry, 58*(Suppl. 11), 19–23.

Pollack, M. H., Worthington, J. J., Otto, M. W., Maki, K. M., Smoller, J. W., Manfro, G. G., Rudolph, R., & Rosenbaum, J. F. (1996). Venlafaxine for panic disorder: Results from a double-blind placebo-controlled study. *Psychopharmacology Bulletin, 32,* 667–670.

Pollard, C. A., Bronson, S. S., & Kenney, M. R. (1989). Prevalence of agoraphobia without panic in clinical settings [Letter to the editor]. *American Journal of Psychiatry, 146,* 559.

Pollard, C. A., & Henderson, J. G. (1988). Four types of social phobia in a community sample. *Journal of Nervous and Mental Disease, 176,* 440–445.

Pollard, C. A., Pollard, H. J., & Corn, K. J. (1989). Panic onset and major events in the lives of agoraphobics: A test of contiguity. *Journal of Abnormal Psychology, 98*(3), 318–321.

Post, R. M., Rubinow, D. R., & Ballenger, J. C. (1986). Conditioning and sensitization in the longitudinal course of affective illness. *British Journal of Psychiatry, 149,* 191–201.

Post, R. M., Rubinow, D. R., Uhde, T. W., Roy-Byrne, P., Linnoila, M., Rosoff, A., & Cowdry, R. (1989). Dysphoric mania: Clinical and biological correlates. *Archives of General Psychiatry, 46,* 353–358.

Poulton, R., Davies, S., Menzies, R. G., Langley, J. D., & Silva, P. A. (1998). Evidence for a nonassociative model of the acquisition of a fear of heights. *Behaviour Research and Therapy, 36,* 537–544.

Poulton, R., Menzies, R. G., Craske, M. G., Langley, J. D., & Silva, P. A. (1999). Water trauma and swimming experiences up to age 9 and fear of water at age 18: A longitudinal study. *Behaviour Research and Therapy, 37,* 39–48.

Pourmotabbed, T., McLeod, D. R., Hoehn-Saric, R., Hipsley, P., & Greenblatt, D. J. (1996). Treatment, discontinuation, and psychomotor effects of diazepam in women with generalized anxiety disorder. *Journal of Clinical Psychopharmacology, 16,* 202–207.

Powell, B. J., Penick, E. C., Othmer, E., Bingham, S. F., & Rice, A. S. (1982). Prevalence of additional psychiatric syndromes among male alcoholics. *Journal of Clinical Psychiatry, 43,* 404–407.

Powell, G. E. (1979). *Brain and personality.* London: Saxon House.

Power, K. G., Jerrom, D. W., Simpson, R. J., Mitchell, M. J., & Swanson, V. (1989). A controlled comparison of cognitive behaviour therapy, diazepam and placebo in the management of generalized anxiety. *Behavioural Psychotherapy, 17,* 1–14.

Power, K. G., Simpson, M. B., Swanson, V., & Wallace, L. A. (1990). A controlled comparison of cognitive-behaviour therapy, diazepam, and placebo, alone and in combination, for the treatment of generalised anxiety disorder. *Journal of Anxiety Disorders, 4,* 267–292.

Prigatano, G. P., & Johnson, H. J. (1974). Autonomic nervous system changes associated with a spider phobic reaction. *Journal of Abnormal Psychology, 83,* 169–177.

Prins, A., Kaloupek, D. G., & Keane, T. M. (1995). Psychophysiological evidence for autonomic arousal and startle in traumatized adult populations. In M. J. Friedman, D. S. Charney, & A. Deutch (Eds.), *Neurobiological and clinical consequences of stress: From normal adaptation to post-traumatic stress disorder.* New York: Raven Press.

Pruzinsky, T., & Borkovec, T. D. (1983, December). *Cognitive characteristics of chronic worriers.* Paper presented at the 17th Annual Convention of the Association for Advancement of Behavior Therapy, Washington, DC.

Purdon, C. (1999). Thought suppression and psychopathology. *Behaviour Research and Therapy, 37,* 1029–1054.

Pury, C. L. S., & Mineka, S. (1997). Covariation bias for blood–injury stimuli and aversive outcomes. *Behaviour Research and Therapy, 35,* 35–47.

Pylyshyn, Z. W. (1973). What the mind's eye tells the mind's brain: A critique of mental imagery. *Psychological Bulletin, 80,* 1–22.

Quitkin, F. M., Rifkin, A., Kaplan, J., & Klein, D. F. (1972). Phobic anxiety syndrome complicated by drug dependence and addiction. *Archives of General Psychiatry, 27,* 159–162.

Rachman, S. J. (1973). Some similarities and differences between obsessional ruminations and morbid preoccupations. *Canadian Psychiatric Association Journal, 18,* 71–74.

Rachman, S. J. (1974). Primary obsessional slowness. *Behaviour Research and Therapy, 12,* 9–18.

Rachman, S. J. (1976a). Obsessional–compulsive checking. *Behaviour Research and Therapy, 14,* 269–277.

Rachman, S. J. (1976b). The passing of the two-stage theory of fear and avoidance: Fresh possibilities. *Behaviour Research and Therapy, 14,* 125–131.

Rachman, S. J. (1977). The conditioning theory of fear acquisition: A critical examination. *Behaviour Research and Therapy, 15,* 375–387.

Rachman, S. J. (1978). *Fear and courage.* San Francisco: Freeman.

Rachman, S. J. (1979). The concept of required helpfulness. *Behaviour Research and Therapy, 17,* 279–293.

Rachman, S. J. (1980). Emotional processing. *Behaviour Research and Therapy, 18,* 51–60.

Rachman, S. J. (1983). The modification of agoraphobic avoidance behaviour. *Behaviour Research and Therapy, 21,* 567–574.

Rachman, S. J. (1984). Agoraphobia: A safety-signal perspective. *Behaviour Research and Therapy, 22,* 59–70.

Rachman, S. J. (1989). The return of fear: Review and prospect. *Clinical Psychology Review, 9,* 147–168.

Rachman, S. J. (1991). Neo-conditioning and the classical theory of fear acquisition. *Clinical Psychology Review, 11,* 155–173.

Rachman, S. J. (1993). Obsessions, responsibility and guilt. *Behaviour Research and Therapy, 31,* 149–154.

Rachman, S. J. (1997). A cognitive theory of obsessions. *Behaviour Research and Therapy, 35,* 793–802.

Rachman, S. J., Cobb, J., Grey, S., McDonald, B., Mawson, D., Sartory, G., & Stern, R. (1979). The behavioural treatment of obsessive–compulsive disorders, with and without clomipramine. *Behaviour Research and Therapy, 17,* 467–478.

Rachman, S. J., Craske, M. G., Tallman, K., & Solyom, C. (1986). Does escape behaviour strengthen agoraphobic avoidance?: A replication. *Behavior Therapy, 17,* 366–384.

Rachman, S. J., & Cuk, M. (1992). Fearful distortions. *Behaviour Research and Therapy, 30,* 583–589.

Rachman, S. J., & de Silva, P. (1978). Abnormal and normal obsessions. *Behaviour Research and Therapy, 16,* 233–248.

Rachman, S. J., & Hodgson, R. J. (1980). *Obsessions and compulsions.* Englewood Cliffs, NJ: Prentice-Hall.

Rachman, S. J., Levitt, K., & Lopatka, C. (1987). Panic: The links between cognitions and bodily symptoms: I. *Behavior Research and Therapy, 25*(5), 411–423.

Rachman, S. J., & Lopatka, C. (1988). Return of fear: Underlearning and overlearning. *Behaviour Research and Therapy, 26,* 99–104.

Rachman, S. J., Robinson, S., & Lopatka, C. (1987). Is incomplete fear reduction followed by a return of fear? *Behaviour Research and Therapy, 25,* 67–69.

Rachman, S. J., & Whittal, M. (1989). The effect of an aversive event on the return of fear. *Behaviour Research and Therapy, 27,* 513–520.

Radomsky, A. S., Teachman, B., Baker, V., & Rachman, S. (1996, November). *Perceptual distortions and cognitions of feared stimuli.* Paper presented at the 30th Annual Convention of the Association for Advancement of Behavior Therapy, New York.

Raguram, R., & Bhide, A. V. (1985). Patterns of phobic neurosis: A retrospective study. *British Journal of Psychiatry, 147,* 557–560.

Rainey, J. M., Ettedgui, E., Pohl, R. B., & Bridges, M. (1985). Effect of acute β-adrenergic blockade on lactate-induced panic. *Archives of General Psychiatry, 42,* 104–105.

Rainey, J. M., Pohl, R. B., Williams, M., Kritter, E., Freedman, R. R., & Ettedgui, E. (1984). A comparison of lactate and isoproterenol anxiety states. *Psychopathology, 17,* 74–82.

Ramsey, G. (1943). The sexual development of boys. *American Journal of Psychology, 56,* 217.

Rao, A. V. A. (1964). A controlled trial with "Valium" in obsessive–compulsive state. *Journal of the Indian Medical Association, 42,* 564–567.

Rapaport, M. H., Frevert, T., Babvior, S., Seymour, S., Zisook, S. Kelsoe, J., & Judd, L. L. (1996). Comparison of descriptive variables for symptomatic volunteers and clinical patients with anxiety disorders. *Anxiety, 2,* 117–122.

Rapee, R. M. (1985). A distinction between panic disorder and generalized anxiety disorder: Clinical presentation. *Australian and New Zealand Journal of Psychiatry, 19,* 227–232.

Rapee, R. M. (1986). Differential response to hyperventilation in panic disorder and generalized anxiety disorder. *Journal of Abnormal Psychology, 95,* 24–28.

Rapee, R. M. (1991). Generalized anxiety disorder: A review of clinical features and theoretical concepts. *Clinical Psychology Review, 11,* 419–440.

Rapee, R. M. (1993). The utilisation of working memory by worry. *Behaviour Research and Therapy*, *31*(6), 617–620.

Rapee, R. M. (1994a). Failure to replicate a memory bias in panic disorder. *Journal of Anxiety Disorders*, *8*, 291–300.

Rapee, R. M. (1994b). Detection of somatic sensations in panic disorder. *Behaviour Research and Therapy*, *32*, 825–831.

Rapee, R. M. (1997). Potential role of childrearing practices in the development of anxiety and depression. *Clinical Psychology Review*, *17*, 47–67.

Rapee, R. M., Ancis, J. R., & Barlow, D. H. (1988). Emotional reactions to physiological sensations: Panic disorder patients and nonclinical subjects. *Behaviour Research and Therapy*, *26*, 265–269.

Rapee, R. M., Brown, T. A., Antony, M. M., & Barlow, D. H. (1992). Response to hyperventilation and inhalation of 5.5% carbon dioxide-enriched air across the DSM-III-R anxiety disorders. *Journal of Abnormal Psychology*, *101*, 538–552.

Rapee, R. M., Craske, M. G., & Barlow, D. H. (1990). Subject described features of panic attacks using a new self-monitoring form. *Journal of Anxiety Disorders*, *4*, 171–181.

Rapee, R. M., Craske, M. G., & Barlow, D. H. (1995). Assessment instrument for panic disorder that includes fear of sensation–producing activities: The Albany Panic and Phobia Questionnaire. *Anxiety*, *1*, 114–122.

Rapee, R. M., Craske, M., Brown, T. A., & Barlow, D. H. (1996). Measurement of perceived control over anxiety-related events. *Behavior Therapy*, *27*, 279–293.

Rapee, R. M., & Heimberg, R. G. (1997). A cognitive-behavioral model of anxiety in social phobia. *Behaviour Research and Therapy*, *35*, 741–756.

Rapee, R. M., & Lim, L. (1992). Discrepancy between self- and observer ratings of performance in social phobics. *Journal of Abnormal Psychology*, *101*, 728–731.

Rapee, R. M., Litwin, E. M., & Barlow, D. H. (1990). Impact of life events on subjects with panic disorder and on comparison subjects. *American Journal of Psychiatry*, *147*, 640–644.

Rapee, R. M., Matttick, R., & Murrell, E. (1986). Cognitive mediation in the affective component of spontaneous panic attacks. *Journal of Behavior Therapy and Experimental Psychiatry*, *17*, 245–253.

Rapee, R. M., McCallum, S. L., Melville, L. F., Ravenscroft, H., & Rodney, J. M. (1994). Memory bias in social phobia. *Behaviour Research and Therapy*, *32*, 89–99.

Rapee, R. M., & Sanderson, W. C. (1998). *Social phobia: Clinical application of evidence-based psychotherapy*. Northvale, NJ: Jason Aronson.

Rapee, R. M., Sanderson, W. C., & Barlow, D. H. (1987, November). *Social phobia symptoms across the DSM-III anxiety disorders categories*. Paper presented at the 21st Annual Convention of the Association for Advancement of Behavior Therapy, Boston.

Rapee, R. M., Sanderson, W. C., & Barlow, D. H. (1988). Social phobia features across the DSM-III-R anxiety disorders. *Journal of Psychopathology and Behavioral Assessment*, *10*, 287–299.

Rapee, R. M., Sanderson, W. C., McCauley, P. A., & Di Nardo, P. A. (1992). Differences in reported symptom profile between panic disorder and other DSM-III-R anxiety disorders. *Behaviour Research and Therapy*, *30*, 45–52.

Rapee, R. M., Telfer, L. A., & Barlow, D. H. (1991). The role of safety cues in mediating response to inhalations of CO_2 in agoraphobics. *Behaviour Research and Therapy*, *29*, 353–355.

Rapoport, J. L. (1989). *Obsessive–compulsive disorder in children and adolescents*. Washington, DC: American Psychiatric Press.

Raskin, M. (1975). Decreased skin conductance response habituation in chronically anxious patients. *Biological Psychology*, *2*, 309–319.

Raskin, M., Peeke, H. V. S., Dickman, W., & Pinkster, H. (1982). Panic and generalized anxiety disorders: Developmental antecedents and precipitants. *Archives of General Psychiatry*, *39*, 687–689.

Rasmussen, S. A., & Eisen, J. L. (1989). Clinical features and phenomenology of obsessive compulsive disorder. *Psychiatric Annuals*, *19*, 67–73.

Rasmussen, S. A., & Eisen, J. (1990). Epidemiology and clinical features of obsessive–compulsive disorder. In M. A. Jenike, L. Baer, & W. E. Minichiello (Eds.), *Obsessive–compulsive disorders: Theory and management.* Chicago: Year Book Medical.

Rasmussen, S. A., & Eisen, J. L. (1991). Phenomenology of obsessive compulsive disorder. In J. Zohar, T. Insel, & S. Rasmussen (Ed.). *Psychobiology of obsessive compulsive disorder.* New York: Springer-Verlag.

Rasmussen, S. A., & Eisen, J. L. (1992a). The epidemiology and clinical features of obsessive compulsive disorder. *Psychiatric Clinics of North America, 15,* 743–758.

Rasmussen, S. A., & Eisen, J. L. (1992b). The epidemiology and differential diagnosis of obsessive compulsive disorder. *Journal of Clinical Psychiatry, 53,* 4–10.

Rasmussen, S. A., & Tsuang, M. T. (1986). Clinical characteristics and family history in DSM-III obsessive–compulsive disorder. *American Journal of Psychiatry, 143,* 317–322.

Rathus, J. H., Sanderson, W. C., Miller, A. L., & Wetzler, S. (1995). Impact of personality functioning on cognitive behavioral treatment of panic disorder: A preliminary report. *Journal of Personality Disorders, 9,* 160–168.

Rauch, S. L., Savage, C. R., Alpert, N. M., Miguel, E. C., Baer, L., Breiter, H. C., Fischman, A. J., Manzo, P. A., Moretti, C., & Jenike, M. A. (1995). A positron emission tomographic study of simple phobic symptom provocation. *Archives of General Psychiatry, 52,* 20–28.

Razran, G. (1961). The observable unconscious and the inferable conscious in current Soviet psychophysiology: Interoceptive conditioning, semantic conditioning, and the orienting reflex. *Psychological Review, 68,* 81–150.

Redd, W. H., & Andrykowski, M. A. (1982). Behavioral interventions in cancer treatment: Controlling aversion reactions to chemotherapy. *Journal of Consulting and Clinical Psychology, 50,* 1018–1029.

Redmond, D. E., Jr. (1977). Alterations in the function of the nucleus locus coeruleus: A possible model for studies of anxiety. In I. Hanin & E. Usdin (Eds.), *Animal models in psychiatry and neurology.* New York: Pergamon Press.

Redmond, D. E., Jr. (1979). New and old evidence for the involvement of a brain norepinephrine system in anxiety. In W. E. Fann, I. Karacan, A. D. Pokorny, & R. L. Williams (Eds.), *Phenomenology and treatment of anxiety.* New York: Spectrum.

Redmond, D. E., Jr., & Huang, V. H. (1979). Current concepts: II. New evidence for a locus coeruleus–norepinephrine connection with anxiety. *Life Sciences, 25,* 2149–2162.

Reed, G. F. (1985). *Obsessional experience and compulsive behavior: A cognitive-structured approach.* New York: Academic Press.

Rees, C. S., Richards, J. C., & Smith, L. M. (1998). Medical utilisation and costs in panic disorder: A comparison with social phobia. *Journal of Anxiety Disorders, 12,* 421–435.

Rehm, L. P., & Marston, A. R. (1968). Reduction of social anxiety through modification of self-reinforcement: An investigation therapy technique. *Journal of Consulting and Clinical Psychology, 32,* 565–574.

Reich, J., Noyes, R., & Troughton, E. (1987). Dependent personality disorder associated with phobic avoidance in patients with panic disorder. *American Journal of Psychiatry, 144,* 323–326.

Reich, J., & Yates, W. (1988). A pilot study of treatment of social phobia with alprazolam. *American Journal of Psychiatry, 145,* 590–594.

Reisenzein, R. (1983). The Schachter theory of emotion: Two decades later. *Psychological Bulletin, 94,* 239–264.

Reiss, D., Hetherington, E. M., Plomin, R., Howe, G. W., Simmens, S. J., Henderson, S. H., O'Connor, T. J., Bussell, D. A., Anderson, E. R., & Law, T. (1995). Genetic questions for environmental studies: Differential parenting and psychopathology in adolescence. *Archives of General Psychiatry, 52,* 925–936.

Reiss, S. (1987). Theoretical perspectives on the fear of anxiety. *Clinical Psychology Review, 7,* 585–596.

Reiss, S. (1991). Expectancy model of fear, anxiety, and panic. *Clinical Psychology Review, 11,* 141–153.

Reiss, S., Peterson, R. A., Gursky, D. M., & McNally, R. J. (1986). Anxiety sensitivity, anxiety frequency, and the prediction of fearfulness. *Behaviour Research and Therapy, 24,* 1–8.

Reiter, S. R., Pollack, M. H., Rosenbaum, J. F., & Cohen, L. S. (1990). Clonazepam for the treatment of social phobia. *Journal of Clinical Psychiatry, 51,* 470–472.

Renfrey, G., & Spates, C. R. (1994). Eye movement desensitization: A partial dismantling study. *Journal of Behavior Therapy and Experimental Psychiatry, 25,* 231–239.

Rescorla, R. A., & Wagner, A. R. (1972). A theory of Pavlovian conditioning: Variations in the effectiveness of reinforcement and non-reinforcement. In A. H. Black & W. F. Prokasy (Eds.), *Classical conditioning II: Current research and theory.* New York: Appleton-Century-Crofts.

Resick, P. A., Nishith, P. & Astin, M. (2000). *A comparison of cognitive processing therapy and prolonged exposure: A randomized controlled clinical trial.* Paper presented at the World Conference of the International Society for Traumatic Stress Studies, Melbourne, Australia.

Resick, P. A., & Schnicke, M. K. (1992). Cognitive processing therapy for sexual assault victims. *Journal of Consulting and Clinical Psychology, 60,* 748–756.

Resnick, H. S., Kilpatrick, D. G., Dansky, B. S., Saunders, B. E., & Best, C. L. (1993). Prevalence of civilian trauma and posttraumatic stress disorder in a representative national sample of women. *Journal of Consulting and Clinical Psychology, 61,* 984–991.

Reynolds, D. (1976). *Morita psychotherapy.* Berkeley: University of California Press.

Rhéaume, J., & Ladouceur, R. (2000). Cognitive and behavioral treatments of checking behaviours: An examination of individual cognitive change. *Clinical Psychology and Psychotherapy, 7,* 118–127.

Rhéaume, J., Freeston, M. H., Dugas, M., Letarte, H., & Ladouceur, R. (1995). Perfectionism, responsibility and obsessive compulsive symptoms. *Behaviour Research and Therapy, 33,* 785–794.

Rhéaume, J., Freeston, M. H., Leger, E., & Ladouceur, R. (1998). Bad luck: An underestimated factor in the development of obsessive–compulsive disorder. *Clinical Psychology and Psychotherapy, 5,* 1–12.

Rice, D. P., & Miller, L. S. (1993). The economic burden of mental disorders. *Advances in Health Economics and Health Services Research, 14,* 37–53.

Richards, D. A., Lovell, K., & Marks, I. M. (1994). Post-traumatic stress disorder: Evaluation of a behavioral treatment program. *Journal of Traumatic Stress, 7,* 669–680.

Richmond, V. P., & McCroskey, J. C. (1992). *Communication: Apprehension, avoidance, and effectiveness* (3rd ed.). Scottsdale, AZ: Gorsuch Scarisbrick.

Rickels, K. (1985). Alprazolam in the management of anxiety. In M. H. Lader & H. C. Davies (Eds.), *Drug treatment of neurotic disorders: Focus on alprazolam.* Edinburgh: Churchill Livingstone.

Rickels, K., Case, W. G., Downing, R. W., & Winokur, A. (1983). Long-term diazepam therapy and clinical outcome. *Journal of the American Medical Association, 250,* 767–771.

Rickels, K., Case, W. G., Schweizer, E. E., Swenson, C., & Fridman, R. B. (1986). Low-dose dependence in chronic benzodiazepine users: A preliminary report on 119 patients. *Psychopharmacology Bulletin, 22,* 407–415.

Rickels, K., DeMartinis, N., & Aufdembrinke, B. (2000). A double-blind, placebo-controlled trial of abecarnil and diazepam in the treatment of patients with generalized anxiety disorder. *Journal of Clinical Psychopharmacology, 20,* 12–18.

Rickels, K., Downing, R., Schweizer, E., & Hassman, H. (1993). Antidepressants for the treatment of generalized anxiety disorder. *Archives of General Psychiatry, 50,* 884–895.

Rickels, K., Pollack, M. H., Sheehan, D. V., & Haskins, J. T. (2000). Efficacy of extended-release venlafaxine in nondepressed outpatients with generalized anxiety disorder. *American Journal of Psychiatry, 157,* 968–974.

Rickels, K., & Schweizer, E. (1998). The spectrum of generalized anxiety in clinical practice: The role of short-term, intermittent treatment. *British Journal of Psychiatry, 173*(Suppl. 34), 49–54.

Rickels, K., Schweizer, E., Csanalosi, I., Case, W. G., & Chung, H. (1988). Long-term treatment of anxiety and risk of withdrawal. *Archives of General Psychiatry, 45,* 444–450.

Rickels, K., Weisman, K., Norstad, N., Singer, M., Stoltz, K., Brown, A., & Danton, J. (1982). Buspirone and diazepam in anxiety: A controlled study. *Journal of Clinical Psychiatry, 43,* 81–86.

Ries, B. J., McNeil, D. W., Boone, M. L., Turk, C. L., Carter, L. E., & Heimberg, R. G. (1998). Assessment of contemporary social phobia verbal report instrument. *Behaviour Research and Therapy, 36,* 983–994.

Rimm, D. C., Janda, L. H., Lancaster, D. W., Nahl, M., & Dittmar, K. (1977). An exploratory investigation of the origin and maintenance of phobias. *Behaviour Research and Therapy, 15,* 231–238.

Riordan, C. (1979). *Interpersonal attraction in aversive situations.* Unpublished doctoral dissertation, State University of New York at Albany.

Riskind, J. H., Beck, A. T., Berchick, R. J., Brown, G., & Steer, R. A. (1987). Reliability of the DSM-III-R diagnoses for major depression and generalized anxiety disorder using the Structured Clinical Interview for DSM-III-R. *Archives of General Psychiatry, 44,* 817–820.

Riskind, J. H., Beck, A. T., Brown, G., & Steer, R. A. (1987). Taking the measure of anxiety and depression: Validity of the reconstructed Hamilton Scales. *Journal of Nervous and Mental Disease, 175,* 474–479.

Riskind, J. H., Moore, R., & Bowley, L. (1995). The looming of spiders: The fearful perceptual distortion of movement and menace. *Behaviour Research and Therapy, 33,* 171–178.

Robins, L. N., Helzer, J. E., Croughan, J. L., & Ratcliff, K. S. (1981). National Institute of Mental Health Diagnostic Interview Schedule: Its history, characteristics, and validity. *Archives of General Psychiatry, 38,* 381–389.

Robins, L. N., Helzer, J. E., Weissman, M. M., Orvaschel, H., Gruenberg, E., Burke, J. D., & Regier, D. A. (1984). Prevalence of specific psychiatric disorders in three sites. *Archives of General Psychiatry, 41,* 949–958.

Robins, S., & Novaco, R. W. (2000). Anger control as a health promotion mechanism. In D. I. Mostofsky & D. H. Barlow (Eds.), *The management of stress and anxiety in medical disorders.* Needham Heights, MA: Allyn & Bacon.

Robinson, J. L., Kagan, J., Reznick, J. S., & Corley, R. (1992). The heritability of inhibited and uninhibited behavior: A twin study. *Developmental Psychology, 28,* 1030–1037.

Rocca, P., Beoni, A. M., Eva, C., Ferrero, P., Zanalda, E., & Ravizza, L. (1998). Peripheral benzodiazepine receptor messenger RNA is decreased in lymphocytes of generalized anxiety disorder patients. *Biological Psychiatry, 43,* 767–773.

Rocca, P., Fonzo, V., Scotta, M., Zanalda, E., & Ravizza, L. (1997). Paroxetine efficacy in the treatment of generalized anxiety disorder. *Acta Psychiatrica Scandinavica, 95,* 444–450.

Rodin, J., & Langer, E. J. (1977). Long-term effects of a control-relevant intervention with the institutionalized aged. *Journal of Personality and Social Psychology, 35*(12), 897–902.

Rodriguez, B. I., & Craske, M. G. (1993). The effects of distraction during exposure to phobic stimuli. *Behaviour Research and Therapy, 31,* 549–558.

Rodriguez, B. I., & Craske, M. G. (1995). Does distraction interfere with fear reduction during exposure? A test among animal-fearful subjects. *Behavior Therapy, 26,* 337–349.

Rodriguez, B. I., Craske, M. G., Mineka, S., & Hladek, D. (1999). Context-specificity of relapse: Effects of therapist and environmental context on return of fear. *Behaviour Research and Therapy, 37,* 845–862.

Roemer, L., & Borkovec, T. D. (1993). Worry: Unwanted cognitive experience that controls unwanted somatic experience. In D. M. Wegner & J. Pennebaker (Eds.), *Handbook of mental control.* Englewood Cliffs, NJ: Prentice-Hall.

Roemer, L., Borkovec, M., Posa, S., & Borkovec, T. D. (1995). A self-report diagnostic measure of generalized anxiety disorder. *Journal of Behavior Therapy and Experimental Psychiatry, 26,* 345–350.

Roemer, L., Molina, S., & Borkovec, T. D. (1997). An investigation of worry content among generally anxious individuals. *Journal of Nervous and Mental Disease, 185*(5), 314–319.

Roemer, L., & Orsillo, S. M. (in press). Expanding our conceptualization of and treatment for generalized anxiety disorder: Integrating mindfulness/acceptance-based approaches with existing cognitive-behavioral models. *Clinical Psychology: Science and Practice.*

Rogers, M., White, K., Warshaw, M., Yonkers, K., Rodriguez-Villa, R, Chang, G., & Keller, M. B. (1994). Prevalence of medical illness in patients with anxiety disorders. *International Journal of Psychiatry in Medicine, 24,* 83–96.

Romach, M. K., Somer, G. R., Sobell, L. C., Sobell, M. B., Kaplan, H. L., & Sellers, E. M. (1992). Characteristics of long-term alprazolam users in the community. *Journal of Clinical Psychopharmacology, 12,* 316–321.

Rose, M. P., & McGlynn, F. D. (1997). Toward a standard experiment for studying post-treatment return of fear. *Journal of Anxiety Disorders, 11,* 263–277.

Rose, M. P., McGlynn, F. D., & Lazarte, A. (1995). Control and attention influence snake phobics' arousal and fear during laboratory confrontations with a caged snake. *Journal of Anxiety Disorders, 9,* 293–302.

Rose, R. J., & Chesney, M. A. (1986). Cardiovascular stress reactivity: A behavior-genetic perspective. *Behavior Therapy, 17,* 314–323.

Rose, R. J., & Ditto, W. B. (1983). A developmental-genetic analysis of common fears from early adolescence to early adulthood. *Child Development, 54,* 361–368.

Rosellini, R. A., Warren, D. A., & DeCola, J. P. (1987). Predictability and controllability: Differential effects upon contextual fear. *Learning and Motivation, 18,* 392–420.

Rosen, J. B., & Schulken, J. (1998). From normal fear to pathological anxiety. *Psychological Review, 105,* 325–350.

Rosenbaum, J. F., Biederman, J., Hirshfeld, D. R., Bolduc, E. A., & Chaloff, J. (1991). Behavioral inhibition in children: A possible precursor to panic disorder and social phobia. *Journal of Clinical Psychiatry, 52,* 5–9.

Rosenbaum, J. F., Biederman, J., Pollack, R. A., & Hirshfeld, D. R. (1994). The etiology of social phobia. *Journal of Clinical Psychiatry, 55,* 10–16.

Rosenbaum, J. F., Fava, M., Pava, J. A., McCarthy, J. K., Steingard, R. J., & Bouffides, E. (1993). Anger attacks in unipolar depression: Part 2. Neuroendocrine correlates and changes following fluoxetine treatment. *American Journal of Psychiatry, 150*(8), 1164–1168.

Rosenberg, A., & Kagan, J. (1987). Iris pigmentation and behavioral inhibition. *Developmental Psychobiology, 20,* 377–392.

Rosenman, R. H., & Swan, G. E. (1988). Some relationships of contrasting emotions to cardiovascular disorders. *Stress Medicine, 4,* 27–32.

Roth, M. (1959). The phobic anxiety–depersonalization syndrome. *Proceedings of the Royal Society of Medicine, 52,* 587–596.

Roth, M. (1960). The phobic anxiety–depersonalization syndrome and some general aetiological problems in psychiatry. *Journal of Neuropsychiatry, 306,* 293–306.

Roth, S., & Friedman, M. J. (Eds.). (1998). Childhood trauma remembered: A report on the current scientific knowledge base and its applications. *Journal of Child Sexual Abuse, 7,* 83–109.

Roth, W. T., Margraf, J., Ehlers, A., Taylor, C. B., Maddock, R. J., Davies, S., & Agras, W. S. (1992). Stress test reactivity in panic disorder. *Archives of General Psychiatry, 49,* 301–310.

Rothbaum, B. O. (1997). A controlled study of eye movement desensitization and reprocessing in the treatment of posttraumatic stress disordered sexual assault victims. *Bulletin of the Menninger Clinic, 61,* 317–334.

Rothbaum, B. O., & Hodges, L. F. (1999). The use of virtual reality exposure in the treatment of anxiety disorders. *Behavior Modification, 23,* 507–525.

Rothbaum, B. O., Hodges, L. F., Kooper, R., Opdyke, D., Williford, J. S., & North, M. (1995a). Virtual reality graded exposure in the treatment of acrophobia: A case report. *Behavior Therapy, 26,* 547–554.

Rothbaum, B. O., Hodges, L. F., Kooper, R., Opdyke, D., Williford, J. S., & North, M. (1995b).

Effectiveness of computer-generated (virtual reality) graded exposure in the treatment of acrophobia. *American Journal of Psychiatry, 152,* 626–628.

Rothbaum, B. O., Hodges, L. F., & Smith, S. (1999). Virtual reality exposure therapy abbreviated treatment manual: Fear of flying application. *Cognitive and Behavioral Practice, 6,* 234–244.

Rothbaum, B. O., Hodges, L. F., Smith, S., Lee, J. H., & Price, L. (2000). A controlled study of virtual reality exposure therapy for the fear of flying. *Journal of Consulting and Clinical Psychology, 68,* 1020–1026.

Rothbaum, B. O., Hodges, L. F., Watson, B. A., Kessler, G. D., & Opdyke, D. (1996). Virtual reality exposure therapy in the treatment of fear of flying: A case report. *Behaviour Research and Therapy, 34,* 477–481.

Rothenberg, A. (1986). Eating disorder as a modern obsessive compulsive syndrome. *Psychiatry, 49,* 45–53.

Rotter, J. B. (1954). *Social learning and clinical psychology.* Englewood Cliffs, NJ: Prentice-Hall.

Rotter, J. B. (1966). Generalized expectancies for internal versus external control of reinforcement. *Psychological Monographs, 80*(1, Whole No. 609).

Rowe, M. K., & Craske, M. G. (1998a). Effects of an expanding–spaced vs. massed exposure schedule on fear reduction and return of fear. *Behaviour Research and Therapy, 36,* 701–717.

Rowe, M. K., & Craske, M. G. (1998b). Effects of varied-stimulus exposure training on fear reduction and return of fear. *Behaviour Research and Therapy, 36,* 719–734.

Rowland, D. L., Cooper, S. E., & Heiman, J. R. (1995). A preliminary investigation of affective and cognitive response to erotic stimulation in men before and after sex therapy. *Journal of Sex and Marital Therapy, 21*(1), 3–20.

Roy, M. A., Neale, M. C., Pedersen, N. L., Mathé, A. A., & Kendler, K. S. (1995). A twin study of generalized anxiety disorder and major depression. *Psychological Medicine, 25,* 1037–1040.

Roy-Byrne, P. P. (1996). Generalized anxiety and mixed anxiety–depression: Association with disability and health care utilization. *Journal of Clinical Psychiatry, 57,* 86–91.

Roy-Byrne, P. P., & Cowley, D. S. (1995). Course and outcome in panic disorder: A review of recent follow-up studies. *Anxiety, 1,* 151–160.

Roy-Byrne, P. P., Geraci, M., & Uhde, T. W. (1986). Life events and the onset of panic disorder. *American Journal of Psychiatry, 143,* 1424–1427.

Roy-Byrne, P. P., & Katon, W. (1997). Generalized anxiety disorder in primary care: The precursor/modifier pathway to increased health care utilization. *Journal of Clinical Psychiatry, 58,* 34–38.

Roy-Byrne, P. P., & Katon, W. (2000). Anxiety management in the medical setting: Rationale, barriers to diagnosis and treatment, and proposed solutions. In D. I. Mostofsky & D. H. Barlow (Eds.). *The management of stress and anxiety in medical disorders.* Boston. Allyn & Bacon.

Roy-Byrne, P. P., Stein, M., Russo, J., Mercier, E., Thomas, R., McQuaid, J., Katon, W., Craske, M., Bystrisky, S., & Sherbourne, C. (1999). Panic disorder in the primary care setting: Comorbidity, disability, service utilization, and treatment. *Journal of Clinical Psychiatry, 60,* 492–499.

Roy-Byrne, P. P., Wingerson, D., Cowley, D., & Dager, S. (1993). Psychopharmacologic treatment of panic, generalized anxiety disorder, and social phobia. *Psychiatric Clinics of North America, 16,* 719–735.

Rusalova, M. N., Izard, C. E., & Simonov, P. V. (1975, September). Comparative analysis of mimical and autonomic components of man's emotional state. *Aviation, Space, and Environmental Medicine,* 1132–1134.

Rush, A. J., & Weissenburger, J. E. (1998). *Melancholic symptom features: A review and commentary for DSM-IV.* Unpublished manuscript.

Russell, J. A. (1980). A circumplex model of affect. *Journal of Personality and Social Psychology, 39,* 1161–1178.

Russell, J. A. (1991). Culture and the categorization of emotions. *Psychological Bulletin, 110,* 426–450.

Russell, J. A., & Carroll, J. M. (1999). On the bipolarity of positive and negative affect. *Psychological Bulletin, 125,* 3–30.

Russell, J. A., & Mehrabian, A. (1977). Evidence for a three-factor theory of emotions. *Journal of Research in Personality, 11,* 273–294.

Rutter, M. (1980). Attachment and the development of social relationships. In M. Rutter (Ed.), *Scientific foundation of developmental psychiatry.* London: Heinemann.

Sachdev, P. S., Hay, P. J., & Cumming, S. (1992). Psychosurgical treatment of obsessive–compulsive disorder. *Archives of General Psychiatry, 49*(7), 582–583.

Sackheim, H. A., & Gur, R. C. (1979). Self-deception, other-deception, and self-reported psychopathology. *Journal of Consulting and Clinical Psychology, 47,* 213–215.

Safran, J. D., & Segal, Z. V. (1990). *Interpersonal process in cognitive therapy.* Northvale, NJ: Jason Aronson.

Safren, S. A., Heimberg, R. G., & Juster, H. R. (1997). Clients' expectancies and their relationship to pretreatment symptomatology and outcome of cognitive-behavioral group treatment for social phobia. *Journal of Consulting and Clinical Psychology, 65,* 694–698.

Saigh, P. A. (1988). The validity of the DSM-III posttraumatic stress disorder classification as applied to adolescents. *Professional School Psychology, 3,* 283–290.

Saigh, P. A. (1989). The validity of the DSM-III posttraumatic stress disorder classification as applied to children. *Journal of Abnormal Psychology, 98,* 189–192.

Sakheim, D. K., Barlow, D. H., Abrahamson, D. J., & Beck, J. G. (1987). Distinguishing between organogenic and psychogenic erectile dysfunction. *Behaviour Research and Therapy, 25,* 379–390.

Salge, R. A., Beck, J. G., & Logan, A. C. (1988). A community survey of panic. *Journal of Anxiety Disorders, 2,* 157–167.

Salkovskis, P. M. (1985). Obsessional–compulsive problems: A cognitive behavioral analysis. *Behaviour Research and Therapy, 23,* 571–583.

Salkovskis, P. M. (1989). Cognitive-behavioral factors and the persistence of intrusive thoughts in obsessional problems. *Behaviour Research and Therapy, 27,* 677–682.

Salkovskis, P. M. (1996). Cognitive-behavioral approaches to understanding obsessional problems. In R. M. Rapee (Ed.), *Current controversies in the anxiety disorders.* New York: Guilford Press.

Salkovskis, P. M., & Campbell, P. (1994). Thought suppression induces intrusion in naturally occurring negative intrusive thoughts. *Behaviour Research and Therapy, 32,* 1–8.

Salkovskis, P. M., Clark, D. M., & Gelder, M. G. (1996). Cognition–behaviour links in the persistence of panic. *Behaviour Research and Therapy, 34,* 453–458.

Salkovskis, P. M., & Harrison, J. (1984). Abnormal and normal obsessions: A replication. *Behaviour Research and Therapy, 22,* 549–552.

Salkovskis, P. M., & Mills, I. (1994). Induced mood, phobic responding and the return of fear. *Behaviour Research and Therapy, 32,* 439–445.

Salkovskis, P. M., Shafran, R., Rachman, S., & Freeston, M. H. (1999). Multiple pathways to inflated responsibility beliefs in obsessional problems: Possible origins and implications for therapy and research. *Behaviour Therapy and Research, 37,* 1055–1072.

Salkovskis, P. M., & Warwick, H. M. C. (1986). Morbid preoccupations, health anxiety and reassurance: A cognitive-behavioural approach to hypochondriasis. *Behaviour Research and Therapy, 24,* 597–602.

Salkovskis, P. M., Warwick, H. M. C., Clark, D. M., & Wessels, D. J. (1986). A demonstration of acute hyperventilation during naturally occurring panic attacks. *Behaviour Research and Therapy, 24,* 91–94.

Salvador-Carulla, L., Segui, J., Fernandez-Cano, P., & Canet, J. (1995). Costs and offset effect in panic disorder. *British Journal of Psychiatry, 116*(27), 23–28.

Salvador-Carulla, S. J., Segui, J., Fernandez-Cano, P., & Canet, J. (1995). Costs and offset effect in panic disorders. *British Journal of Psychiatry, 166*(Suppl. 27), 23–28.

Sanavio, E. (1988). Obsessions and compulsions: The Padua Inventory. *Behaviour Research and Therapy, 26,* 169–177.

Sanavio, E., & Vidotto, G. (1985). The components of the Maudsley Obsessional–Compulsive Questionnaire. *Behaviour Research and Therapy, 23,* 659–662.

Sanderson, A., & Carpenter, R. (1992). Eye movement desensitization versus image confrontation: A single-session crossover study of 58 phobic subjects. *Journal of Behavior Therapy and Experimental Psychiatry, 23,* 269–275.

Sanderson, W. C., & Barlow, D. H. (1990). A description of patients diagnosed with DSM-III-R generalized anxiety disorder. *Journal of Nervous and Mental Disease, 178*(9), 588–591.

Sanderson, W. C., Di Nardo, P. A., Rapee, R. M., & Barlow, D. H. (1990). Syndrome comorbidity in patients diagnosed with a DSM-III-R anxiety disorder. *Journal of Abnormal Psychology, 99,* 308–312.

Sanderson, W. C., Rapee, R. M., & Barlow, D. H. (1989). The influence of an illusion of control on panic attacks induced via inhalation of 5.5% carbon dioxide-enriched air. *Archives of General Psychiatry, 46,* 157–164.

Sanderson, W. C., & Wetzler, S. (1990). Five percent carbon dioxide challenge: Valid analogue and marker of panic disorder? *Biological Psychiatry, 27,* 689–701.

Sanderson, W. C., & Wetzler, S. (1993). Observations on the cognitive behavioral treatment of panic disorder: Impact of benzodiazepines. *Psychotherapy, 30,* 125–132.

Sapolsky, R. M. (1990). Stress in the wild. *Scientific American,* 116–123.

Sapolsky, R. M. (1992). *Stress, the aging brain, and the mechanisms of neuron death.* Cambridge, MA: MIT Press.

Sapolsky, R. M., Alberts, S. C., & Altman, J. (1997). Hypercortisolism associated with social subordinance or social isolation among wild baboons. *Archives of General Psychiatry, 54,* 1137–1143.

Sapolsky, R. M., & Ray, J. C. (1989). Styles of dominance and their endocrine correlates among wild olive baboons (*Papio anubis*). *American Journal of Primatology, 18*(1), 1–13.

Sarason, I. G. (1982). *Stress, anxiety and cognitive interference: Reactions to tests.* Arlington, VA: Office of Naval Research.

Sarason, I. G. (1984). Stress, anxiety, and cognitive interference: Reactions to tests. *Journal of Personality and Social Psychology, 46,* 929–938.

Sarason, I. G. (1985). Cognitive processes, anxiety, and the treatment of anxiety disorders. In A. H. Tuma & J. D. Maser (Eds.), *Anxiety and the anxiety disorders.* Hillsdale, NJ: Erlbaum.

Sarason, I. G., Pierce, G. R., & Sarason, B. R. (Eds.). (1996). *Cognitive interference: Theories, methods, and findings.* Mahwah, NJ: Erlbaum.

Sarbin, T. R. (1964). Anxiety: Reification of a metaphor. *Archives of General Psychiatry, 10,* 630–638.

Sarrel, D. M., & Masters, W. H. (1982). Sexual molestation of men by women. *Archives of Sexual Behavior, 11,* 117–131.

Sartorius, N., Ustun, T., Lecrubier, Y., & Wittchen, H.-U. (1996). Depression comorbid with anxiety: Results from the WHO Study on Psychological Disorders in Primary Health Care. *British Journal of Psychiatry, 168*(Suppl. 30), 38–43.

Sass, K. J., Sass, A., Westerveld, M., Lencz, T., Novelly, R. A., Kim, J. H., & Spencer, D. D. (1992). Specificity in the correlation of verbal memory and hippocampal neuron loss: Dissociation of memory, language, and verbal intellectual ability. *Journal of Clinical and Experimental Neuropsychology, 14*(5), 662–672.

Saudino, K. J., & Cherny, S. S. (2001). Sources of continuity and change in observed temperament. In R. N. Emde & J. K. Hewitt (Eds.), *Infancy to early childhood: Genetic and environmental influences on developmental change.* New York: Oxford University Press.

Saunders, B., Arata, C., & Kilpatrick, D. G. (1990). Development of a crime-related posttraumatic stress disorder scale for women with the Symptom Checklist 90-R. *Journal of Traumatic Stress, 3,* 439–448.

Savage, C. R., Baer, L., Keuthen, N. J., Brown, H. D., Rauch, S. L., & Jenike, M. A. (1999). Organizational strategies mediate nonverbal memory impairment in obsessive–compulsive disorder. *Biological Psychiatry, 45,* 909–916.

Savron, G., Fava, G. A., Grandi, S., Rafanelli, C., Raffi, A. R., & Belluardo, P. (1996). Hypochondriacal fears and beliefs in obsessive–compulsive disorder. *Acta Psychiatrica Scandinavica, 93*, 345–348.

Sawchuk, C. N., Lee, T. C., Tolin, D. F., & Lohr, J. M. (1997, November). *Generalized disgust sensitivity in blood–injection–injury phobia.* Paper presented at the 31st Annual Convention of the Association for Advancement of Behavior Therapy, Miami Beach, FL.

Sawchuk, C. N., Lohr, J. M., Lee, T. C., & Tolin, D. F. (1999). Exposure to disgust-evoking imagery and information processing biases in blood–injection–injury phobia. *Behaviour Research and Therapy, 37*, 249–257.

Sawchuk, C. N., Lohr, J. M., Tolin, D. F., Lee, T. C., & Kleinknecht, R. A. (2000). Disgust sensitivity and contamination fears in spider and blood–injection–injury phobias. *Behaviour Research and Therapy, 38*, 753–762.

Schachter, S. (1964). The interaction of cognitive and physiological determinants of emotional state. In L. Berkowitz (Ed.), *Advances in experimental social psychology* (Vol. 1). New York: Academic Press.

Schachter, S., & Singer, J. (1962). Cognitive, social and physiological determinants of emotional state. *Psychological Review, 69*, 379–397.

Schatzberg, A. F. (2000). New indications for antidepressants. *Journal of Clinical Psychiatry, 61*(Suppl. 11), 9–17.

Schatzberg, A. F., Samson, J. A., Rothschild, A. J., Bond, T. C., & Regier, D. A. (1998). McLean Hospital Depression Research Facility: Early-onset phobic disorders and adult-onset major depression. *British Journal of Psychiatry, 173*(Suppl. 34), 29–34.

Scheier, M. F., &Carver, C. S. (1983). Two sides of the self: One for you and one for me. In J. Suls & A. G. Greenwald (Eds.), *Psychological perspectives on the self* (Vol. 2). Hillsdale, NJ: Erlbaum.

Scheier, M. F., Carver, C. S., & Gibbons, F. X. (1981). Self-focused attention and reactions to fear. *Journal of Research in Personality, 15*, 1–15.

Scheier, M. F., Carver, C. S., & Matthews, K. A. (1983). Attentional factors in the perception of bodily states. In J. T. Cacioppo & R. E. Petty (Eds.), *Social psychophysiology: A sourcebook.* New York: Guilford Press.

Schlenker, B. R. (1987). Threats to identity: Self-identification and social stress. In C. R. Snyder & C. Ford (Eds.), *Coping with negative life events: Clinical and social psychology perspectives.* New York: Plenum Press.

Schmidt, N. B., Lerew, D. R., & Jackson, R. J. (1997). The role of anxiety sensitivity in the pathogenesis of panic: Prospective evaluation of spontaneous panic attacks during acute stress. *Journal of Abnormal Psychology, 106*(3), 355–364.

Schmidt, N. B., Lerew, D. R., & Jackson, R. J. (1999). Prospective evaluation of anxiety sensitivity in the pathogenesis of panic: Replication and extension. *Journal of Abnormal Psychology, 108*(3), 532–537.

Schmidt, N. B., Lerew, D. R., & Trakowski, J. H. (1997). Body vigilance in panic disorder: Evaluating attention to bodily perturbations. *Journal of Consulting and Clinical Psychology, 65*, 214–220.

Schmidt, N. B., & Telch, M. J. (1994). Role of fear of fear and safety information in moderating the effects of voluntary hyperventilation. *Behavior Therapy, 25*, 197–208.

Schmidt, N. B., Telch, M. J., & Jaimez, T. L. (1996). Biological challenge manipulation of PCO_2 levels: A test of Klein's (1993) suffocation alarm theory of panic. *Journal of Abnormal Psychology, 105*, 446–454.

Schmidt, N. B., Trakowski, J. H., & Staab, J. P. (1997). Extinction of panicogenic effects of a 35% CO_2 challenge in patients with panic disorder. *Journal of Abnormal Psychology, 106*, 630–638.

Schmidt, N. B., Wollaway-Bickel, K., Trakowski, J., Santiago, H., Storey, J., Koselka, M., & Cook, J. (2000). Dismantling cognitive-behavioral treatment for panic disorder: Questioning the utility of breathing retraining. *Journal of Consulting and Clinical Psychology, 68*, 417–424.

Schmidt, R. A., & Bjork, R. A. (1992). New conceptualizations of practice: Common principles in three paradigms suggest new concepts for training. *Psychological Science, 3*, 207–217.

Schmidt, S. M., Zoega, T., & Crowe, R. R. (1993). Excluding linkage between panic disorder and the gamma-aminobutyric acid beta 1 receptor locus in five Icelandic pedigrees. *Acta Psychiatrica Scandinavica, 88,* 225–228.

Schneewind, K. A. (1995). Impact of family processes on control beliefs. In A. Bandura (Ed.), *Self-efficacy in changing societies.* New York: Cambridge University Press.

Schneewind, K. A., & Pfeiffer, P. (1978). Elteriches Eziehungsverhalten und kindliche Selbsver-standwortlichkeit [Parenting and children's self-responsibility]. In K. A. Schneewind & H. Lukesch (Eds.), *Familiare Sozialisation [Family Socialization].* Stuttgart, Germany: Klett-Cotta.

Schneier, F. R., Chin, S. J., Hollander, E., & Liebowitz, M. R. (1992). Fluoxetine in social phobia [Letter to the editor]. *Journal of Clinical Psychopharmacology, 12,* 62–64.

Schneier, F. R., Heckelman, L. R., Garfinkel, R., Campeas, R., Fallon, B., Gitow, A., Street, L., DelBene, D., & Liebowitz, M. R. (1994). Functional impairment in social phobia. *Journal of Clinical Psychiatry, 55,* 322–331.

Schneier, F. R., Johnson, J., Hornig, C. D., Liebowitz, M. R., & Weissman, M. M. (1992). Social phobia: Comorbidity and morbidity in an epidemiological sample. *Archives of General Psychiatry, 49,* 282–288.

Schneier, F. R., Saoud, J. B., Campeas, R., Fallon, B. A., Hollander, E., Coplan, J., & Liebowitz, M. R. (1993). Buspirone in social phobia. *Journal of Clinical Psychopharmacology, 13,* 251–256.

Schneier, F. R., Spitzer, R. L., Gibbon, M., Fyer, A. J., & Liebowitz, M. R. (1991). The relation-ship of social phobia subtypes and avoidant personality disorder. *Comprehensive Psychiatry, 32,* 496–502.

Schneier, F. R., & Welkowitz, L. (1996). *The hidden face of shyness: Understanding and overscoming social anxiety.* New York: Avon Books.

Schnoll, S. H., & Daghestani, A. N. (1986). Treatment of marijuana abuse. *Psychiatric Annals, 16,* 249–254.

Schnurr, P. P., Friedman, M. J., Sengupta, A., Jankowski, M. K., & Holmes, T. (2000). PTSD and utilization of medical treatment services among male Vietnam veterans. *Journal of Nervous and Mental Disease, 188,* 496–504.

Schuckit, M. A., & Hesselbrock, V. (1994). Alcohol dependence and anxiety disorders: What is the relationship? *American Journal of Psychiatry, 151*(12), 1723–1734.

Schwalberg, M. D., Barlow, D. H., Alger, S. A., & Howard, L. J. (1992). Comparison of bulimics, obese binge eaters, social phobics and individuals with panic disorder on comorbidity across the DSM-III-R anxiety disorders. *Journal of Abnormal Psychology, 101,* 675–681.

Schwartz, C. E., Snidman, N., & Kagan, J. (1999). Adolescent social anxiety as an outcome of inhibited behavior in childhood. *Journal of the American Academy of Child and Adolescent Psychiatry, 38,* 1008–1015.

Schwartz, G. E. (1976). Self-regulation of response patterning: Implications for psychophysiologi-cal research and therapy. *Biofeedback and Self-Regulation, 1,* 7–30.

Schwartz, G. E., Fair, P. L., Salt, P., Mandel, M. R., & Klerman, G. L. (1976). Facial muscle pat-terning to affective imagery in depressed and nondepressed subjects. *Science, 192,* 489–491.

Schwartz, G. E., Goetz, R. R., Klein, D. F., Endicott, J., & Gorman, J. M. (1996). Tidal volume of respiration and "sighing" as indicators of breathing irregularities in panic disorder patients. *Anxiety, 2,* 145–148.

Schwartz, G. E., Weinburger, D. A., & Singer, B. A. (1981). Cardiovascular differentiation of hap-piness, sadness, anger, and fear following imagery and exercise. *Psychosomatic Medicine, 43,* 343–364.

Schwartz, J. M., Stoessel, P. W., Baxter, L. R., Martin, K. M., & Phelps, M. E. (1996). Systematic changes in cerebral glucose metabolic rate after successful behavior modification treatment of obsessive–compulsive disorder. *Archives of General Psychiatry, 53,* 109–113.

Schwartz, M. S., & Schwartz, N. M. (1995). Problems with relaxation and biofeedback: Assisted relaxation and guidelines for management. In M. S. Schwartz & Associates, *Biofeedback: A practitioner's guide* (2nd ed.). New York: Guilford Press.

Schwartz, R. M., & Garamoni, G. L. (1989). Cognitive balance and psychopathology: Evaluation of an information processing model of positive and negative states of mind. *Clinical Psychology Review*, *9*, 271–294.

Schwartz, S. G., Adler, P. S. J., & Kaloupek, D. G. (1987, November). *Sources of variation in human fear responding: Subtypes, cue content, and coping*. Paper presented at the 21st Annual Convention of the Association for Advancement of Behavior Therapy, Boston.

Schwarzer, R., & Wicklund, R. A. (Eds.). (1991). *Anxiety and self-focused attention*. New York: Harwood.

Schweizer, E., Patterson, W., Rickels, K., & Rosenthal, M. (1993). Double-blind, placebo-controlled study of a once-a-day, sustained-release preparation of alprazolam for the treatment of panic disorder. *American Journal of Psychiatry*, *150*, 1210–1215.

Schweizer, E., Pohl, R., Balon, R., Fox, I., Rickels, K., & Yeragani, V. K. (1990). Lorazepam vs. alprazolam in the treatment of panic disorder. *Pharmacopsychiatry*, *23*, 90–93.

Schweizer, E., & Rickels, K. (1996). Pharmacological treatment for generalized anxiety disorder. In M. R. Mavissakalian & R. F. Prien (Eds.), *Long-term treatments of anxiety disorders*. Washington, DC: American Psychiatric Press.

Schweizer, E., & Rickels, K. (1997). Placebo response in generalized anxiety: Its effect on the outcome of clinical trials. *Journal of Clinical Psychiatry*, *58*(Suppl. 11), 30–38.

Schweizer, E., Rickels, K., & Lucki, I. (1986). Resistance to the anti-anxiety effect of buspirone in patients with a history of benzodiazepine use. *New England Journal of Medicine*, *314*, 719–720.

Schweizer, E., Rickels, K., Weiss, S., & Zavodnick, S. (1993). Maintenance drug treatment of panic disorder: Results of a prospective, placebo-controlled comparison of alprazolam and imipramine. *Archives of General Psychiatry*, *50*, 51–60.

Segal, D. L., Hersen, M., & Van Hesselt, V. B. (1994). Reliability of the Structured Interview for DSM-III-R: An evaluative review. *Comprehensive Psychiatry*, *35*, 316–327.

Segal, M., & Bloom, F. (1976). The action of norepinephrine in the rat hippocampus: III. Hippocampal cellular responses to locus coeruleus stimulation in the awake rate. *Brain Research*, *107*, 499–501.

Seidel, W. F., Cohen, S. A., Bliwise, N. G., & Dement, W. C. (1985). Buspirone: An anxiolytic without sedative effect. *Psychopharmacology*, *87*, 371–373.

Seligman, M. E. P. (1968). Chronic fear produced by unpredictable electric shock. *Journal of Comparative and Physiological Psychology*, *66*, 402–411.

Seligman, M. E. P. (1971). Phobias and preparedness. *Behavior Therapy*, *2*, 307–320.

Seligman, M. E. P. (1975). *Helplessness: On depression, development, and death*. San Francisco: Freeman.

Seligman, M. E. P., & Johnston, J. (1973). A cognitive theory of avoidance learning. In J. McGuigan & B. Lumsden (Eds.), *Contemporary approaches to conditioning and learning*. New York: Wiley.

Seligman, M. E. P., Peterson, C., Kaslow, N. J., Tanenbaum, R. L., Alloy, L. B., & Abramson, L. Y. (1984). Attributional style and depressive symptoms among children. *Journal of Abnormal Psychology*, *93*, 235–238.

Sellers, E. M., Schneiderman, J. F., Romach, M. K., Kaplan, H. L, & Somer, G. R. (1992). Comparative drug effects and abuse liability of lorazepam, buspirone, and secobarbital in nondependent subjects. *Journal of Clinical Psychopharmacology*, *12*, 79–85.

Shader, R. I., & Greenblatt, D. J. (1993). Use of benzodiazepines in anxiety disorder. *New England Journal of Medicine*, *328*, 1398–1405.

Shafran, R., Booth, R., & Rachman, S. (1993). The reduction of claustrophobia: II. Cognitive analyses. *Behaviour Research and Therapy*, *31*, 75–85.

Shafran, R., Thordarson, D., & Rachman, S. (1996). Thought action fusion in obsessive compulsive disorder. *Journal of Anxiey Disorders*, *5*, 379–391.

Shagass, C. (1955). Differentiation between anxiety and depression by the photically activated electroencephalogram. *American Journal of Psychiatry*, *112*, 41–46.

Shalev, A. Y., Peri, T., Brandes, D., Freedman, S., Orr, S. P., & Pitman, R. (2000). Auditory startle responses in trauma survivors with PTSD: A prospective study. *American Journal of Psychiatry, 157,* 255–261.

Shapiro, D. (1974). Operant-feedback control of human blood pressure: Some clinical issues. In P. A. Obrist, A. H. Black, J. Brener, & L. V. DiCara (Eds.), *Cardiovascular psychophysiology: Current issues in response mechanisms, biofeedback, and methodology.* Chicago: Aldine.

Shapiro, F. (1989). Eye movement desensitization: A new treatment for post-traumatic stress disorder. *Journal of Behavior Therapy and Experimental Psychiatry, 20,* 211–217.

Shapiro, F. (1995). *Eye movement desensitization and reprocessing: Basic principles, protocols, and procedures.* New York: Guilford Press.

Shapiro, F. (1999). Eye movement desensitization and reprocessing (EMDR) and the anxiety disorders: Clinical and research implications of an integrated psychotherapy treatment. *Journal of Anxiety Disorders, 13,* 35–67.

Shay, J. (1992). Fluoxetine reduces explosiveness and elevates mood of Vietnam combat veterans with PTSD. *Journal of Traumatic Stress, 5,* 97–101.

Shear, M. K. (1986). Pathophysiology of panic: A review of pharmacologic provocative tests and naturalistic monitoring data. *Journal of Clinical Psychiatry, 47,* 18–26.

Shear, M. K. (1991). The concept of uncontrollability. *Psychological Inquiry, 2*(1), 88–93.

Shear, M. K. (1996). Factors in the etiology and pathogenesis of panic disorder: Revisiting the attachment–separation paradigm. *American Journal of Psychiatry, 153,* 125–136.

Shear, M. K., & Maser, J. D. (1994). Standardized assessment for panic disorder research: A conference report. *Archives of General Psychiatry, 51,* 346–354.

Shear, M. K., Brown, T. A., Barlow, D. H., Money, R., Sholomskas, D. E., Woods, S. W., Gorman, J. M., & Papp, L. A. (1997). Multicenter Collaborative Panic Disorder Severity Scale. *American Journal of Psychiatry, 154,* 1571–1575.

Shear, M. K., Cooper, A. M., Klerman, G. L., & Busch, F. N. (1993). A psychodynamic model of panic disorder. *American Journal of Psychiatry, 150*(6), 859–866.

Shear, M. K., Devereux, R. B., & Kramer-Fox, R. (1991). Mitral valve prolapse and anxiety: How close is the association? In A. P. Shapiro & A. Baum (Eds.), *Behavioral aspects of cardiovascular disease.* Hillsdale, NJ: Erlbaum.

Shear, M. K., Houck, P., Greeno, C., & Masters, B. S. (in press). Emotion-focused psychotherapy for panic disorder: A randomized treatment study. *American Journal of Psychiatry.*

Shear, M. K., Pilkonis, P. A., Cloitre, M., & Leon, A. C. (1994). Cognitive behavioral treatment compared with nonprescriptive treatment of panic disorder. *Archives of General Psychiatry, 51,* 395–401.

Shear, M. K., Polan, J. J., Harshfield, G., Pickering, T., Mann, J. J., Frances, A., & James, G. (1992). Ambulatory monitoring of blood pressure and heart rate in panic patients. *Journal of Anxiety Disorders, 6,* 213–221.

Shear, M. K., Vander Bilt, J., Rucci, P., Endicott, J., Lydiard, R., Otto, M. W., Pollack, M. H., Chandler, L., Williams, J., Ali, A., & Frank, D. (2001). Reliability and validity of a structured interview guide for the Hamilton Anxiety Rating Scale (SIGH-A). *Depression and Anxiety, 13,* 166–178.

Sheehan, D. (1982). Current concepts in psychiatry: Panic attacks and phobias. *New England Journal of Medicine, 307,* 156–158.

Sheehan, D. V. (1999). Venlafaxine extended release (XR) in the treatment of generalized anxiety disorder. *Journal of Clinical Psychiatry, 60*(Suppl. 22), 23–28.

Sheline, Y., Wang, P., Gado, M., Csernansky, J., & Vannier, M. (1996). Hippocampal atrophy in major depression. *Proceedings of the National Academy of Sciences USA, 93,* 3908–3913.

Shelton, M. R., & Garber, J. (1987, August). *Development and validation of a children's pleasant and unpleasant events schedule.* Paper presented at the 95th Annual Convention of the American Psychological Association, New York.

Sher, K. J., Frost, R. O., & Otto, R. (1983). Cognitive deficits in compulsive checks: An exploratory study. *Behaviour Research and Therapy, 21,* 357–363.

Sher, K. J., Mann, B., & Frost, R. O. (1984). Cognitive dysfunction in compulsive checkers: Further explorations. *Behaviour Research and Therapy*, 22, 493–502.

Sherbourne, C. D., Wells, K. B., & Judd, L. (1996). Functioning and well being of patients with panic disorder. *American Journal of Psychiatry*, 153, 213–218.

Sherbourne, C. D., Wells, K. B., Meredith, L. S., Jackson, C. A., & Camp, P. (1996). Comorbid anxiety disorder and the functioning and well-being of chronically ill patients of general medical providers. *Archives of General Psychiatry*, 53, 889–894.

Shields, J. (1962). *Monozygotic twins brought up apart and together*. London: Oxford University Press.

Shilik, J., Aluoja, A. V., Vasar, E. P., & Bradwejn, J. (1997). Effects of citalopram treatment on behavioural, cardiovascular, amd neuroendocrine response to cholecystokinin tetrapeptide challenge in panic disorder patients. *Journal of Psychiatric Neuroscience*, 22, 332–340.

Shiller, V. M., Izard, C. E., & Hembree, E. A. (1986). Patterns of emotion expression during separation in the strange-situation procedure. *Developmental Psychology*, 22, 378–382.

Shively, C. A. (1998). Social subordination stress, behavior, and central monoaminergic function in female cynomolgus monkeys. *Biological Psychiatry*, 44, 882–891.

Shrout, P. E., Spitzer, R. L., & Fleiss, J. L. (1987). Quantification of agreement in psychiatric diagnosis revisited. *Archives of General Psychiatry*, 44, 172–177.

Siegel, L., Jones, W. C., & Wilson, J. O. (1990). Economic and life consequences experienced by a group of individuals with panic disorder. *Journal of Anxiety Disorders*, 4, 201–211.

Siegel, L. J., & Griffin, N. J. (1984). Correlates of depressive symptoms in adolescents. *Journal of Youth and Adolescence*, 13, 475–487.

Siitonen, L., & Tanne, J. (1976). Effect of beta-blockade during bowling competitions. *Annals of Clinical Research*, 8, 393–398.

Silove, D., Manicavasagar, V., O'Connell, D., & Morris-Yates, A. (1995). Genetic factors in early separation anxiety: Implications for the genesis of adult anxiety disorders. *Acta Psychiatrica Scandinavica*, 92, 17–24.

Silove, D., Parker, G., Hadzi-Pavlovic, D., Manicavasgar, V., & Blaszczynski, A. (1991). Parental representations of patients with panic disorder and centralized anxiety disorder. *British Journal of Psychiatry*, 159, 835–841.

Silverman, W. K., La Greca, A. M., & Wasserstein, S. (1995). What do children worry about?: Worries and their relation to anxiety. *Child Development*, 66, 671–686.

Silverman, W. K., & Nelles, W. B. (1988). Anxiety Disorders Interview Schedule for Children. *Journal of the American Academy of Child and Adolescent Psychiatry*, 27, 772–778.

Simeon, D., Hollander, E., Stein, D., Cohen, L., & Aronowitz, B. (1995). Body dysmorphic disorder in the DSM-IV field trial for obsessive compulsive disorder. *American Journal of Psychiatry*, 152, 1207–1209.

Simon, G., Ormel, J., Von Korff, M., & Barlow, W. (1995). Health care costs associated with depressive and anxiety disorders in primary care. *American Journal of Psychiatry*, 152, 352–357.

Simpson, H. B., Gorfinkle, K. S., & Liebowitz, M. R. (1999). Cognitive behavioral therapy as an adjunct to serotonin reuptake inhibitors in obsessive–compulsive disorder: An open trial. *Journal of Clinical Psychiatry*, 60, 584–590.

Simpson, H. B., Schneier, F. R., Campeas, R. B., Marshall, R. D., Fallon, B. A., Davies, S., Klein, D. F., & Liebowitz, M. R. (1998). Imipramine in the treatment of social phobia. *Journal of Clinical Psychopharmacology*, 18, 132–135.

Sims, C. (2000, March 17.) Behold, the fragrant Japanese man. *New York Times*, A8.

Singer, J. L., & Antrobus, J. S. (1972). Daydreaming, imaginal processes, and personality: A normative study. In P. Sheehan (Ed.), *The function and nature of imagery*. New York: Academic Press.

Singer, M. I., Anglin, T. M., Song, L.-Y., & Lunghofer, L. (1995). Adolescents' exposure to violence and associated symptoms of psychological trauma. *Journal of the American Medical Association*, 273, 477–482.

Singh, A. N. (1996). Mitral valve prolapse syndrome. *International Medical Journal*, 3, 101–106.

Sinnott, A., Jones, R. B., Scott-Fordham, A., & Woodward, R. (1981). Augmentation of in vivo exposure treatment for agoraphobia by the formation of neighborhood self-help groups. *Behaviour Research and Therapy, 19,* 339–347.

Siqueland, L., Kendall, P. C., & Steinberg, L. (1996). Anxiety in children: Perceived family environments and observed family interaction. *Journal of Clinical Child Psychology, 25,* 225–237.

Skinner, E. A. (1986). The origin of young children's perceived control: Mother contingent and sensitive behavior. *International Journal of Behavioral Development, 9,* 359–382.

Skinner, E. A., Chapman, M., & Baltes, P. B. (1988). Control, means–ends and agency beliefs: A new conceptualization and its measurement during childhood. *Journal of Personality and Social Psychology, 54,* 117–133.

Skolnick, P., & Paul, S. M. (1982). Molecular pharmacology of the benzodiazepines. *International Review of Neurobiology, 23,* 103.

Skoog, G., & Skoog, I. (1999). A 40-year follow-up of patients with obsessive–compulsive disorder. *Archives of General Psychiatry, 56,* 121–127.

Skre, I., Onstad, S., Torgersen, S., & Kringlen, E. (1991). High interrater reliability for the Structured Clinical Interview for DSM-III-R Axis I (SCID-I). *Acta Psychiatric Scandinavica, 84,* 167–173.

Skre, I., Onstad, S., Torgersen, S., Lygren, S., & Kringlen, E. (1993). A twin study of DSM-III-R anxiety disorders. *Acta Psychiatrica Scandinavica, 88,* 85–92.

Slater, E., & Shields, J. (1969). Genetical aspects of anxiety. *British Journal of Psychiatry, 3,* 62–71.

Sloan, E. P., Natarajan, M., Baker, B., Dorian, P., Mironov, D., Barr, A., Newman, D., & Shapiro, C. M. (1999). Nocturnal and daytime panic attacks: Comparison of sleep architecture, heart rate variability, and response to sodium lactate challenge. *Biological Psyhciatry, 45,* 1313–1320.

Smail, P., Stockwell, T., Canter, S., & Hodgson, R. (1984). Alcohol dependence and phobic anxiety states: I. A prevalence study. *British Journal of Psychiatry, 144,* 53–57.

Smith, J. S., & Kiloh, L. G. (1980). The psychosurgical treatment of anxiety. In G. D. Burrows & B. Davies (Eds.), *Handbook of studies on anxiety.* Amsterdam: Elsevier/North-Holland.

Smith, K. L., Kirkby, K. C., Montgomery, I. M., & Daniels, B. A. (1997). Computer-delivered modeling of exposure for spider phobia: Relevant versus irrelevant exposure. *Journal of Anxiety Disorders, 11,* 489–497.

Smith, L. C., Friedman, S., & Nevid, J. (1999). Clinical and sociocultural differences in African American and European American patients with panic disorder and agoraphobia. *The Journal of Nervous and Mental Disease, 187,* 549–561.

Smith, S. M., Rothbaum, B. O., & Hodges, L. (1999). Treatment of fear of flying using virtual reality exposure therapy: A single case study. *The Behavior Therapist, 22,* 154–160.

Smoller, J. W., Pollack, M., Otto, M., Rosenbaum, J., & Kradin, R. (1996). Panic, anxiety, dyspnea, and respiratory disease: Theoretical and clinical considerations. *American Journal of Respiratory Critical Care Medicine, 154,* 6–17.

Smoller, J. W., & Tsuang, M. T. (1998). Panic and phobic anxiety: Defining phenotypes for genetic studies. *American Journal of Psychiatry, 155,* 1152–1162.

Snaith, R. P. (1968). A clinical investigation of phobia. *British Journal of Psychiatry, 114,* 673–697.

Solomon, S. D., Gerrity, E. T., & Muff, A. M. (1992). Efficacy of treatments for posttraumatic stress disorder. *Journal of the American Medical Association, 265,* 633–637.

Solyom, L., Beck, P., Solyom, C., & Hugel, R. (1974). Some etiological factors in phobic neurosis. *Canadian Journal of Psychiatry, 19,* 69–78.

Solyom, L., DiNicola, V. F., Sookman, D., & Luchins, D. (1985). Is there an obsessive psychosis?: Aetiological and prognostic factors of an atypical form of obsessive–compulsive neurosis. *Canadian Journal of Psychiatry, 30,* 372–379.

Souêtre, E., Lozet, H., Cimarosti, I., Martin, P., Chignon, J. M., Adès, J., Tignol, J., & Dacourt, G. (1994). Cost of anxiety disorders: Impact of comorbidity. *Journal of Psychosomatic Research, 38*(Suppl. 1), 151–160.

Spence, J. (1997). Structure of anxiety symptoms among children: A confirmatory factor-analytic study. *Journal of Abnormal Psychology, 106,* 280–297.

Sperry, R. (1982). Some effects of disconnecting the cerebral hemispheres. *Science, 217,* 1223–1226.

Spiegel, D. A. (1998a). Efficacy studies of alprazolam in panic disorder. *Psychopharmacology Bulletin, 34,* 191–195.

Spiegel, D. A., & Barlow, D. H. (2000a, November). *Eight-day treatment of panic disorder with moderate to severe agoraphobia: Preliminary outcome data.* Poster presented at the 34th Annual Convention of the Association for Advancement of Behavior Therapy, New Orleans, LA.

Spiegel, D. A., & Barlow, D. H. (2000b, November). Intensive treatment for panic disorder and agoraphobia. In M. G. Craske (Chair), *Brief cognitive behavioral therapy for anxiety: Intervention and prevention.* Symposium conducted at the 34th Annual Convention of the Association for Advancement of Behavior Therapy, New Orleans, LA.

Spiegel, D. A., & Barlow, D. H. (2000c). Generalized anxiety disorders. In M. G. Gelder, J. J. Lopez-Ibor, & N. C. Andreasen (Eds.), *The new Oxford textbook of psychiatry.* New York: Oxford University Press.

Spiegel, D. A., & Bruce, T. J. (1997). Benzodiazepines and exposure-based cognitive behavior therapies for panic disorder: Conclusions from combined treatment trials. *American Journal of Psychiatry, 154,* 773–780.

Spiegel, D. A., Bruce, T. J., Gregg, S. F., & Nuzzarello, A. (1994). Does cognitive behavior therapy assist slow taper alprazolam discontinuation in panic disorder? *American Journal of Psychiatry, 151,* 876–881.

Spiegel, D. A., Wiegel, M., Baker, S. L., & Greene, K. A. I. (2000). Pharmacotherapy of anxiety disorders. In D. I. Mostofsky & D. H. Barlow (Eds.), *The management of stress and anxiety in medical disorders.* Boston: Allyn & Bacon.

Spielberger, C. D. (1966). Theory and research on anxiety. In C. D. Spielberger (Ed.), *Anxiety and behavior.* New York: Academic Press.

Spielberger, C. D. (1972). Anxiety as an emotional state. In C. D. Spielberger (Ed.), *Anxiety: Current trends in theory and research* (Vol. 1). New York: Academic Press.

Spielberger, C. D. (1979). *Understanding stress and anxiety.* New York: Harper & Row.

Spielberger, C. D. (1985). Anxiety, cognition, and affect: A state–trait perspective. In A. H. Tuma & J. D. Maser (Eds.), *Anxiety and the anxiety disorders.* Hillsdale, NJ: Erlbaum.

Spielberger, C. D., Gorsuch, R. L., & Lushene, R. E. (1970). *Manual for the State–Trait Anxiety Inventory.* Palo Alto, CA: Consulting Psychologists Press.

Spielberger, C. D., Gorsuch, R. L., Lushene, R., Vagg, P. R., & Jacobs, G. A. (1983). *Manual for the State–Trait Anxiety Inventory (Form Y Self-Evaluation Questionnaire).* Palo Alto, CA: Consulting Psychologists Press.

Spielberger, C. D., Johnson, E. H., Russell, S. F., Crane, R. J., Jacobs, G. A., & Worden, T. J. (1985). The experience and expression of anger: Construction and validation of an anger expression scale. In M. A. Chesney & R. H. Rosenman (Eds.), *Anger and hostility in cardiovascular and behavioral disorders.* New York: Hemisphere/McGraw-Hill.

Spielberger, C. D., Krasner, S. S., & Solomon, E. P. (1988). The experience, expression, and control of anger. In M. E. Janisse (Ed.), *Health psychology: Individual differences and stress.* New York: Springer-Verlag.

Spinhoven, P., Onstein, E. J., Sterk, P. J., & le Haen-Versteijnen, D. (1992). The hyperventilation provocation test in panic disorder. *Behaviour Research and Therapy, 30,* 453–461.

Spitzer, R. L., Kroenke, K., Linzer, M., Hahn, S. R., Williams, J. B. W., deGruy, F. V., III, Brody, D., & Davies, M. (1995). Health related quality of life in primary care patients with mental disorders: Results from the PRIME MD 1000 Study. *Journal of American Medical Association, 274*(19), 1511–1517.

Spitzer, R. L., & Williams, J. B. W. (1985). Proposed revisions in the DSM-III classification of anxiety disorders based on research and clinical experience. In A. H. Tuma & J. D. Maser (Eds.), *Anxiety and the anxiety disorders.* Hillsdale, NJ: Erlbaum.

Spitzer, R., Williams, J. W., Gibbon, M., & First, M. (1985). Structured Clinical Interview for DSM. New York State Psychiatric Institute, Biometrics Department.

Spitzer, R. L., Williams, J. B. W., Gibbon, M., & First, M. B. (1994). *Structured Clinical Interview for DSM-IV (SCID-IV)*. New York: Biometric Research Department, New York State Psychiatric Institute.

Spitzer, R. L., Williams, J. B. W., Kroenke, K., Linzer, M., deGruy, F. V., III, Hahn, S. R., Brody, D., & Johnson, J. G. (1994). Utility of a new procedure for diagnosing mental disorders in primary care: The PRIME-MD 1000 study. *Journal of the American Medical Association, 272,* 1749–1756.

Squires, R. F., & Braestrup, C. (1970). Benzodiazepine receptors in rat brain. *Nature (London), 226,* 732–734.

Sramek, J. J., Tansman, M., Suri, A., Hornig-Rohan, M., Amsterdam, J. D., Stahl, S. M., Weisler, R. H., & Cutler, N. R. (1996). Efficacy of buspirone in generalized anxiety disorder with co-existing mild depressive symptoms. *Journal of Clinical Psychiatry, 57,* 287–291.

Sroufe, L. A. (1990). Considering the normal and abnormal together: The essence of developmental psychopathology. *Development and Psychopathology, 2,* 335–347.

Stahl, S. M. (1996). *Essential psychopharmacology*. Cambridge, England: Cambridge University Press.

Stanley, M. A., Beck, J. G., & Glassco, J. D. (1996). Treatment of generalized anxiety in older adults: A preliminary comparison of cognitive-behavioral and supportive approaches. *Behavior Therapy, 27,* 565–581.

Stanley, M. A., & Novy, D. M. (2000). Cognitive-behavior therapy for generalized anxiety in late life: An evaluation overview. *Journal of Anxiety Disorders, 14,* 191–207.

Starcevic, V. (1995). Pathological worry in major depression: A preliminary report. *Behaviour Research and Therapy, 33,* 55–56.

Starcevic, V., Fallon, S., & Uhlenhuth, E. H. (1994). The frequency and severity of generalized anxiety disorder symptoms: Toward a less cumbersome conceptualization. *Journal of Nervous and Mental Disease, 182,* 80–84.

Starcevic, V., Uhlenhuth, E. H., Kellner, R., & Pathak, D. (1993). Comorbidity in panic disorder: II. Chronology of appearance and pathogenic comorbidity. *Psychiatry Research, 46,* 285–293.

Stark, K. D., Humphrey, L. L., Crook, K., & Lewis, K. (1990). Perceived family environments of depressed and anxious children: Child's and maternal figure's perspectives. *Journal of Abnormal Child Psychology, 18,* 527–547.

Starkman, M. N., Giordani, B., Gebarski, S. S., Berent, S., Schork, M. A., & Schteingart, D. E. (1999). Decrease in cortisol reverses human hippocampal atrophy following treatment of Cushing's disease. *Biological Psychiatry, 46,* 1595–1602.

Staub, E., Tursky, B., & Schwartz, G. E. (1971). Self-control and predictability: Their effects on reactions to aversive stimulation. *Journal of Personality and Social Psychology, 18*(2), 157–162.

Stegen, K., de Bruyne, K., Rasschaert, W., van de Woestijne, K., & van den Bergh, O. (1999). Fear-relevant images as conditioned stimuli for somatic complaints, respiratory behavior, and reduced end-tidal pCO2. *Journal of Abnormal Psychology, 108,* 143–152.

Stein, D. J., & Bouwer, C. (1997). A neuro-evolutionary approach to the anxiety disorders. *Journal of Anxiety Disorders, 11*(4), 409–429.

Stein, J. M., Papp, L. A., Klein, D. F., Cohen, S., Simon, J., Ross, D., Martinez, J., & Gorman, J. M. (1992). Exercise intolerance in panic disorder patients. *Biological Psychiatry, 32,* 281–287.

Stein, M. B. (1995). *Social phobia: Clinical and research perspectives*. Washington, DC: American Psychiatric Press.

Stein, M. B., Asmundson, G. J., Ireland, D., & Walker, J. D. (1994). Panic disorder in patients attending a clinic for vestibular disorders. *American Journal of Psychiatry, 151,* 1697–1700.

Stein, M. B., Koverola, C., Hanna, C., Torchia, M. G., & McClarty, B. (1997). Hippocampal volume in women victimized by childhood sexual abuse. *Psychological Medicine, 27,* 951–959.

Stein, M. B., Liebowitz, M. R. Lydiard, R. B., Pitts, C. D., Bushnell, W., & Gergel, I. (1998). Paroxetine treatment of generalized social phobia (social anxiety disorder): A randomized clinical trial. *Journal of the American Medical Association, 280,* 708–713.

Stein, M. B., Tancer, M. E., & Uhde, T. W. (1992). Heart rate and plasma norepinephrine responsivity to orthostatic challenge in anxiety disorders: Comparison of patients with panic disorder and social phobia and normal control subjects. *Archives of General Psychiatry, 49,* 311–317.

Stein, M. B., Walker, J. R., & Forde, D. R. (1996). Public speaking fears in a community sample. Prevalence, impact on functioning, and diagnostic classification. *Archives of General Psychiatry, 53,* 169–174.

Steketee, G. (1993). *Treatment of obsessive compulsive disorder.* New York: Guilford Press.

Steketee, G. (1998). Judy: A compelling case of obsessive–compulsive disorder. In R. P. Halgin & S. K. Whitbourne (Eds.), *A casebook in abnormal psychology.* Oxford: Oxford University Press.

Steketee, G., Bransfield, S., Miller, S. M., & Foa, E. B. (1989). The effect of information and coping style on the reduction of phobic anxiety during exposure. *Journal of Anxiety Disorders, 3,* 69–85.

Steketee, G., Chambless, D. L., & Tran, G. Q. (2001). Effects of Axis I and II comorbidity on behavior therapy outcome for obsessive compulsive disorder and agoraphobia. *Comprehensive Psychiatry, 42,* 76–86.

Steketee, G., Chambless, D. L., Tran, G. Q., Worden, H., & Gillis, M. M. (1995). Behavioral avoidance test for obsessive compulsive disorder. *Behaviour Research and Therapy, 34,* 73–83.

Steketee, G., & Frost, R. O. (1998). Obsessive–compulsive disorder. In A. S. Bellack & M. Hersen (Eds.), *Comprehensive clinical psychology: Vol. 6. Adults: Clinical formulation and treatment.* Oxford: Pergamon Press.

Steketee, G., Frost, R. O., & Bogart, K. (1996). Yale–Brown Obsessive Compulsive Scale: Interview versus self-report. *Behavioral Assessment, 34,* 675–684.

Steketee, G., Grayson, J. B., & Foa, E. B. (1985). Obsessive–compulsive disorder: Differences between washers and checkers. *Behaviour Research and Therapy, 23,* 197–201.

Steketee, G., Grayson, J. B., & Foa, E. B. (1987). A comparison of characteristics of obsessive–compulsive disorder and anxiety disorder. *Journal of Anxiety Disorders, 1,* 325–335.

Steketee, G., Quay, S., & White, K. (1991). Religion and guilt in OCD patients. *Journal of Anxiety Disorders, 5,* 359–367.

Steketee, G., & Shapiro, L. J. (1995). Predicting behavioral treatment outcome for agoraphobia and obsessive compulsive disorder. *Clinical Psychology Review, 15,* 317–346.

Stemberger, R. T., Turner, S. M., Beidel, D. C., & Calhoun, K. S. (1995). Social phobia: An analysis of possible developmental factors. *Journal of Abnormal Psychology, 104,* 526–531.

Stern, R. S., & Cobb, J. P. (1978). Phenomenology of obsessive–compulsive neurosis. *British Journal of Psychiatry, 132,* 233–239.

Stern, R. S., & Marks, I. (1973). Brief and prolonged flooding: A comparison in agoraphobic patients. *Archives of General Psychiatry, 28,* 270–276.

Sternbach, H. (1990). Fluoxetine treatment of social phobia. *Journal of Clinical Psychopharmacology, 10,* 230–231.

Stevenson, J., Batten, N., & Cherner, M. (1992). Fears and fearfulness in children and adolescents: A genetic analysis of twin data. *Journal of Child Psychology and Psychiatry, 33,* 977–985.

Stewart, S. H., Samoluk, S. B., & MacDonald, A. B. (1999). Anxiety sensitivity and substance use and abuse. In S. Taylor (Ed.), *Anxiety sensitivity: Theory, research, and treatment of the fear of anxiety.* Mahwah, NJ: Erlbaum.

Stewart, W., Linet, M., & Cenentano, D. (1989). Migraine headaches and panic attacks. *Psychosomatic Medicine, 51,* 559–569.

Stöber, J. (1998). Worry, problem elaboration and suppression of imagery: The role of concreteness. *Behaviour Research and Therapy, 36,* 751–756.

Stock, W. E., & Geer, J. H. (1982). A study of fantasy-based sexual arousal in women. *Archives of Sexual Behavior, 11*(1), 33–47.

Stockwell, R., Smail, P., Hodgson, R., & Canter, S. (1984). Alcohol dependence and phobic anxiety states: II. A retrospective study. *British Journal of Psychiatry, 144,* 58–63.

Stokes, P. (1985). The neuroendocrinology of anxiety. In A. H. Tuma & I. D. Maser (Eds.), *Anxiety and the anxiety disorders.* Hillsdale, NJ: Erlbaum.

Stopa, L., & Clark, D. M. (1993). Cognitive processes in social phobia. *Behaviour Research and Therapy, 31,* 255–267.

Stopa, L., & Clark, D. M. (2000). Social phobia and interpretation of social events. *Behaviour Research and Therapy, 38,* 273–283.

Storms, M. D., & Nisbett, R. E. (1970). Insomnia and the attribution process. *Journal of Personality and Social Psychology, 16,* 319–328.

Strand, M., Hetta, J., Rosen, A., Sörenson, S., Malmström, R., Fabian, C., Marits, K., Vetterskog, K., Liljestrand, A. G., & Hegen, C. (1990). A double-blind, controlled trial in primary care patients with generalized anxiety: A comparison between buspirone and oxazepam. *Journal of Clinical Psychiatry, 51*(Suppl. 9), 40–45.

Stravynski, A., & Greenberg, D. (1989). Behavioural psychotherapy for social phobia and dysfunction. *International Review of Psychiatry, 1,* 207–218.

Street, L. L., Craske, M. G., & Barlow, D. H. (1989). Sensation, cognitions, and the perception of cues associated with expected and unexpected panic attacks. *Behaviour Research and Therapy, 27,* 189–198.

Stroop, J. R. (1935). Studies of interference in serial verbal reactions. *Journal of Experimental Psychology, 18,* 643–661.

Stuart, G. L., Treat, T. A., & Wade, W. A. (2000). Effectiveness of an empirically based treatment for panic disorder delivered in a service clinic setting: 1-year follow-up. *Journal of Consulting and Clinical Psychology, 68,* 506–512.

Sturges, L. V., & Goelsch, V. L. (1996). Psychophysiological reactivity and heartbeat awareness in anxiety sensitivity. *Journal of Anxiety Disorders, 10*(4), 283–294.

Sturt, E. (1981). Hierarchical patterns in the distribution of psychiatric symptoms. *Psychological Medicine, 11,* 783–794.

Suarez, S. D., & Gallup, G. G., Jr. (1979). Tonic immobility as a response to rape in humans: A theoretical note. *Psychological Record, 29,* 315–320.

Sullivan, G. M., Kent, J. M., & Coplan, J. D. (2000). The neurobiology of stress and anxiety. In D. I. Mostofsky & D. H. Barlow (Eds.), *The management of stress and anxiety in medical disorders.*

Suls, J., & Fletcher, B. (1985a). The relative efficacy of avoidant and nonavoidant coping strategies: A meta-analysis. *Health Psychology, 4,* 249–288.

Suls, J., & Fletcher, B. (1985b). Self-attention, life stress, and illness: A prospective study. *Psychosomatic Medicine, 47,* 469–481.

Summerfelt, L. J., Richter, M. A., Antony, M. M., & Swinson, R. P. (1999). Symptom structure in obsessive–compulsive disorder: A confirmatory factor-analytic study. *Behaviour Research and Therapy, 37,* 297–311.

Suomi, S. J. (1986). Anxiety-like disorders in young nonhuman primates. In R. Gittelman (Ed.), *Anxiety disorders of childhood.* New York: Guilford Press.

Suomi, S. J. (1991). Early stress and adult emotional reactivity in rhesus monkeys. *Ciba Foundation Symposiums, 156,* 171–183.

Suomi, S. J. (1999). Attachment in rhesus monkeys. In J. Cassidy & P. R. Shaver (Eds.), *Handbook of attachment: Theory, research, and clinical applications.* New York: Guilford Press.

Suomi, S. J. (2000). A biobehavioral perspective on developmental psychopathology. In A. J. Sameroff, M. Lewis, & S. M. Miller (Eds.), *Handbook of Developmental Psychopathology.* New York: Kluwer Academic/Plenum.

Suomi, S. J., Kraemer, G. W., Baysinger, C. M., & DeLizio, R. D. (1981). Inherited and experimental factors assocaited with individual differences in anxious behavior displayed by rhesus monkeys. In D. F. Klein & J. Rabkin (Eds), *Anxiety: New research and changing concepts.* New York: Raven Press.

Surtees, P. G., & Kendell, R. E. (1979). The hierarchy model of psychiatric symptomatology: An investigation based on Present State Examination ratings. *British Journal of Psychiatry, 135,* 438–443.

Sutker, P. B., & Allain, A. N. (1996). Assessment of PTSD and other mental disorders in World War II and Korean conflict POW survivors and combat veterans. *Psychological Assessment, 8,* 18–25.

Sutker, P. B., Uddo, M., Brailey, K., & Allain, A. N. (1993). War-zone trauma and stress-related symptoms in Operation Desert Shield/Storm (ODS) returnees. *Journal of Social Issues, 49,* 33–50.

Sutker, P. B., Uddo-Crane, M., & Allain, A. N. (1991). Clinical and research assessment of post-traumatic stress disorder: A conceptual overview. *Psychological Assessment, 3,* 520–530.

Swedo, S. E., & Kiessling, L. S. (1994). Specultions on antineuronal antibody-mediated neuropsy-chiatric disorders of childhood. *Pediatrics, 93,* 323–326.

Swedo, S. E., Rapaport, J. L., Cheslow, D. L., & Leonard, H. L. (1989). High prevalence of obsessive compulsive symptoms in patients with Sydenham's chorea. *American Journal of Psychiatry, 146,* 246–249.

Swendsen, J. D., Merikangas, K. R., Canino, G. J., Kessler, R. C., Rubio-Stipec, M., & Angst, J. (1998). The comorbidity of alcoholism with anxiety and depressive disorders in four geographic communities. *Comprehensive Psychiatry, 39*(4), 176–184.

Swinson, R. P. (1986). Reply to Kleiner. *The Behavior Therapist, 9,* 110–128.

Swinson, R. P., Fergus, K. D., Cox, B. J., & Wickwire, K. (1995). Efficacy of telephone-administered behavioral therapy for panic disorder with agoraphobia. *Behaviour Research and Therapy, 33,* 465–469.

Szuster, R. R., Pontius, E. B., & Campos, P. E. (1988). Marijuana sensitivity and panic anxiety. *Journal of Clinical Psychiatry, 49,* 427–429.

Takahashi, T. (1989). Social phobia syndrome in Japan. *Comprehensive Psychiatry, 30,* 45–52.

Tallis, F. (1995). The characteristics of obsessional thnking: Difficulty demonstrating the obvious? *Clinical Psychology and Psychotherapy, 2,* 24–39.

Tallis, F., Davey, G. C. L., & Bond, A. (1994). The Worry Domains Questionnaire. In G. C. L. Davey & F. Tallis (Eds.), *Worrying: Perspectives on theory, assessment, and treatment.* New York: Wiley.

Tallis, F., Davey, G. C. L., & Capuzzo, N. (1994). The phenomenology of non-pathological worry: A preliminary investigation. In G. C. L. Davey & F. Tallis (Eds.), *Worrying: Perspectives on theory, assessment, and treatment.* New York: Wiley.

Tallis, F., Eysenck, M. W., & Mathews, A. (1991). Elevated evidence requirements and worry. *Personality and Individual Differences, 12,* 21–27.

Tallis, F., Eysenck, M. W., & Mathews, A. (1992a). A questionnaire for the measurement of non-pathological worry. *Personality and Individual Differences, 13,* 161–168.

Tallis, F., Eysenck, M. W., & Mathews, A. (1992b). Worry: A critical analysis of some theoretical approaches. *Anxiety Research, 4,* 97–108.

Tan, E. S. (1969). The symptomatology of anxiety in west Malaysia. *Australian and New Zealand Journal of Psychiatry, 3,* 271–276.

Tan, E. S. (1980). Transcultural aspects of anxiety. In G. D. Burrows & B. Davies (Eds.), *Handbook of studies on anxiety.* Amsterdam: Elsevier/North-Holland.

Tancer, M. E. (1993). Neurobiology of social phobia. *Journal of Clinical Psychiatry, 54,* 26–30.

Tarrier, N., Pilgrim, H., Sommerfield, C., Faragher, B., Reynolds, M., Graham, E., & Barrowclough, C. (1999). A randomized trial of cognitive therapy and imaginal exposure in the treatment of chronic posttraumatic stress disorder. *Journal of Consulting and Clinical Psychology, 67,* 13–18.

Tata, P. R., Leibowitz, J. A., Prunty, M. J., Cameron, M., & Pickering, A. D. (1996). Attentional bias in obsessional compulsive disorder. *Behaviour Research and Therapy, 34,* 53–60.

Taylor, C. B., King, R., Ehlers, A., Margraf, J., Clark, D., Hayward, C., Roth, W. T., & Agras, S. (1987). Treadmill exercise test and ambulatory measures in panic attacks. *American Journal of Cardiology, 60,* 48J–52J.

Taylor, C. B., Sheikh, J., Agras, W. S., Roth, W. T., Margraf, J., Ehlers, A., Maddock, R. J., & Gossard, D. (1986). Self-report of panic attacks: Agreement with heart rate changes. *American Journal of Psychiatry, 143,* 478–482.

Taylor, C. B., Telch, M. J., & Haavik, D. (1983). Ambulatory heart rate changes during panic attacks. *Journal of Psychosomatic Research, 17,* 1–6.

Taylor, J. E., Deane, F. P., & Podd, J. V. (1999). Stability of driving fear acquisition pathways over one year. *Behaviour Research and Therapy, 37,* 927–939.

Taylor, S. (1996). Meta-analysis of cognitive-behavioral treatments for social phobia. *Journal of Behaviour Therapy and Experimental Psychiatry, 27,* 1–9.

Taylor, S. (Ed.). (1999). *Anxiety sensitivity: Theory, research, and treatment of the fear of anxiety.* Mahwah, NJ: Erlbaum.

Taylor, S., & Cox, B. J. (1998). An expanded Anxiety Sensitivity Index: Evidence for a hierarchic structure in a clinical sample. *Journal of Anxiety Disorders, 12,* 463–483.

Taylor, S., Koch, W. J., & McNally, R. J. (1992). How does anxiety sensitivity vary across the anxiety disorders? *Journal of Anxiety Disorders, 6,* 249–259.

Taylor, S., Koch, W. J., McNally, R. J., & Crockett, D. J. (1992). Conceptualizations of anxiety sensitivity. *Psychological Assessment, 4,* 245–250.

Taylor, S., Koch, W. J., Woody, S., & McLean, P. (1997). Reliability and validity of the Cognition Checklist with psychiatric outpatients. *Assessment, 4,* 9–16.

Taylor, S., & Rachman, S. J. (1991). Fear of sadness. *Journal of Anxiety Disorders, 5,* 375–381.

Taylor, S., & Rachman, S. J. (1992). Fear and avoidance of aversive affective states: Dimensions and causal relations. *Journal of Anxiety Disorders, 6,* 15–25.

Taylor, S., & Rachman, S. J. (1994). Klein's suffocation theory of panic. *Archives of General Psychiatry, 51,* 505–506.

Taylor, S. E., & Brown, J. D. (1988). Illusion and well-being: A social psychological perspective on mental health. *Psychological Bulletin, 103*(2), 193–210.

Taylor, S. E., & Brown, J. D. (1994). Positive illusions and well-being revisited: Separating fact from fiction. *Psychological Bulletin, 116,* 21–27.

Taylor, S. E., Kemeny, M. E., Reed, G. M., Bower, J. E., & Gruenewald, T. L. (2000). Psychological resources, positive illusions, and health. *American Psychologist, 55,* 99–109.

Teasdale, J. D. (1983). Negative thinking in depression: Cause, effect, or reciprocal relationship. *Advances in Behaviour Research and Therapy, 5,* 3–25.

Teasdale, J. D. (1985). Psychophysiological treatments for depression: How do they work? *Behaviour Research and Therapy, 23,* 157–165.

Teasdale, J. D. (1993). Emotion and two kinds of meaning: Cognitive therapy and applied cognitive science. *Behaviour Research and Therapy, 31,* 339–354.

Teghtsoonian, R., & Frost, R. O. (1982). The effects of viewing distance on fear of snakes. *Journal of Behavior Therapy and Experimental Psychiatry, 13,* 181–190.

Telch, M. J., Agras, W. S., Taylor, C. B., Roth, W. T., & Gallen, C. (1985). Combined pharmacological and behavioral treatment for agoraphobia. *Behaviour Research and Therapy, 23,* 325–335.

Telch, M. J., Brouillard, M., Telch, C. F., Agras, W. S., & Taylor, C. B. (1989). Role of cognitive appraisal in panic-related avoidance. *Behaviour Research and Therapy, 27,* 373–383.

Telch, M. J., Ilai, D., Valentiner, D., & Craske, M. G. (1994). Match–mismatch of fear, panic and performance. *Behaviour Research and Therapy, 32,* 691–700.

Telch, M. J., & Lucas, J. A. (1994). Combined pharmacological and psychological treatment for panic disorder: Current status and future directions. In B. E. Wolfe & J. D. Maser (Eds.), *Treatment of panic disorder: A consensus development conference.* Washington, DC: American Psychiatric Press.

Telch, M. J., Lucas, J. A., & Nelson, P. (1989). Nonclinical panic in college students: An investigation of prevalence and symptomatology. *Journal of Abnormal Psychology, 98,* 300–306.

Telch, M. J., Lucas, J. A., Schmidt, N. B., Hanna, H. H., Jaimcz, T. S., & Lucas, R. A. (1993). Group cognitive-behavioral treatment of panic disorder. *Behaviour Research and Therapy, 31*, 279–287.

Telch, M. J., Schmidt, N. B., Jaimez, T. L., Jacquin, K. M., & Harrington, P. J. (1995). Impact of cognitive-behavioral treatment on quality of life in panic disorder patients. *Journal of Consulting and Clinical Psychology, 63*, 823–830.

Telch, M. J., Shermis, M. D., & Lucas, J. A. (1989). Anxiety sensitivity: Unitary personality trait or domain-specific appraisals. *Journal of Anxiety Disorders, 3*, 25–32.

Telch, M. J., Silverman, A., & Schmidt, N. B. (1996). Effects of anxiety sensitivity and perceived control on emotional responding to caffeine challenge. *Journal of Anxiety Disorders, 10*, 21–35.

Tellegen, A. (1982). *Brief manual for the Multidimensional Personality Questionnaire.* Unpublished manuscript, University of Minnesota.

Tellegen, A. (1985). Structures of mood and personality and their relevance to assessing anxiety, with an emphasis on self-report. In A. H. Tuma & J. D. Maser (Eds.), *Anxiety and the anxiety disorders.* Hillsdale, NJ: Erlbaum.

Tellegen, A., Lykken, D. T., Bouchard, T. J., Wilcox, K. J., Segal, N. L., & Rich, S. (1988). Personality similarity in twins reared apart and together. *Journal of Personality and Social Psychology, 54*, 1031–1039.

Tennant, C., Hurry, J., & Bebbington, P. (1982). The relation of childhood separation experiences to adult depressive and anxiety states. *British Journal of Psychiatry, 141*, 175–182.

Terhune, W. B. (1949). The phobic syndrome. *Archives of Neurology and Psychiatry, 62*, 162–172.

Thase, M. E. (1990). Relapse and recurrence in unipolar major depression: Short-term and long-term approaches. *Journal of Clinical Psychiatry, 51*(Suppl. 6), 51–57.

Thayer, J. F., Friedman, B. H., & Borkovec, T. D. (1996). Autonomic characteristics of generalized anxiety disorder and worry. *Biological Psychiatry, 39*, 255–266.

Thayer, J. F., Friedman, B. H., Borkovec, T. D., Johnsen, B. H., & Molina, S. (2000). Phasic heart period reactions to cued threat and nonthreat stimuli in generalized anxiety disorder. *Psychophysiology, 37*, 361–368.

Thom, A., Sartory, G., & Jöhren, P. (2000). Comparison between one-session psychological treatment and benzodiazepine in dental phobia. *Journal of Consulting and Clinical Psychology, 68*, 378–387.

Thompson, A. H., Bland, R. C., & Orn, H. T. (1989). Relationship and chronology of depression, agoraphobia, and panic disorder in the general population. *Journal of Nervous and Mental Disease, 177*, 456–463.

Thompson, R. A. (1998). Early sociopersonality development. In W. Damon (Series Ed.) & N. Eisenberg (Vol. Ed.), *Handbook of child psychology: Vol. 3. Social, emotional, and personality development* (5th ed., pp. 25–104). New York: Wiley.

Thompson, S. C. (1999). Illusions of control: How we overestimate our personal influence. *Current Directions in Psyhological Science, 8*(6), 187–190.

Thompson, S. C., Armstrong, W., & Thomas, C. (1998). Illusions of control, underestimations, and accuracy: A control heuristic explanation. *Psychological Bulletin, 123*, 143–161.

Thorén, P., Äsberg, M., Cronholm, B., Jörnestedt, L., & Träskman, L. (1980). Clomipramine treatment of obsessive–compulsive disorder: A controlled clinical trial. *Archives of General Psychiatry, 37*, 1281–1289.

Thornicroft, G., Colson, L., & Marks, I. (1991). An in-patient behavioral psychotherapy unit description and audit. *British Journal of Psychiatry, 158*, 362–367.

Thorpe, C. L., & Burns, L. E. (1983). *The agoraphobic syndrome.* New York: Wiley.

Thorpe, S. J., & Salkovskis, P. M. (1995). Phobic beliefs: Do cognitive factors play a role in specific phobias? *Behaviour Research and Therapy, 33*, 805–816.

Thorpe, S. J., & Salkovskis, P. M. (1997a). Information processing in spider phobics: The Stroop colour naming task may indicate strategic but not automatic attentional bias. *Behaviour Research and Therapy, 35*, 131–144.

Thorpe, S. J., & Salkovskis, P. M. (1997b). The effect of one-session treatment for spider phobia on attentional bias and beliefs. *British Journal of Clinical Psychology, 36,* 225–241.

Thorpe, S. J., & Salkovskis, P. M. (1998a). Studies on the role of disgust in the acquisition and maintenance of specific phobias. *Behaviour Research and Therapy, 36,* 877–893.

Thorpe, S. J., & Salkovskis, P. M. (1998b). Selective attention to real phobic and safety stimuli. *Behaviour Research and Therapy, 36,* 471–481.

Thyer, B. A., & Curtis, G. C. (1984). The effects of ethanol intoxication on phobic anxiety. *Behaviour Research and Therapy, 22,* 559–610.

Thyer, B. A., & Curtis, G. C. (1985). On the diphasic nature of vasovagal fainting associated with blood–injury–illness phobia. *Pavlovian Journal of Biological Science, 20,* 84–87.

Thyer, B. A., & Himle, J. (1985). Temporal relationship between panic attack onset and phobic avoidance in agoraphobia. *Behaviour Research and Therapy, 23,* 607–608.

Thyer, B. A., & Himle, J. (1987). Phobic anxiety and panic anxiety: How do they differ? *Journal of Anxiety Disorders, 1,* 59–67.

Thyer, B. A., Himle, I., Curtis, G. C., Cameron, O. G., & Nesse, R. M. (1985). A comparison of panic disorder and agoraphobia with panic attacks. *Comprehensive Psychiatry, 26,* 208–214.

Thyer, B. A., Nesse, R. M., Cameron, O. G., & Curtis, G. C. (1985). Agoraphobia: A test of the separation anxiety hypotheses. *Behaviour Research and Therapy, 23,* 75–78.

Thyer, B. A., Nesse, R. M., Curtis, G. C., & Cameron, O. G. (1986). Panic disorder: A test of the separation anxiety hypothesis. *Behaviour Research and Therapy, 24,* 209–211.

Thyer, B. A., Papsdorf, J. D., & Wright, P. (1984). Physiological and psychological effects of acute intentional hyperventilation. *Behaviour Research and Therapy, 22,* 587–590.

Thyer, B. A., Parrish, R. T., Curtis, G. C., Nesse, R. M., & Cameron, O. G. (1985). Ages of onset of DSM-III anxiety disorders. *Comprehensive Psychiatry, 26,* 113–122.

Thyer, B. A., Parrish, R. T., Himle, J., Cameron, O. G., Curtis, G. C., & Nesse, R. M. (1986). Alcohol abuse among clinically anxious patients. *Behaviour Research and Therapy, 24,* 357–359.

Tolin, D. F., Lohr, J. M., Lee, T. C., & Sawchuk, C. N. (1999). Visual avoidance in specific phobia. *Behaviour Research and Therapy, 37,* 63–70.

Tolin, D. F., Lohr, J. M., Sawchuk, C. N., & Lee, T. C. (1997). Disgust and disgust sensitivity in blood–injection–injury and spider phobia. *Behaviour Research and Therapy, 35,* 949–953.

Tollefson, G. D. (1993). Major depression. In D. I. Dunner (Ed.), *Current psychiatric therapy.* Philadelphia: Saunders.

Tollefson, G. D., & Rosenbaum, J. F. (1998). Selective serotonin reuptake inhibitors. In A. F. Schatzberg & C. B. Nemeroff (Eds.), *Textbook of psychopharmacology* (2nd ed.). Washington, DC: American Psychiatric Press.

Tomarken, A. J., Davidson, R. J., Wheeler, R. E., & Doss, R. C. (1992). Individual differences in anterior brain asymmetry and fundamental dimensions of emotion. *Journal of Personality and Social Psychology, 62,* 676–687.

Tomarken, A. J., Mineka, S., & Cook, M. (1989). Fear-relevant selective associations and covariation bias. *Journal of Abnormal Psychology, 98,* 381–394.

Toren, P., Eldar, S., Cendorf, D., Wolmer, L., Weizman, R., Zubadi, R., Koren, S., & Laor, N. (1999). The prevalence of mitral valve prolapse in children with anxiety disorders. *Journal of Psychiatric Research, 33,* 357–361.

Torgersen, S. (1979). The nature and origin of common phobic fears. *British Journal of Psychiatry, 134,* 343–351.

Torgersen, S. (1983a). Genetic factors in anxiety disorders. *Archives of General Psychiatry, 40,* 1085–1089.

Torgersen, S. (1983b). Genetics of neurosis: The effects of sampling variation upon the twin concordance ratio. *British Journal of Psychiatry, 142,* 126–132.

Townend, E., Dimigen, G., & Fung, D. (2000). A clinical study of child dental anxiety. *Behaviour Research and Therapy, 38,* 31–46.

Tracey, S. A., Chorpita, B. F., Douban, J., & Barlow, D. H. (1997). Empirical evaluation of DSM-IV generalized anxiety disorder criteria in children and adolescents. *Journal of Clinical Child Psychology, 26,* 404–414.

Tran, G. Q., & Chambless, D. L. (1995). Psychopathology of social phobia: Effects of subtype and of avoidant personality disorder. *Journal of Anxiety Disorders, 9,* 489–501.

Troisi, J. R., Critchfield, T. S., & Griffith, J. (1993). Buspirone and lorazepam abuse liability in humans: Behavioural effects, subjective effects, and choice. *Behavioural Pharmacology, 4,* 217–230.

Trower, P., Bryant, B., & Argyle, M. (1978). *Social skills and mental health.* London: Methuen.

Trower, P., & Gilbert, P. (1989). New theoretical conceptions of social anxiety and social phobia. *Clinical Psychology Review, 9,* 19–35.

True, W. R., Rice, J., Eisen, S. A., Heath, A. C., Goldberg, J., Lyons, M. J., & Nowak, J. (1993). A twin study of genetic and environmental contributions to liability for posttraumatic stress symptoms. *Archives of General Psychiatry, 50,* 257–264.

Trull, T. J., & Sher, K. J. (1994). Relationship between the five-factor model of personality and Axis I disorders in a nonclinical sample. *Journal of Abnormal Psychology, 103*(2), 350–360.

Tsao, J. C. I., & Craske, M. G. (2000). Timing of treatment and return of fear: Effects of massed, uniform-, and expanding–spaced exposure schedules. *Behavior Therapy, 31,* 479–497.

Tsao, J. C. I., Lewin, M. R., & Craske, M. G. (1998). The effects of cognitive-behavior therapy for panic disorder on comorbid conditions. *Journal of Anxiety Disorders, 12,* 357–371.

Turkat, I. D. (1982). An investigation of parental modeling in the etiology of diabetic illness behavior. *Behaviour Research and Therapy, 20,* 547–552.

Turner, J. E., & Cole, D. A. (1994). Developmental differences in cognitive diatheses for child depression. *Journal of Abnormal Child Psychology, 22,* 15–32.

Turner, S. M., & Beidel, D. C. (1988). Some further comments on the measurement of social phobia. *Behaviour Research and Therapy, 26,* 411–413.

Turner, S. M., Beidel, D. C., Cooley, M. R., Woody, S. R., & Messer, S. C. (1994). A multicomponent behavioral treatment of social phobia: Social Effectiveness Therapy. *Behaviour Research and Therapy, 32,* 381–390.

Turner, S. M., Beidel, D. C., & Cooley-Quille, M. R. (1995). Two year follow-up of social phobics treated with Social Effectiveness Therapy. *Behaviour Research and Therapy, 33,* 553–556.

Turner, S. M., Beidel, D. C., & Costello, A. (1987). Psychopathology in the offspring of anxiety disorders patients. *Journal of Consulting and Clinical Psychology, 55,* 229–235.

Turner, S. M., Beidel, D. C., Dancu, C. V., & Stanley, M. A. (1989). An empirically derived inventory to measure social fears and anxiety: The Social Phobia and Anxiety Inventory. *Psychological Assessment, 1,* 35–40.

Turner, S. M., Beidel, D. C., & Jacob, R. G. (1988). Assessment of panic. In S. J. Rachman & J. D. Maser (Eds.), *Panic: Psychological perspectives.* Hillsdale, NJ: Erlbaum.

Turner, S. M., Beidel, D. C., & Jacob, R. G. (1994). Social phobia: A comparison of behavior therapy and atenolol. *Journal of Consulting and Clinical Psychology, 62,* 350–358.

Turner, S. M., Beidel, D. C., Long, P. J., & Townsley, R. M. (1993). A composite measure to determine the functional status of treated social phobics: The Social Phobia Endstate Functioning Index. *Behavior Therapy, 24,* 265–275.

Turner, S. M., Beidel, D. C., & Nathan, R. S. (1985). Biological factors in obsessive–compulsive disorders. *Psychological Bulletin, 97,* 451–461.

Turner, S. M., Beidel, D. C., & Stanley, M. A. (1992). Are obsessional thoughts and worry different cognitive phenomena? *Clinical Psychology Review, 12,* 257–270.

Turner, S. M., Beidel, D. C., & Townsley, R. M. (1990). Social phobia: Relationship to shyness. *Behaviour Research and Therapy, 28,* 497–505.

Turner, S. M., Beidel, D. C., & Townsley, R. M. (1992). Social phobia: A comparison of specific and generalized subtypes and avoidant personality disorder. *Journal of Abnormal Psychology, 101,* 326–331.

Turner, S. M., Beidel, D. C., & Wolff, P. L. (1994). A composite measure to determine improvement following treatment for social phobia: The Index of Social Phobia Improvement. *Behaviour Research and Therapy, 4,* 471–476.

Turner, S. M., Beidel, D. C., & Wolff, P. L. (1996). Is behavioral inhibition related to the anxiety disorders? *Clinical Psychology Review, 16,* 157–172.

Turner, S. M., Beidel, D. C., Wolff, P. L., Spaulding, S., & Jacob, R. G. (1996). Clinical features affecting treatment outcome in social phobia. *Behaviour Research and Therapy, 34,* 795–804.

Turner, S. M., Cooley-Quille, M. R., & Beidel, D. C. (1996). Behavioral and pharmacological treatment for social phobia. In M. R. Mavissakalian & R. F. Prien (Eds.), *Long-term treatments of anxiety disorders.* Washington, DC: American Psychiatric Press.

Turner, S. M., Hersen, M., Bellack, A. S., Andrasik, F., & Capparell, H. V. (1980). Behavioral and pharmacological treatment of obsessive–compulsive disorders. *Journal of Nervous and Mental Disease, 168,* 651–657.

Turner, S. M., Hersen, M., Bellack, A. S., & Wells, K. C. (1979). Behavioural treatment of obsessive-compulsive nerurosis. *Behaviour Research and Therapy, 17,* 95–106.

Turner, S. M., McCanna, M., & Beidel, D. C. (1987). Discriminative validity of the Social Avoidance and Distress and Fear of Negative Evaluation Scale. *Behaviour Research and Therapy, 25,* 113–115.

Turner, S. M., Stanley, M. A., Beidel, D. C., & Bond, L. (1989). The Social Phobia and Anxiety Inventory: Construct validity. *Journal of Psychopathology and Behavioral Assessment, 11,* 221–234.

Turner, S. M., Williams, S. L., Beidel, D. C., & Mezzich, J. E. (1986). Panic disorder and agoraphobia with panic attacks: Covariation along the dimensions of panic and agoraphobic fear. *Journal of Abnormal Psychology, 95,* 384–388.

Tyrer, P. J. (1973). Relevance of bodily feelings in emotion. *Lancet, i,* 915–916.

Tyrer, P. J. (1976). *The role of bodily feelings in anxiety.* London: Oxford University Press.

Tyrer, P. J. (1984). Classification of anxiety. *British Journal of Psychiatry, 144,* 78–93.

Tyrer, P. J. (1989). *Classification of neurosis.* Chichester, England: Wiley.

Tyrer, P. J., Seivewright, N., Murphy, S., Ferguson, B., Kingdon, D., Barczak, B., Brothwell, J., Darling, C., Gregory, S., & Johnson, A. L. (1988). The Nottingham study of neurotic disorder: Comparison of drug and psychological treatments. *Lancet, ii,* 235–240.

Udelman, H. D., & Udelman, D. L. (1990). Concurrent use of buspirone in anxious patients during withdrawal from alprazolam therapy. *Journal of Clinical Psychiatry, 51*(Suppl. 9), 46–50.

Uhde, T. W. (1994). The anxiety disorders: Phenomenology and treatment of core symptoms and associated sleep disturbance. In M. Kryger, T. Roth, & W. Dement (Eds.), *Principles and practice of sleep medicine.* Philadelphia: Saunders.

Uhde, T. W., Boulenger, J. P., Post, R. M., Siever, L. J., Vittone, B. J., Jimerson, D. C., & Roy-Byrne, P. P. (1984). Fear and anxiety: Relationship to noradrenergic function. *Psychopathology, 17,* 8–23.

Uhde, T. W., Boulenger, J. P., Roy-Byrne, P. P., Geraci, M. P., Vittone, B. J., & Post, R. M. (1985). Longitudinal course of panic disorder: Clinical and biological considerations. *Progressive Neuro-Psychopharmacology and Biological Psychiatry, 9,* 39–51.

Uhde, T. W., Boulenger, J. P., Vittone, B., Siever, L., & Post, R. M. (1985). Human anxiety and nonadrenergic function: Preliminary studies with caffeine, clonidine and yohimbine. In *Proceedings of the Seventh World Congress of Psychiatry.* New York: Plenum Press.

Uhde, T., Siever, L., & Post, R. M. (1984). Clonidine: Acute challenge and clinical trial paradigms for the investigation and treatment of anxiety disorders, affective illness, and pain syndromes. In R. M. Post & J. C. Ballenger (Eds.), *Neurobiology of mood disorders.* Baltimore: Williams & Wilkins.

Uhde, T., Siever, L., Post, R. M., Jimerson, D., Boulenger, J. P., & Buchsbaum, M. (1982). The relationship of plasma-free MHPG to anxiety and psychophysical pain in normal volunteers. *Psychopharmacological Bulletin, 18,* 129–132.

Uhlenhuth, E. H. (1998). Treatment strategies in panic disorder: Recommendations of an expert panel [Abstract]. *Psiquiatria Biologica*, 6(Suppl. 1), 96.

Uhlenhuth, E. H., Matuzas, W., Warner, T. D., & Thompson, P. M. (1997). Methodological issues in psychopharmacological research: Growing placebo response rate: The problem in recent therapeutic trials. *Psychopharmacology Bulletin*, 33, 31–39.

Ulett, G. A., Gleser, G., Winokur, G., & Lawler, A. (1953). The EEG and reaction to phobic stimulation as an index of anxiety-proneness. *Electroencephalography and Clinical Neurophysiology*, 5, 23–32.

Unrug-Neervoort, A., van Luijtelaar, G., & Coenen, A. M. (1992). Cognition and vigilance: Differential effects of diazepam and buspirone on memory and psychomotor performance. *Neuropsychobiology*, 26, 146–150.

Valentiner, D. P., Telch, M. J., Ilai, D., & Hehmsoth, M. M. (1993). Claustrophobic fear behavior: A test of the expectancy model of fear. *Behaviour Research and Therapy*, 31, 395–402.

Valentiner, D. P., Telch, M. J., Petruzzi, D. C., & Bolte, M. C. (1996). Cognitive mechanisms in claustrophobia: An examination of Reiss and McNally's expectancy model and Bandura's self-efficacy theory. *Cognitive Therapy and Research*, 20, 593–612.

van Ameringen, M., Mancini, C., & Streiner, D. L. (1993). Fluoxetine efficacy in social phobia. *Journal of Clinical Psychiatry*, 54, 27–32.

van Balkom, A. J. L. M., Bakker, A., Spinhoven, P., Blaauw, B. M. J. W., Smeenk, S., & Ruesink, B. (1997). A meta-analysis of the treatment of panic disorder with or without agoraphobia: A comparison of psychopharmacological, cognitive-behavioral, and combination treatments. *Journal of Nervous and Mental Disease*, 185, 510–516.

van Balkom, A. J. L. M., de Haan, E., van Oppen, P., Spinhoven, P., Hoogduin, K. A. L., Vermeulen, A. W. A., & van Dyck, R. (1998). Cognitive and behavioral therapies alone and in combination with fluvoxamine in the treatment of obsessive compulsive disorder. *Journal of Nervous and Mental Disease*, 186, 492–499.

van Balkom, A. J. L. M., van Oppen, P., Vermeulen, A. W. A., van Dyck, R., Nauta, M. C. E., & Vorst, H. C. M. (1994). A meta-analysis on the treatment of obsessive–compulsive disorder: A comparison of antidepressants, behavior, and cognitive therapy. *Clinical Psychology Review*, 14, 359–381.

van den Hout, M. A. (1988). The explanation of experimental panic. In S. Rachman & J. D. Maser (Eds.), *Panic: Psychological perspectives*. Hillsdale, NJ: Erlbaum.

van den Hout, M. A., & Griez, E. (1982). Cardiovascular and subjective responses to inhalation of carbon dioxide. *Psychotherapy and Psychosomatics*, 37, 75–82.

van den Hout, M., Tenney, N., Huygens, K., & de Jong, P. (1997). Preconscious processing bias in specific phobia. *Behaviour Research and Therapy*, 35, 29–34.

van der Does, A. J. W., Antony, M. M., Ehlers, A., & Barsky, A. J. (2000). Heartbeat perception in panic disorder: A reanalysis. *Behaviour Research and Therapy*, 38, 47–62.

van der Kolk, B. A., Dreyfuss, D., Michaels, M., Berkowitz, R., Saxe, G., & Goldenberg, I. (1994). Fluoxetine in posttraumatic stress disorder. *Journal of Clinical Psychiatry*, 55, 517–522.

van der Molen, M. A., van den Hout, M. A., van Dieren, A. C., & Griez, E. (1989). Childhood separation anxiety and adult-onset panic disorders. *Journal of Anxiety Disorders*, 3, 97–106.

van Megan, H., Westenberg, M., & den Boer, J. A. (1997). Effect of the selective serotonin reuptake inhibitor fluvoxamine of CCK-4 induced panic attacks. *Psychopharmacology*, 129, 357–364.

van Noppen, B., Steketee, G., McCorkle, B., & Pato, M. T. (1997). Group and multi-family behavioral treatment for OCD: A pilot study. *Journal of Anxiety Disorders*, 11, 431–446.

van Oppen, P., de Haan, E., van Balkom, A., Spinhoven, P., Hoogduin, K., & van Dyck, R. (1995). Cognitive therapy and exposure in vivo in the treatment of obsessive compulsive disorder. *Behaviour Research and Therapy*, 4, 379–390.

van Oppen, P., Hoekstra, R. J., & Emmelkamp, P. M. G. (1995). The structure of obsessive–compulsive symptoms. *Behaviour Research and Therapy*, 33, 15–23.

van Vliet, I. M., den Boer, J. A., & Westenberg, H. G. M. (1994). Psychopharmacological treatment of social phobia: A double-blind, placebo-controlled study with fluvoxamine. *Psychopharmacology, 115,* 128–134.

van Zijderveld, G. A., TenVoorde, B. J., Veltman, D. J., van Doornen, L. J., Orlebeke, J. F., van Dyck, R., & Tilders, F. J. H. (1997). Cardiovascular, respiratory, and panic reactions to epinephrine in panic disorder patients. *Biological Psychiatry, 41,* 249–251.

van Zijderveld, G. A., van Doornen, L. J. P., Orlebeke, J. F., & Snieder, H. (1992). The psychophysiological effects of adrenaline infusions as a function of trait anxiety and aerobic fitness. *Anxiety Research, 4,* 257–274.

van Zijderveld, G. A., van Doornen, L. J. P., van Faassen, I., Orlebeke, J. F., van Dyck, R., & Tilders, F. J. H. (1993). Adrenaline and the relationship between neurosomatism, aerobic fitness and mental task performance. *Biological Psychology, 36,* 157–181.

Vasey, M. W., & Borkovec, T. D. (1992). A catastrophizing assessment of worrisome thoughts. *Cognitive Therapy and Research, 16,* 505–520.

Vasey, M. W., Crnic, K. A., & Carter, W. G. (1994). Worry in childhood: Developmental perspective. *Cognitive Therapy and Research, 18,* 529–549.

Vasterling, J. J., Brailey, K., Constans, J. I., & Sotker, P. B. (1998). Attention and memory dysfunction in posttraumatic stress disorders. *Neuropsychology, 12*(1), 125–133.

Vaughan, K., Armstrong, M. S., Gold, R., O'Connor, N., Jenneke, W., & Tarrier, N. (1994). A trial of eye movement desensitization compared to image habituation training and applied muscle relaxation in post-traumatic stress disorder. *Journal of Behavior Therapy and Experimental Psychiatry, 25,* 283–291.

Vega, W. A., Kolody, B., Aguilar-Gaxiola, S., Alderete, E., Catalano, R., & Caraveo-Anduaga, J. (1998). Lifetime prevalence of DSM-III-R psychiatric disorders among urban and rural Mexican Americans in California. *Archives of General Psychiatry, 55,* 771–778.

Verburg, K., Griez, E., & Meijer, J. (1994). A 35% carbon dioxide challenge in simple phobias. *Acta Psychiatrica Scandinavica, 90,* 420–423.

Verburg, K., Griez, E., Meijer, J., & Pols, H. (1995). Respiratory disorders as a possible predisposing factor for panic disorder. *Journal of Affective Disorders, 33,* 129–134.

Vermilyea, J. A., Boice, R., & Barlow, D. H. (1984). Rachman and Hodgson (1974) a decade later: How do desynchronous response systems relate to the treatment of agoraphobia? *Behaviour Research and Therapy, 22,* 615–621.

Versiani, M., Mundim, F. D., Nardi, A. E., & Liebowitz, M. R. (1988). Tranylcypromine in social phobia. *Journal of Clinical Psychopharmacology, 8,* 279–283.

Versiani, M., Nardi, A. E., Mundim, F. D., Alves, A. B., Liebowitz, M. R., & Amrein, R. (1992). Pharmacotherapy of social phobia: A controlled study with moclobemide and phenelzine. *British Journal of Psychiatry, 161,* 353–360.

Versiani, M., Nardi, A. E., Mundim, F. D., Pinto, S., Saboya, E., & Kovacs, R. (1996). The long-term treatment of social phobia with moclobemide. *International Journal of Psychopharmacology, 11,* 83–33.

Vrana, S. R., Cuthbert, B. N., & Lang, P. J. (1986). Fear imagery and text processing. *Psychophysiology, 23,* 247–253.

Waddell, M. T., Barlow, D. H., & O'Brien, G. T. (1984). A preliminary investigation of cognitive and relaxation treatment of panic disorder: Effects on intense anxiety vs. "background" anxiety. *Behaviour Research and Therapy, 22,* 393–402.

Wade, A. G., Lepola, U., Koponen, H. J., Pedersen, V., & Pedersen, T. (1997). The effect of citalopram in panic disorder. *British Journal of Psychiatry, 170,* 549–553.

Wade, W. A., Treat, T. A., & Stuart, G. L. (1998). Transporting an empirically supported treatment for panic disorder to a service clinic setting: A benchmarking strategy. *Journal of Consulting and Clinical Psychology, 66,* 231–239.

Wagner, A. R. (1981). SOP: A model of automatic memory processing in animal behavior. In N. E. Spear & R. R. Miller (Eds.), *Information processing in animals: Memory mechanisms.* Hillsdale, NJ: Erlbaum.

Waikar, S. V., Bystritsky, A., Craske, M. G., & Murphy, K. (1994–1995). Etiological beliefs and treatment preferences in anxiety-disordered patients. *Anxiety, 1*, 134–137.

Wallace, C. S., Kilman, V. L., Withers, G. S., & Greenough, W. T. (1992). Increases in dendritic length in occipital cortex after 4 days of differential housing in weanling rats. *Behavioral and Neural Biology, 58*, 64–68.

Wallace, S. T., & Alden, L. E. (1991). A comparison of social standards and perceived ability in anxious and nonanxious men. *Cognitive Therapy and Research, 15*, 237–254.

Wallace, S. T., & Alden, L. E. (1995). Social anxiety and standard setting following social success or failure. *Cognitive Therapy and Research, 19*, 613–631.

Wallace, S. T., & Alden, L. E. (1997). Social phobia and positive social events: The price of success. *Journal of Abnormal Psychology, 106*, 416–424.

Waller, N. G., & Meehl, P. E. (1997). *Multivariate taxometric procedures: Distinguishing types from continua.* Newbury Park, CA: Sage.

Wallnau, L. H., & Gallup, G. G., Jr. (1977). A serotonergic, midbrain–raphe model of tonic immobility. *Biobehavioral Reviews, 1*, 35–43.

Walls, M. M., & Kleinknecht, R. A. (1996, April). *Disgust factors as predictors of blood–injury fear and fainting.* Paper presented at the annual meeting of the Western Psychological Association, San José, CA.

Walter, D. A., & Ziegler, C. A. (1980). The effects of birth order on locus of control. *Bulletin of the Psychonomic Society, 15*, 293–294.

Walter, W. G. (1964). Slow potential waves in the human brain assodated with expectancy, attention and decision. *Archives für Psychiatrie und Nervenkrankheiten, 206*, 309–322.

Walters, K. S., & Hope, D. A. (1998). Analysis of social behavior in individuals with social phobia and nonanxious participants using a psychobiological model. *Behavior Therapy, 29*, 387–407.

Walton, D. (1960). The relevance of learning theory to the treatment of an obsessive–compulsive state. In H. J. Eysenck (Ed.), *Behaviour therapy and the neuroses.* Oxford: Pergamon Press.

Wamboldt, M. Z., & Insel, T. R. (1988). Pharmacologic models. In C. G. Last & M. Hersen (Eds.), *Handbook of anxiety disorders.* New York: Pergamon Press.

Wang, Z. W., Crowe, R. R., & Noyes, R. (1992). Adrenergic receptor genes as candidate genes for panic disorder: A linkage study. *American Journal of Psychiatry, 149*, 470–474.

Wardle, J., Hayward, P., Higgitt, A., Stabi, M., Blizard, R., & Gray, J. (1994). Effects of concurrent diazepam treatment on the outcome of exposure therapy in agoraphobia. *Behaviour Research and Therapy, 32*, 203–215.

Ware, J., Jain, K., Burgess, I., & Davey, G. C. L. (1994). Disease-avoidance model: Factor analysis of common animal fears. *Behaviour Research and Therapy, 32*, 57–63.

Warshaw, M. G., Massion, A. O., Peterson, L. G., Pratt, L. A., & Keller, M. B. (1995). Suicidal behavior in patients with panic disorder: Retrospective and prospective data. *Journal of Affective Disorders, 34*, 235–247.

Washington, R. A. (1974). The relationship between children's school performances and parent participation as a function of the movement toward community control of the schools. *Dissertation Abstracts International, 35*, 4202B.

Watari, K. F., & Brodbeck, C. (2000). Culture, health, and financial appraisals: Comparison of worry in older Japanese Americans and European Americans. *Journal of Clinical Geropsychology, 6*, 25–39.

Watson, C. G., Juba, M. P., Manifold, V., Kucala, T., & Anderson, P. (1991). The PTSD Interview: Rationale, description, reliability, and concurrent validity of a DSM-III-based technique. *Journal of Clinical Psychology, 47*, 179–188.

Watson, C. G., Kucala, T., & Manifold, V. (1986). A cross-validation of the Keane and Penk MMPI scales as measures of post-traumatic stress disorder. *Journal of Clinical Psychology, 42*, 727–732.

Watson, D., & Clark, L. A. (1984). Negative affectivity: The disposition to experience negative emotional states. *Psychological Bulletin, 96*, 465–490.

Watson, D., & Clark, L. A. (1991). *Manual for the Positive and Negative Affect Schedule—Expanded Form*. Iowa City: University of Iowa.

Watson, D., Clark, L. A., & Carey, G. (1988). Positive and negative affectivity and their relation to the anxiety and depressive disorders. *Journal of Abnormal Psychology, 97*, 346–353.

Watson, D., Clark, L. A., & Harkness, A. R. (1994). Structures of personality and their relevance to psychopathology. *Journal of Abnormal Psychology, 103*, 18–31.

Watson, D., Clark, L. A., & Tellegen, A. (1988). Development and validation of brief measures of Positive and Negative Affect: The PANAS Scales. *Journal of Personality and Social Psychology, 54*, 1063–1070.

Watson, D., Clark, L. A., Weber, K., Assenheimer, J. S., Strauss, M. E., & McCormick, R. A. (1995). Testing a tripartite model: II. Exploring the symptom structure of anxiety and depression in student, adult, and patient samples. *Journal of Abnormal Psychology, 104*, 15–25.

Watson, D., & Friend, R. (1969). Measurement of social-evaluative anxiety. *Journal of Consulting and Clinical Psychology, 33*, 448–457.

Watson, D., Weber, K., Assenheimer, J. S., Clark, L. A., Strauss, M. E., & McCormick, R. A. (1995). Testing a tripartite model: I. Evaluating the convergent and discriminant validity of anxiety and depression symptom scales. *Journal of Abnormal Psychology, 104*, 3–14.

Watson, J., & Raynor, R. (1920). Conditioned emotional reactions. *Journal of Genetic Psychology, 37*, 394–419.

Watson, J. P., & Marks, I. M. (1971). Relevant and irrelevant fear in flooding: A crossover study of phobic patients. *Behavior Therapy, 2*, 275–293.

Watts, F. N., McKenna, F. P., Sharrock, R., & Trezise, L. (1986). Colour naming of phobia-related words. *British Journal of Psychology, 77*, 97–108.

Watts, F. N., Trezise, L., & Sharrock, R. (1986). Processing of phobic stimuli. *British Journal of Clinical Psychology, 25*, 253–259.

Wearn, J. T., & Sturgis, C. C. (1919). Studies on epinephrine: I. Effects of the injection of epinephrine in soldiers with "irritable heart." *Archives of Internal Medicine, 24*, 247–268.

Weathers, F. W., Blake, D. D., Krinsley, K. E., Haddad, W., Huska, J. A., & Keane, T. M. (1992). *The Clinician-Administered PTSD Scale: Reliability and construct validity*. Paper presented at the 26th Annual Convention of the Association for Advancement of Behavior Therapy, Boston.

Weathers, F. W., Keane, T. M., & Davidson, J. R. T. (2001). The Clinician-Administered PTSD Scale: A review of the first ten years of research. *Depression and Anxiety, 13*, 132–156.

Weathers, F. W., Litz, B. T., Herman, D., Huska, J., & Keane, T. M. (1993). *The PTSD Checklist (PCL): Reliability, validity and diagnostic utility*. Paper presented at the meeting of the International Society for Traumatic Stress Studies, San Antonio, TX.

Weathers, F. W., Ruscio, A. M., & Keane, T. M. (1999). Psychometric properties of nine scoring rules for the Clinician-Administered Posttraumatic Stress Disorder Scale. *Psychological Assessment, 11*, 124–133.

Webster, A. S. (1953). The development of phobias in married women. *Psychological Monographs, 67*, 367.

Weems, C. F., Silverman, W. K., & La Greca, A. M. (2000). What do youth referred for anxiety problems worry about?: Worry and its relation to anxiety and anxiety disorders in children and adolescents. *Journal of Abnormal Child Psychology, 28*, 63–72.

Wegner, D. M. (1989). *White bears and other unwanted thoughts*. New York: Viking.

Wegner, D. M. (1994). Ironic processes of mental control. *Psychological Review, 101*, 34–52.

Wegner, D. M., & Giuliano, T. (1980). Arousal-induced attention to the self. *Journal of Personality and Social Psychology, 38*, 719–726.

Wegner, D. M., & Zanakos, S. (1994). Chronic thought suppression. *Journal of Personality, 62*, 615–640.

Weilner, A., Reich, T., Robins, I., Fishman, R., & van Doren, T. (1976). Obsessive–compulsive neurosis. *Comprehensive Psychiatry, 17*, 527–539.

Weiner, H. (1985). The psychobiology and pathophysiology of anxiety and fear. In A. H. Tuma & J. D. Maser (Eds.), *Anxiety and the anxiety disorders*. Hillsdale, NJ: Erlbaum.

Weir, R. O., & Marshall, W. L. (1980). Relaxation and distraction in experimental desensitization. *Journal of Clinical Psychology, 36,* 246–252.

Weisberg, R. B., Brown, T. A., Wincze, J. P., & Barlow, D. H. (2001). Causal attributions and male sexual arousal: The impact of attributions for a bogus erectile difficulty on sexual arousal, cognitions, and affect. *Journal of Abnormal Psychology, 110*(2), 324–334.

Weisberg, R. B., Sbrocco, T. A., & Barlow, D. H. (1994, November). *A comparison of sexual fantasy use between men with situational erectile disorder, generalized erectile disorder, and sexually functional males: Preliminary results.* Paper presented at the 28th Annual Convention of the Association for Advancement of Behavior Therapy, San Diego, CA.

Weiss, D. (1997). Structured clinical interview techniques. In J. P. Wilson & T. M. Keane (Eds.), *Assessing psychological trauma and PTSD.* New York: Guilford Press.

Weiss, D., & Marmar, C. (1997) The Impact of Event Scale—Revised. In J. P. Wilson & T. M. Keane (Eds.) *Assessing psychological trauma and PTSD.* New York: Guilford Press.

Weiss, J. M. (1971a). Effects of coping behavior in different warning signal conditions on stress pathology in rats. *Journal of Comparative and Physiological Psychology, 77,* 1–13.

Weiss, J. M. (1971b). Effects of punishing the coping response (conflict) on stress pathology in rats. *Journal of Comparative and Physiological Psychology, 77,* 14–21.

Weiss, J. M., Bailey, W. H., Goodman, P. A., Hoffman, L. I., Ambrose, M. I., Salman, S., & Charry, I. M. (1982). A model for neurochemical study of depression. In M. Y. Spiegelstein & A. Levy (Eds.), *Behavioral models and the analysis of drug action.* Amsterdam: Elsevier.

Weiss, J. M., Glazer, H. I., & Poherecky, L. A. (1976). Coping behavior and neurochemical changes: An alternative explanation for the original "learned helplessness" experiments. In A. Serban & A. Kling (Eds.), *Animal models in human psychobiology.* New York: Plenum Press.

Weiss, K. J., & Rosenberg, D. J. (1985). Prevalence of anxiety disorders among alcoholics. *Journal of Clinical Psychiatry, 46,* 3–5.

Weissman, M. M. (1985). The epidemiology of anxiety disorders: Rates, risks and familial patterns. In A. H. Tuma & I. D. Maser (Eds.), *Anxiety and the anxiety disorders.* Hillsdale, NJ: Erlbaum.

Weissman, M. M. (1991). Panic disorder: Impact on quality of life. *Journal of Clinical Psychiatry, 52*(Suppl. Feb), 6–8.

Weissman, M. M. (1993). Family genetic studies of panic disorder. *Journal of Psychiatric Research, 27*(Suppl. 1), 69–78.

Weissmann, M. M., Bland, R., Canino, G., Greenwald, S., Hwo, H., Lee, C., Newman, S., Oakley-Browne, M., Rubio-Stipek, M., Wickramaratne, P., Wittchen, H., & Eng-Kung, Y. (1994). The cross national epidemiology of obsessive compulsive disorder. *Journal of Clinical Psychiatry, 55,* 5–10.

Weissman, M. M., Klerman, G. L., Markowitz, J. S., & Ouellette, R. (1989). Suicidal ideation and suicide attempts in panic disorder and attacks. *New England Journal of Medicine, 321,* 1209–1214.

Weissman, M. M., Leaf, P. I., Blazer, D. G., Boyd, J. H., & Florio, L. (1986). The relationship between panic disorder and agoraphobia: An epidemiologic perspective. *Psychopharmacology Bulletin, 43,* 787–791.

Weissman, M. M., Leckman, J. F., Merikangas, K. R., Gammon, G. D., & Prusoff, B. A. (1984). Depression and anxiety disorders in parents and children. *Archives of General Psychiatry, 41,* 845–852.

Weisz, J. R., & Stipek, D. J. (1982). Competence, contingency, and the undevelopment of perceived control. *Human Development, 25,* 250–281.

Welkowitz, L. A., Papp, L., Martinez, J., Browne, S., & Gorman, J. M. (1999). Instructional set and physiological response to CO_2 inhalation. *American Journal of Psychiatry, 156,* 745–748.

Wells, A. (1990). Panic disorder in association with relaxation induced anxiety: An attentional training approach to treatment. *Behavior Therapy, 21,* 273–280.

Wells, A. (1994a). Attention and the control of worry. In G. C. L. Davey & F. Tallis (Eds.), *Worrying: Perspectives on theory, assessment, and treatment.* New York: Wiley.

Wells, A. (1994b). A multi-dimensional measure of worry: Development and preliminary validation of the Anxious Thoughts Inventory. *Anxiety, Stress, and Coping, 6*, 289–299.

Wells, A. (1995). Meta-cognition and worry: A cognitive model of generalized anxiety disorder. *Behavioural and Cognitive Psychotherapy, 23*, 301–320.

Wells, A. (1997). *Cognitive therapy of anxiety disorders: A practice manual and conceptual guide.* New York: Wiley.

Wells, A. (1999). A metacognitive model and therapy for generalized anxiety disorder. *Clinical Psychology and Psychotherapy, 6*, 86–95.

Wells, A., & Carter, K. (1999). Preliminary tests of a cognitive model of generalized anxiety disorder. *Behaviour Research and Therapy, 37*, 585–594.

Wells, A., & Clark, D. M. (1997). Social phobia: A cognitive approach. In G. C. L. Davey (Ed.), *Phobias: A handbook of theory, research, and treatment.* Chichester, England: Wiley.

Wells, A., Clark, D. M., & Ahmad, S. (1998). How do I look with my mind's eye?: Perspective taking in social phobic imagery. *Behaviour Research and Therapy, 36*, 631–634.

Wells, A., Clark, D. M., Salkovskis, P. M., Ludgate, J., Hackmann, A., & Gelder, M. (1995). Social phobia: The role of in-situation safety behaviors in maintaining anxiety and negative beliefs. *Behavior Therapy, 26*, 153–161.

Wells, A., & Davies, M. (1994). The Thought Control Questionnaire: A measure of individual differences in the control of unwanted thoughts. *Behaviour Research and Therapy, 32*, 871–878.

Wells, A., & Papageorgiou, C. (1995). Worry and the incubation of intrusive images following stress. *Behaviour Research and Therapy, 33*, 579–583.

Wells, A., & Papageorgiou, C. (1998a). Relationships between worry, obsessive–compulsive symptoms and meta-cognitive beliefs. *Behaviour Research and Therapy, 36*, 899–913.

Wells, A., & Papageorgiou, C. (1998b). Social phobia: Effects of external attention on anxiety, negative beliefs, and perspective taking. *Behavior Therapy, 29*, 357–370.

Wells, A., & Papageorgiou, C. (1999). The observer perspective: Biased imagery in social phobia, agoraphobia, and blood–injury phobia. *Behaviour Research and Therapy, 37*, 653–658.

Wells, K., Goldberg, G., Brook, R., & Leake, B. (1986). Quality of care of psychotropic drug use in internal medicine group practices. *Western Journal of Medicine, 14*, 710–714.

Wenzel, A., & Holt, C. S. (1999). Dot probe performance in two specific phobias. *British Journal of Clinical Psychology, 38*, 407–410.

Wessel, I., & Merckelbach, H. (1997). The impact of anxiety on memory for details in spider phobics. *Applied Cognitive Psychology, 11*, 223–231.

Wessel, I., & Merckelbach, H. (1998). Memory for threat-relevant and threat-irrelevant cues in spider phobics. *Cognitions and Emotion, 12*, 93–104.

Westphal, C. (1871). Die agoraphobia: Eine neuropathische Eischeinung. *Archives für Psychiatrie und Nervenkrankheiten, 3*, 384–412.

Wheeler, E. O., White, P. D., Reed, E., & Cohen, M. E. (1948). Familial incidence of neurocirculatory asthenia ("anxiety neurosis," "effort syndrome"). *Journal of Clinical Investigation, 27*, 562.

White, B. V., & Gildea, E. F. (1937). "Cold pressor test" in tension and anxiety: A cardiochronographic study. *Archives of Neurology and Psychiatry, 38*, 964–984.

Whitehead, W. E., Robinson, A., Blackwell, B., & Stutz, R. M. (1978). Flooding treatment of phobias: Does chronic diazepam increase effectiveness? *Journal of Behavior Therapy and Experimental Psychiatry, 9*, 219–225.

Whitehead, W. E., Winget, C., Fedoravicius, A. S., Wooley, S., & Blackwell, B. (1982). Learned illness behavior in patients with irritable bowel syndrome and peptic ulcer. *Digestive Diseases and Sciences, 27*, 202–208.

Whitehead, W. W., Bush, C., Heller, G., & Costa, P. (1986). Social learning influences of menstrual symptoms and illness behavior. *Health Psychology, 5*, 13–23.

Wiborg, I. M., & Dahl, A. V. (1996). Does brief dynamic psychotherapy reduce the relapse rate of panic disorder? *Archives of General Psychiatry, 53*, 689–694.

Widom, C. S. (1989). The cycle of violence. *Science, 244*, 160–166.

Wiedemann, G., Pauli, P., Dengler, W., Lutzenberger, W., Birbaumer, N., & Buchkremer, G. (1999).

Frontal brain asymmetry as a biological substrate of emotions in patients with panic disorders. *Archives of General Psychiatry, 56,* 78–84.

Wiersma, A., Baauw, A. D., Bohus, B., & Koolhaas, J. M. (1995). Behavioural activation produced by CRH but not a-helical CRH (CRH-receptor antagonist) when microinfused into the central nucleus of the amygdala under stress-free conditions. *Psychoneuroendocrinology, 20,* 423–432.

Wik, G., Fredrikson, M., & Fischer, H. (1997). Evidence of altered cerebral blood-flow relationships in acute phobia. *International Journal of Neuroscience, 91,* 253–263.

Wilhelm, F. H., & Roth, W. T. (1996, November). *Acute and delayed effects of alprazolam on flight phobics during exposure.* Paper presented at the 30th Annual Convention of the Association for Advancement of Behavior Therapy, New York.

Wilkinson, D. J. C., Thompson, J. M., Lambert, G. W., Jennings, G. L., Schwarz, R. G., Jeffreys, D., Turner, A. G., & Esler, M. D. (1998). Sympathetic activity in patients with panic disorder at rest, under laboratory mental stress, and during panic attacks. *Archives of General Psychiatry, 55,* 511–520.

Wilkinson, G., Balestrieri, M., Ruggeri, M., & Bellantuono, C. (1991). Meta-analysis of double-blind placebo-controlled trials of antidepressants and benzodiazepines for patients with panic disorders. *Psychological Medicine, 21,* 991–998.

Williams, J., Mathews, A., & MacLeod, C. (1996). The emotional Stroop task and psychopathology. *Psychological Bulletin, 120*(1), 3–24.

Williams, J., Watts, F. N., MacLeod, C., & Mathews, A. (1988). *Cognitive psychology and emotional disorders.* Chichester, England: Wiley.

Williams, J. B. W., Gibbon, M., First, M. B., Spitzer, R. L., Davies, M., Borus, J., Howes, M. J., Kane, J., Pope, H. G., Rounsaville, B., & Wittchen, H. (1992). The Structured Clinical Interview for DSM-III-R (SCID): II. Multisite test–retest reliability. *Archives of General Psychiatry, 49,* 630–636.

Williams, K. E., Chambless, D. L., & Ahrens, A. (1997). Are emotions frightening?: An extension of the fear of fear construct. *Behaviour Research and Therapy, 35*(3), 239–248.

Williams, S. L. (1985). On the nature and measurement of agoraphobia. *Progress in Behavior Modification, 19,* 109–144.

Williams, S. L., Kinney, P. J., Harap, S. T., & Liebmann, M. (1997). Thoughts of agoraphobic people during scary tasks. *Journal of Abnormal Psychology, 106,* 511–520.

Williams, S. L., & Rappoport, A. (1983). Cognitive treatment in the natural environment for agoraphobics. *Behavior Therapy, 14,* 299–313.

Williams, S. L., Turner, S. M., & Peer, D. F. (1985). Guided mastery and performance desensitization treatments for severe acrophobia. *Journal of Consulting and Clinical Psychology, 53,* 237–247.

Wilson, G. D., & Priest, H. F. (1968). The principal components of phobic stimuli. *Journal of Clinical Psychology, 24,* 191.

Wilson, J. P., & Keane, T. M. (Eds.). (1997). *Assessing psychological trauma and PTSD.* New York: Guilford Press.

Wilson, S. A., Becker, L. A., & Tinker, R. H. (1995). Eye movement desensitization and reprocessing (EMDR) treatment for psychologically traumatized individuals. *Journal of Consulting and Clinical Psychology, 63,* 928–937.

Wincze, J. P., Venditti, E., Barlow, D. H., & Mavissakalian, M. R. (1980). The effects of a subjective monitoring task in the physiological measure of genital response to erotic stimulation. *Archives of Sexual Behavior, 9*(6), 533–545.

Wing, J. K., Cooper, J. E., & Sartorius, N. (1974). *The measurement and classification of psychiatric symptoms: An instruction manual for the PSE and Catego program.* Cambridge, England: Cambridge University Press.

Wirtz, P. W., & Harrell, A. V. (1987). Effects of post assault exposure to attack-similar stimuli on long-term recovery of victims. *Journal of Consulting and Clinical Psychology, 55,* 10–16.

Wisner, K. L., Peindl, K. s., Gigliotti, T., & Hanusa, B. H. (1999). Obsessions and compulsions in women with postpartum depression. *Journal of Clinical Psychiatry, 60,* 176–180.

Wisocki, P. A. (1988). Worry as a phenomenon relevant to the elderly. *Behavior Therapy, 19,* 369–379.

Wittchen, H.-U. (1986). Epidemiology of panic attacks and panic disorders. In L. Hand & H.-U. Wittchen (Eds.), *Panic and phobias: Empirical evidence of theoretical models and long-term effects of behavioral treatments.* Berlin: Springer-Verlag.

Wittchen, H.-U., & Essau, C. A. (1991). The epidemiology of panic attacks, panic disorder, and agoraphobia. In J. R. Walker, G. R. Norton, & C. A. Ross (Eds.), *Panic disorder and agoraphobia.* Monterey, CA: Brooks/Cole.

Wittchen, H.-U., Essau, C. A., Von Zerssen, D., Krieg, J.-C., & Zaudig, M. (1992). Lifetime and six-month prevalence of mental disorders in the Munich follow-up study. *European Archives of Psychiatry and Clinical Neuroscience, 241,* 247–258.

Wittchen, H.-U., Nelson, C. B., & Lachner, G. (1998). Prevalence of mental disorders and psychosocial impairments in adolescents and young adults. *Psychological Medicine, 28,* 109–126.

Wittchen, H.-U., Reed, V., & Kessler, R. C. (1998). The relationship of agoraphobia and panic in a community sample of adolescents and young adults. *Archives of General Psychiatry, 55,* 1017–1024.

Wittchen, H.-U., Zhao, S., Kessler, R. C., & Eaton, W. W. (1994). DSM-III-R generalized anxiety disorder in the National Comorbidity Survey. *Archives of General Psychiatry, 51,* 355–364.

Wolchik, S. A., Beggs, V. E., Wincze, J. P., Sakheim, D. K., Barlow, D. H., & Mavissakalian, M. R. (1980). The effect of emotional arousal on subsequent sexual arousal in men. *Journal of Abnormal Psychology, 89,* 595–599.

Wolfe, D. A., Sas, L., & Wekerle, C. (1994). Factors associated with the development of posttraumatic stress disorder among child victims of sexual abuse. *Child Abuse and Neglect, 18,* 37–50.

Wolfe, J., Brown, P. J., & Kelley, J. M. (1993). Reassessing war stress: Exposure and the Persian Gulf War. *Journal of Social Issues, 49,* 15–31.

Wolpe, J. (1952). Experimental neurosis as learned behavior. *British Journal of Psychology, 43,* 243–268.

Wolpe, J. (1954). Reciprocal inhibition as the main basis of psychotherapeutic effects. *Archives of Neurology and Psychiatry, 72,* 205.

Wolpe, J. (1958). *Psychotherapy by reciprocal inhibition.* Stanford, CA: Stanford University Press.

Wolpe, J. (1973). *The practice of behavior therapy* (2nd ed.). New York: Pergamon Press.

Wolpe, J. (1978). Cognition and causation in human behavior and its therapy. *American Psychologist, 33,* 437–446.

Woodman, C. L., Noyes, R., Black, D. W., Schlosser, S., & Yagla, S. J. (1999). A 5-year follow-up study of generalized anxiety disorder and panic disorder. *Journal of Nervous and Mental Disease, 187,* 3–9.

Woodruff, M. L., & Lippincott, W. I. (1976). Hyperemotionality and enhanced tonic immobility after septal lesions in the rabbit. *Brain, Behavior and Evolution, 13,* 22–33.

Woodruff, R. H., Guze, S. B., & Clayton, P. J. (1972). Anxiety neurosis among psychiatric outpatients. *Comprehensive Psychiatry, 13,* 165–170.

Woods, S. W., Charney, D. S., Silver, J. M., Krystal, J. H., & Heninger, G. R. (1991). Behavioral, biochemical, and cardiovascular responses to the benzodiazepene receptor antagonist flumazenil in panic disorder. *Psychiatric Research, 36,* 115–127.

Woods, S. W., Charney, D. S., Goodman, W. K., & Heninger, G. R. (1987). Carbon dioxide-induced anxiety: Behavioral, physiologic, and biochemical effects of 5% CO_2 in panic disorder patients and 5 and 7. 5% CO_2 in healthy subjects. *Archives of General Psychiatry, 44,* 365–375.

Woods, S. W., Charney, D. S., Loke, J., Goodman, W. K., Redmond, D. E., & Heninger, G. R. (1986). Carbon dioxide sensitivity in panic anxiety. *Archives of General Psychiatry, 43,* 900–909.

Woods, S. W., Charney, D. S., McPherson, C. A., Gradman, A. H., & Heninger, G. R. (1987).

Situational panic attacks: Behavioral, physiological, and biochemical characterization. *Archives of General Psychiatry, 44,* 365–375.

Woody, S. R. (1996). Effects of focus of attention on anxiety levels and social performance of individuals with social phobia. *Journal of Abnormal Psychology, 105,* 61–69.

Woody, S. R., Chambless, D. L., & Glass, C. R. (1997). Self-focused attention in the treatment of social phobia. *Behaviour Research and Therapy, 35,* 117–129.

Woody, S. R., McLean, P., Taylor, S., & Koch, W. J. (1999). Treatment of major depression in the context of panic disorder. *Journal of Affective Disorders, 53,* 163–174.

Woody, S. R., Steketee, G., & Chambless, D. L. (1995). Reliability and validity of the Yale–Brown Obsessive Compulsive Scale. *Behaviour Research and Therapy, 33,* 597–605.

Woody, S. R., & Teachman, B. (2000). Intersection of disgust and fear: Normative and pathological views. *Clinical Psychology: Science and Practice, 7,* 291–311.

World Health Organization. (1990). *Composite International Diagnostic Interview.* Geneva: Author.

Worthington, J. J., Pollack, M. H., Otto, M. W., McLean, R. Y. S., Moroz, G., & Rosenbaum, J. F. (1998). Long-term experience with clonazepam in patients with a primary diagnosis of panic disorder. *Psychopharacology Bulletin, 34,* 199–205.

Wulsin, L. R., Arnold, L. M., & Hillard, J. R. (1991). Axis I disorders in ER patients with atypical chest pain. *International Journal of Psychiatry in Medicine, 21,* 37–46.

Wundt, W. (1896). *Grundriss der psychologie.* Leipzig: Engelman.

Yang, S., Tsai, T. H., Hou, Z. Y., Chen, C. Y., & Sim, C. B. (1997). The effect of panic attack on mitral valve prolapse. *Acta Psychiatrica Scandinavica, 96,* 408–411.

Yaryura-Tobias, J. A., Grunes, M. S., Todaro, J., McKay, D., Neziroglu, F. A., & Stockman, R. (2000). Nosological insertion of Axis I disorders in the etiology of obsessive–compulsive disorder. *Journal of Anxiety Disorders, 14,* 19–30.

Yeh, S. R., Fricke, R. A., & Edwards, D. H. (1996). The effect of social experience on serotonergic modulation of the escape circuit of crayfish. *Science, 271,* 366–369.

Yehuda, R. (1997). Sensitization of the hypothalamic–pituitary–adrenal axis in posttraumatic stress disorder. *Annals of the New York Academy of Sciences, 821,* 57–75.

Yehuda, R., Boisoneau, D., Lowy, M. T., & Giller, E. L. (1995). Dose–response changes in plasma cortisol and lymphocyte glucocorticoid receptors following dexamethasone administration in combat veterans with and without posttraumatic stress disorder. *Archives of General Psychiatry, 52,* 538–593.

Yehuda, R., Giller, E. L., Jr., Levengood, R. A., Southwick, S. M., & Siever, L. J. (1995). Hypothalamic–pituitary–adrenal functioning in post-traumatic stress disorder: Expanding the concept of the stress response spectrum. In M. J. Friedman, D. S. Charney, & A. Y. Deutch (Eds.), *Neurobiological and clinical consequences of stress: From normal adaptation to post-traumatic stress disorder.* Philadelphia: Lippincott–Raven.

Yehuda, R., Levengood, R. A., Schmeidler, J., Wilson, S., Guo, L. S., & Gerber, D. (1996). Increased pituitary activation following metyrapone administration in post-traumatic stress disorder. *Psychoneuroendocrinology, 21,* 1–16.

Yehuda, R., Lowy, M. T., Southwick, S. M., Shaffer, D., & Giller, E. L. (1991). Increased number of glucocorticoid receptors in post-traumatic stress disorder. *American Journal of Psychiatry, 148,* 499–504.

Yehuda, R., & McFarlane, A. C. (1995). Conflict between current knowledge about posttraumatic stress disorder and its original conceptual basis. *American Journal of Psychiatry, 152,* 1705–1713.

Yehuda, R., Teicher, M. H., Trestman, R. L., Levengood, R. A., & Siever, R. J. (1996). Cortisol regulation in posttraumatic stress disorder and major depression: A chronobiological analysis. *Biological Psychiatry, 40,* 79–88.

Yelin, E., Mathias, S., Buesching, D., Rowland, C., Caluscin, R., & Fifer, S. (1996). The impact of employment of an intervention to increase recognition of previously untreated anxiety among primary care physicians. *Social Sciences and Medicine, 42,* 1069–1075.

Yeragani, V. K., Pohl, R., Srinivasan, K., Balon, R., Ramesh, C., & Berchou, R. (1995). Effects of isoproterenol infusions on heart rate variability in patients with panic disorder. *Psychiatry Research, 56,* 289–293.

Yerkes, R. M., & Dodson, J. D. (1908). The relation of strength of stimulus to rapidity of habit-formation. *Journal of Comparative Neurology and Psychology, 18,* 459–482.

Yinglin, K., Wulsin, L., Arnold, L., & Rouan, G. (1993). Estimated prevalences of panic disorder and depression among consecutive patients seen in an emergency department with acute chest pain. *Journal of General Internal Medicine, 8,* 231–235.

Yonkers, K. A., Warshaw, M. R., Massion, A. O., & Keller, M. B. (1996). Phenomenology and course of generalised anxiety disorder. *British Journal of Psychiatry, 168,* 308–313.

Yonkers, K. A., Zlotnick, C., Allsworth, J., Warshaw, M., Shea, T., & Keller, M. B. (1998). Is the course of panic disorder the same in men and women? *American Journal of Psychiatry, 155,* 596–602.

Young, J. E., Weinberger, A. D., & Beck, A. T. (2001). Cognitive therapy for depression. In D. H. Barlow (Ed.), *Clinical handbook of psychological disorders: A step-by-step treatment manual* (3rd ed.). New York: Guilford Press.

Young, J. P. R., Fenton, G. W., & Lader, M. H. (1971). Inheritance of neurotic traits: A twin study of the Middlesex Hospital Questionnaire. *British Journal of Psychiatry, 119,* 393–398.

Zajecka, J. M. (1996). The effect of nefazodone on co-morbid anxiety symptoms associated with depression: Experience in family practice and psychiatric outpatient clinics. *Journal of Clinical Psychiatry, 57*(Suppl. 2), 10–14.

Zajonc, R. B. (1980). Feeling and thinking: Preferences need no inferences. *American Psychologist, 35,* 151–175.

Zajonc, R. B. (1984). On the primacy of affect. *American Psychologist, 39,* 117–123.

Zaubler, T. S., & Katon, W. (1996). Panic disorder and medical comorbidity: A review of the medical and psychiatric literature. *Bulletin of the Menninger Clinic, 60*(2, Suppl. A), A12–A38.

Zevon, M. A., & Tellegen, A. (1982). The structure of mood change: Anidrographic/nomothetic analysis. *Journal of Personality and Social Psychology, 43,* 111–122.

Zillmann, D. (1983a). Arousal and aggression. In R. G. Geen & E. Donnerstein (Eds.), *Aggression: Theoretical and empirical reviews* (Vol. 1). New York: Academic Press.

Zillmann, D. (1983b). Transfer of excitation in emotional behavior. In J. T. Cacioppo & R. E. Petty (Eds.), *Social psychophysiology: A sourcebook.* New York: Guilford Press.

Zimbardo, P. G. (1977). *Shyness: What it is and what to do about it.* Reading, MA: Addison-Wesley.

Zinbarg, R. E., & Barlow, D. H. (1991). Mixed anxiety–depression: A new diagnostic category? In R. M. Rapee & D. H. Barlow (Eds.), *Chronic anxiety: Generalized anxiety disorder and mixed anxiety–depression.* New York: Guilford Press.

Zinbarg, R. E., & Barlow, D. H. (1996). Structure of anxiety and the anxiety disorders: A hierarchical model. *Journal of Abnormal Psychology, 105*(2), 181–193.

Zinbarg, R. E., Barlow, D. H., & Brown, T. A. (1997). Hierarchical structure and general factor saturation of the Anxiety Sensitivity Index: Evidence and implications. *Psychological Assessment, 9,* 277–284.

Zinbarg, R. E., Barlow, D. H., Liebowitz, M. R., Street, L., Broadhead, E., Katon, W., Roy-Byrne, P., Lepine, J.-P., Teherani, M., Richards, J., Brantley, P. J., & Kraemer, H. (1994). The DSM-IV field trial for mixed anxiety–depression. *American Journal of Psychiatry, 151,* 1153–1162.

Zinbarg, R. E., Barlow, D. H., Liebowitz, M. R., Street, L., Broadhead, E., Katon, W., Roy-Byrne, P. Lepine, J.-P., Teherani, M., Richards, J., Brantly, P. J., & Kraemer, H. (1998). The DSM-IV field trial for mixed anxiety–depression. In T. A. Widiger, A. J. Frances, H. A. Pincus, R. Ross, M. B. First, Davis, W., & Kline, M. (Eds.), *DSM-IV sourcebook* (Vol. 4). Washington, DC: American Psychiatric Association.

Zinbarg, R. E., Craske, M. G., & Barlow, D. H. (1993). *Therapist's guide for the mastery of your anxiety and worry.* San Antonio, TX: Psychological Corporation/Graywind Publications Incoporated.

Zitrin, C. M., Klein, D. F., Woerner, M. G., & Ross, D. C. (1983). Treatment of phobias: I. Comparison of imipramine hydrochloride and placebo. *Archives of General Psychiatry, 40,* 125–138.

Zoellner, L. A., & Craske, M. G. (1999). Interoceptive accuracy and panic. *Behaviour Research and Therapy, 37*, 1141–1158.

Zoellner, L. A., Craske, M. G., Hussain, A., Lewis, M., & Echeveri, A., (1996, November). *Contextual effects of alprazolam during exposure therapy.* Paper presented at the 30th Annual Convention of the Association for Advancement of Behavior Therapy, New York.

Zola-Morgan, S. M., & Squire, L. R. (1990). The primate hippocampal formation: Evidence for a time-limited role in memory storage. *Science, 250*, 288–290.

Zuckerman, M., & Lubin, B. (1965). *Manual for the Multiple Affect Adjective Checklist.* San Diego, CA: Educational and Industrial Testing Service.

Zung, W. W. (1965). A self-rating depression scale. *Archives of General Psychiatry, 12*, 63–70.

Zvolensky, M. J., Eifert, G. H., Lejuez, C. W., & McNeil, D. W. (1999). The effects offset control over 20% carbon dioxide-enriched air on anxious responding. *Journal of Abnormal Psychology, 108*, 624–632.

Zvolensky, M. J., Lejuez, C. W., & Eifert, G. H. (1998). The role of offset control in anxious responding: An experimental test using repeated administrations of 20% carbon dioxide-enriched air. *Behavior Therapy, 29*, 193–209.

Zwi, A. B. (1991). Militarism, militarization, health, and the Third World. *Medicine and War, 7*, 262–268.

Author Index

Subject Index